AF811936

Evolution

Contemporary Protocols for Anterior Single-Tooth Implants

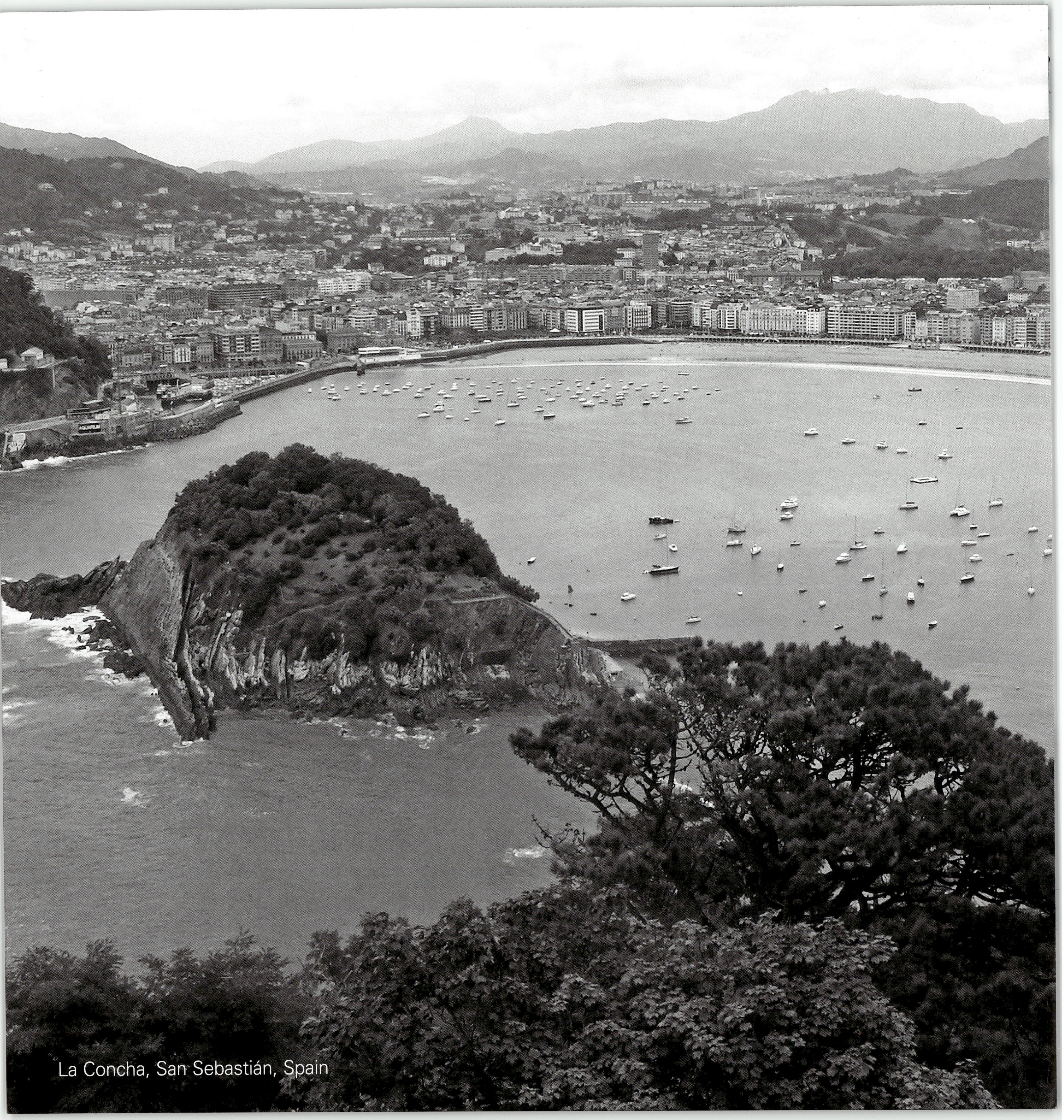

La Concha, San Sebastián, Spain

evolution

Contemporary Protocols for Anterior Single-Tooth Implants

Iñaki Gamborena, DMD, MSD
Private Practice
San Sebastián, Spain

Markus B. Blatz, DMD, PhD
Professor and Chairman
Department of Preventive and Restorative Sciences
University of Pennsylvania School of Dental Medicine
Philadelphia, Pennsylvania

quintessence books
Quintessence Publishing Co, Inc
Chicago, Berlin, Tokyo, London, Paris, Milan, Barcelona, Beijing, Istanbul, Moscow, New Delhi, Prague, São Paulo, Seoul, and Warsaw

Library of Congress Cataloging-in-Publication Data

Gamborena, Iñaki, author.
Evolution : contemporary protocols for anterior single-tooth implants / Iñaki Gamborena and Markus B. Blatz.
p. ; cm.
Includes bibliographical references.
ISBN 978-0-86715-496-2
I. Blatz, Markus B., author. II. Title.
[DNLM: 1. Dental Implants, Single-Tooth. 2. Clinical Protocols. 3. Dental Implantation--methods. WU 640]
RK667.I45
617.6'93--dc23
2014026922

5 4 3 2 1

quintessence books

© 2015 Quintessence Publishing Co Inc

Quintessence Publishing Co Inc
4350 Chandler Drive
Hanover Park, IL 60133
www.quintpub.com

All rights reserved. This book or any part thereof may not be reproduced, stored in a retrieval system, or transmitted in any form or by any means, electronic, mechanical, photocopying, or otherwise, without prior written permission of the publisher.

Editor: Leah Huffman
Design and production: Ted Pereda

Printed in China

Dedication

To Mila

— Iñaki Gamborena

To Ulrike, Anna, Linus, Lillian, and Amelie

— Markus B. Blatz

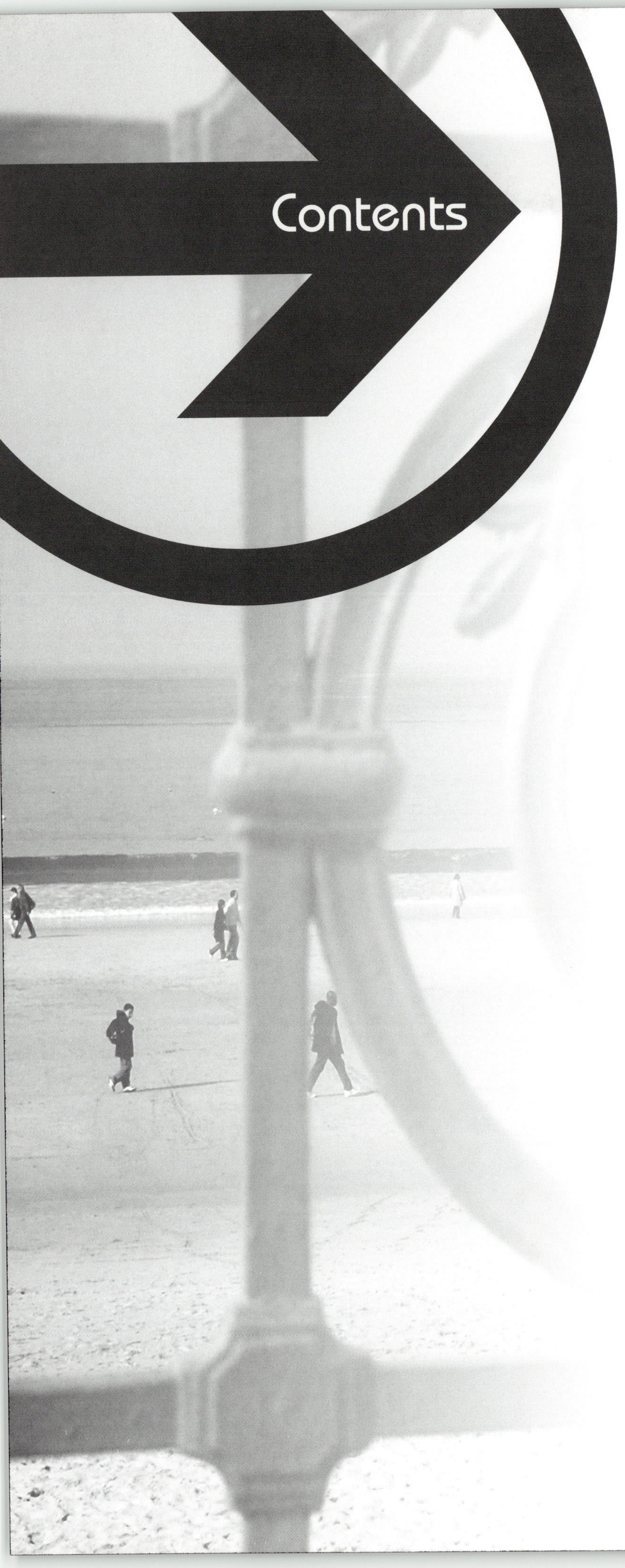

Contents

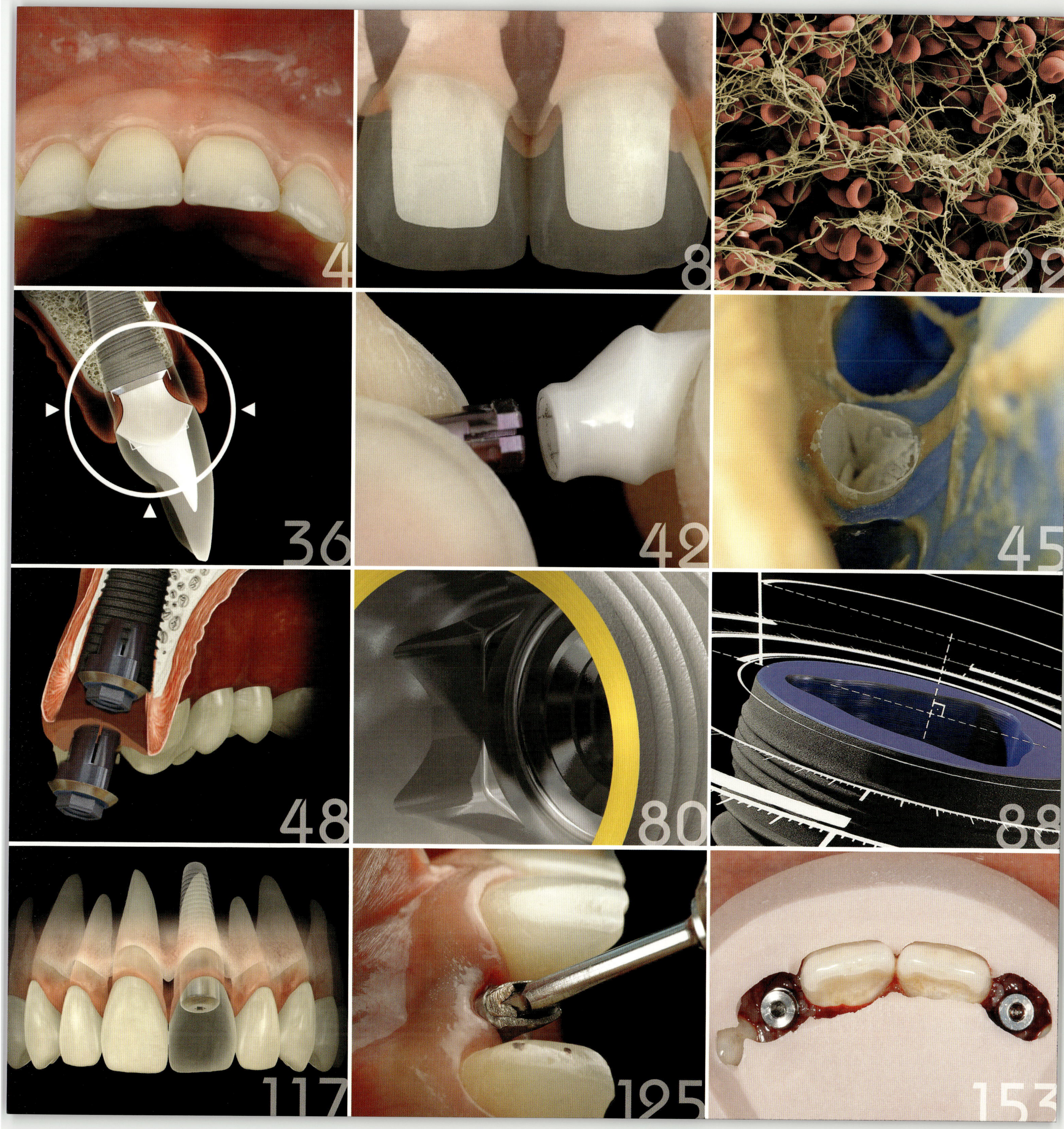
4
8
22
36
42
45
48
80
88
117
125
153

Contents

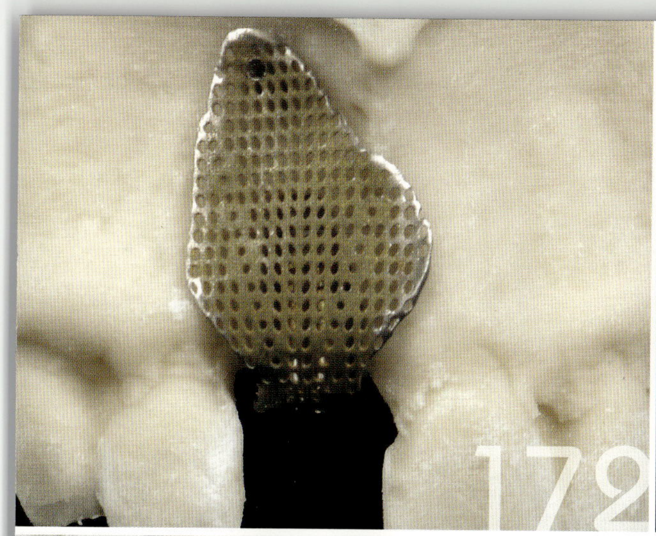
172

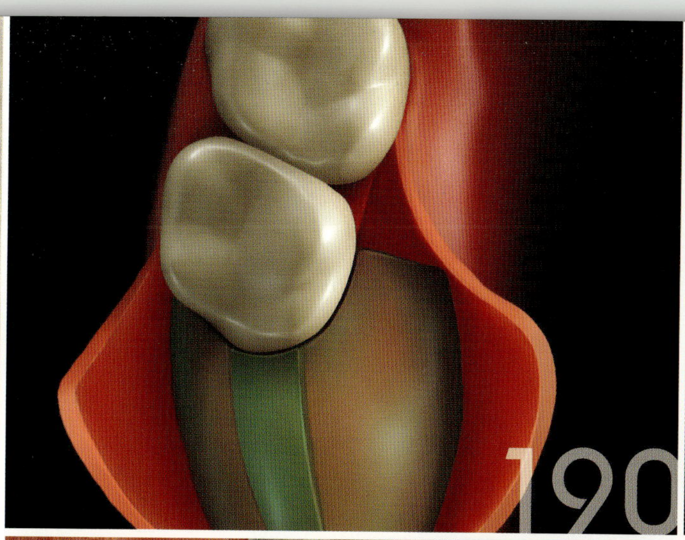
190

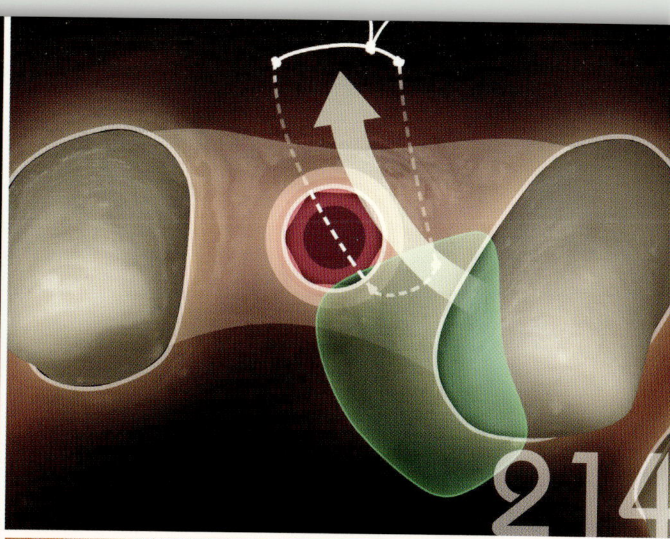
214

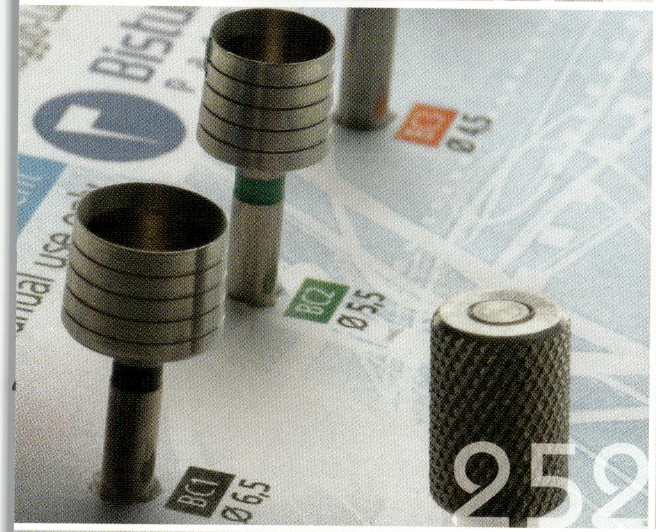
BC1
Ø6,5
BC2
Ø5,5
Ø4,5
252

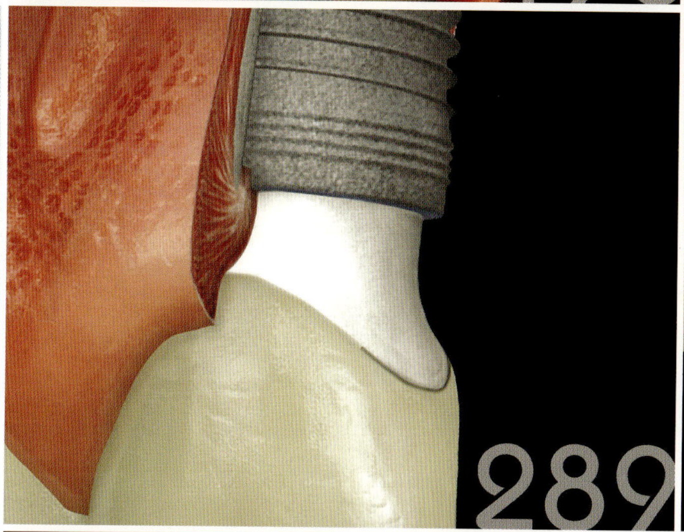
289

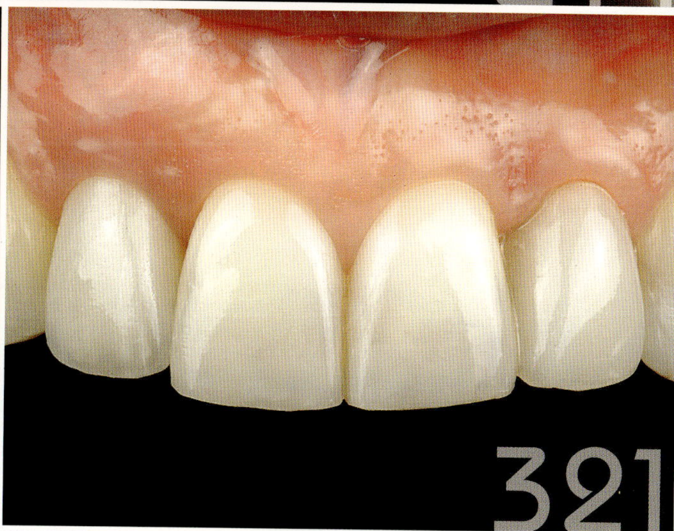
321

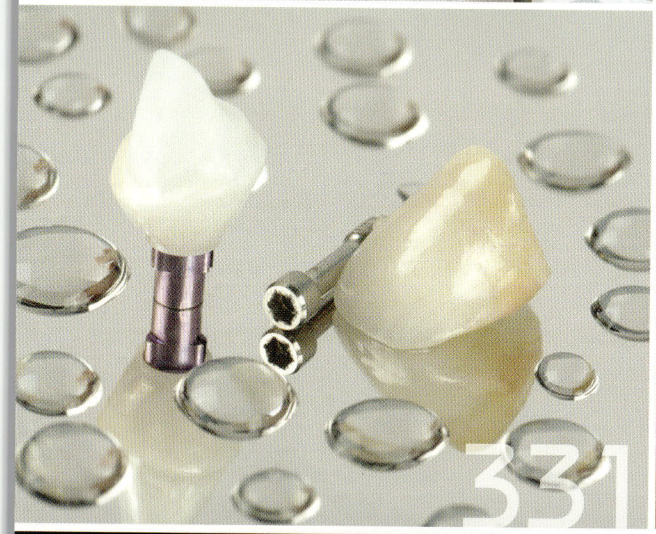
331

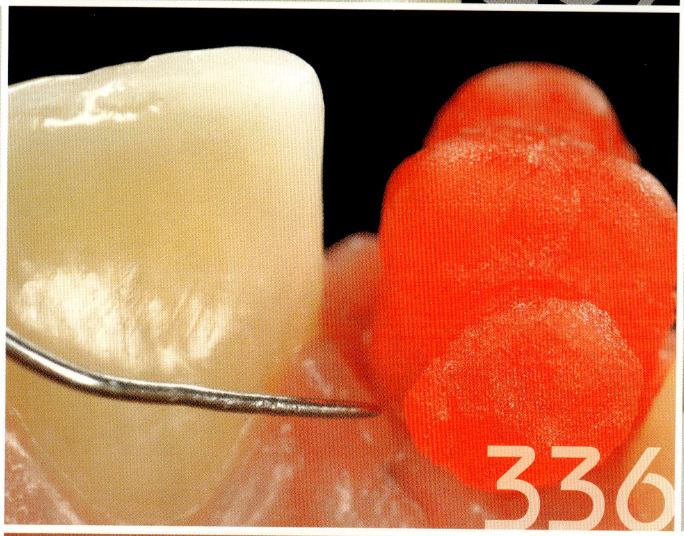
336

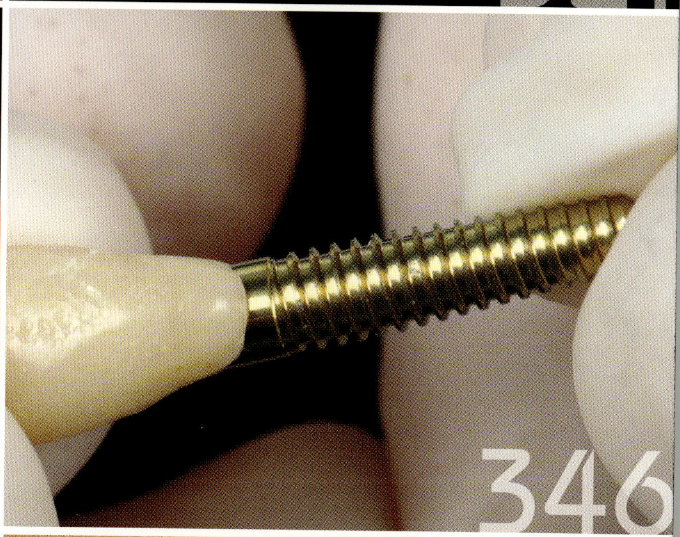
346

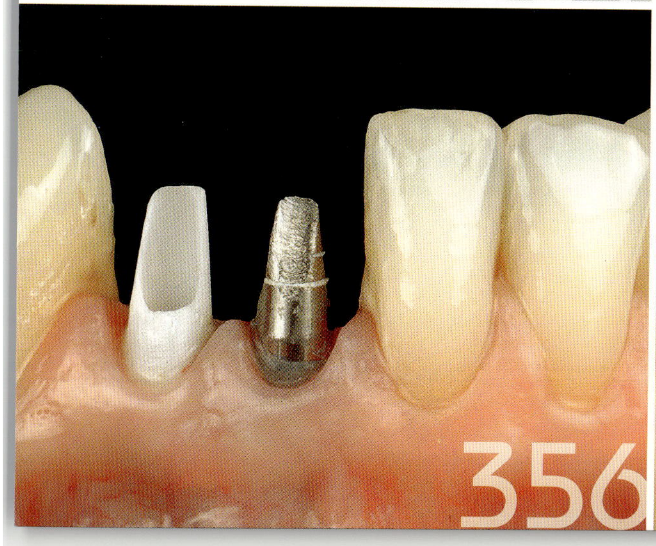
356

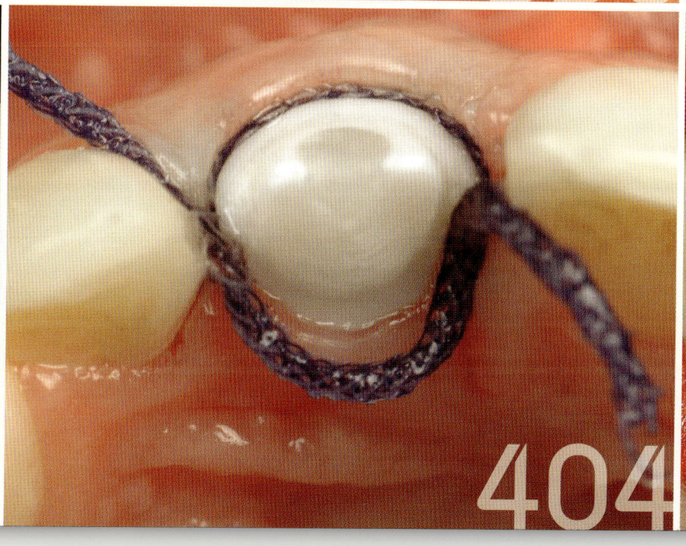
404

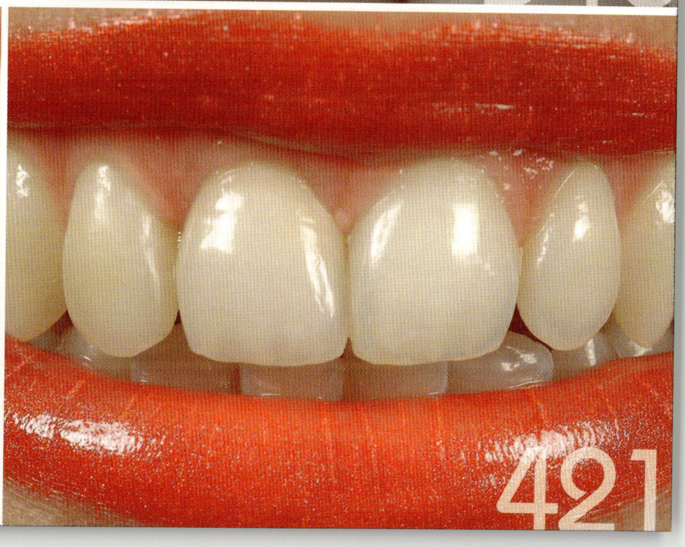
421

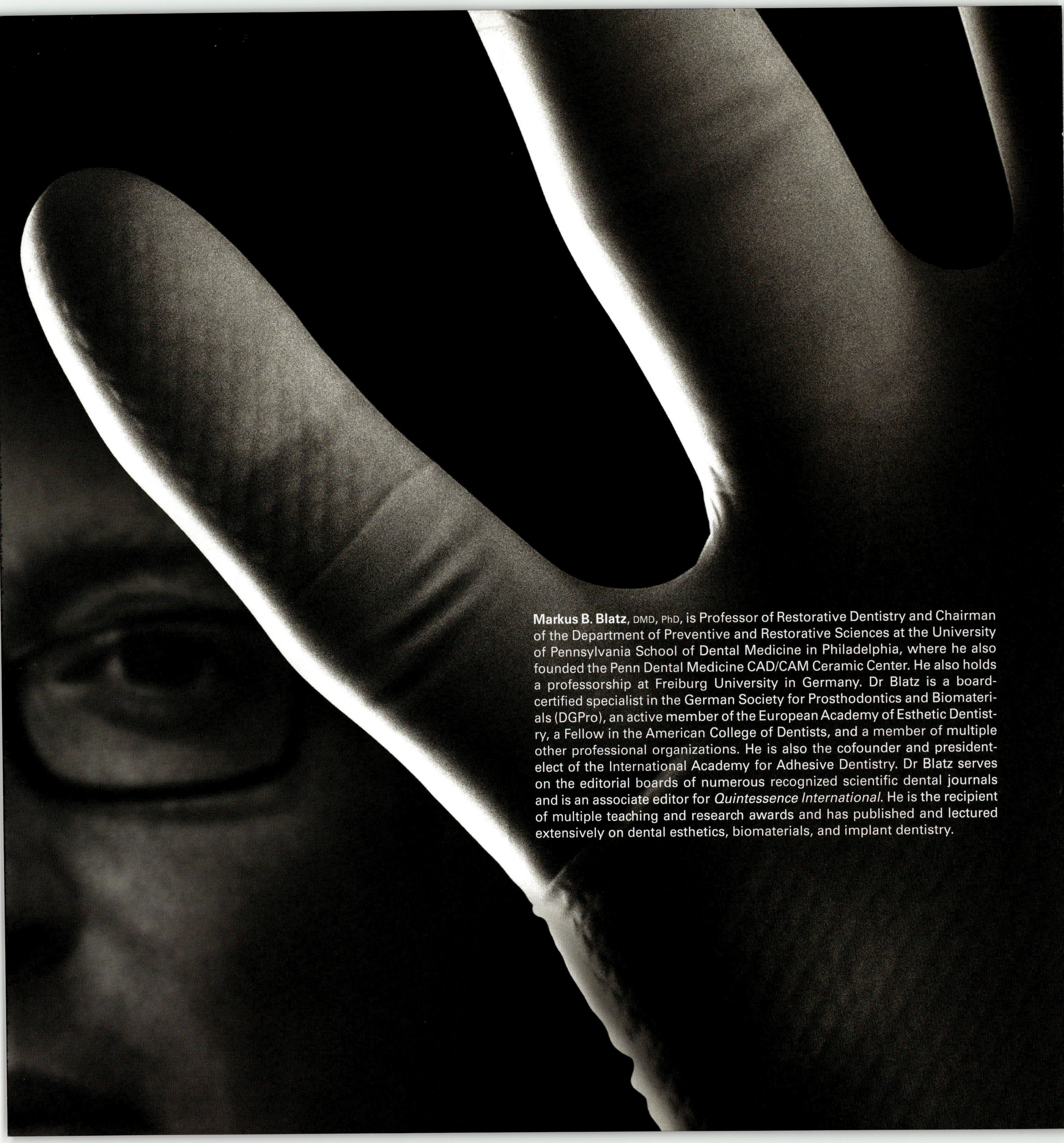

Markus B. Blatz, DMD, PhD, is Professor of Restorative Dentistry and Chairman of the Department of Preventive and Restorative Sciences at the University of Pennsylvania School of Dental Medicine in Philadelphia, where he also founded the Penn Dental Medicine CAD/CAM Ceramic Center. He also holds a professorship at Freiburg University in Germany. Dr Blatz is a board-certified specialist in the German Society for Prosthodontics and Biomaterials (DGPro), an active member of the European Academy of Esthetic Dentistry, a Fellow in the American College of Dentists, and a member of multiple other professional organizations. He is also the cofounder and president-elect of the International Academy for Adhesive Dentistry. Dr Blatz serves on the editorial boards of numerous recognized scientific dental journals and is an associate editor for *Quintessence International*. He is the recipient of multiple teaching and research awards and has published and lectured extensively on dental esthetics, biomaterials, and implant dentistry.

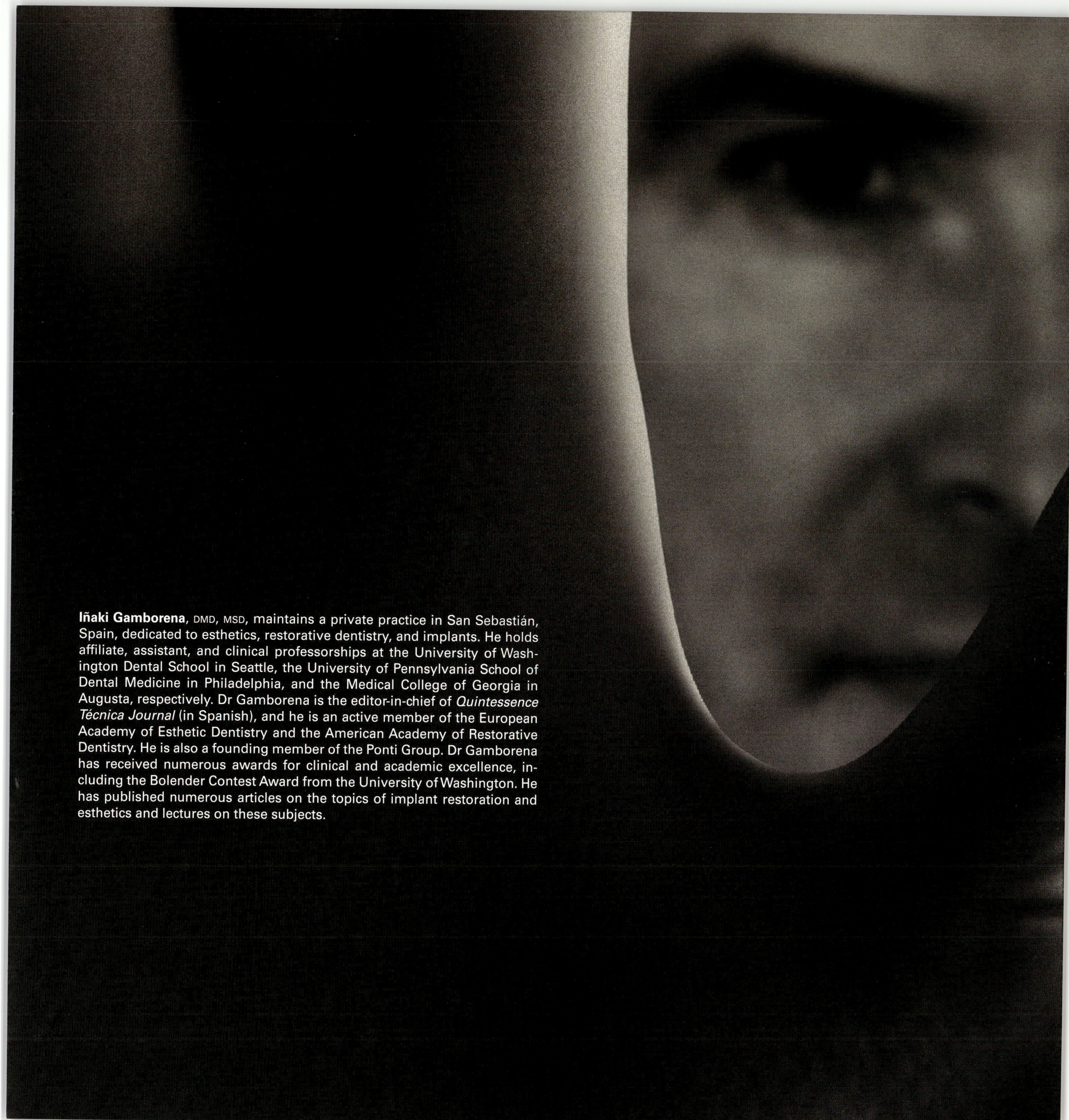

Iñaki Gamborena, DMD, MSD, maintains a private practice in San Sebastián, Spain, dedicated to esthetics, restorative dentistry, and implants. He holds affiliate, assistant, and clinical professorships at the University of Washington Dental School in Seattle, the University of Pennsylvania School of Dental Medicine in Philadelphia, and the Medical College of Georgia in Augusta, respectively. Dr Gamborena is the editor-in-chief of *Quintessence Técnica Journal* (in Spanish), and he is an active member of the European Academy of Esthetic Dentistry and the American Academy of Restorative Dentistry. He is also a founding member of the Ponti Group. Dr Gamborena has received numerous awards for clinical and academic excellence, including the Bolender Contest Award from the University of Washington. He has published numerous articles on the topics of implant restoration and esthetics and lectures on these subjects.

Introduction

"I believe in intuition and inspiration. Imagination is more important than knowledge. For knowledge is limited, whereas imagination embraces the entire world, stimulating progress, giving birth to EVOLUTION. It is, strictly speaking, a real factor in scientific research."
— Albert Einstein

There is a constant **evolution** of dental treatment concepts, techniques, technologies, and materials continuously pushing the borders of what is possible and the envelope of clinical excellence for the ultimate goal: the best possible care for our patients. One of the areas with the most palpable and rapid developments is implant dentistry, enhanced through the implementation of minimally invasive surgical techniques, novel implant designs, esthetic restorative materials, and innovative CAD/CAM technologies. The single-tooth implant has become a very popular treatment option in the anterior dentition. However, while the key to success in this demanding and challenging treatment lies in the very fine details, there is little detailed guidance in the dental literature to assist the clinician in achieving optimal long-lasting esthetic and functional outcomes. The intention of this book is to provide exactly that and to present a snapshot of current techniques and technologies, purposely pushing the boundaries with some of these novel concepts beyond common ideas with the goal of instilling imagination, creativity, and curiosity for what lies ahead.

In this technology-driven age, we are experiencing a drastic change in how information and knowledge are being perceived, collected, and processed by the new generation of learners. Our pedagogical methods and teaching tools have to adapt to this fast **evolution** to remain relevant and to ensure that the proper information reaches our current and future clinicians. While the general concept of writing a book still has some traditional connotations, we intentionally created a novel concept that recognizes the needs of a fast-paced, visually oriented readership. Some of it is probably due to our own impatience with some classic textbooks that may provide excellent content but force the reader to skip between different and usually separated sections of extensive text, illustrations, figure legends, and literature references. Because the focus of this book is clinical technique, we decided to present step-by-step procedures in the format of comic strips with the explanatory text in immediate proximity. One could also view them as video clips played in adjustable slow motion to allow readers to follow every step at their own pace and to stop whenever they feel necessary to review what they find important and observe the small details that may make the difference between failure and success. Some of these sequences are continued and spread across two or more pages. This format may initially be confusing, so we added small and large arrows that indicate sequences of clinical illustrations displayed on one page (vertical arrows pointing down) or spread across two pages (horizontal arrows pointing from left to right).

Another area of great **evolution** is dental research. Over the past years, we have made great strides in the understanding and implementation of evidence-based dentistry in the clinical decision-making process. As we strive to gain relevant scientific information from high-level clinical trials and systematic literature reviews, we often find ourselves left with very little conclusive evidence and realize how early we are in this process and how much more clinical research is necessary. In this digital age, an abundance of scientific literature, publications, and references is easily accessible and quickly updated with a few keystrokes. Conversely, some of the literature cited in printed textbooks may be outdated rather quickly. Therefore, instead of loosely collecting and listing as many references as possible and filling pages with narrative literature reviews, our aim was to be as concise as possible. We targeted some key topics and presented the findings of our in-depth literature searches in the various "Research" sections throughout the book. Each section was purposely confined to one written page and supported by a limited number of the most relevant references, starting with current systematic reviews where available. The "Research" sections have a consistent layout and are therefore easy to identify. The reference lists are placed immediately adjacent to the respective text, so flipping between pages is not necessary.

And last but not least, this entire book has been nothing short of an **evolution**. It started with a simple conversation between two friends, who had worked together and published articles for some years, about the need for a clinically oriented booklet that focuses exclusively on single-tooth implant esthetics from a surgical and restorative standpoint. What was planned to be a brief clinical manual and technical guide for the dental practitioner has morphed into this book. Along the way, we realized that a general description of implant procedures was not sufficient enough to give the clinician meaningful guidance and that we had to provide a much greater level of detail of our concepts, techniques, and materials that, based on many years of experience and research, facilitate success. For example, we initially kept the description and explanation of the actual implant selection very generic. However, the attributes, dimensions, surface, geometry, thread configuration, and design of a specific implant directly influence how an implant is selected, placed, and ultimately restored. While some may view the detailed description of the implants as well as the fact that only one implant manufacturer was used as commercially biased, this information is important for the reader to understand the rationale for our implant selection and treatment philosophies. The results shown may well be achievable with other implant systems. In addition, due to the constant and progressive developments, some of the implants used in the earlier cases may not be available anymore, and even current ones may be modified or replaced in the future.

It is important to understand the fundamental concepts of implant hard and soft tissue integration to comprehend the basic implant selection and placement principles. The importance of soft tissue esthetics and minimally invasive surgical procedures along with optimized restorative protocols are the key aspects demonstrated in this book. However, these are steps in the **evolution** of implant dentistry that will be modified and improved in the future.

We sincerely hope that this book will stimulate your imagination and serve as an inspiration for your work. Enjoy, and keep the curiosity!

Iñaki Gamborena

Markus B. Blatz

Acknowledgments

We would like to thank all of our mentors and teachers throughout the years who have encouraged us to ask questions and be creative, our dental technicians and staff for their support and effort to always strive for the best, Dr Peter Schüpbach for the stunning illustrations and explanation of peri-implant tissues, and the most important people in our lives: our family and friends—the ones who are still with us and the ones who are at peace.

"The important thing is not to stop questioning. Curiosity has its own reason for existing. One cannot help but be in awe when he contemplates the mysteries of eternity, of life, of the marvelous structure of reality. It is enough if one tries merely to comprehend a little of this mystery every day. Never lose a holy curiosity."

— Albert Einstein

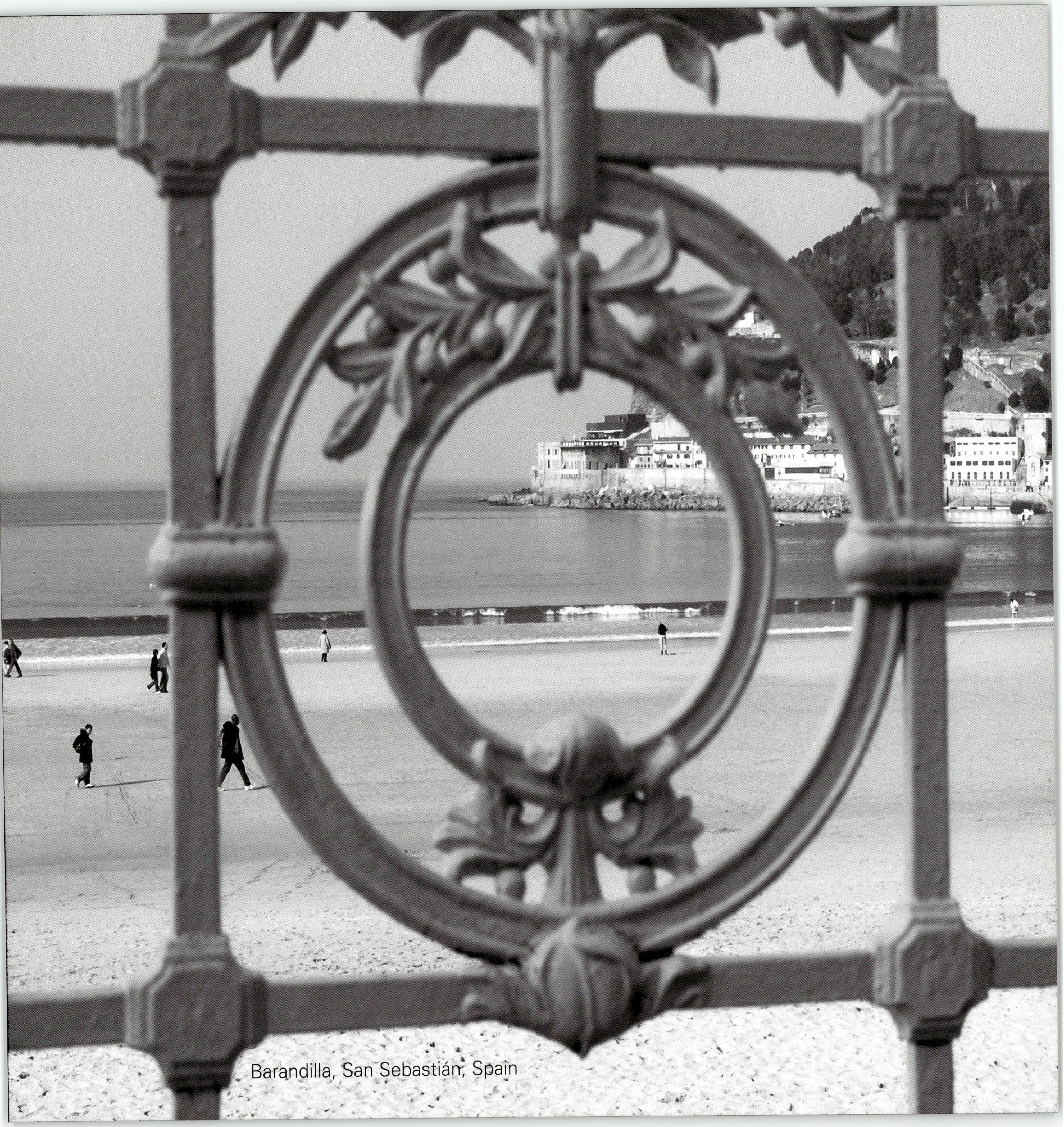

Barandilla, San Sebastián, Spain

Contemporary Approach to Dental Implantology

1. Esthetic and Soft Tissue Considerations
    - Esthetic Parameters for Anterior Single-Tooth Implant Restorations
    - Soft Tissue Characteristics Around Implants

2. Biologic Impact of Implant, Abutment, and Prosthetic Design
    - Clinical Protocol with Platform Shift Concept: Delayed Implant Placement
    - Clinical Protocol with Platform Shift Concept: Immediate Implant Placement
    - Clinical Results with Platform Shift Concept

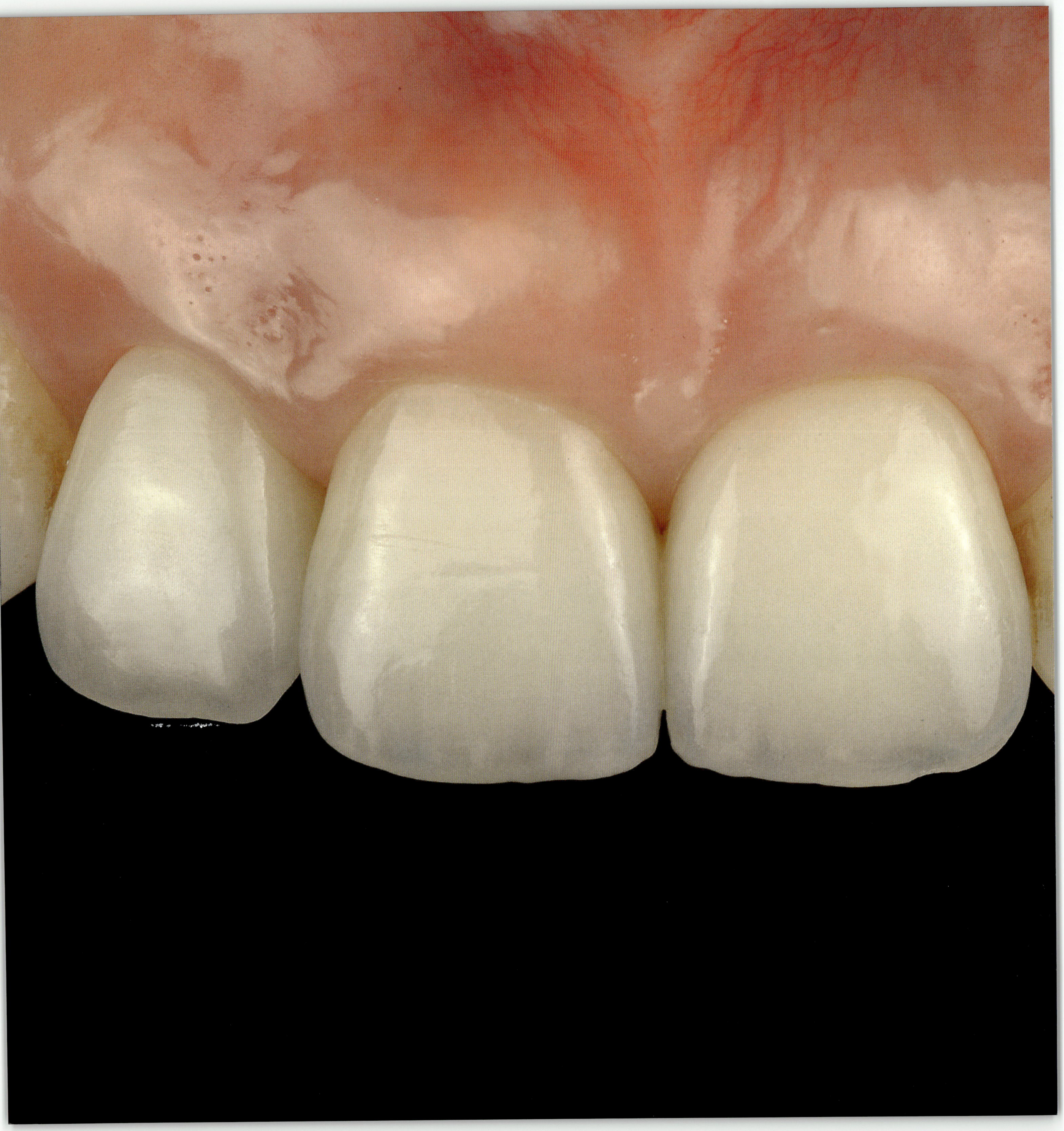

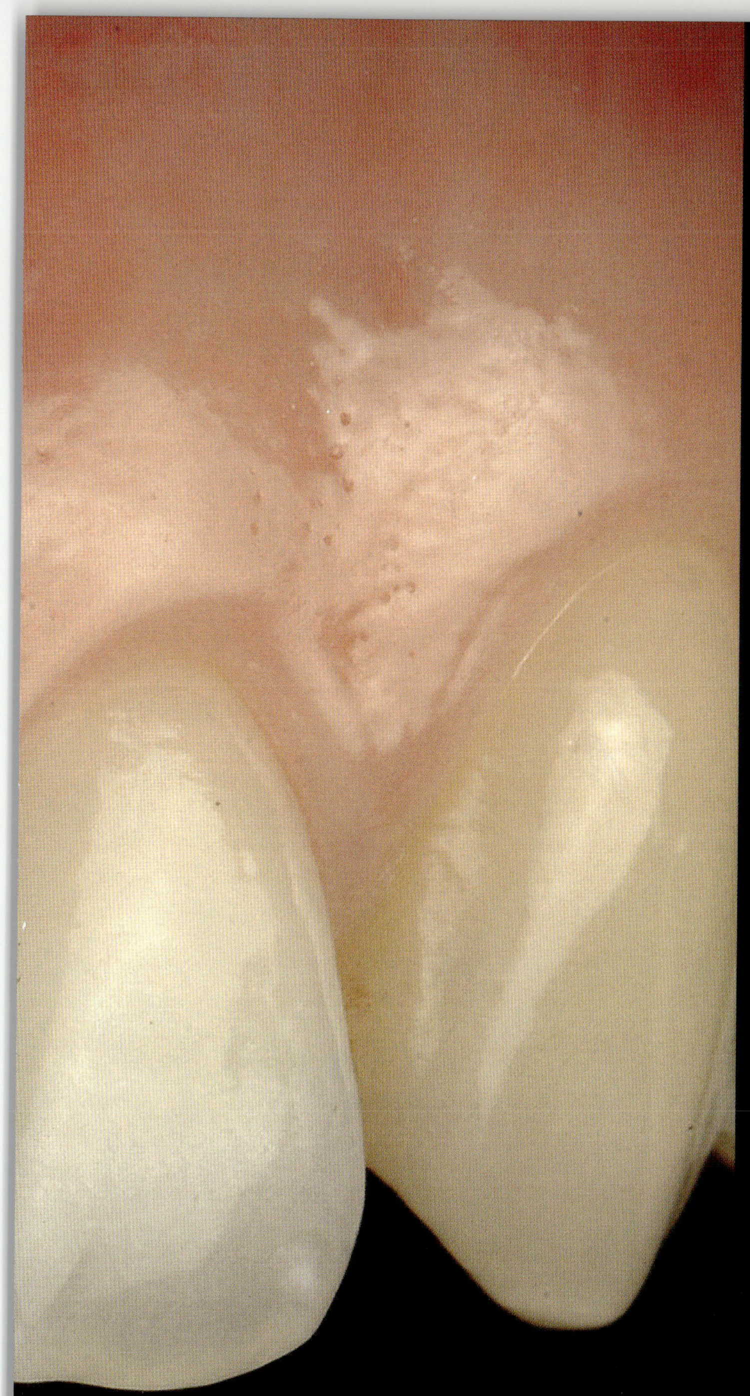

Esthetic and Soft Tissue Considerations

- Esthetic Parameters for Anterior Single-Tooth Implant Restorations
  → Research: Esthetic parameters
- Soft Tissue Characteristics Around Implants
  → Research: Peri-implant soft tissue

Chapter 1

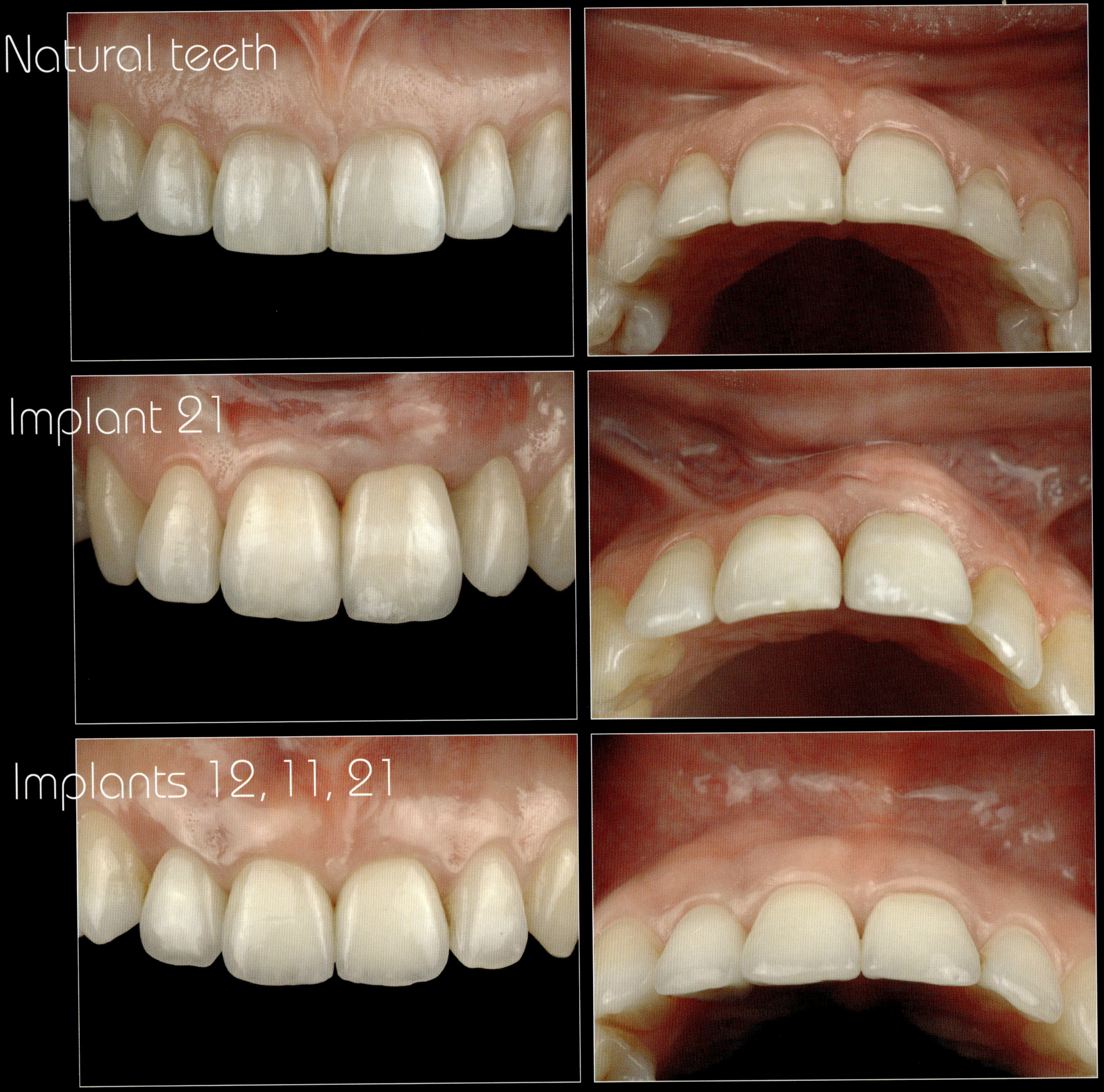
Natural teeth
Implant 21
Implants 12, 11, 21

Esthetic Parameters for Anterior Single-Tooth Implant Restorations

Esthetic success of a tooth restoration or replacement is judged by its "invisible" and perfect integration with the surrounding dentition. These "white esthetics" relate to the shape, surface morphology, dimensions, proportions, shade, position, and angulation of anterior teeth. Other crucial esthetic parameters that are often overlooked are the morphology, texture, and color of the surrounding gingiva—the "pink" or "red esthetics." The soft tissues serve as the "natural frame" of the teeth and are essential for esthetic success.

The photos on the top depict ideal natural teeth and their surrounding soft tissues with symmetric and even gingival scalloping, complete interproximal papillae, and a uniform light pink color. The occlusal view illustrates the natural and symmetric hard and soft tissue support of the teeth.

The patient situation in the middle reveals an implant-supported restoration of the maxillary left central incisor. The soft tissue situation is less than ideal: deficient papillae, nonsymmetric contour and texture, discoloration, and insufficient three-dimensional support. It demonstrates that a nice restoration alone does not imply esthetic success without adequate soft tissue conditions.

The three implant crowns shown in the bottom photos blend perfectly with the remaining teeth, not just from a restorative standpoint but also in respect to soft tissue integration and harmony: ideal tissue scallop, symmetry, color, morphology, texture, three-dimensional contour, and papillary heights.

Successful implementation of these esthetic parameters should be the goal for all restorative and surgical treatments. They are especially difficult to achieve with dental implant restorations, where the initial situation is usually already highly compromised.

Research

Esthetic parameters

Esthetic success of a dental restoration in the anterior maxilla is greatly judged by its indiscernible integration with the surrounding dentition. Therefore, the ultimate esthetic guides for a single-tooth implant-supported restoration are the adjacent and contralateral teeth.

Among the most critical esthetic parameters are tooth position, angulation, dimensions, proportions, shape, surface morphology, and shade.[1–3] These have to be viewed in context with the overall appearance, face, and lips of the patient.[4] Length and dominance of the central incisors, the incisal profile, a convex smile line, symmetry, and tooth display at rest are fundamental parameters that must be idealized for ultimate esthetic success and a pleasing outcome.[1]

Esthetics, however, is not an exact science, and existing clinical studies can only provide average values and common guidelines that must be viewed in context of cultural and individual preferences. Many of the studies on esthetic guidelines presented in the classic literature use two-dimensional assessment tools such as photographs to provide measurements and average values and to assist in the esthetic treatment-planning process. With the increasing use of three-dimensional (3D) scanning and computer-aided design/computer-assisted manufacture technologies, clinical studies on 3D assessments and verification of esthetic parameters have become available[5] and provide extremely helpful tools for the design and fabrication of the "invisible" restoration.

Crucial esthetic parameters that are often overlooked are the morphology, texture, and color of the surrounding gingiva.[6,7] The hard and soft tissues provide the natural frame for the teeth and any dental restoration and are therefore pivotal for esthetic success.[1,6,7] Soft tissue esthetics are also referred to as "pink" or "red esthetics."[1,7] They are often ignored because their handling, manipulation, healing, and ultimate outcome are very demanding, time intensive, and highly unpredictable.[7] Esthetic soft tissue guidelines refer to various parameters, including symmetry, contour, scallop, biotype, papillary height, morphology, texture, and color.[7]

A prevalence of grayish soft tissue discolorations around full-coverage porcelain-fused-to-metal and even all-ceramic restorations was described in the literature.[8] In addition, facial features such as the position of the upper lip and the height of the smile line[8–10] seem to influence the color appearance of the gingiva. It was noted that "this problem is particularly evident in the presence of the upper lip, which can generate an 'umbrella effect' characterized by gray marginal gingivae and dark interdental papillae."[8] This negative "umbrella effect" is magnified with dental implant restorations in the anterior maxilla, due to the fact that the supporting hard and soft tissues are often already compromised before treatment. Esthetic outcomes are influenced by the surgical procedures, the selection and placement of the implants, as well as the design and color of the prosthetic components and the definitive restorations.[11–18]

Ideal surgical and restorative success with maxillary anterior implant-supported restorations presents a great challenge for the entire dental team.[12] However, the best and most esthetic treatment should always be the ultimate goal for our patients, who are greatly affected by the appearance of their teeth and the attractiveness of their smiles.[19]

References

1. Chiche G, Pinault A. Esthetics of Anterior Fixed Prosthodontics. Chicago: Quintessence, 1994.

2. Matthews TG. The anatomy of a smile. J Prosthet Dent 1978; 39:128–134.

3. Fradeani M. Esthetic Analysis: A Systematic Approach to Prosthetic Treatment. Chicago: Quintessence, 2005.

4. Passia N, Blatz MB, Strub JR. Is the smile line a valid parameter for esthetic evaluation? A review of the literature. Eur J Esthet Dent 2011;6:338–351.

5. Horvath SD, Wegstein PG, Luethi M, Blatz MB. The correlation between anterior tooth form and gender—A 3D analysis in humans. Eur J Esthet Dent 2012;7:334–343.

6. Bitter RN. The periodontal factor in esthetic smile design—Altering gingival display. Gen Dent 2007;55:616–622.

7. Blatz MB, Hürzeler MB, Strub JR. Reconstruction of the lost interproximal papilla—Presentation of some surgical and non-surgical procedures. Int J Periodontics Restorative Dent 1999;19:395–406.

8. Magne P, Magne M, Belser U. The esthetic width in fixed prosthodontics. J Prosthodont 1999;8:106–118.

9. Vig RG, Brundo GC. The kinetics of anterior tooth display. J Prosthet Dent 1978;39:502–504.

10. Fradeani M. Evaluation of dentolabial parameters as part of a comprehensive esthetic analysis. Eur J Esthet Dent 2006;1:62–69.

11. Gamborena I, Blatz MB. Current clinical and technical protocols for single-tooth immediate implant procedures. Quintessence Dent Technol 2008;31:49–60.

12. Gamborena I, Blatz MB. The grey zone around dental implants—Keys to esthetic success. Am J Esthet Dent 2011; 1:26–46.

13. Holst S, Blatz MB, Hegenbarth E, Wichmann M, Eitner S. Prosthodontic considerations for predictable single-implant esthetics in the anterior maxilla. J Oral Maxillofac Surg 2005;63(9 suppl 2):89–96.

14. Kois JC, Kan JY. Predictable peri-implant gingival aesthetics: Surgical and prosthodontic rationales. Pract Proced Aesthet Dent 2001;13:691–698.

15. Blatz MB, Bergler M, Holst S, Block M. Zirconia abutments for single-tooth implants—Rationale and clinical guidelines. J Oral Maxillofac Surg 2009;67(11 suppl):74–81.

16. Yildirim M, Edelhoff D, Hanish O, Spiekermann H. Ceramic abutments—A new era in achieving optimal esthetics in implant dentistry. Int J Periodontics Restorative Dent 2000;20:81–91.

17. Jung RE, Sailer I, Hämmerle CH, Attin T, Schmidlin P. In vitro color changes of soft tissues caused by restorative materials. Int J Periodontics Restorative Dent 2007;27:251–257.

18. Jung RE, Holderegger C, Sailer I, Khraisat A, Suter A, Hämmerle CH. The effect of all-ceramic and porcelain-fused-to-metal restorations on marginal peri-implant soft tissue color: A randomized controlled clinical trial. Int J Periodontics Restorative Dent 2008;28:357–365.

19. Van der Geld P, Oosterveld P, Van Heck G, Kuijpers-Jagtman AM. Smile attractiveness. Self-perception and influence on personality. Angle Orthod 2007;77:759–765.

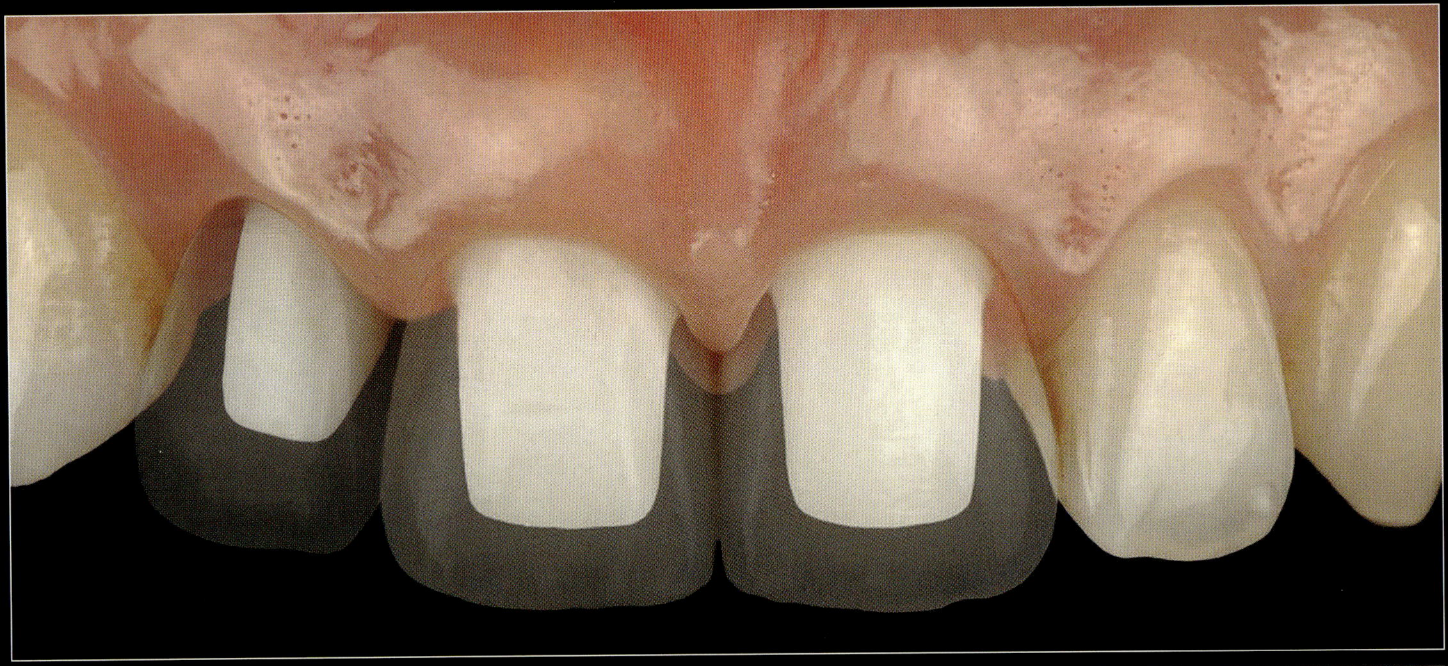

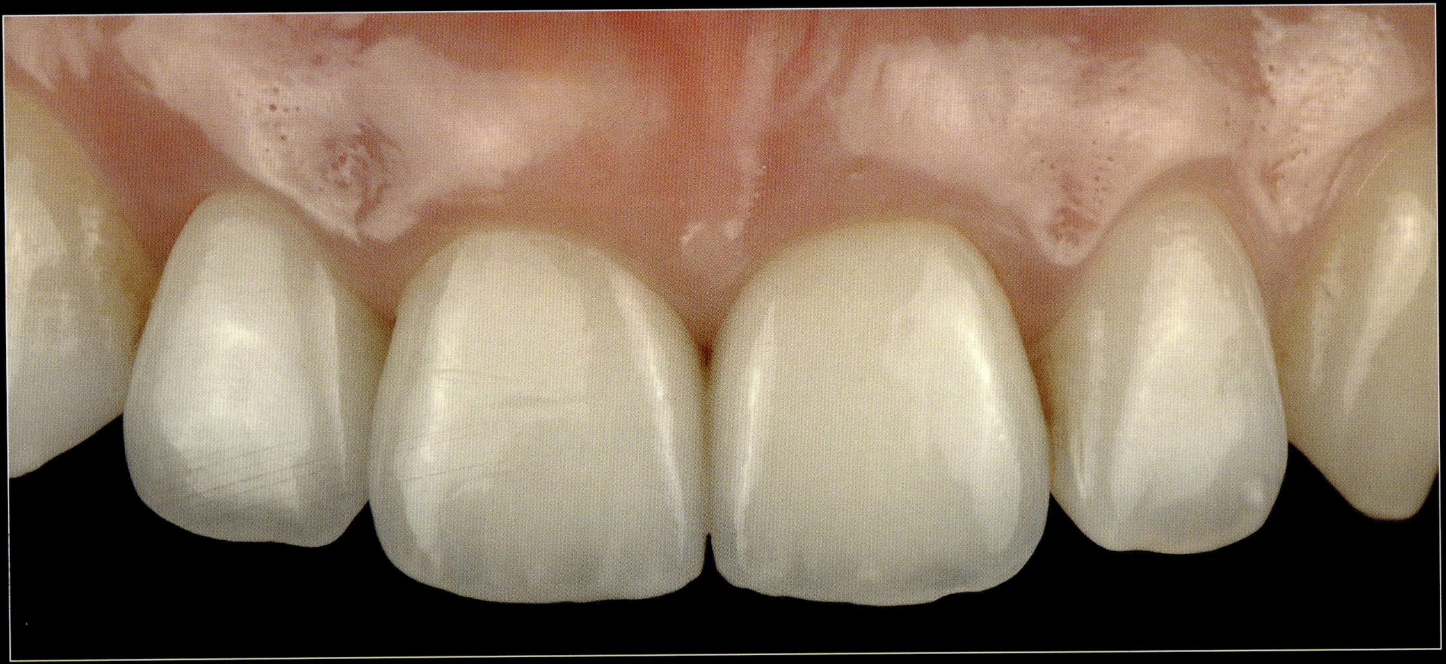

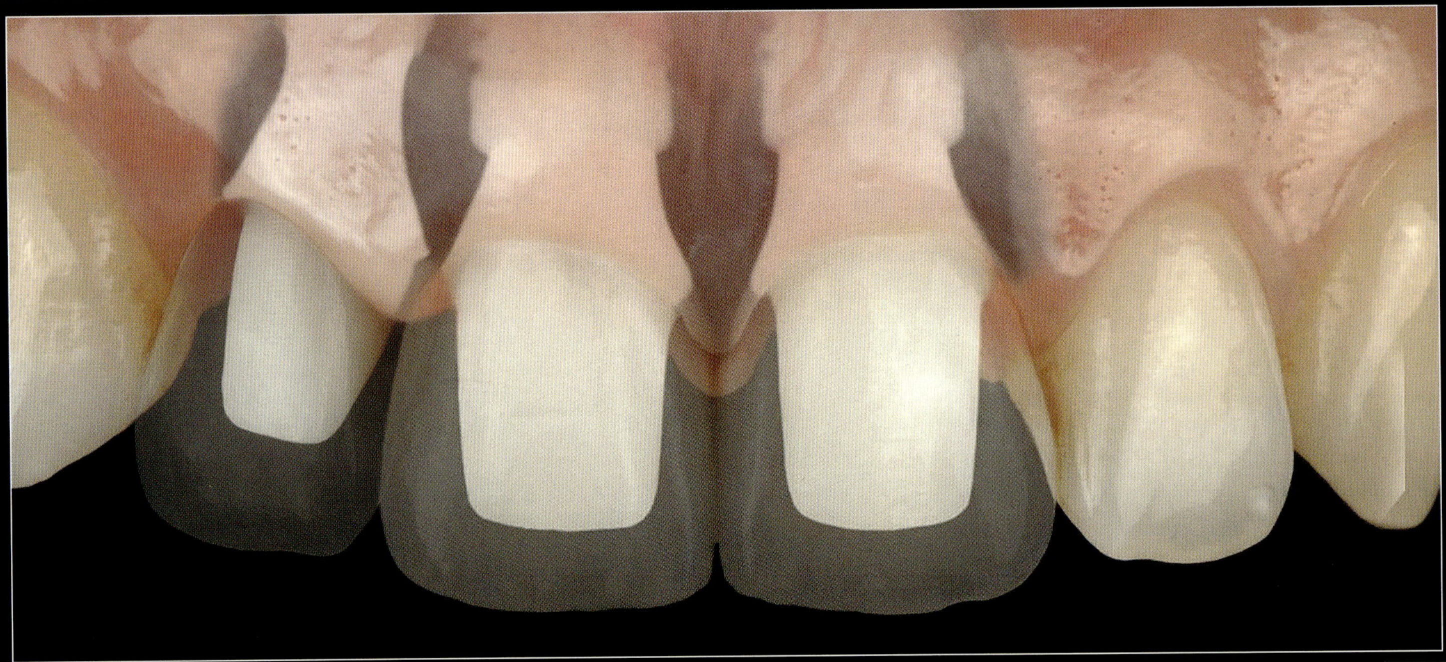

Soft Tissue Characteristics Around Implants

This section was contributed by Peter Schüpbach, Dr sc Nat ETH, Zurich, Switzerland.

Research

Peri-implant soft tissue

When dental implants are placed into alveolar bone, it is expected that they will osseointegrate and, perhaps more importantly, that the peri-implant mucosa will heal to the abutment surface. In doing so, the primary functions of the periodontal tissues are fulfilled, which are the attachment and protection of the soft tissue and the underlying bone. For this to happen, the structural framework of the peri-implant mucosa must match the architecture of the gingiva.

Brånemark, Zarb, and Albrektsson et al[1–3] were pioneers who demonstrated that the sophisticated, suspension-like anchorage of a tooth in alveolar bone by the periodontal ligament can be successfully replaced by a rigid, ankylotic-like, direct structural and functional connection between ordered living bone and an implant surface. From their research, the mechanisms of peri-implant endosseous wound healing have become better understood.[4–6]

Today, it is generally accepted that bone forms adjacent to smooth, machined (turned) implant surfaces, a phenomenon called *distance osteogenesis*.[4] Conversely, bone also forms directly on and along moderately rough implant surfaces, a phenomenon called *contact osteogenesis*.[6] Surface roughness, surface coating, biomimetic approaches, and growth factor delivery may also accelerate osseointegration.[4,7,8]

The peri-implant mucosa surrounding successful endosseous implants is in many ways analogous to the mucosa surrounding natural dentition. Gould et al[9,10] were the first to show in vitro that epithelial cells attach to titanium in a similar way to how epithelium attaches to teeth. Subsequent animal and human studies[11,12] have shown histologically that the epithelial structures and the lamina propria of implants cannot be differentiated from the structures around teeth.

A basal lamina together with hemidesmosomes form an interface, called the *epithelial attachment*, between the tooth surface and the junctional epithelium.[13–15] In 2005, Bosshardt and Lang[12] demonstrated that junctional epithelium around implants originates from epithelial cells of the oral mucosa, as opposed to originating from the reduced enamel epithelium of teeth.

Despite the similarity of epithelial attachment, important differences exist in the way connective tissue interfaces with implant surfaces in the absence of root cementum. With teeth, dentogingival fibers are directed perpendicularly/obliquely to root surfaces and are firmly anchored in the mineralized cementum, whereas with implant surfaces, only an adaptation of connective tissue occurs.

Because of the absence of a cementum layer, collagen fibers run approximately parallel to abutment/implant surfaces and are oriented either coronoapically or circumferentially.[15–18]

However, in terms of granulocyte transmigration through the junctional epithelium to the sulcus, the inflammatory response around abutments/implants has been found to be identical to the inflammatory response around teeth.[18,19]

References

1. Brånemark PI, Hansson BO, Adell R, et al. Osseointegrated implants in the treatment of the edentulous jaw. Experience from a 10-year period. Scand J Plast Reconstr Surg Suppl 1977;16:1–132.

2. Brånemark PI, Zarb GA, Albrektsson T (eds). Tissue-Integrated Prostheses: Osseointegration in Clinical Dentistry. Chicago: Quintessence, 1985.

3. Albrektsson T, Zarb GA (eds). The Brånemark Osseointegrated Implant. Chicago: Quintessence, 1989.

4. Puleo DA, Nanci A. Understanding and controlling the bone-implant interface. Biomaterials 1999;20:2311–2321.

5. Puleo DA, Thomas MV. Implant surfaces. Dent Clin North Am 2006;50:323–338.

6. Davies JE. Understanding peri-implant endosseous healing. J Dent Educ 2003;67:932–949.

7. Chang PC, Lang NP, Giannobile WV. Evaluation of functional dynamics during osseointegration and regeneration associated with oral implants. Clin Oral Implants Res 2010;21:1–12.

8. Stanford CM. Surface modifications of dental implants. Aust Dent J 2008;53(suppl 1):S26–S33.

9. Gould TR, Brunette DM, Westbury L. The attachment mechanism of epithelial cells to titanium in vitro. J Periodontal Res 1981;16:611–616.

10. Gould TR, Westbury L, Brunette DM. Ultrastructural study of the attachment of human gingiva to titanium in vivo. J Prosthet Dent 1984;52:418–420.

11. Pöllänen MT, Salonen JI, Uitto VJ. Structure and function of the tooth-epithelial interface in health and disease. Periodontol 2000 2003;31:12–31.

12. Bosshardt DD, Lang NP. The junctional epithelium: From health to disease. J Dent Res 2005;84:9–20.

13. Listgarten MA. Electron microscopic study of the gingivo-dental junction of man. Am J Anat 1966;119:147–177.

14. Schroeder HE. Ultrastructure of the junctional epithelium of the human gingiva. Helv Odontol Acta 1969;13:65–83.

15. Listgarten MA, Lang NP, Schroeder HE, Schroeder A. Periodontal tissues and their counterparts around endosseous implants. Clin Oral Implants Res 1991;2:1–19.

16. Buser D, Weber HP, Donath K, Fiorellini JP, Paquette DW, Williams RC. Soft tissue reactions to non-submerged unloaded titanium implants in beagle dogs. J Periodontol 1992;63:225–235.

17. Abrahamsson I, Berglundh T, Glantz PO, Lindhe J. The mucosal attachment at different abutments. An experimental study in dogs. J Clin Periodontol 1998;25:721–727.

18. Berglundh T, Lindhe J, Ericsson I, Marinello CP, Liljenberg B, Thomsen P. The soft tissue barrier at implants and teeth. Clin Oral Implants Res 1991;2:81–90.

19. Schüpbach P, Glauser R. The defense architecture of the human periimplant mucosa: A histological study. J Prosthet Dent 2007;97(suppl):S15–S25.

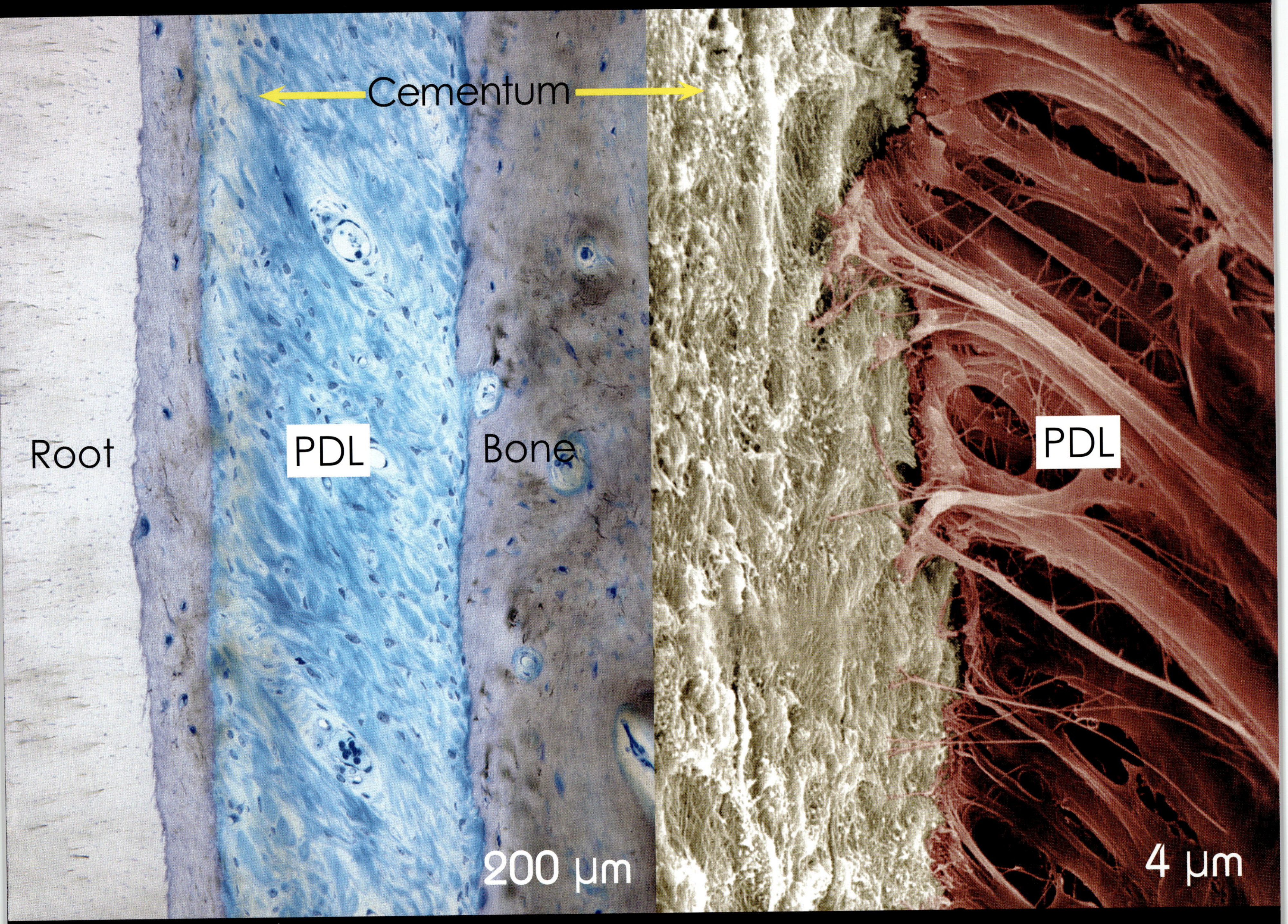
Cementum
Root
PDL
Bone
200 µm
PDL
4 µm

Our teeth are anchored in alveolar bone in a truly spectacular way. A dense connective tissue called the *periodontal ligament (PDL)*, comprising strong collagen fibers, connects the root surface with the alveolar bone. These collagen fibers, each composed of hundreds of densely packed single fibrils, cross the space between root and bone. Fibrils are deeply buried and anchored in the mineralized matrix of root cementum and bone. The periodontal ligament network functions like a flexible suspension that resists displacement forces during mastication and protects our teeth against excessive occlusal load.

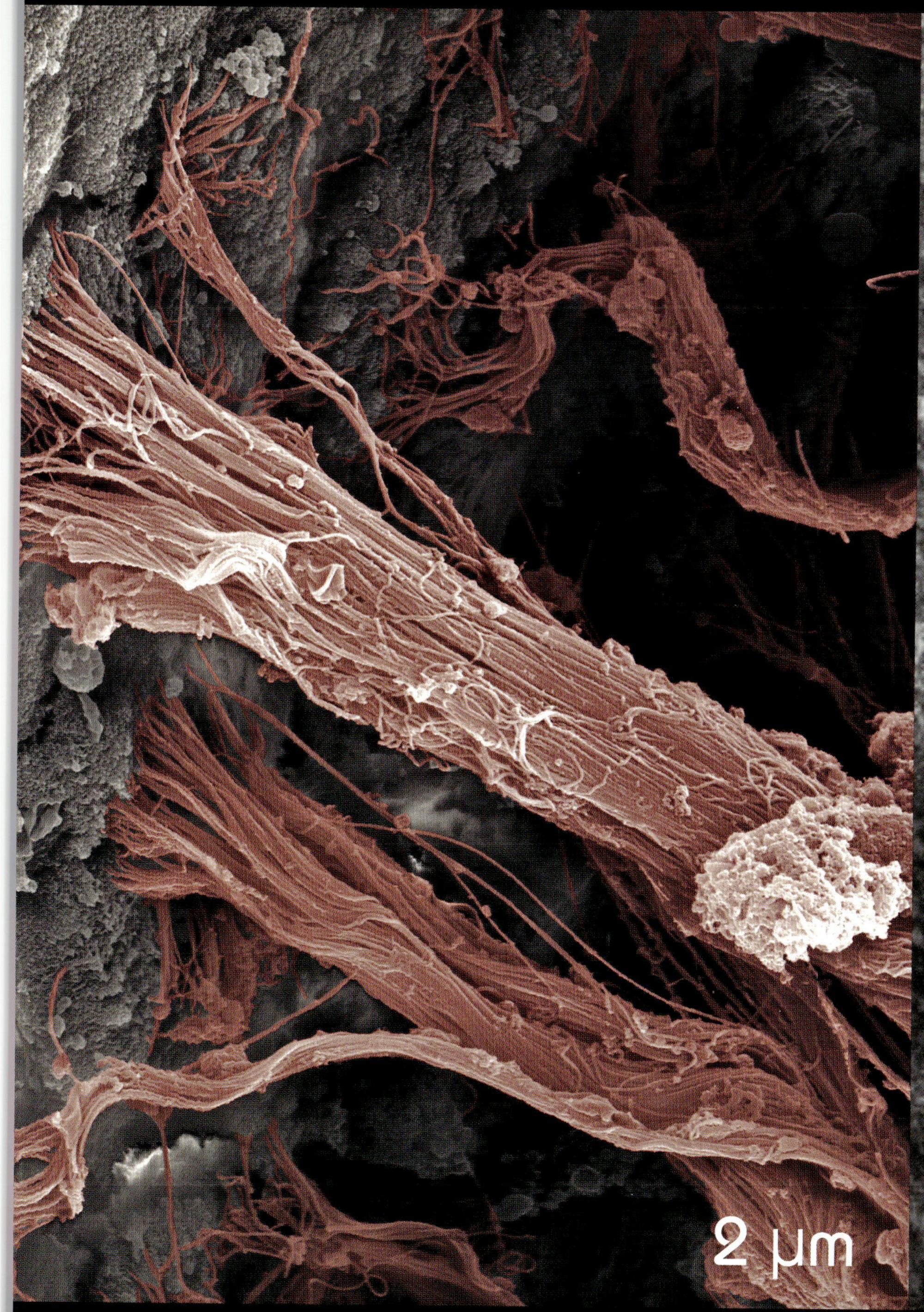

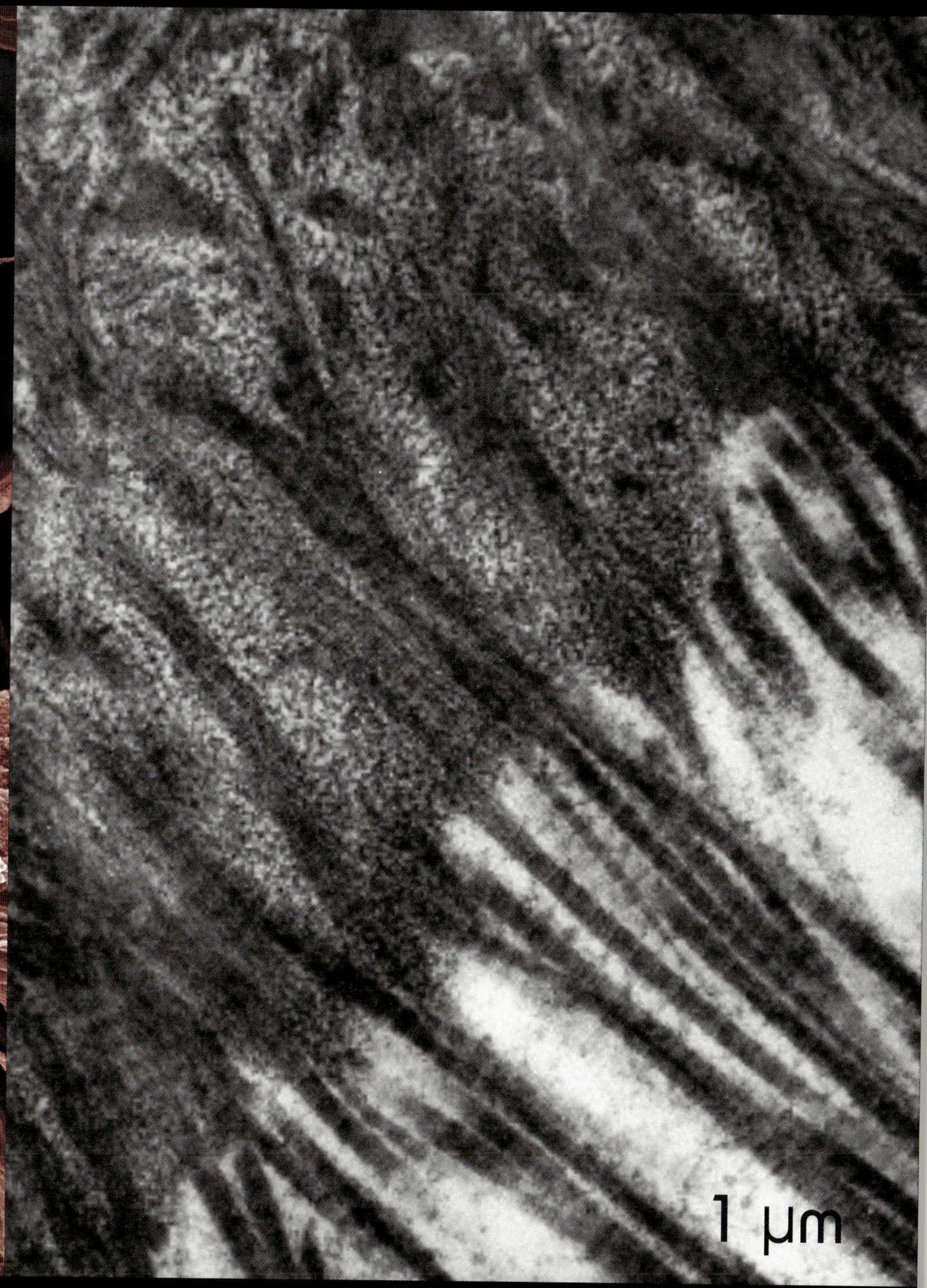

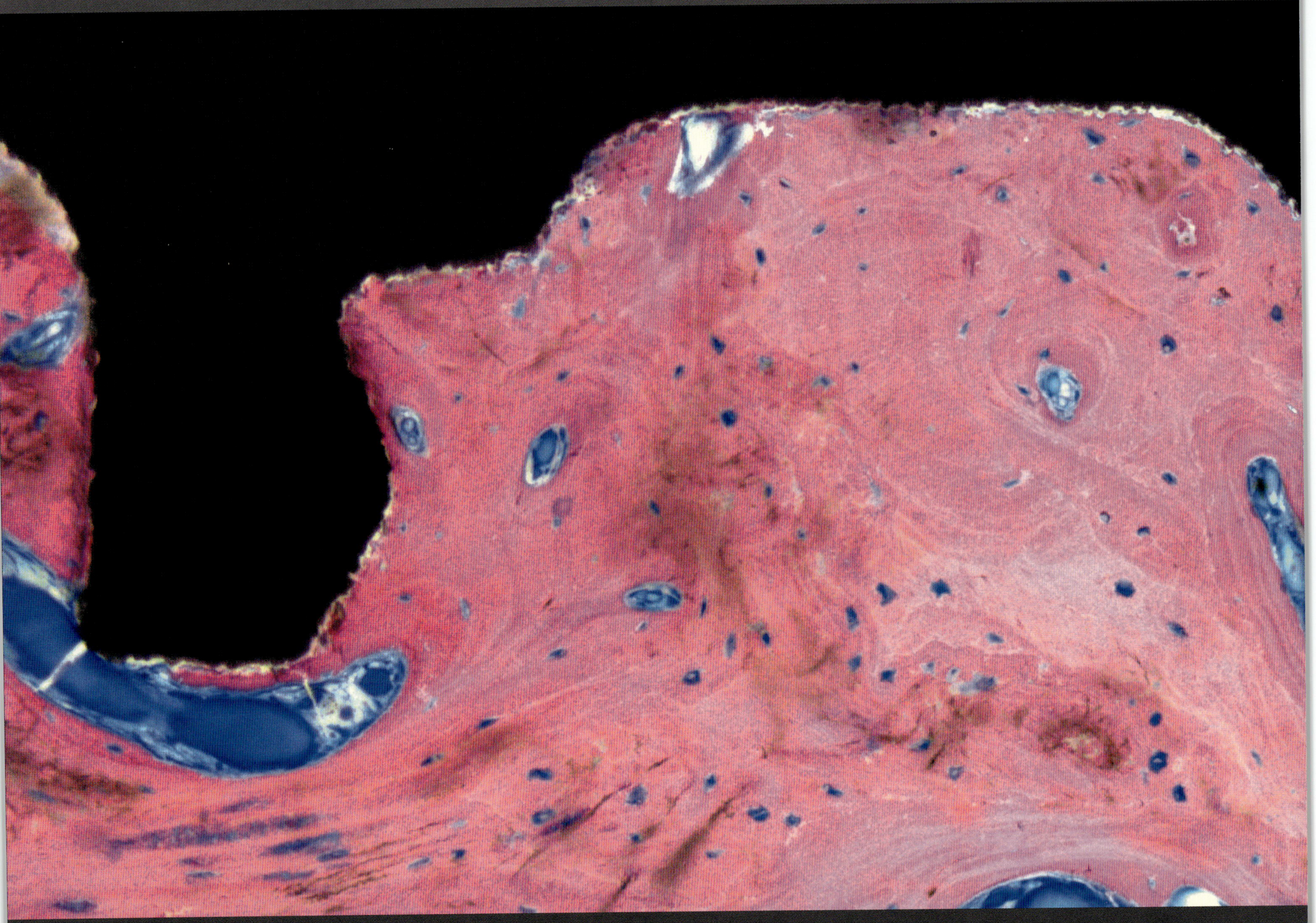

In contrast to the sophisticated way natural teeth are anchored in the alveolar bone, dental implants are osseointegrated in a rather ankylotic way.

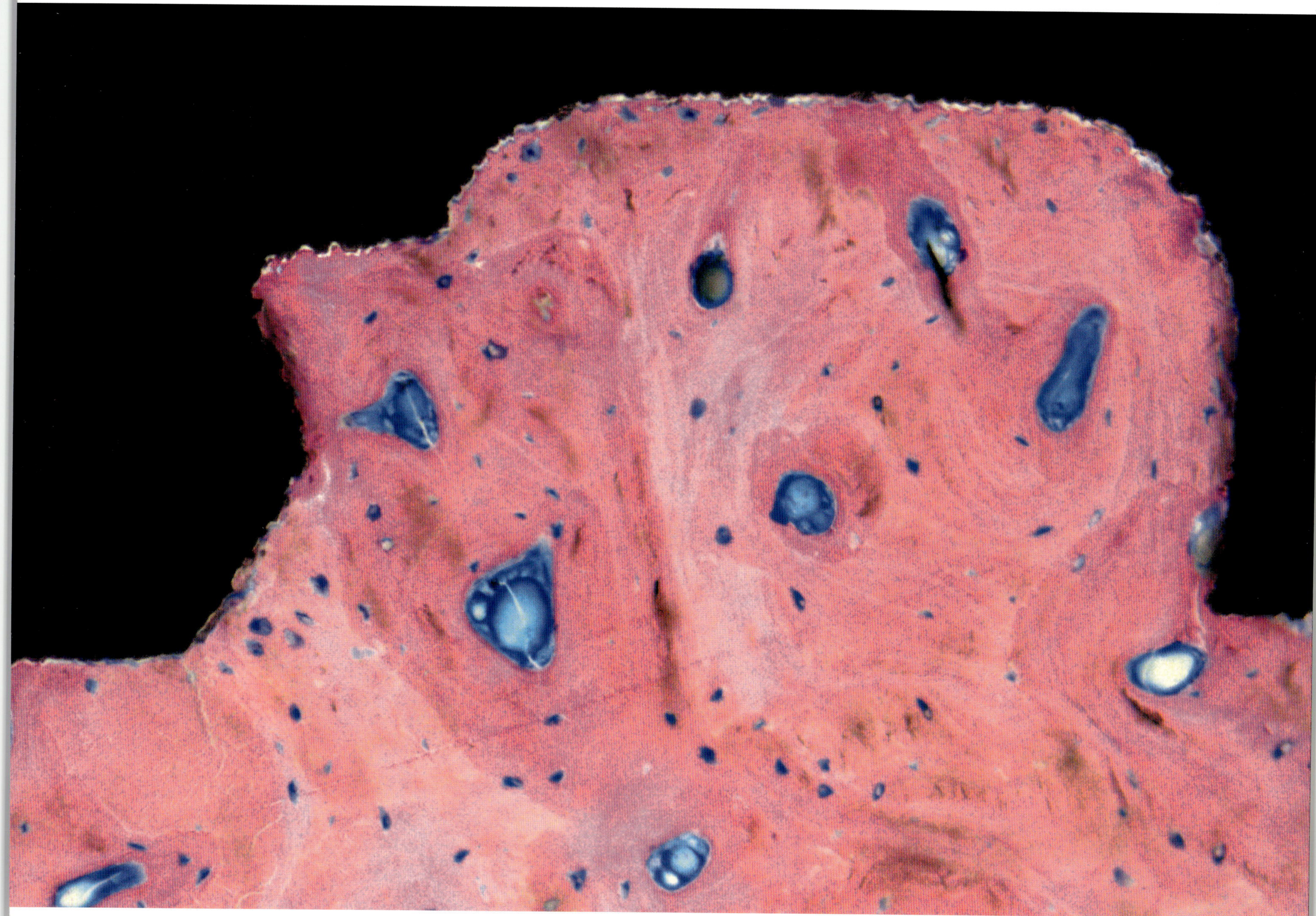

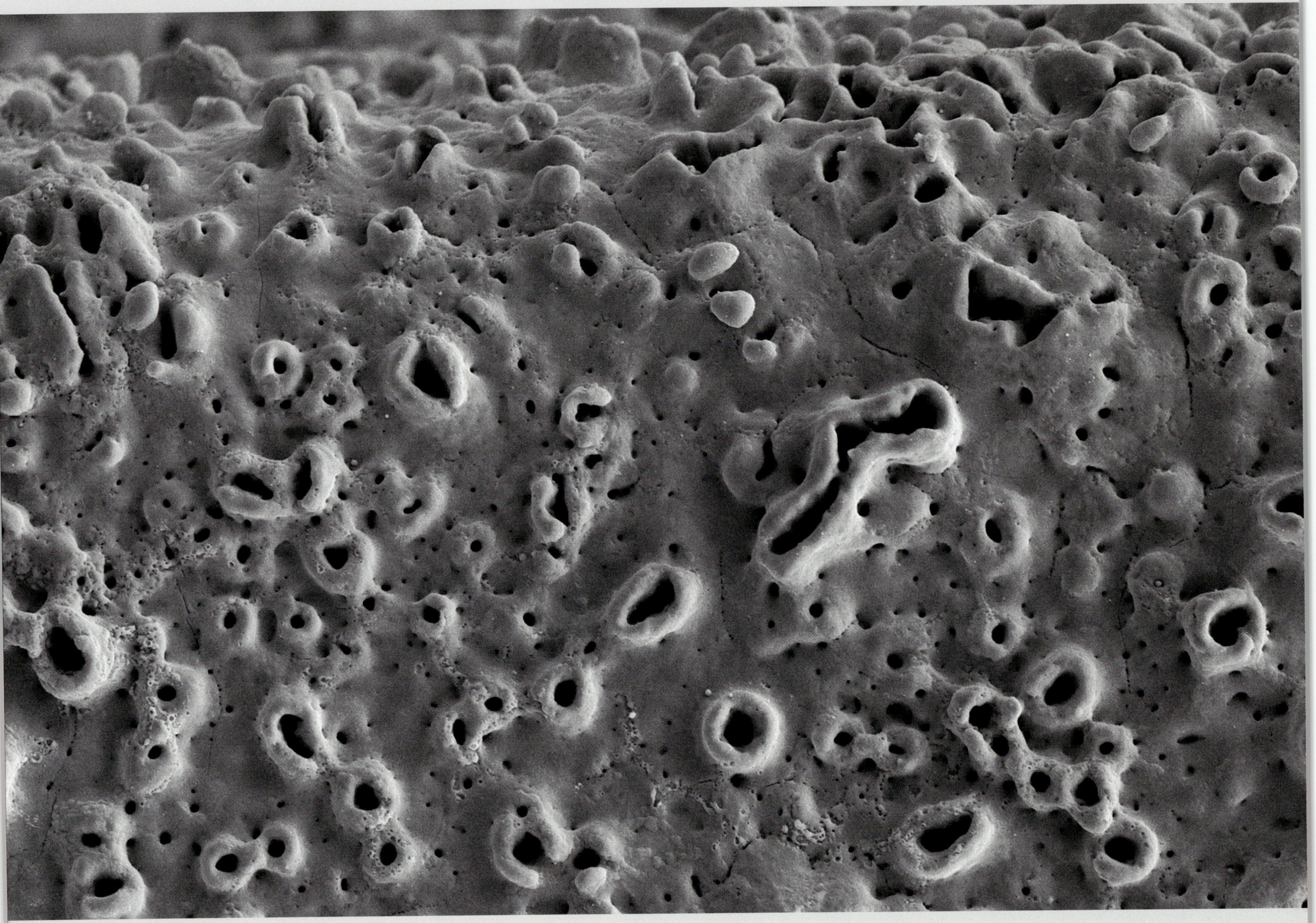

In implant therapy, blood is the first tissue to interact with an implant surface. In 1 mL of blood, there are 5 billion red blood cells, 8 million white blood cells, and 30 million platelets. Platelets are crucial for wound healing. Immediately following placement of an implant, high numbers of flat, inactive platelets *(white arrows)* are attracted to the implant surface.

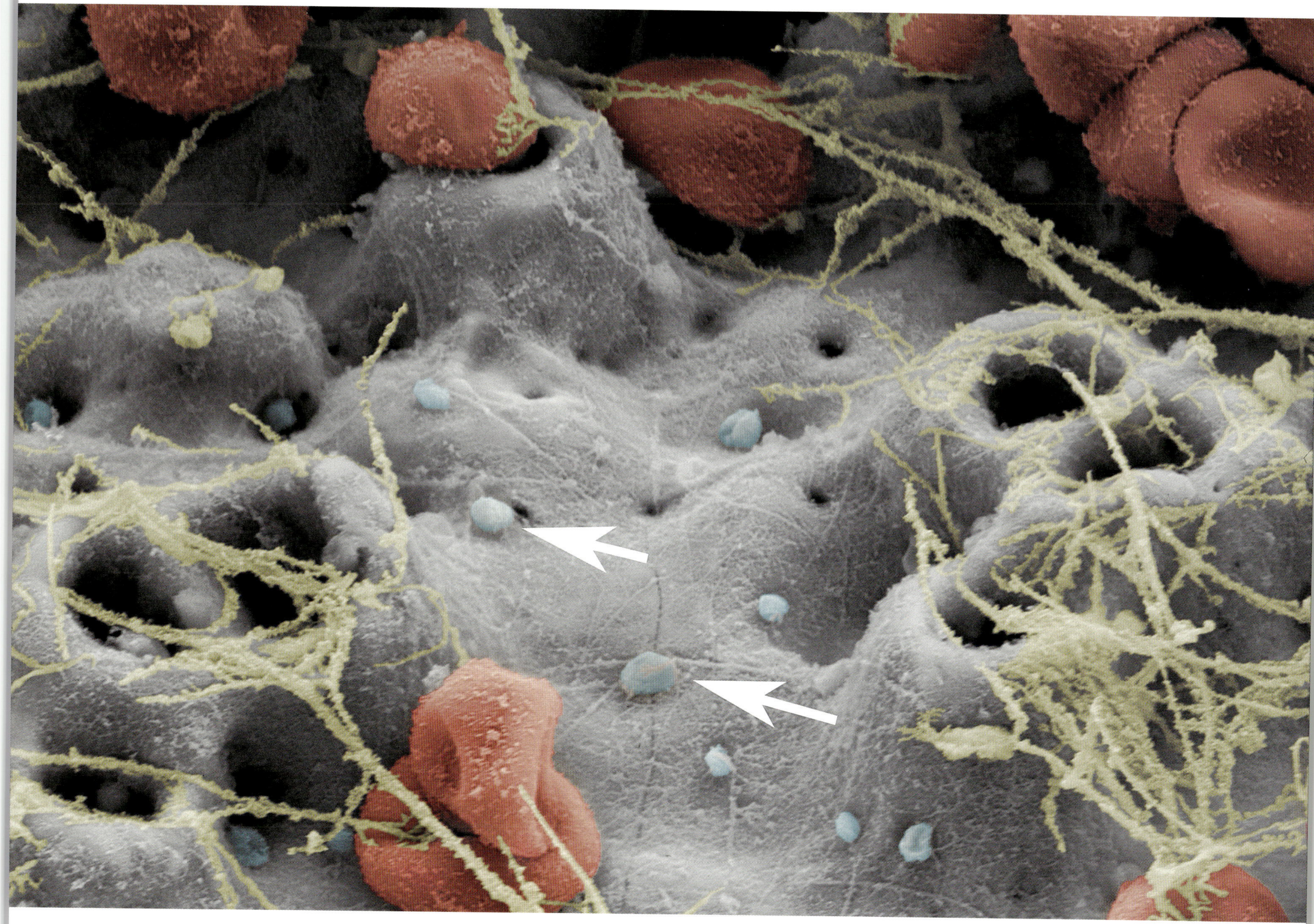

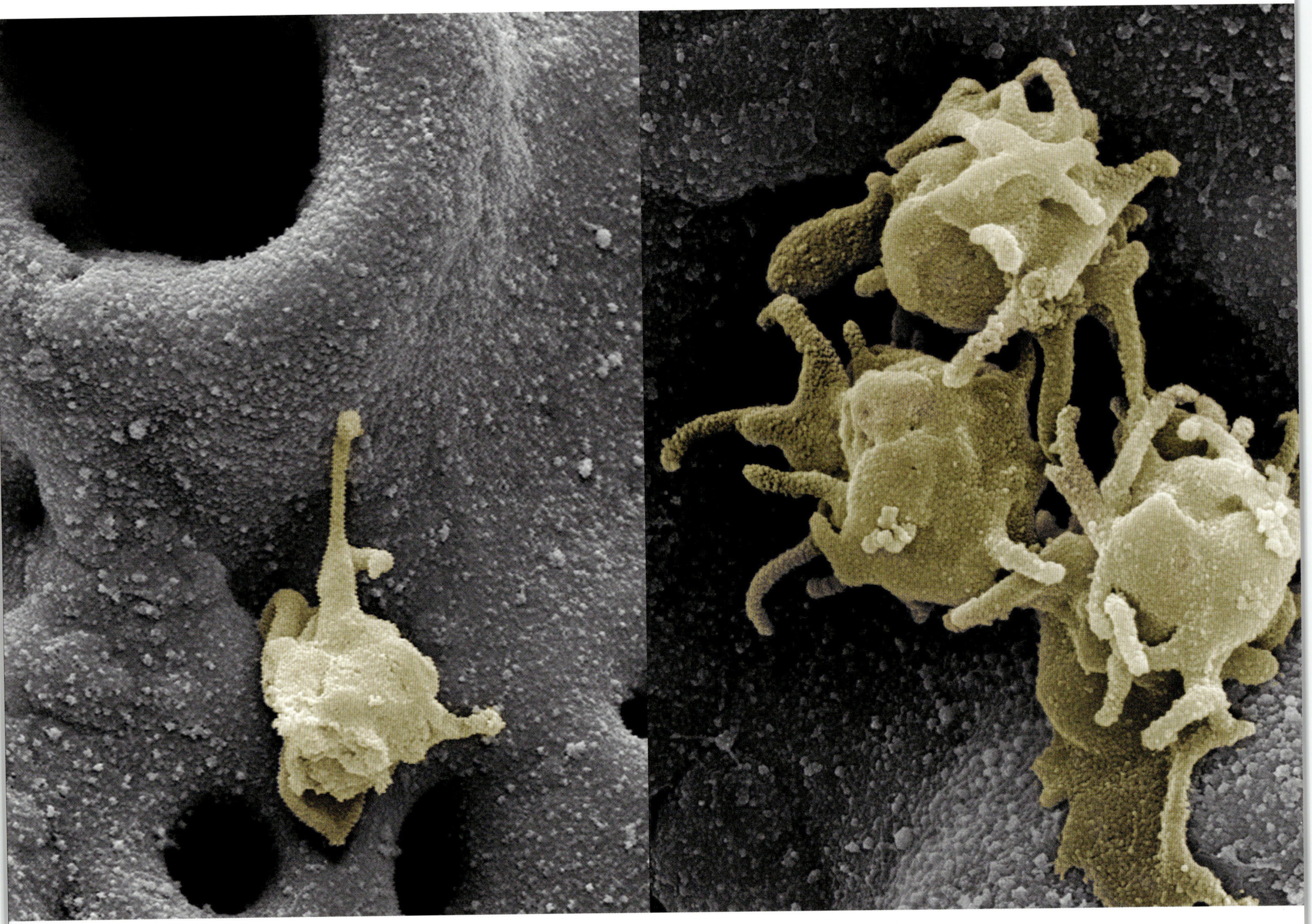

On the implant surface, platelets become immediately activated, their shapes become more spherical, and pseudopods begin to form on their surfaces. They assume stellate shapes with a considerably enlarged surface area. Chemical reactions make the platelet surface sticky. Platelets clump together to form aggregates, which plug the small blood vessels in the periphery of the wound, and bleeding slows.

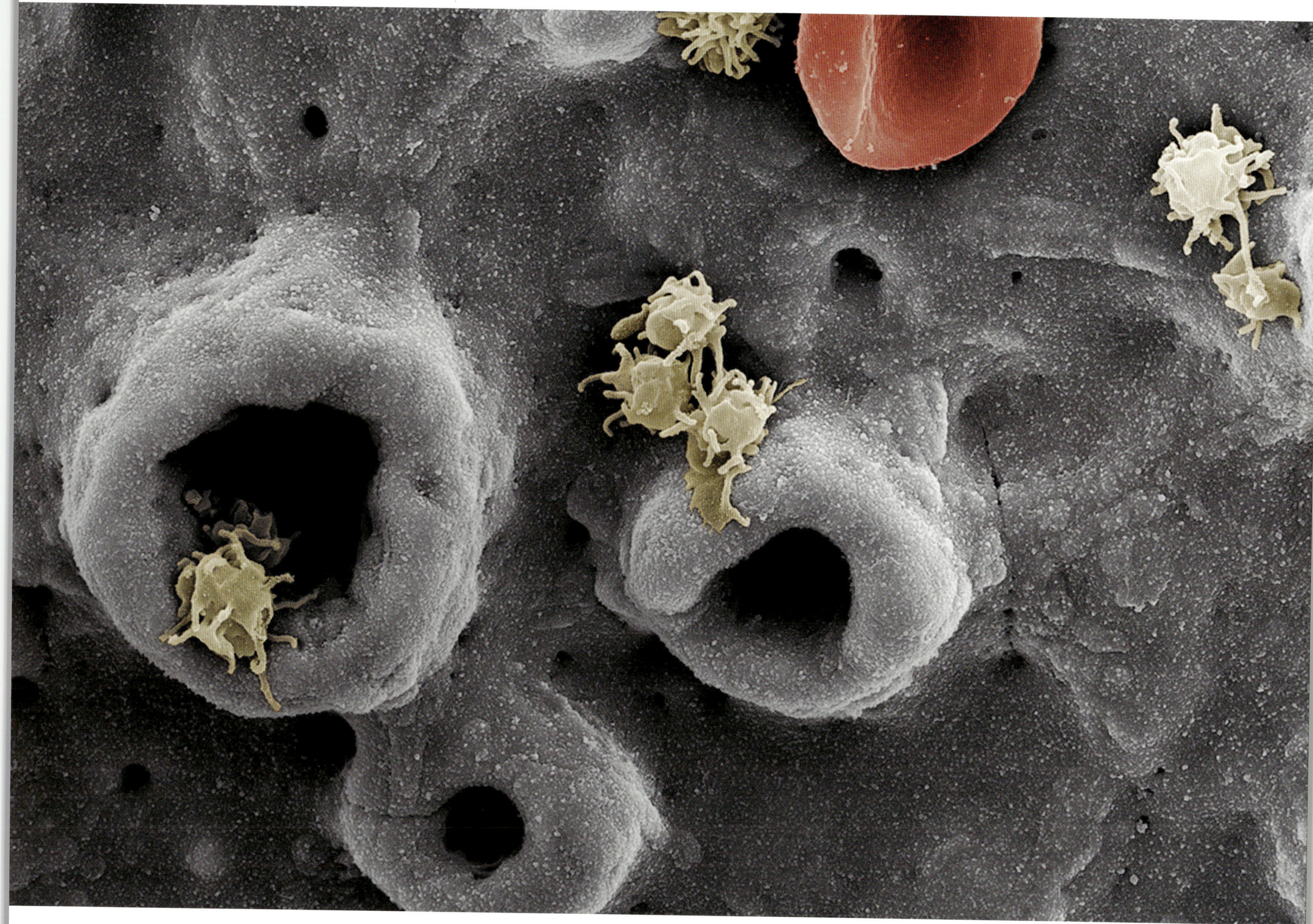

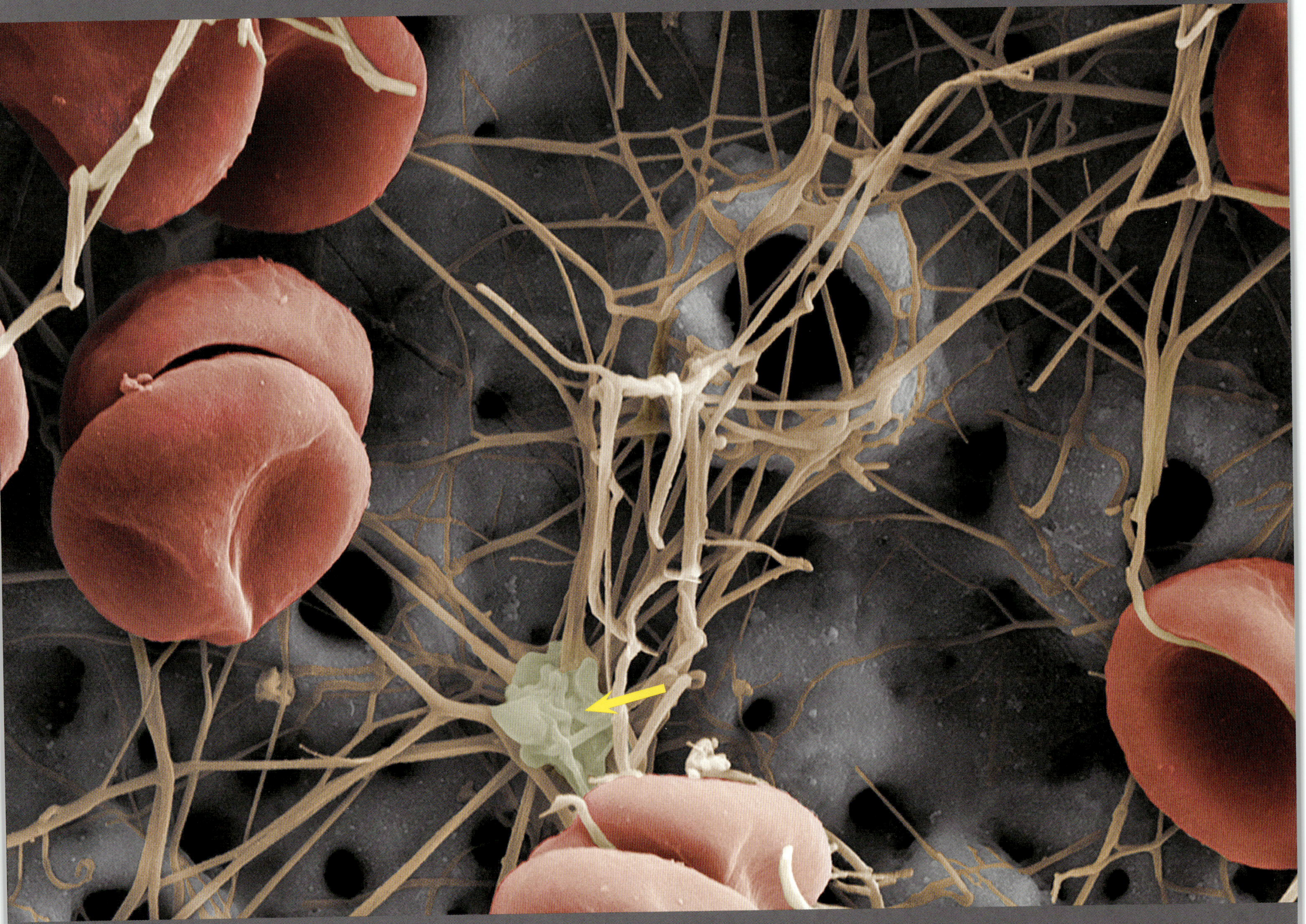

From fibrinogen, clotting proteins form long sticky strands, called *fibrin*. These fibrin strands trap activated platelets *(yellow arrow)* and create a fibrin mesh. At higher magnification, granules filled with batteries of enzymes and growth factors can be seen on the platelets. The activated platelets release these growth factors, which attract various cells types needed for wound healing and subsequent bone formation.

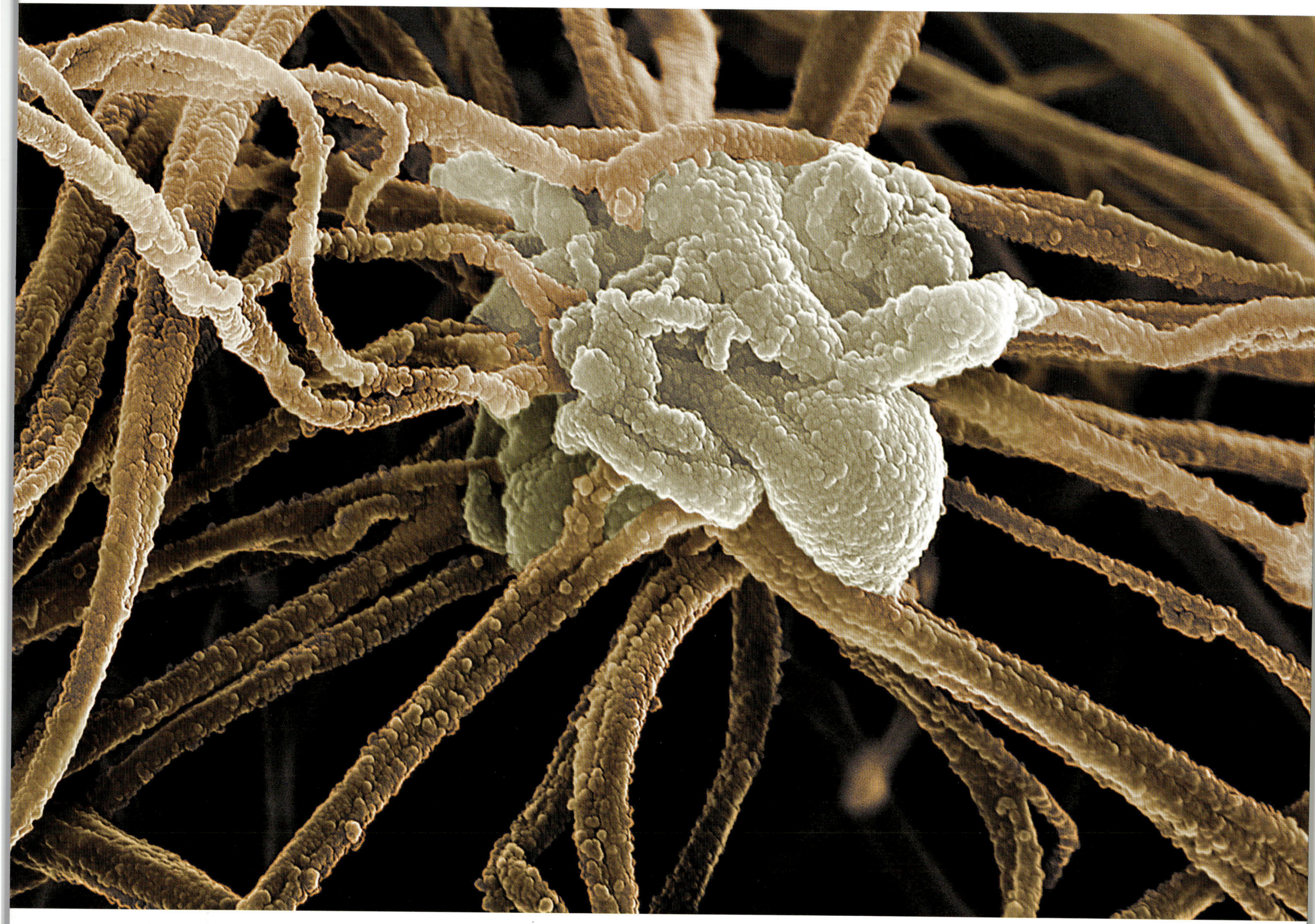

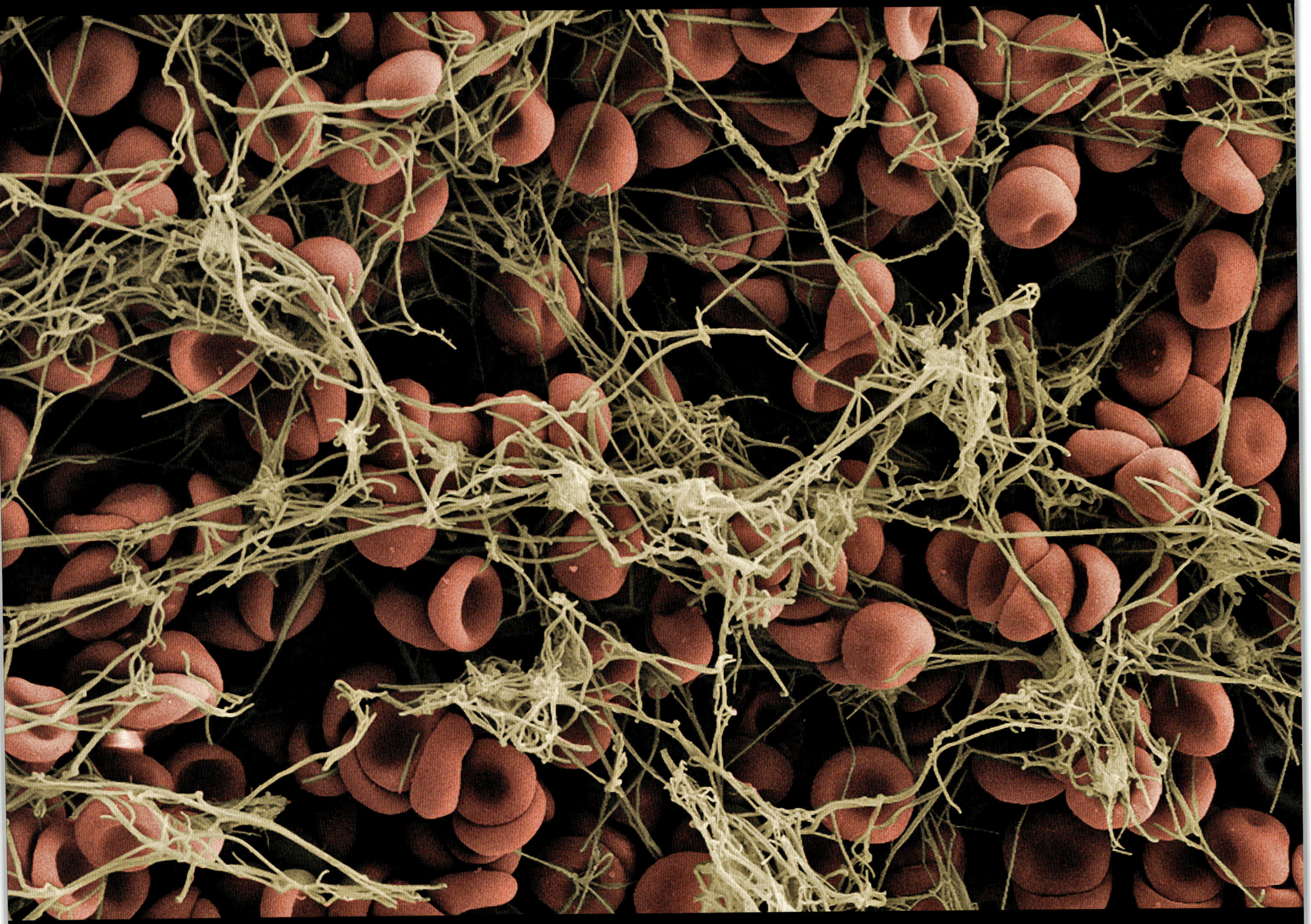

Within minutes following implant placement, a blood clot (seen as a complex mesh) composed of fibrin strands, activated platelets, and red blood cells is formed and becomes firmly attached to the implant surface. The retention of the blood clot is critical for subsequent wound healing steps. Bleeding has now stopped, and the first phase of wound healing, *hemostasis*, is complete.

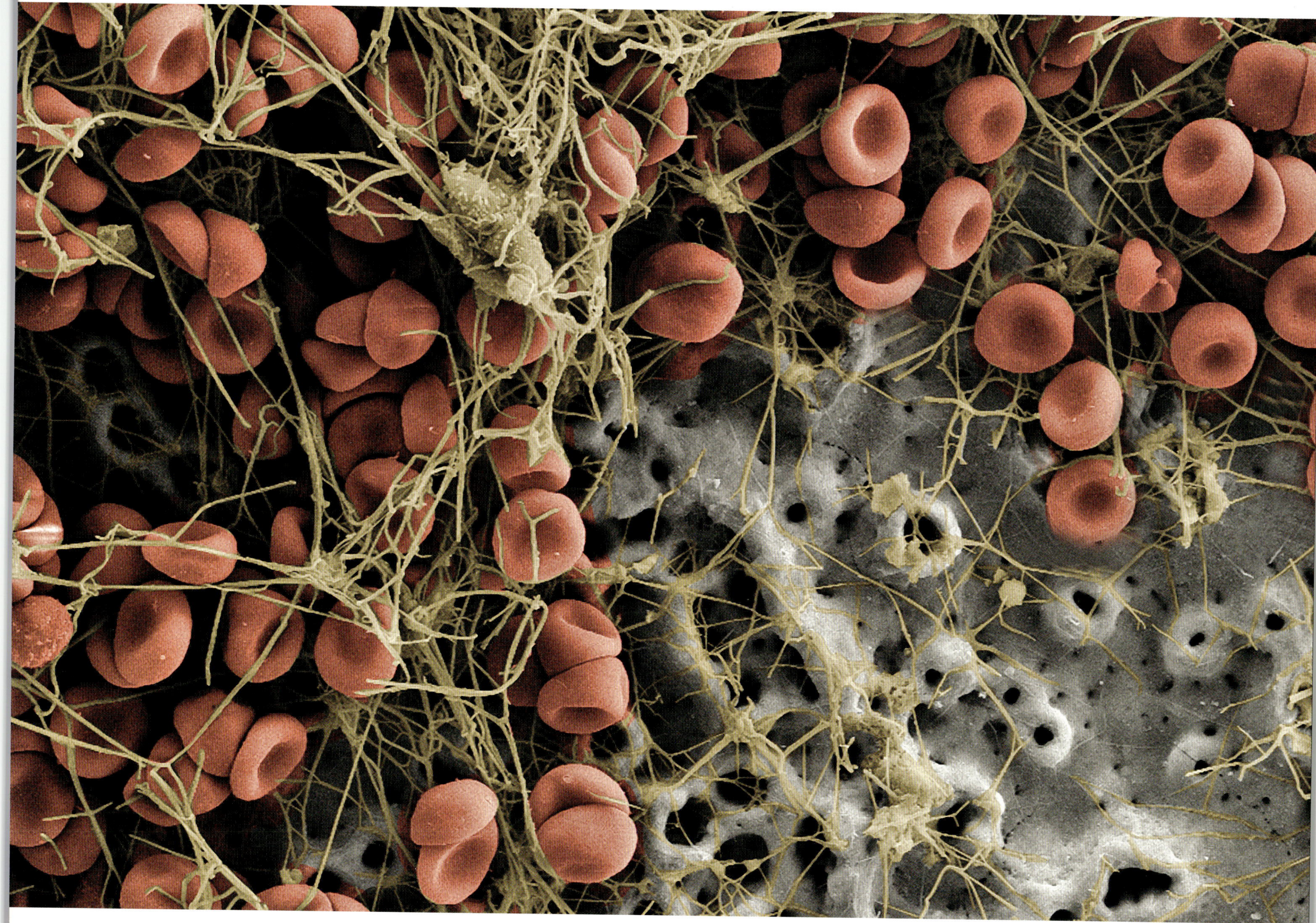

Clinical implication: While important during drilling, irrigation should be avoided during implant placement. Undiluted blood on the implant surface is necessary for effective hemostasis.

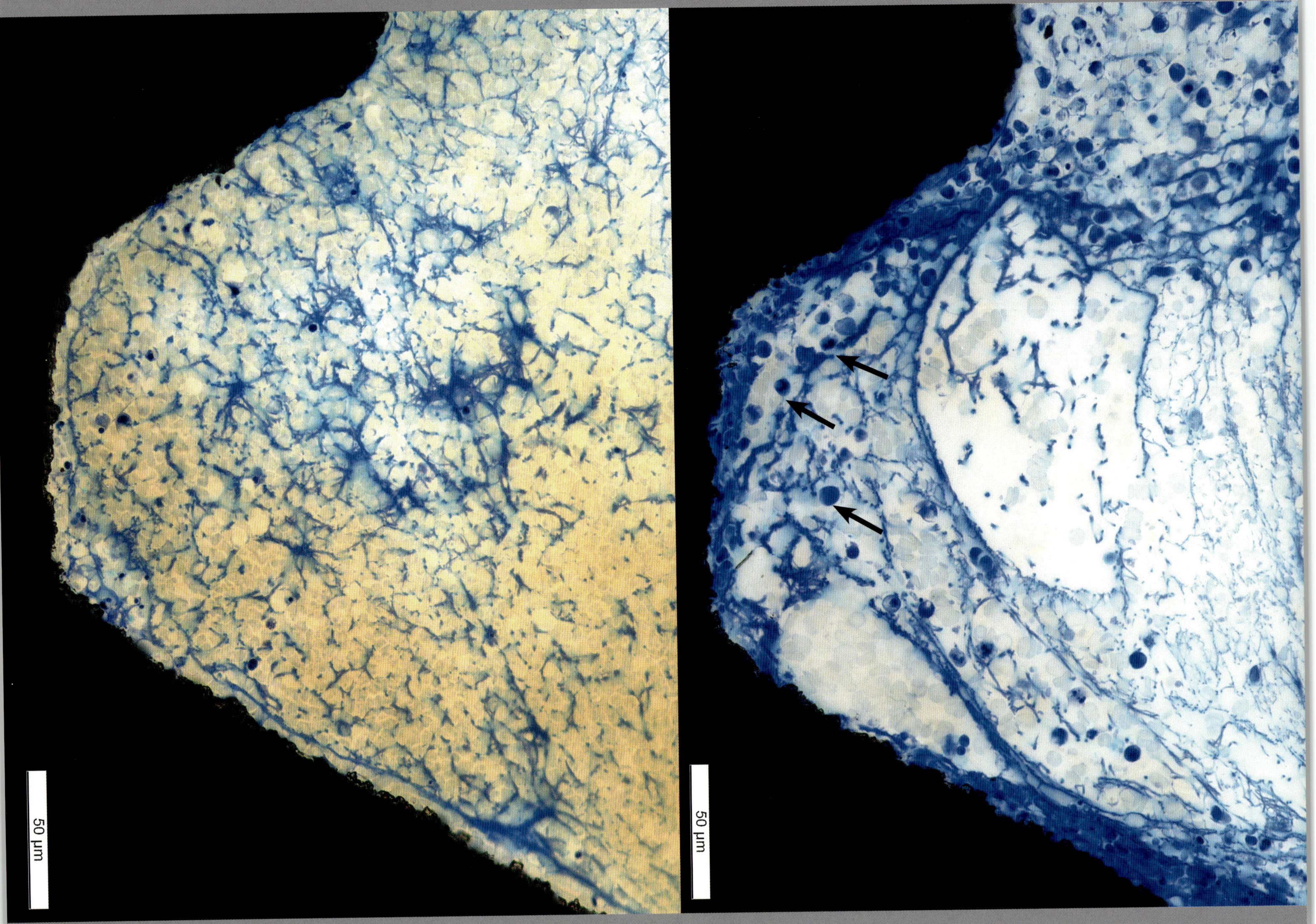
50 µm
50 µm

Once bleeding is controlled, inflammatory cells are attracted and migrate to the wound to promote the inflammatory phase. Initially, leukocytes *(black arrows in SEM micrograph at right on opposite page)* are the most numerous cells. Their numbers usually peak 48 hours following implant placement. Leukocytes are critical for degradation of the fibrin clot (mesh) and help clear the wound of invading bacteria and debris.

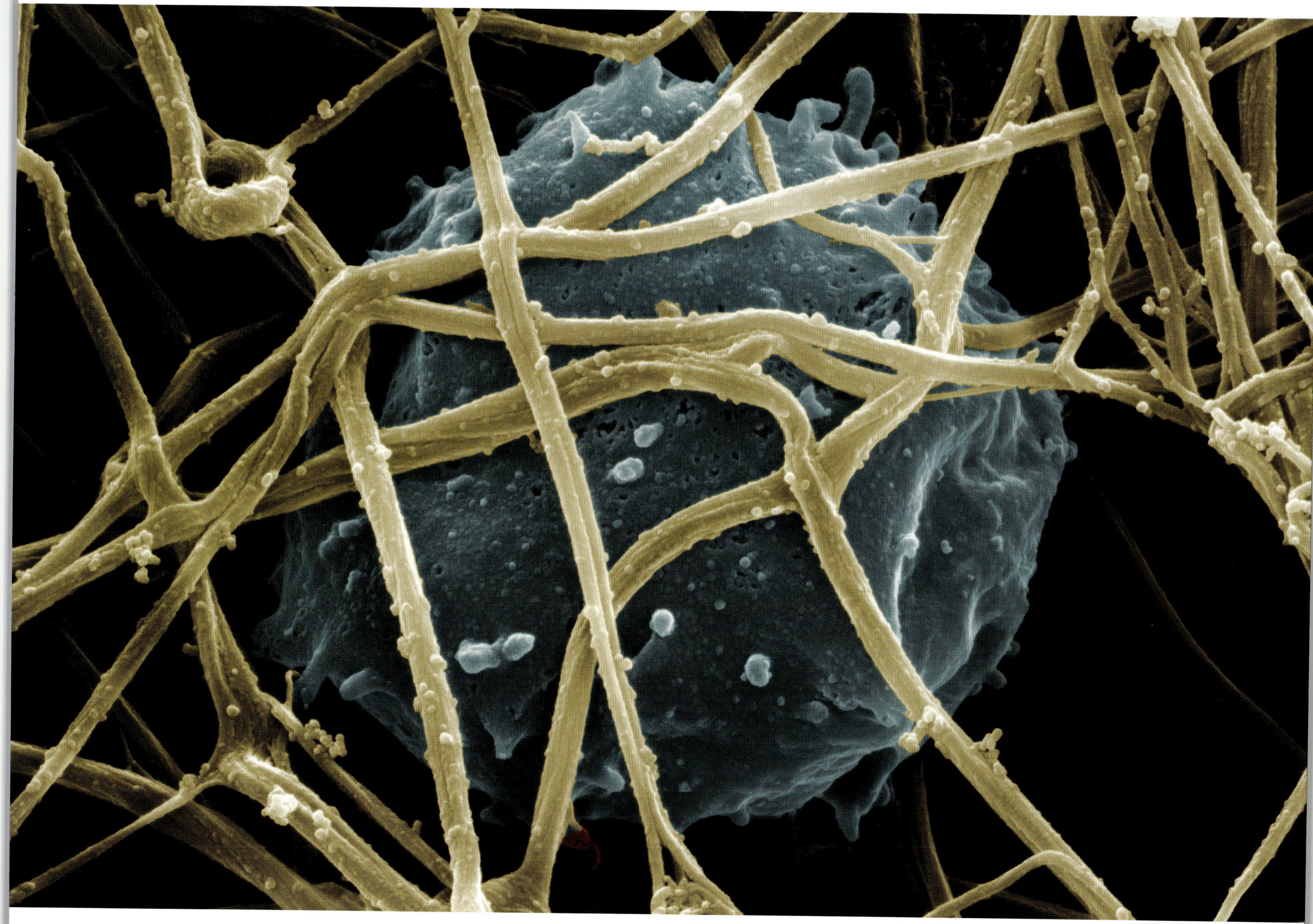

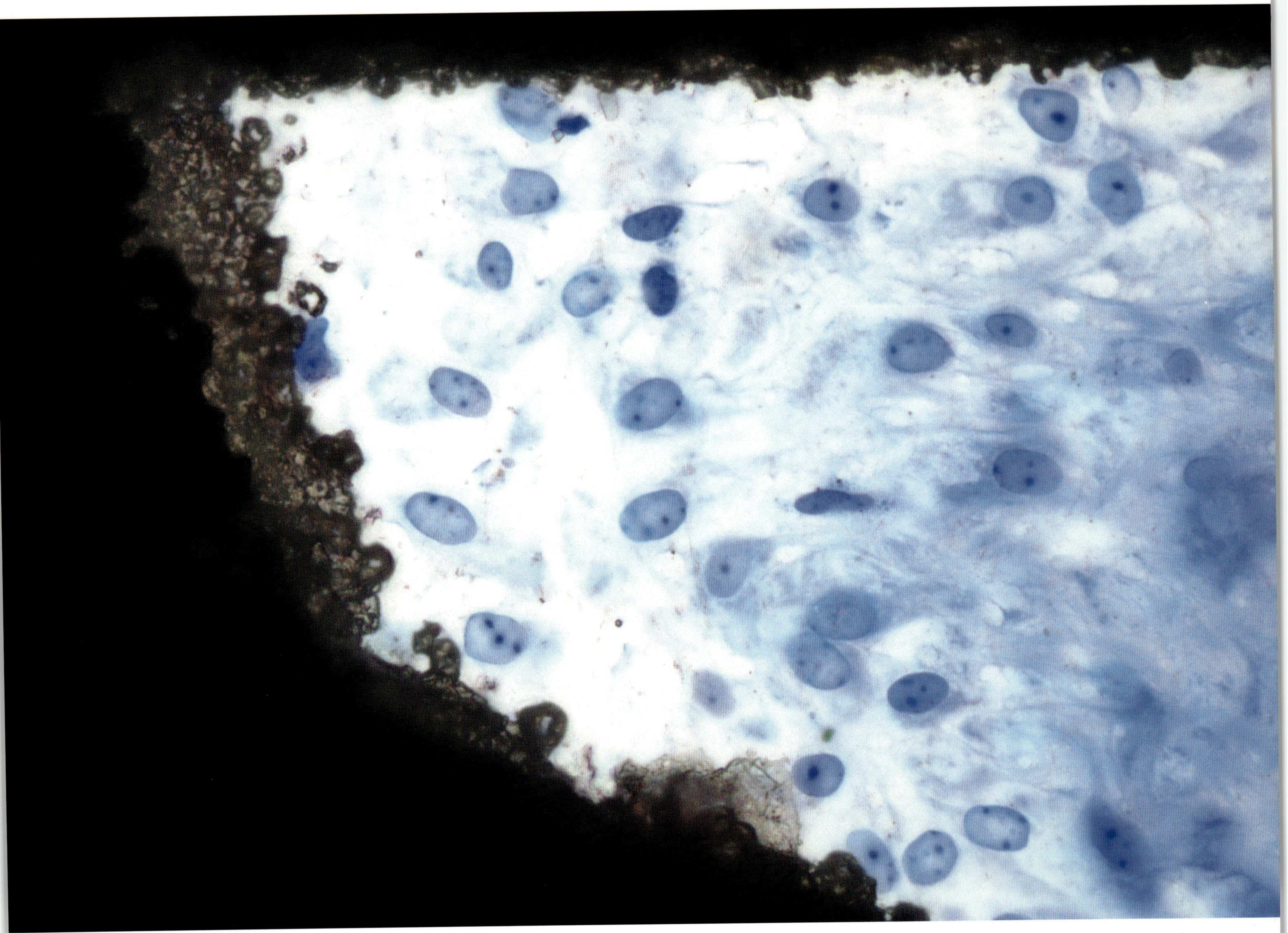

Out of the provisional matrix, osteogenic cells migrate toward the implant surface to start bone formation. If they reach the surface, they differentiate into osteoblasts *(black arrows)*. Osteoblasts secrete an organic collagen matrix, called *osteoid*, that will eventually become mineralized bone.

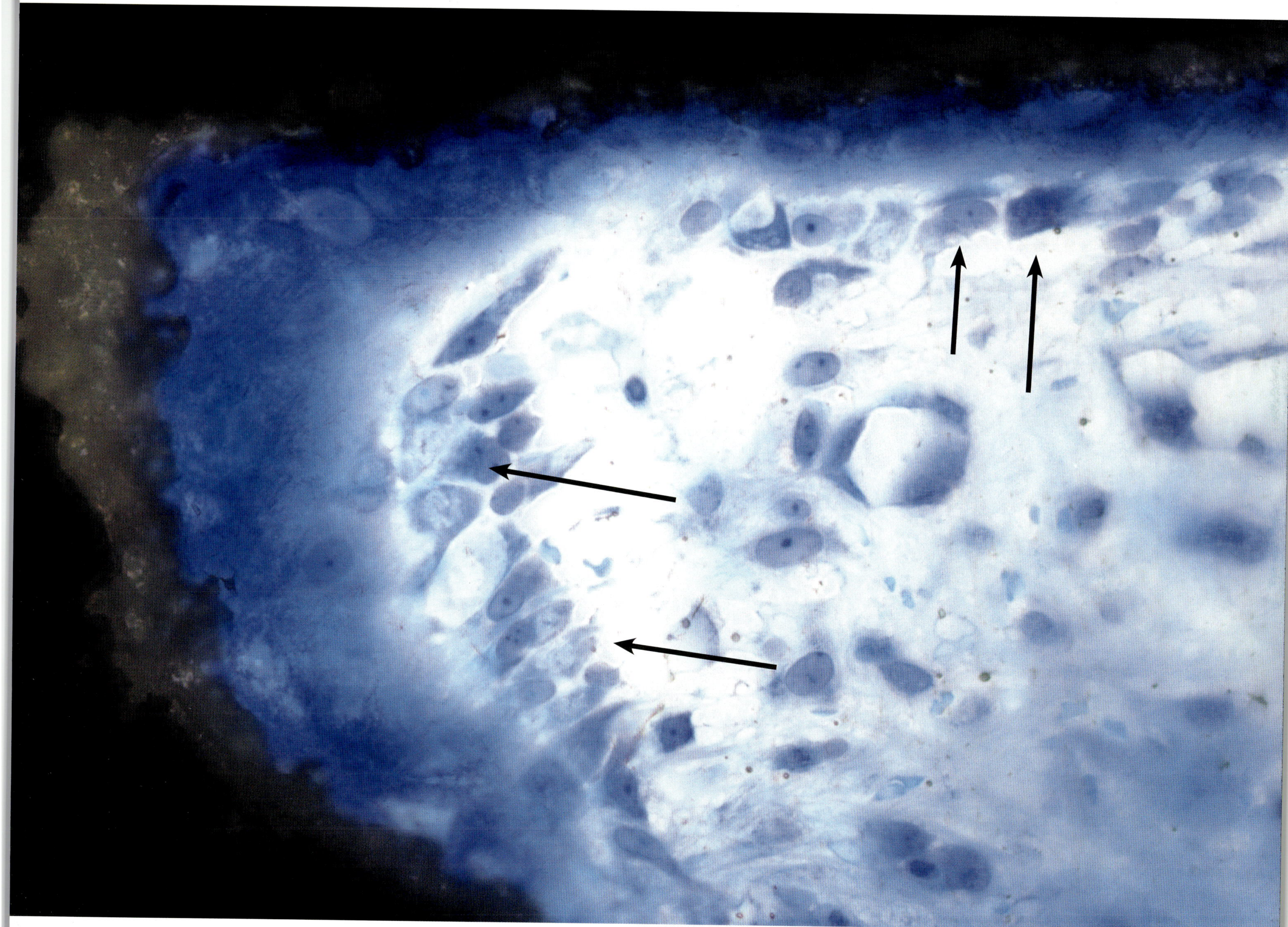

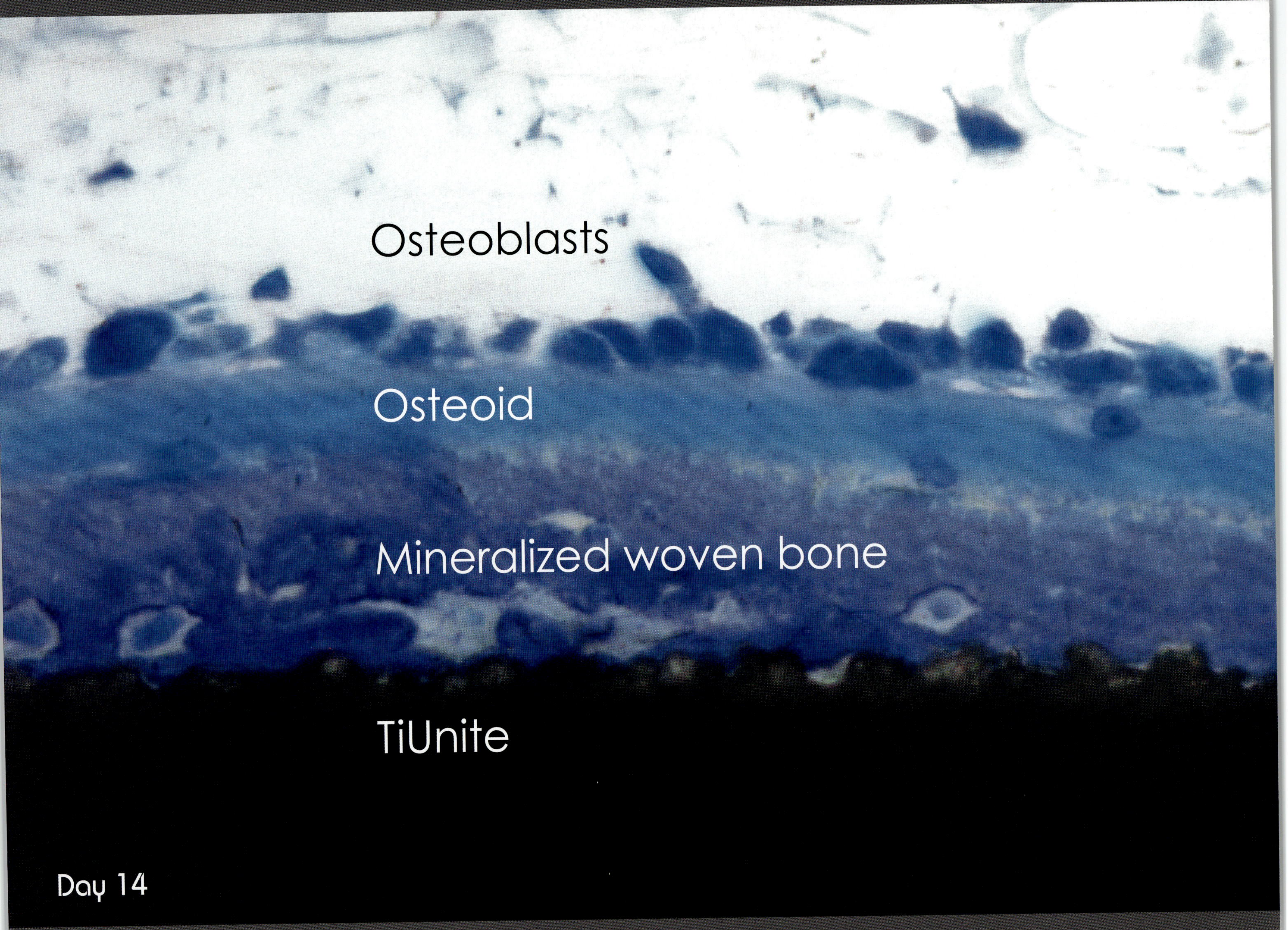
Osteoblasts
Osteoid
Mineralized woven bone
TiUnite
Day 14

New bone formed by contact osteogenesis is initially spread as a thin band along an implant surface. It is important to understand that bone is not actively moving along the surface. The only cells moving are the osteogenic cells, or *preosteoblasts*. These cells migrate by active locomotion to the leading edge of bone formation and become differentiated into osteoblasts. Once there, they begin secreting and mineralizing new bone.

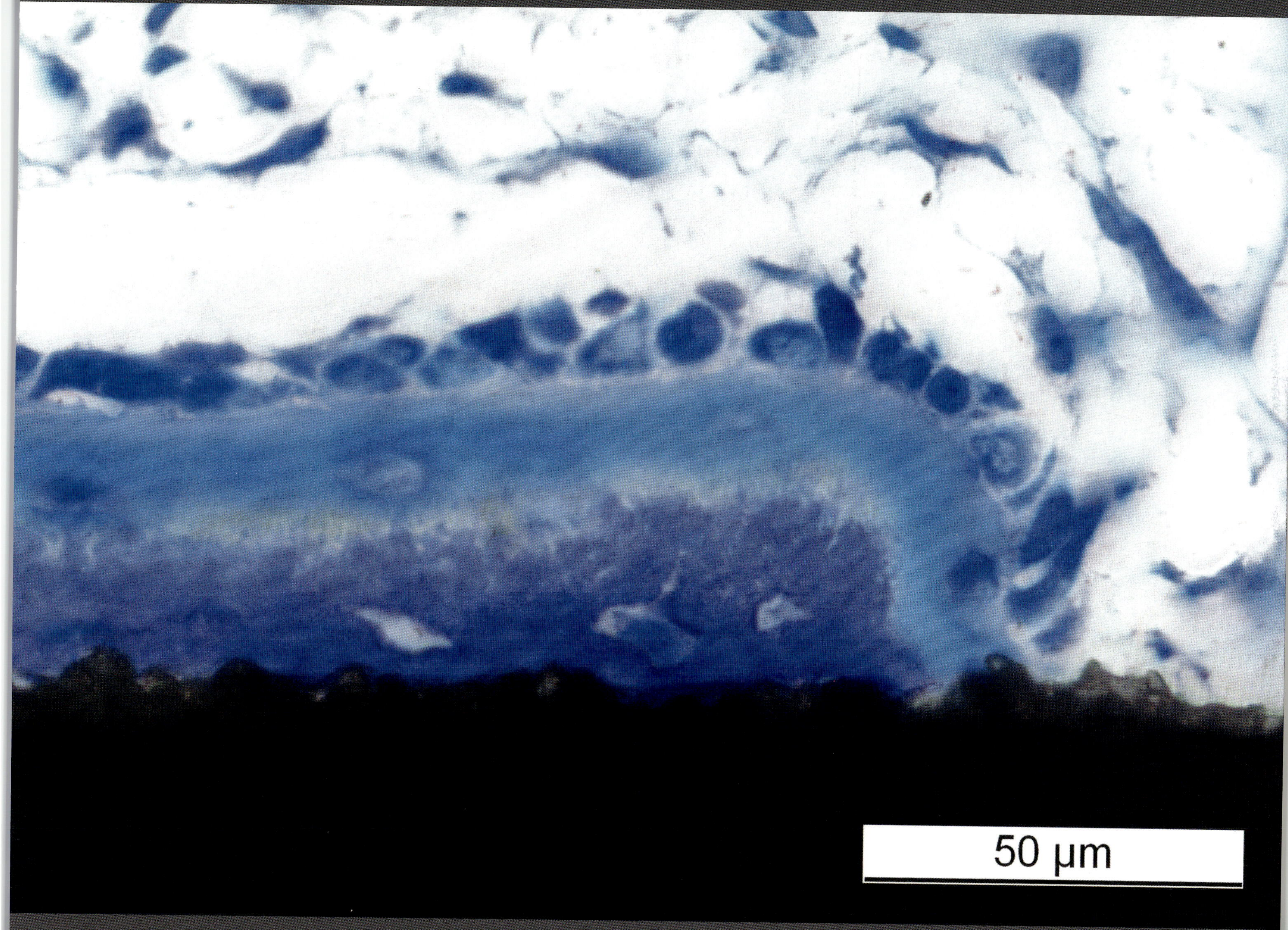

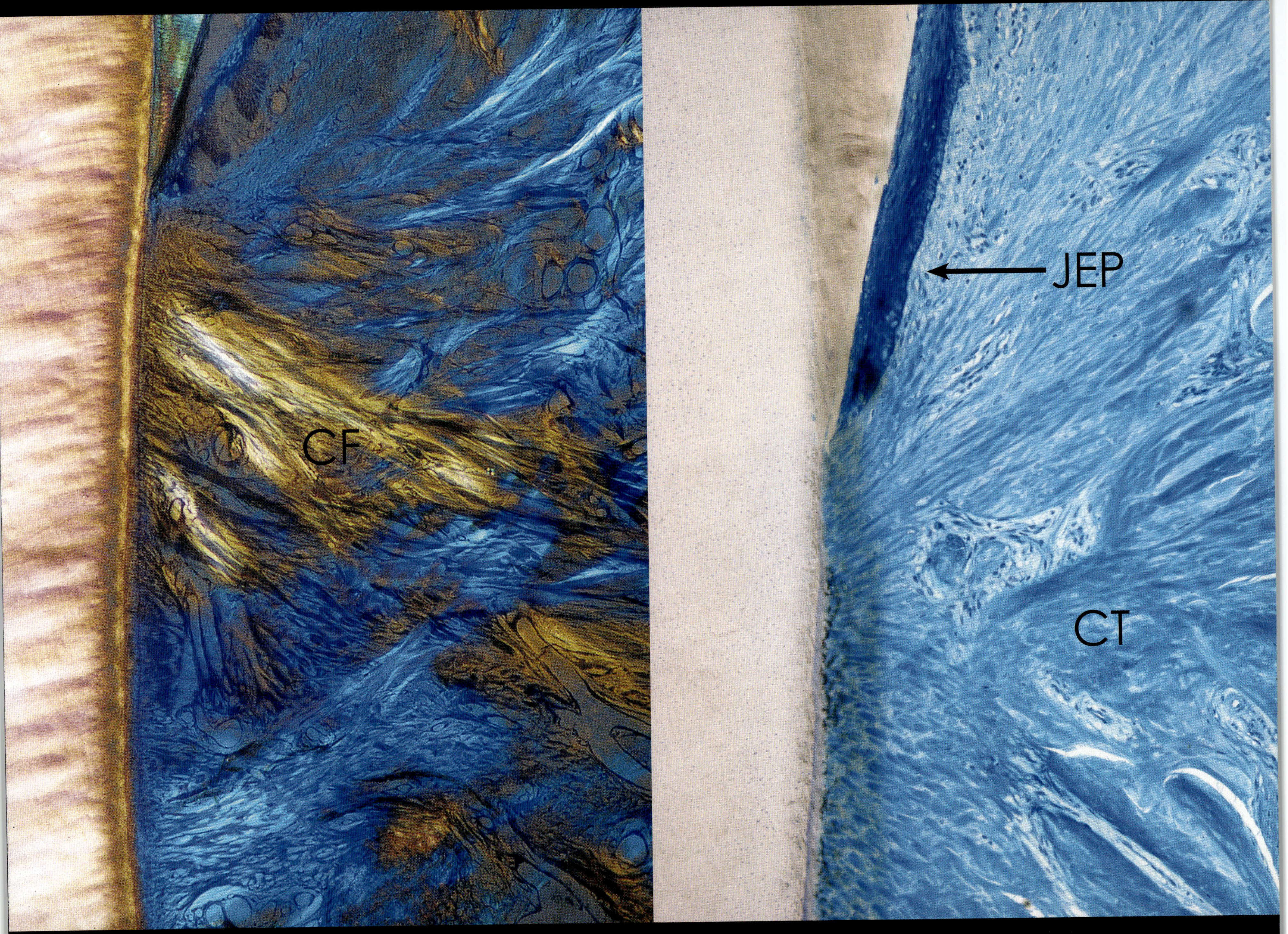
CF
JEP
CT

Besides contributing to anchoring teeth in the jaw, the primary function of the marginal periodontium, or *gingiva*, around natural dentition is protection. Gingiva provides a seal against the contaminated environment of the oral cavity, stabilizes the position of teeth in the alveolar bone, withstands the frictional forces of mastication, and defends the interface between teeth and soft tissue against bacterial ingress.

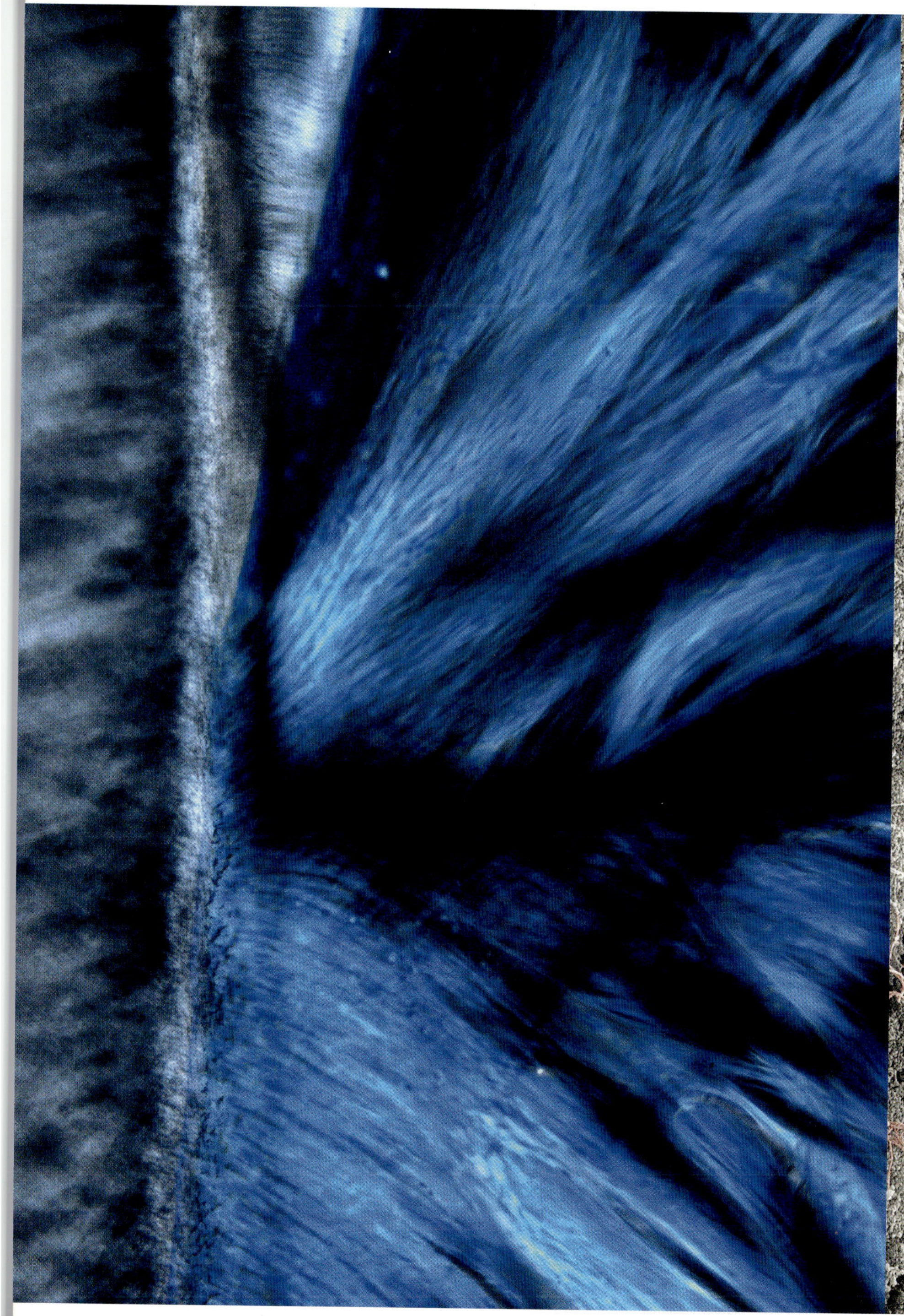

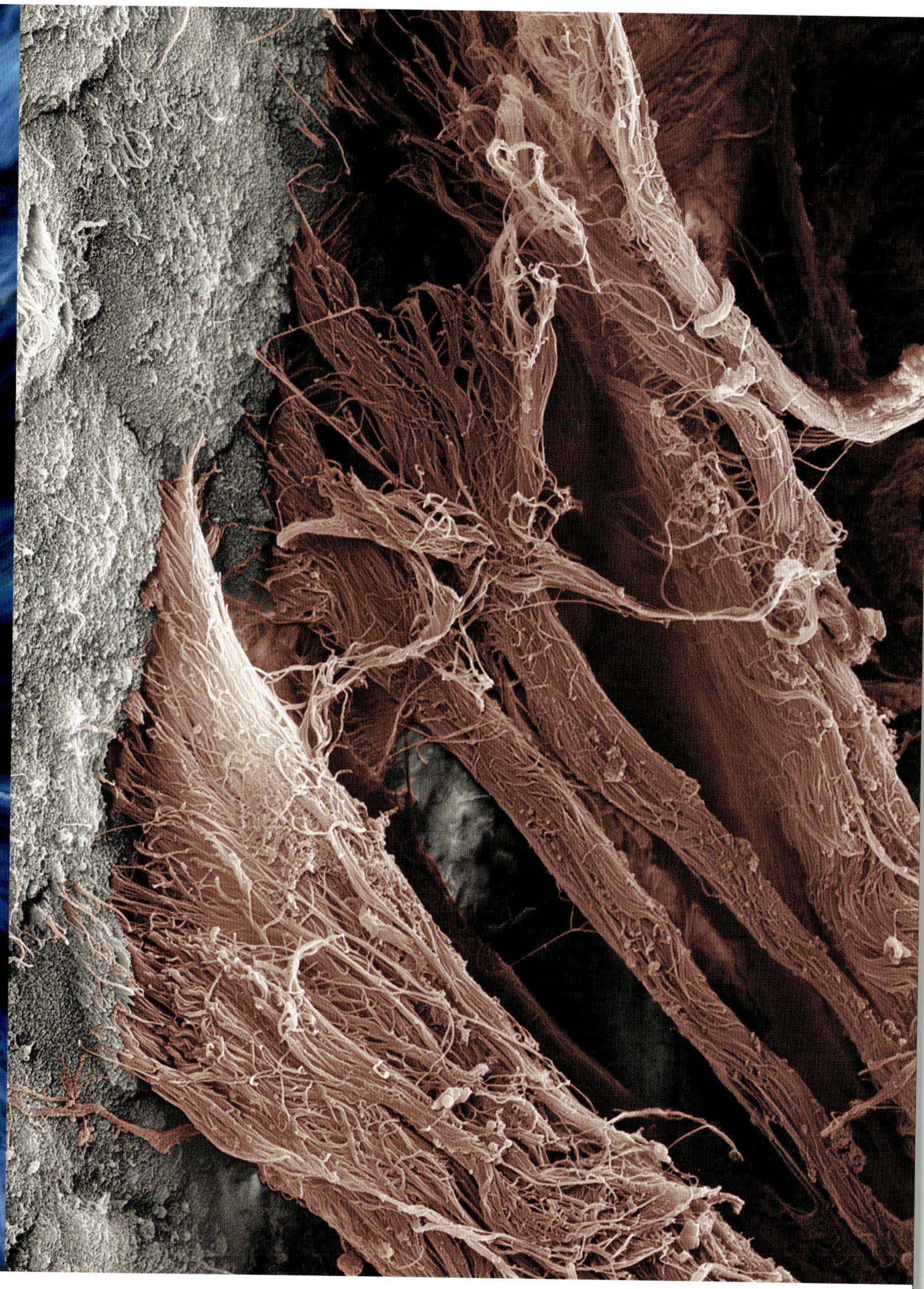

The framework that accomplishes these tasks is comprised of a variety of unique structures. Among these is a highly specialized tissue called *junctional epithelium* (JEP), which protects and seals the gingiva. Another is the way the connective tissue (CT) of the gingiva is anchored in the mineralized cementum of the root, characterized by the strong collagenous fibers (CF) of the supracrestal fiber apparatus.

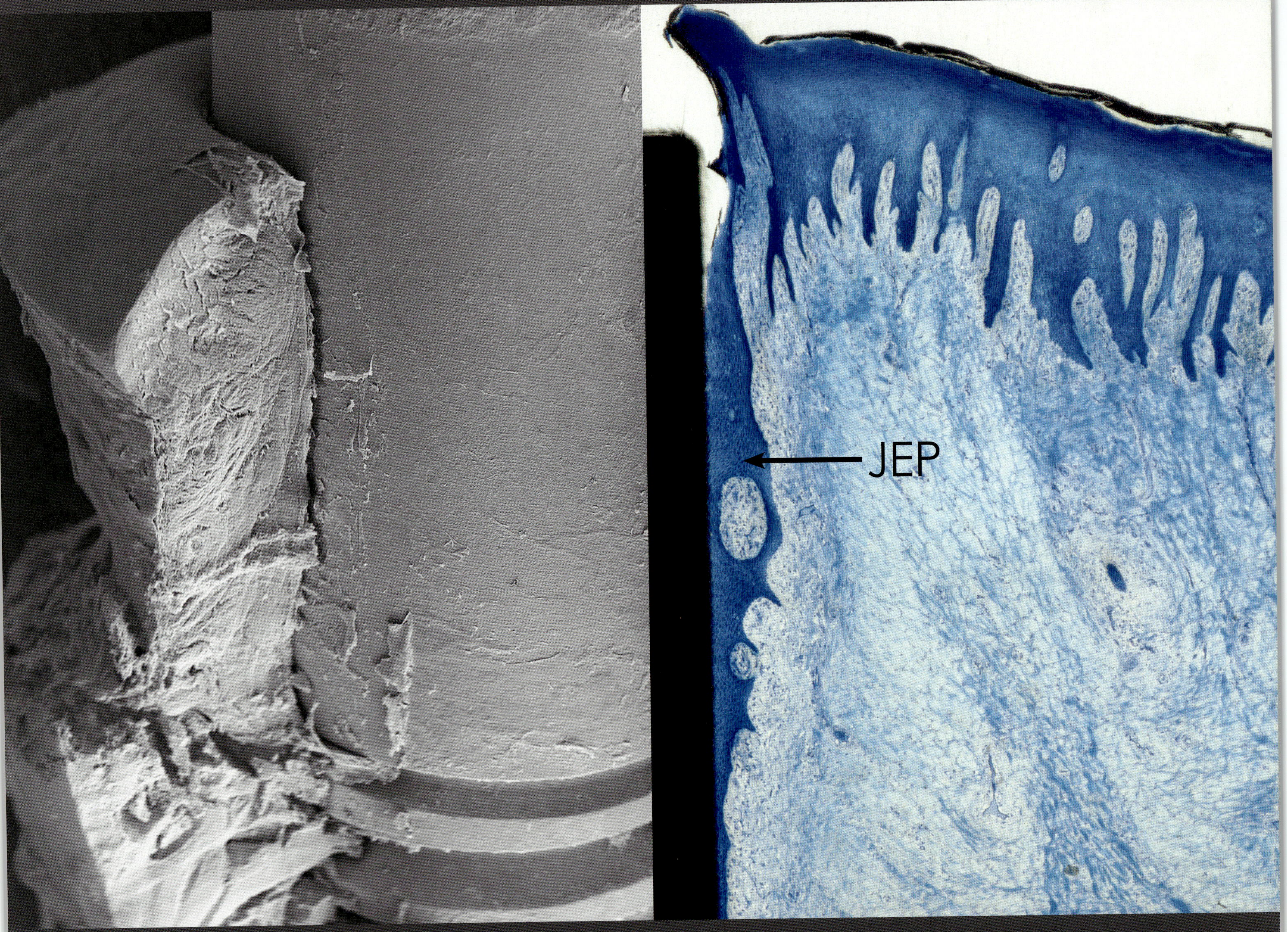
JEP

The peri-implant mucosa surrounding successful endosseous implants is in many ways analogous to gingiva surrounding natural dentition. Of the tissues in contact with implants, the JEP most closely matches the structures around natural dentition. It forms an epithelial sleeve around the tooth collar and preserves the continuity of the epithelial coating of the oral cavity. It is located at the strategically important interface between the contaminated oral cavity and the marginal periodontium, which needs protection from bacteria and their by-products. The epithelial cells of the innermost cell layer are firmly attached to a machined abutment surface *(SEM micrograph below)*.

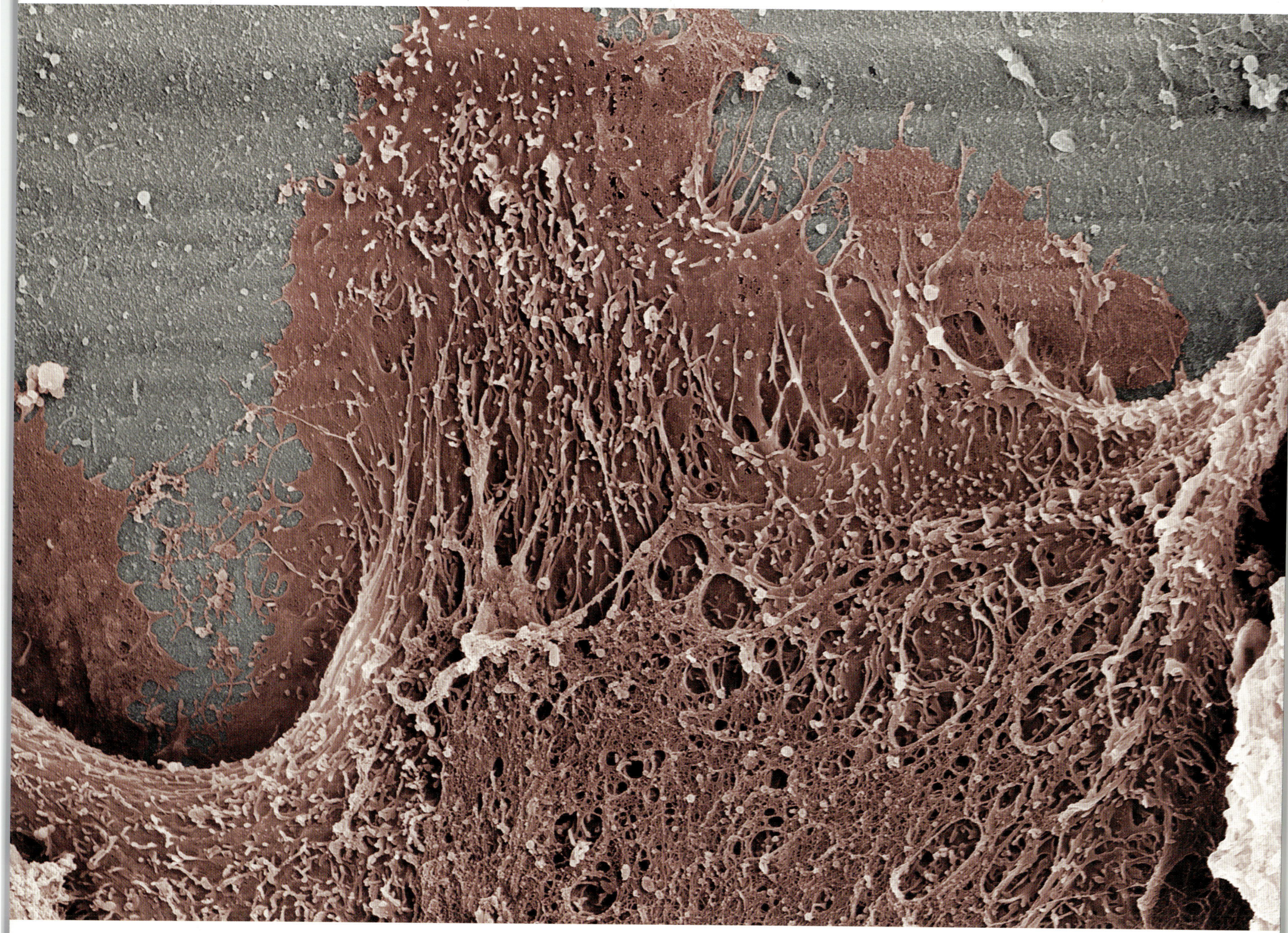

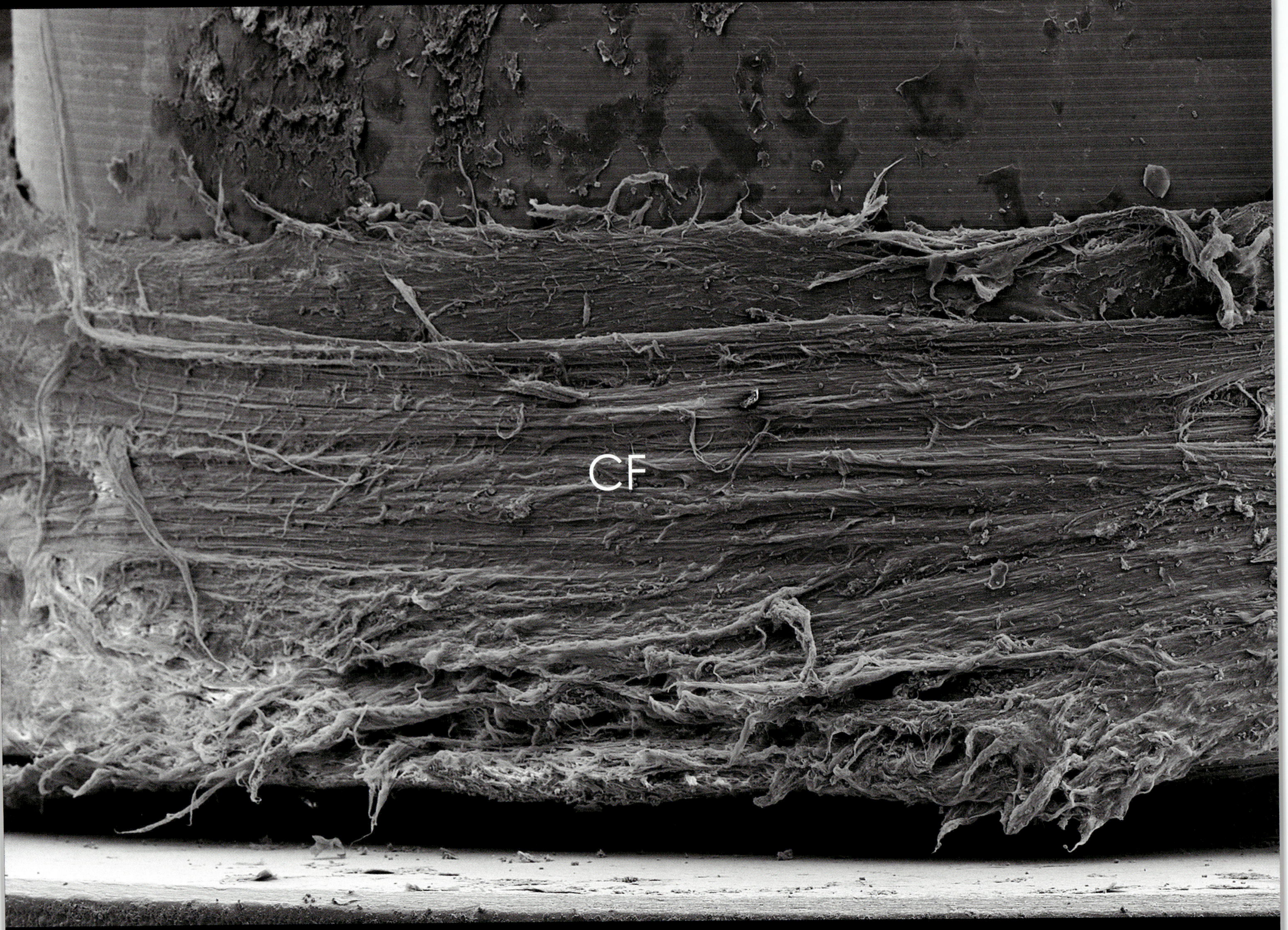
CF

Despite the similarities of the junctional epithelium, important differences exist in the way the connective tissue interfaces with implant surfaces. With implants, functionally oriented CFs anchored in the surface are completely absent and replaced by circumferentially oriented CFs as seen in the SEM micrograph at left and indicated by the *black arrows* in the image below.

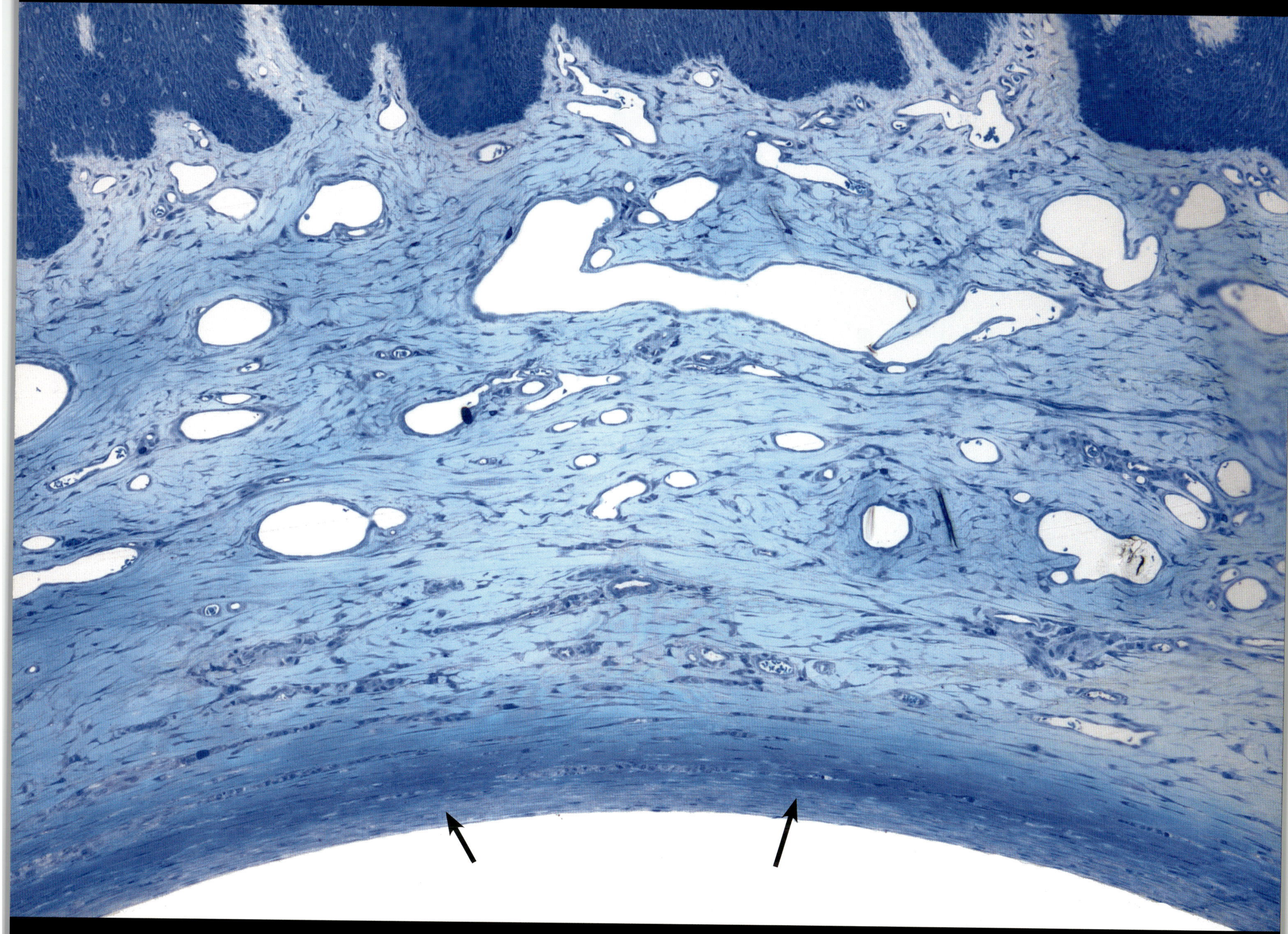

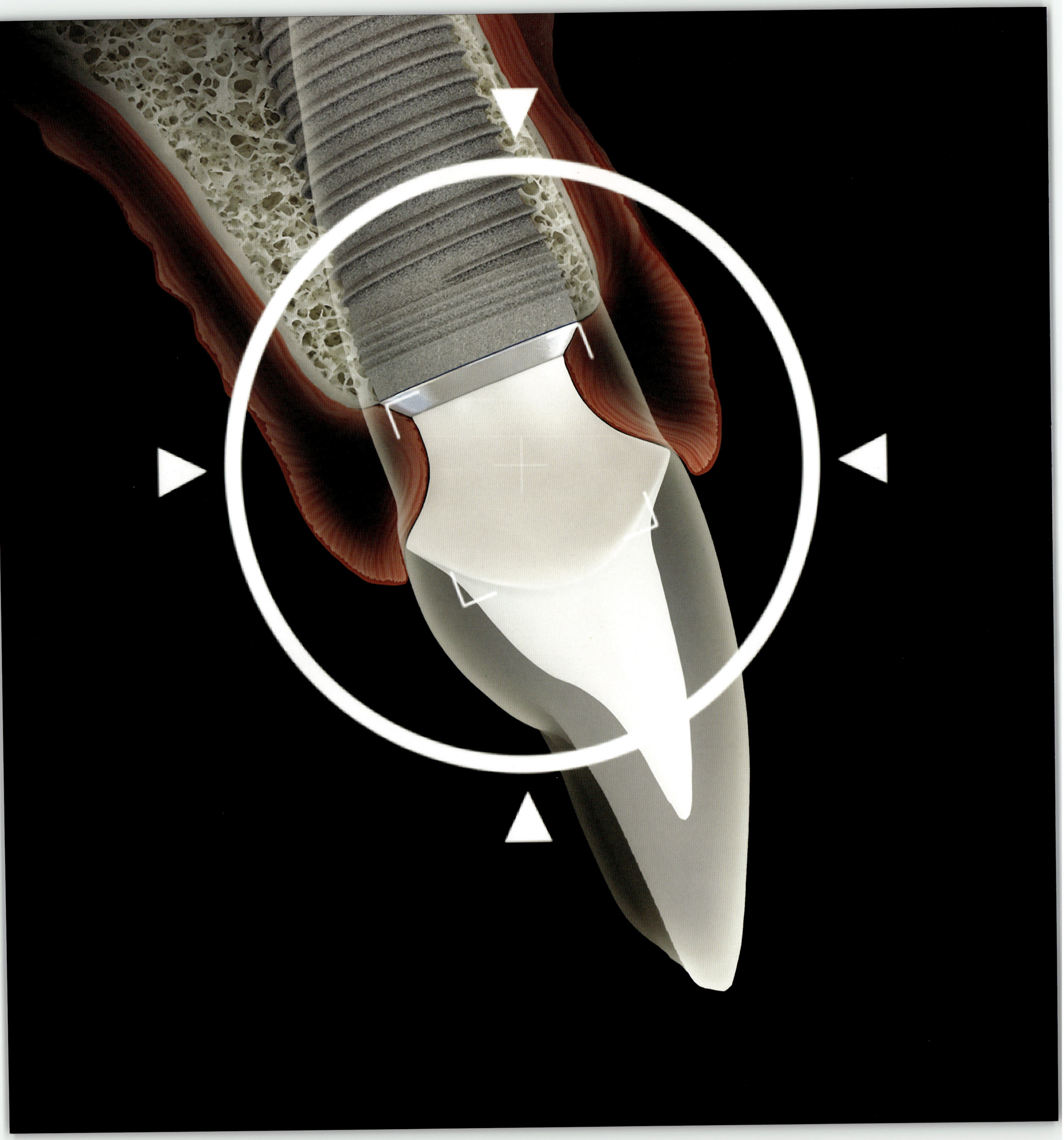

Biologic Impact of Implant, Abutment, and Prosthetic Design

- Clinical Protocol with Platform Shift Concept: Delayed Implant Placement
- Clinical Protocol with Platform Shift Concept: Immediate Implant Placement
  → Research: Platform shifting
- Clinical Results with Platform Shift Concept
  – PS adapter results
  – Disconnection effect
  → Research: Disconnection effect
  – Original PS results
  – Different results with PS adapter
  – PS results with NobelActive
  – PS results with NobelReplace Conical

Chapter 2

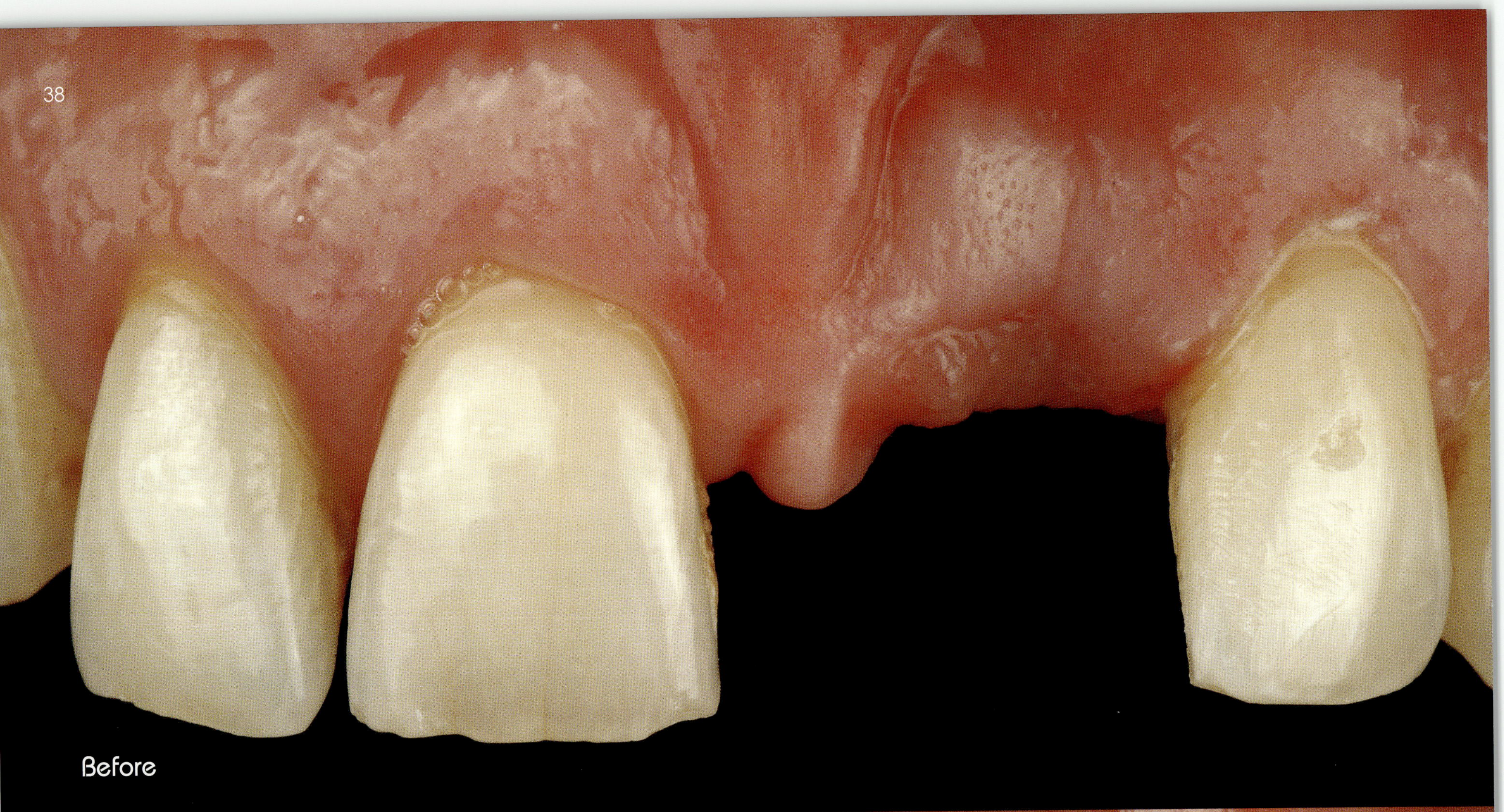

Before

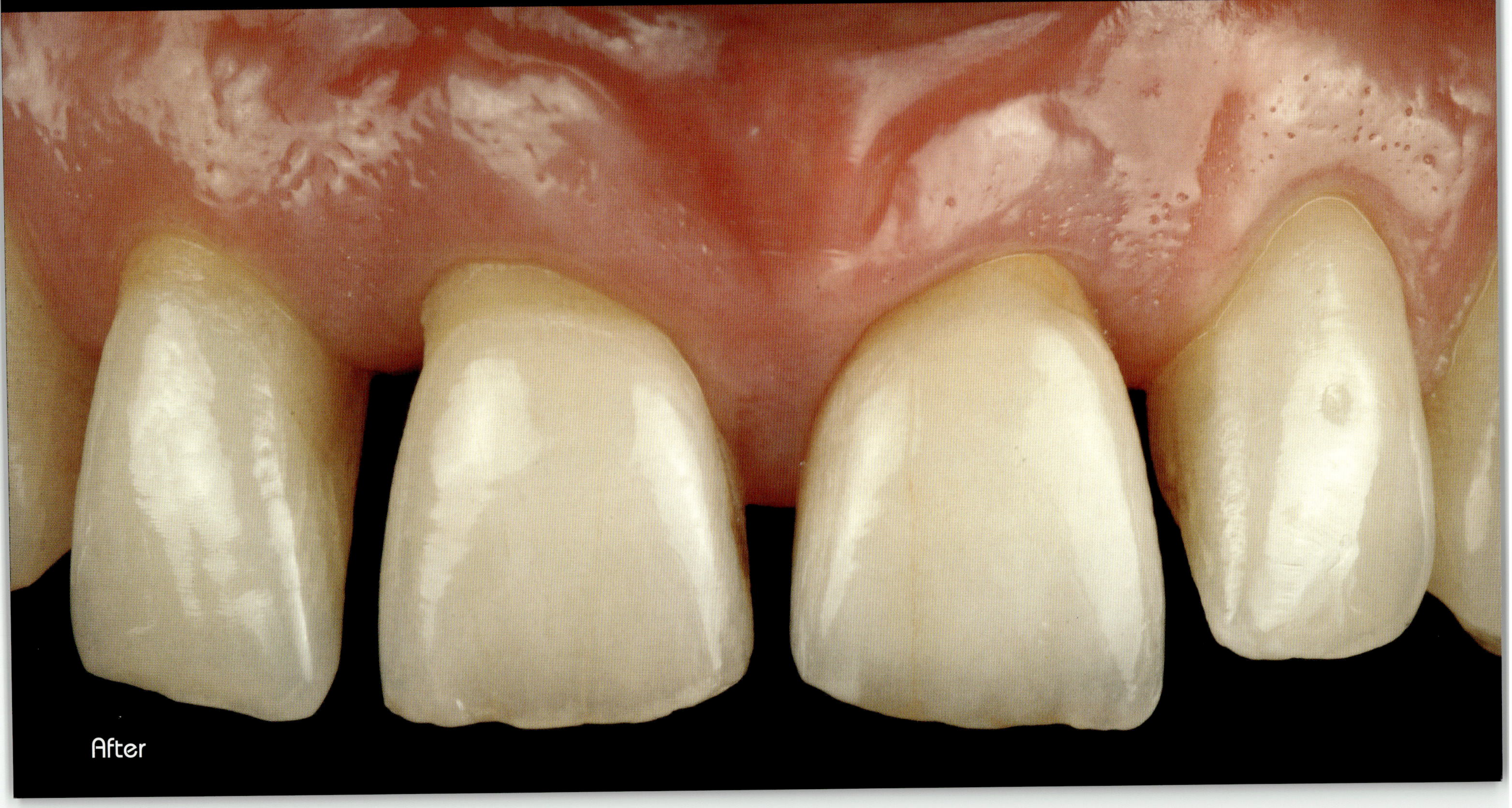

After

2

Clinical Protocol with Platform Shift Concept: Delayed Implant Placement

Delayed implant placement

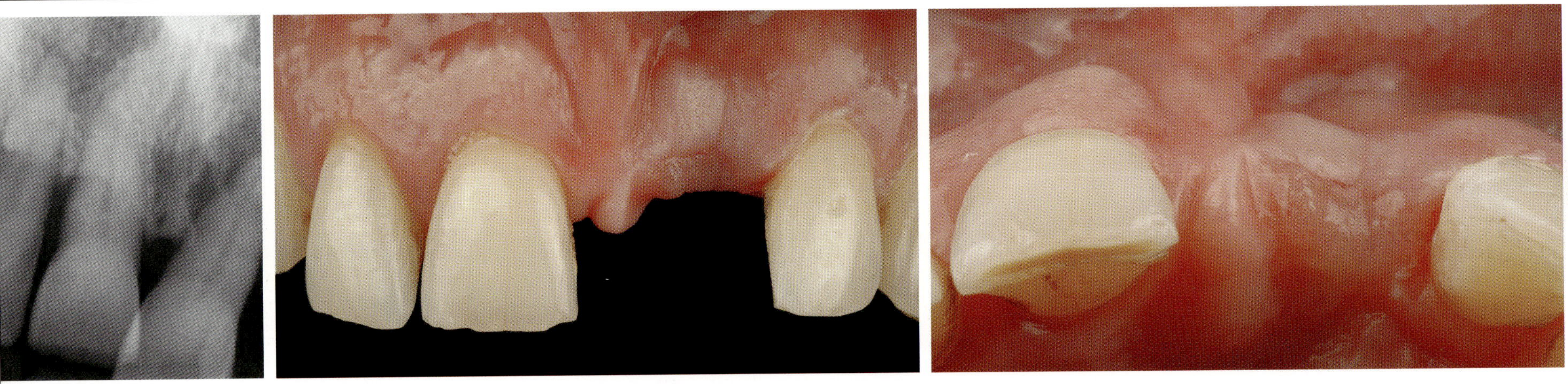

Initial situation 3 months after extraction of the maxillary left central incisor.

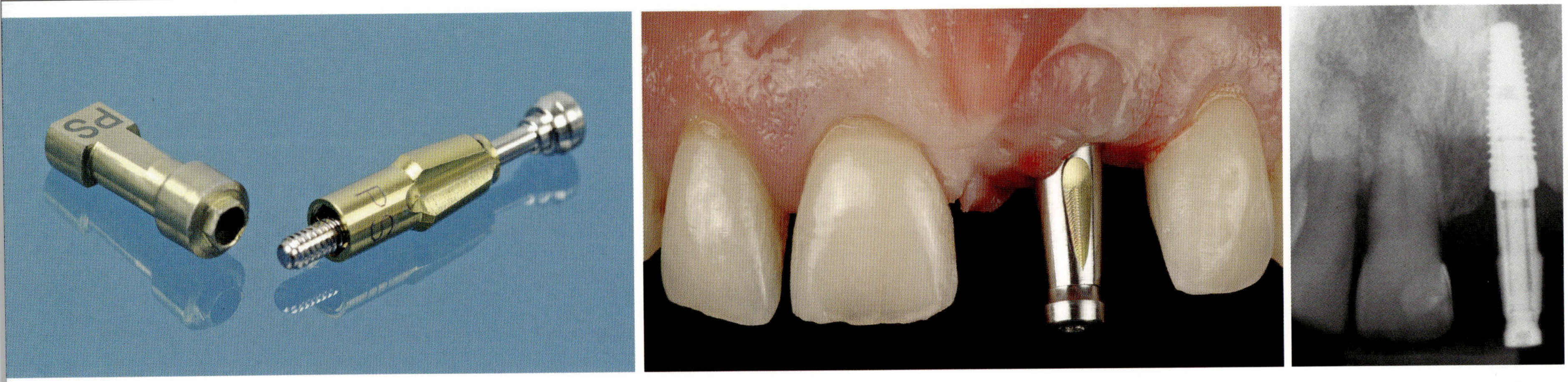

Implant impression with the corresponding impression coping and laboratory analog.

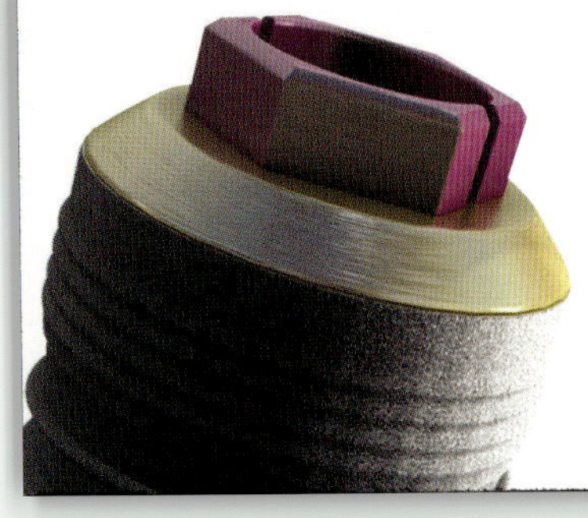

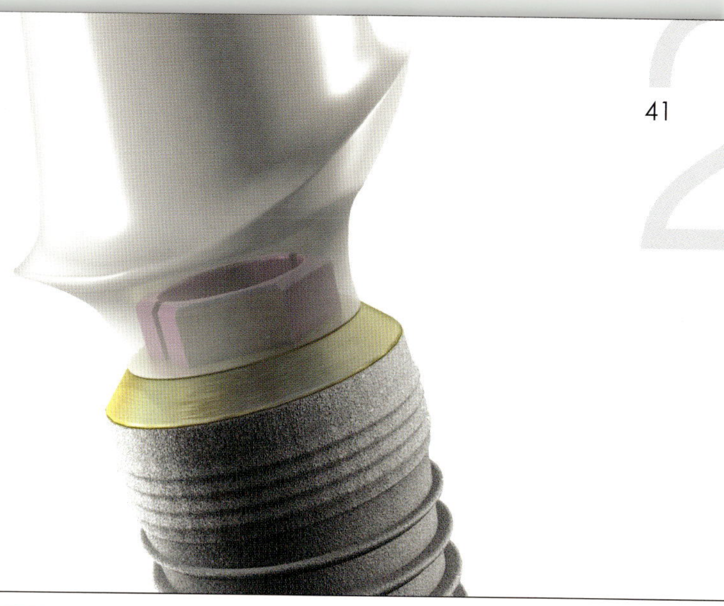

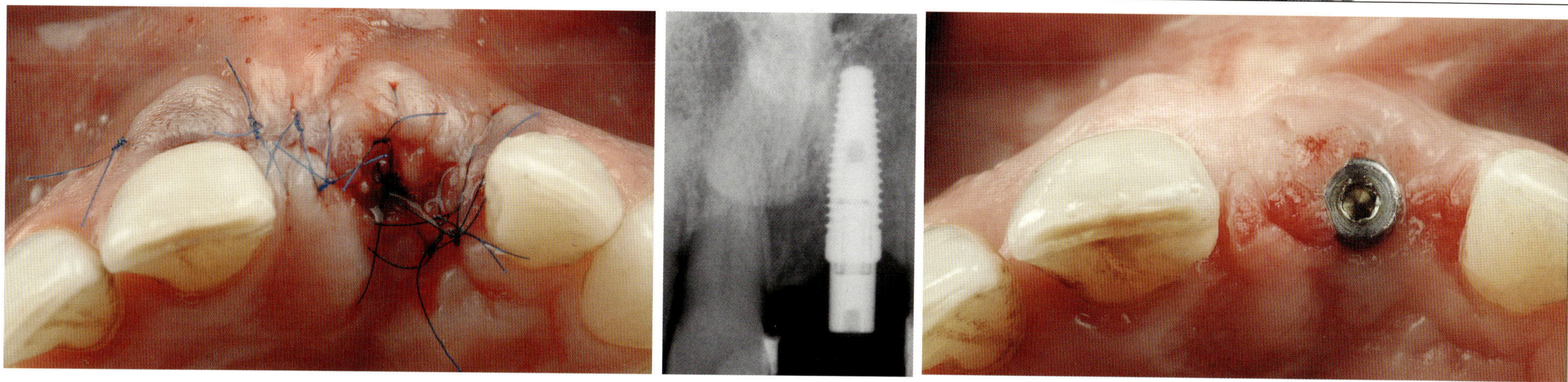

Placement of an implant (4.3 × 13–mm NobelReplace Select Tapered Groovy, Nobel Biocare) and a connective tissue graft with a narrow platform (NP) adapter and NP healing abutment (5 mm high).

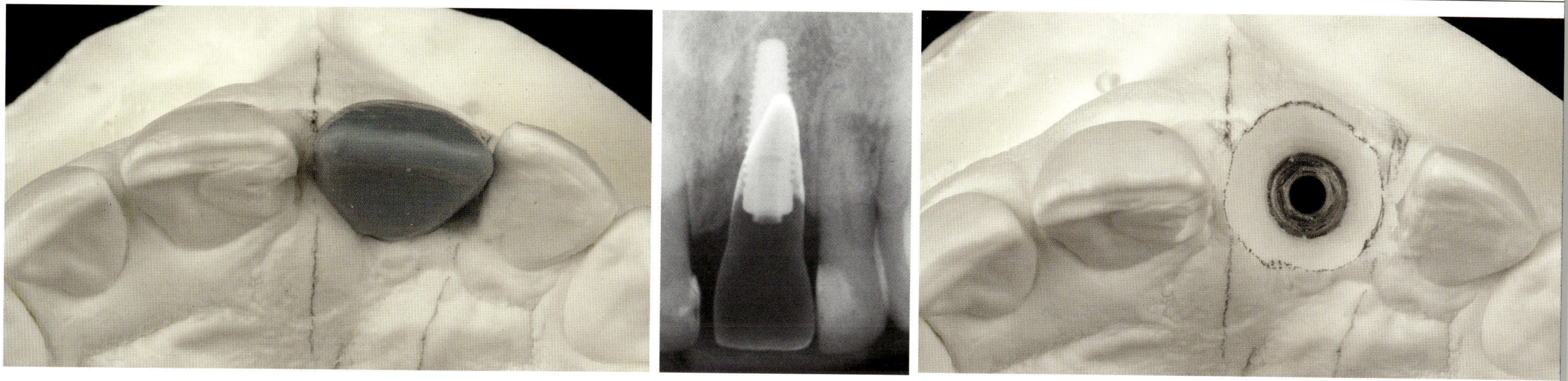

Emergence profile design in the laboratory. The wax-up is designed to re-create the diameter of the root of the original tooth. Superimposed radiographs of the original tooth and the implant serve as indicators for the design of the emergence profile of the implant abutment. A line is drawn on the stone cast around the full-contour wax-up as a guide for the emergence profile, which is then carved into the stone from the head of the implant to this line in a divergent or conical manner.

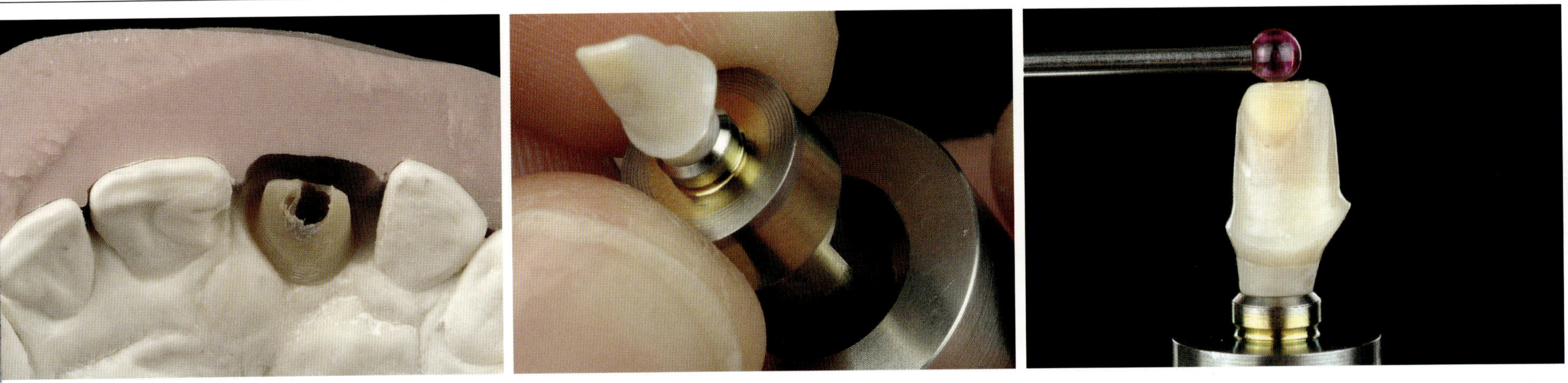

A composite implant abutment is fabricated and designed based on silicone indices from the full-contour wax-up. The final shape of the composite abutment is scanned to fabricate the definitive zirconia abutment.

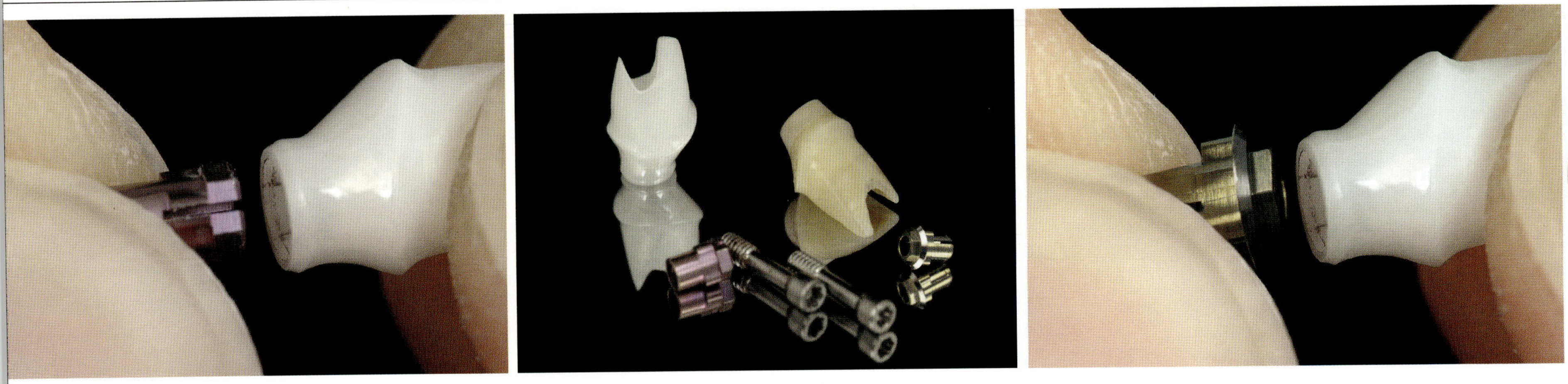

Shift of the connection with implant adapters. To shift from an NP prosthetic connection to a regular platform (RP) implant connection, a longer screw is necessary to connect the new abutment through the NP–RP adapter into the internal implant connection.

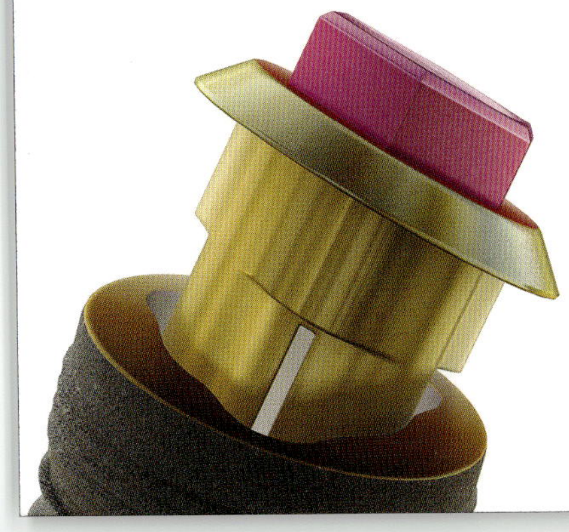

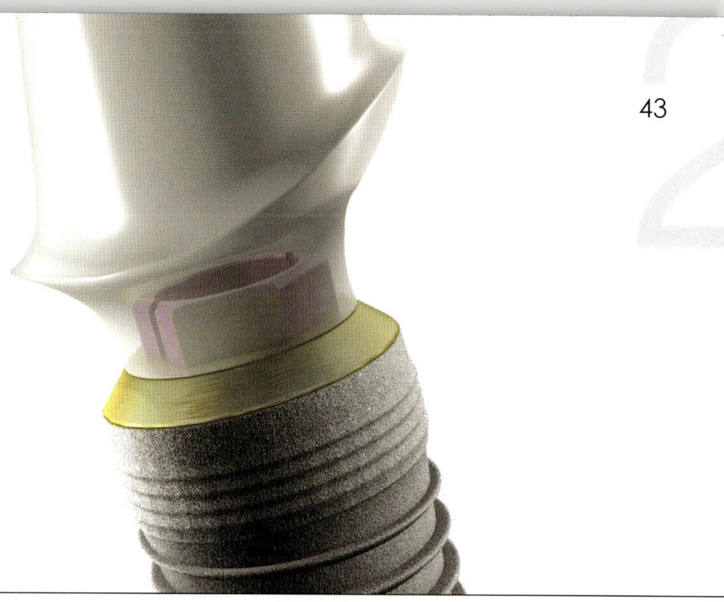

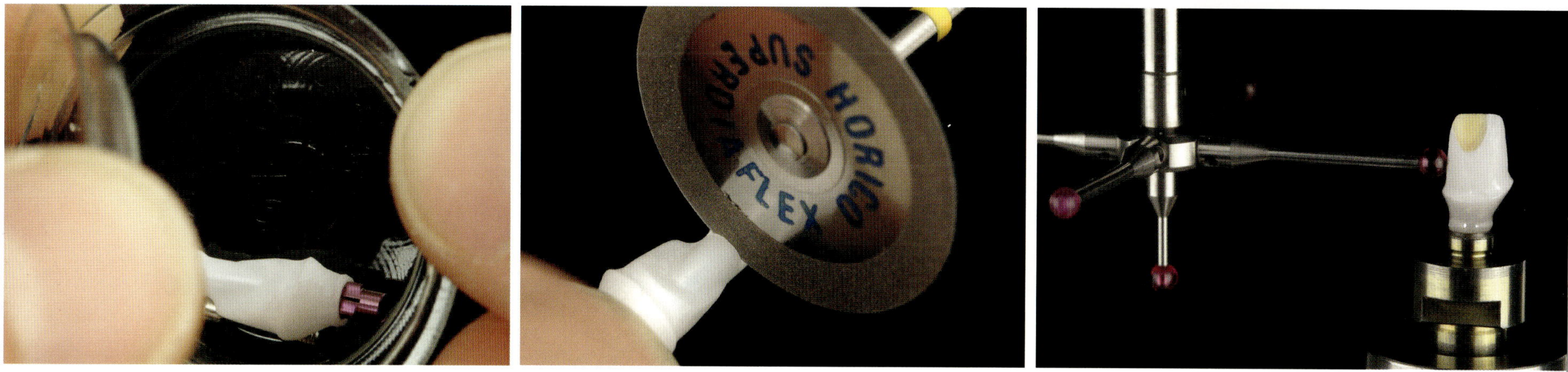

The definitive zirconia abutment is rescanned to fabricate the alumina coping for the definitive crown restoration.

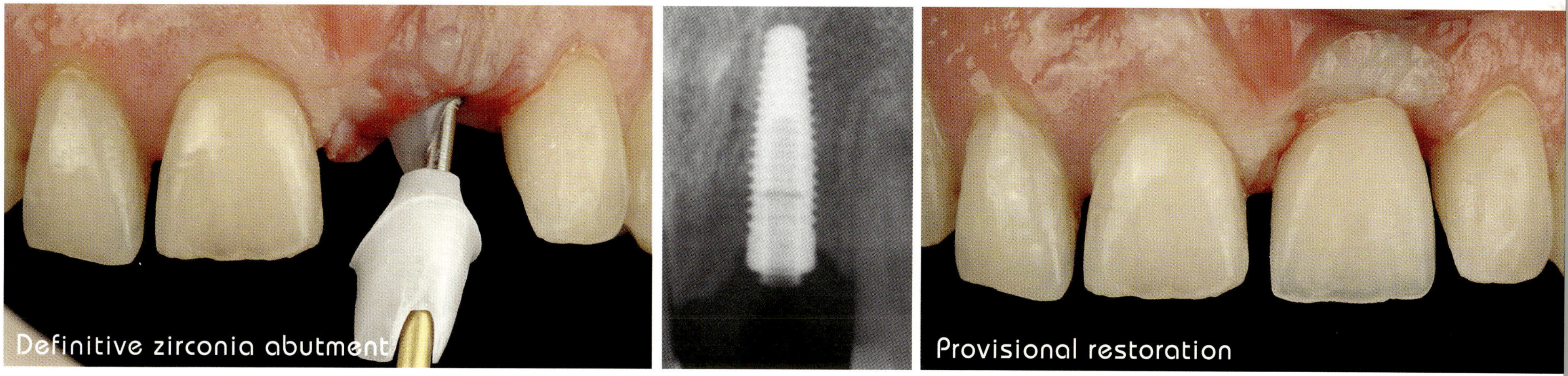

Insertion of the definitive zirconia implant abutment with a provisional crown restoration. First, the NP–RP adapter is inserted for simplified abutment manipulation. Afterward, the abutment is screwed in, and the provisional crown is relined and provisionally cemented.

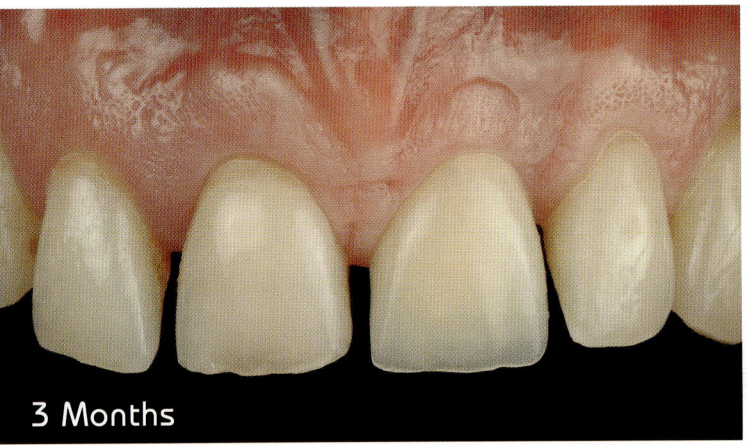

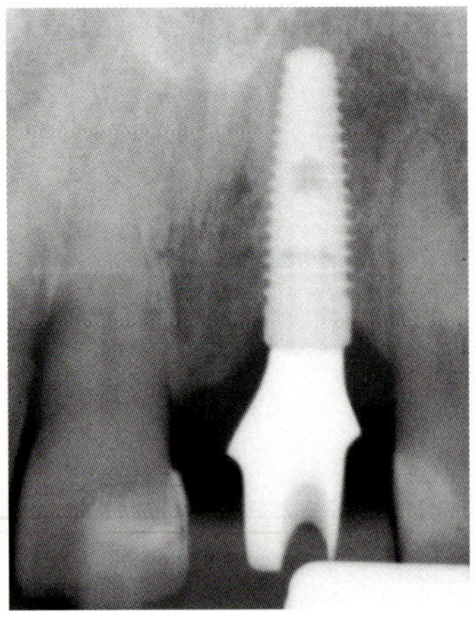

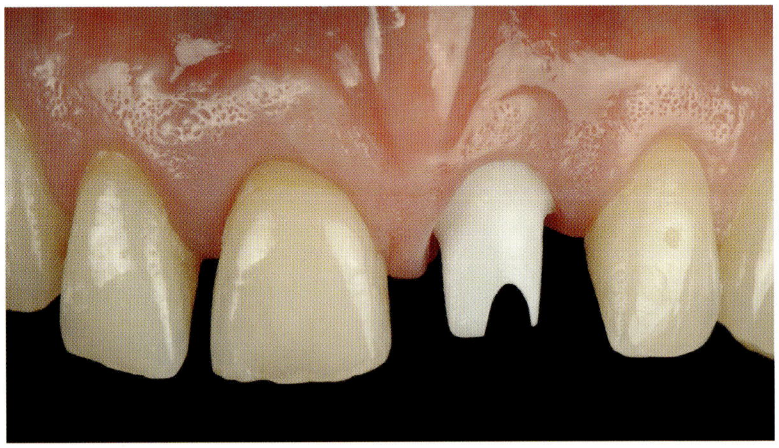

The soft tissue response to the emergence profile created earlier is re-evaluated after at least 3 months have passed.

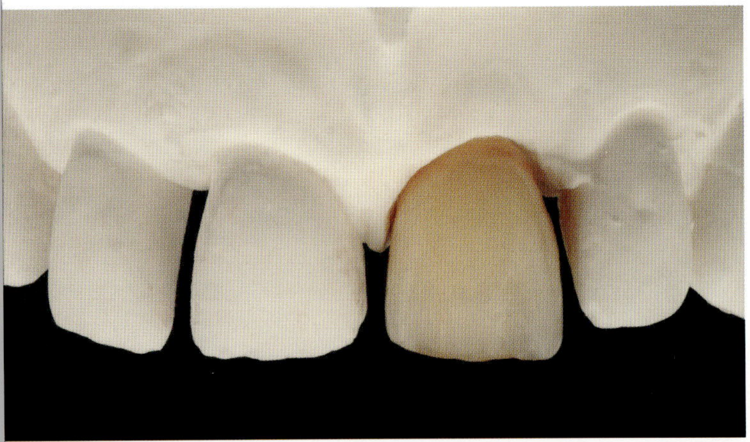

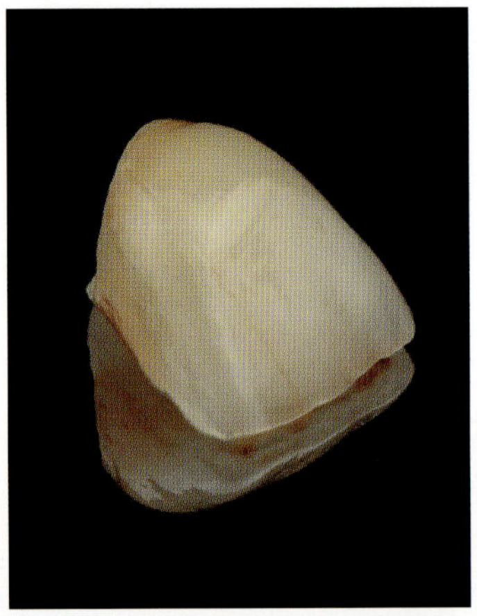

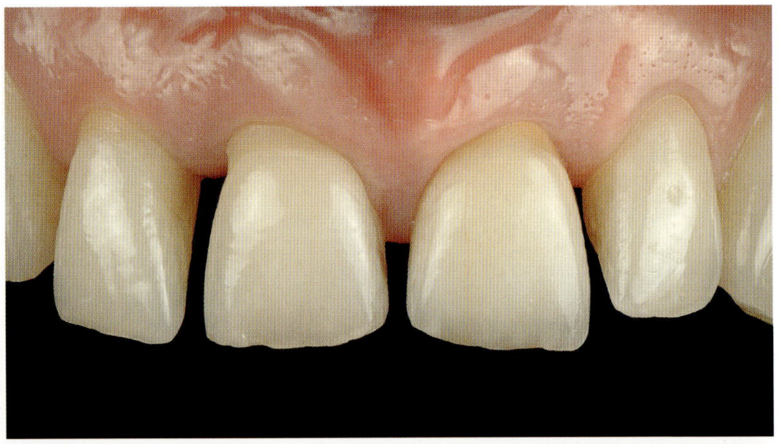

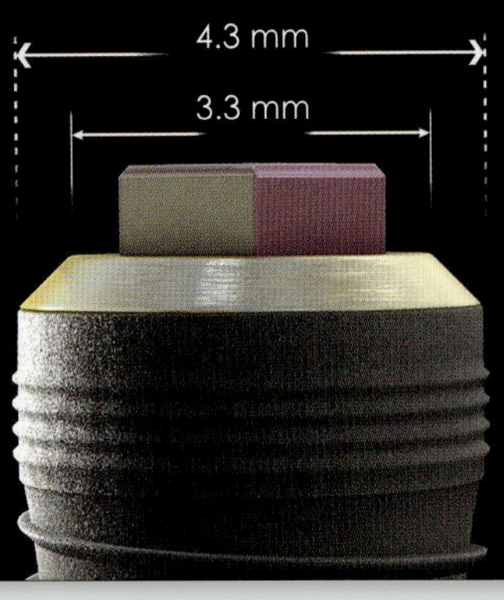

From the laboratory to the final result. The alumina-based crown restoration is cemented with a universal self-adhesive resin cement.

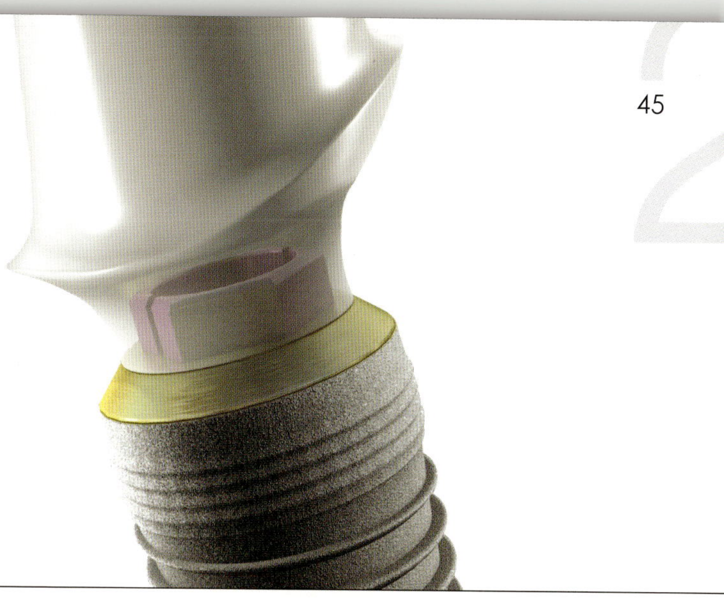

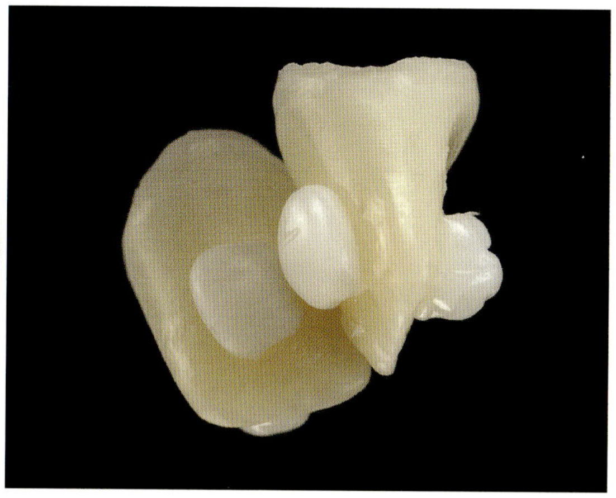

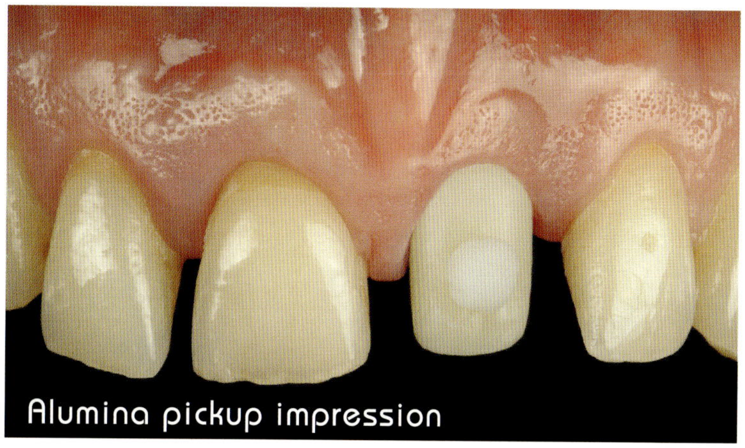

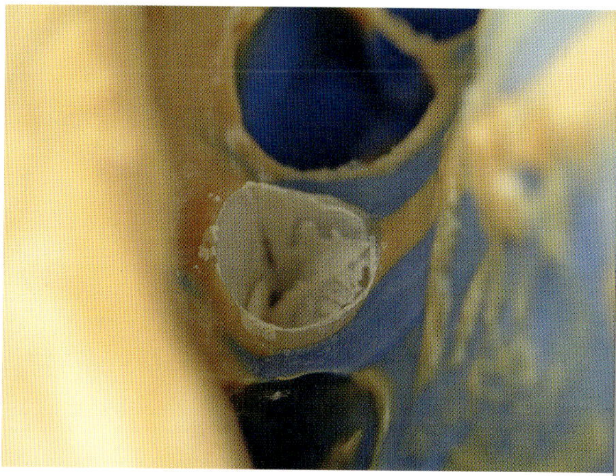

Final impression. A pickup impression is made with the definitive alumina coping to avoid damage to the peri-implant soft tissues through conventional retraction cords. Two composite balls are bonded to the coping for increased retention in the final silicone impression. The coping is cemented to the abutment with provisional cement mixed with petroleum jelly for coping stability and impression accuracy.

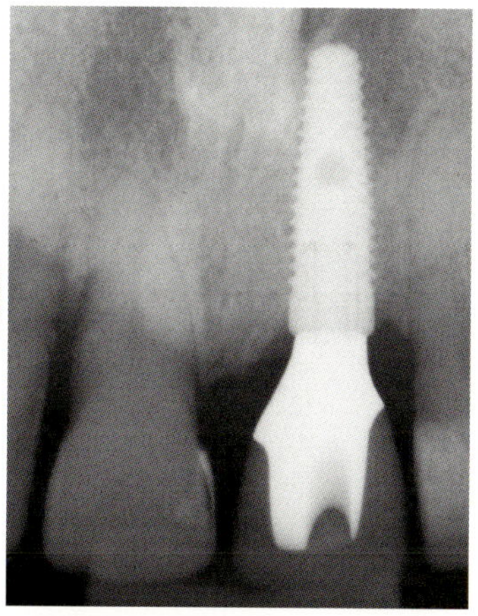

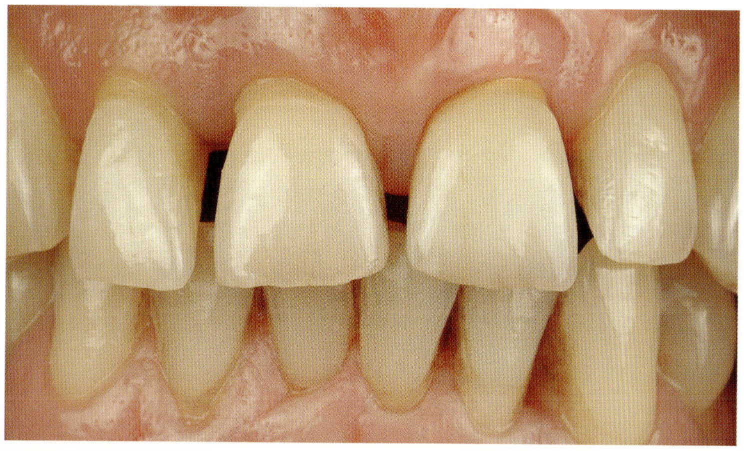

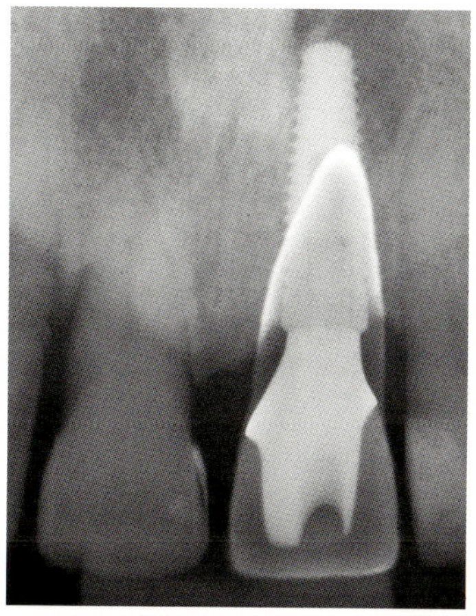

Definitive implant-supported restoration. The platform shift (PS) concept was applied, and the emergence profile and diameter of the original tooth were replicated prosthetically.

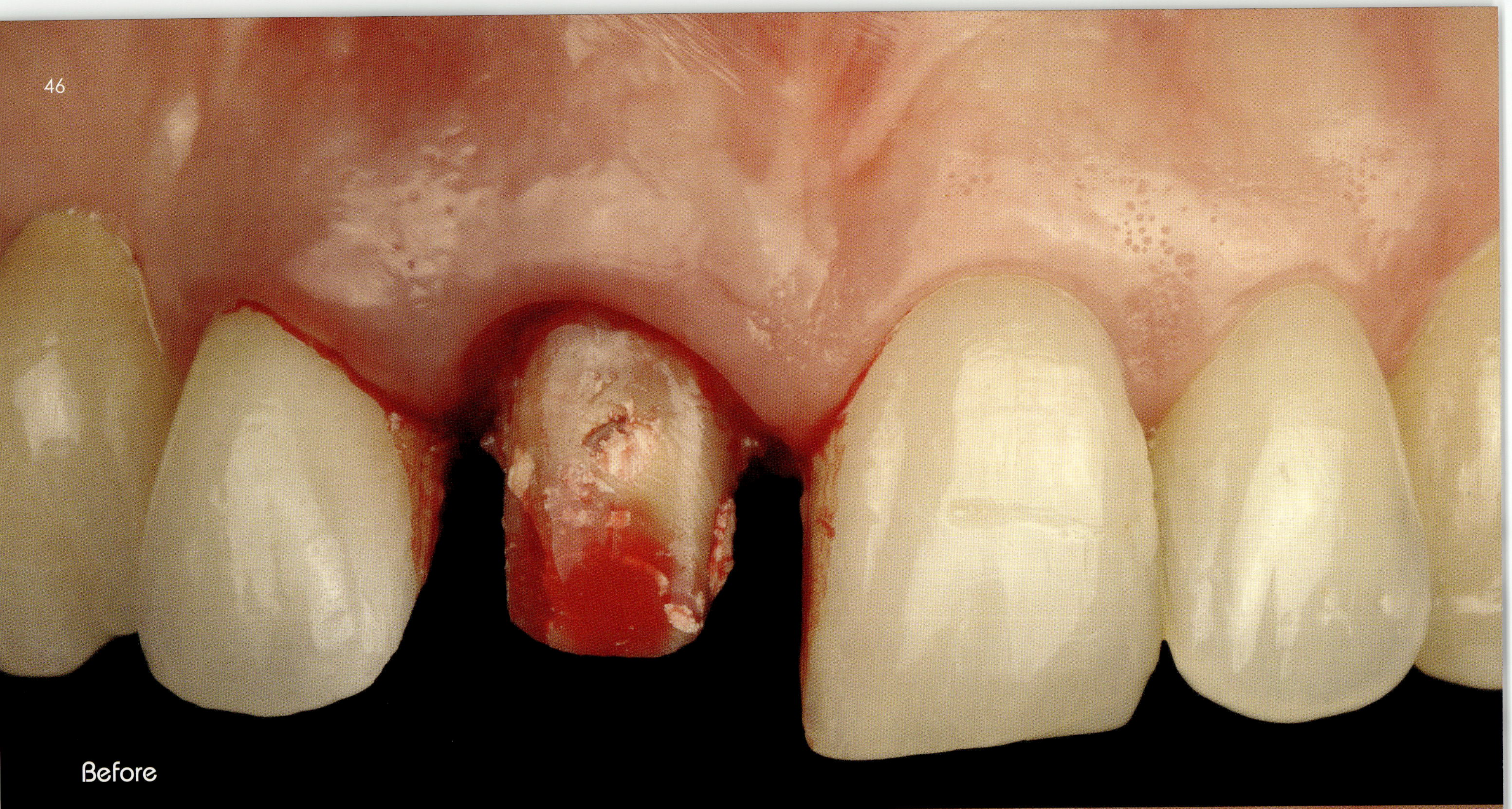

Before

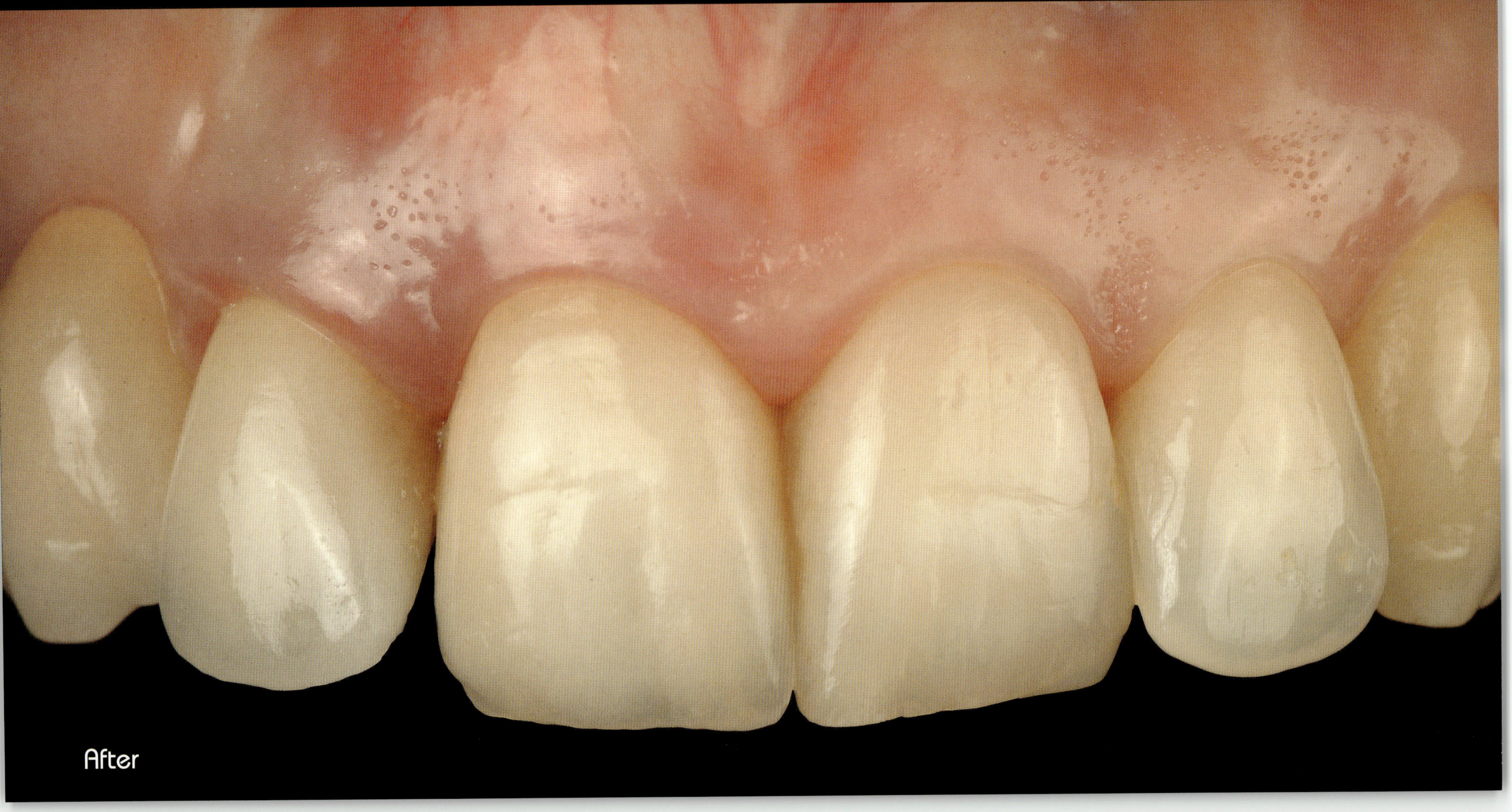

After

Clinical Protocol with Platform Shift Concept: Immediate Implant Placement

Immediate implant placement

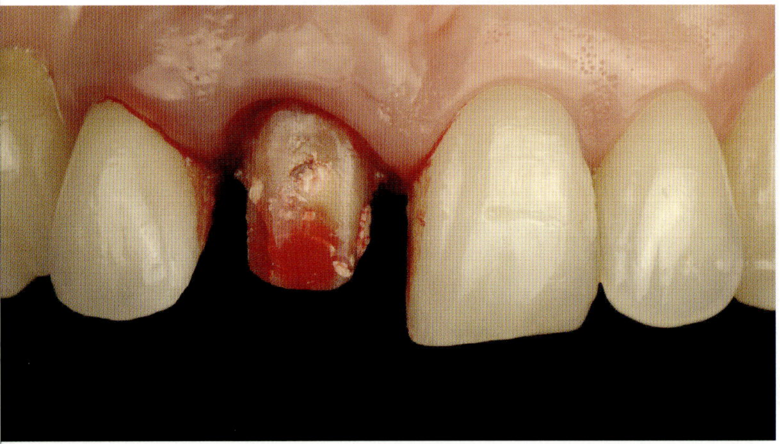

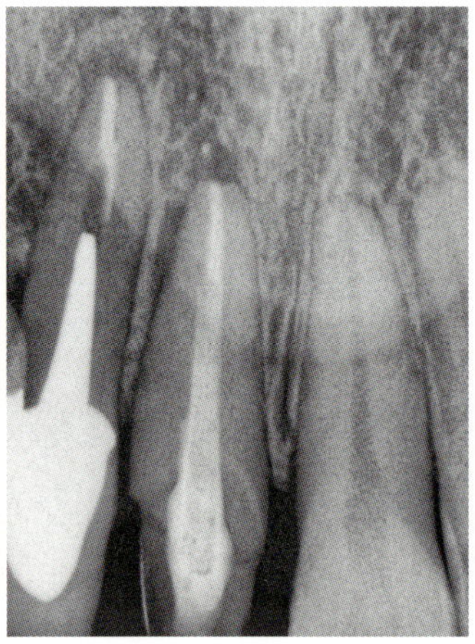

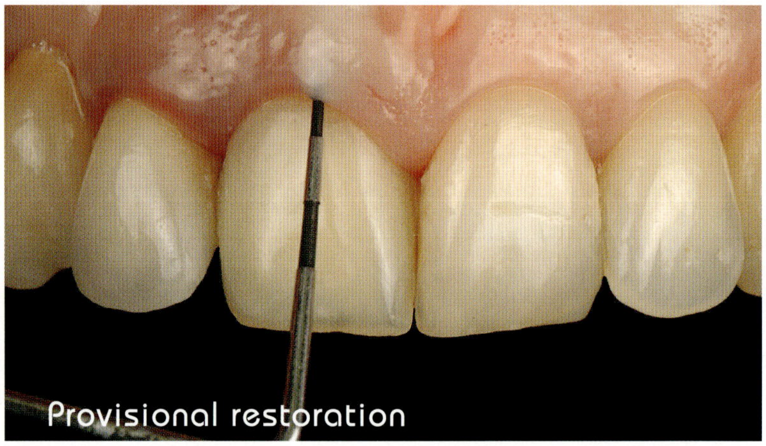

Initial situation with a vertically fractured maxillary right central incisor. A provisional crown was inserted before the immediate implant placement to visualize the soft tissue scalloping and crown support. The soft tissue surrounding the natural tooth is ideal because of its natural attachment complex, and it serves as an indicator and planning tool for the immediate implant placement and prosthetic design.

Immediate implant placement (5 × 13-mm NobelReplace Select Tapered Groovy) following tooth extraction with a flapless procedure and insertion of an RP–wide platform (WP) shift adapter.

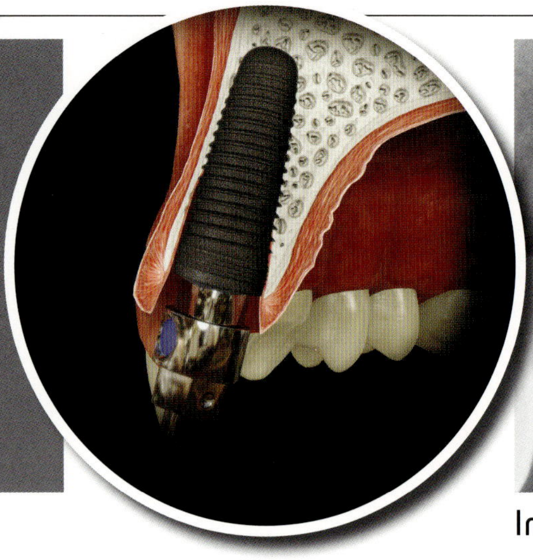

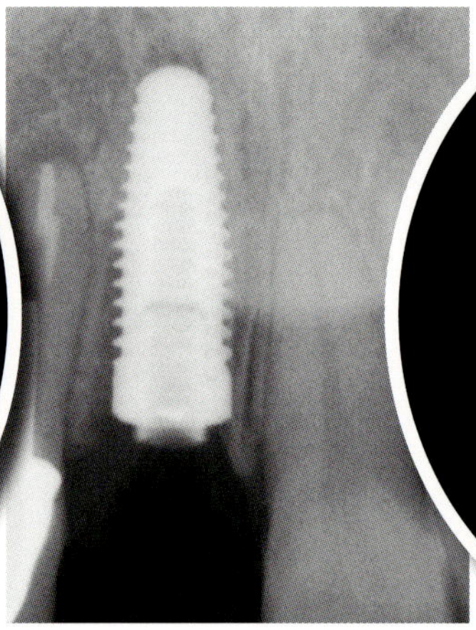

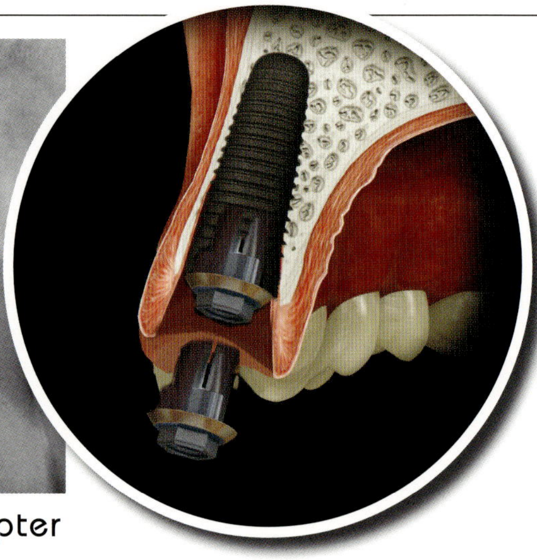

Implant and adapter

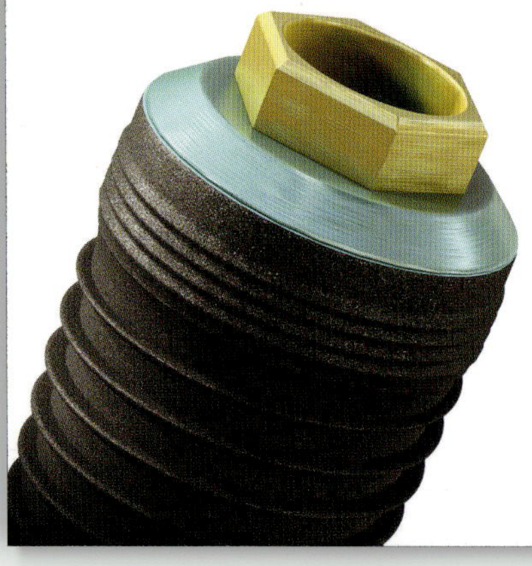

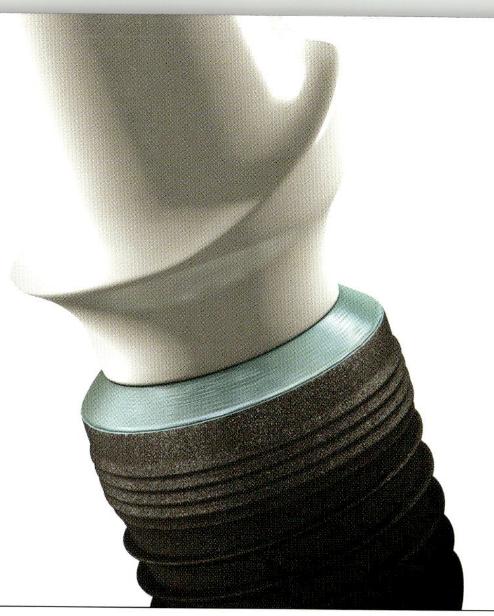

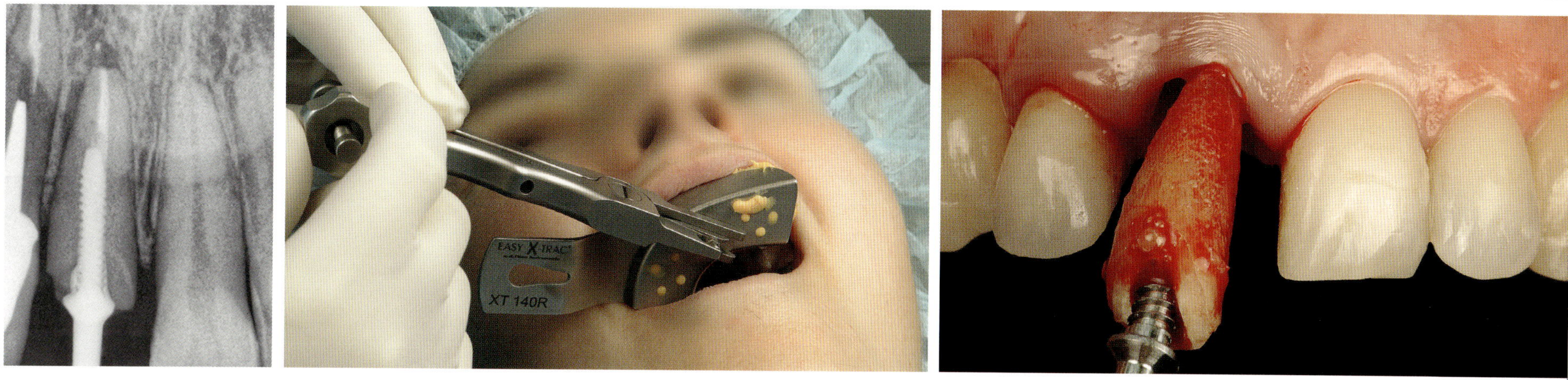

Atraumatic tooth extraction (Easy X-Trac System, A-Titan Instruments).

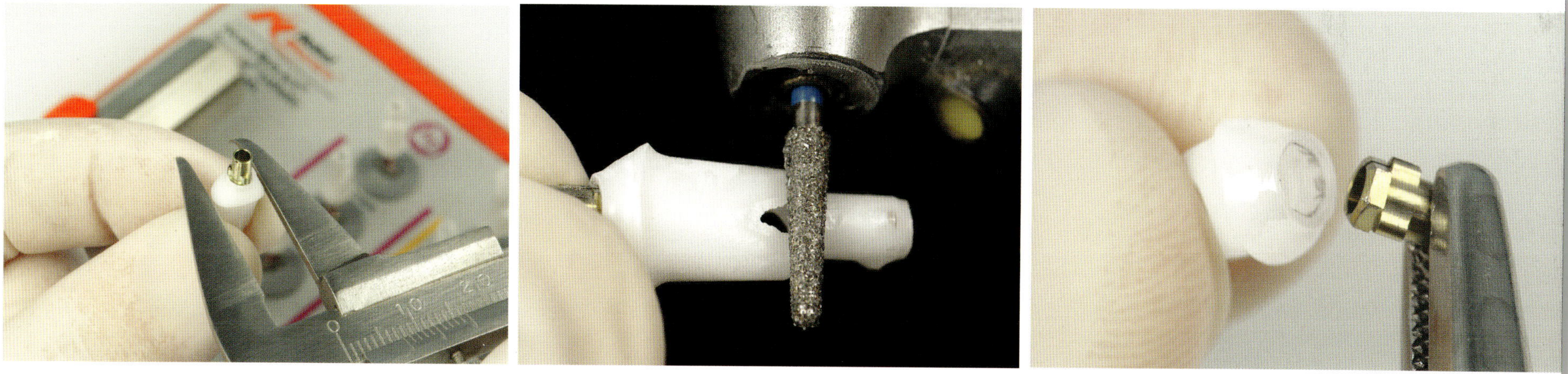

A prefabricated zirconia abutment is selected (NobelReplace Procera Esthetic Abutment Kit) by measuring the mesiodistal width of the original root in the preoperative periapical radiograph. The sprue and the internal RP adapter are removed.

Adaptation and verification. Proper fit and proper seating of the prefabricated zirconia abutment are verified with a periapical radiograph.

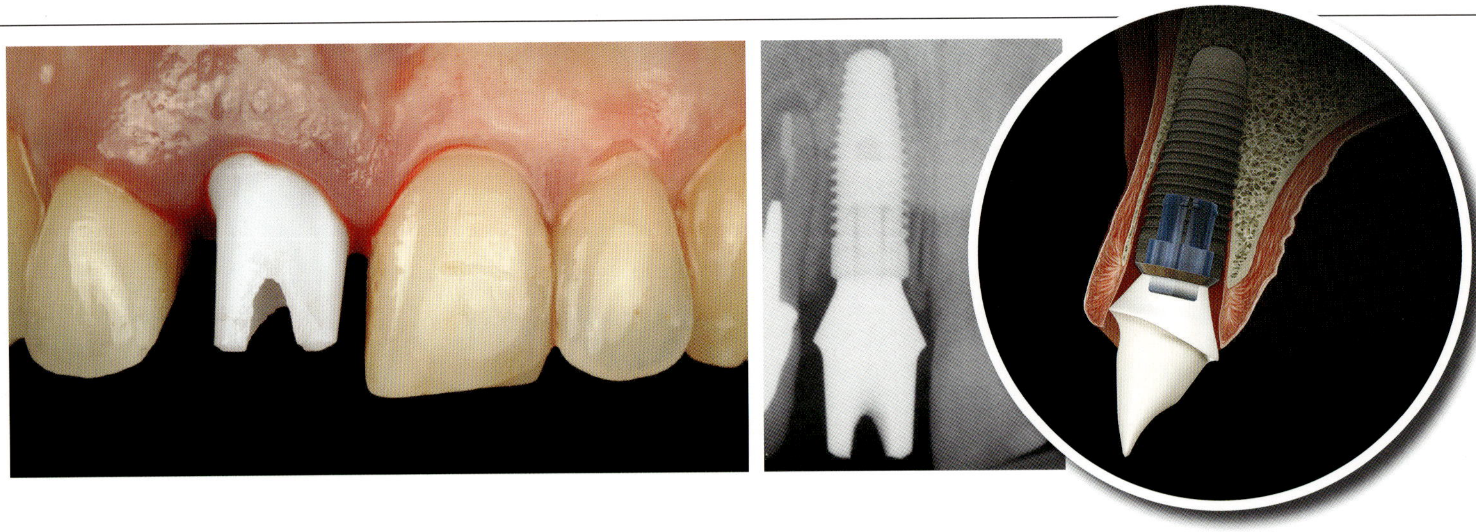

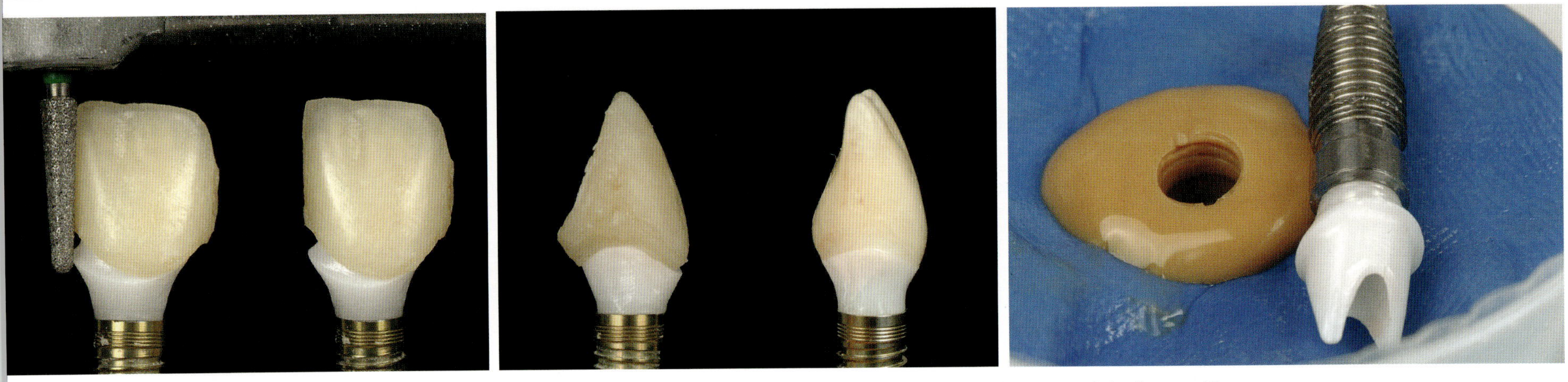

Recontouring of the abutment based on the original crown contour with respect to the position of the implant. Note the subgingival concavity to allow space for tissue grafting and improve soft tissue thickness. A final impression is made at this stage to fabricate the coping for the definitive crown restoration. The need for an additional impression at a later stage is eliminated, thus preventing further trauma to the peri-implant soft tissue.

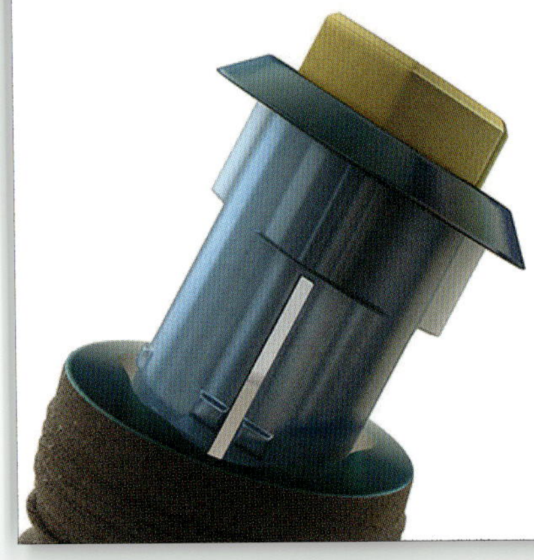

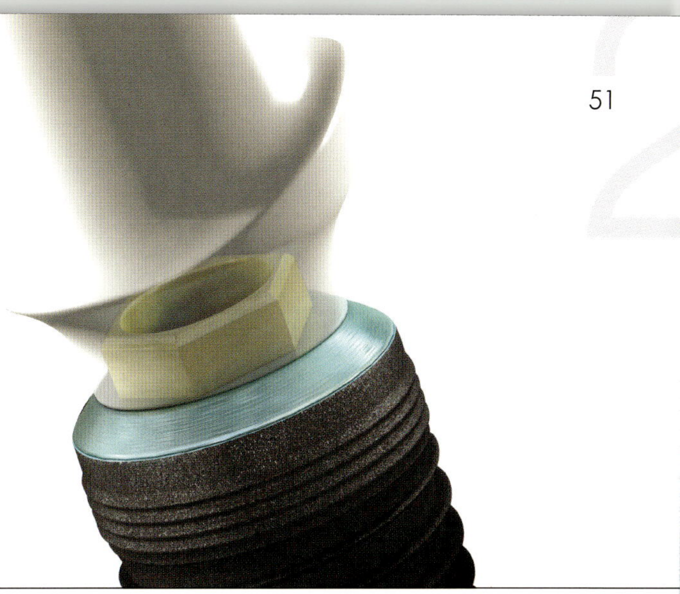

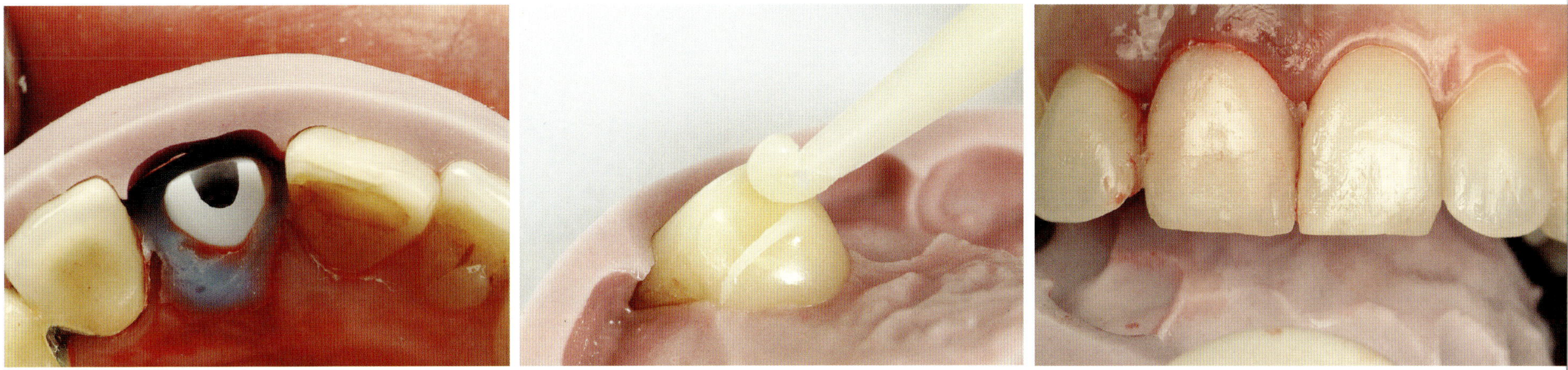

Intraoral preparation of the prefabricated zirconia abutment and relining of the provisional crown. Silicone indices assist with sufficient abutment reduction and ensure proper positioning for provisional crown reline.

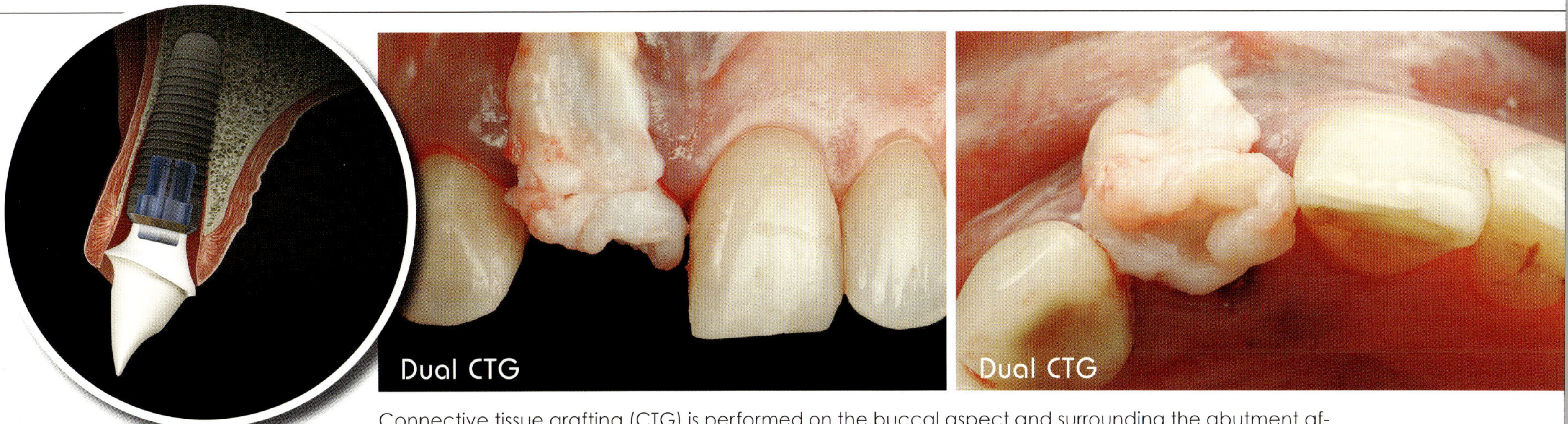

Connective tissue grafting (CTG) is performed on the buccal aspect and surrounding the abutment after the prosthetic phase. Prosthetic adjustments can be made according to the thickness of the grafted tissue.

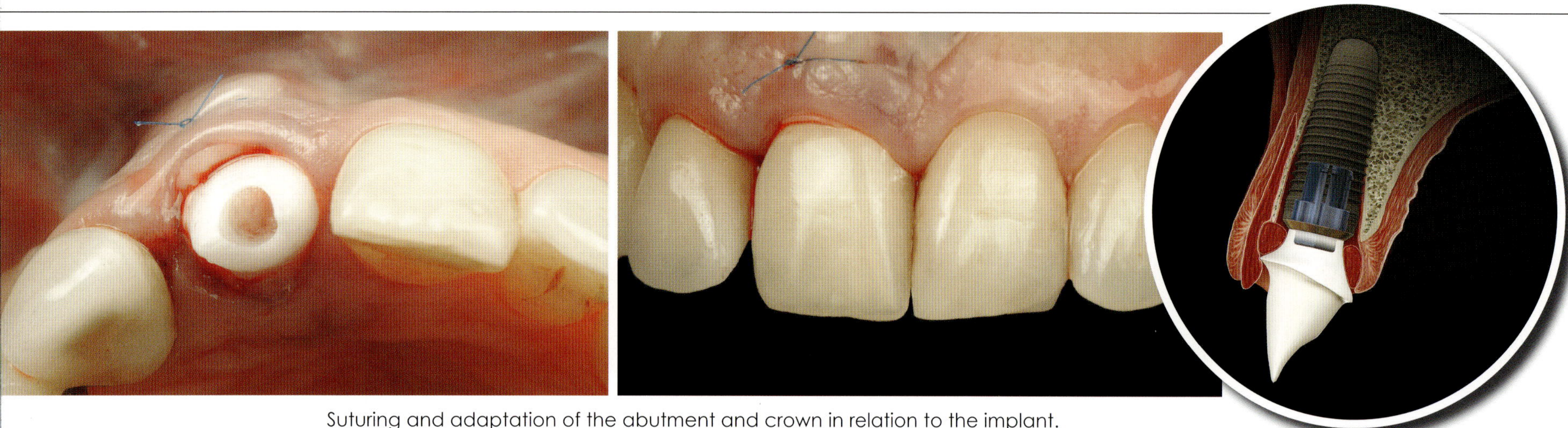

Suturing and adaptation of the abutment and crown in relation to the implant.

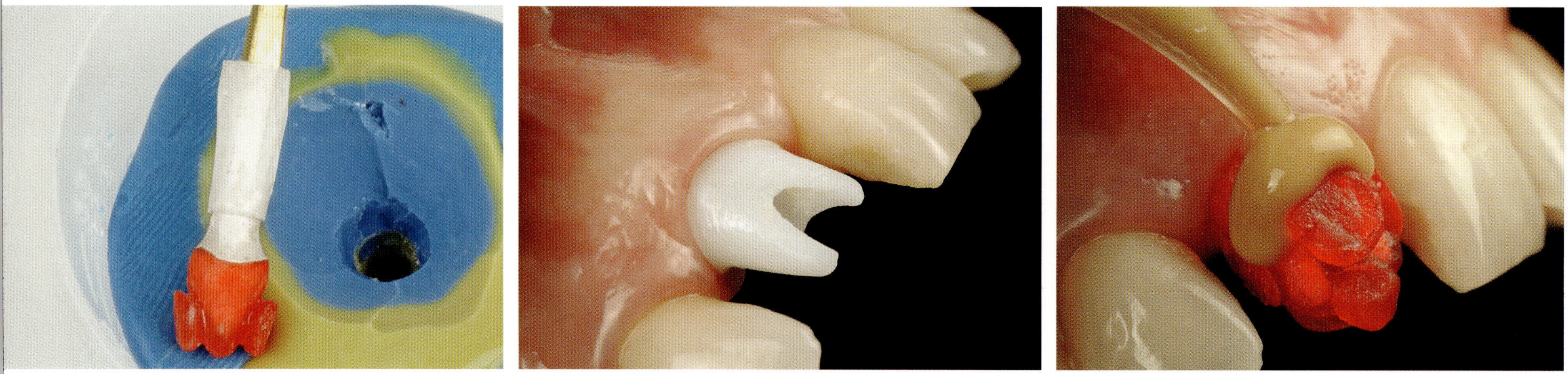

Final impression with a custom acrylic impression coping made from the impression at the time of implant placement, leaving the peri-implant soft tissue undisturbed.

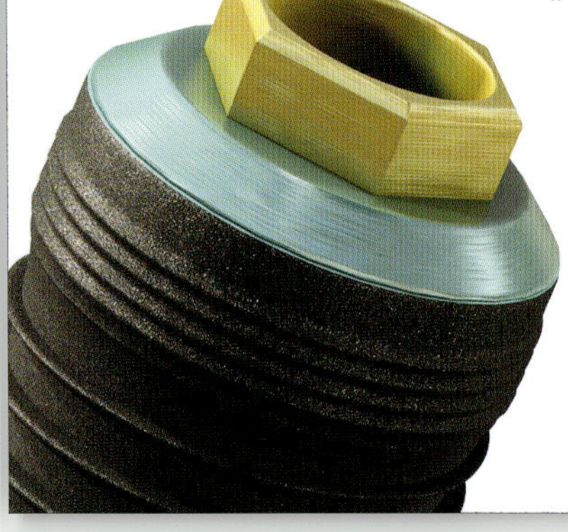

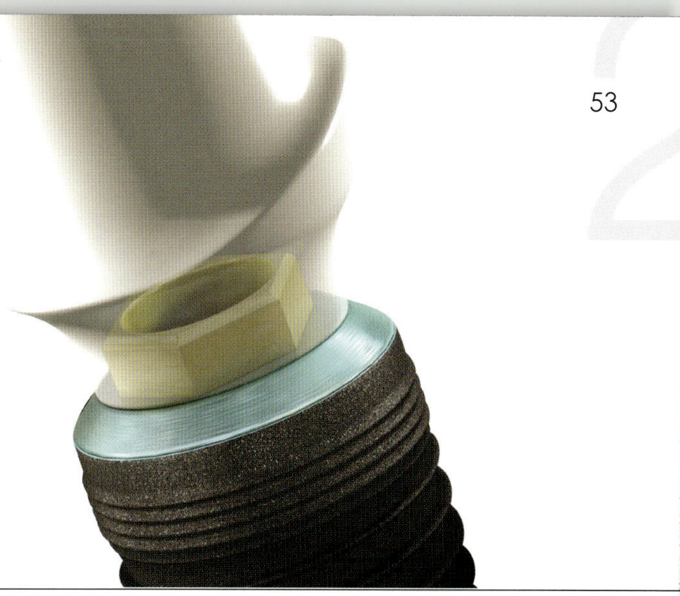

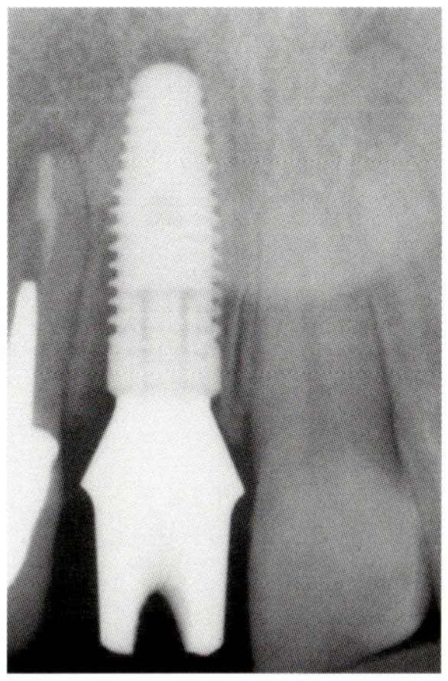

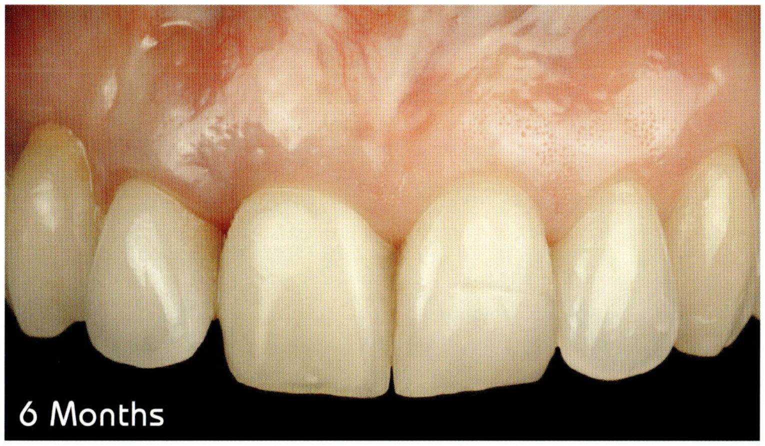

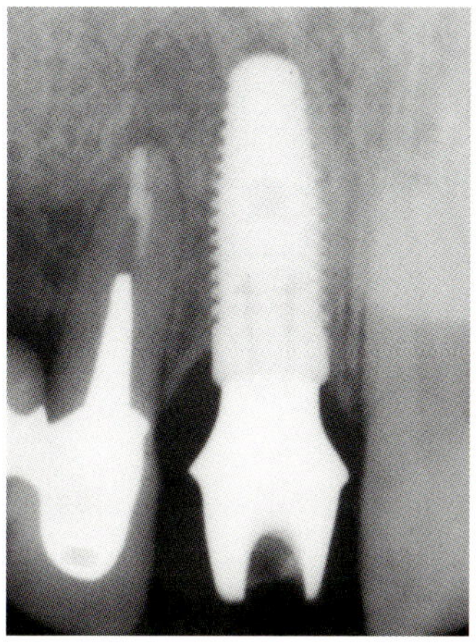

Healing process from day 0 to 6 months postoperative.

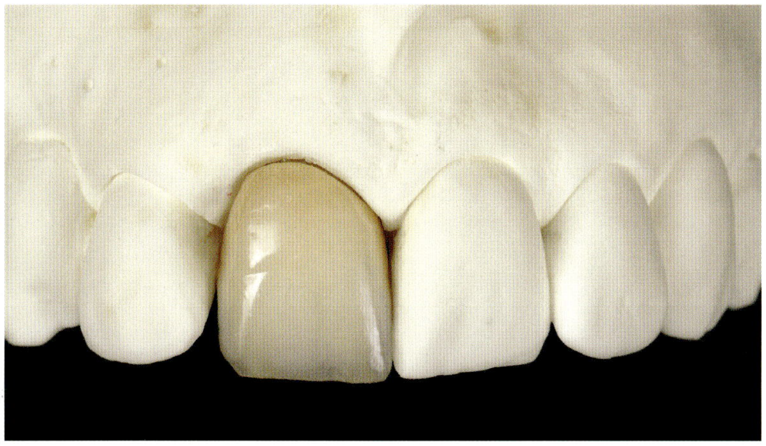

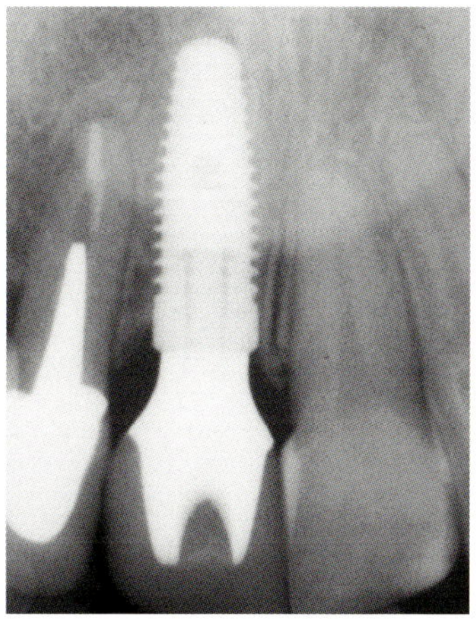

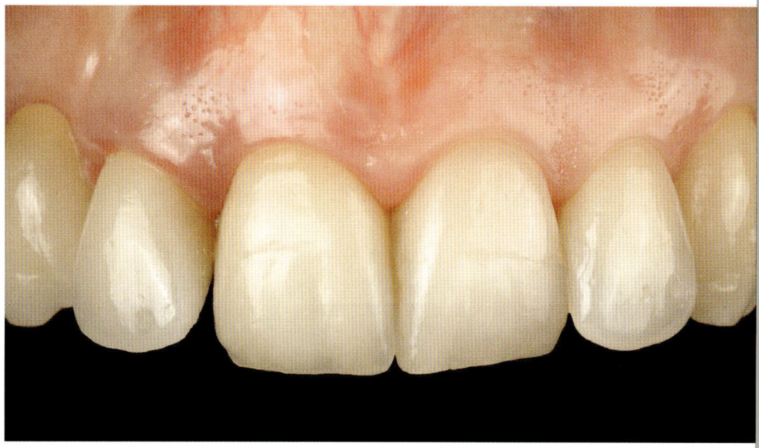

Final result after immediate implant therapy and application of the PS concept.

Platform shifting

The effects of *platform switching* or, more accurately, *platform shifting* on implant success and peri-implant marginal bone levels are continuously discussed. The scientific evidence as demonstrated in clinical trials and analyzed in systematic reviews has long been considered inconclusive but indicative of the potential benefits of PS concepts as well as cautiously supportive.[1–5] One systematic review assessed the difference between implants conventionally restored with the platform-matching or PS technique in terms of implant survival and marginal bone loss based on the available evidence (randomized controlled clinical trials) but also took into account both the patient-cluster effect and the impact of study design.[4] Meta-analysis of 10 randomized controlled trials that fulfilled the inclusion criteria confirmed the effectiveness of the PS concept in limiting marginal bone loss around dental implants. Bone-preserving effects were greater with increasing implant-abutment diameter mismatch and seemed stable over time.[4] In a most recent systematic review, Strietzel et al[5] concluded that, within the limits of the available studies, there is a tendency in favor of the PS technique to prevent or minimize peri-implant marginal bone loss, compared with implants with platform-matching abutments. However, because of the heterogeneity of the 22 studies included in the review, the authors admit that the findings must be interpreted with caution and that the question as to whether PS impacts marginal bone loss around endosseous implants remains largely unanswered. Consequently, there seems to be a need for further clinical trials to provide conclusive evidence.

Animal studies[6] are equally split on the subject, but the lack of significant and conclusive findings in some of those studies seems more related to limitations in study design, selection of (too many) influencing variables, methods, and sample size than actual effects of tested parameters.

Peri-implant bone loss, which to a certain extent is a common occurrence after functional loading of dental implants,[7–9] has become an important parameter to evaluate implant success.[10] Various causal and contributing factors for crestal bone remodeling[1–5] are currently being discussed in the literature: peri-implantitis,[11] biomechanical stresses[12] and occlusal overload,[13,14] ill-fitting prostheses[15] and micromovement of the abutment,[16] surgical trauma,[17] inflammatory response to the implant-abutment microgap,[18] and three-dimensional position of the implant[19] and its shoulder in respect to adjacent anatomical structures such as teeth, implants, and bone crests.

Besides less invasive surgical and immediate placement protocols, PS concepts seem to play an increasingly important role in limiting marginal bone loss.[1–5] The first clinical observation of this phenomenon was actually mostly accidental in nature and due to the unavailability of WP abutments for wide-diameter implants at the time.[20] The logical concept of shifting the unavoidable implant-abutment microgap[21] away from the crestal bone toward the center of the implant platform (by attaching abutments with smaller diameters to RP and WP implants) quickly drew the attention of clinicians and researchers alike. And while further well-designed and long-term clinical studies are needed to support the existing scientific evidence, most current findings cautiously support the benefits of the PS concept.[1–5]

The PS concept seems to have more pronounced effects on marginal bone stability in combination with immediate implant placement as compared with delayed implant placement protocols.[1–5] Also, current implant designs with internal connections, especially Morse tapers, seem more favorable to prevent marginal bone loss when combined with the PS concept.[22]

References

1. Atieh MH, Ibrahim HM, Atieh AH. Platform switching for marginal bone preservation around dental implants: A systematic review and meta-analysis. J Periodontol 2010;81:1350–1366.

2. Stafford GL. Evidence supporting platform-switching to preserve marginal bone levels not definitive. Evid Based Dent 2012;13:56–57.

3. Al-Nsour MM, Chan HL, Wang HL. Effect of the platform-switching technique on preservation of peri-implant marginal bone: A systematic review. Int J Oral Maxillofac Implants 2012;27:138–145.

4. Annibali S, Bignozzi I, Cristalli MP, Graziani F, La Monaca G, Polimeni A. Peri-implant marginal bone level: A systematic review and meta-analysis of studies comparing platform switching versus conventionally restored implants. J Clin Periodontol 2012;39:1097–1113.

5. Strietzel FP, Neumann K, Hertel M. Impact of platform switching on marginal peri-implant bone-level changes. A systematic review and meta-analysis [epub ahead of print 20 Jan 2014]. Clin Oral Implants Res doi:10.1111/clr.12339.

6. Lee J, Fiorini T, Gamborena I, et al. Effect of platform shift/switch on crestal bone levels and mucosa profile following flapless surgery and crestal/subcrestal implant placement [epub ahead of print 29 May 2014]. Clin Implant Dent Relat Res doi:10.1111/cid.12243.

7. Hermann JS, Buser D, Schenk RK, Cochran DL. Crestal bone changes around titanium implants. A histometric evaluation on unloaded non-submerged and submerged implants in the canine mandible. J Periodontol 2000;71:1412–1424.

8. Laurell L, Lundgren D. Marginal bone level changes at dental implants after 5 years in function: A meta-analysis. Clin Implant Dent Relat Res 2011;13:19–28.

9. Hermann JS, Buser D, Schenk RK, Schoolfield JD, Cochran DL. Biologic width around one- and two-piece titanium implants. Clin Oral Implants Res 2001;12:559–571.

10. Albrektsson T, Zarb G, Worthington P, Eriksson AR. The long-term efficacy of currently used dental implants: A review and proposed criteria of success. Int J Oral Maxillofac Implants 1986;1:11–25.

11. Lang NP, Berglundh T. Peri-implant diseases: Where are we now? Consensus of the Seventh European Workshop on Periodontology. J Clin Periodontol 2001;38(suppl 11):178–181.

12. Maeda Y, Miura J, Taki I, Sogo M. Biomechanical analysis on platform switching: Is there any biomechanical rationale? Clin Oral Implants Res 2007;18:581–584.

13. Naert I, Duyck J, Vandamme K. Occlusal overload and bone/implant loss. Clin Oral Implants Res 2012;23(suppl 6):95–107.

14. Zhang X, Duyck J, Vandamme K, Naert I, Carmeliet G. Ultrastructural characterization of the implant interface response to loading. J Dent Res 2014;93:313–318.

15. Assunção WG, Gomes EA, Rocha EP, Delben JA. Three-dimensional finite element analysis of vertical and angular misfit in implant-supported fixed prostheses. Int J Oral Maxillofac Implants 2011;26:788–796.

16. Yamanishi Y, Yamaguchi S, Imazato S, Nakano T, Yatani H. Influences of neck design and implant-abutment joint type on peri-implant bone stress and abutment micromovement: Three-dimensional finite element analysis. Dent Mater 2012;28:1126–1133.

17. Oh HJ, Wikesjö UM, Kang HS, Ku Y, Eom TG, Koo KT. Effect of implant drill characteristics on heat generation in osteotomy sites: A pilot study. Clin Oral Implants Res 2011;22:722–726.

18. Ericsson I, Persson LG, Berglundh T, Marinello CP, Lindhe J, Klinge B. Different types of inflammatory reactions in peri-implant soft tissues. J Clin Periodontol 1995;22:255–261.

19. Baggi L, Cappelloni I, Di Girolamo M, Maceri F, Vairo G. The influence of implant diameter and length on stress distribution of osseointegrated implants related to crestal bone geometry: A three-dimensional finite element analysis. J Prosthet Dent 2008;100:422–431.

20. Lazzara RJ, Porter SS. Platform switching: A new concept in implant dentistry for controlling postrestorative crestal bone levels. Int J Periodontics Restorative Dent 2006;26:9–17.

21. Koutouzis T, Neiva R, Nonhoff J, Lundgren T. Placement of implants with platform-switched Morse taper connections with the implant-abutment interface at different levels in relation to the alveolar crest: A short-term (1-year) randomized prospective controlled clinical trial. Int J Oral Maxillofac Implants 2013;28:1553–1563.

22. Larrucea Verdugo C, Jaramillo Núñez G, Acevedo Avila A, Larrucea San Martín C. Microleakage of the prosthetic abutment/implant interface with internal and external connection: In vitro study [epub ahead of print 4 Jul 2013]. Clin Oral Implants Res doi:10.1111/clr.12217.

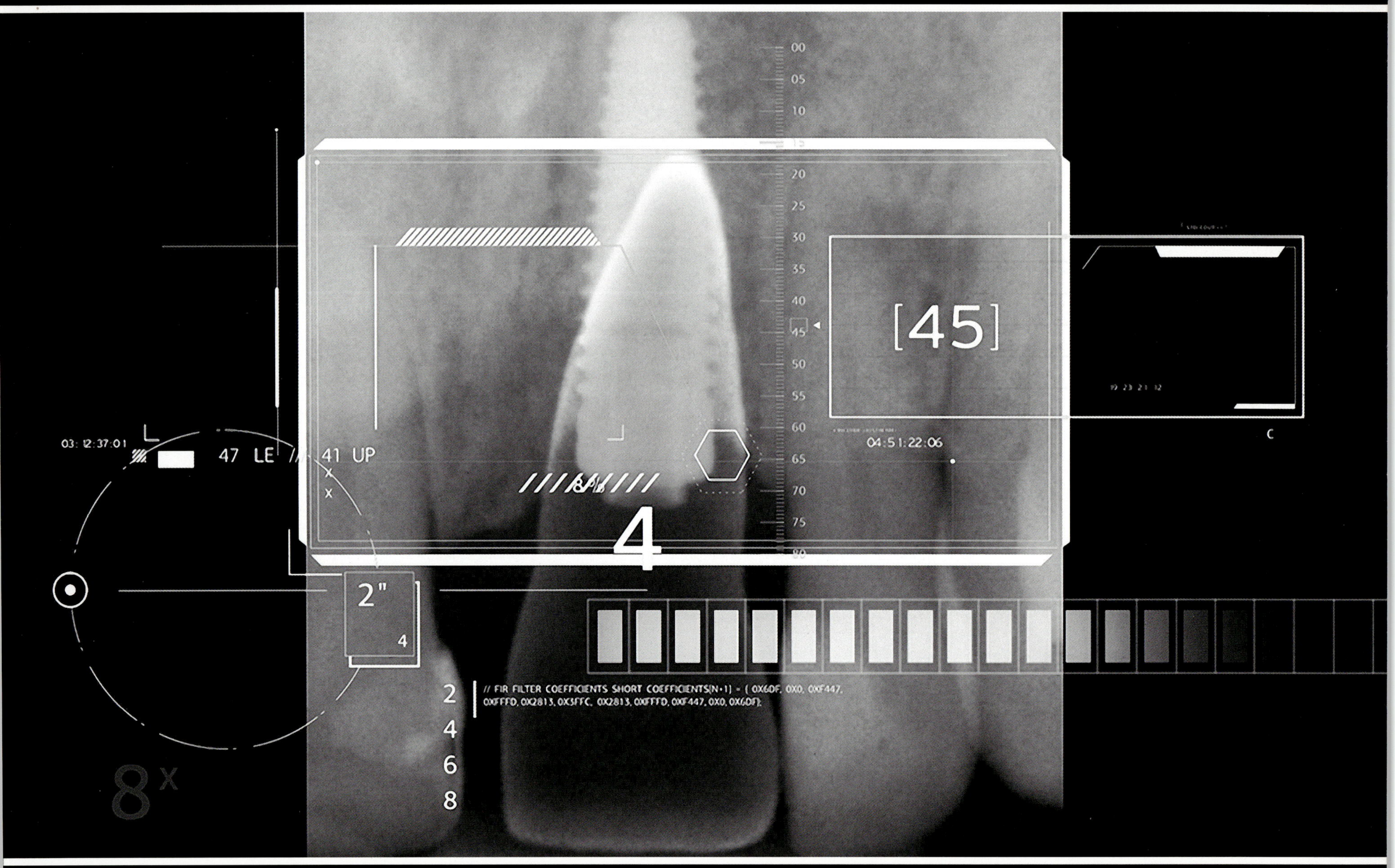

03: 12:37:01
47 LE
41 UP
[45]
04:51:22:06
4
2"
2
4
6
8
// FIR FILTER COEFFICIENTS SHORT COEFFICIENTS[N+1] = { 0X6DF, 0X0, 0XF447, 0XFFFD, 0X2813, 0X3FFC, 0X2813, 0XFFFD, 0XF447, 0X0, 0X6DF};
8x

Clinical Results with Platform Shift Concept

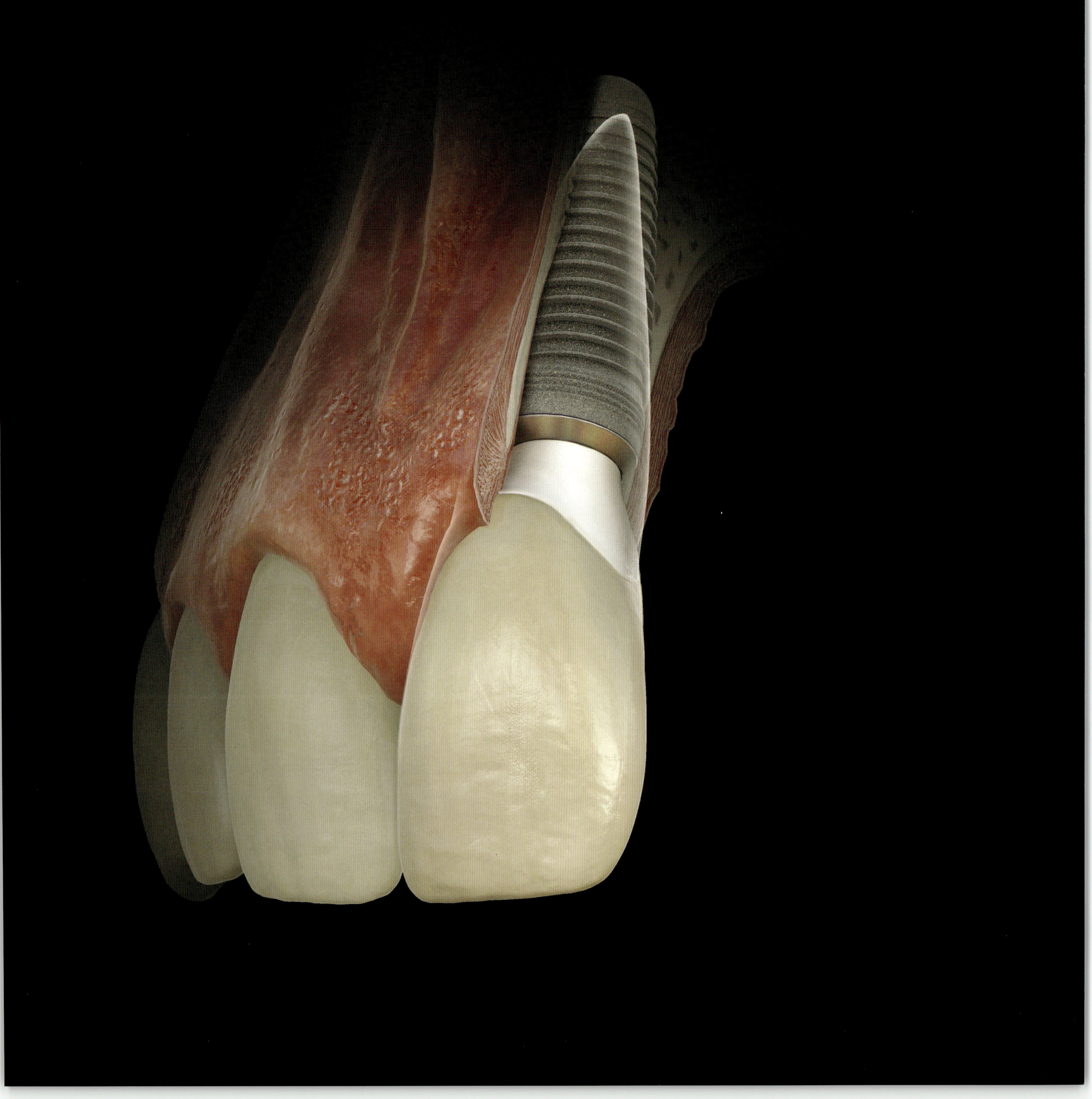

PS adapter results

Delayed implant placement long term (6 years)

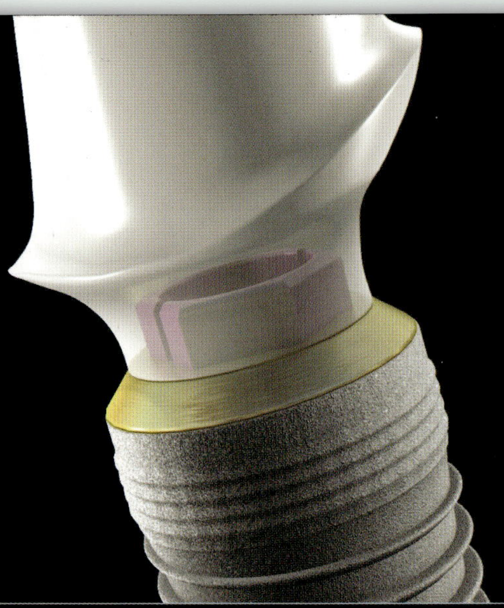

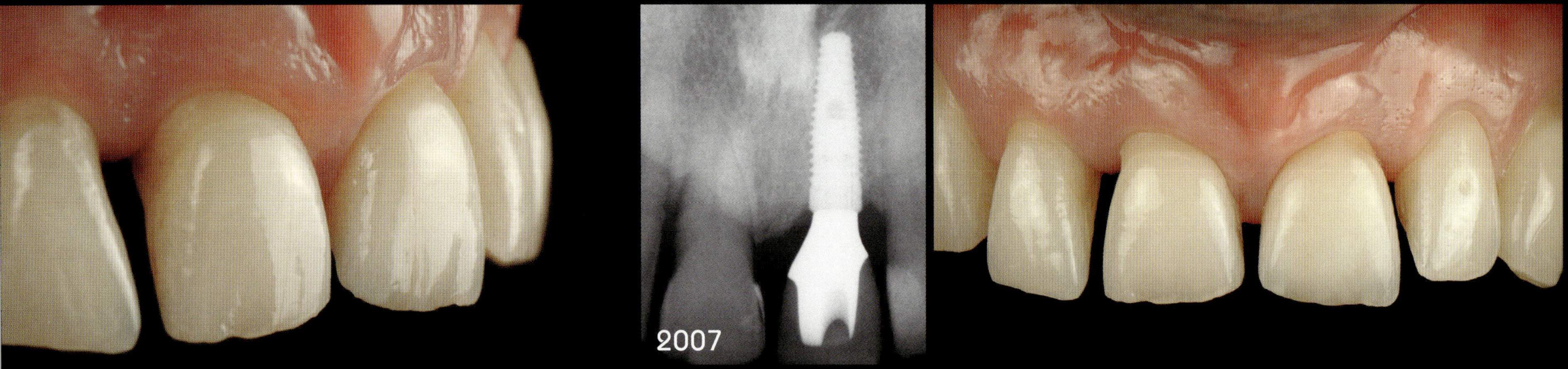

Final outcome of an implant-supported crown in the area of the maxillary left central incisor after delayed implant placement. A CTG was placed during implant surgery, and the PS concept was applied with a PS adapter and the definitive abutment. Clinical views reveal ideal soft tissue morphology, while the radiograph indicates adequate bone support at the time of treatment completion.

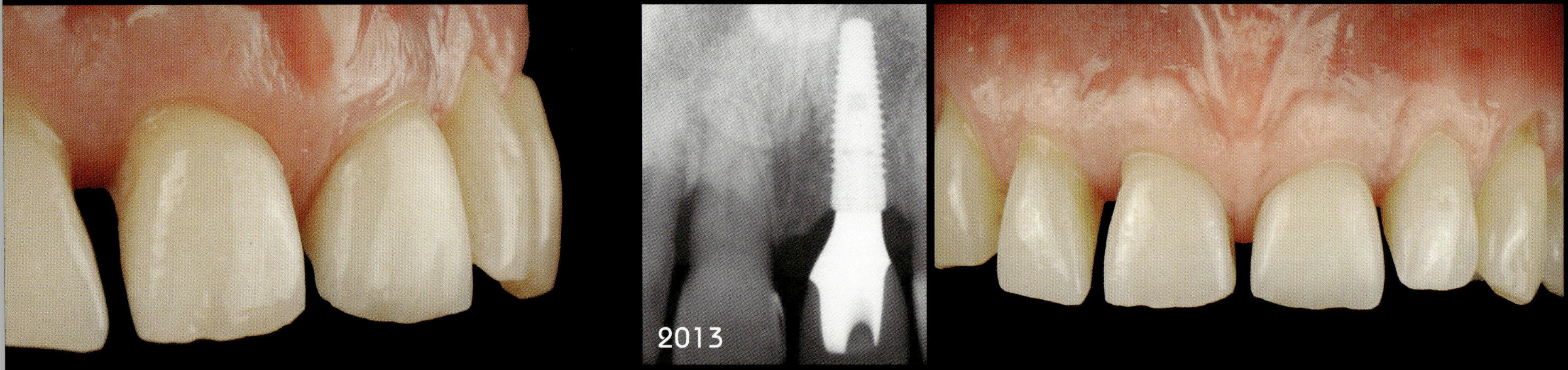

Six years later, the bone levels remained quite stable with only minimal changes in height, as depicted in the periapical radiograph. The clinical situation and especially the soft tissue contour did not change dramatically either. If anything, the maturation of the soft tissues may be viewed to have a positive effect on the long-term result. There are several contributing factors for the long-term success and stability: one-stage surgery with a CTG and the PS concept at the same time as well as a minimally invasive impression technique for the definitive restoration.

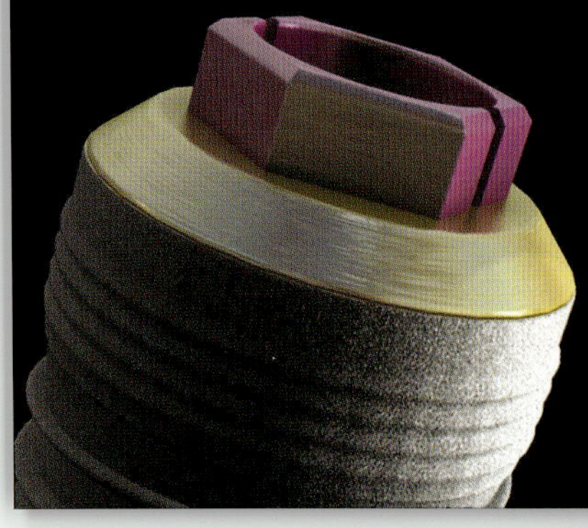

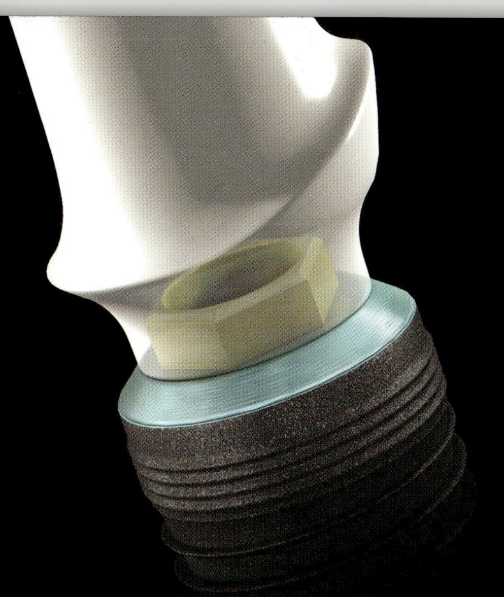

Immediate implant placement long term (5 years)

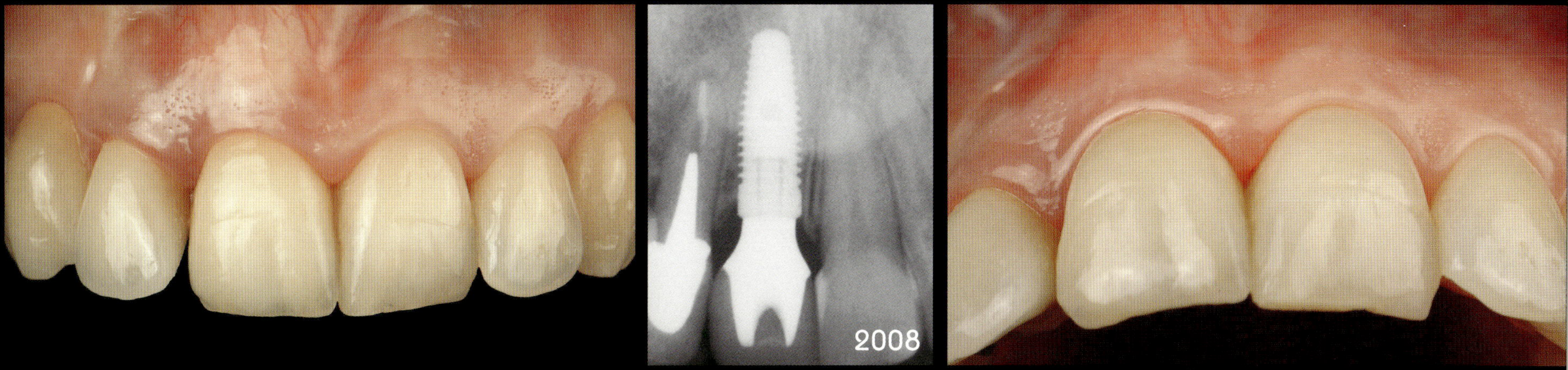

Postoperative clinical situation after completion of an implant-supported crown in the area of the maxillary right central incisor. The implant was placed immediately after tooth extraction. At the same time, the definitive, concave abutment was inserted with a PS adapter, and a CTG was placed to fill the created additional space and thicken the soft tissue biotype. The soft tissue contour, support, thickness, and morphology resembled the gingiva around the natural left central incisor.

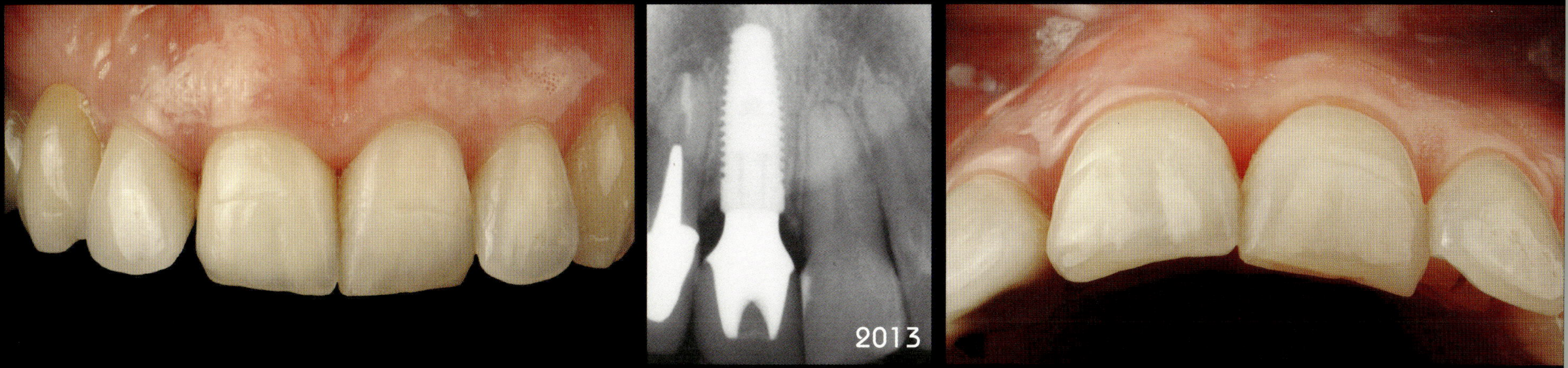

Minimal bone loss after 5 years of function on the distal aspect of the implant collar. The soft tissues remained stable in all dimensions even after the long observation period, which may be attributed to the surgical and restorative techniques: immediate application of the PS concept with PS adapters and a concave abutment as well as CTG placement.

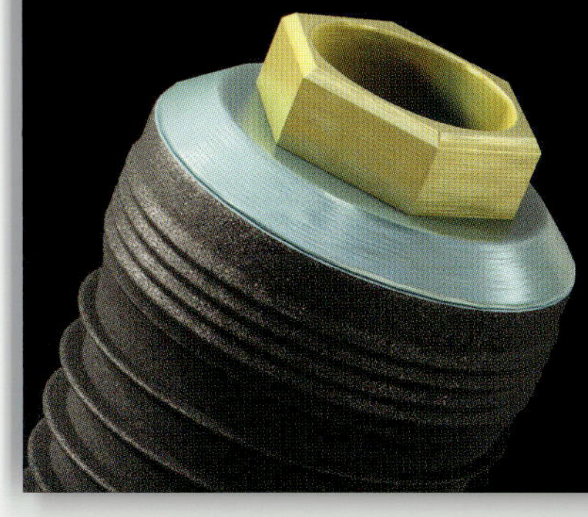

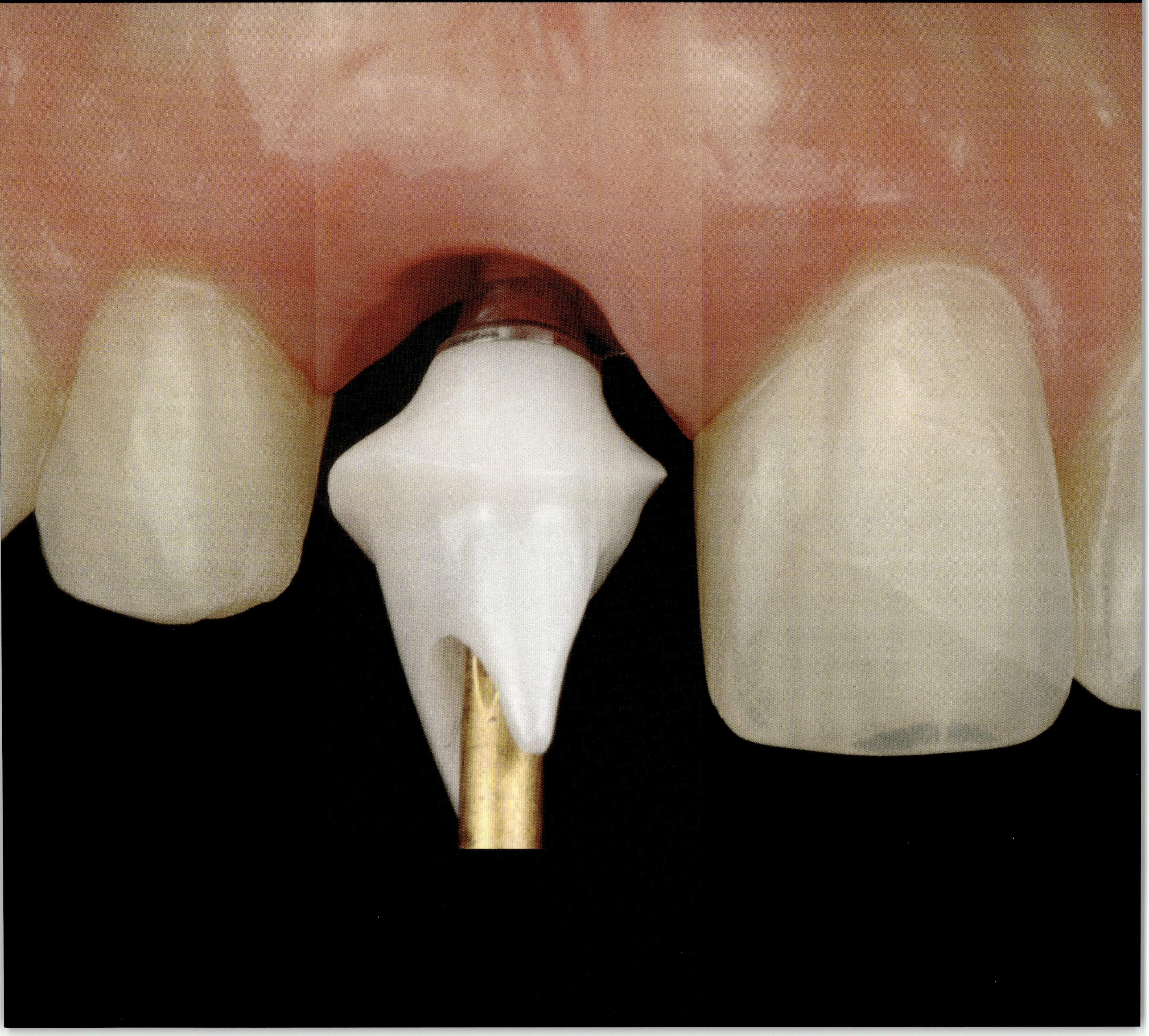

Disconnection effect

This patient case illustrates that violation and disturbance of the peri-implant biologic width affects bone remodeling and may eventually lead to bone loss. Keeping the implant-abutment interface undisturbed by avoiding any disconnection of the prosthetic components is important after immediate implant placement, especially when no CTG is placed to compensate for the resorption of the buccal plate after tooth extraction. The clinical documentation spans over 6 years. As in other cases, a pronounced thinning of the soft tissue was observed 3 years postsurgery. Three years seems to be the crucial time frame for thinning of the peri-implant soft tissue and maturation into mucosa. This often becomes obvious in cases with normal tissue thickness and a type 1 socket, which initially seem ideal.

The patient complained about a "black space" between the central incisors with "saliva coming out" and a "funny feeling" when touching the buccal tissue around the implant. At the time, the authors did not follow any strategy to compensate for the subsequent bone loss at an early stage and rather addressed these problems when they occurred. In this case, a buccal CTG with a tunnel incision on the buccal was placed after 5 years of treatment. The definitive abutment was disconnected during the CTG surgery to allow for a proper incision and the split-thickness flap dissection. Note that bone levels were stable within the first 5 years but resorbed to the first thread once the abutment was disconnected and surgery was performed. Even with the most atraumatic and minimally invasive surgical approach, the combination of implant component disconnection and surgical trauma created bone loss.

Research

Disconnection effect

Several factors influence the soft tissue stability around dental implants and implant-supported prosthetic components and restorations.[1,2] Clinical experience and long-term observations in clinical practice settings have led to the hypothesis that frequent disconnection of prosthetic implant components, such as healing abutments, screw-retained provisional restorations, and definitive abutments or restorations causes inferior peri-implant soft tissue conditions and should therefore be avoided. Several animal studies and histologic investigations support this hypothesis and indicate a correlation between mechanical disruption of the peri-implant soft tissue interface and marginal bone as well as soft tissue loss.[3–5] It remains unclear, however, how many disruptive events or "disconnections" are necessary to cause significant bone loss.[6,7]

More recent clinical studies provide at least some evidence that, indeed, a "one abutment, one time" concept, where the definitive implant abutment is placed at the time of implant surgery and not removed afterward, causes less marginal bone loss.[8–11] This seems especially true for implants placed immediately into fresh extraction sockets.

Canullo et al[8] reported on a randomized clinical trial conducted in private practices to evaluate the influence of restoration on marginal bone loss with immediately placed definitive abutments versus provisional abutments that were later replaced by definitive abutments. Three-year follow-up data indicated significantly lower bone loss in the "one abutment, one time" test group as compared with the control group. In a similar randomized controlled trial with multiple, up to 24-month follow-up visits, Degidi et al[9] concluded that nonremoval of abutments placed at the time of the surgery improved the stability of healed soft and hard tissues around the immediately restored, subcrestally placed tapered single maxillary implants. Comparable studies in various sites, such as the posterior mandible, revealed similar outcomes.[10,11] One long-term study on immediately loaded PS implants placed in heavy smokers found comparable success to those in nonsmokers when the abutments were placed on the day of surgery and never removed thereafter.[12]

While the limited existing evidence indicates that frequent disconnection of implant components is detrimental to bone and soft tissue stability, further studies are needed to support specific clinical protocols and document their outcomes in the long term.

References

1. Rompen E. The impact of the type and configuration of abutments and their (repeated) removal on the attachment level and marginal bone. Eur J Oral Implantol 2012;5(suppl):S83–S90.

2. Rompen E, Touati B, Van Dooren E. Factors influencing marginal tissue remodeling around implants. Pract Proced Aesthet Dent 2003;15:754–761.

3. Abrahamsson I, Berglundh T, Lindhe J. The mucosal barrier following abutment dis/reconnection. An experimental study in dogs. J Clin Periodontol 1997;24:568–572.

4. Hermann JS, Schoolfield JD, Schenk RK, Buser D, Cochran DL. Influence of the size of the microgap on crestal bone changes around titanium implants. A histometric evaluation of unloaded non-submerged implants in the canine mandible. J Periodontol 2001;72:1372–1383.

5. King GN, Hermann JS, Schoolfield JD, Buser D, Cochran DL. Influence of the size of the microgap on crestal bone levels in non-submerged dental implants: A radiographic study in the canine mandible. J Periodontol 2002;73:1111–1117.

6. Abrahamsson I, Berglundh T, Sekino S, Lindhe J. Tissue reactions to abutment shift: An experimental study in dogs. Clin Implant Dent Relat Res 2003;5:82–88.

7. Hermann JS, Jones AA, Bakaeen LG, Buser D, Schoolfield JD, Cochran DL. Influence of a machined collar on crestal bone changes around titanium implants: A histometric study in the canine mandible. J Periodontol 2011;82:1329–1338.

8. Canullo L, Bignozzi I, Cocchetto R, Cristalli MP, Iannello G. Immediate positioning of a definitive abutment versus repeated abutment replacements in post-extractive implants: 3-year follow-up of a randomised multicentre clinical trial. Eur J Oral Implantol 2010;3:285–296.

9. Degidi M, Nardi D, Daprile G, Piattelli A. Nonremoval of immediate abutments in cases involving subcrestally placed postextractive tapered single implants: A randomized controlled clinical study [epub ahead of print 4 Mar 2013]. Clin Implant Dent Relat Res doi:10.1111/cid.12051.

10. Degidi M, Nardi D, Piattelli A. One abutment at one time: Nonremoval of an immediate abutment and its effect on bone healing around subcrestal tapered implants. Clin Oral Implants Res 2011;22:1303–1307.

11. Grandi T, Guazzi P, Samarani R, Garuti G. Immediate positioning of definitive abutments versus repeated abutment replacements in immediately loaded implants: Effects on bone healing at the 1-year follow-up of a multicentre randomized controlled trial. Eur J Oral Implantol 2012;5:9–16.

12. Romanos GE, Gaertner K, Aydin E, Nentwig GH. Long-term results after immediate loading of platform-switched implants in smokers versus nonsmokers with full-arch restorations. Int J Oral Maxillofac Implants 2013;28:841–845.

2005

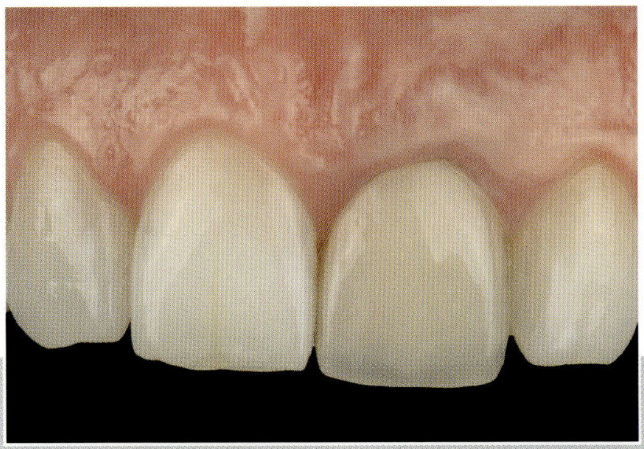

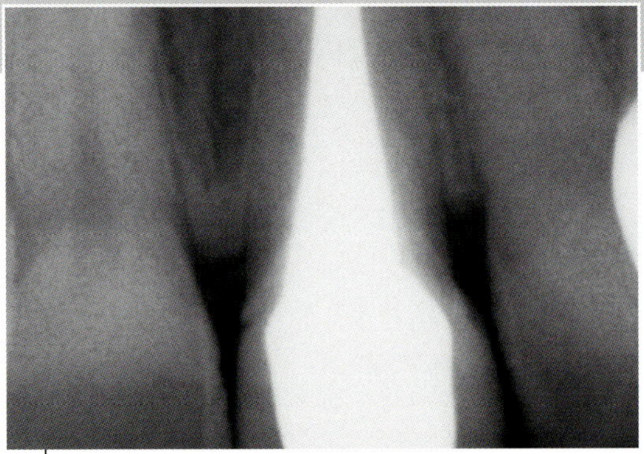

The initial situation reveals an ideal immediate implant case, with a normal crest, socket type 1, and normal biotype. It was decided to place an implant immediately after extraction of the tooth because of prosthetic failures and lack of a sufficient ferrule.

Day 0

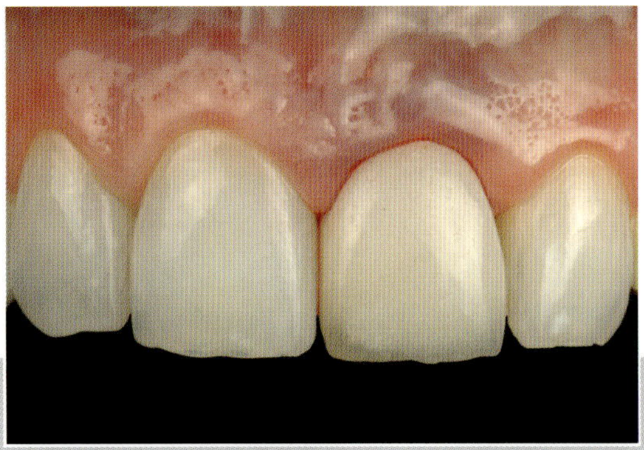

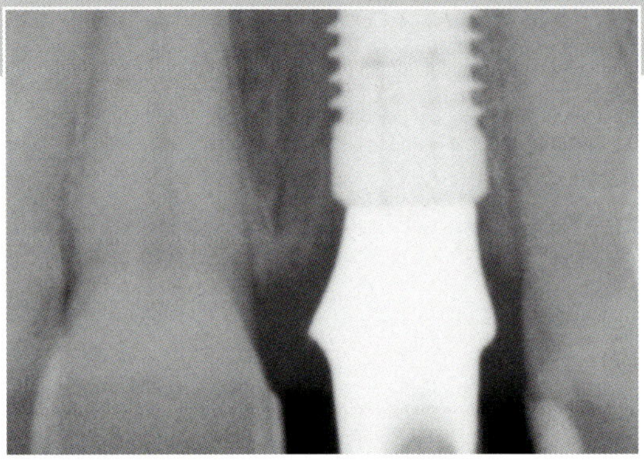

2006

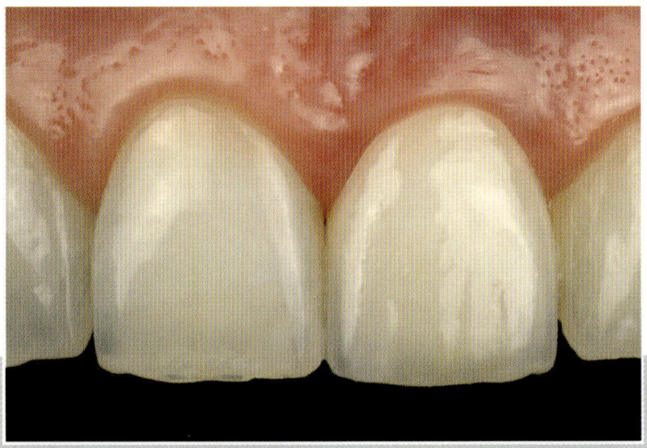

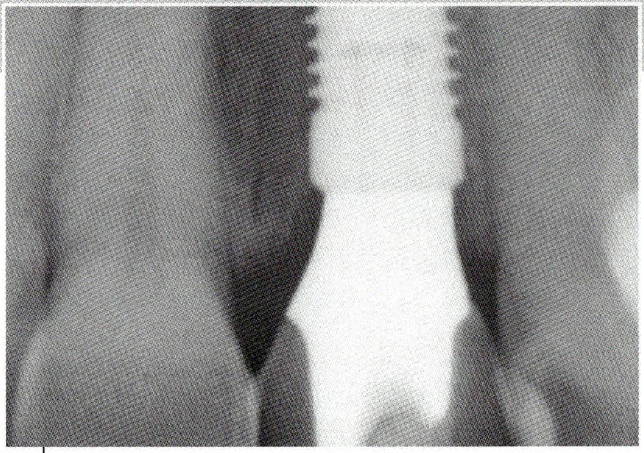

The definitive implant abutment and crown restoration were inserted the day of implant placement. The periapical radiograph reveals stability of the bone and soft tissues, following the PS concept.

1 Year (2007)

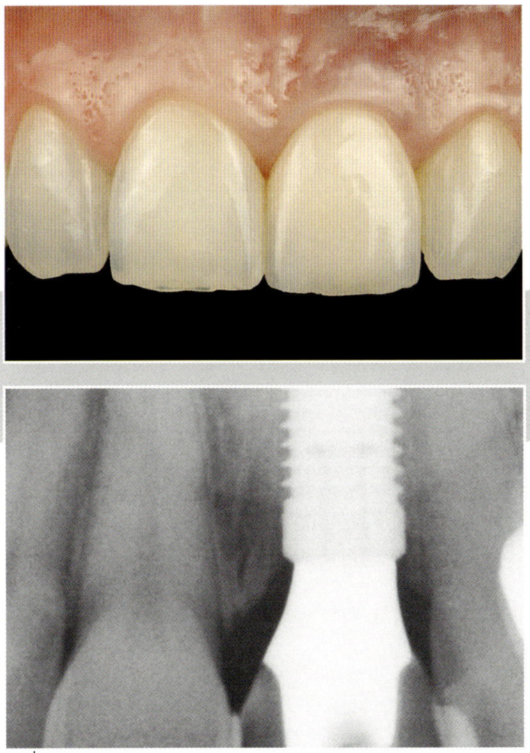

One-year re-evaluation demonstrates only slight soft tissue recession and minimal vertical bone loss adjacent to the abutment but above the implant interface.

2 Years (2008)

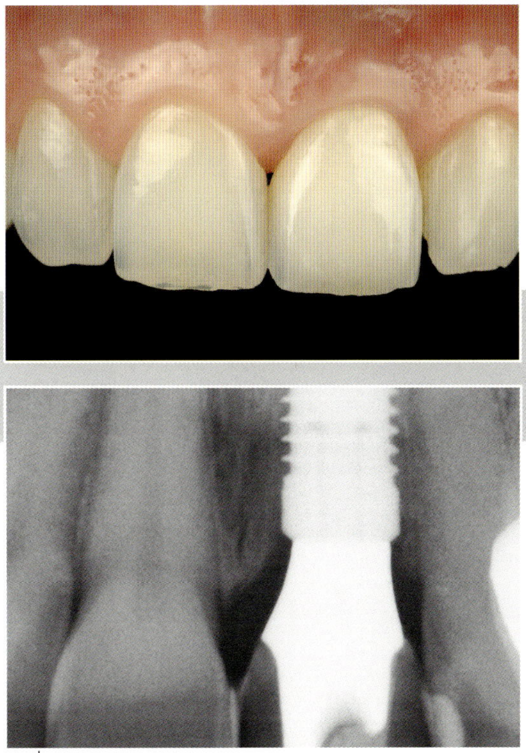

The situation remained similar 2 years postsurgery. However, the patient started complaining about the "black space" between central incisors. Composite resin was applied directly to fill the space to the satisfaction of the patient.

3 Years (2009)

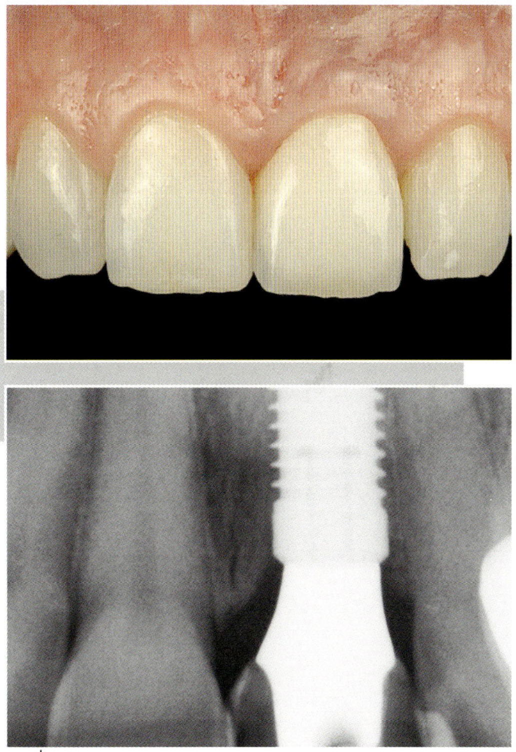

Composite resin restoration 1 year after placement.

4 Years (2010)

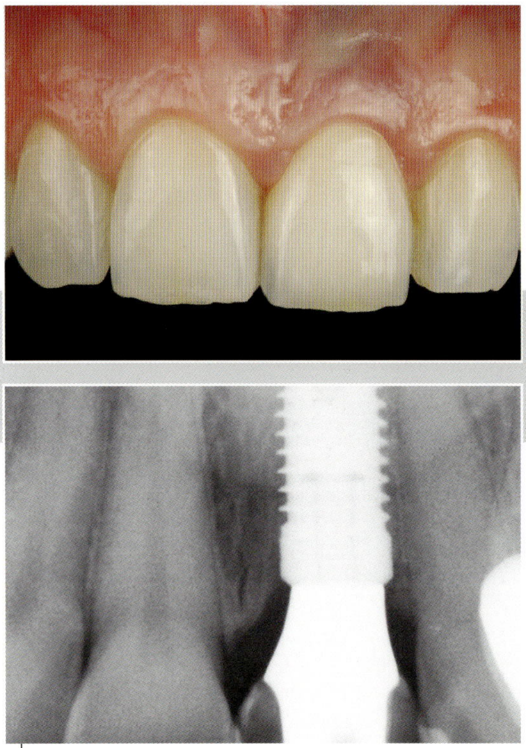

Peri-implant bone and soft tissue remained stable, but a dark shadow of the implant became noticeable.

5 Years (2011)

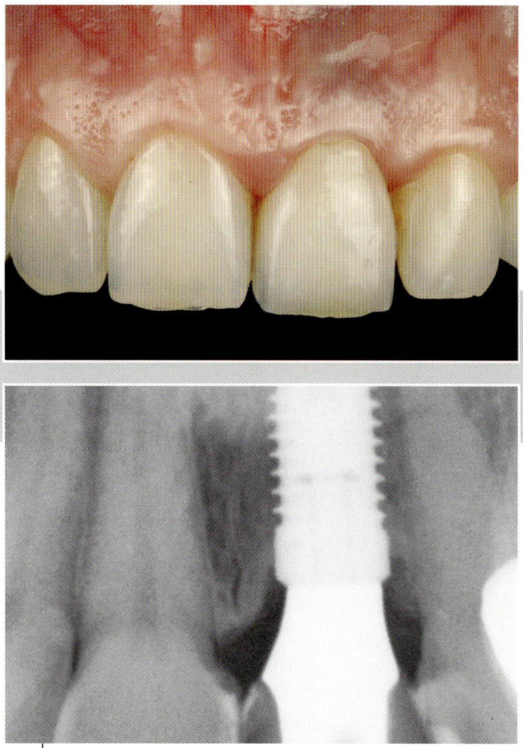

The composite resin restoration fractured 1 year later, leaving the interproximal contact unstable. Bone levels seemed unchanged, but the darkening shadow on the buccal soft tissue had become more pronounced. It was decided to remove the crown and place a CTG with a flapless procedure.

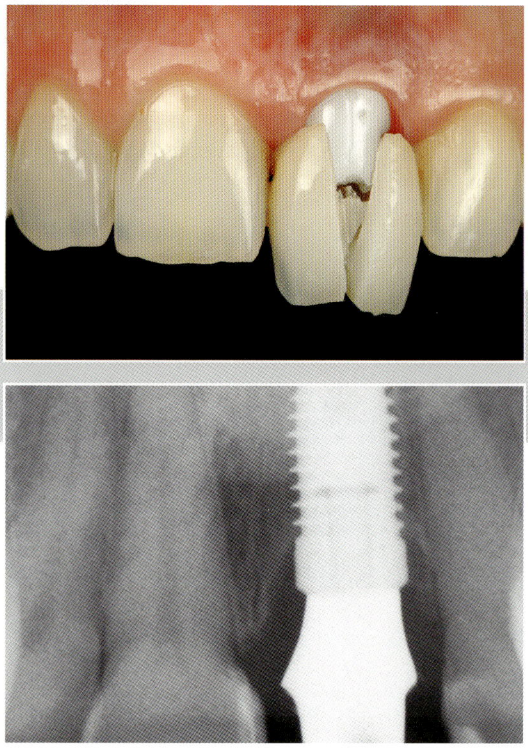

2011

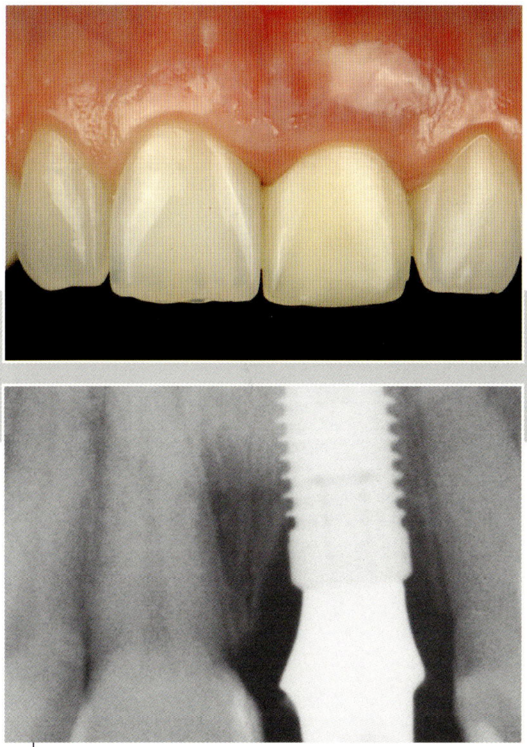

Situation 3 months after placing the CTG and a provisional restoration. The implant abutment had to be removed to facilitate the surgery, and bone resorption to the first implant thread was observed subsequently.

2012

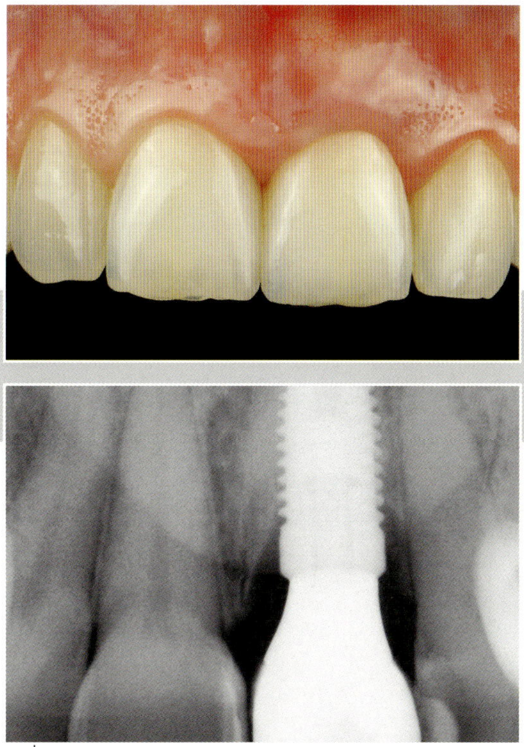

Delivery of the new zirconia crown. While the soft tissue was acceptable, the bone resorbed to the first thread of the implant.

2013

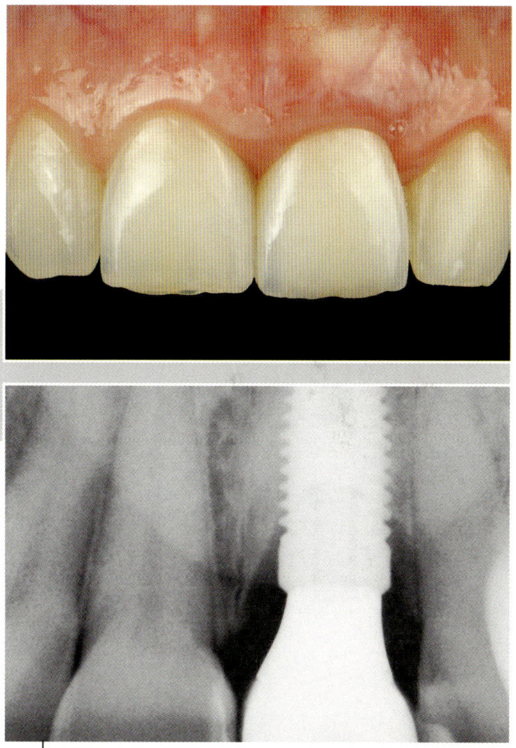

The situation 1 year after the CTG was placed revealed a favorable soft tissue reaction with no changes to the bone height.

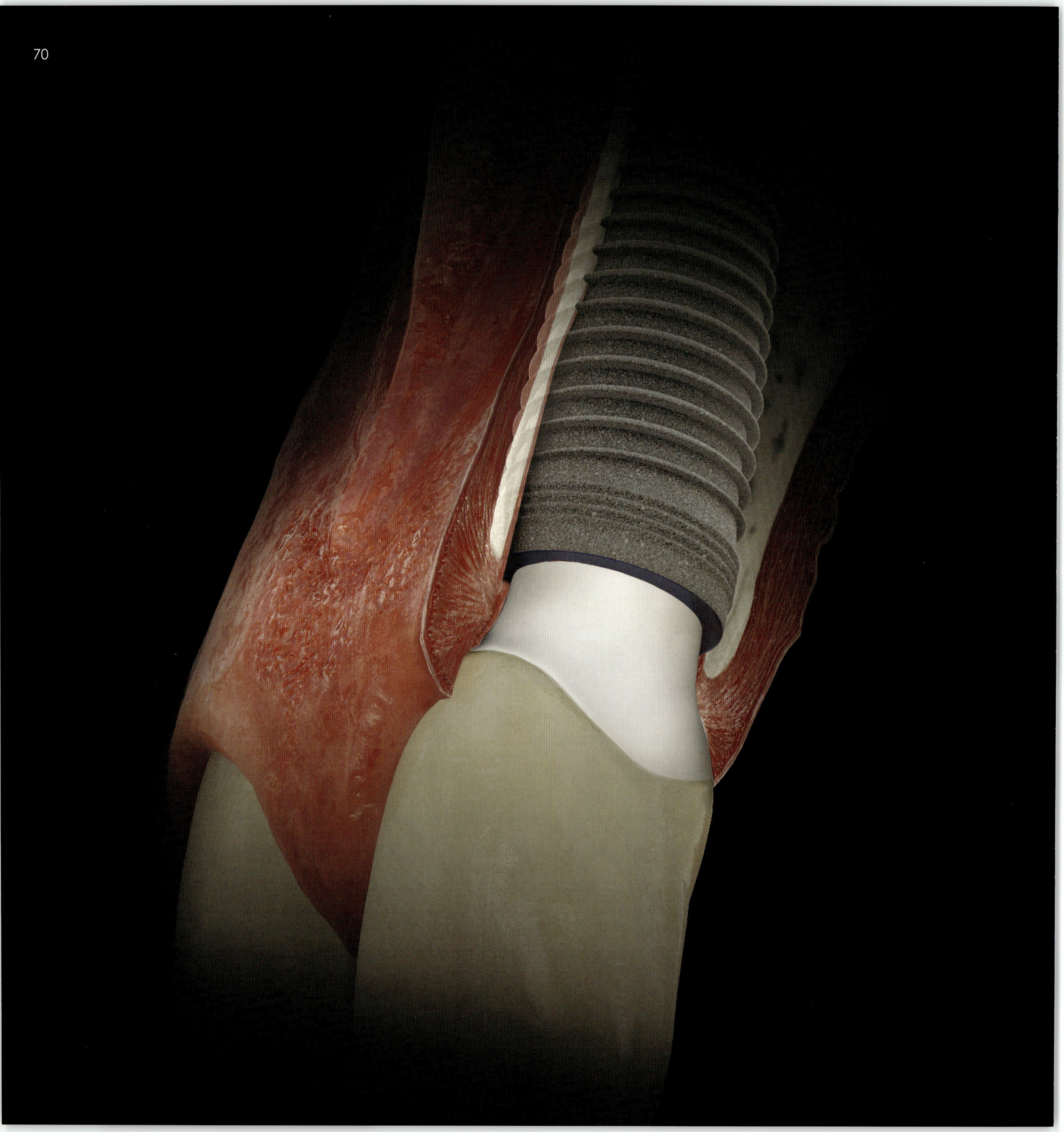

Original PS results

The idea behind PS adapters—to fabricate and place a smaller connection on the internal NobelReplace connection to fit a smaller abutment on a wider implant—was first discussed with the implant manufacturer (Nobel Biocare) in 2004. The original PS adapter had a slight gap between the abutment and the internal connection because of a mismatch in sizes. To avoid this gap and possible contamination at this critical interface, the next generation of PS adapters incorporated a bevel to cover the gap between the smaller abutment and the wider tri-lobe internal connection. However, the PS adapters were not available in all countries around the world. The NobelReplace Conical Connection and NobelReplace Platform Shift were introduced most recently, allowing connection of a smaller abutment and application of the PS concept without adapters.

Clinical outcomes were greatly improved with the second, gapless generation of PS adapters, as illustrated in the following patient cases (Case 3 treated with the original and Case 4 with the improved PS adapters). Independent from the adapters, a tendency toward greater bone loss was consistently noticed after delayed as compared with immediate implant placement. A contributing factor seems to be the timing of placement of the definitive abutment. In immediate implant placement cases, the definitive abutment is usually placed on the day of surgery. On the other hand, delayed implant placement often requires shaping of the ideal emergence profile and soft tissue with provisional implant abutments and crowns before the implant components and restorations can be finalized in a functional and esthetic manner.

Delayed implant placement

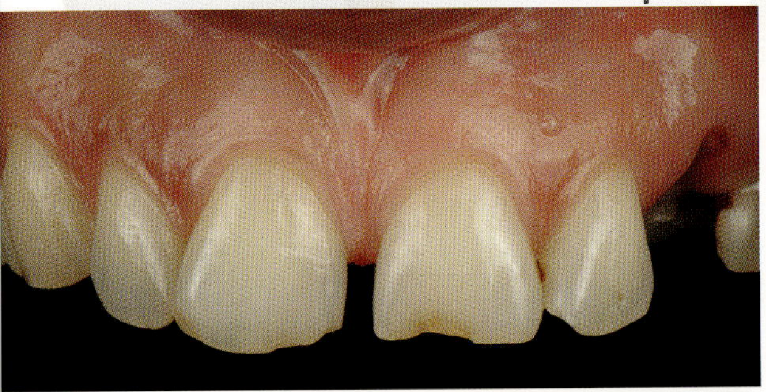

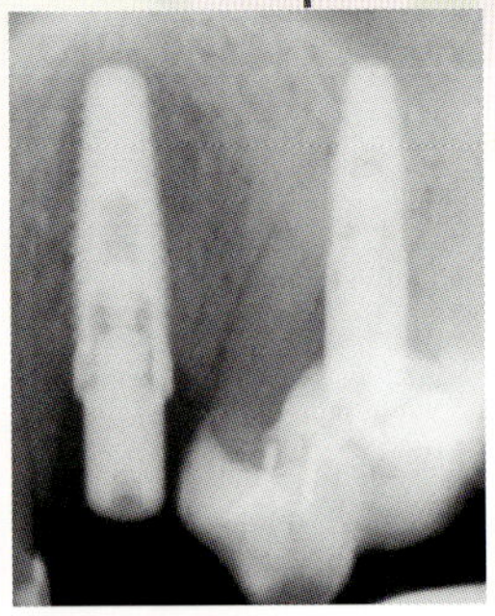

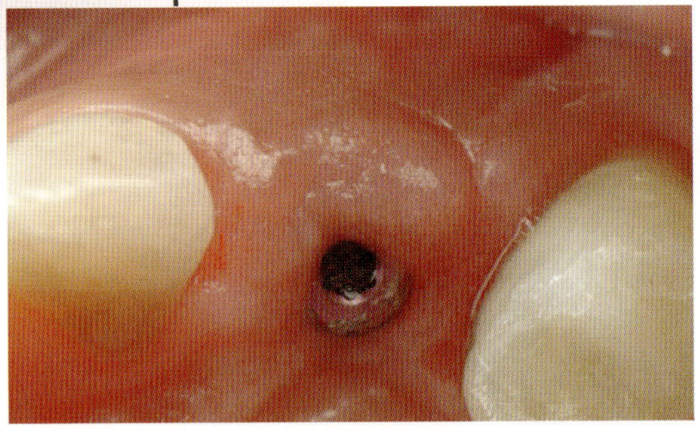

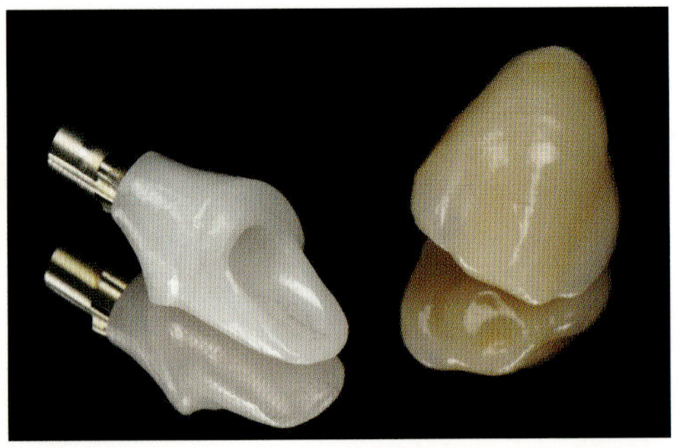

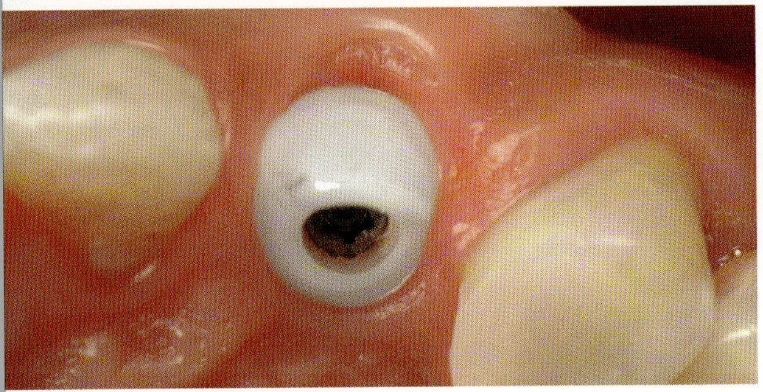

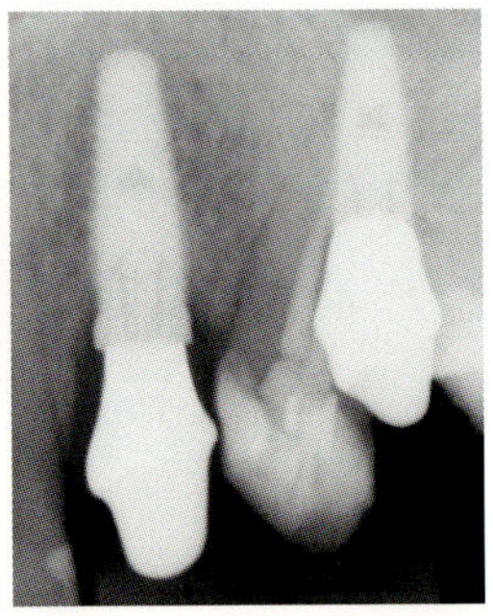

The root of the left maxillary canine was extracted and the site allowed to heal for 3 months. Afterward, implant surgery was performed, and an NP healing abutment as well as a CTG were placed at the same time. A provisional crown and composite abutment were inserted 4 months later. After another 3 months of tissue stabilization, the definitive crown and abutment (NobelProcera Zirconia) were delivered. The periapical radiograph taken after insertion of the definitive abutment already exhibits some bone loss, which may be due to the repeated removal and insertion of implant components during the provisional stage and possible effects created by the gap between the PS adapter and the internal implant connection. Micromovement of the components may be more pronounced because of this gap, the resulting lack of fit, and increased functional load on a canine. Six-year follow-up demonstrates stable esthetic conditions but noticeable bone loss.

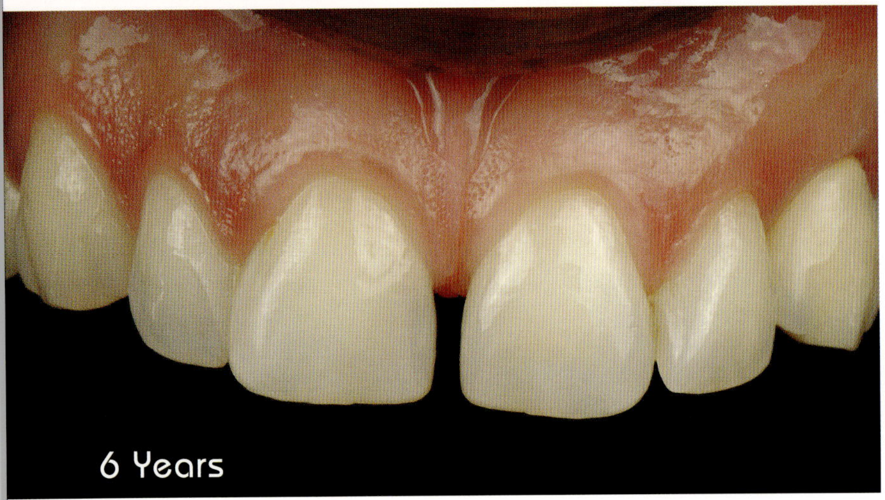

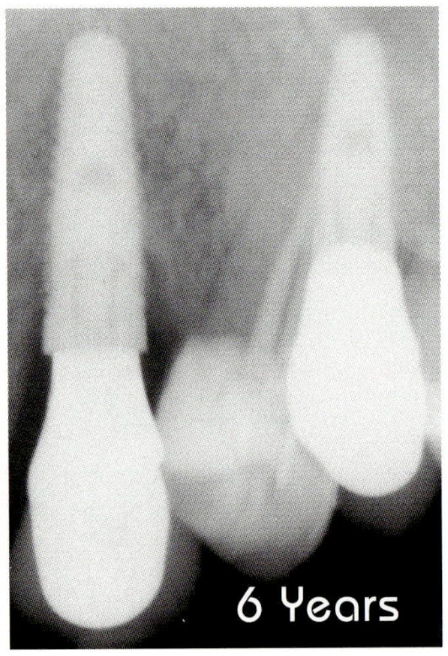

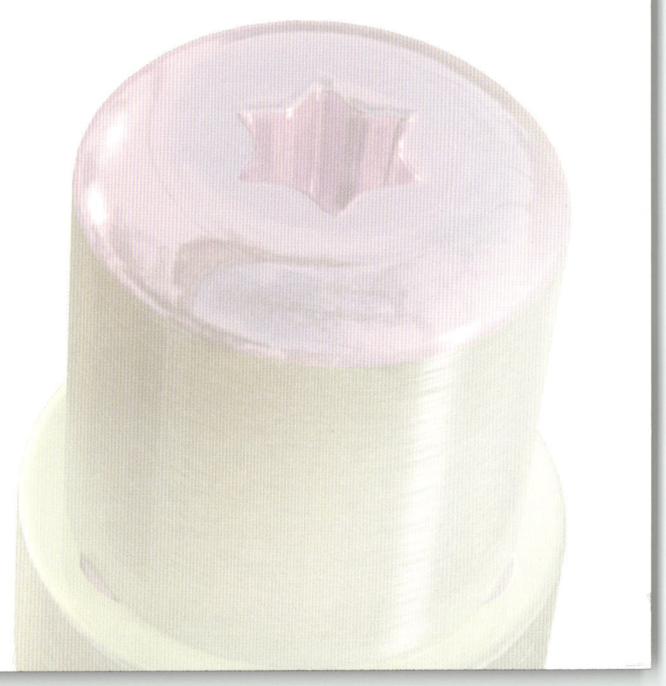

Immediate implant placement

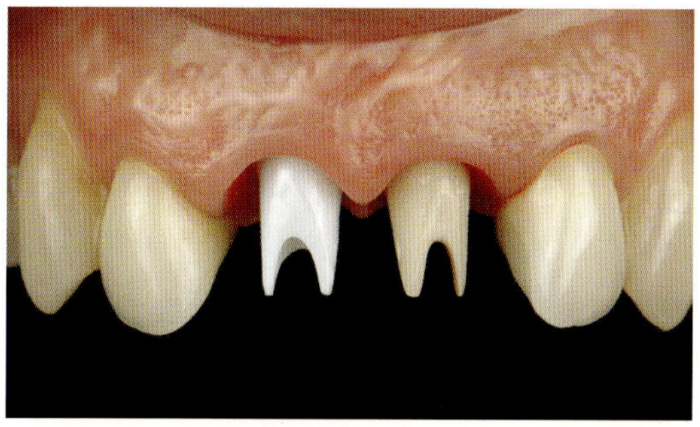

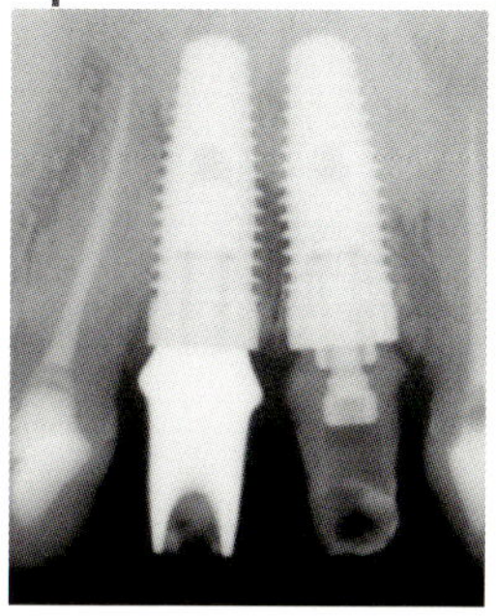

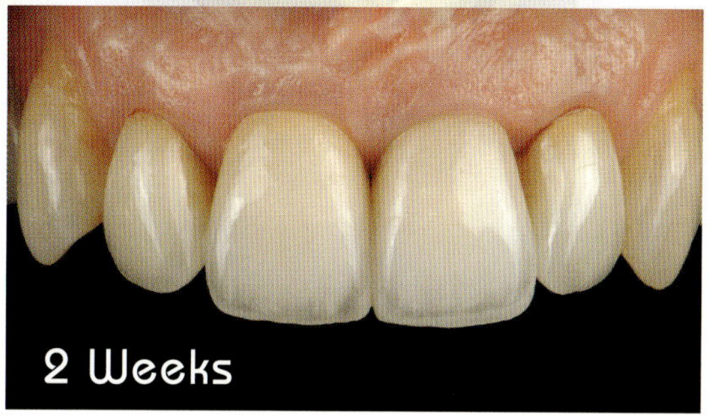

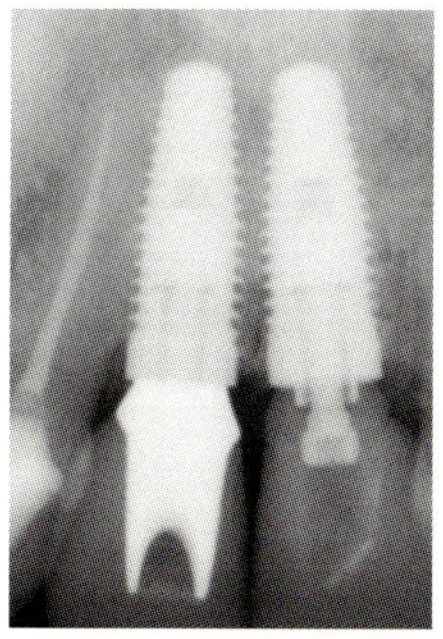

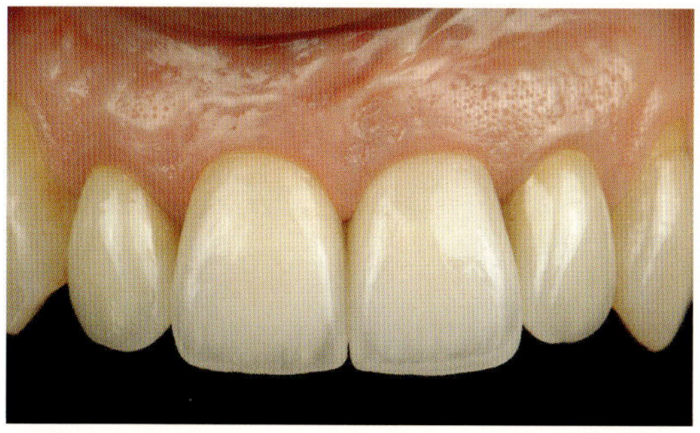

Implants were placed immediately to replace the two maxillary central incisors. However, they were placed subsequently at different times to decrease the amount of surgical trauma and better control the final result. When the first implant was placed in the area of the left maxillary central incisor, prefabricated zirconia abutments were not yet available. But when the second implant was placed 6 months later, a prefabricated zirconia abutment was placed immediately in the site of the right maxillary central incisor. Two alumina crowns were inserted after complete implant integration. Despite the proximity of the implants, favorable bone levels can be observed 7 years postoperatively without any hard or soft tissue augmentation. One supporting factor is the thick tissue biotype in this patient. The discrepancy between hard and soft tissue losses is quite obvious.

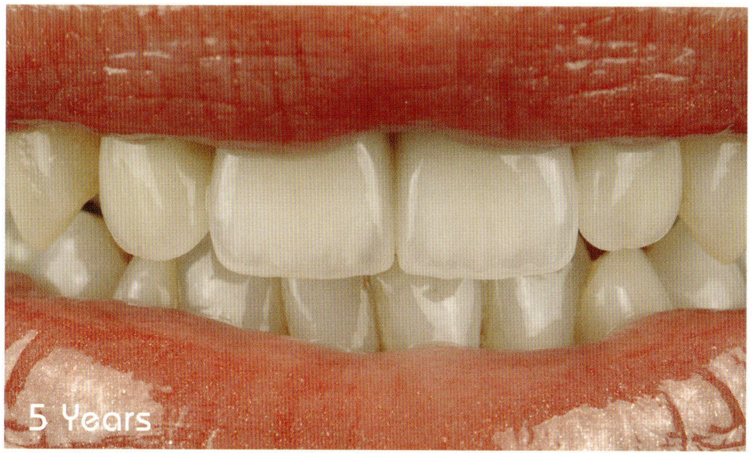

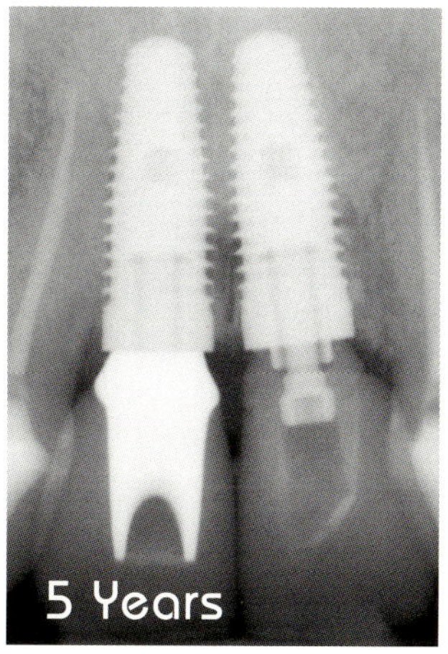

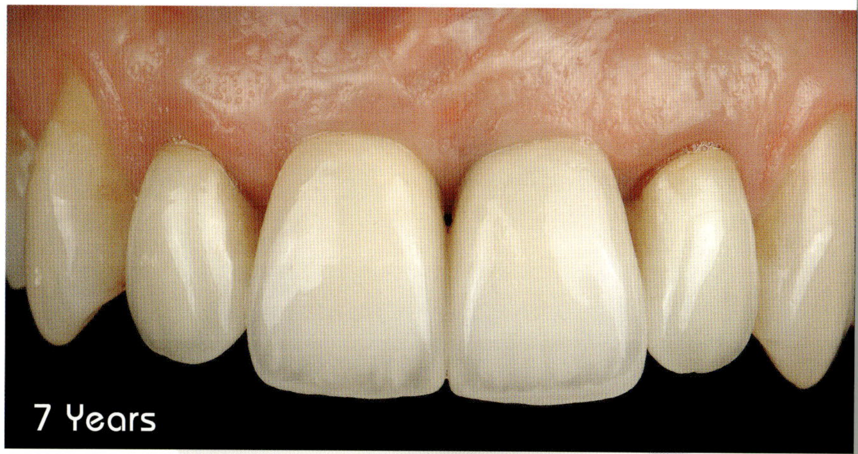

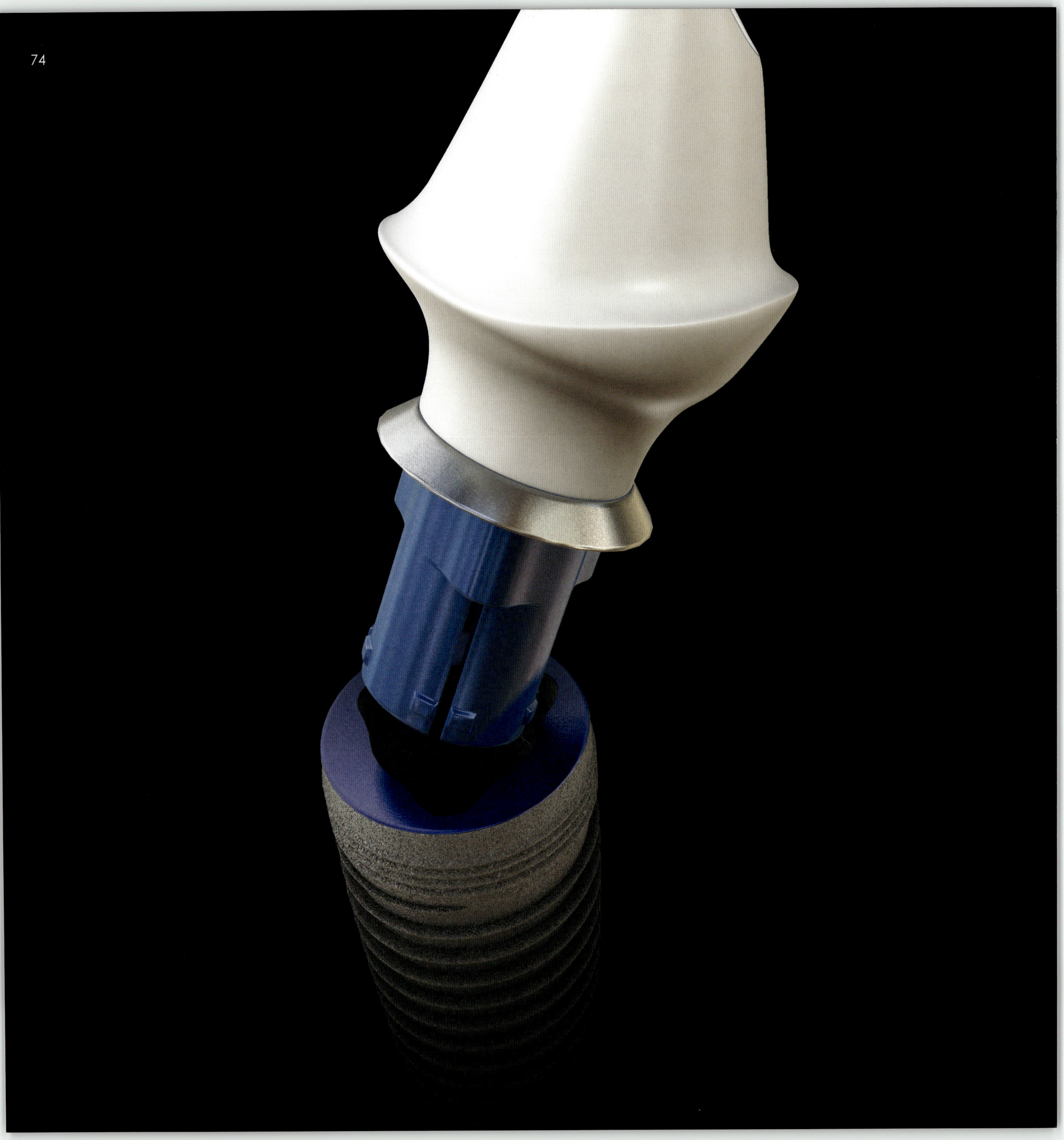

Different results with PS adapter

Soft and especially hard tissue remodeling around the implant-prosthetic interface is a multifactorial phenomenon that is not yet fully understood. It is fair to say that many of our explanations and interventions are based on long-term clinical observations rather than scientific evidence, which itself remains highly inconclusive.

The following patient cases illustrate differing results with the PS concept, which become especially obvious when comparing delayed versus immediate implant and restoration protocols.

The "one abutment one time" concept for improved soft tissue integration requires that the definitive abutment and a provisional crown be placed on the first day of the prosthetic phase, as illustrated in the delayed implant case. To mimic the specific soft tissue scallop of the contralateral lateral incisor and create a better emergence profile, the definitive zirconia abutment had to be disconnected twice (during two separate visits) to reprepare and place the buccal finish line more apically. While soft tissue levels remained rather stable and resulted in an acceptable emergence profile, the bone loss may be attributed to the prosthetic manipulation phase. However, some bone loss can already be seen before the prosthetic phase, which may be due to the compromised quality of the surrounding bone before the implant was placed or the surgical trauma during stage-one surgery, which was combined with a CTG. Implementation of the PS concept with first-generation PS adapters may not be ideal because of the imperfect fit, which may cause fatigue on the components, and because of the gap, which may cause bacterial contamination. In this case, while not detrimental to the esthetic outcome, the PS concept could not prevent peri-implant bone loss. Placement of a CTG during stage-one surgery was key to preserving adequate soft tissue levels despite the loss of bone.

The immediate implant placement case reveals stable bone levels over time. Application of the "one abutment one time" concept and normal biotype and buccal plate/socket configuration were contributing factors.

Delayed implant placement

Delayed implant placement (NobelReplace Groovy RP 4.3 × 13 mm) with a PS adapter and 5-mm NP healing abutment as well as CTG performed in one surgery. Clinical situation after 6 months of healing, before the prosthetic phase. The periapical radiographs reveal bone remodeling and resorption over time, before and after completion of the prosthetic phase.

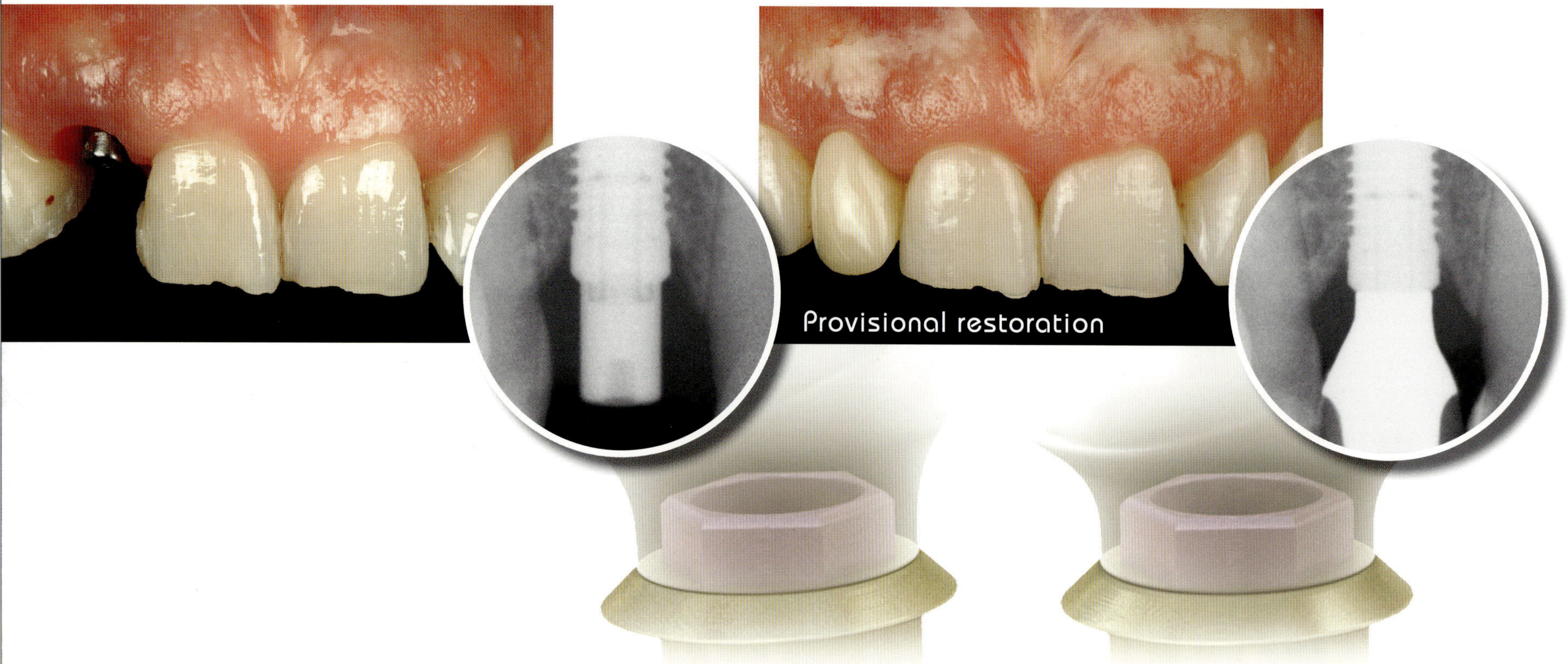

Immediate implant placement

The esthetic results and long-term stability of soft tissue levels are consistent in all cases treated with an immediate implant placement protocol and the PS concept, realized with the PS adapters. In this case, without bone or soft tissue augmentation, the situation remained stable even after 5 years.

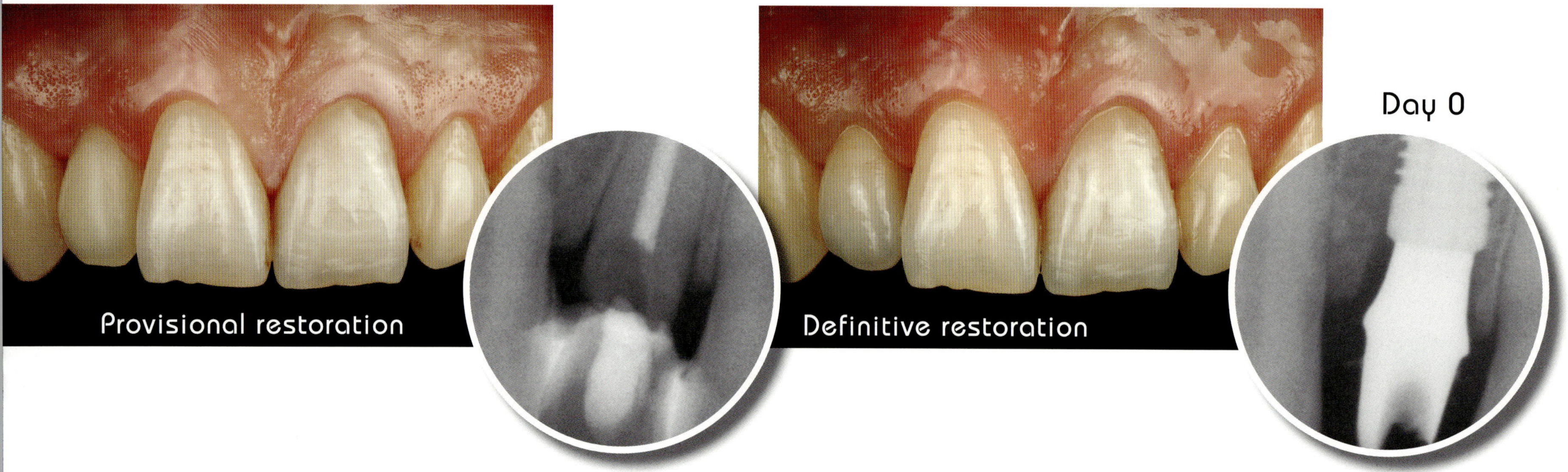

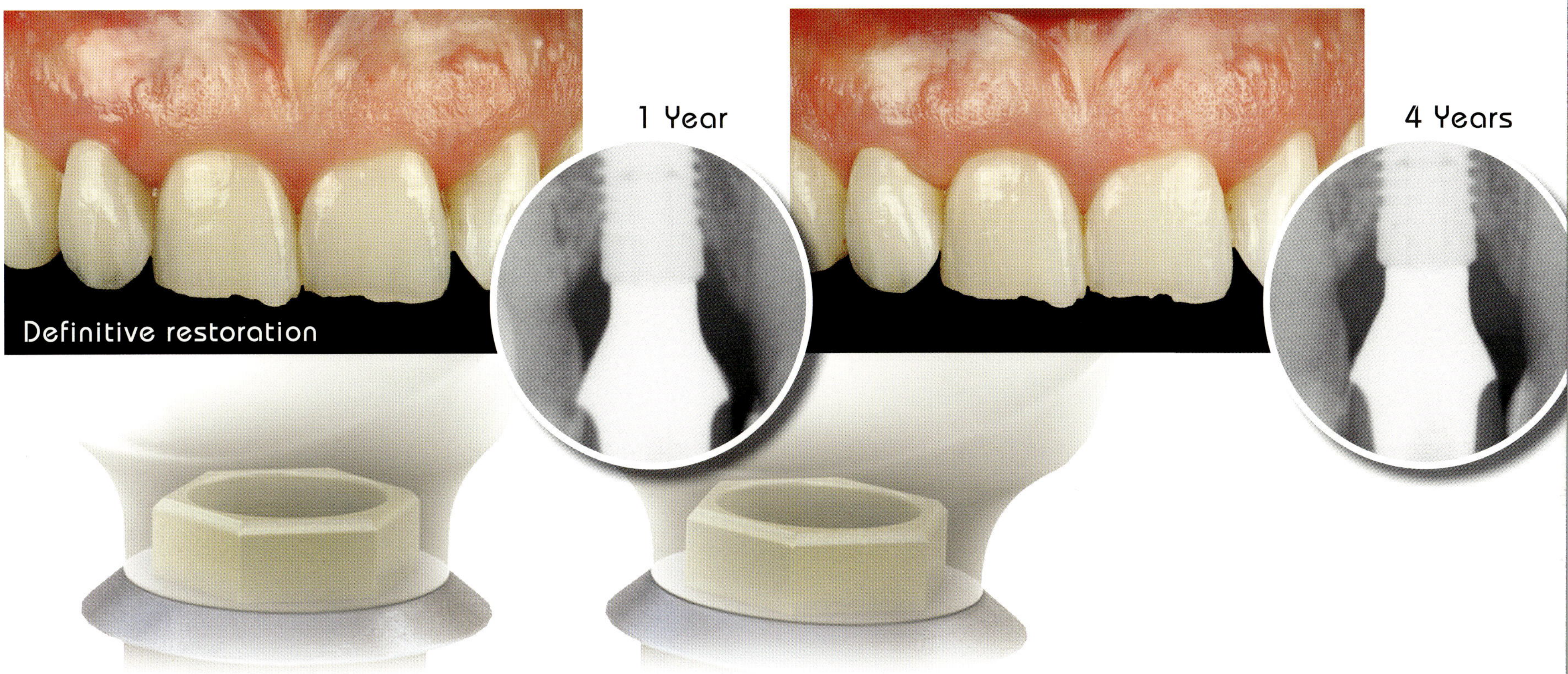
1 Year
4 Years
Definitive restoration

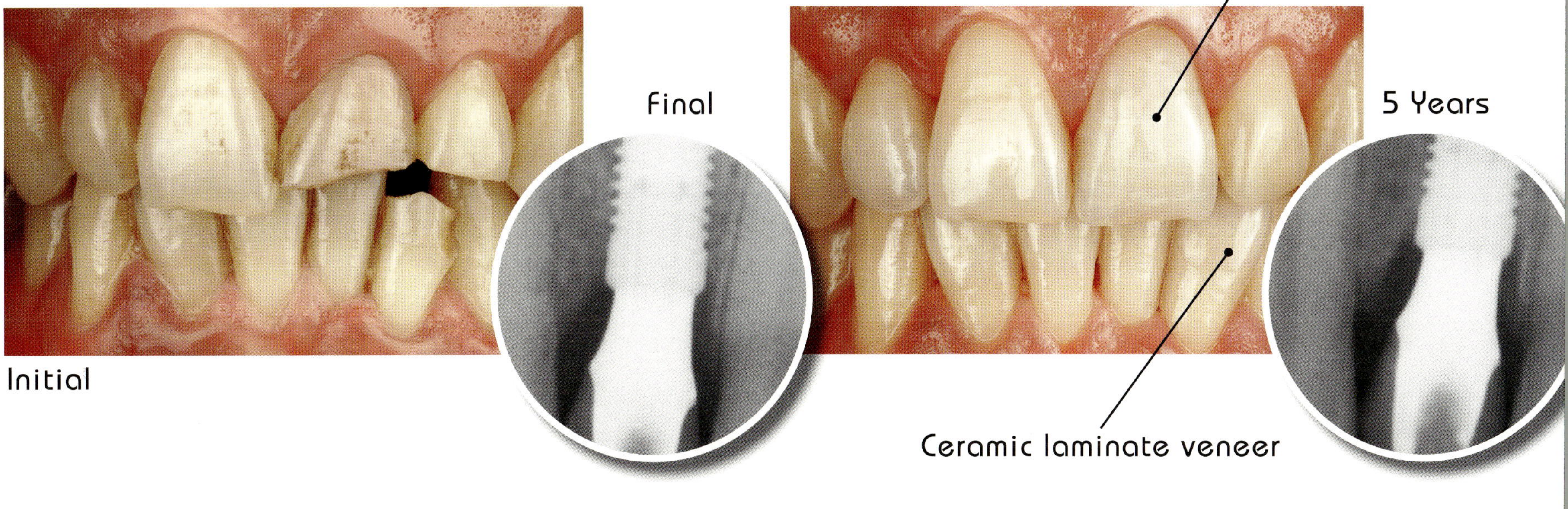
Ceramic laminate veneer
Final
5 Years
Initial
Ceramic laminate veneer

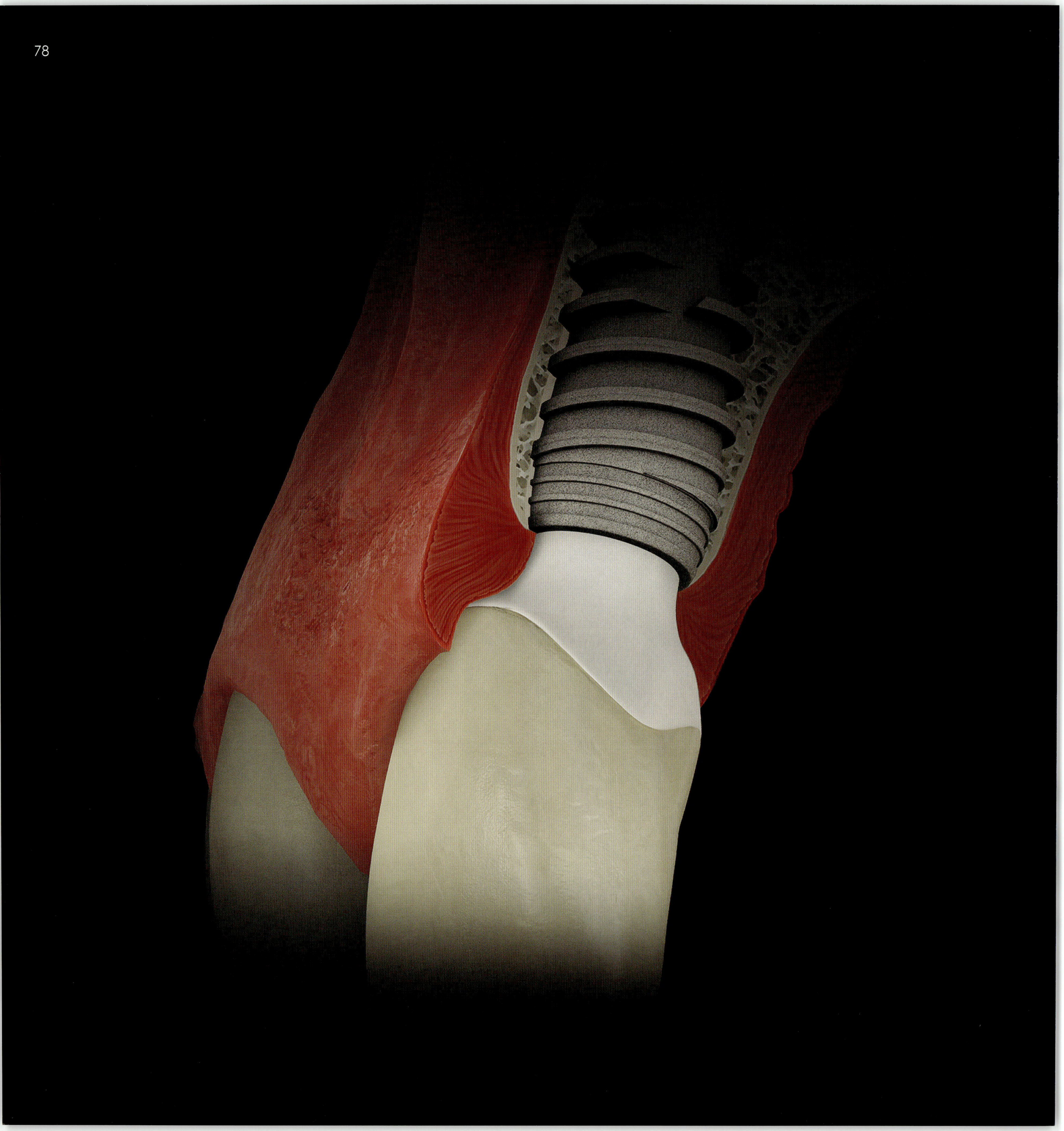

PS results with NobelActive

The NobelActive self-tapping implant with its unique tip and thread design allows for high initial stability and ideal implant placement. The conical internal connection has an internal hex at its most apical area for easy indexing. It provides a tight seal and incorporates the PS concept by design. Improved bone remodeling at the implant-abutment interface has been observed in numerous cases, and bone levels seem more stable than those attained with the use of two components (PS adapters). Greater bone loss at the implant-prosthetic interface was still experienced with a delayed implant placement approach compared with an immediate placement protocol. The clinical results are promising, but further long-term clinical trials are necessary before definitive conclusions can be drawn.

Delayed implant placement

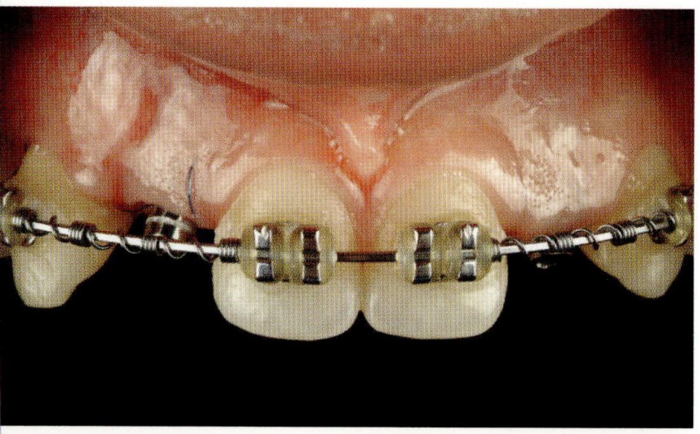

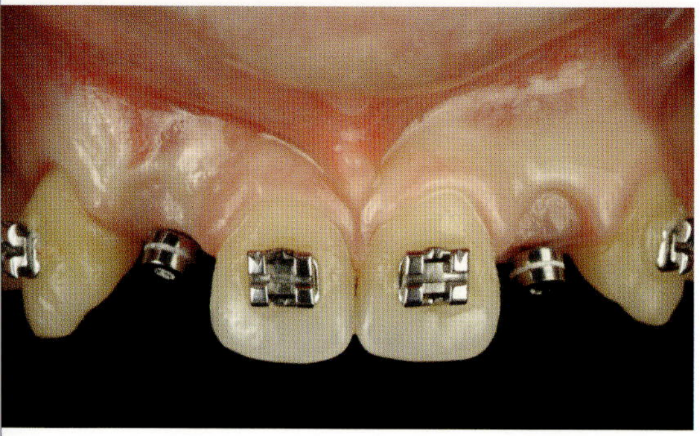

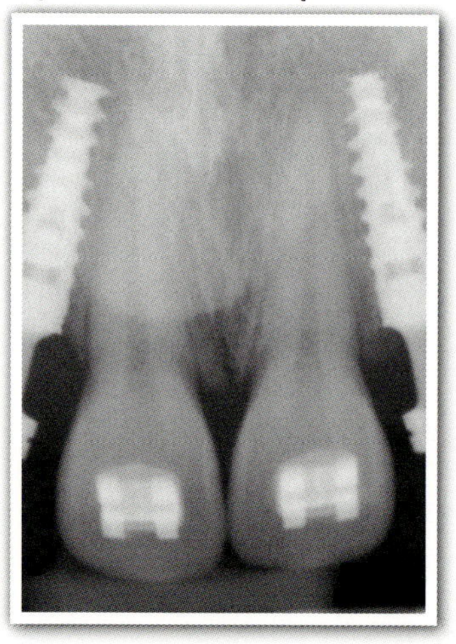

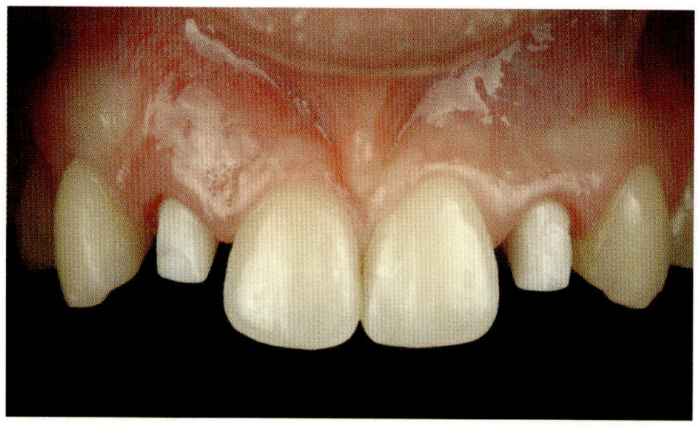

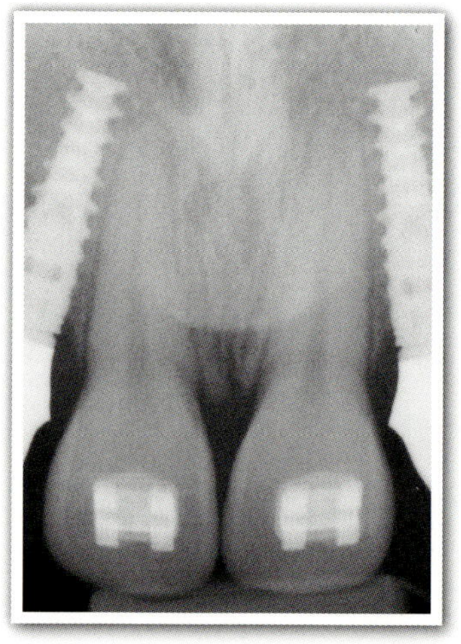

The general treatment philosophy is the same as that for a conventional implant. NobelActive NP 3.5 × 13–mm implants were placed to restore the congenitally missing maxillary lateral incisors. Narrow healing abutments were placed during the implant surgery to provide space for a CTG and ideal wound closure.

During the prosthetic phase, definitive zirconia abutments and provisional crown restorations were inserted for soft tissue manipulation and creation of a natural emergence profile.

Orthodontist: Dr Gorka Loyola

Immediate implant placement

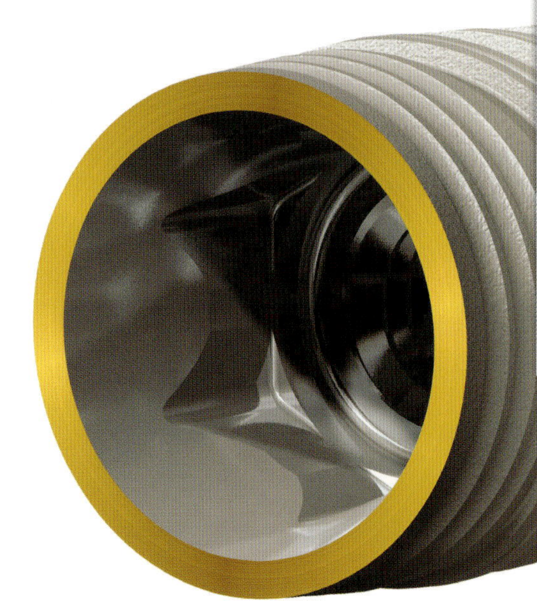

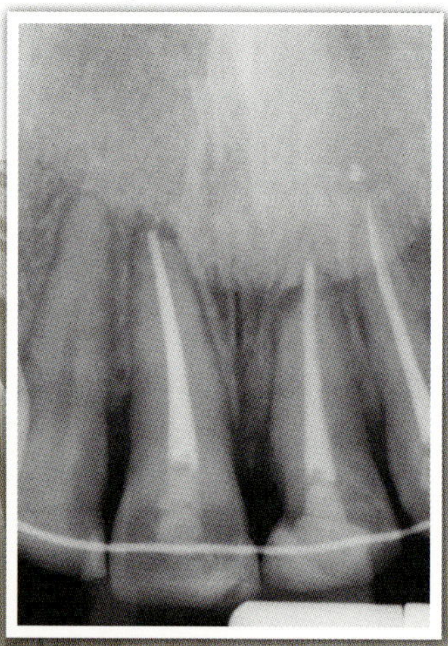

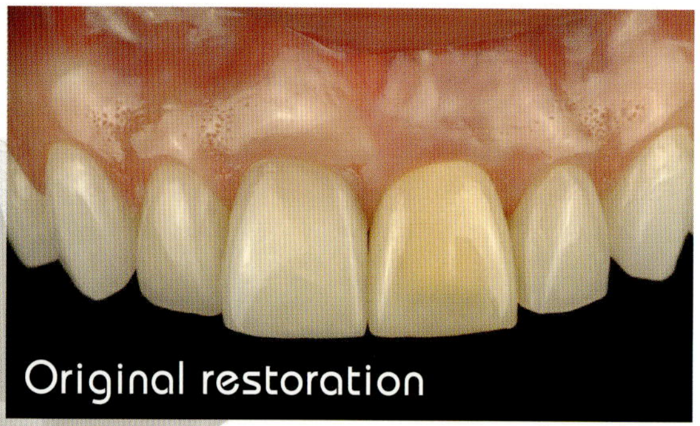

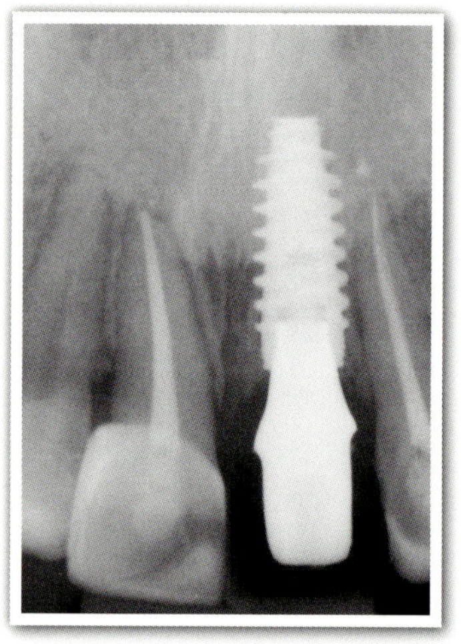

Immediate implant placement after extraction of the left maxillary central incisor. A bone substitute material (Bio-Oss, Geistlich) was placed in the space between the implant and the extraction socket, followed by a CTG, which was harvested from the tuberosity. The definitive zirconia abutment was placed at the same time and restored with a provisional crown.

Clinical situation after insertion of the definitive crowns and gingivectomy on the right maxillary central incisor 1 year postoperative.

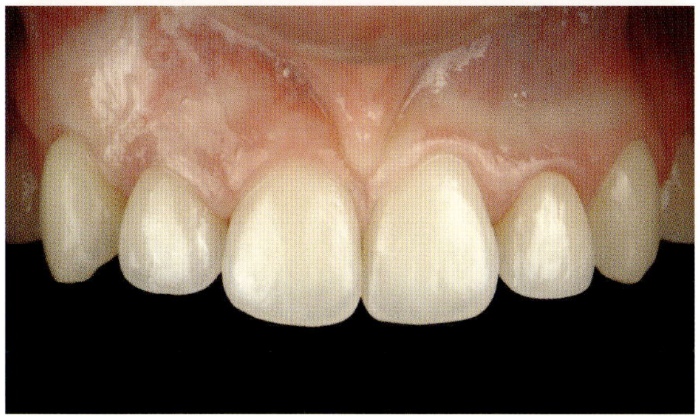

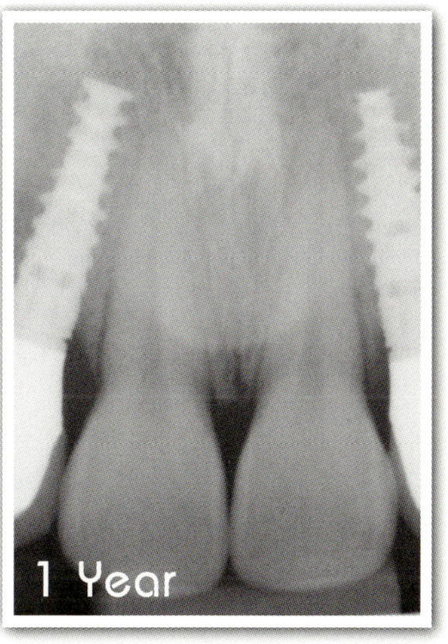

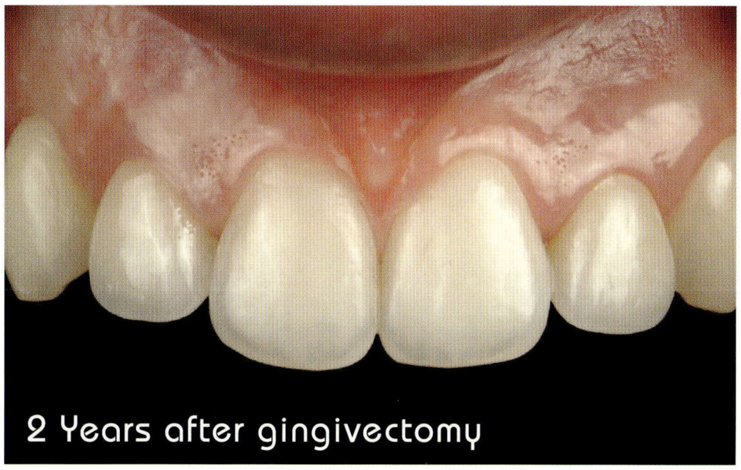

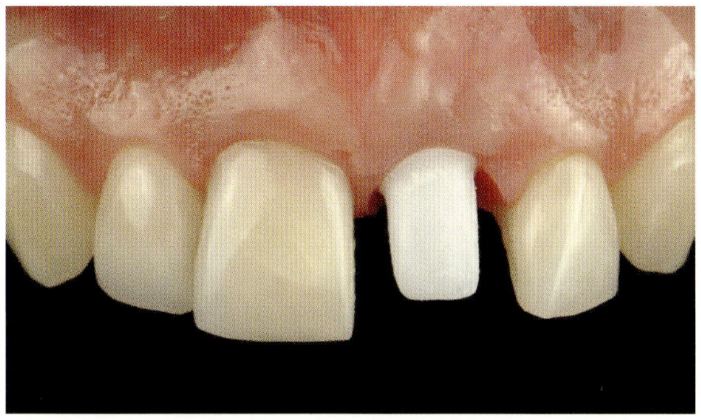

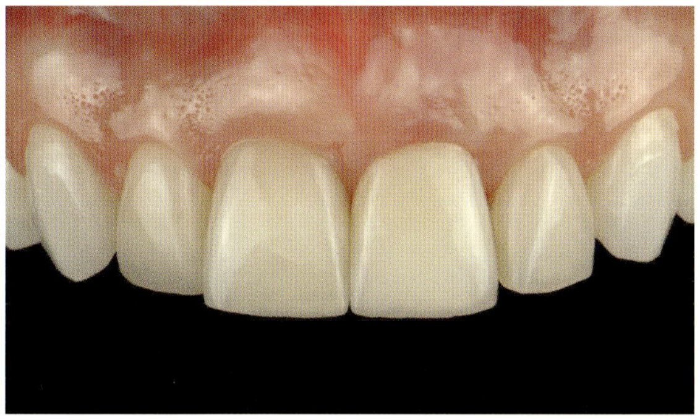

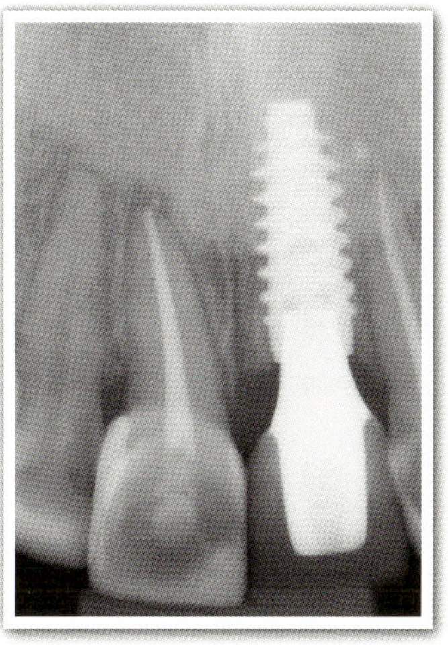

Clinical situation after restoration of the right maxillary central incisor and both maxillary lateral incisors with composite resin and final insertion of the definitive alumina crown.

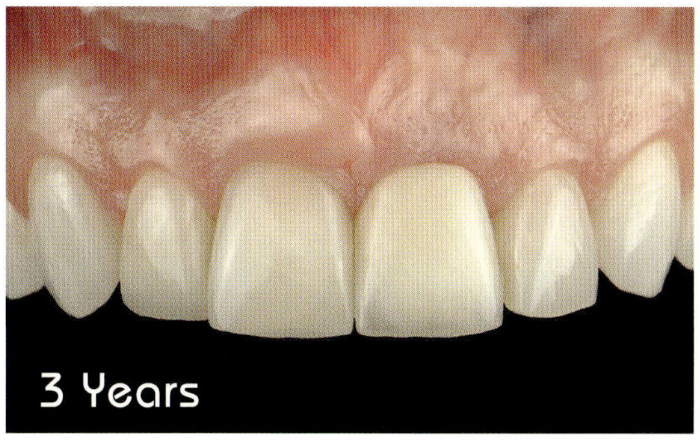

Three-year postoperative situation reveals stable hard and soft tissue conditions.

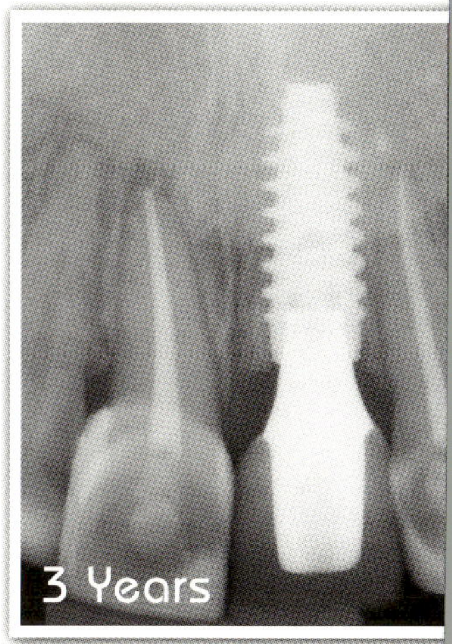

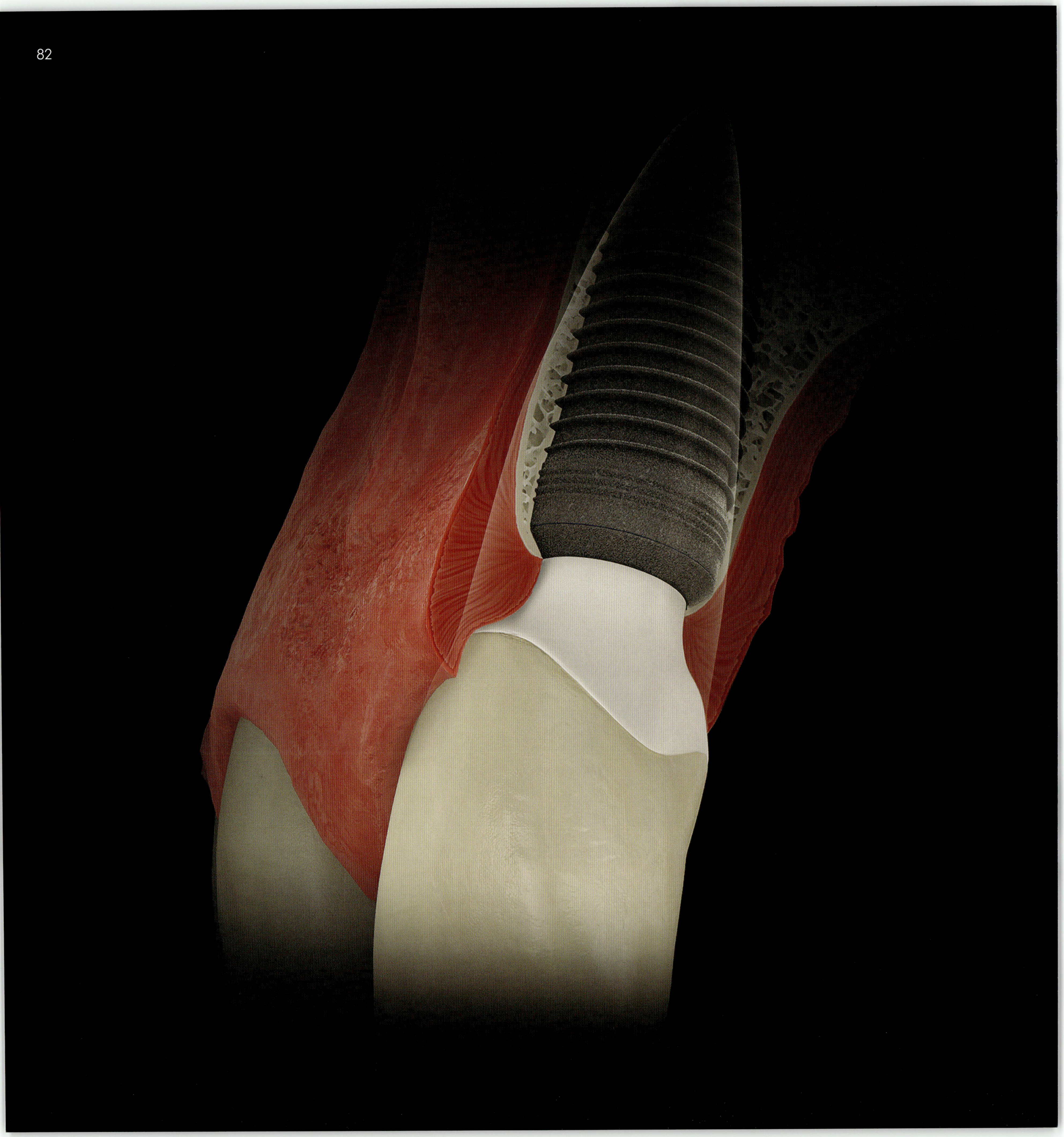

PS results with NobelReplace Conical

The more recently released NobelReplace Conical Connection combines the popular NobelReplace implant body design with the unique internal conical connection of the NobelActive implant. The PS concept is already integrated by design. Short-term clinical experience indicates similar results to those achieved with the NobelActive implant. In delayed implant placement cases, results seem even better, which may be associated with the less pronounced implant thread design and, therefore, less aggressive insertion procedure.

Delayed implant placement

Provisional restoration of the right maxillary lateral incisor is cantilevered off the canine and rests on top of the narrow temporary healing abutment. NobelReplace Conical Connection 4.3 × 13–mm implant with a narrow temporary healing abutment and CTG after 6 months.

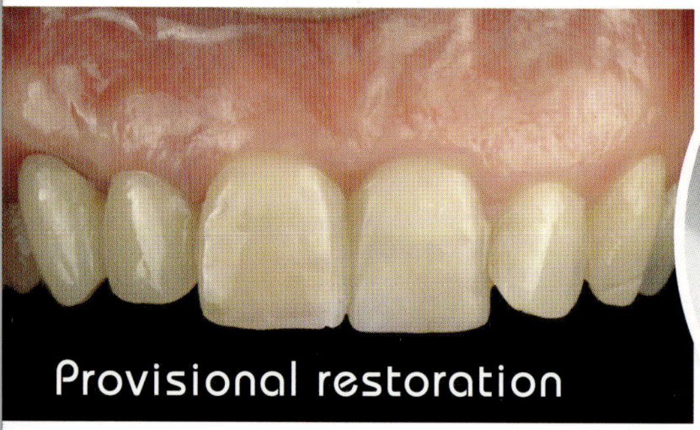

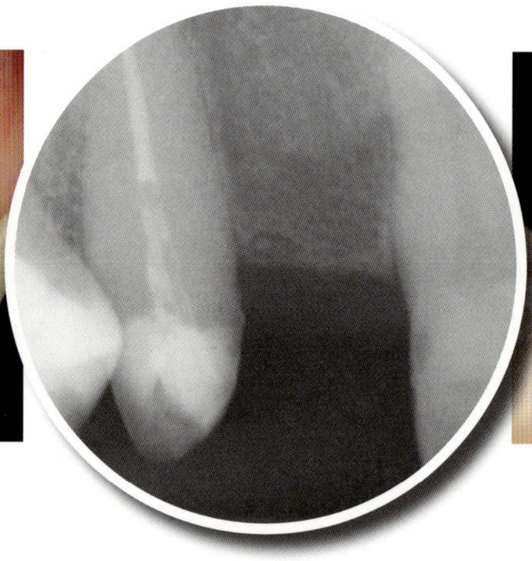

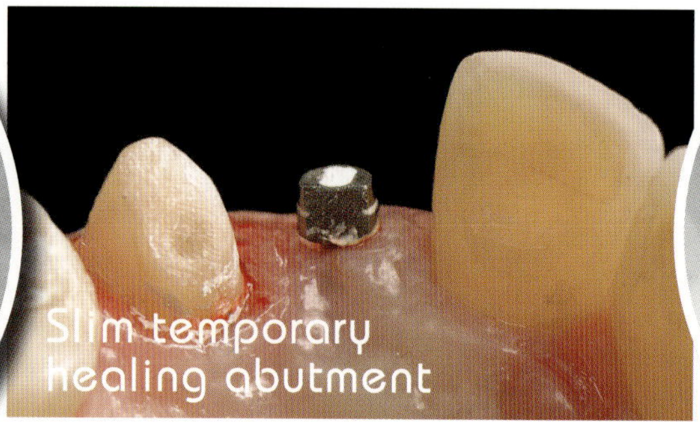

2011

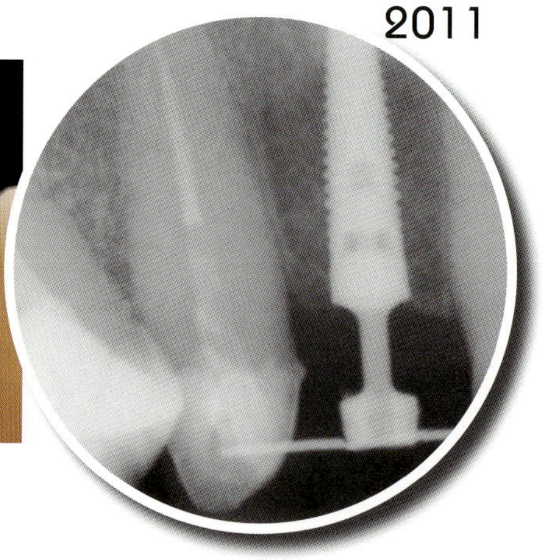

Immediate implant placement

Ideal case for an immediate implant placement after tooth extraction. A bone substitute graft material (Bio-Oss) and CTG were placed to compensate for the resorption typically seen after this type of treatment. Prosthetically, a prefabricated zirconia abutment was customized and adapted to the site. A provisional crown restoration was delivered at the same time.

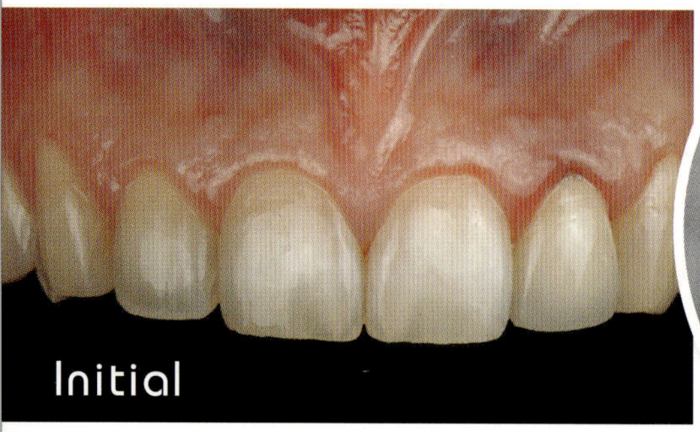

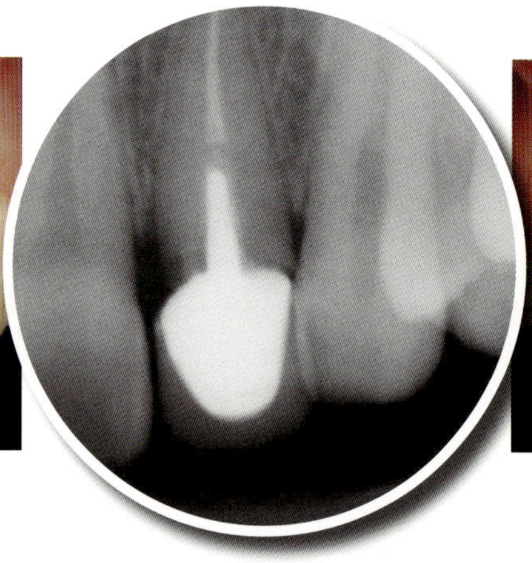

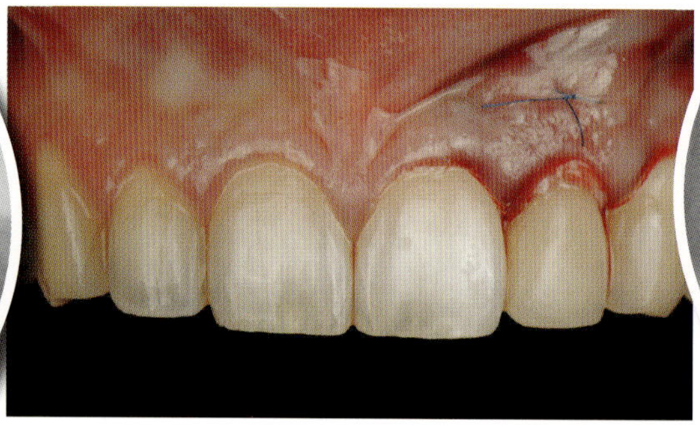

Day 0

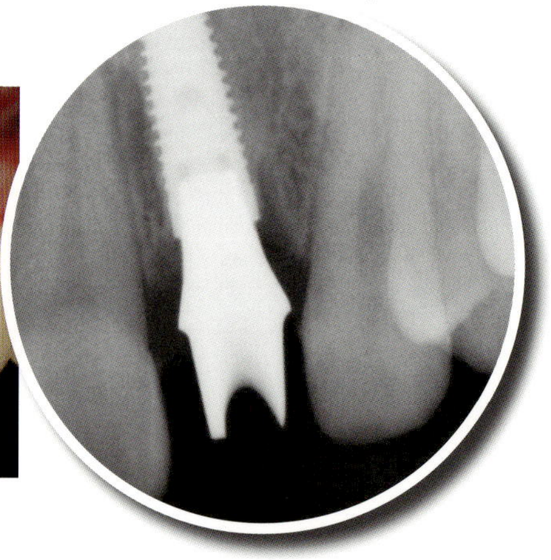

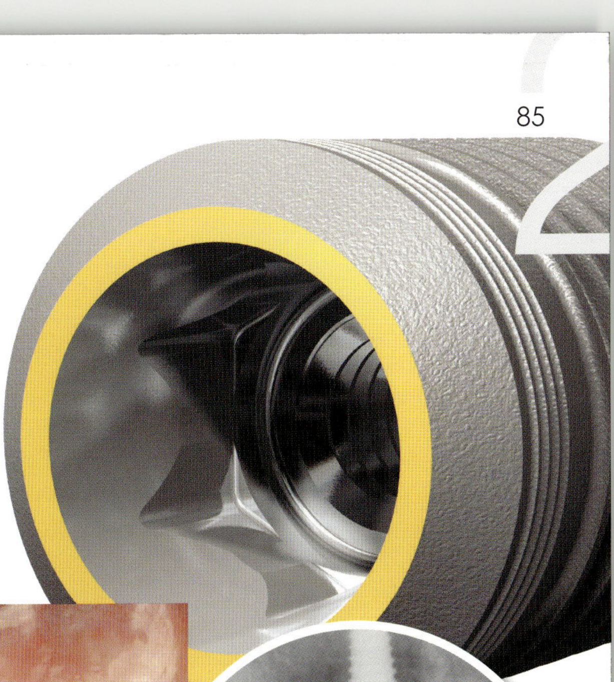

The definitive zirconia (Zr) abutment was inserted on the first day of the prosthetic phase. The existing provisional restoration was relined until the desired soft tissue configuration was achieved. Final impression was then made after placing conventional retraction cords around the tooth and the implant.

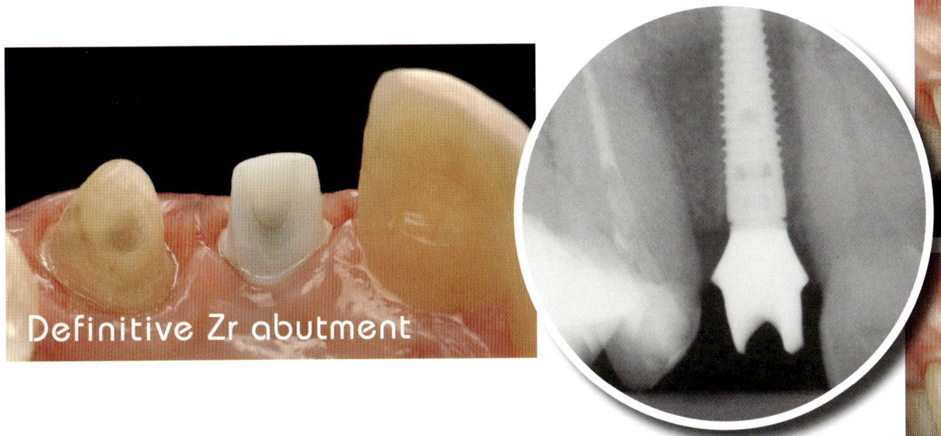

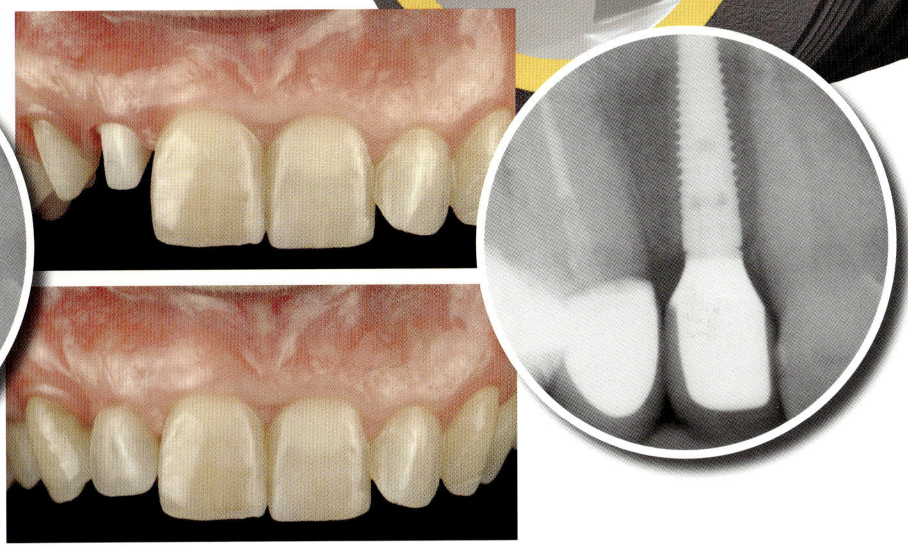

Postoperative situation and the definitive zirconia abutment and crown after 1 year. Bone levels remained stable throughout the treatment.

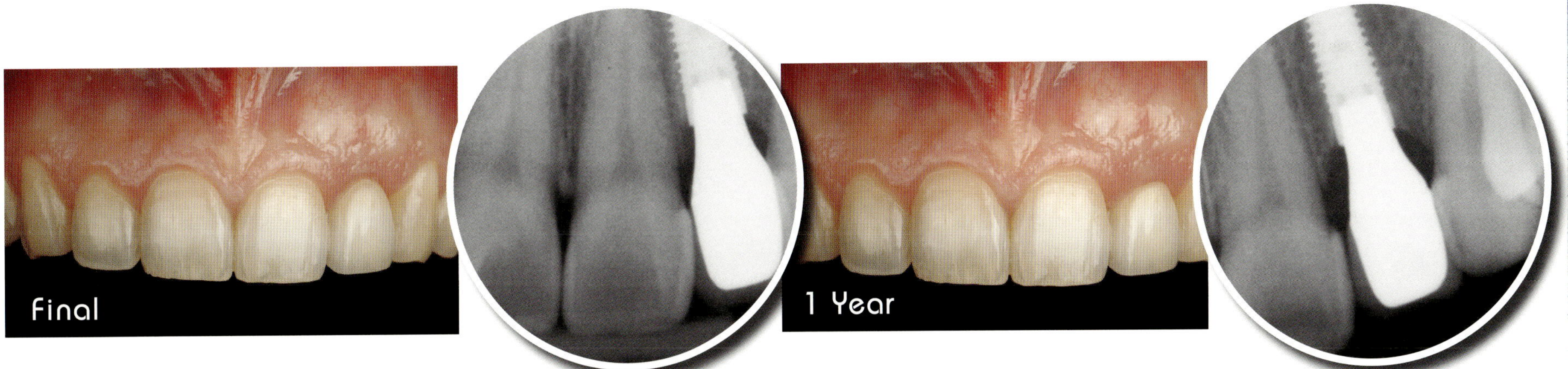

Comparison of the situation a few weeks after final cementation of the definitive zirconia crown with the situation 1 year posttreatment reveals stable bone levels and tissue conditions. The outcome looks promising, but longer follow-up times will be needed.

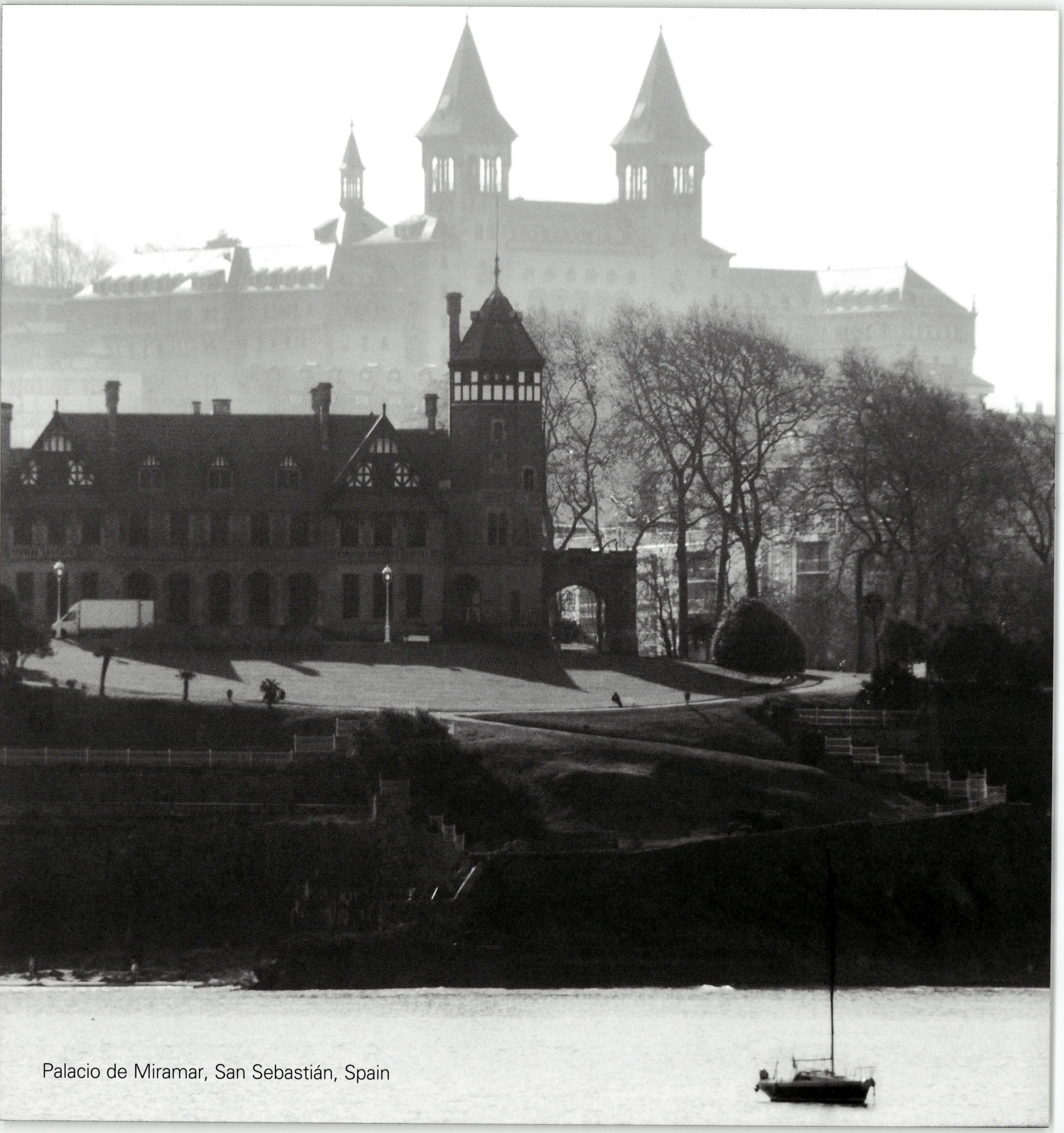

Palacio de Miramar, San Sebastián, Spain

Natural Oral Peri-implant Esthetics

3. Ideal 3D Implant Placement
    - General Considerations
    - Guided Surgery

4. Creating a Natural Soft Tissue Contour
    - Bone Grafting
    - Soft Tissue Grafting Procedures
    - Creating a Soft Tissue Contour Prosthetically Through Provisional Restoration
    - Orthodontics to Maximize Soft Tissue Esthetics

5. Laboratory Communication for Definitive Restoration
    - Impressions
    - Without Removing the Abutment
    - 3D Emergence Profile and Tooth Contour
    - Color and Coping Selection
    - Abutment Material Selection

6. Definitive Restoration
    - Contemporary Concept

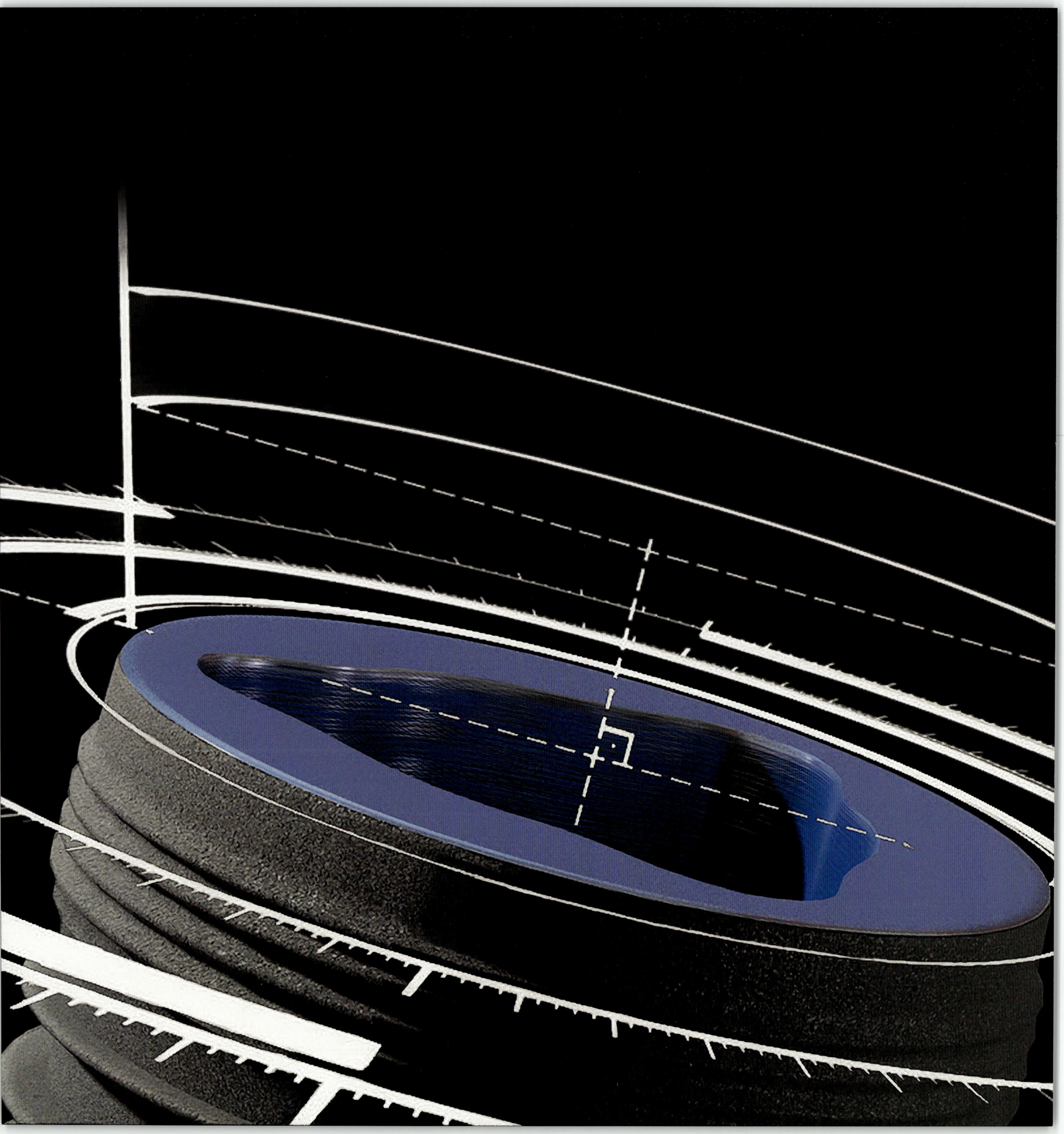

Ideal 3D Implant Placement

→ Research: 3D implant placement

- General Considerations
  - Implant selection
  - Buccolingual position
  - Mesiodistal position and distance requirements
  - Angulation
  - Depth and orientation
  - Dentogingival angle and emergence profile
  - Interim restorations
- Guided Surgery

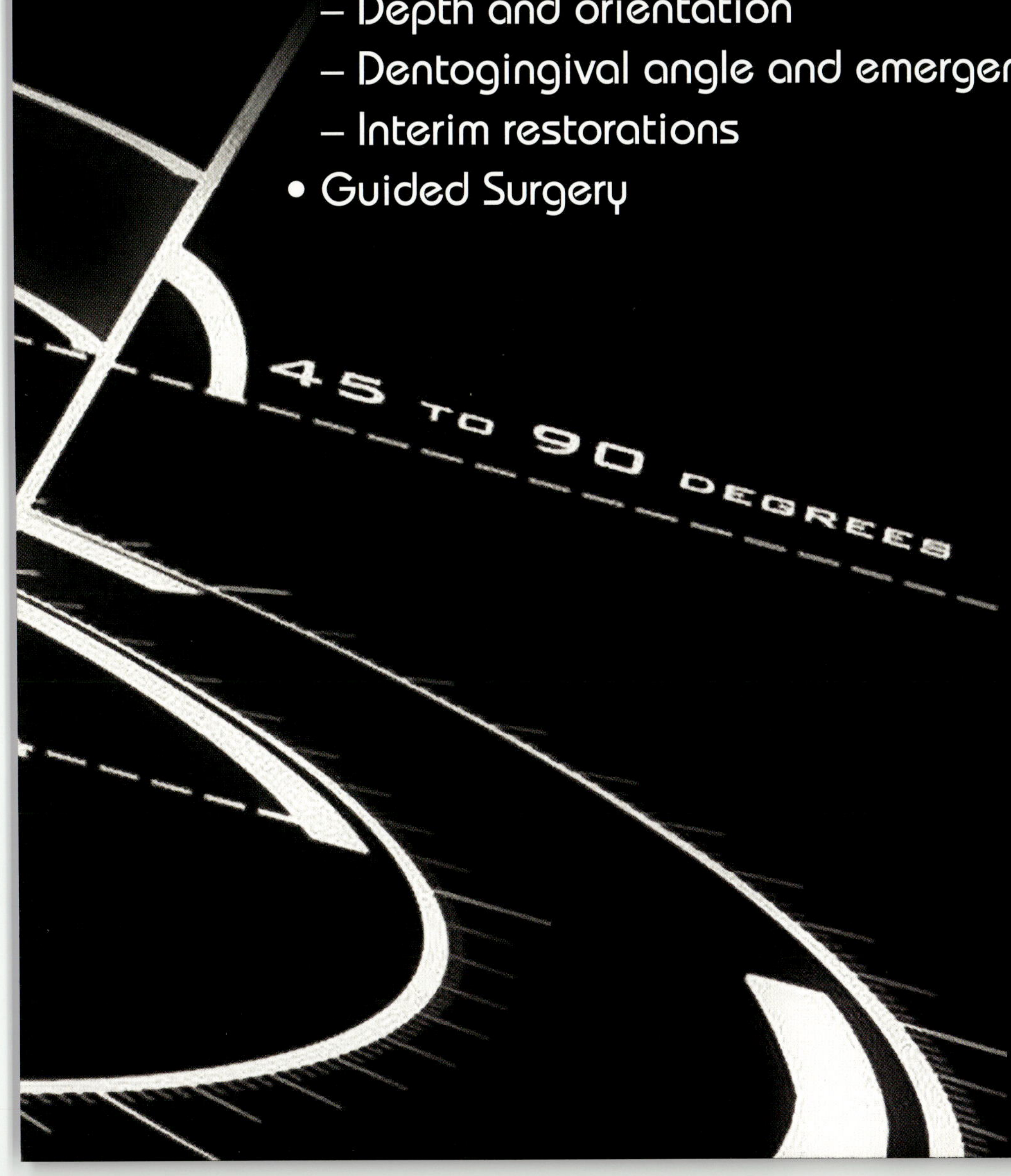

Chapter 3

Research

3D implant placement

The fundamental prerequisites for a natural and esthetic implant-supported restoration as well as ideal soft tissue contour, color, and stability are proper implant selection followed by optimal implant placement and angulation in all three dimensions: buccolingual, mesiodistal, and apicocoronal.[1–6] The current scientific evidence from high-level clinical trials, compiled in a systematic review,[7] fails to provide much guidance in respect to implant selection and does not confirm any particular implant type, shape, or surface to be superior to others but suggests further studies. Some of these important factors may never have been properly investigated or cannot be isolated and confirmed in randomized clinical trials. Nevertheless, proper implant selection is a critical step to a successful outcome.[1–5] It should be based on the available three-dimensional (3D) space; the type, shape, and dimensions of the restored tooth; and the supporting bone density, anatomy, and morphology.[8]

The soft tissue contour is a crucial factor in the outcome and is determined by the underlying bone and peri-implant soft tissue architecture.[9] The interproximal bone height as well as the height and thickness of the buccal bone crest are two of the most important anatomical factors.[1] The soft tissue biotype and thickness directly affect the soft and hard tissue stability after implant placement.[10,11] Conversely, the soft tissue thickness is, to a certain degree, influenced by the 3D position of the implant. In the buccolingual dimension, for example, an implant positioned or angulated too far to the labial aspect may lead to a thinner or coronally displaced labial soft tissue margin.[12]

The presence and volume of the interproximal papilla is determined by the supporting bone on the adjacent teeth[9,13] but also influenced by the position and angulation of the implant, especially the implant shoulder.[1–5] A 5-mm or smaller vertical distance between the interproximal bone crest and the interdental contact point seems to ensure the presence of a complete interproximal papilla.[14] Vertical distances of 6 mm and greater mean significantly and increasingly lower probabilities of a complete papilla that fills the entire space up to the contact point. The mesiodistal horizontal distance between an implant and a tooth should be about 1.5 to 2.0 mm.[15] It should ideally be about 3.0 to 3.5 mm between adjacent implants.[16,17] An implant placed too close to the adjacent tooth may cause resorption of the interproximal alveolar crest to the level of the crest on the implant and possibly lead to papilla loss.[18,19] A similar but more dramatic effect is seen between implants placed too close together.[15] However, when implants are restored according to the platform shift (PS) concept and the prosthetic connection is moved away from the bone, interimplant distances of 2 mm may still be acceptable.[20] On the other hand, implants placed too far from each other or the adjacent teeth may also lead to insufficient soft and hard tissue support.[15] In respect to depth, the implant should be placed about 3 to 4 mm apical to the prospective gingival margin.[1–4] An implant placed too far apically may lead to unnecessary bone loss and soft tissue resorption, while a "shallow" implant poses severe restorative difficulties in the attempt to create a natural emergence profile.[1] Placement or angulation of the implant too far to the labial aspect may cause soft tissue recession.[12] However, a palatally displaced or angulated implant may be difficult or impossible to restore with a natural emergence profile.[1–5,21]

Therefore, the implant placement must be restoratively driven in all three dimensions.[5] The greater the 3D mismatch between the crown and the implant body positions, the poorer and less stable the final outcome will be.[1–5]

References

1. Buser D, Martin W, Belser UC. Optimizing esthetics for implant restorations in the anterior maxilla: Anatomic and surgical considerations. Int J Oral Maxillofac Implants 2004;19:43–61.

2. Belser U, Buser D, Higginbottom F. Consensus statements and recommended clinical procedures regarding esthetics in implant dentistry. Int J Oral Maxillofac Implants 2004;19:73–74.

3. Higginbottom F, Belser U, Jones JD, Keith SE. Prosthetic management of implants in the esthetic zone. Int J Oral Maxillofac Implants 2004;19:62–72.

4. Belser UC, Schmid B, Higginbottom F, Buser D. Outcome analysis of implant restorations located in the anterior maxilla: A review of the recent literature. Int J Oral Maxillofac Implants 2004;19:30–42.

5. Garber DA. The esthetic dental implant: Letting the restoration be the guide. J Am Dent Assoc 1995;126:319–325.

6. Gamborena I, Blatz MB. Current clinical and technical protocols for single-tooth immediate implant procedures. Quintessence Dent Technol 2008;31:49–60.

7. Esposito M, Murray-Curtis L, Grusovin MG, Coulthard P, Worthington HV. Interventions for replacing missing teeth: Different types of dental implants. Cochrane Database Syst Rev 2007;(4):CD003815.

8. Schropp L, Stavropoulos A, Gotfredsen E, Wenzel A. Comparison of panoramic and conventional cross-sectional tomography for preoperative selection of implant size. Clin Oral Implants Res 2011;22:424–429.

9. Kan JY, Rungcharassaeng K, Umezu K, Kois JC. Dimensions of peri-implant mucosa: An evaluation of maxillary anterior single implants in humans. J Periodontol 2003;74:557–562.

10. Fu JH, Lee A, Wang HL. Influence of tissue biotype on implant esthetics. Int J Oral Maxillofac Implants 2011;26:499–508.

11. Puisys A, Linkevicius T. The influence of mucosal tissue thickening on crestal bone stability around bone-level implants. A prospective controlled clinical trial [epub ahead of print 9 Dec 2013]. Clin Oral Implants Res doi:10.1111/clr.12301.

12. Peng M, Fei W, Hosseini M, Gotfredsen K. Influence of implant position on clinical crown length and peri-implant soft tissue dimensions at implant-supported single crowns replacing maxillary central incisors. Int J Periodontics Restorative Dent 2013;33:785–793.

13. Blatz MB, Hürzeler MB, Strub JR. Reconstruction of the lost interproximal papilla—Presentation of some surgical and non-surgical procedures. Int J Periodontics Restorative Dent 1999;19:395–406.

14. Choquet V, Hermans M, Adriaenssens P, Daelemans P, Tarnow DP, Malevez C. Clinical and radiographic evaluation of the papilla level adjacent to single-tooth dental implants. A retrospective study in the maxillary anterior region. J Periodontol 2001;72:1364–1371.

15. Tarnow DP, Cho SC, Wallace SS. The effect of inter-implant distance on the height of inter-implant bone crest. J Periodontol 2000;71:546–549.

16. Tarnow D, Elian N, Fletcher P, et al. Vertical distance from the crest of bone to the height of the interproximal papilla between adjacent implants. J Periodontol 2003;74:1785–1788.

17. Kois JC. Predictable single-tooth peri-implant esthetics: Five diagnostic keys. Compend Contin Educ Dent 2004;25:895–896,898,900.

18. Esposito M, Ekestubbe A, Gröndahl K. Radiological evaluation of marginal bone loss at tooth surfaces facing single Brånemark implants. Clin Oral Implants Res 1993;4:151–157.

19. Thilander B, Odman J, Jemt T. Single implants in the upper incisor region and their relationship to the adjacent teeth. An 8-year follow-up study. Clin Oral Implants Res 1999;10:346–355.

20. Elian N, Bloom M, Dard M, Cho SC, Trushkowsky RD, Tarnow D. Effect of interimplant distance (2 and 3 mm) on the height of interimplant bone crest: A histomorphometric evaluation. J Periodontol 2011;82:1749–1756.

21. Tarnow DP, Eskow RN. Considerations for single-unit esthetic implant restorations. Compend Contin Educ Dent 1995;16:778,780,782–784.

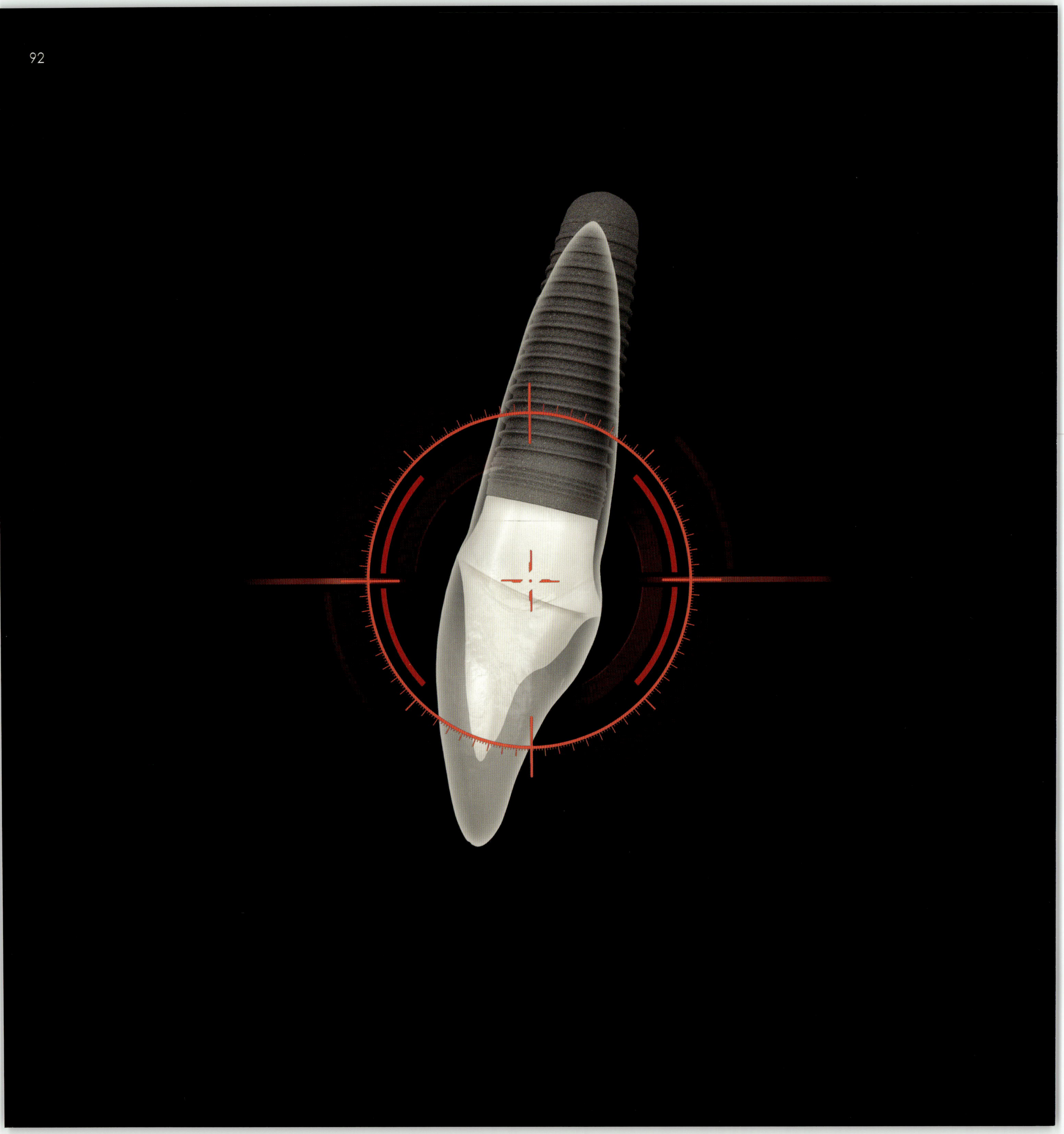

General Considerations

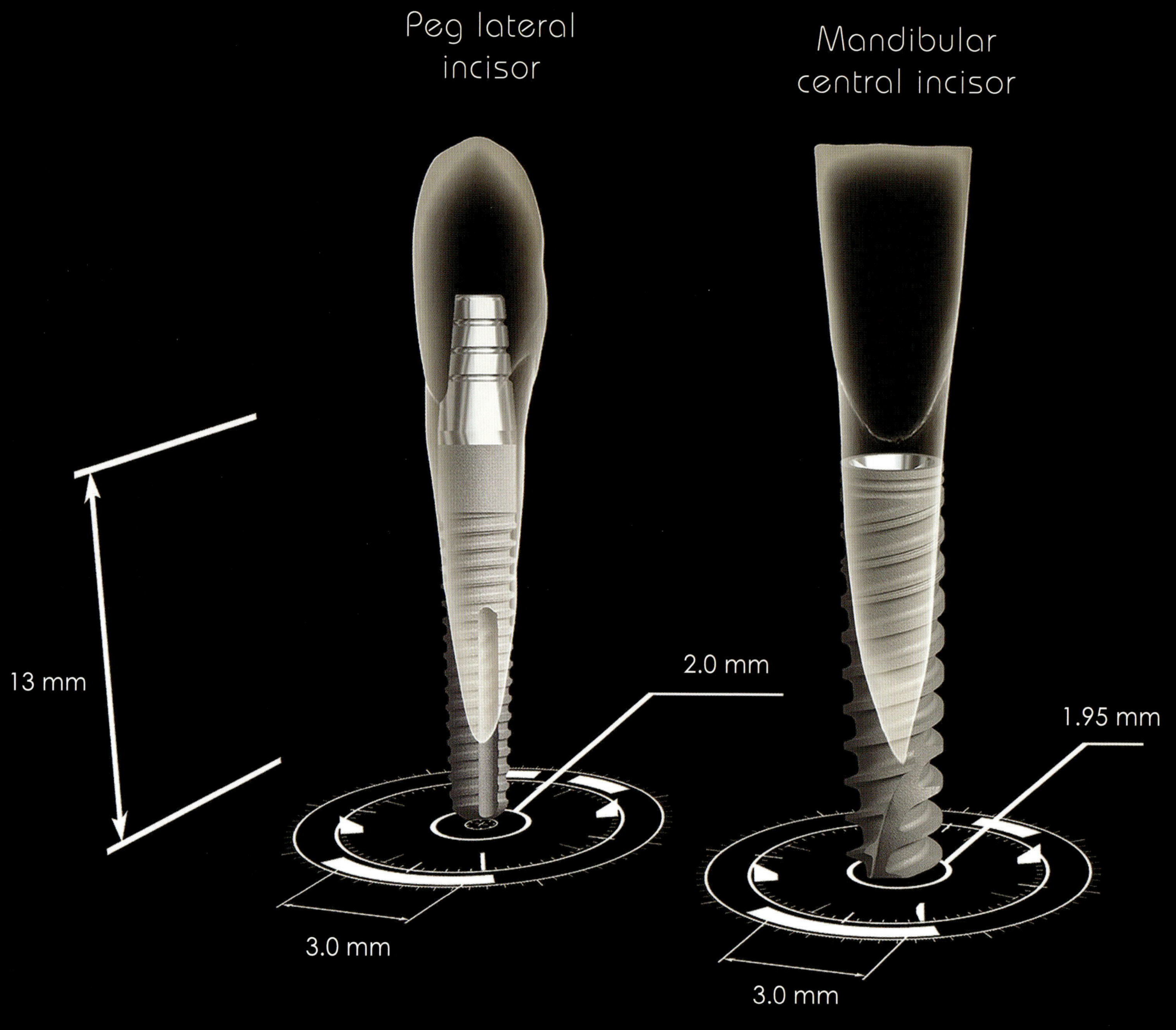
Peg lateral incisor
Mandibular central incisor
13 mm
2.0 mm
1.95 mm
3.0 mm
3.0 mm

Implant selection

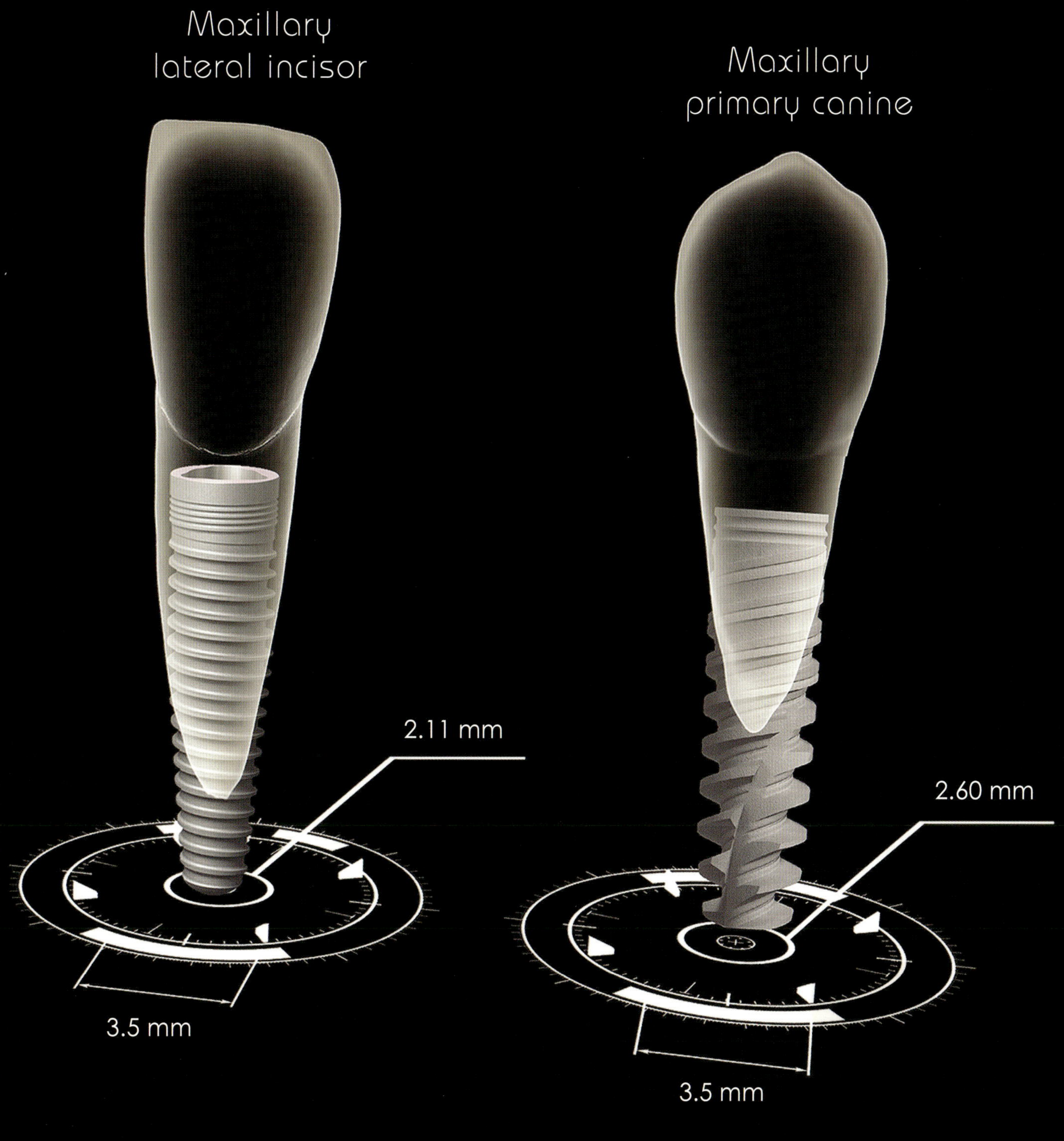

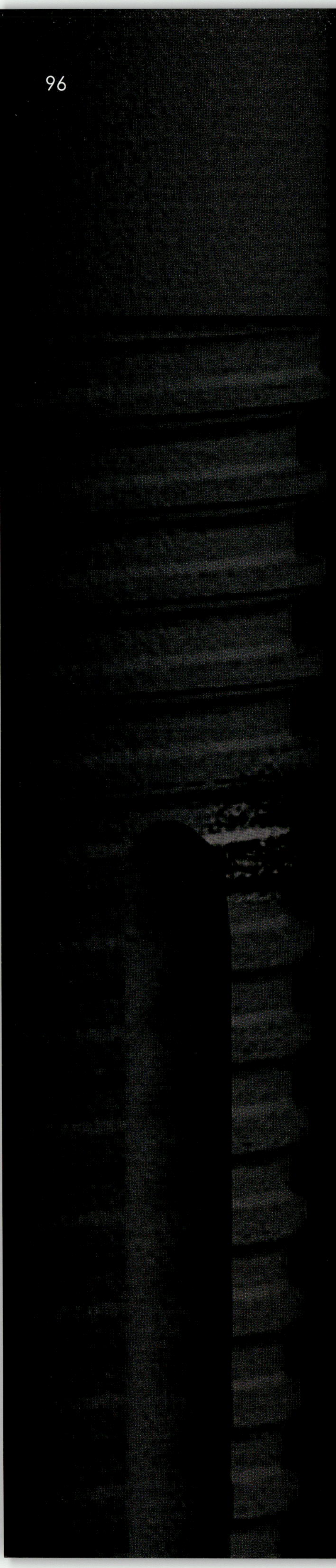

Implant dimensions

The dimensions of an implant are critical to consider during the implant selection, yet these dimensions are not always made readily available by implant manufacturers. For example, while dimensions for the neck of the implant, which are necessary for papillary esthetics around implants, are often specified by manufacturers, the body and tip dimensions often are not. These two aspects are important to consider given the proximity of the implant to the adjacent roots; a minimum of 1 mm is necessary to avoid osseointegration problems and damage to the tip of the root. Proper implant selection is therefore crucial. Because implant dentistry is a prosthetic discipline that includes a surgical component, the first step of selection is to measure the mesiodistal space at the edentulous site for the definitive crown and then to measure the apical space between the roots. The final step is to replace the missing crown, which requires careful attention to the pink esthetic parameters, papillary height, scalloping, thickness, and color of the natural dentition.

This section presents information regarding the measurements of the neck and tip of the implants used for the clinical cases presented in this book so that the ideal implant can be selected for each specific case. Note that the NobelActive 3.0 (Nobel Biocare) has the narrowest tip and that the NobelReplace has a narrower tip than the NobelActive NP. All implants shown are conical so that no emphasis on the body dimensions is necessary during the planning and implant-selection process.

NECK AND TIP MEASUREMENTS (mm)	IMPLANT TYPE	MINIMUM MD SPACE	IDEAL MD SPACE	INDICATIONS
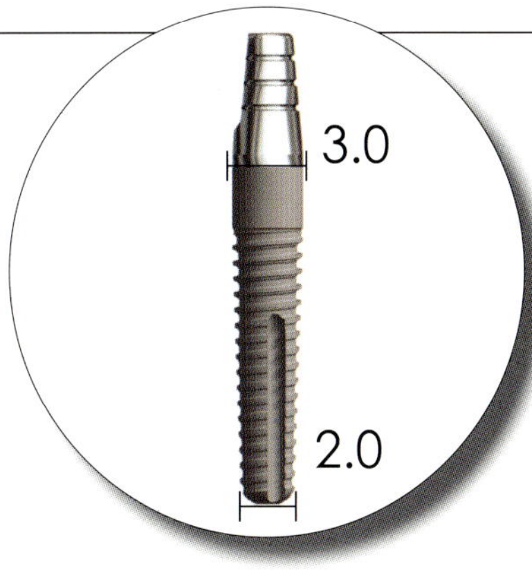	**NobelDirect 3.0** (one piece)	5.0 mm	5.5–6.0 mm	• Small maxillary lateral incisors (peg laterals) • Mandibular central incisors
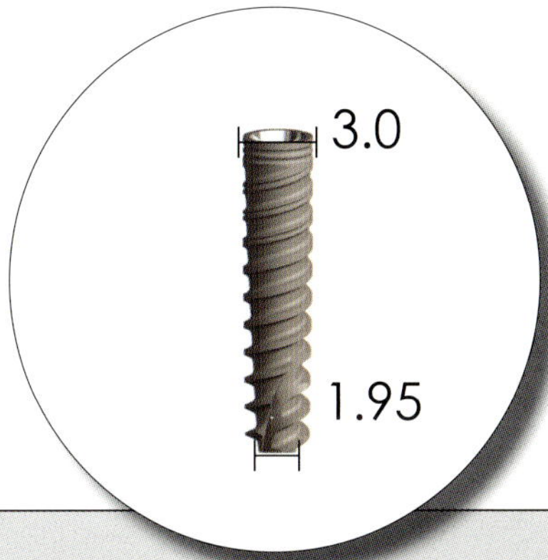	**NobelActive 3.0**	5.0 mm	5.5–6.0 mm	
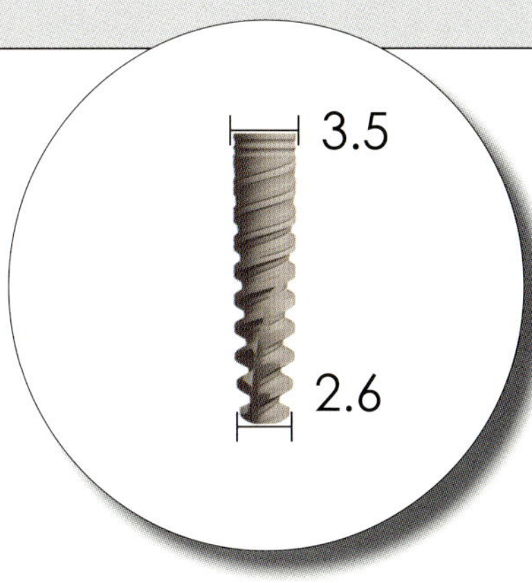	**NobelActive NP**	5.5 mm	6.0–7.0 mm	• Maxillary lateral incisors • Mandibular lateral incisors
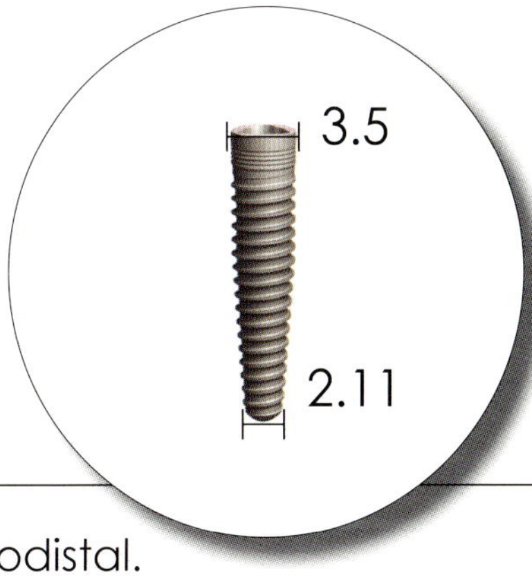	**NobelReplace Tapered NP**	5.0 mm	6.0–7.0 mm	

MD, mesiodistal.

NobelDirect 3.0

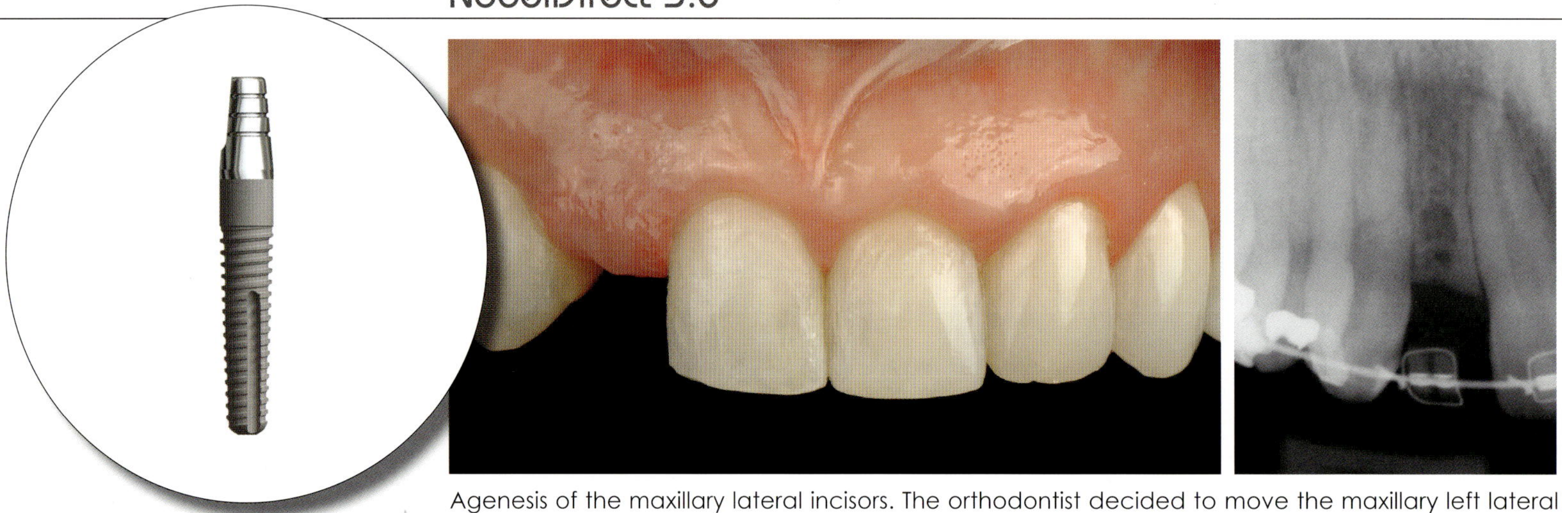

Agenesis of the maxillary lateral incisors. The orthodontist decided to move the maxillary left lateral incisor mesially and restore the first premolar in the canine position through a composite restoration. The space for implant placement was opened in the position of the maxillary right lateral incisor.

NobelActive 3.0

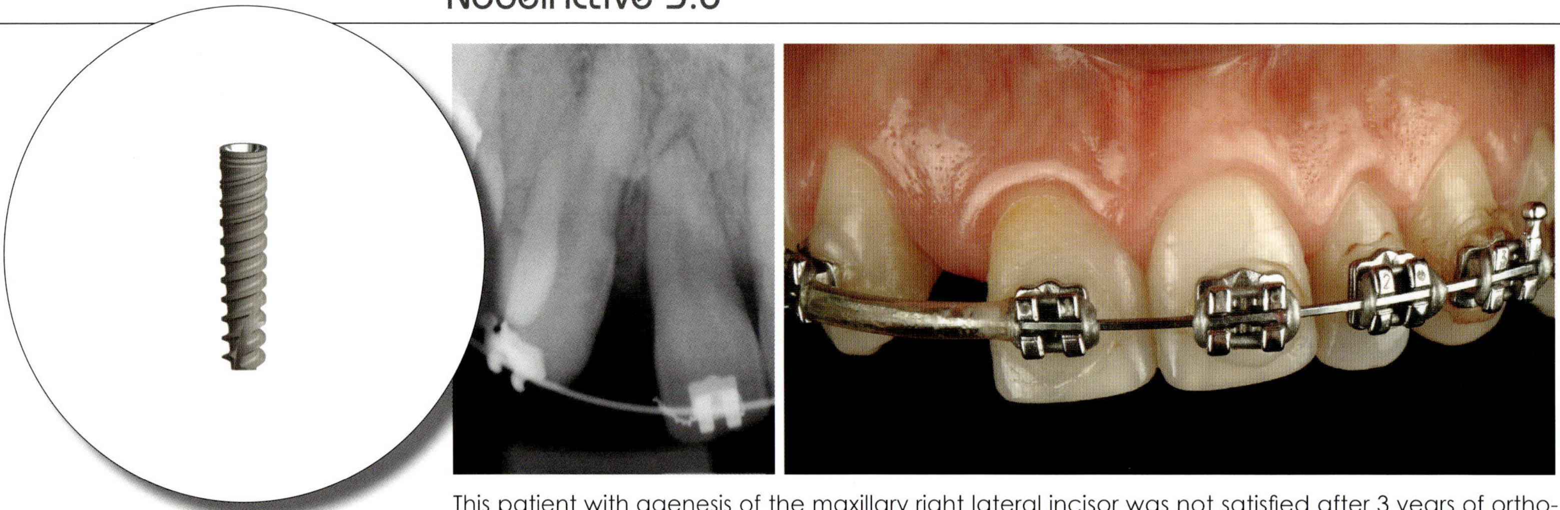

This patient with agenesis of the maxillary right lateral incisor was not satisfied after 3 years of orthodontic treatment, during which no apical space was created for implant placement. Additional orthodontic treatment was planned to restore space prosthetically and surgically. A NobelActive 3.0 implant was selected because it is the smallest two-piece implant and offers great stability.

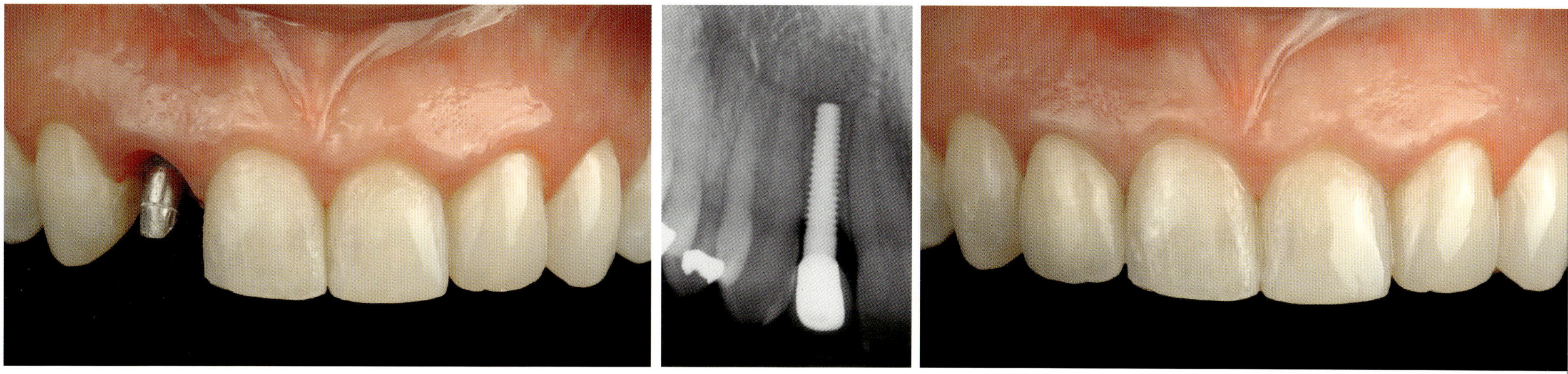

The maximum space that could be created mesiodistally was 5 mm, the absolute minimum amount needed for a 3-mm implant. At that time, the only 3-mm implant available was the NobelDirect 3.0 one-piece implant. Besides its small size, its main benefit is that it incorporates the abutment. This one-piece design, however, presents some difficulties during creation of the emergence profile and during placement when a lack of bone requires angulation of the implant.

Orthodontist: Dr Alvaro Larriu

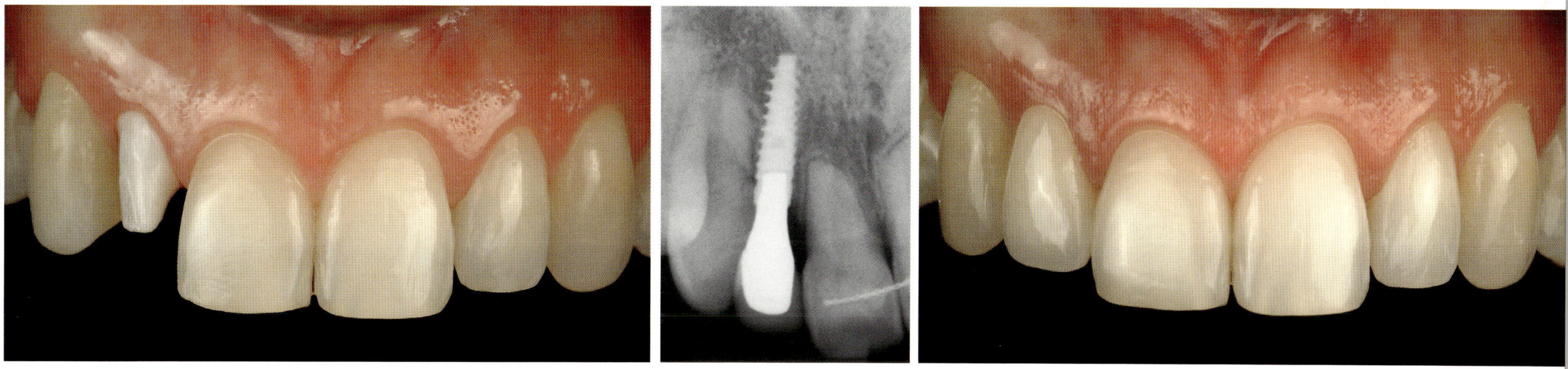

Final situation after prosthetically and surgically restoring space for implant placement. Apart from the complex gingival scalloping of the contralateral lateral incisor, the resulting restoration appears natural.

Orthodontist: Dr Domingo Martín

NobelReplace Tapered NP

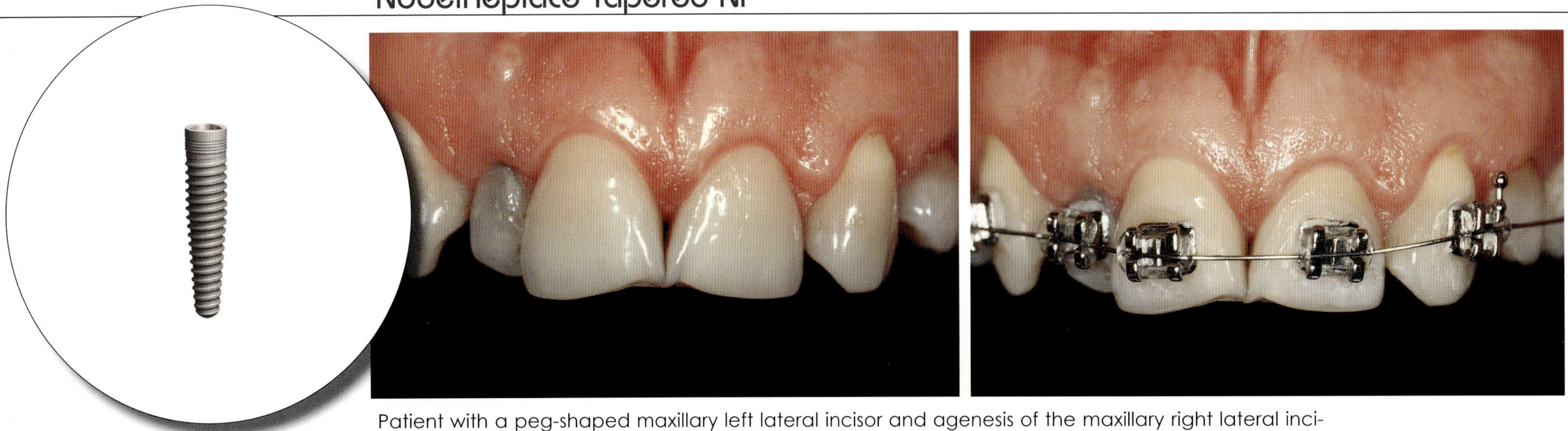

Patient with a peg-shaped maxillary left lateral incisor and agenesis of the maxillary right lateral incisor. It was decided to slightly reposition the canines to make room for restoration of the lateral incisors with bilateral implants. Because of the arch characteristics of the anterior maxilla and the tooth sizes in that region, conventional narrow platform (NP) implants could be inserted. NobelReplace Tapered NP implants were selected because their threads are smooth and allow for ideal stability for delayed implant placement.

NobelActive NP

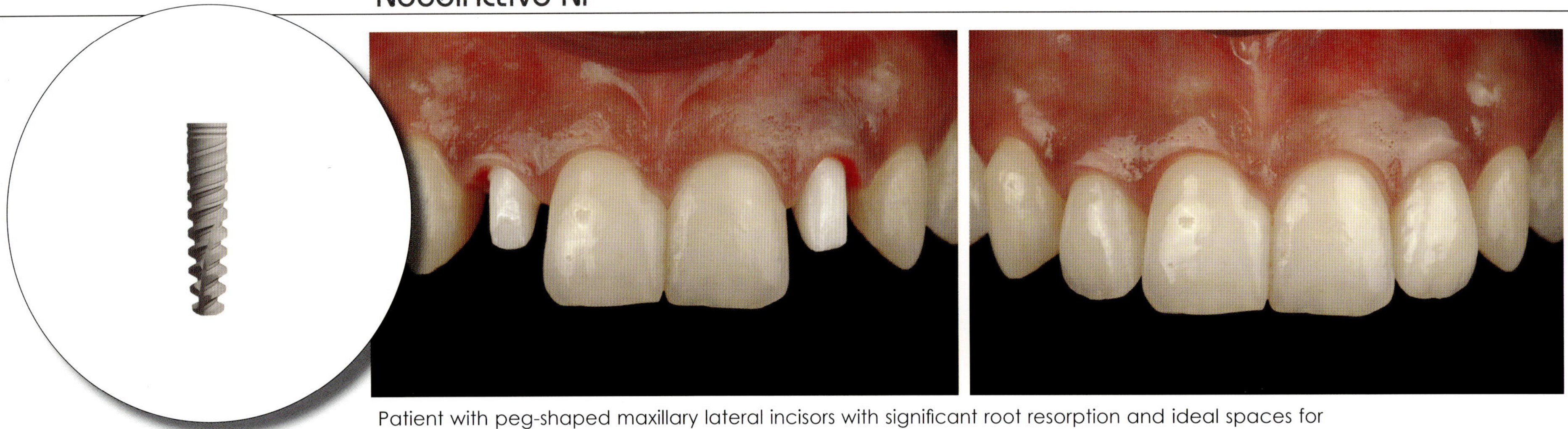

Patient with peg-shaped maxillary lateral incisors with significant root resorption and ideal spaces for implant placement. In this situation, conventional NobelActive NP implants were used because their threads allow initial torque and stability ideal for immediate implant placement.

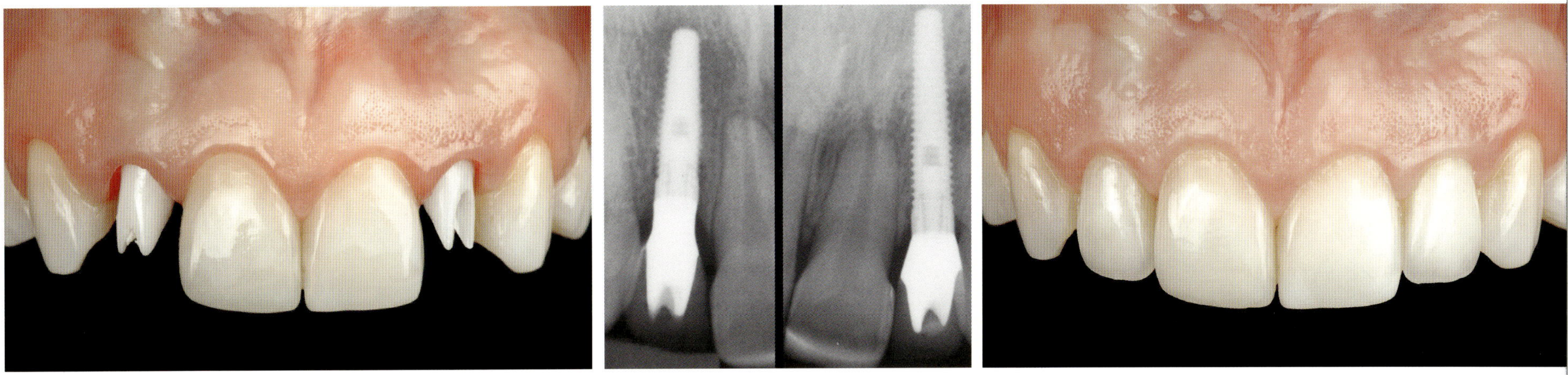

Ideal spaces were provided by the orthodontist (6 mm mesiodistally), which allowed for excellent papillary height configuration around the peri-implant restorations. Minor tooth stripping and movements had to be performed to achieve the esthetic goals: center the dental midline, open 6 mm of mesiodistal space, and create adequate anterior interdental proportions and a Class I canine relationship.

Orthodontist: Dr Domingo Martín

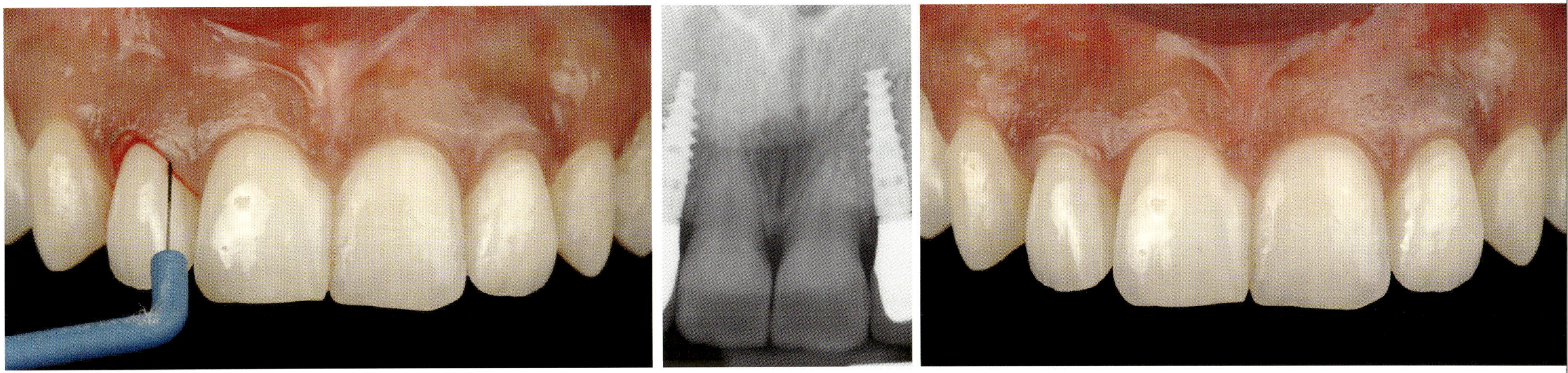

Three months after final cementation, a gingivectomy was performed on the implant in the right lateral incisor position to correct gingival heights and control soft tissue scalloping.

Combination case

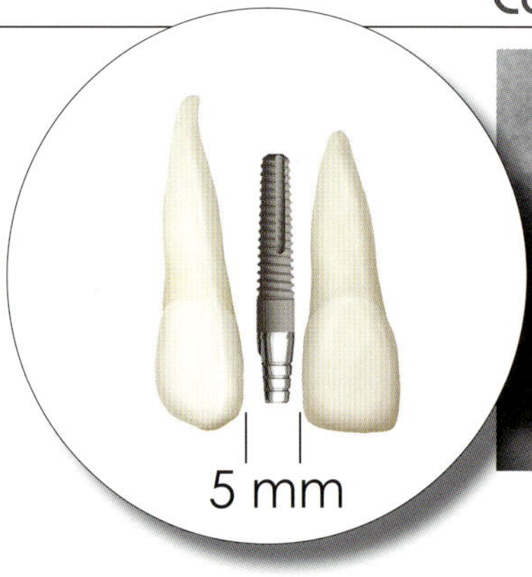

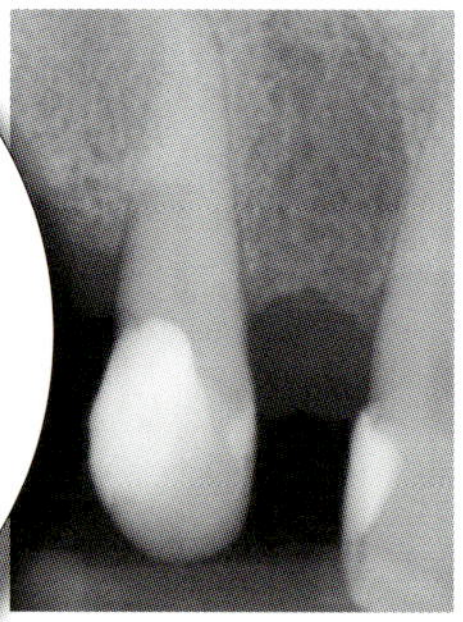
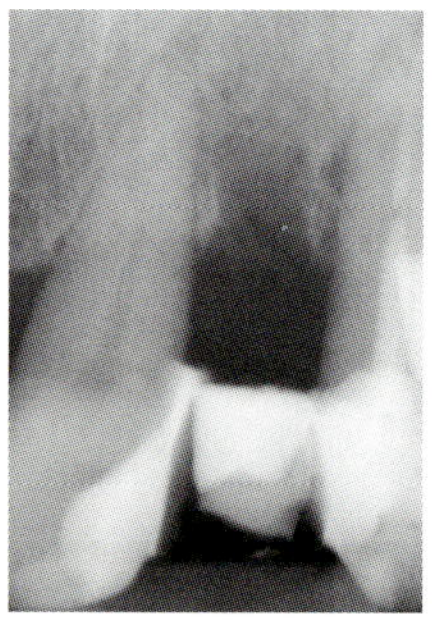
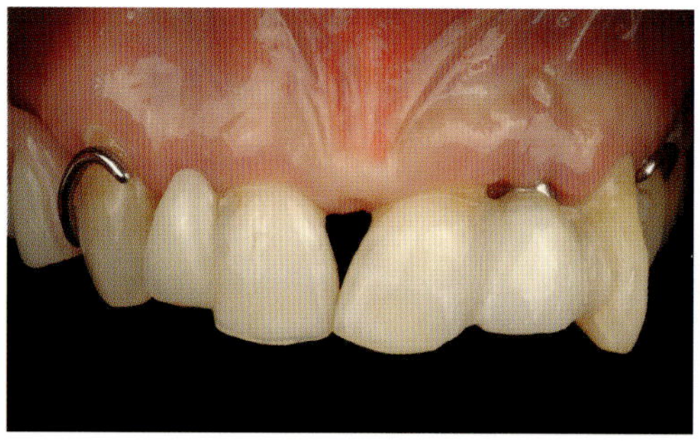
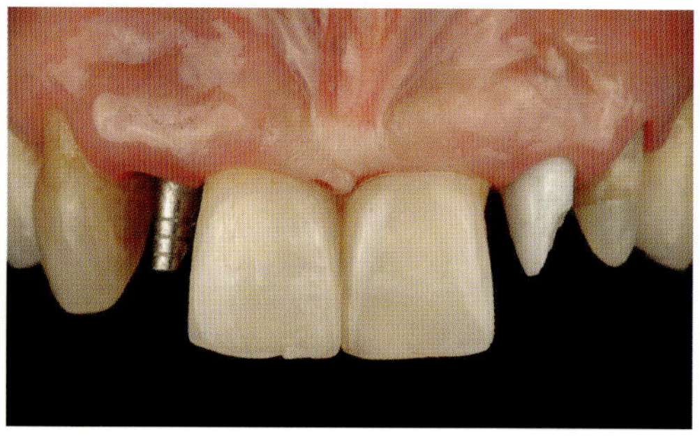

The importance of implant selection is demonstrated in this case with missing lateral incisors. The site of the maxillary right lateral incisor had a mesiodistal space of only 4.5 mm. Therefore, stripping of the adjacent teeth was necessary to at least slightly increase the space. NobelDirect 3.0 was the only implant available at the time to replace the missing tooth. The site of the maxillary left lateral incisor had a normal mesiodistal space and was restored with a two-piece NobelReplace Tapered NP implant.

Adjacent mandibular anterior teeth

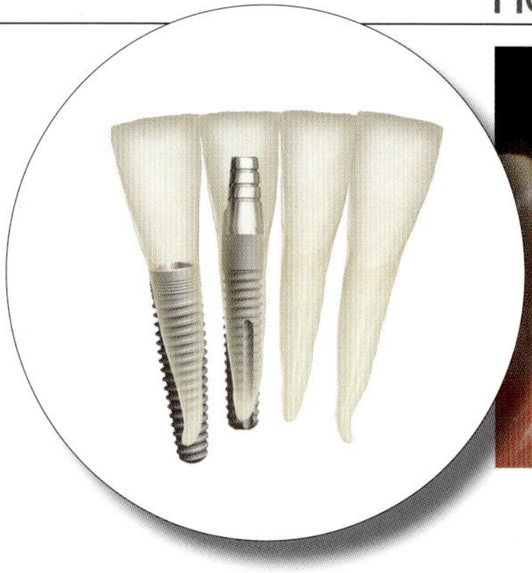
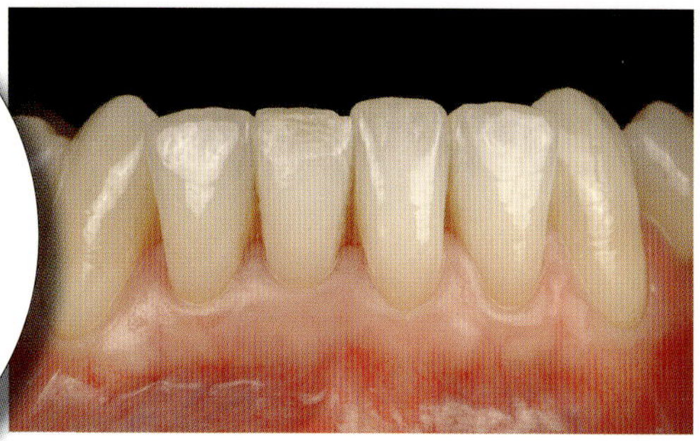
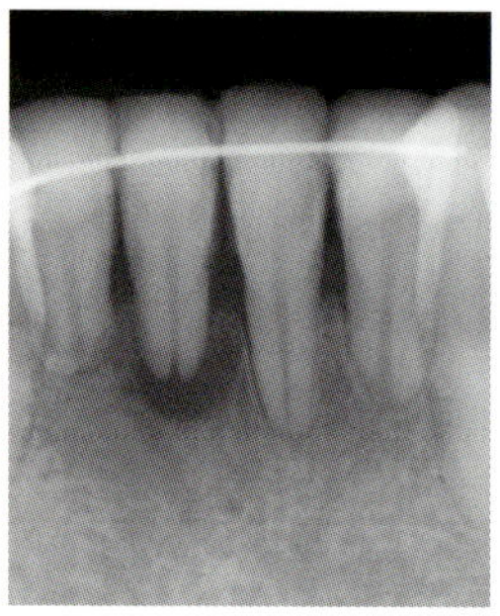
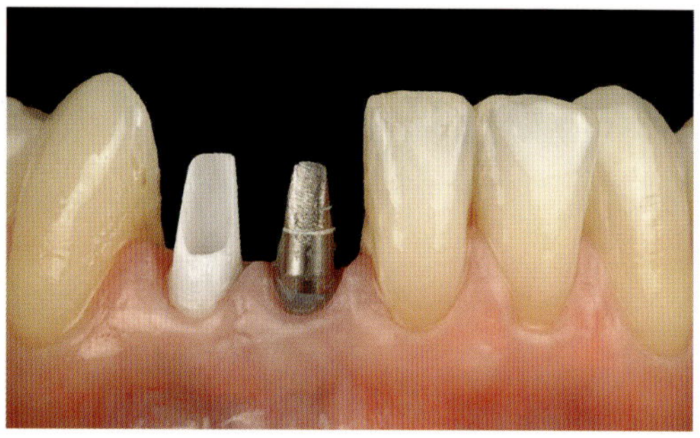

Perhaps the most challenging implant restoration is that of adjacent mandibular anterior teeth. Two NobelDirect 3.0 implants were originally planned to restore the missing mandibular right central incisor and its adjacent lateral incisor to allow more space for peri-implant tissue esthetics, especially in respect to papillary height. However, alternative implant placement therapy was performed to reduce the trauma and bone resorption. A connective tissue graft (CTG) was placed at the site of the mandibular right central incisor, and 3 months later one was placed at the site of the adjacent lateral incisor. A two-piece NobelReplace Tapered NP implant was inserted in the site of the lateral incisor because of the lack of torque and stability of the previous NobelDirect 3.0.

Adjacent mandibular central incisors

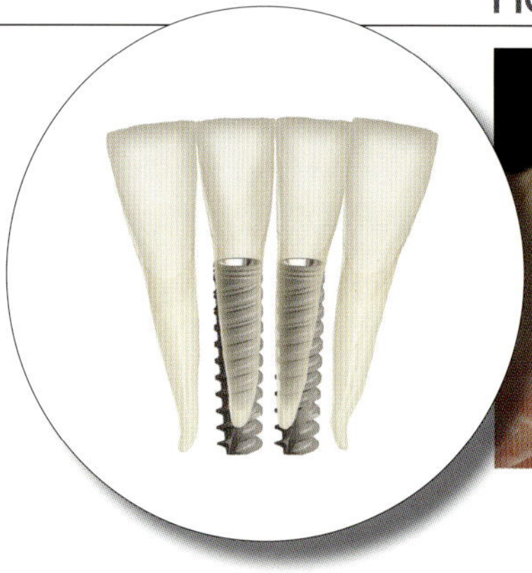
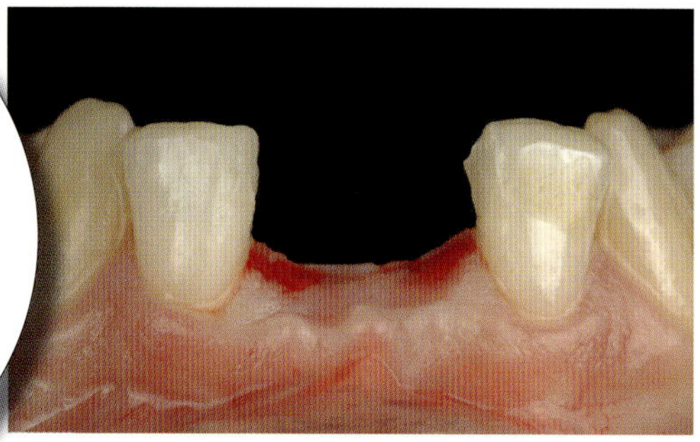
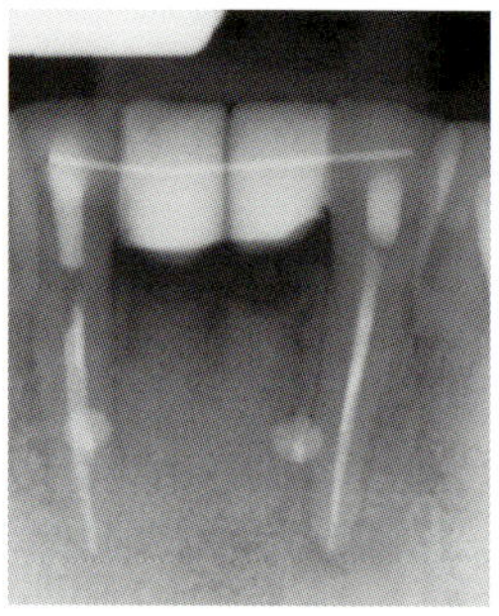
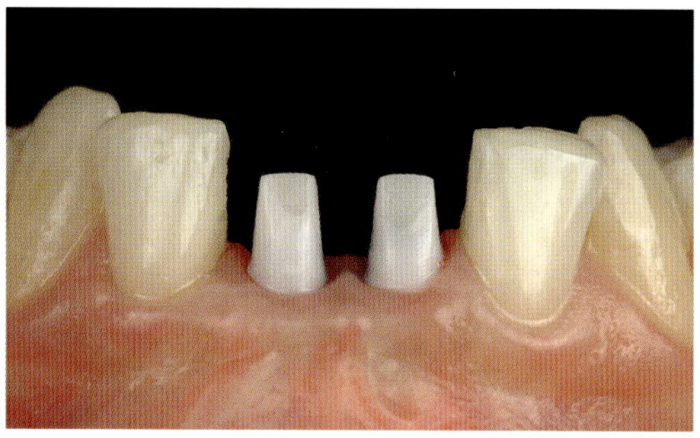

NobelDirect 3.0 implants would not have been the ideal choice in this situation because of the limited grip during insertion in dense bone. The NobelActive 3.0 implant was just released when this patient presented to our office. With very limited space available, there was no room for error in respect to implant location and angulation. The existing defect and delayed implant placement protocol make it almost impossible to re-create the interproximal papilla height.

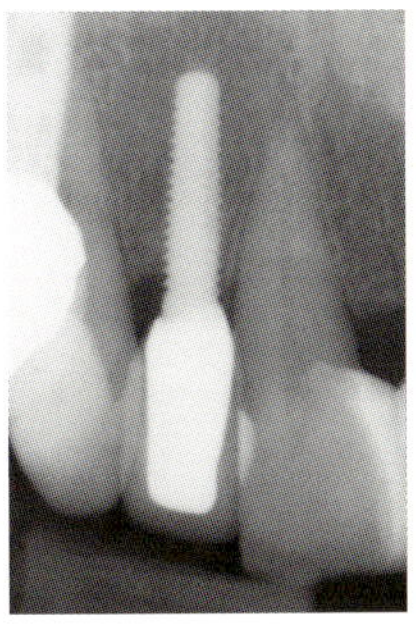

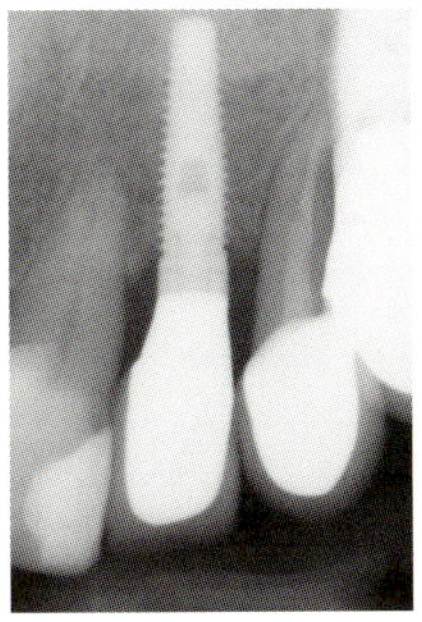

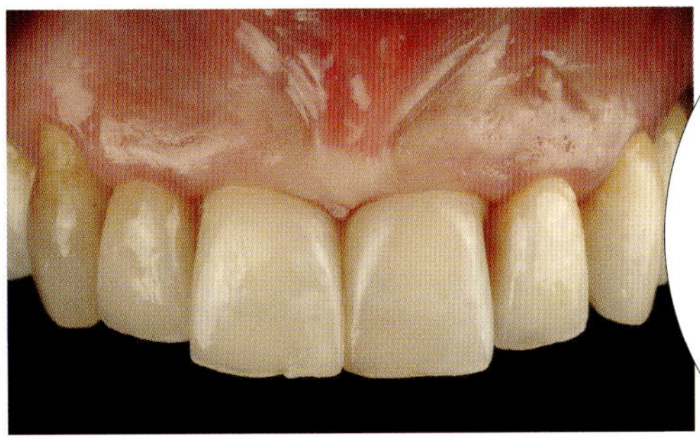

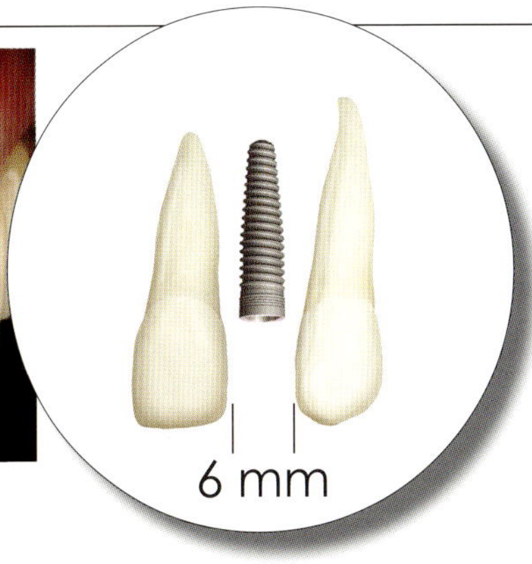

The patient declined orthodontic treatment, so composite restorations were fabricated and placed on both central incisors to close the large black triangle with a long contact point, which blended with the flat gingival scalloping of the peri-implant soft tissue topography.

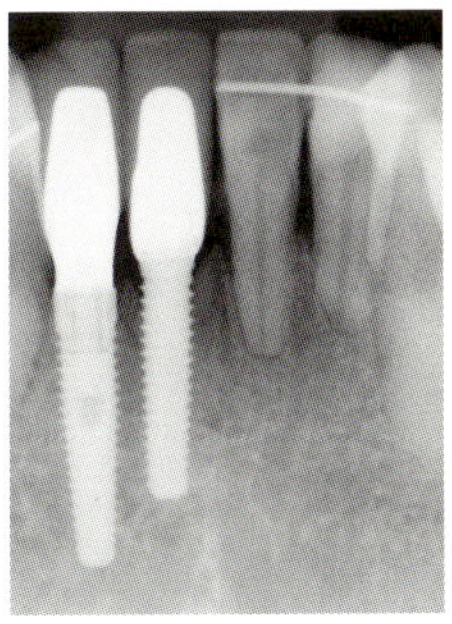

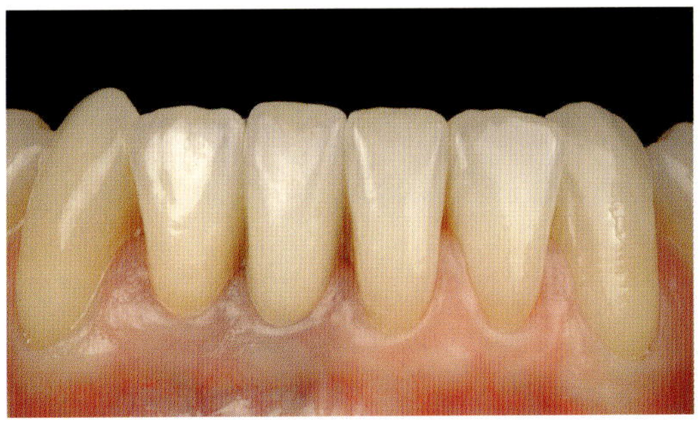

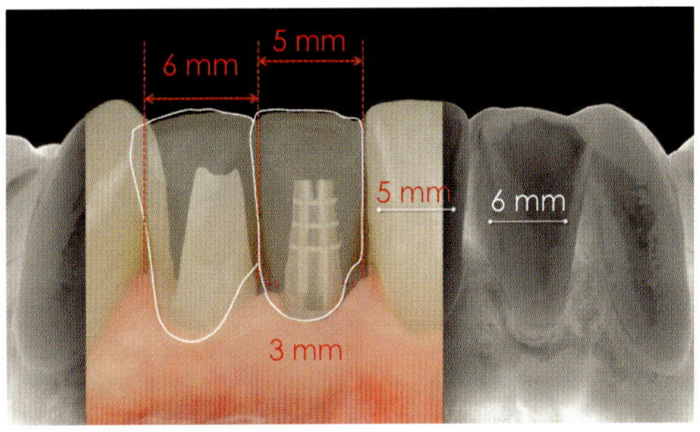

Definitive implant restoration with limited space. The soft tissue characteristics were maintained with the exception of the loss of papillary height between the adjacent implants.

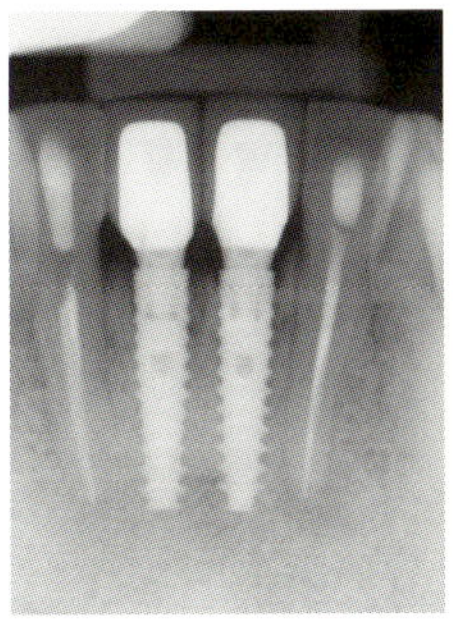

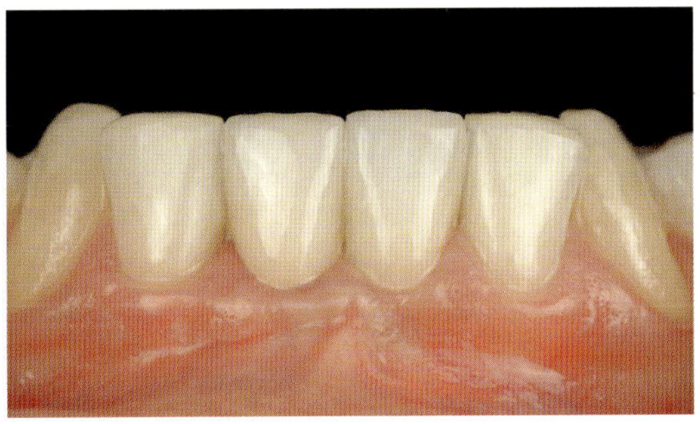

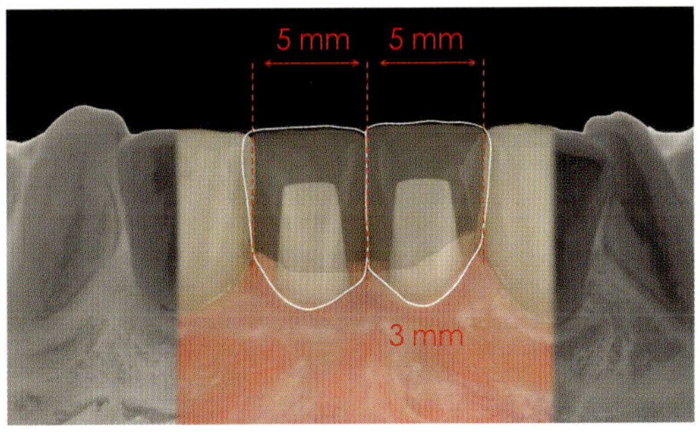

Final outcome after the placement of two adjacent NobelActive 3.0 implants incorporating the platform shift concept, which allowed for extra soft tissue thickness and long-term tissue stability. The implants have close proximity but a relatively short central papilla compared with the adjacent papillae.

Adjacent implants

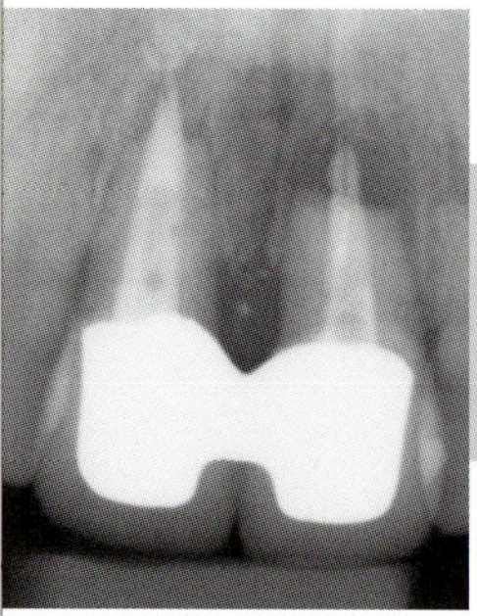

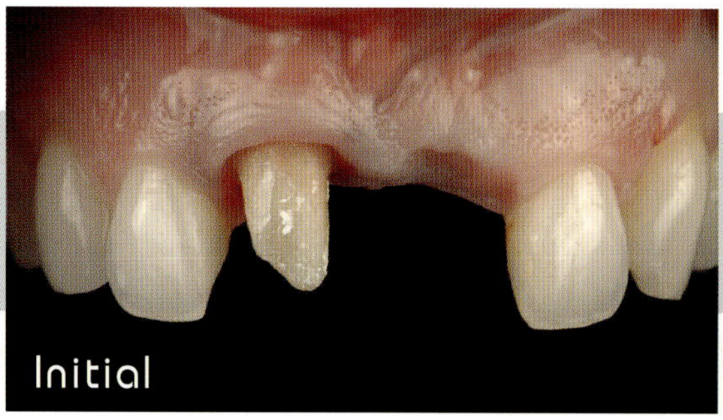

Initial

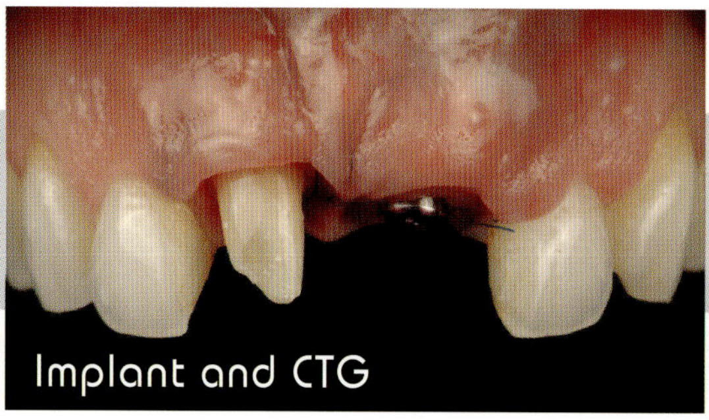

Implant and CTG

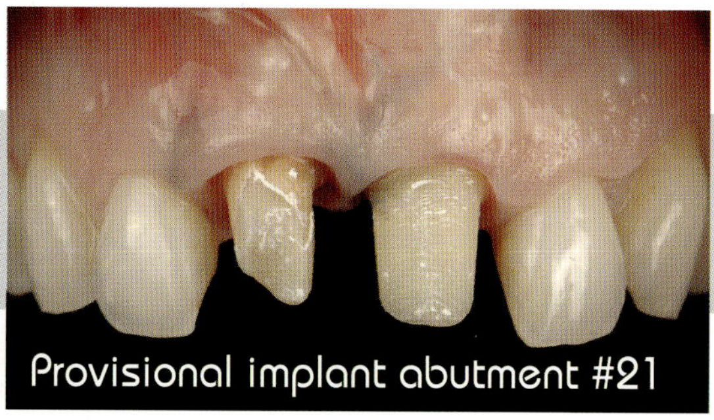

Provisional implant abutment #21

When placing adjacent implants, always start with the most difficult one. This is important in situations where, for example, one tooth requires a delayed implant placement approach because of extensive periapical inflammation while the adjacent tooth can be replaced following the immediate implant placement and restoration concept. In this case, the implant replacing the infected tooth should be restored first. When the adjacent implant is restored subsequently, both implant sites should receive CTGs to compensate for and control any vertical bone and tissue recession, which will enhance peri-implant soft tissue esthetics.

The diameter of the implants selected will differ between delayed implant placement and immediate implant placement. Implants for a delayed site always need to be small in diameter to allow

Adjacent implants

The patient presented with failing maxillary central incisors, each with periapical lesions. The sequence of treatment was carefully planned to avoid as much soft tissue recession as possible and prevent uneven gingival levels and long central incisors. The left central incisor was extracted first, and the implant, a 3.5 × 13–mm NobelReplace Tapered NP, was placed with a CTG after 3 months of bone healing. After healing, the provisional abutment and crown were fabricated and placed to control the buccal volume and soft tissue architecture.

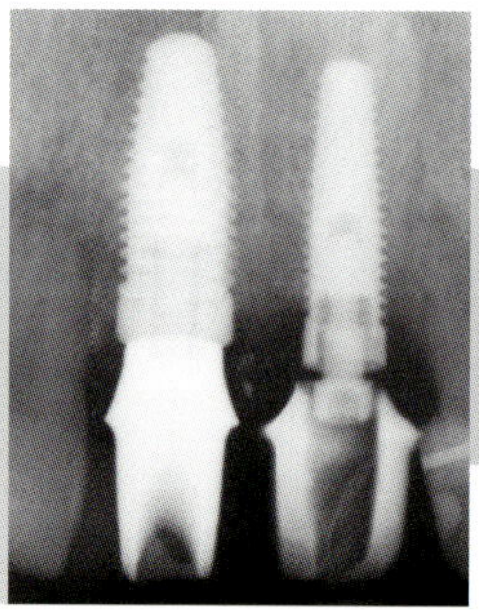

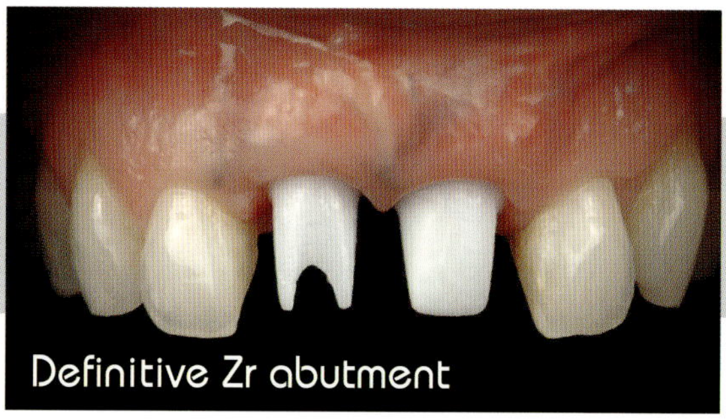

Definitive Zr abutment

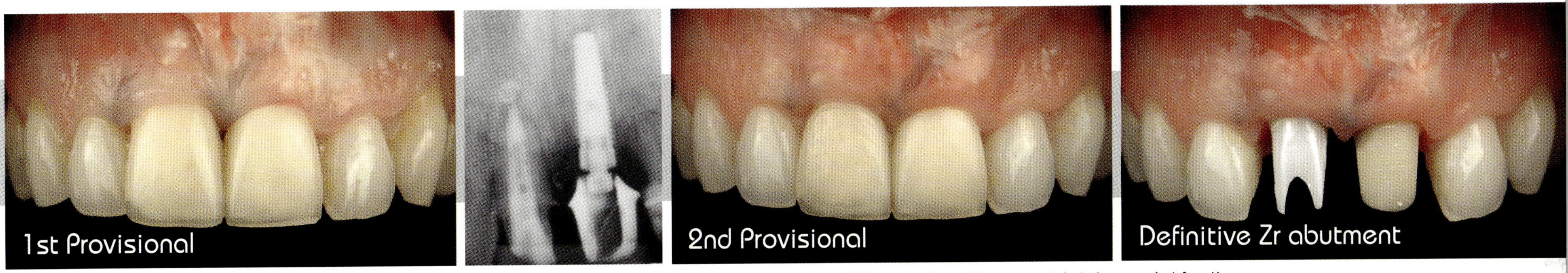

greater distance between the implant and the adjacent interproximal bone, which is crucial for the height of the interproximal papilla. The smaller diameter allows for perfect placement within the confines of the buccolingual bone, retaining a maximum thickness of bone on the labial aspect for long-term stability and leaving more space for tissue thickness and blood supply as well as prosthetic soft tissue management.

For immediate implant placement, on the other hand, wider-diameter implants make it easier to achieve the necessary initial torque and implant stability. Proper abutment selection and application of the platform shift concept are necessary to create sufficient space for connective tissue grafting and an ideal emergence profile with adequate and long-term stable soft tissue support.

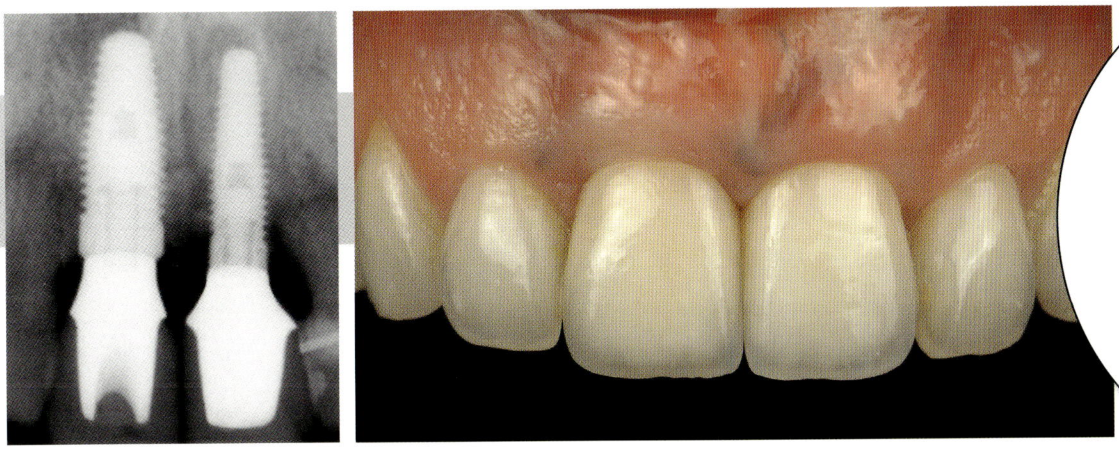

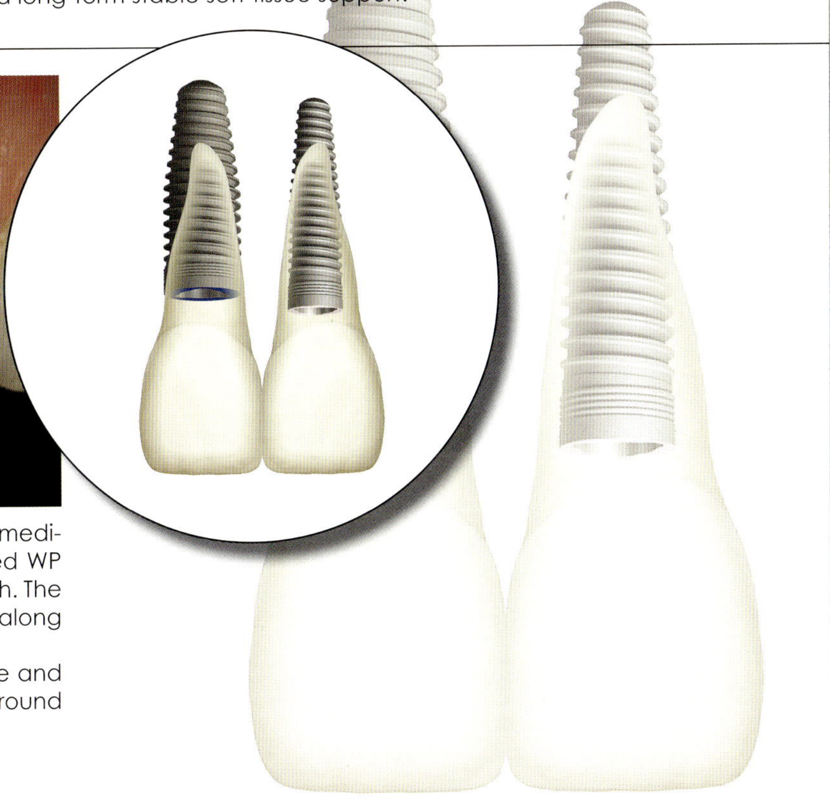

One month after tissue stability was achieved with the left central incisor, an implant was immediately placed in the right central incisor position after tooth extraction. NobelReplace Tapered WP (wide platform) (5 × 13 mm) was selected because of the large diameter of the extracted tooth. The definitive prefabricated zirconia (Zr) abutment was placed at the time of implant placement along with a CTG.

The definitive Procera zirconia abutment for the left central incisor followed the same shape and contour as the previous composite provisional abutment. Bone remodeling and cratering around that implant was obvious.

Hard and soft tissue stability was adequate 1 year after final cementation.

Adjacent implants and three-unit fixed partial dentures

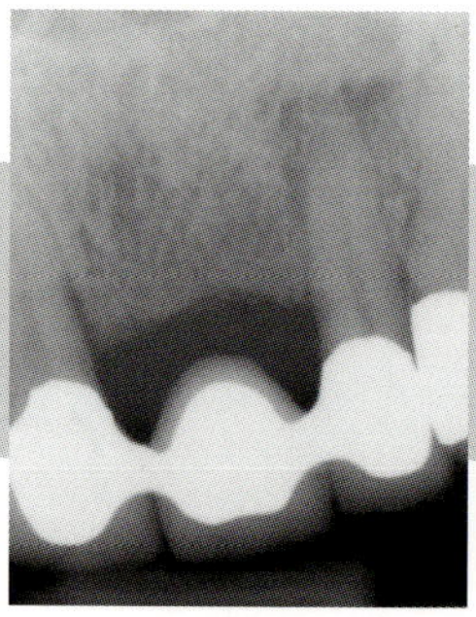

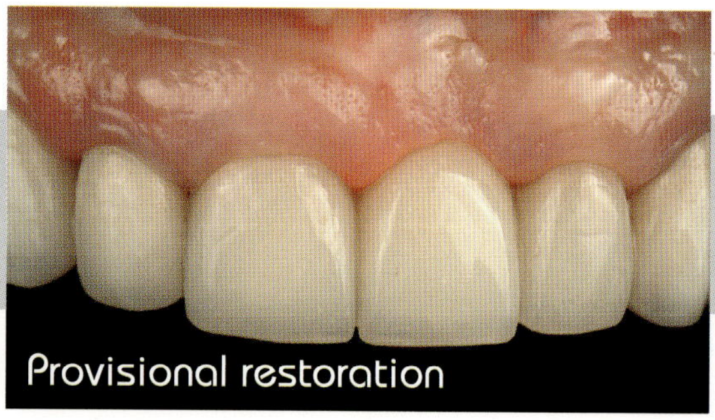

Provisional restoration

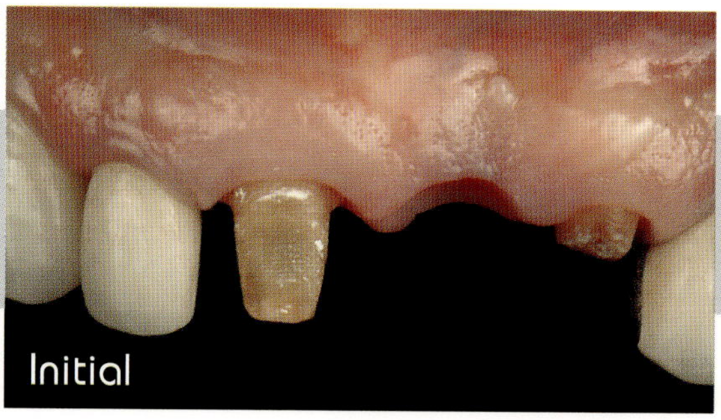

Initial

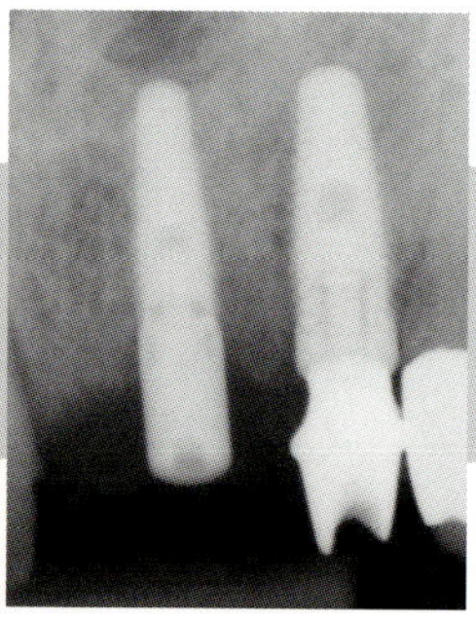

This patient presented with a fractured abutment on the maxillary left lateral incisor of a three-unit porcelain-fused-to-metal fixed partial denture (FPD). A provisional FPD was inserted to evaluate the tooth to be extracted. The treatment plan was to extract the left lateral incisor first. The implant chosen was a 4.3 × 13–mm NobelReplace Tapered RP (regular platform) with PS adapter and zirconia prefabricated esthetic abutment followed by a CTG, splinted to the natural tooth. After 3 months of healing, delayed implant placement was performed on the left central incisor; a narrow implant (NobelReplace Tapered NP 3.5 × 13 mm) was chosen to create more space for prosthetic management of the surrounding tissues. Care was taken at the incision level to avoid elevating or cutting the mesial aspect of the papillae of the left central incisor to avoid trauma and postoperative soft tissue recession.

Soft tissue contour and support are created during the provisional phase through provisional-guided soft tissue manipulation to provide an ideal framework for the definitive restoration, in this case made with Procera alumina.

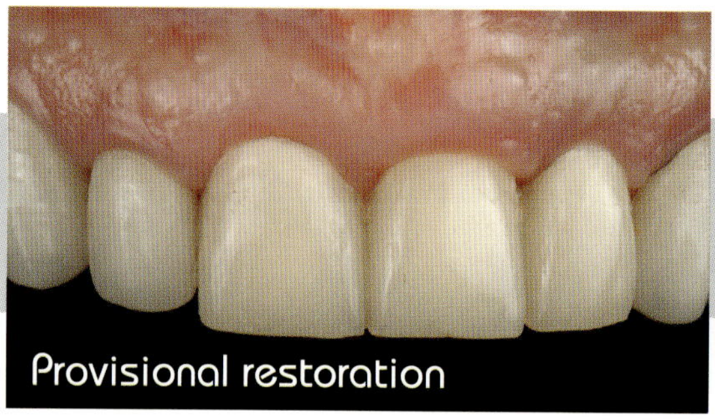

Provisional restoration

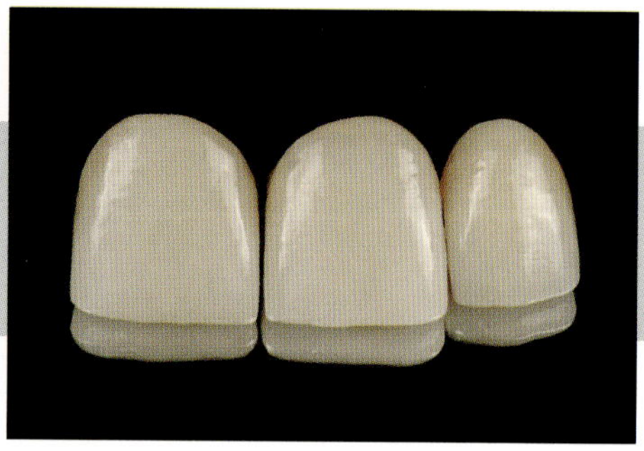

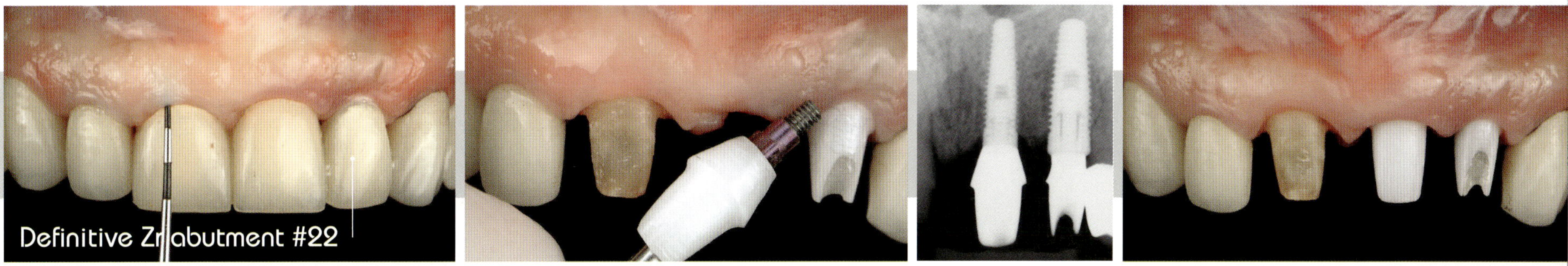

Three months after the final surgery of the delayed implant placement, some recession occurred that affected the papillary height between the two adjacent implants. Control of the soft tissue levels is essential for the final outcome. The definitive zirconia abutment was delivered, and the provisional restoration was adjusted in height to support the soft tissue from the abutment tooth to the implants.

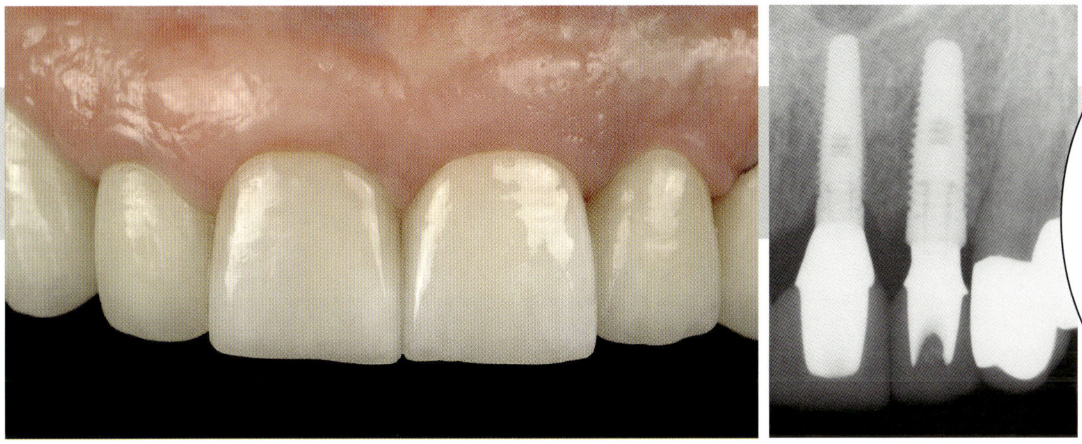

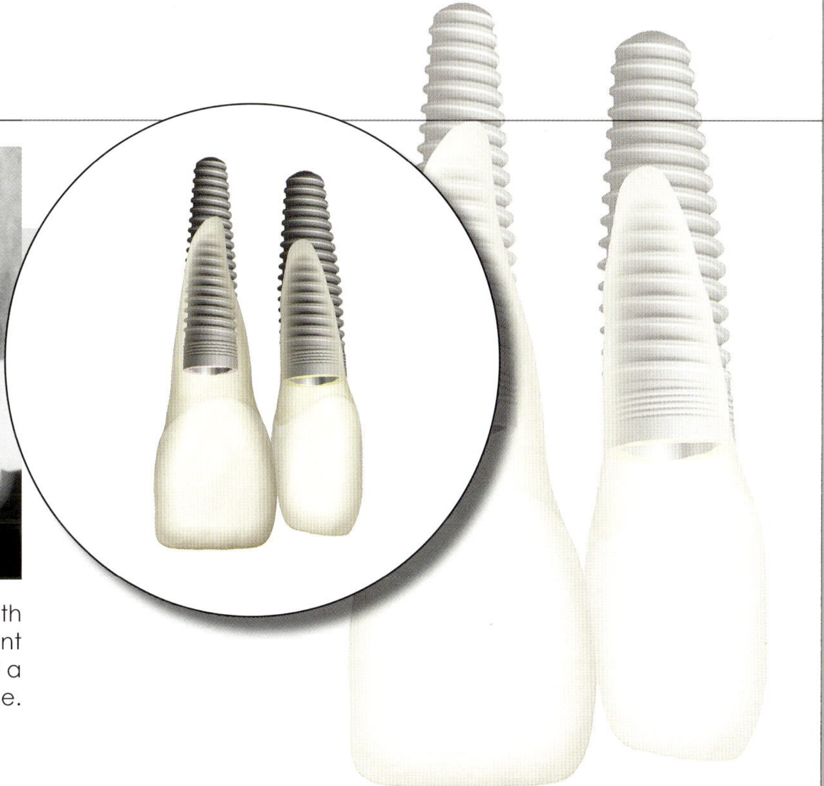

The definitive restorations were placed on two adjacent implants with minimal resorption. Clinical success depends on sequential implant placement, selection of the implant diameters, and placement of a definitive abutment on the first day of the restorative treatment phase.

Adjacent implants and two-unit fixed partial dentures

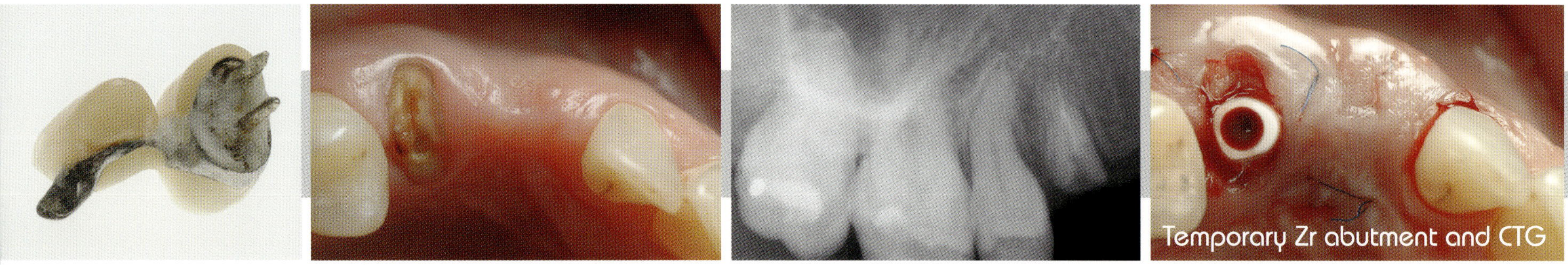

The patient presented with a failing cantilevered FPD from the maxillary right first premolar to the right canine, with a pontic in the canine area and an occlusal rest on the adjacent lateral incisor. The first phase of treatment included immediate implant placement for the right first premolar. A NobelActive WP (5 × 10 mm) implant was placed to provide adequate initial torque and stability. A CTG and a definitive prefabricated zirconia abutment were placed concurrently. The edentulous ridge was also augmented with a CTG to minimize trauma during placement of the second implant in the canine area.

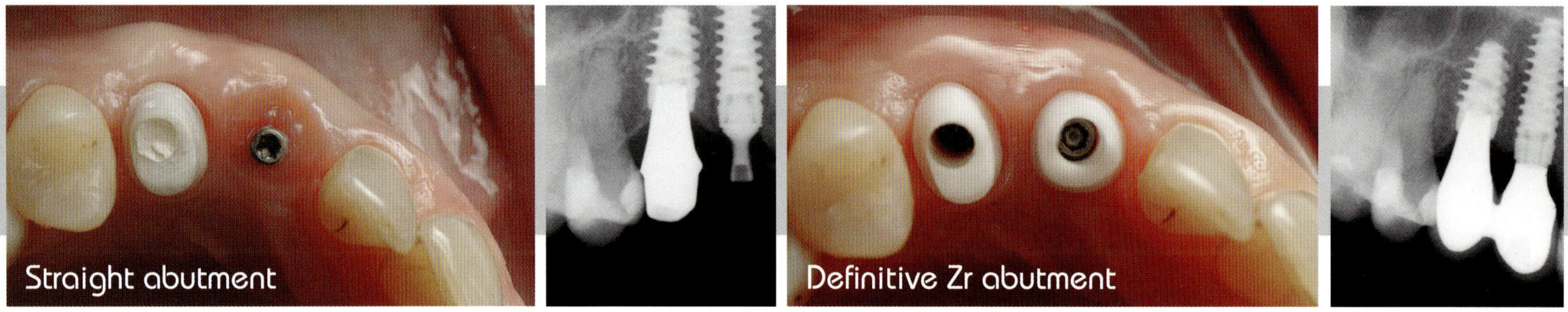

In contrast to the immediate protocol, which requires insertion of the definitive abutment at the time of implant placement, a straight healing abutment was connected to the implant during the delayed placement. The healing abutment allows greater space for the soft tissue during its maturation phase. Subsequently, instead of using a prefabricated abutment, the definitive zirconia abutment was custom fabricated for optimal soft tissue support. The final outcome reveals only minimal loss of interproximal tissue height.

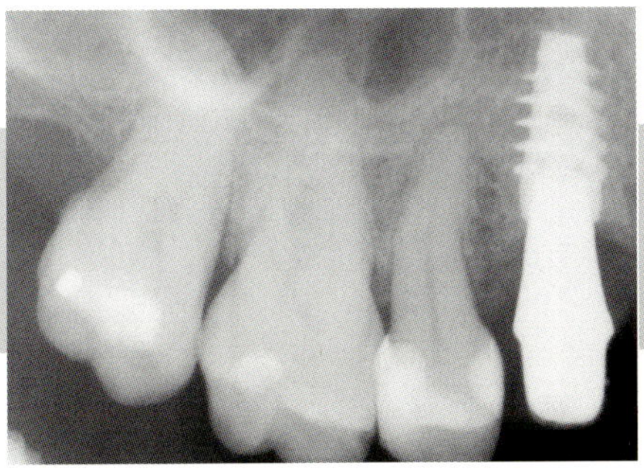
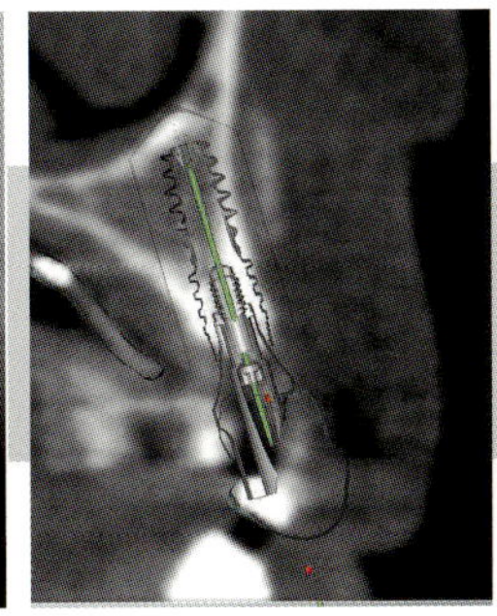
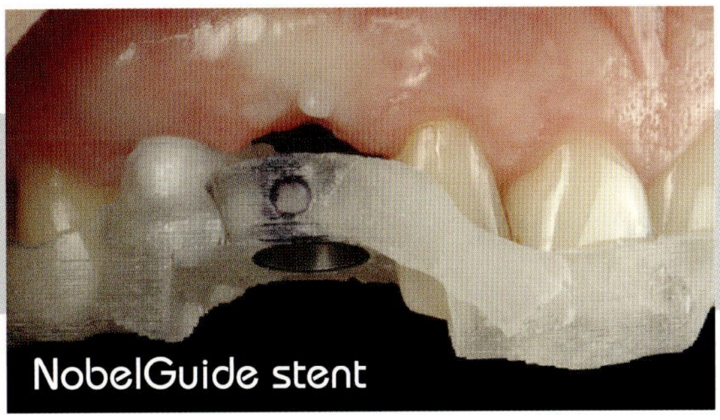

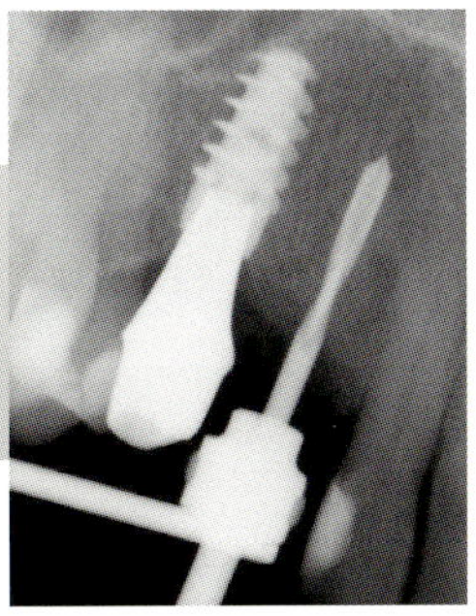

The delayed implant surgery in the area of the right canine was carried out with as minimal invasiveness as possible to maintain the interproximal papillae and avoid compromising the esthetic outcome. Guided surgery (NobelGuide) was used for ideal implant placement (NobelActive RP 4.3 × 15 mm) and minimal trauma.

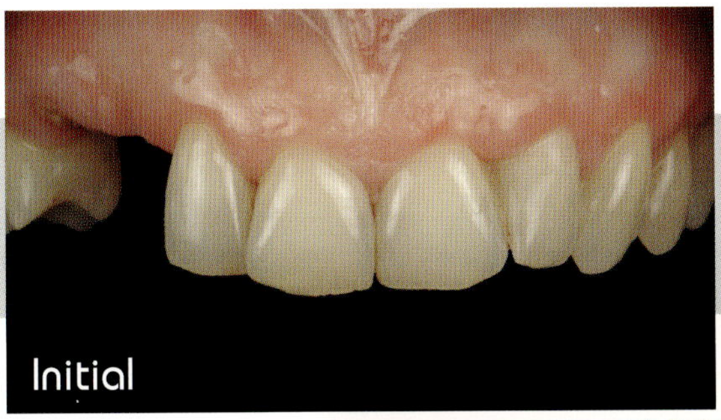

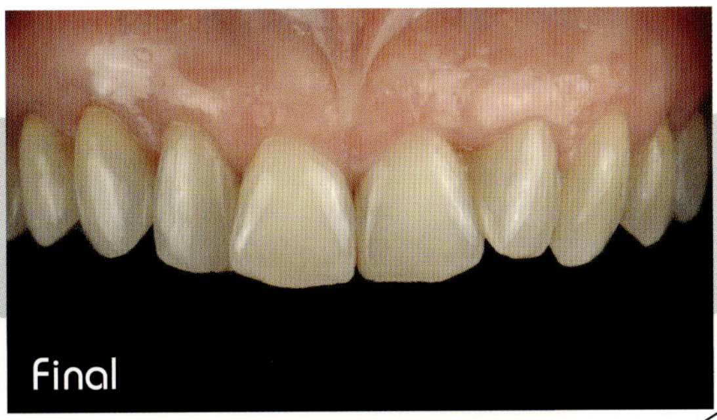

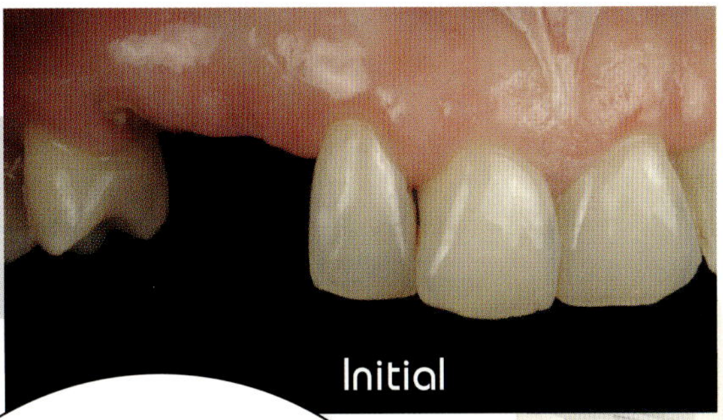

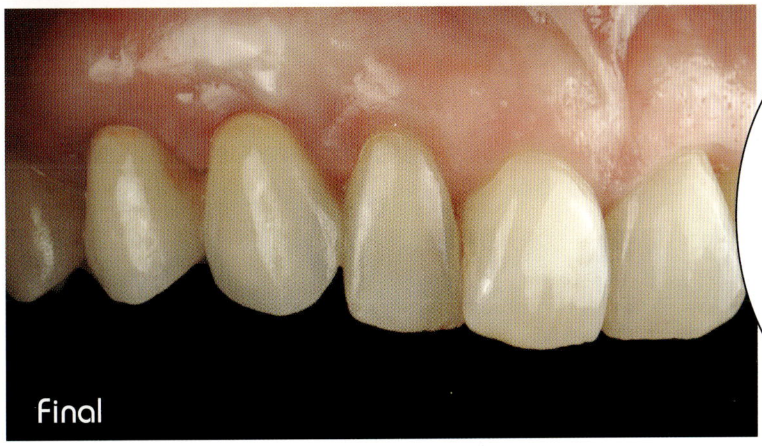

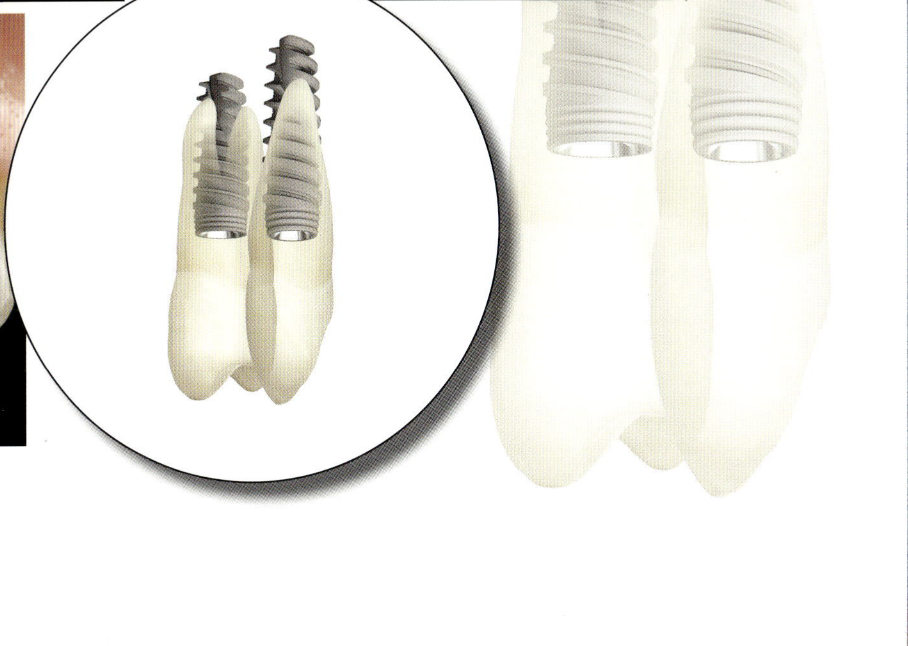

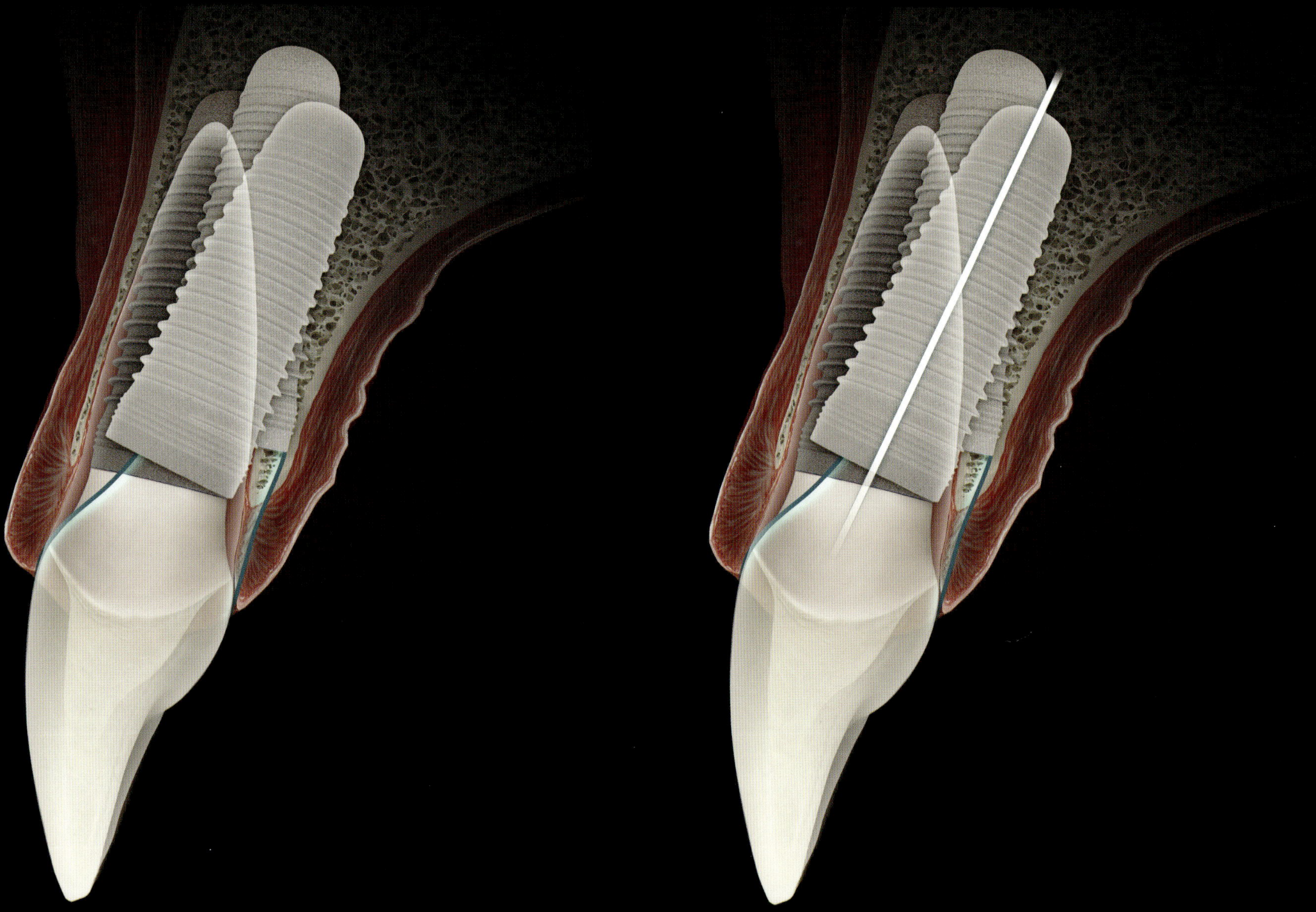

Buccolingual position

Buccolingual position

Implants should be placed as far buccal as possible in order to create a smooth transition between the crown and the implant. The idea is to be as facial as possible while remaining centered in reference to the incisal edge of the tooth to provide the same emergence profile as that of the tooth.

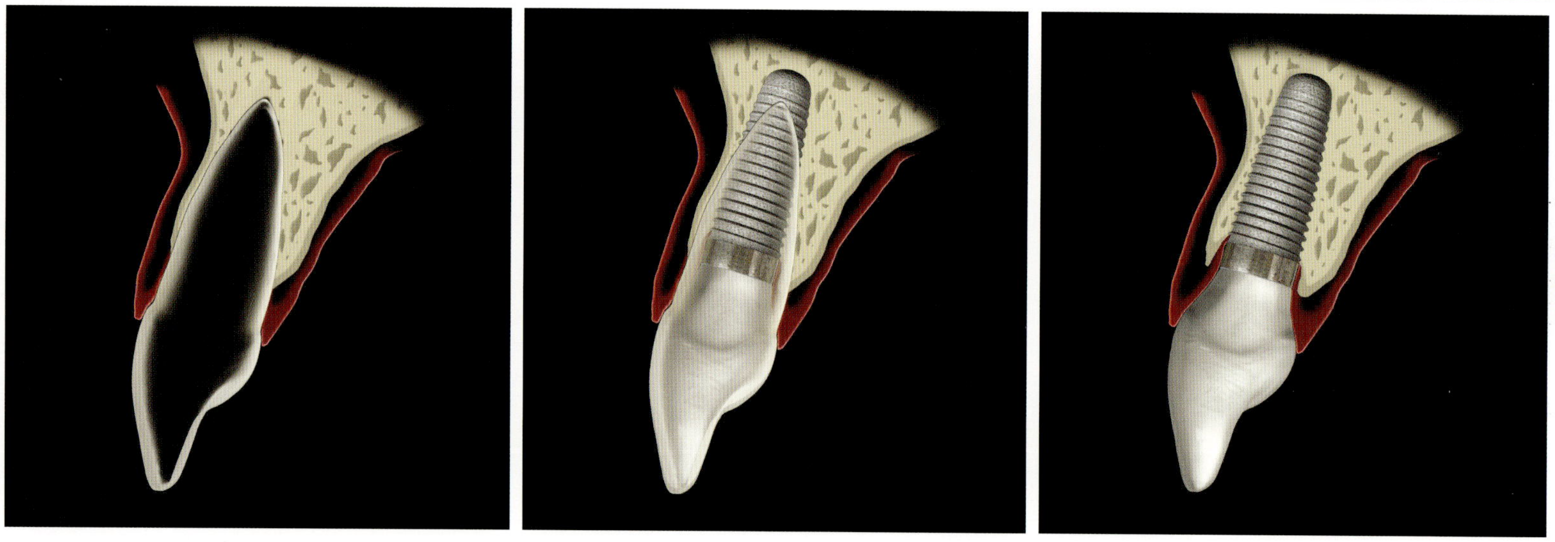

Screw-retained restoration

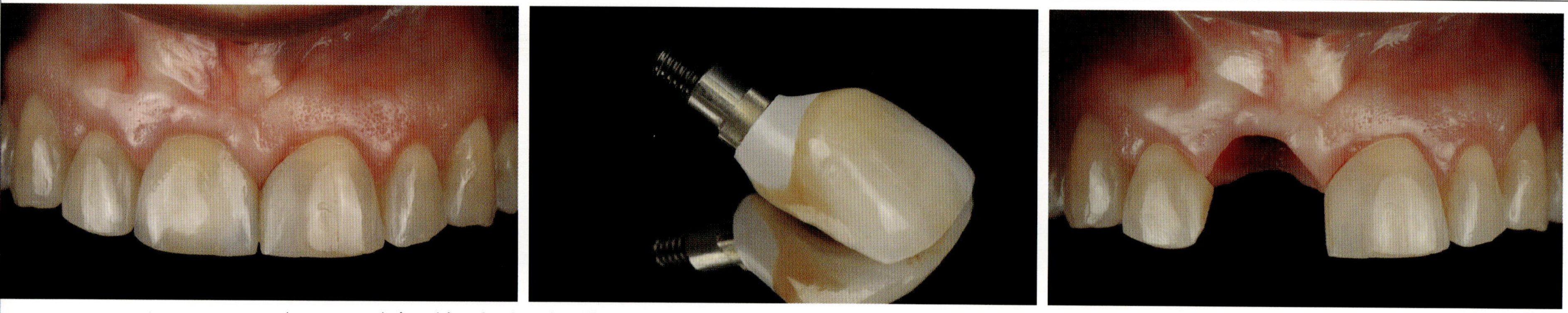

A screw-retained implant restoration on the maxillary right central incisor is directed toward the cingulum because of the lack of buccal bone volume. A CTG was placed during implant surgery to augment the buccal defect. The zirconia restoration was left in direct contact with the tissue to promote soft tissue integration.

Cemented restoration

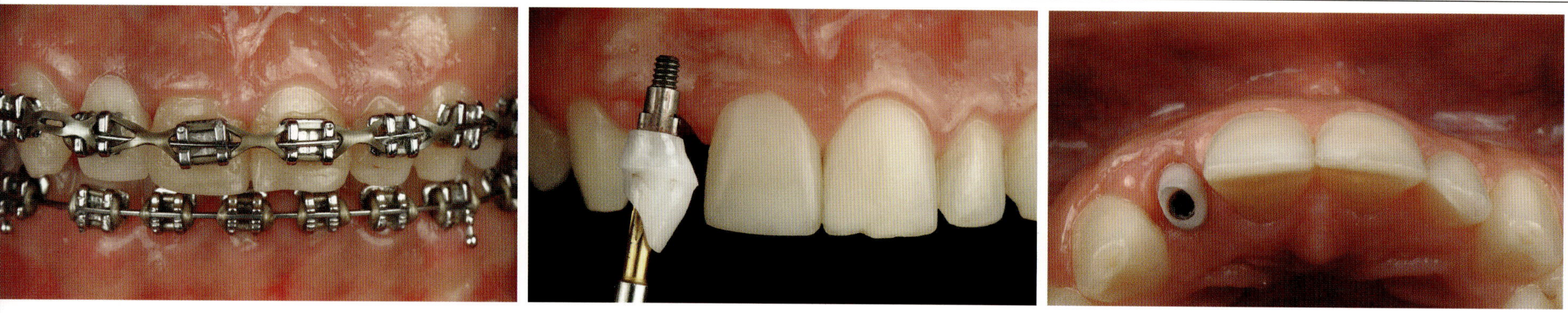

Agenesis of the maxillary right lateral incisor and palatal placement of the implant due to lack of bone. A cement-retained implant restoration provides an enhanced biologic response to the peri-implant bone and soft tissue.

Orthodontist: Dr Domingo Martín

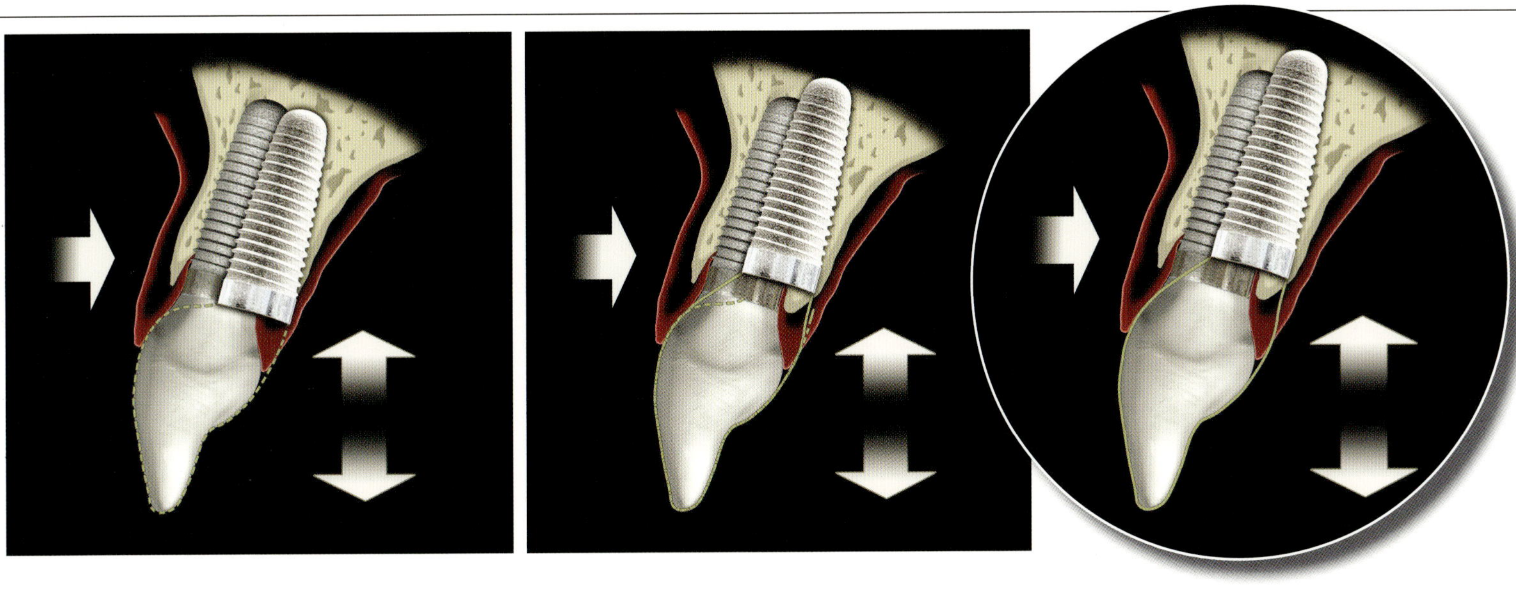

This placement concept provides long-term soft tissue stability and esthetics. The long axis of the implant should be directed between the incisal edge and the cingulum to avoid problems during the restorative phase. This implant position favors a cement-retained restoration.

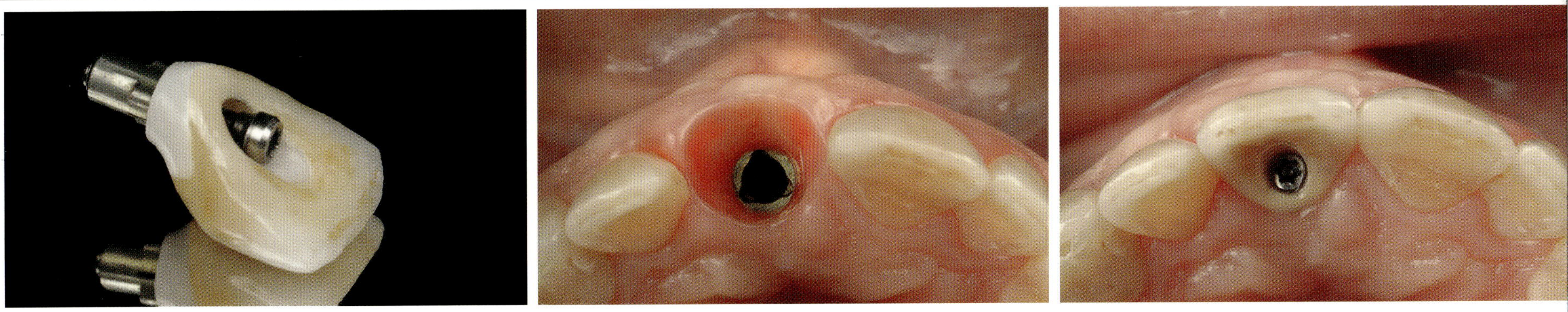

The occlusal view reveals the augmented site and the palatal position of the implant directed to the cingulum.

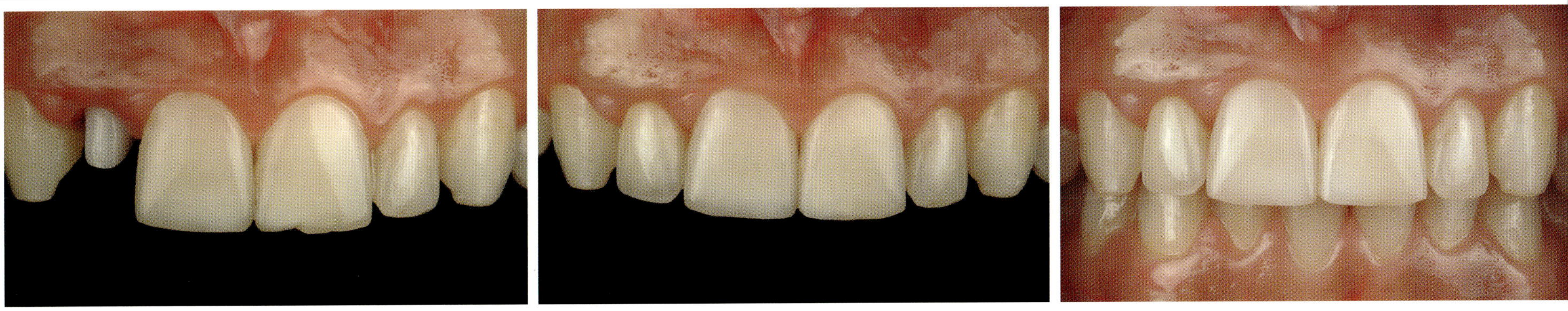

The final outcome reveals successful implant integration.

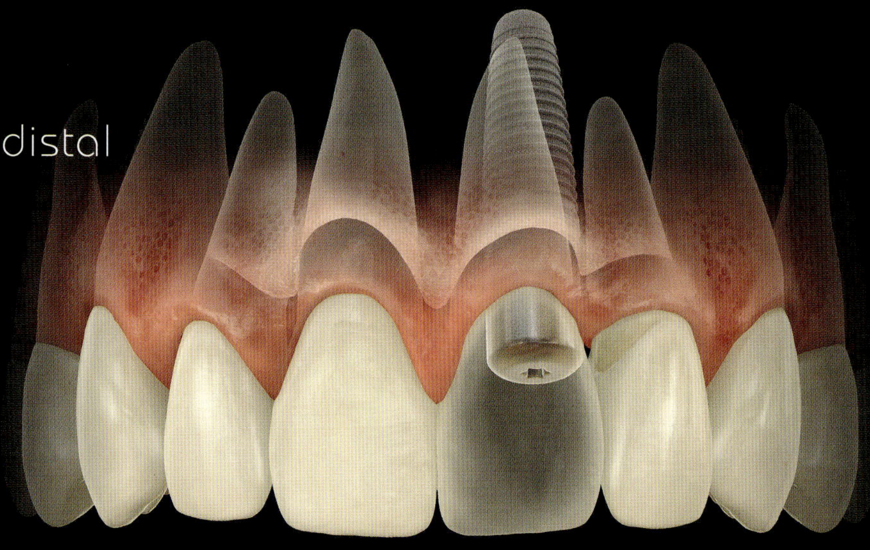
Too distal

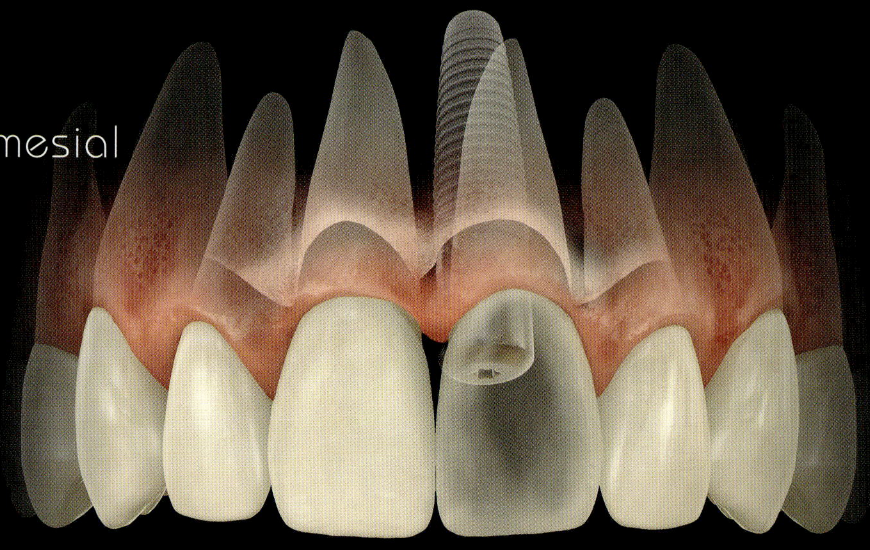
Too mesial

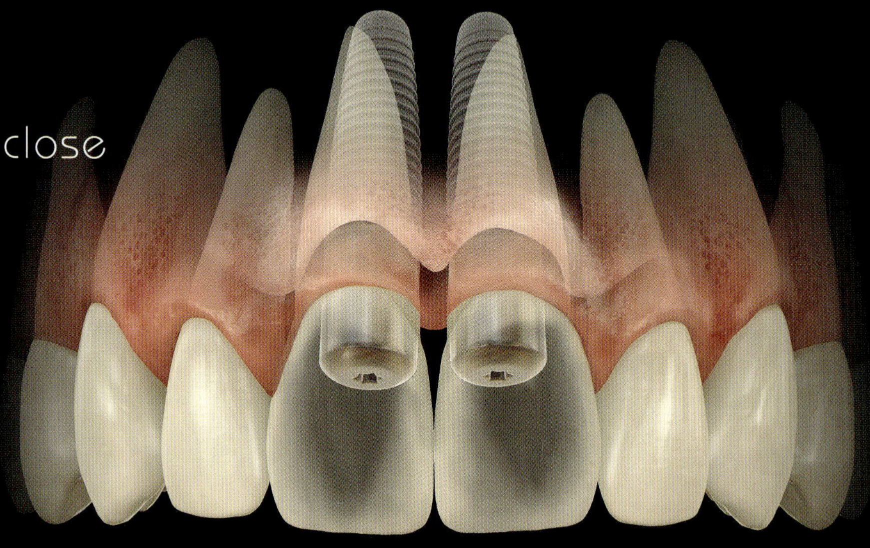
Too close

Mesiodistal position and distance requirements

The fundamental rule is that the implant should be placed in the center of the available mesiodistal space. In situations where this rule cannot be followed, implant placement slightly toward the distal provides some esthetic advantages, because the distal papillae will be hidden by the buccal contour of the tooth restoration. Mesial positioning always causes esthetic problems because it places the implant too close to the adjacent tooth, which leads to insufficient prosthetic space, encroachment of the dentogingival complex, and destruction of the interproximal bone of the adjacent tooth, resulting in a flat and unesthetic papilla. The minimum distance from the tooth to the implant should be 1.5 mm (ideally 2.0 mm). Greater distance between the tooth and the implant means better blood supply and bone support for the interproximal papilla and, consequently, a better esthetic result. Ultimately, the height of the papilla is determined by the height of the crestal bone around the adjacent tooth and not the implant.

Esthetic consequences of implant placement too mesial

In this challenging situation, the maxillary left lateral incisor had to be extracted, and the four anterior porcelain-fused-to-metal crowns needed replacement because of leakage and esthetic failure. Orthodontic treatment was performed to level the interproximal bone between the right central and lateral incisors and between the left central and lateral incisors. The left lateral incisor was then extracted, and after a 3-month healing period for bone maturation, the implant (NobelReplace Tapered with PS adapter and NP healing

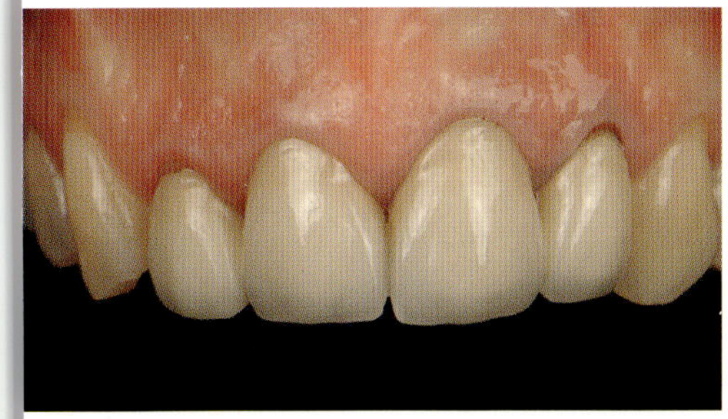
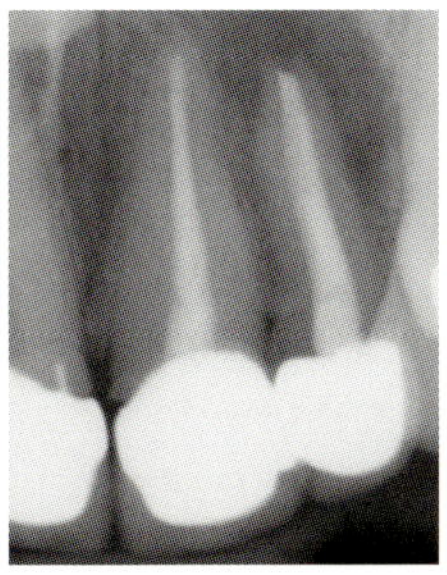
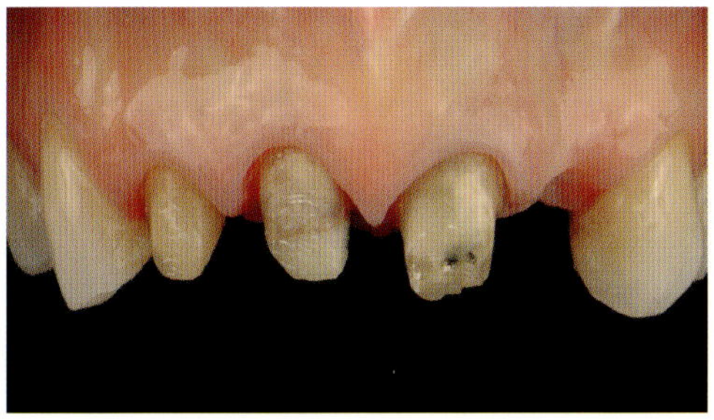
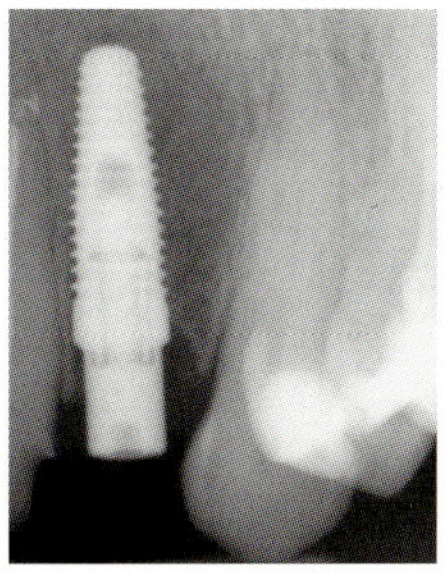
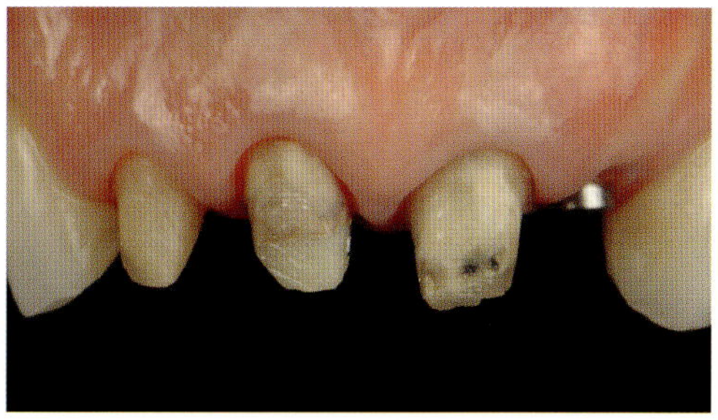

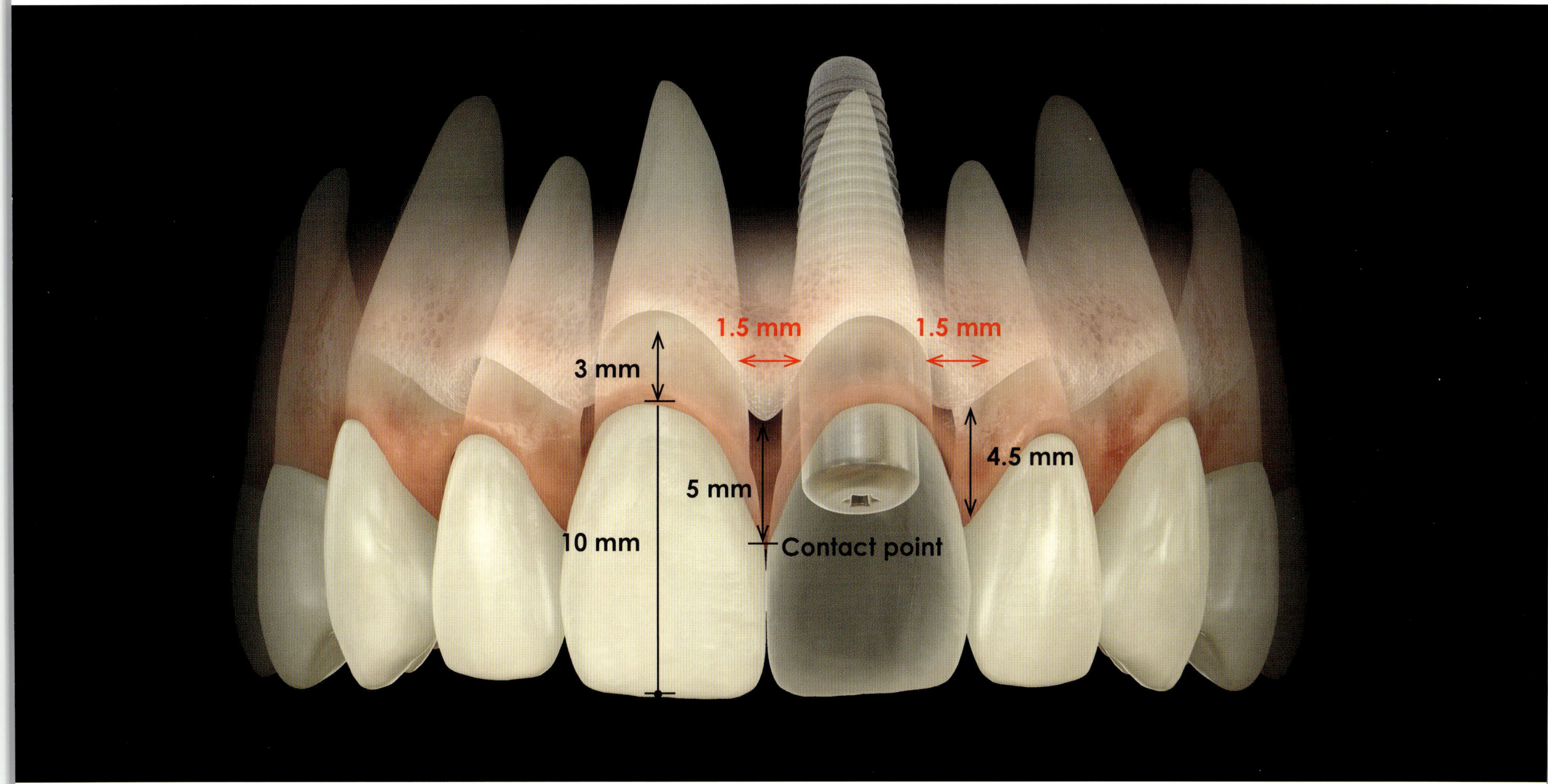

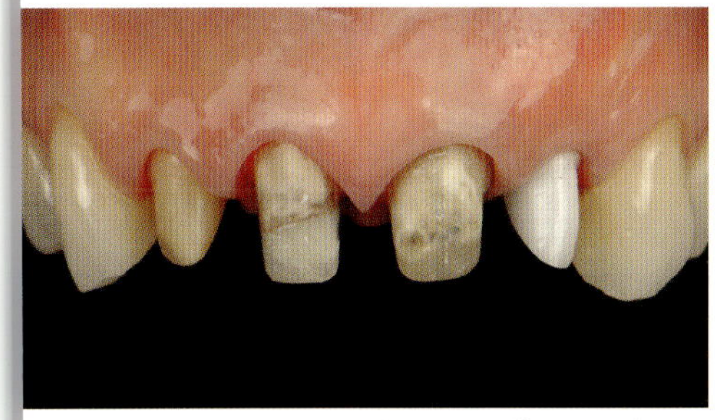
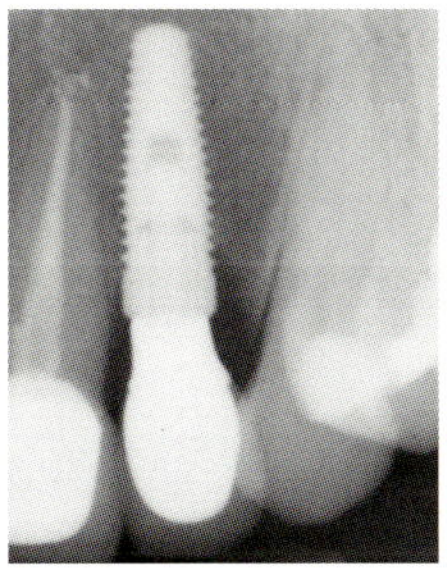
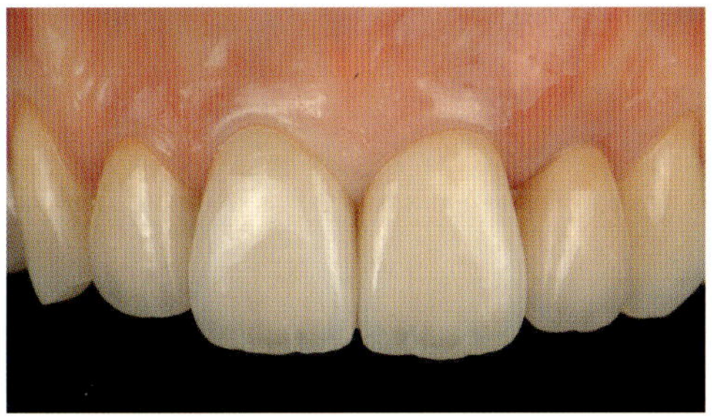
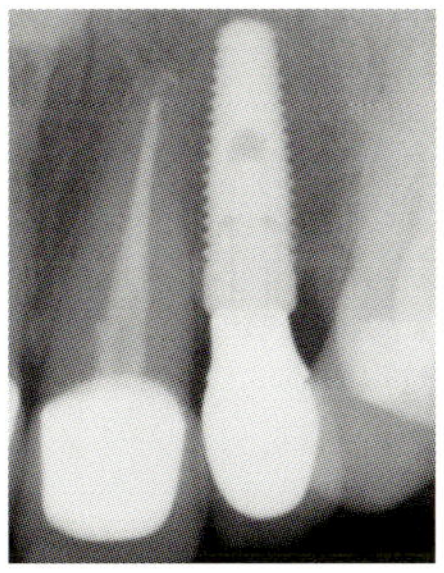
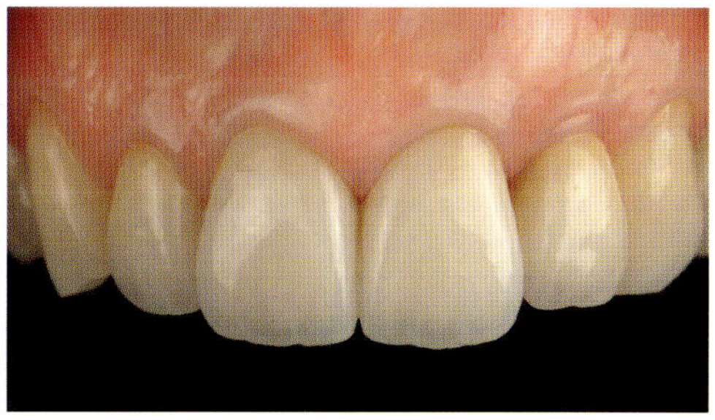

abutment) was placed together with a CTG. The implant was not placed ideally; it was positioned too close to the distal aspect of the left central incisor.

Between final cementation and the 5-year follow-up, the distal papilla lost both height and volume. One can speculate that without application of the PS concept, the papilla loss may have been even more severe. PS relieves the stress on the crestal bone of the adjacent tooth and, therefore, seems to limit its resorption.

Esthetic consequences of adjacent implants placed too close together

Both central incisors were extracted due to excessive loss of tooth structure. A staged immediate implant placement sequence was applied to limit bone and soft tissue resorption typical for this type of treatment. First, an implant was placed in the position of the left central incisor. This implant, how-

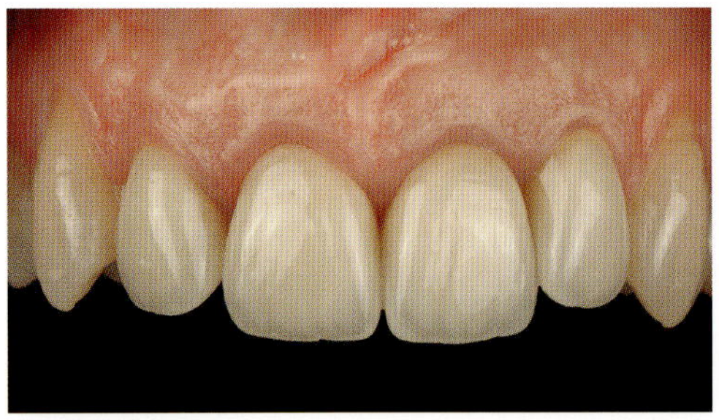

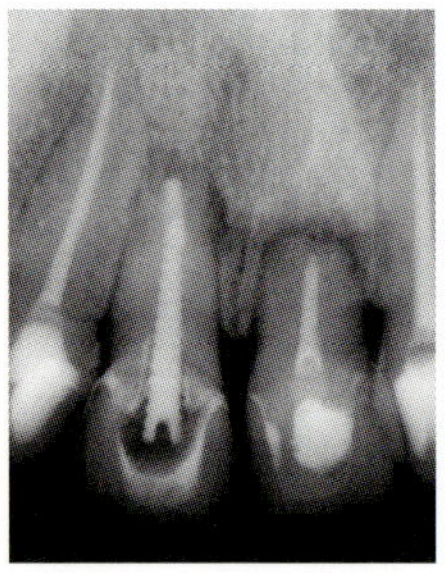

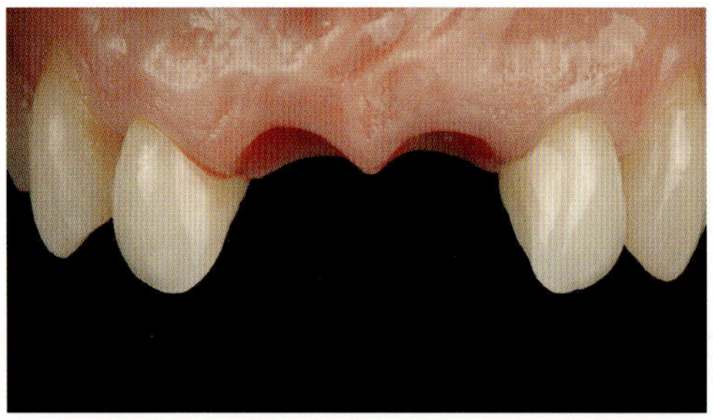

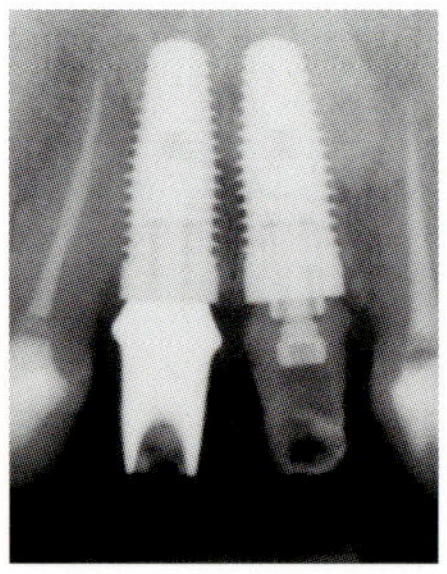

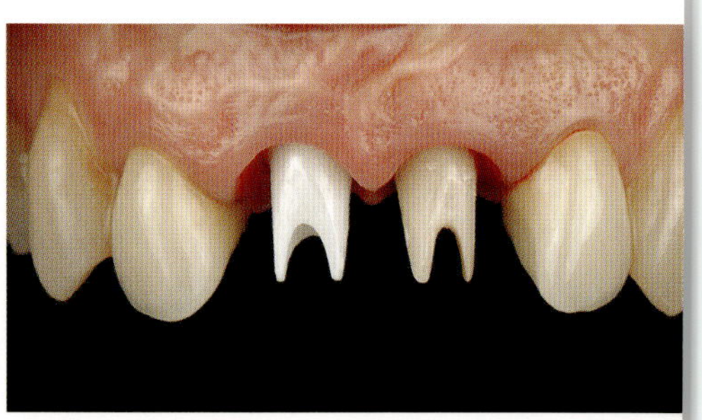

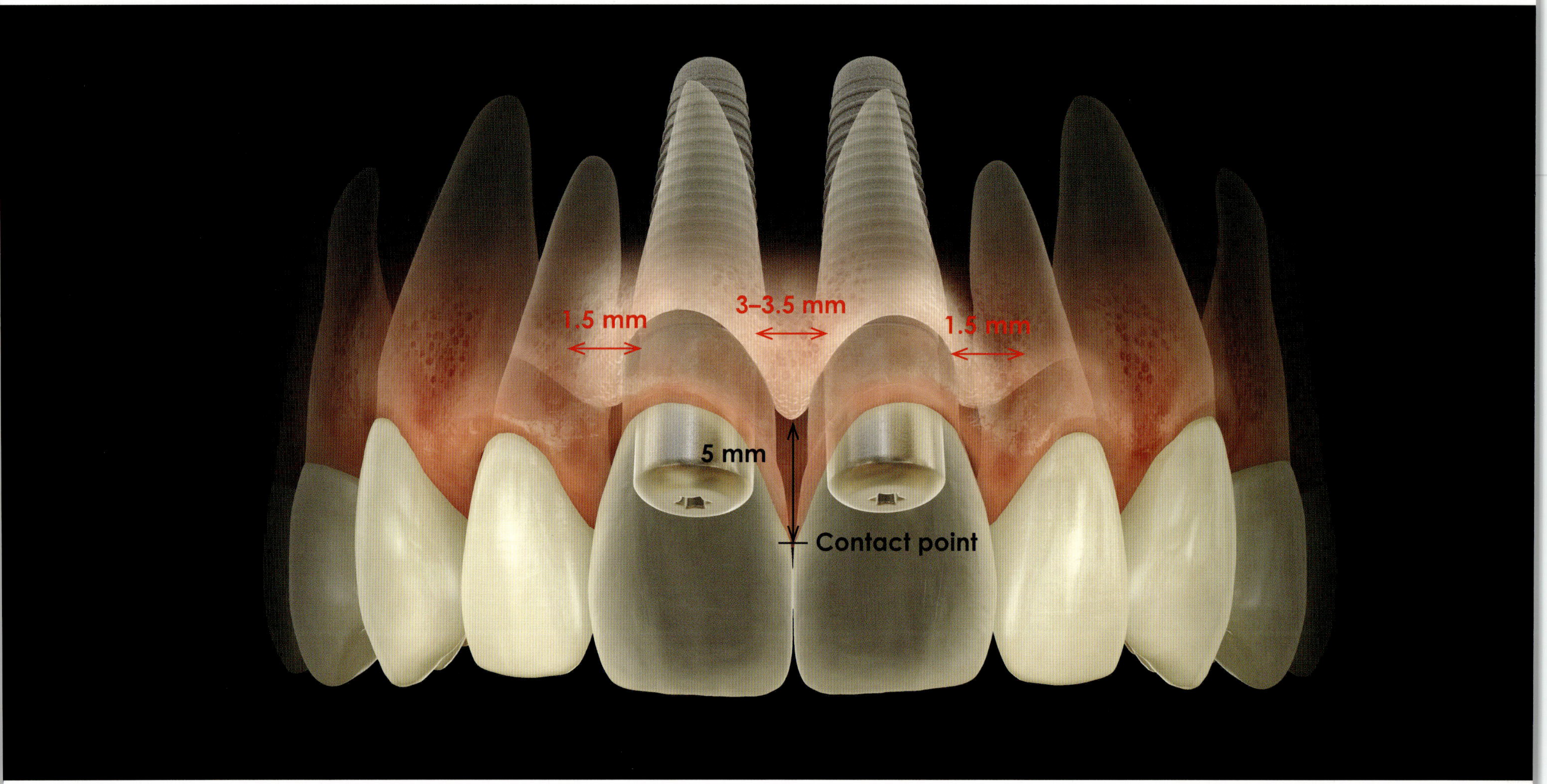

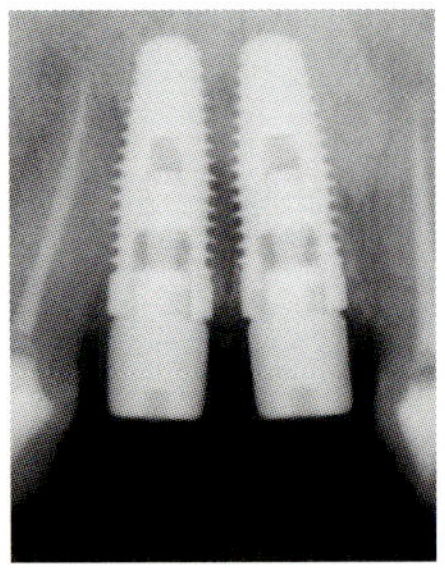

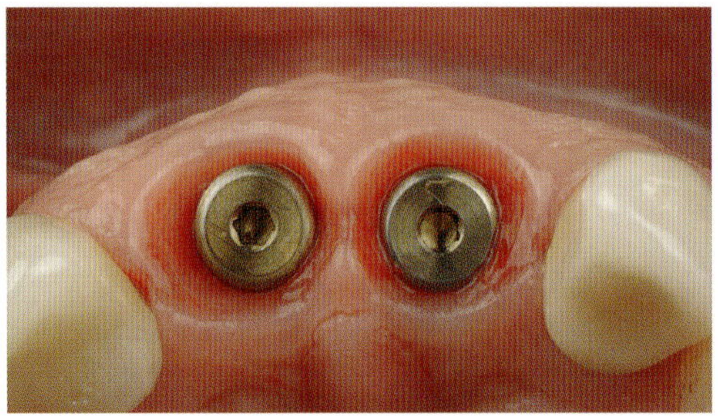

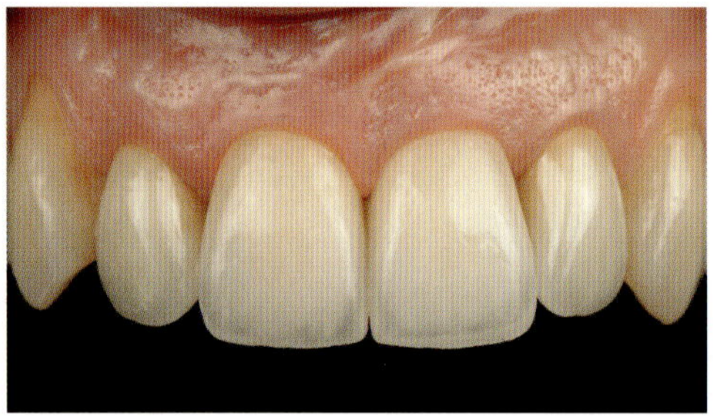

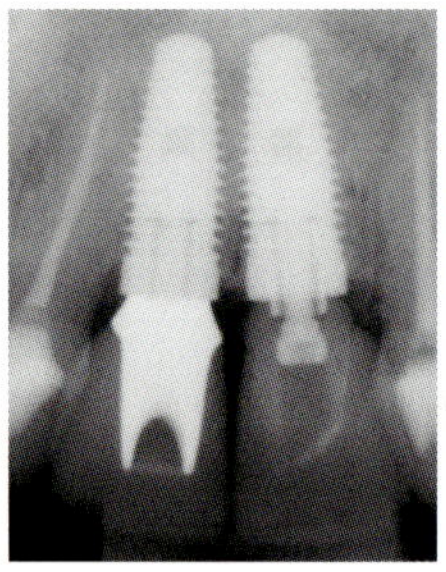

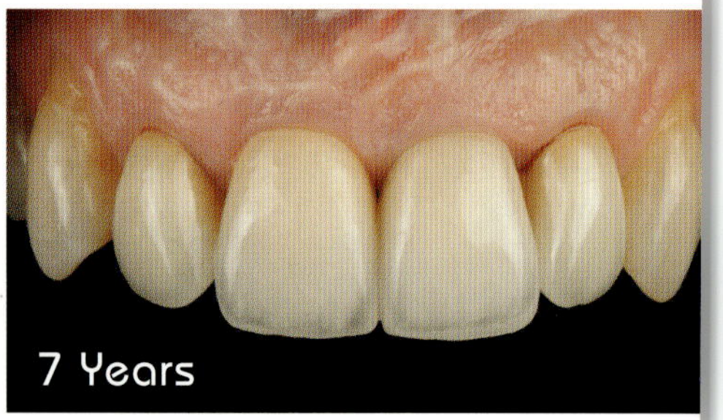

ever, was inclined too mesially, making the insertion of the second implant in the position of the right central incisor 6 months later very difficult. Consequently, the implants were positioned too close to each other. The definitive restorations were delivered after 1 year of provisionalization. The 7-year postoperative photograph and periapical radiograph show the magnitude of the resorption and the flattening of the interproximal papillae.

Mandibular central incisors

Both mandibular central incisors had to be extracted because of periodontal problems. With an immediate implant placement protocol, two NobelActive 3.0 implants were inserted with customized

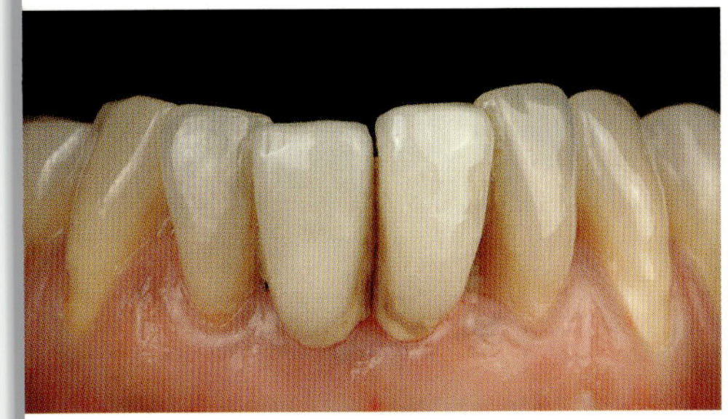
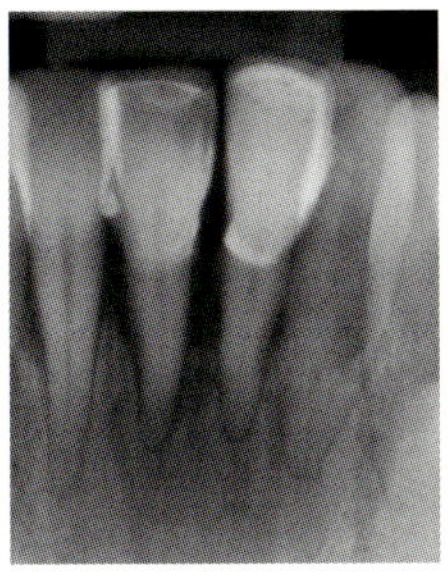
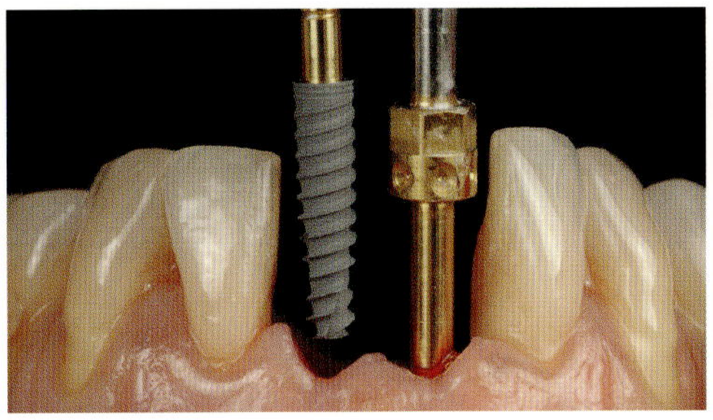
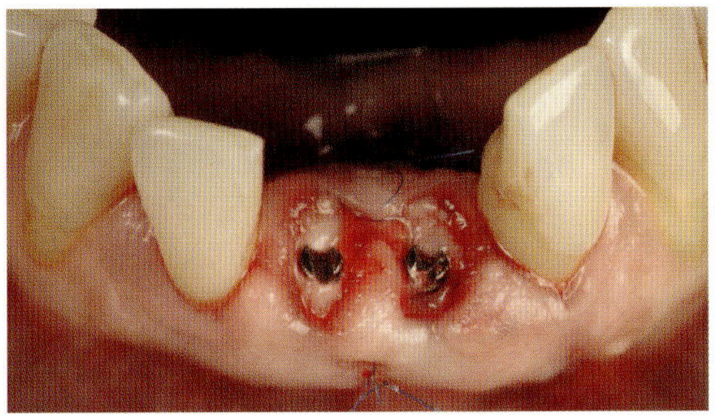
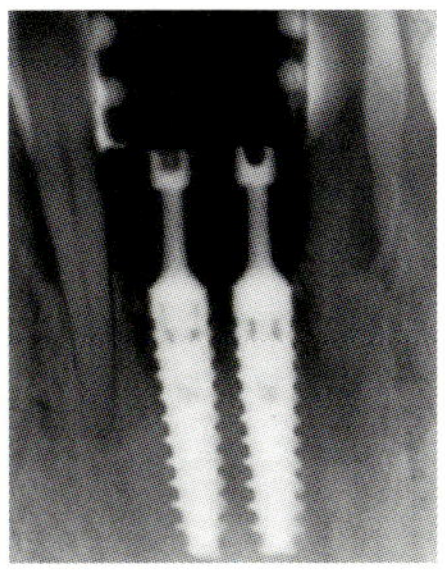

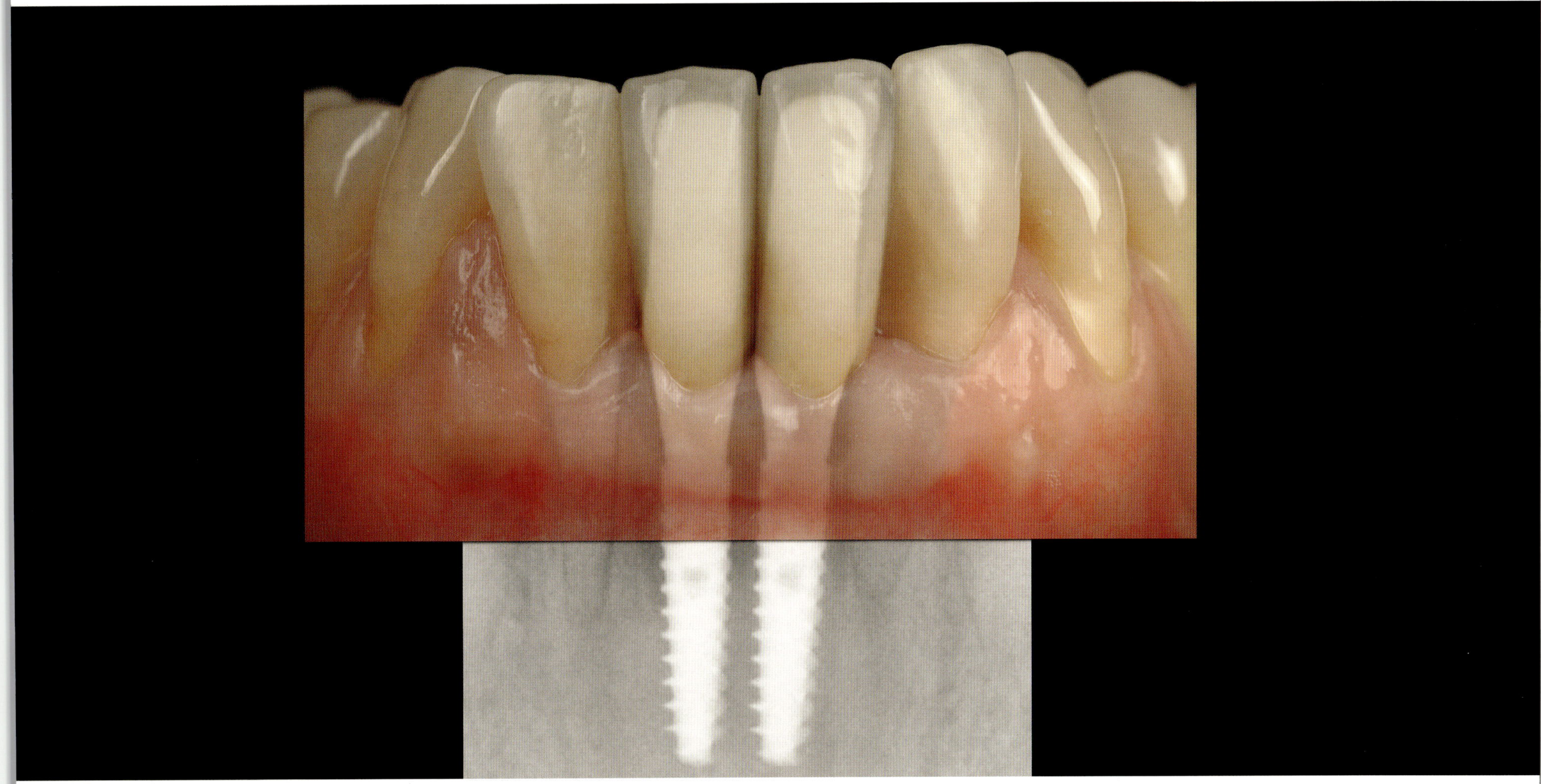

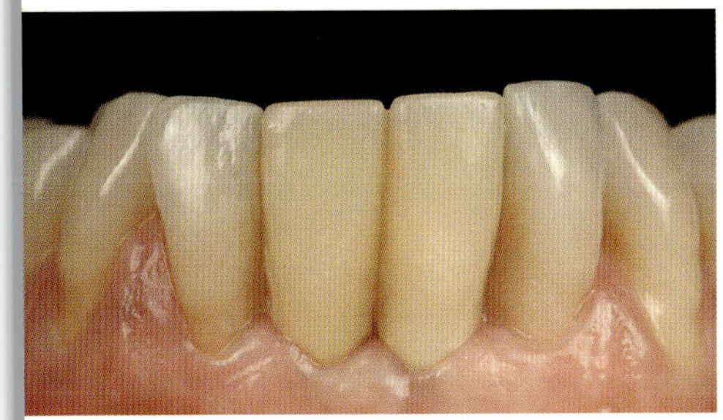
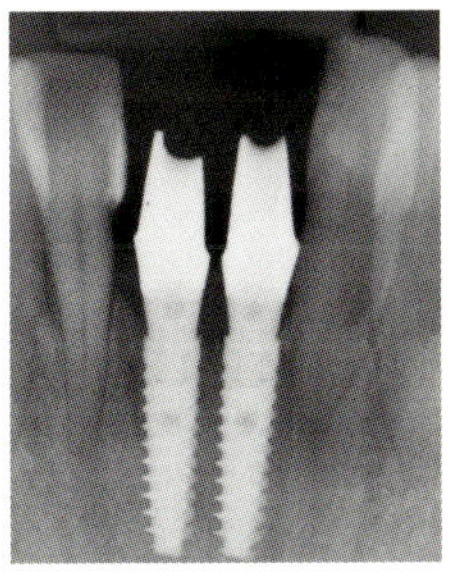
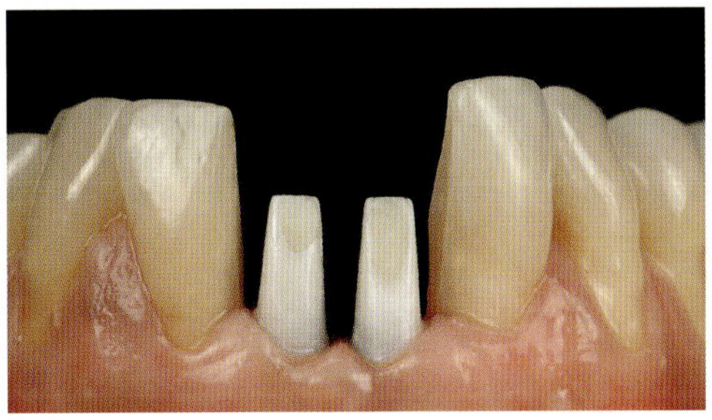
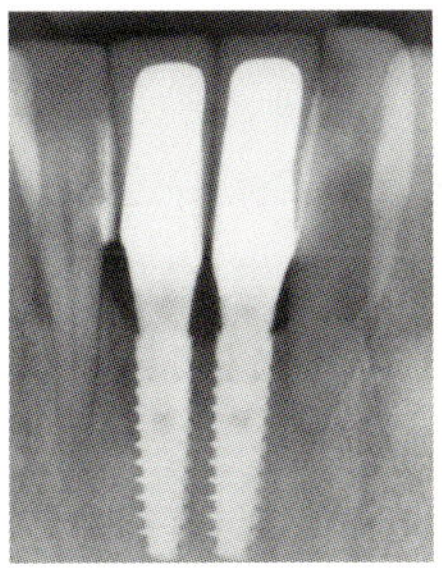
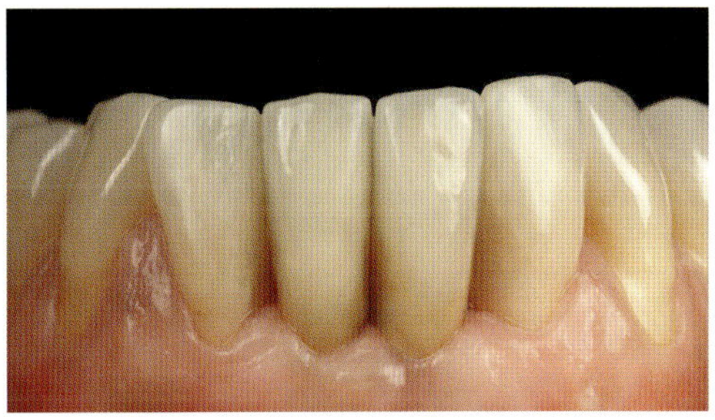

provisional healing abutments to provide maximum space for the CTG. Definitive zirconia abutments were inserted on the first day of the provisional phase and not removed thereafter, which led to a satisfactory outcome.

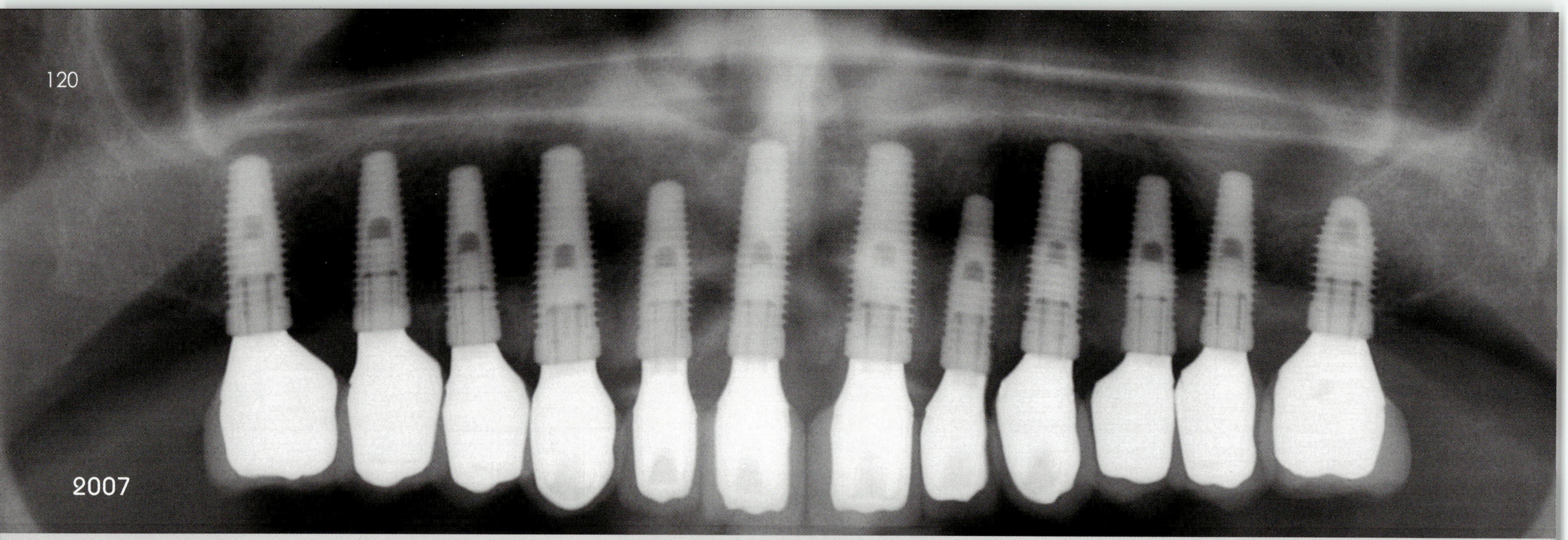

Placement of multiple implants

Especially in situations where full-arch rehabilitations are necessary, proper case selection during the treatment-planning stage becomes a crucial factor. Better outcomes are typically achieved in patients with a thick tissue biotype and thick buccal plates. This patient presented with biomechanical problems resulting from insufficient remaining tooth structure and functional complications. One implant (NobelReplace Tapered) was placed per tooth. PS adapters and definitive custom zirconia abutments were inserted the same day, while augmentative procedures were not employed. The only obvious recession was on the maxillary left central and lateral incisors.

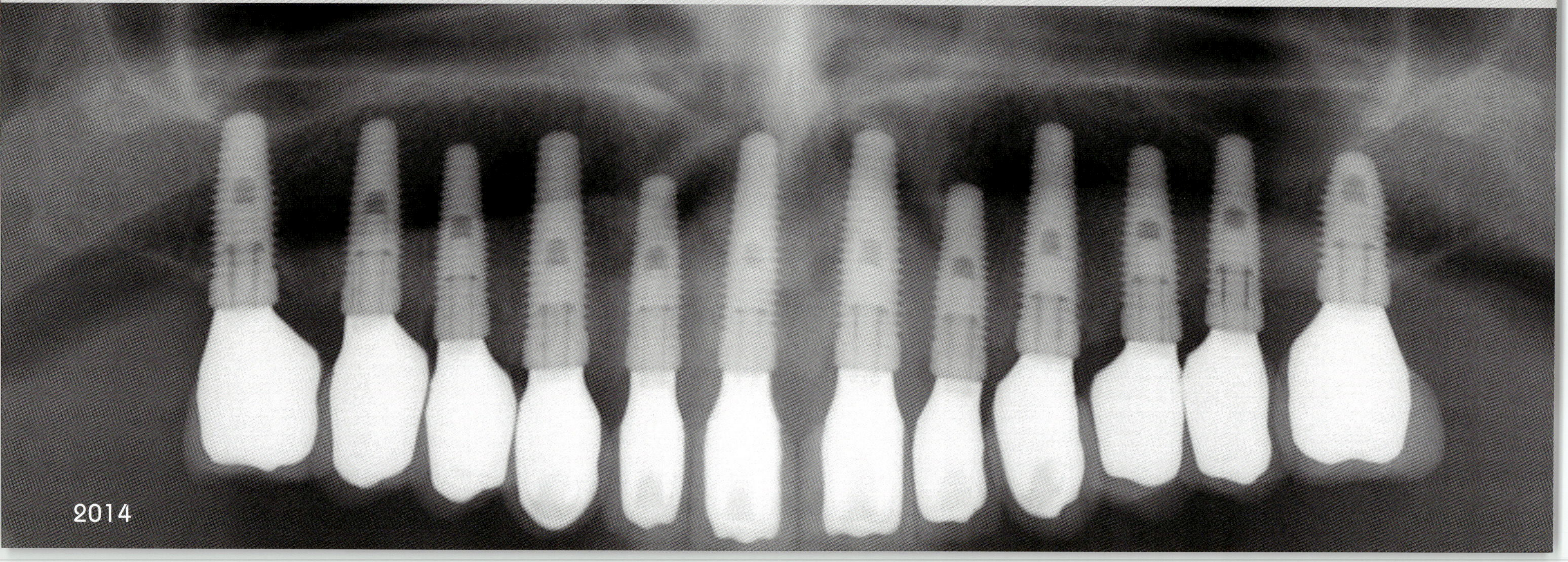

The 1-year and 5-year recall radiographs and clinical photographs reveal that a combination of proper patient selection, atraumatic surgery with a flapless immediate implant placement, and same-day abutment placement with the PS concept seems to be pertinent for a satisfactory outcome.

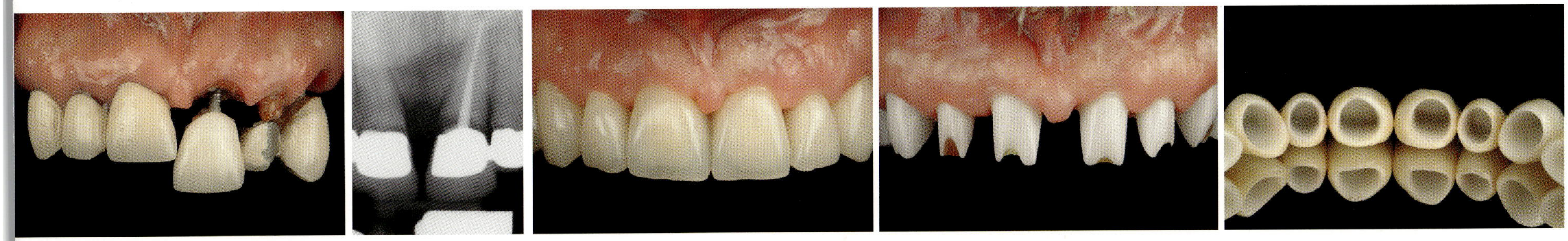

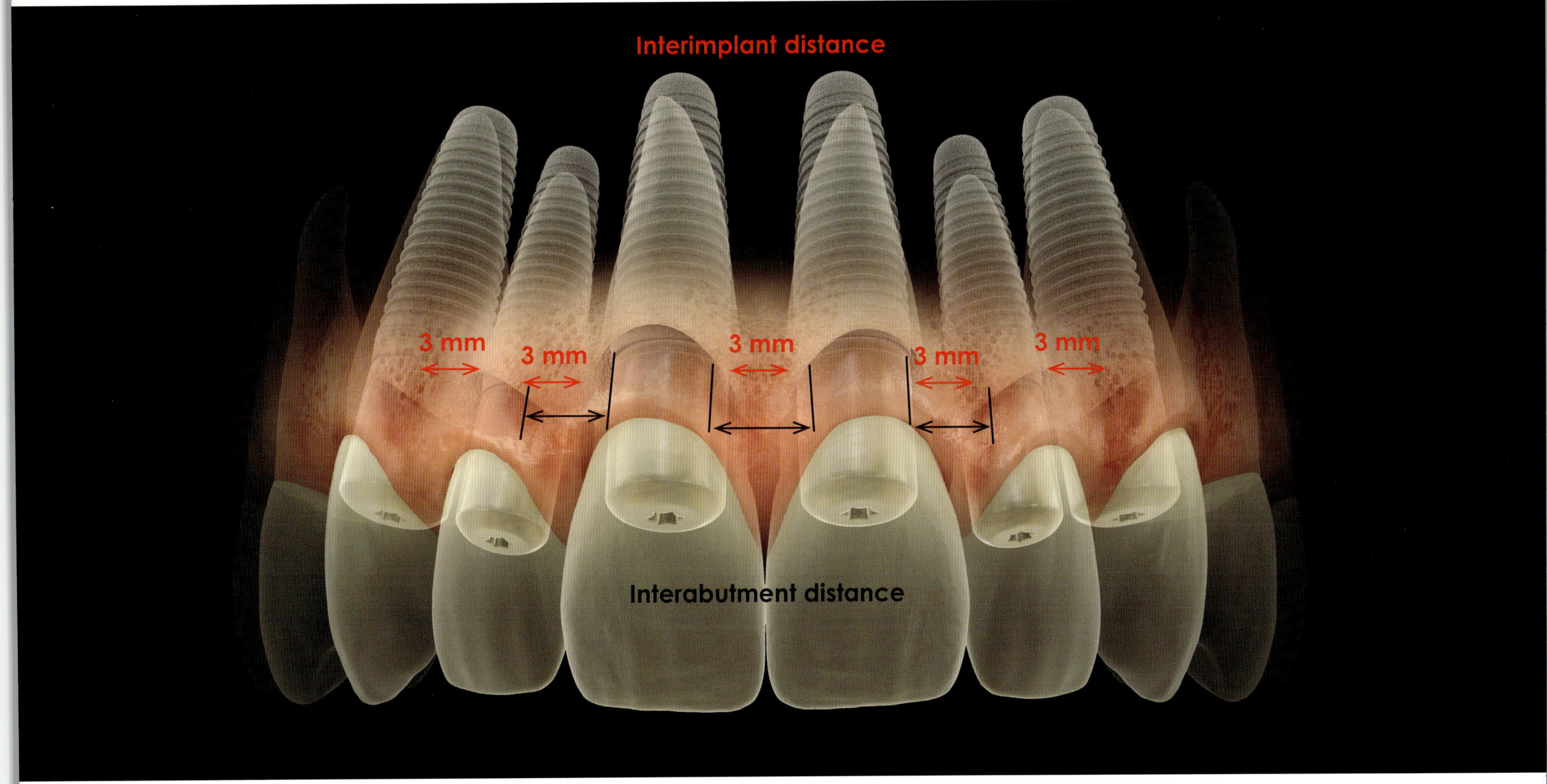

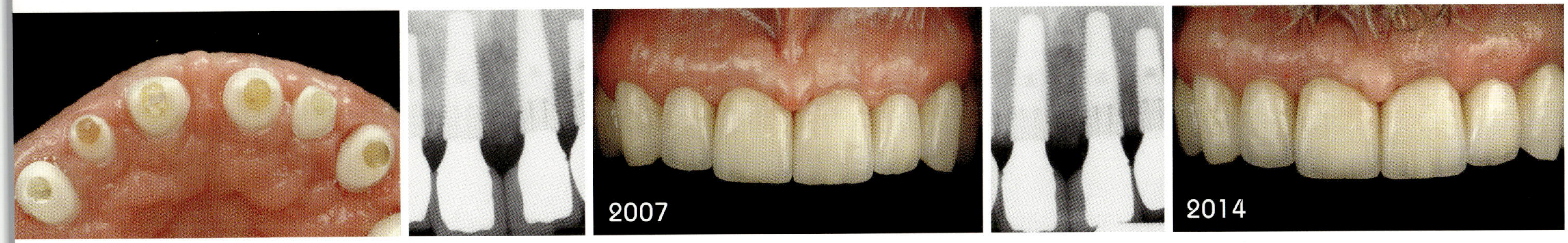

Even though the interimplant distances were minimal, the interabutment distances were increased with the PS concept, which allows for greater soft tissue volume and, therefore, reduced stresses on the tissue at the abutment-implant interface and enhanced soft tissue vascularization.

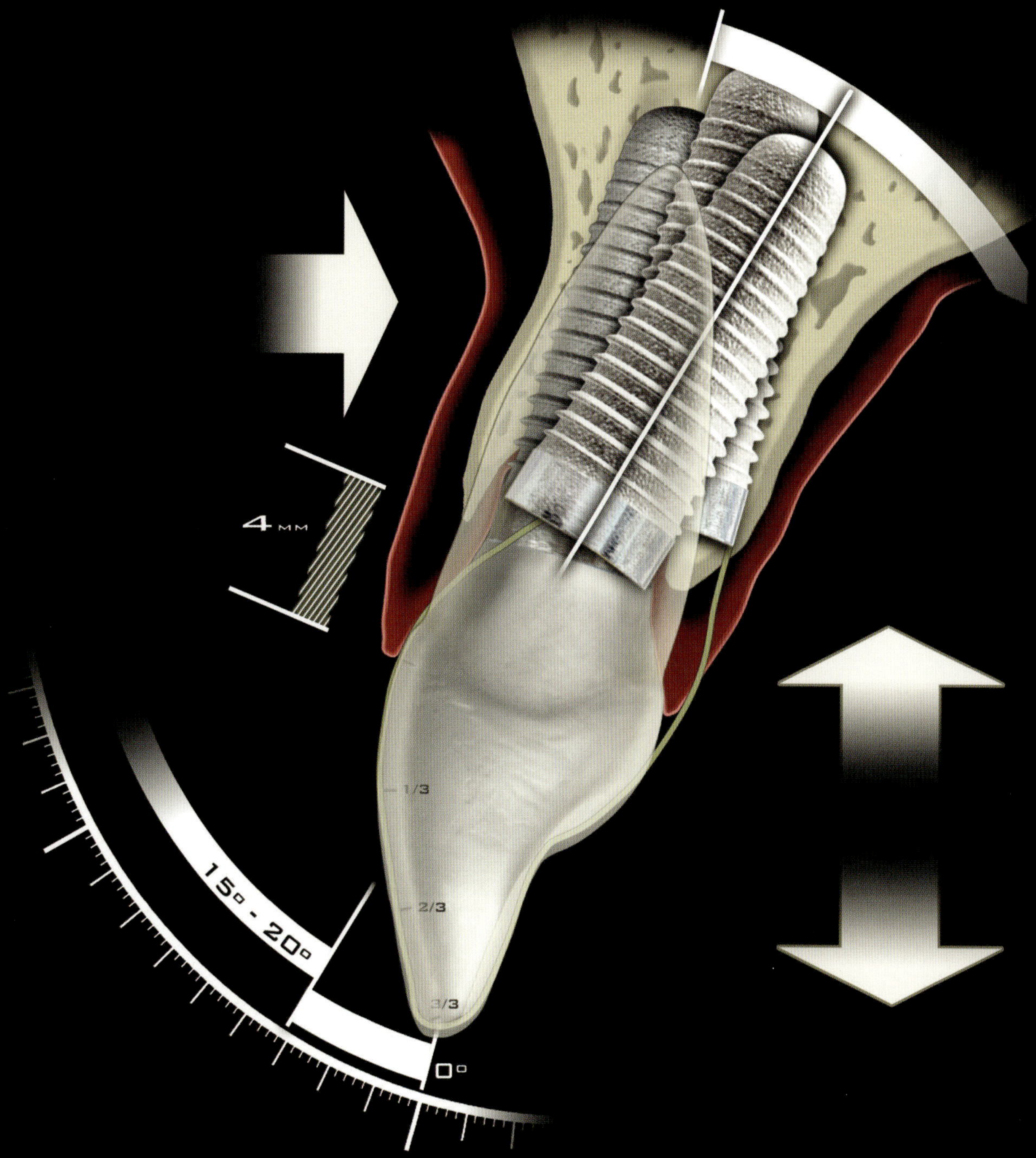
4 MM
1/3
2/3
3/3
15° - 20°
0°

Angulation

The reference for implant placement angulation is the incisal edge of the tooth to be restored or that of the neighboring teeth present. Angulation is probably the most difficult position to visualize once a flap is opened. As a hint, one of the best ways to visualize the angulation while placing the implant is to "virtually" divide the buccal contour of the tooth to be replaced or the adjacent ones into thirds: incisal, middle, and gingival. The long axis of the implant should be directed as closely as possible to the incisal edge as an extension of the crown. This resembles the morphology of natural anterior teeth and, therefore, facilitates the creation of a natural emergence profile.

In the event that the angulation and inclination axis of the implant is oriented too far buccally and more toward the middle than the incisal third of the tooth, a prosthetic compensation is easily possible, as the angulation will be between 15 and 20 degrees from the ideal, incisal edge–oriented position. However, when the long axis of the implant points toward the gingival third of the buccal contour, compensation with prosthetic components and an acceptable outcome are not possible.

This simple and imaginary division of the tooth into thirds and sagittal verification while placing the implant is a helpful way to control the correct implant positioning during surgery.

An implant placed with the long axis toward the palatal aspect of the prospective tooth makes it more difficult to create an adequate emergence profile. In the event of a palatal angulation, the depth of the implant becomes a crucial factor for the possibility to compensate for such a mistake through prosthetic means. A common approach to compensate for nonideal implant angulation and depth due to surgical errors is the use of implant components made from nonmetallic esthetic materials (eg, zirconia abutments). Structural, morphologic, and mechanical considerations need to be understood before using this type of abutment. Zirconia, for example, needs a minimum thickness of about 0.8 mm to withstand occlusal functional loads without fracture. These fundamental material thickness requirements are often not followed, especially in the area of the screw access hole, where supporting walls can be rather thin. Understanding these basic concepts suggests that if a screw access hole is located too far buccally within the gingival third, the minimal thickness requirement for zirconia may be compromised. In such cases, titanium abutments should be used for biomechanical reasons and strength. Screw-retained implant-supported restorations are not as limited by material thickness requirements because they do not involve a separate abutment. Here, the screw access hole should be located slightly further to the palatal aspect, ideally in the area of the cingulum of the prospective tooth.

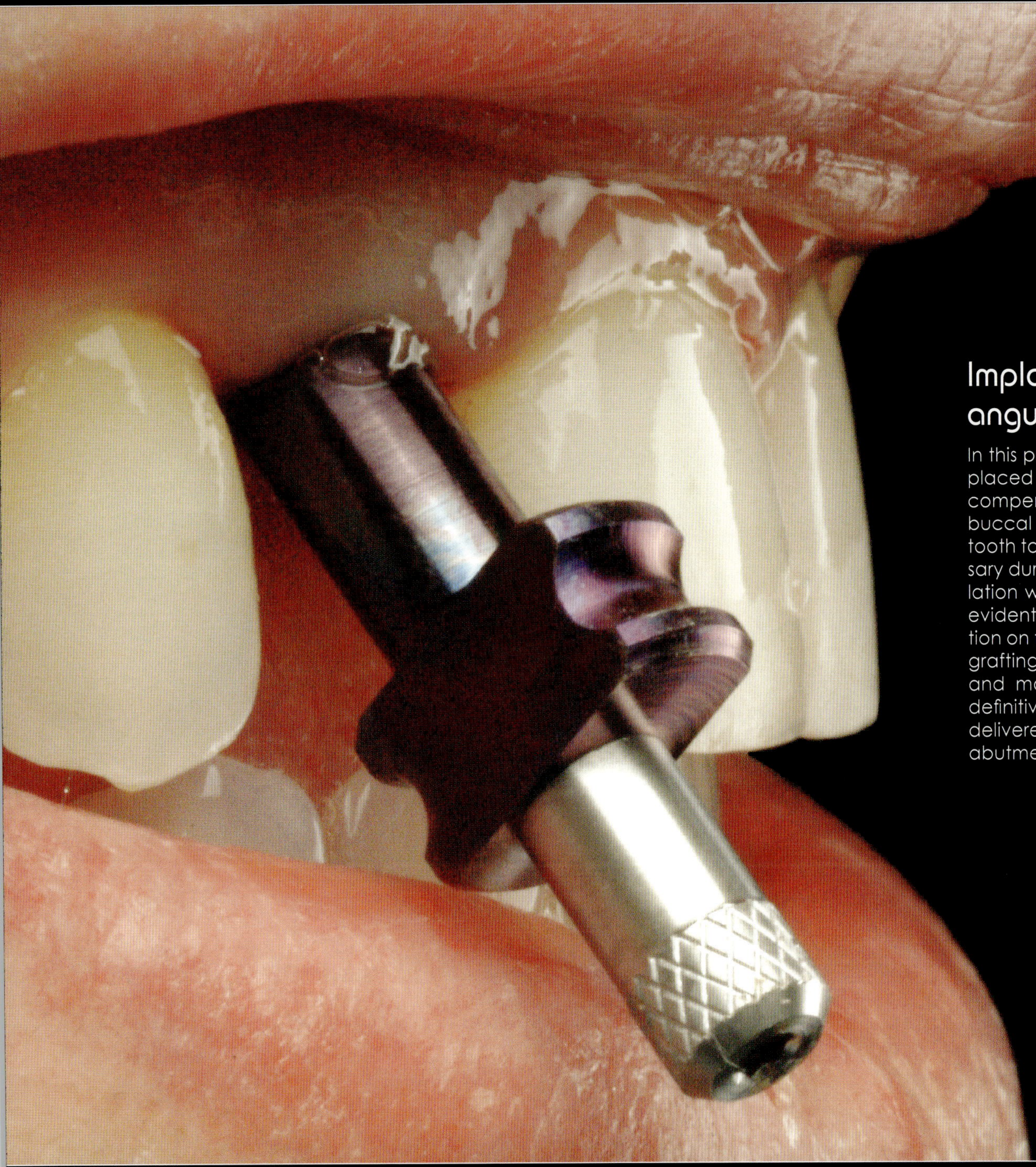

Implant with too much angulation

In this patient with dental agenesis, implants were placed in an angulated manner with a CTG to compensate for deficient tissue volume. The three buccal planes (thirds) are marked on the adjacent tooth to visualize the amount of angulation necessary during implant placement. The implant angulation with respect to the prosthetic angulation is evident during relining of the provisional restoration on the prepared abutment. Connective tissue grafting was performed to provide tissue volume and mask the abutment-implant interface. The definitive zirconia-based crown restoration was delivered with the intention to block out the dark abutment substructure.

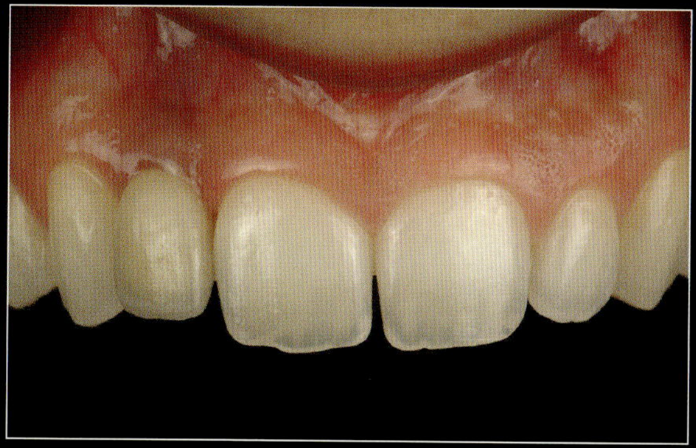

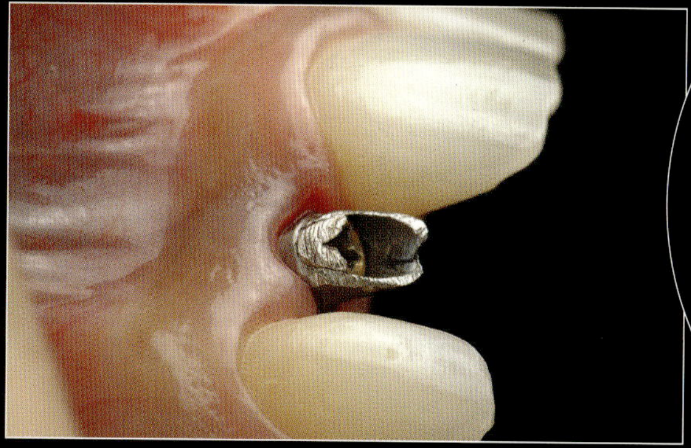

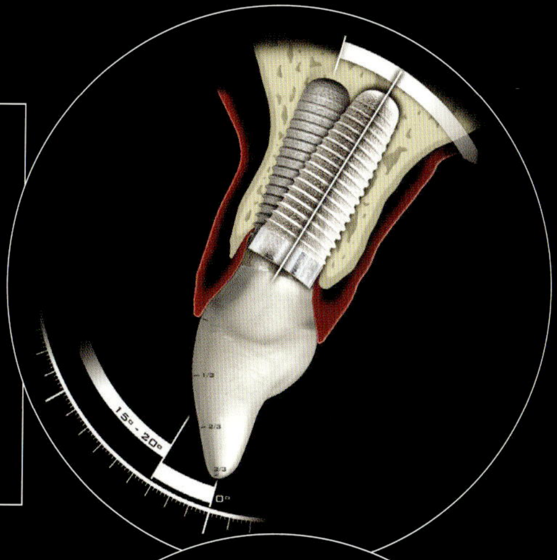
15° - 20°
0°

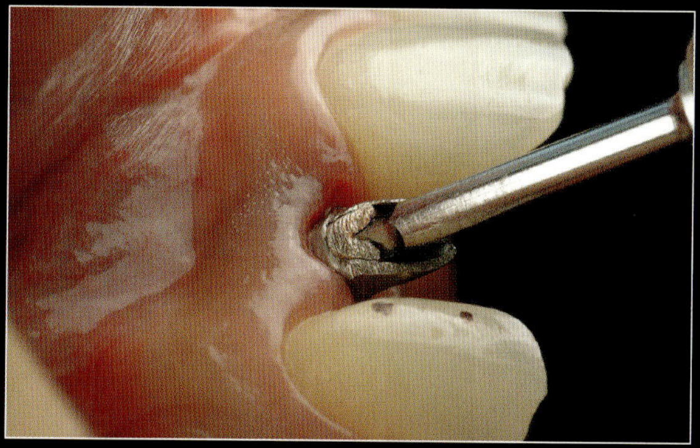

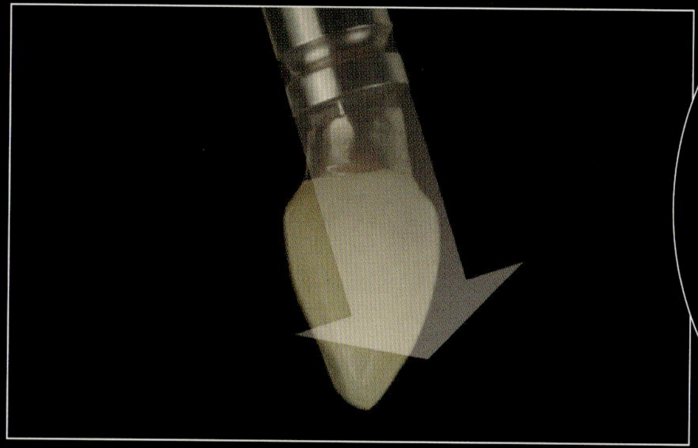

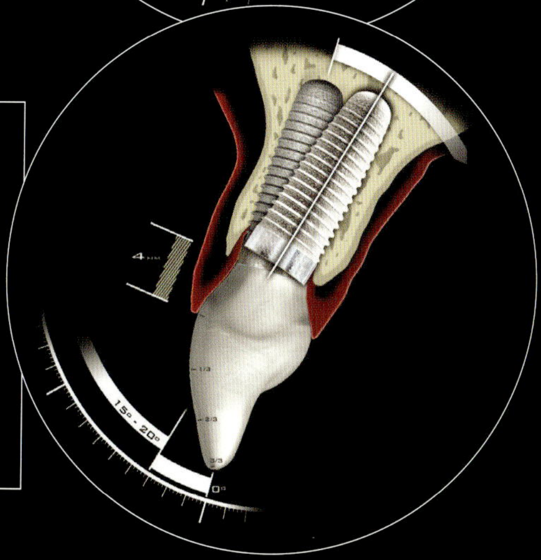
15° - 20°
0°

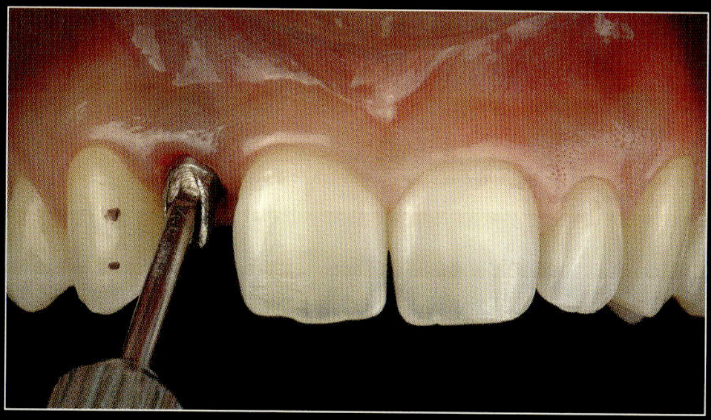

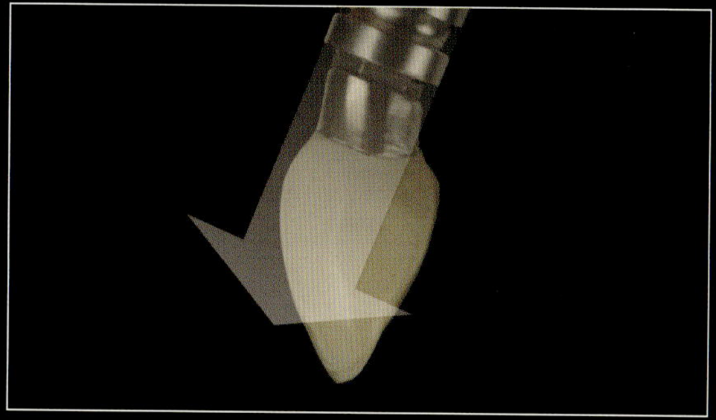

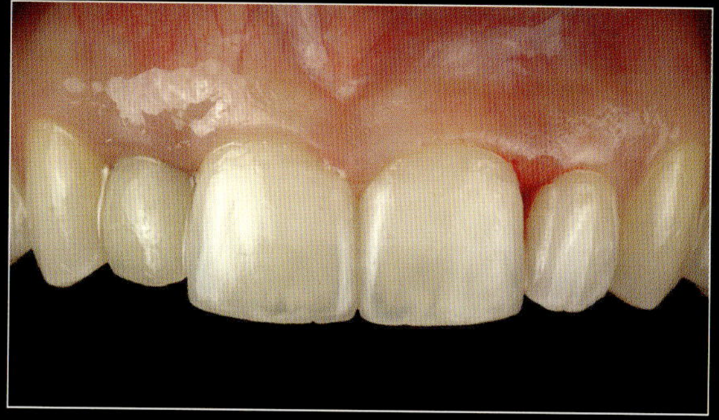

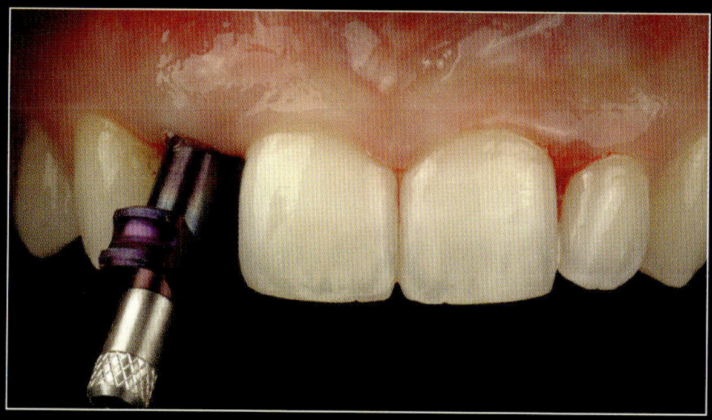

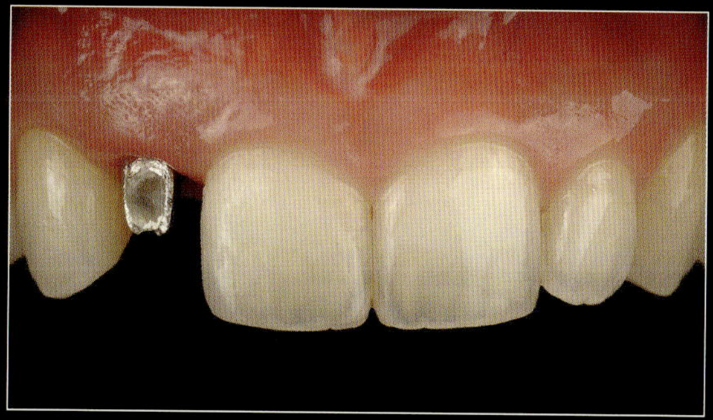

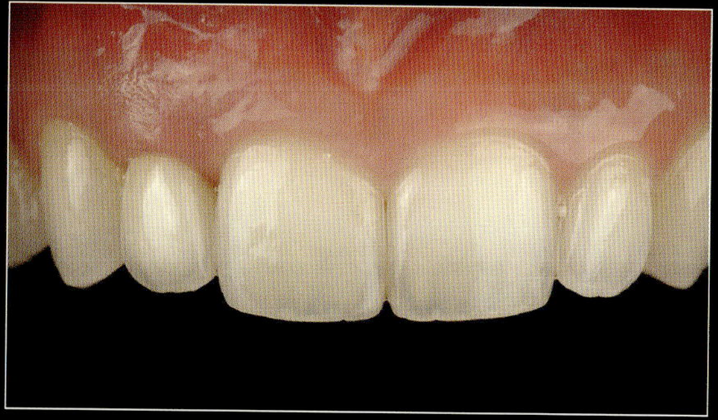

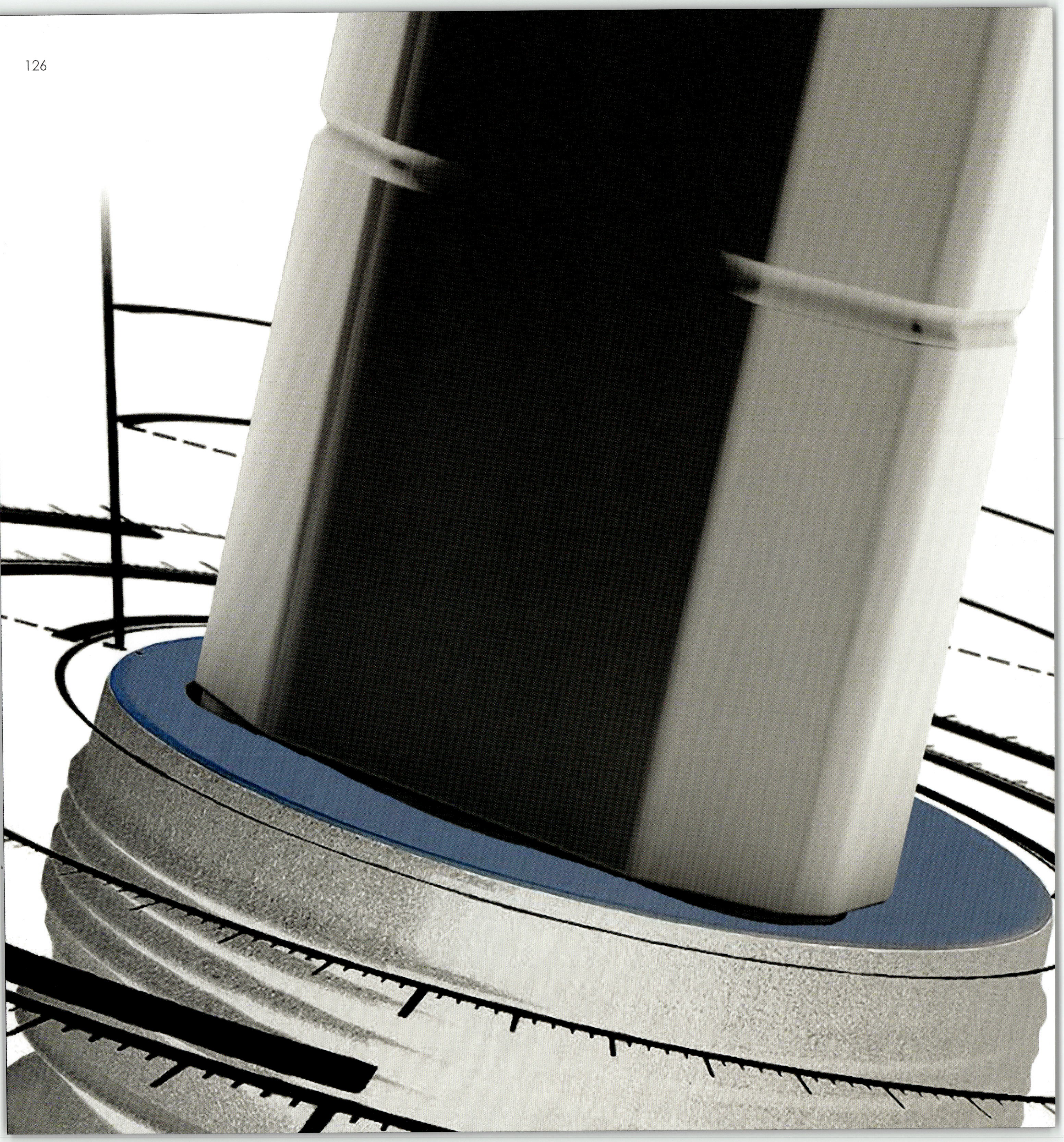

Depth and orientation

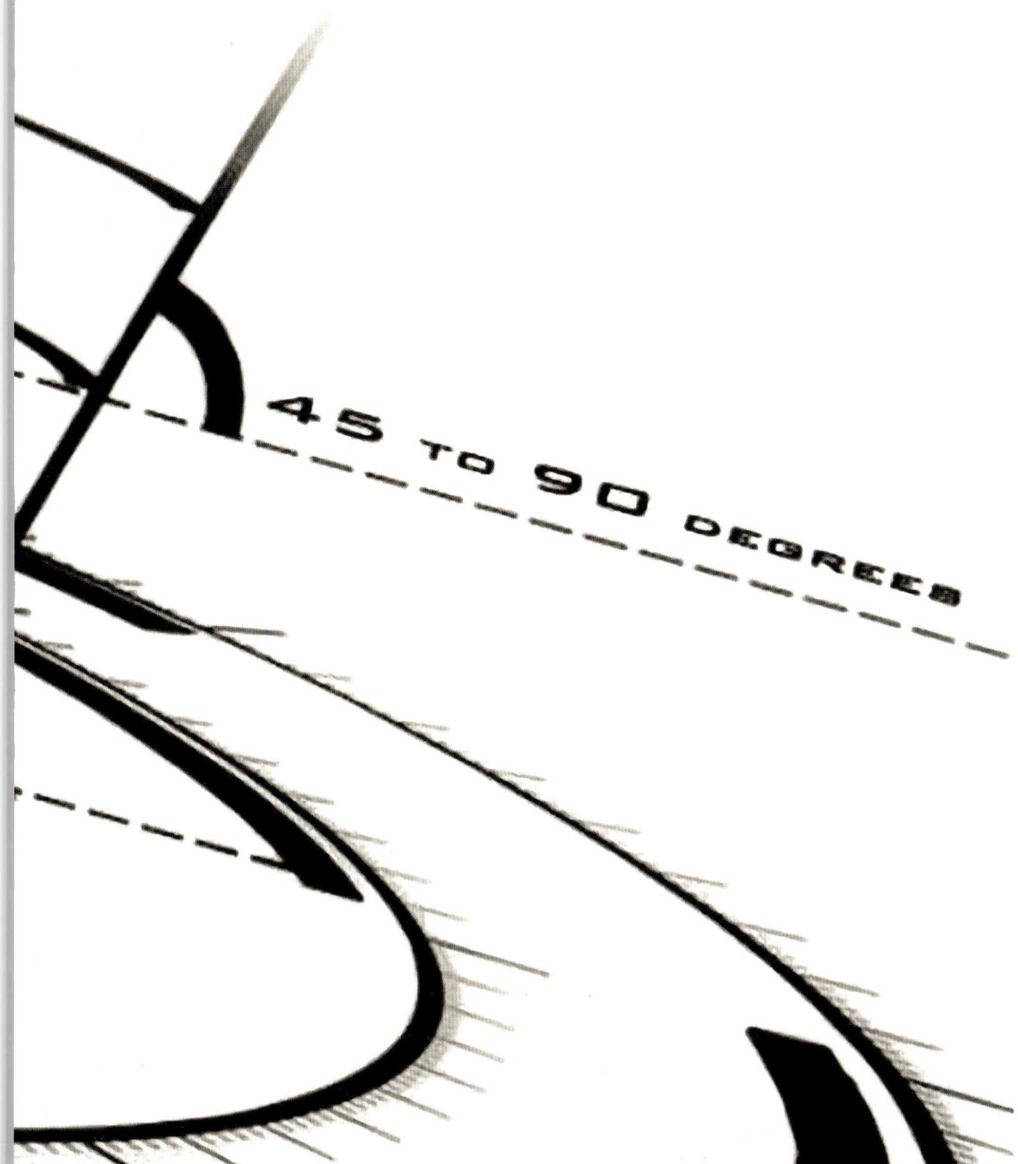

Implant depth

Depth of the implant is one of the most important parameters for functional and esthetic success and must be determined during treatment planning because it dictates the type of implant connection design selected. The implant should be placed below tissue in the "comfortable zone" or "safe zone" to hide and mask the restoration–implant connection interface. Implant connections (internal or external) and the type of design allow different implant positioning depths. While an internal Morse taper connection can be placed subcrestally, conventional internal or external connections must be placed crestally or supracrestally, depending on the macrodesign of the implant collar.

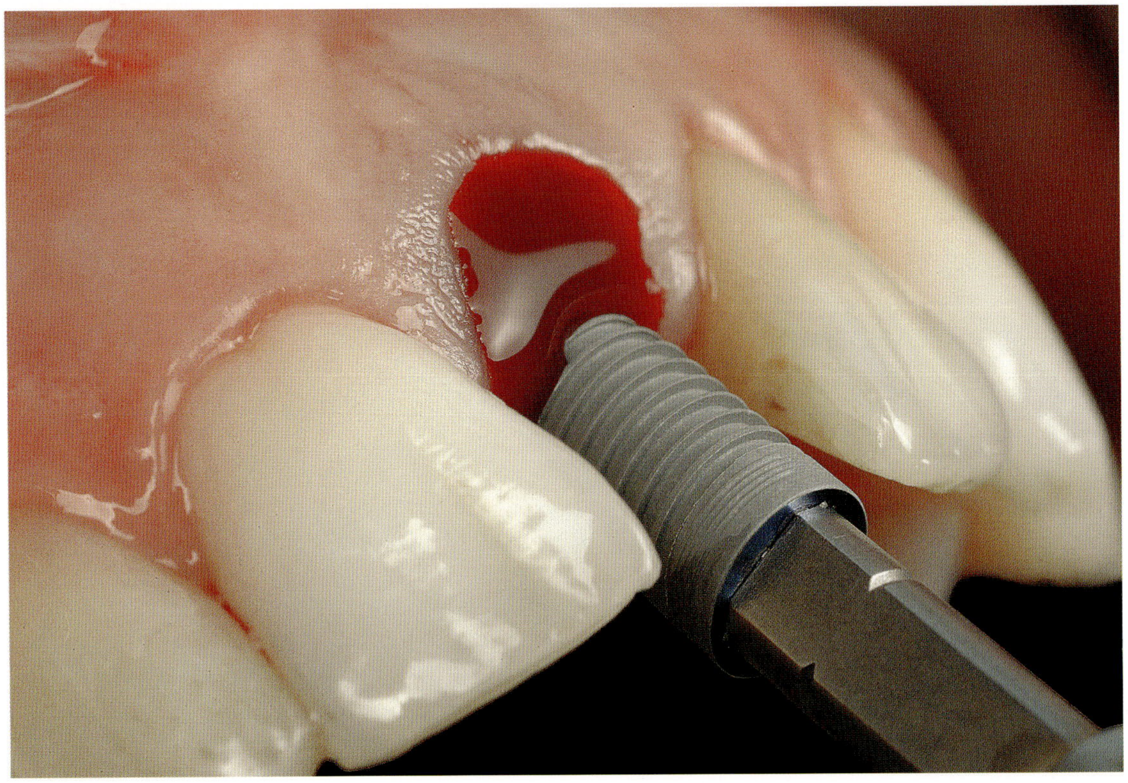

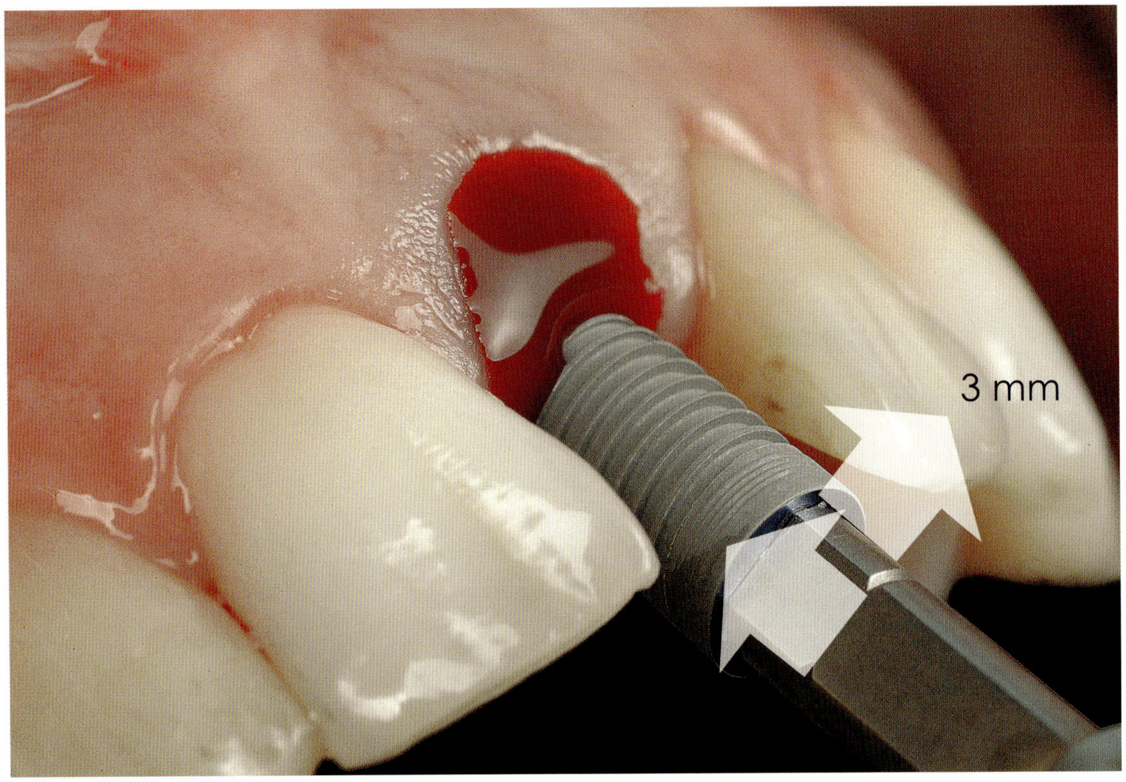

The deeper the implant, the more complex the restorative phase because of the interaction with the interproximal bone. Ideally, the implant shoulder should be placed 3 to 4 mm apical to the prospective gingival margin, which has to be created through the provisional restoration. The reference used during implant placement is the adjacent tooth for the central incisors or the contralateral tooth for canines and lateral incisors. Bone level can also serve as a reference for the lateral incisors. However, because the gingival margin around lateral incisors is typically positioned more coronal than that on central incisors, it is important not to position implants replacing lateral incisors at the same level as the central incisors when attempting to re-create the horizontal symmetry seen in nature.

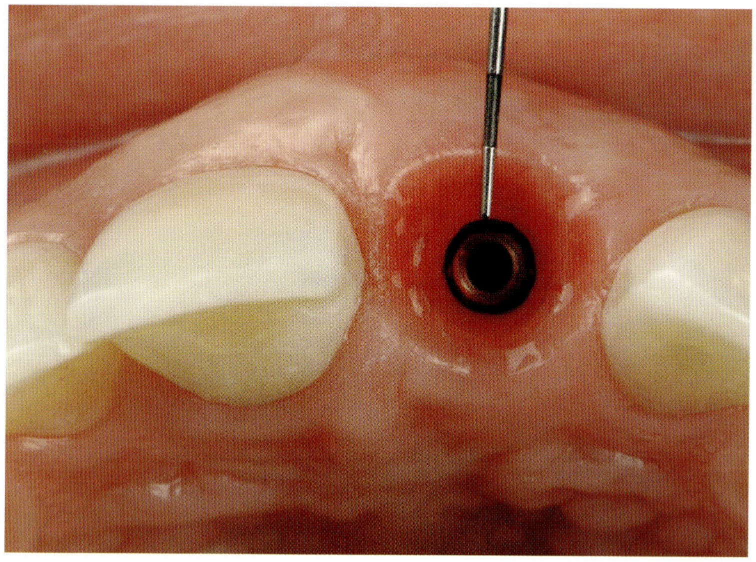

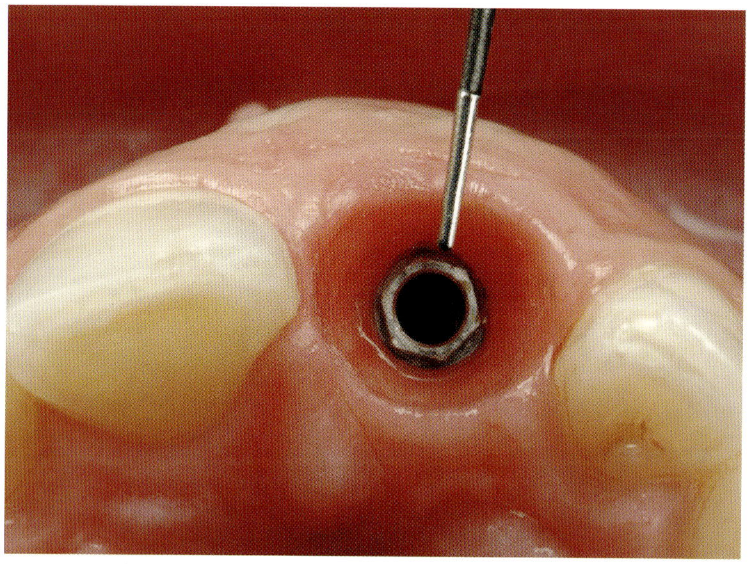

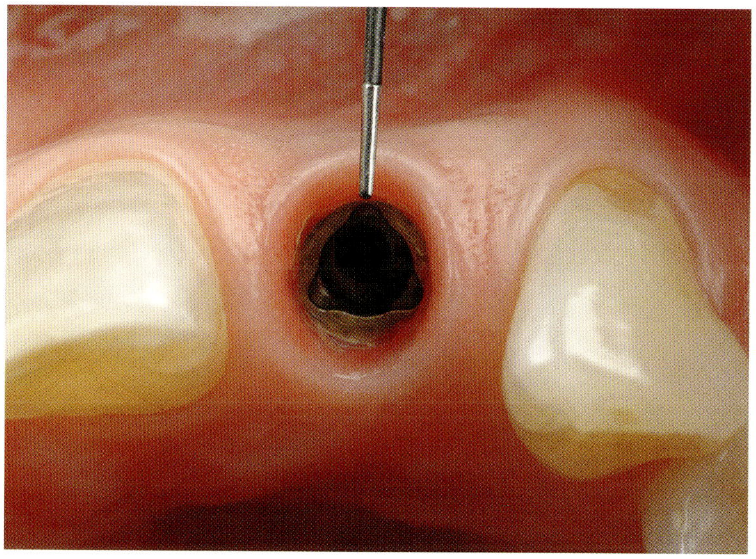

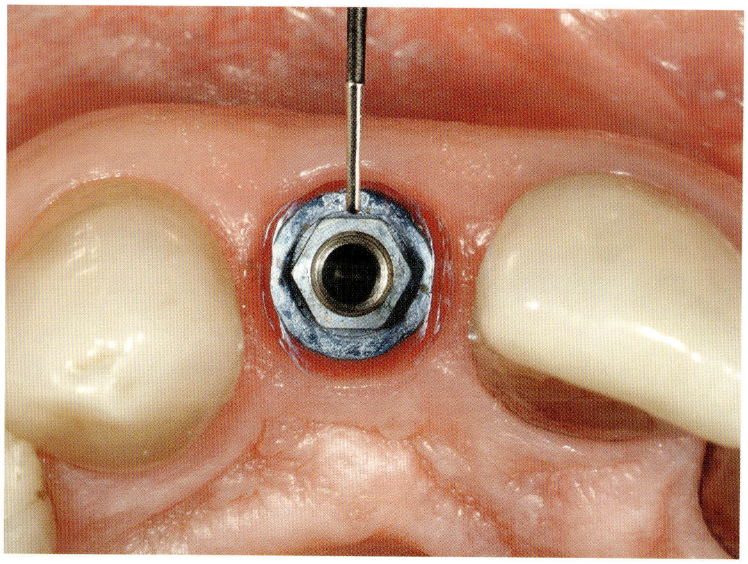

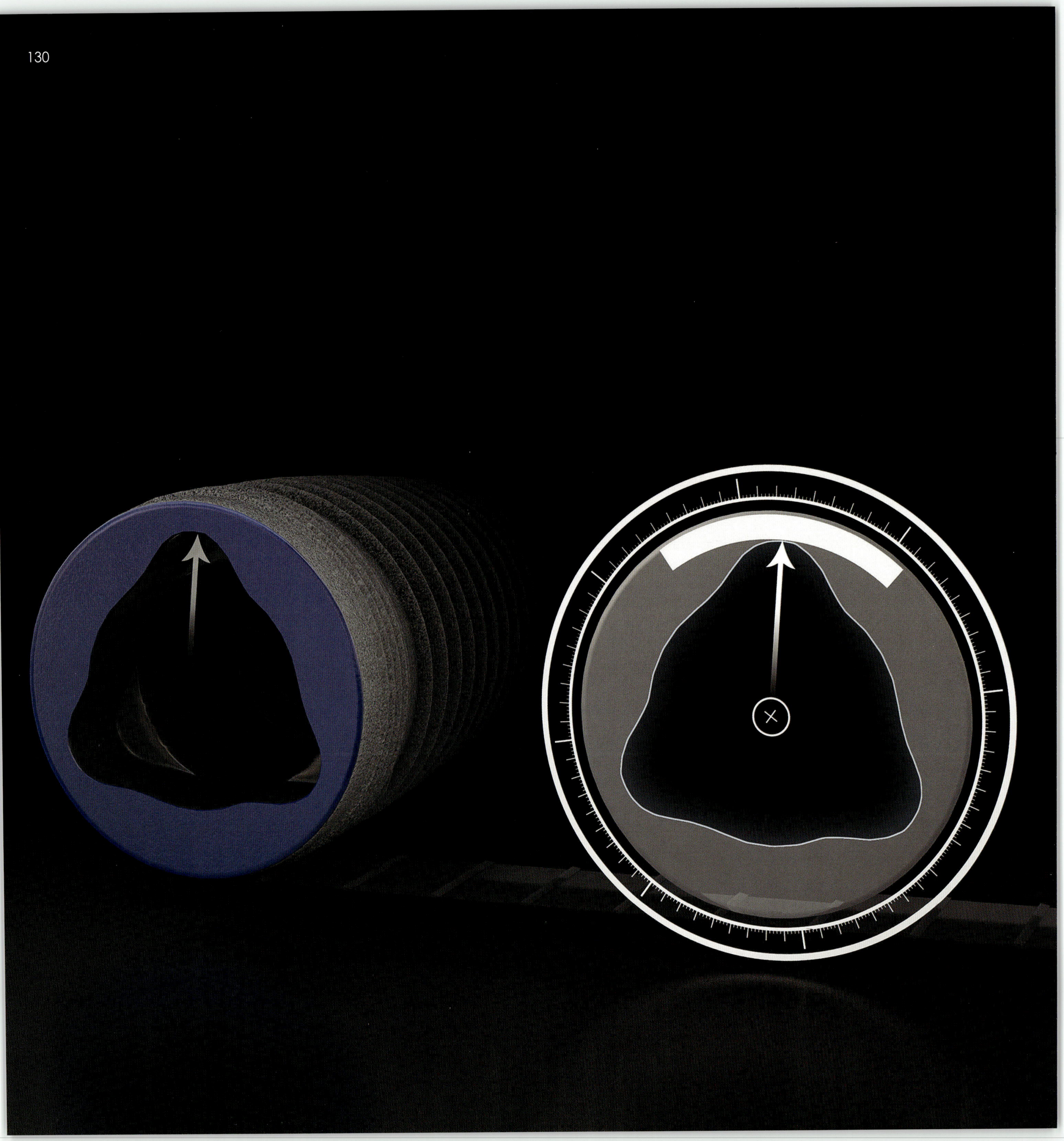

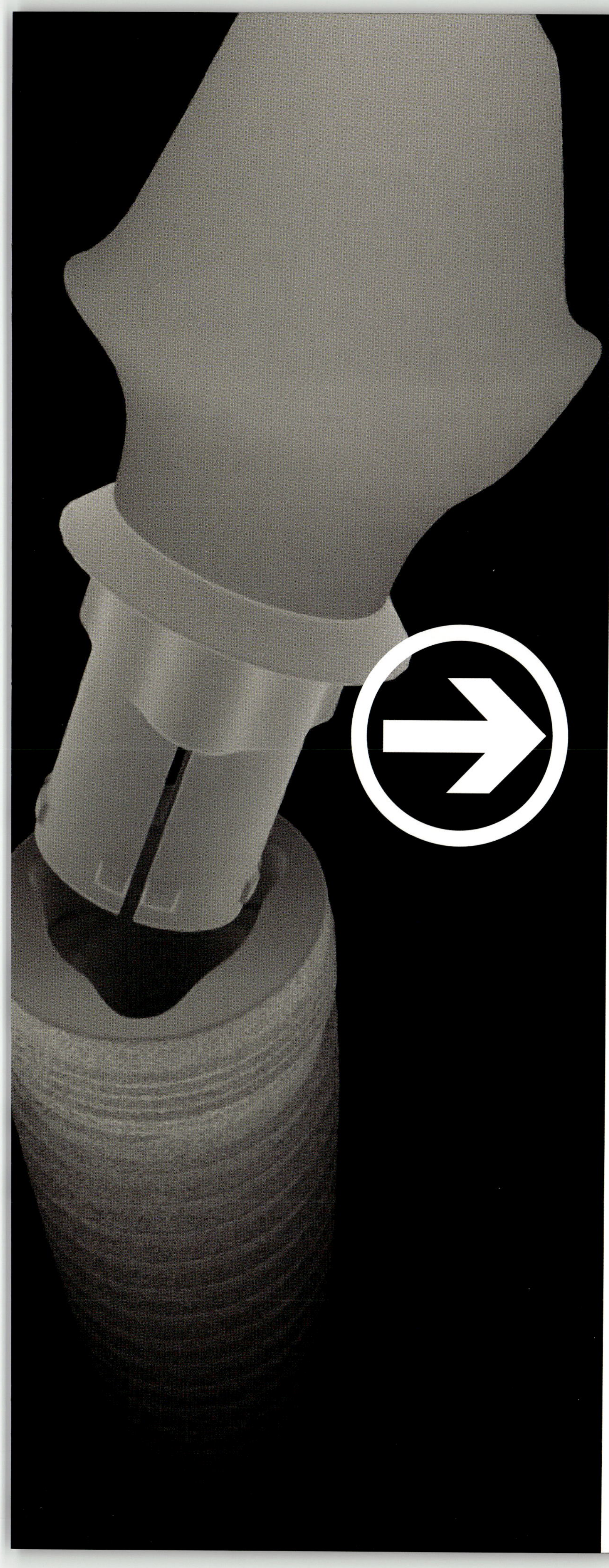

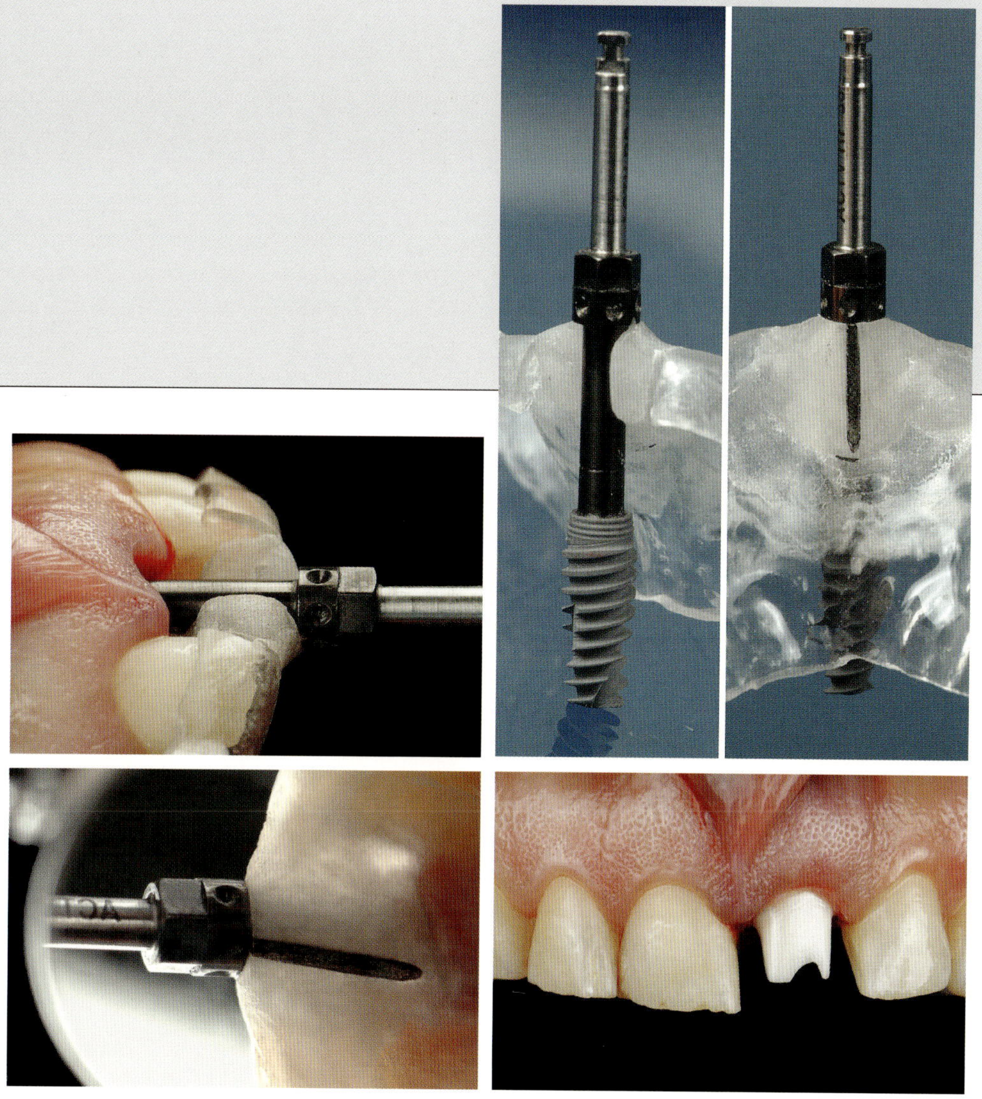

Implant head orientation

Proper orientation of the implant head connection is critical for ideal implant placement, no matter the brand of implant placed. With NobelReplace implants, for example, one of the three lobes of the internal connection should be oriented toward the buccal aspect. The orientation of the implant head in one specific direction allows for detection of transfer mistakes from the impression to the dental laboratory and also during fabrication of the master cast and subsequent prosthetic restoration. One of the biggest advantages of proper orientation is the ability to fabricate a customized abutment or individually adjust a prefabricated abutment before the surgery, allowing the surgeon to provide a provisional restoration on the day of implant placement. This is shown above with a NobelActive implant with customized definitive zirconia abutment.

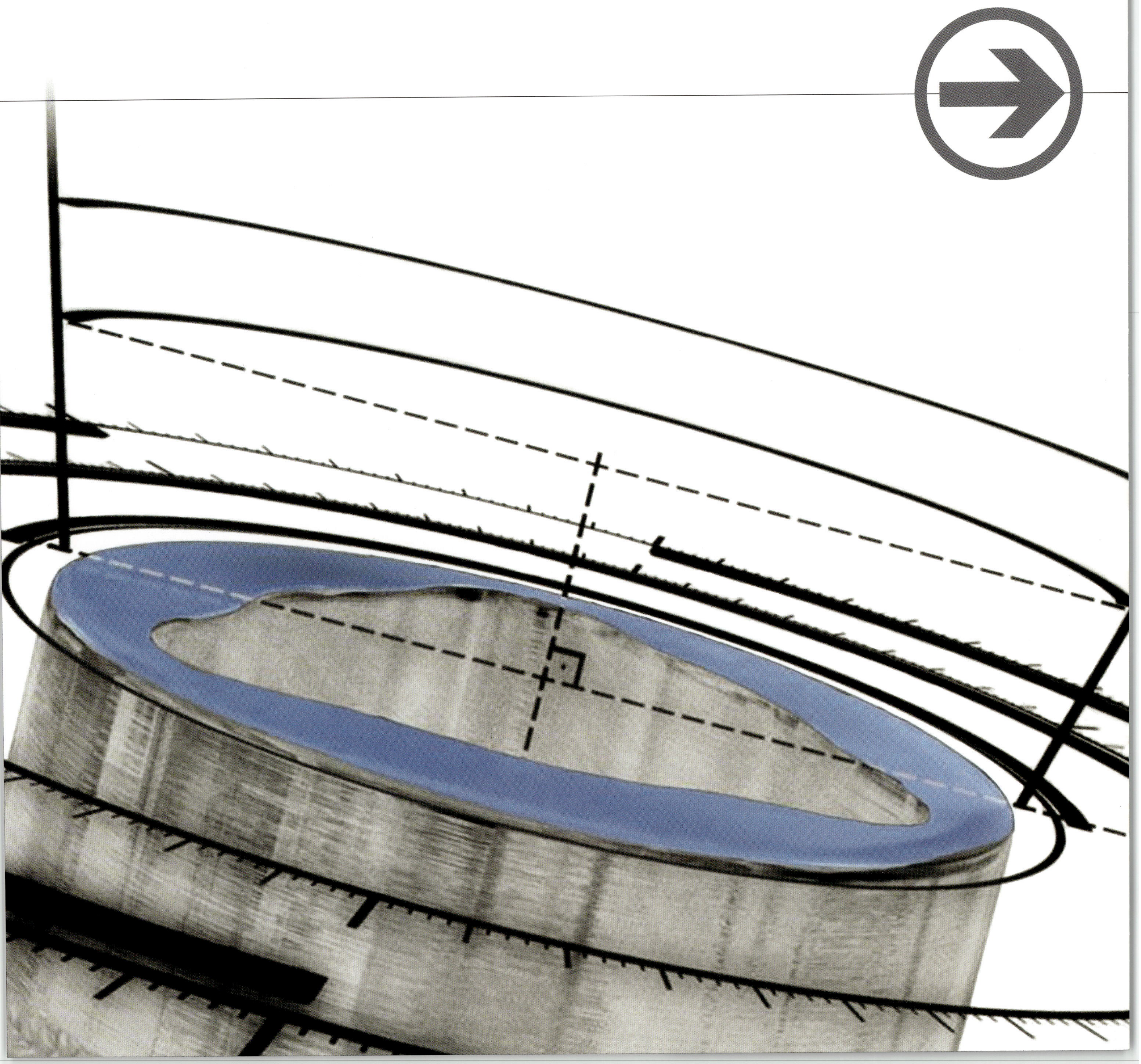

No matter the type of implant selected, the head of the implant connection should be oriented in a certain manner as a guide during the restorative phase. This method simplifies the delivery of the definitive custom or prefabricated abutment on the day of the implant placement to provide the patient with immediate function and esthetics.

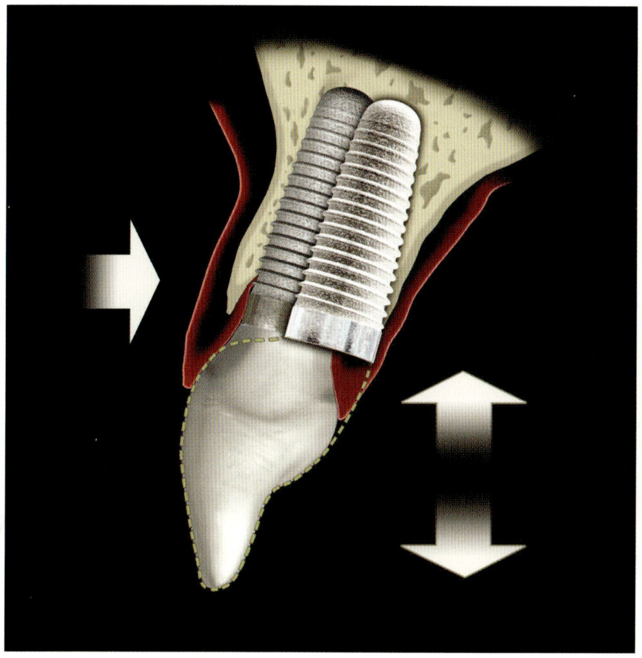

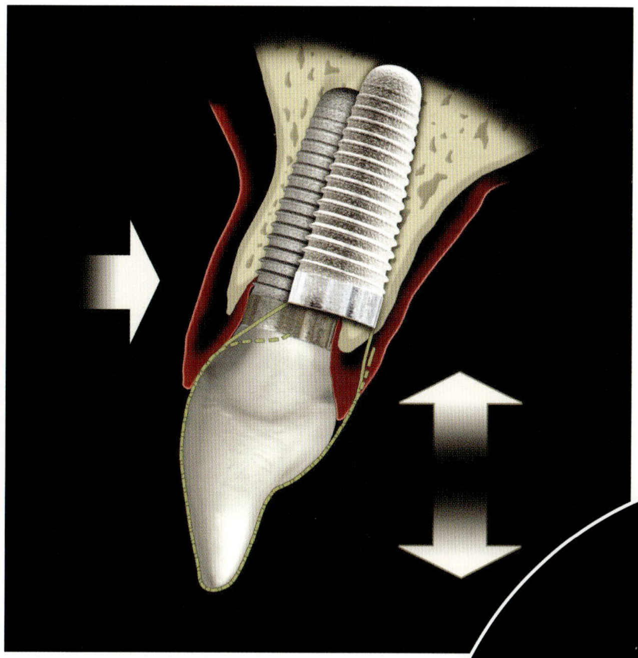

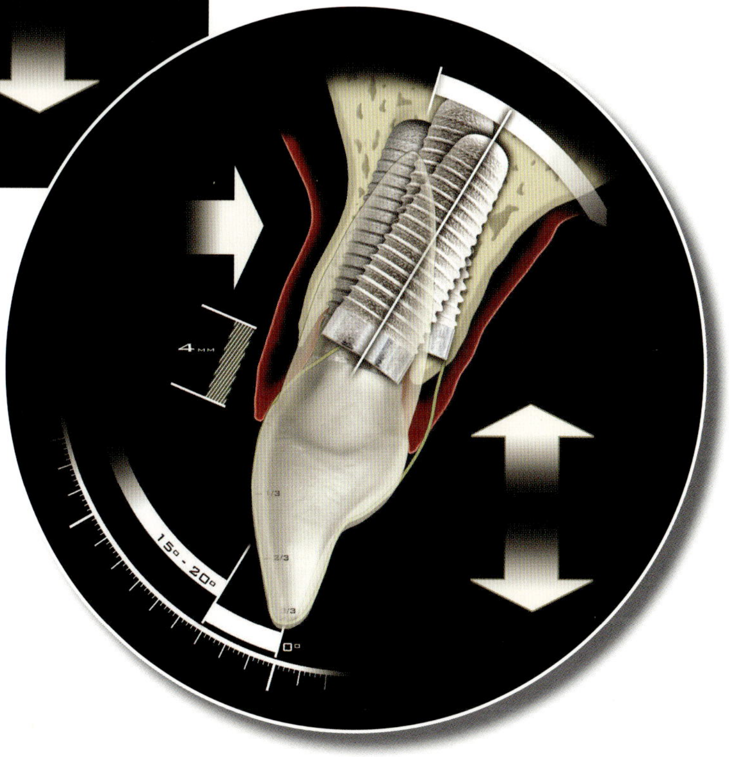

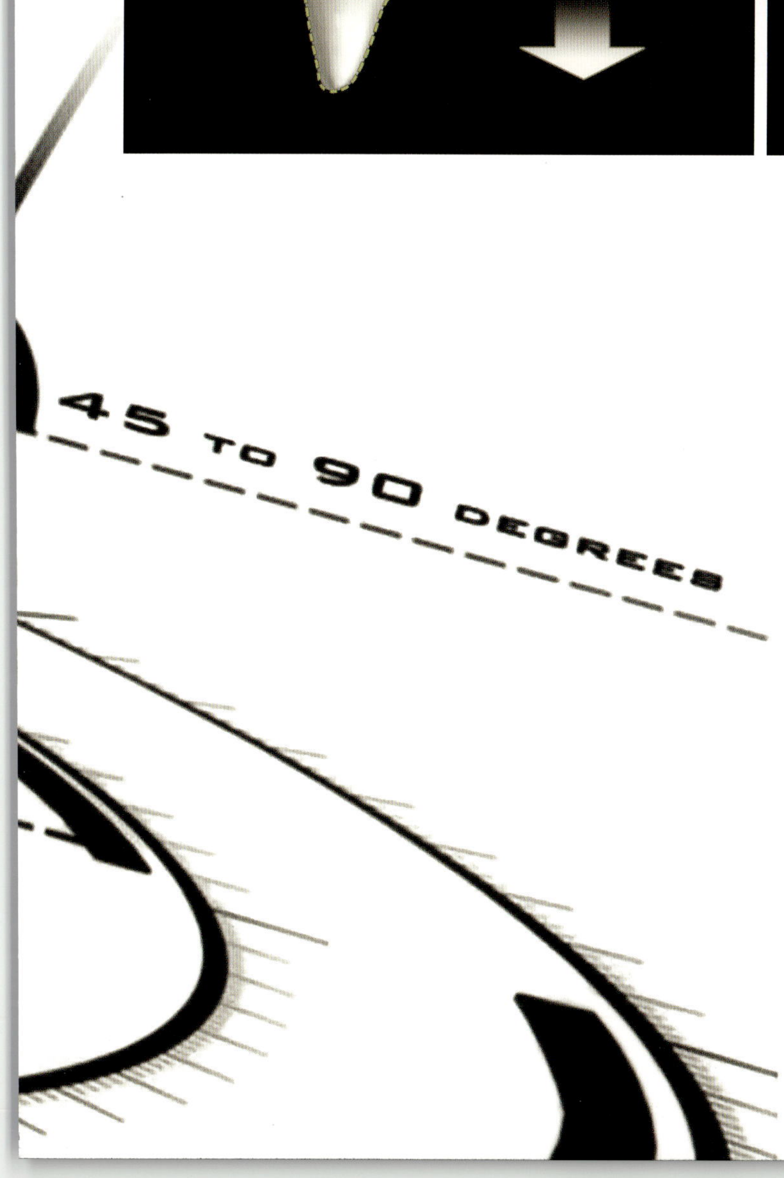

Depth is perhaps the most crucial aspect to take into consideration while placing an implant. If the implant is not placed deep enough, it will be impossible to generate an ideal emergence profile to match the scalloping of the adjacent teeth. This vertical problem is difficult to treat due to the lack of space to hide the prosthetic connection. An implant placed too deep, on the other hand, can cause unnecessary bone loss due to the positive bone defect and bacteria ingrowth, especially with external connections. When the implant is placed just deep enough, a smooth emergence profile can be created to better integrate the implant prosthesis with the surrounding teeth. The comfortable zone is from 3 to 4 mm apical to the prospective gingival margin. The buccolingual position has a crucial impact on the emergence profile; for example, the illustration shows that the more palatal the implant is positioned, the deeper it must be placed to satisfy an ideal emergence profile.

Initial

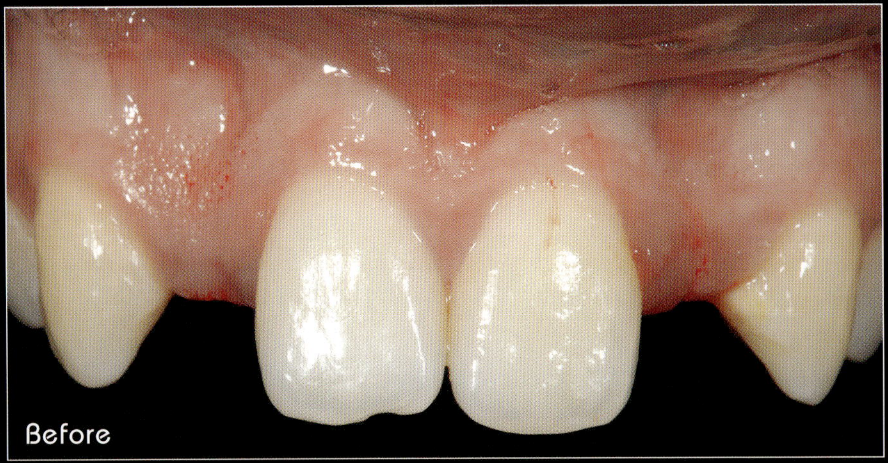

Before

Creating peri-implant soft tissue volume

• 3 Months after surgery

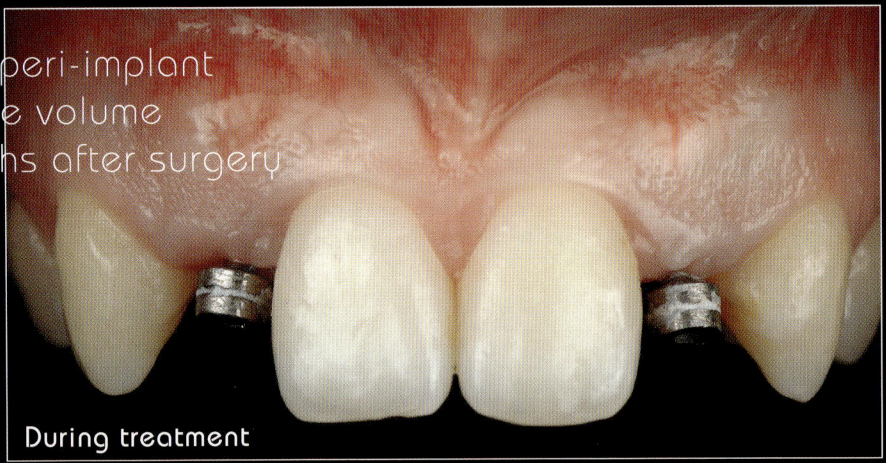

During treatment

Leveling finishing lines

• Emergence profile designs

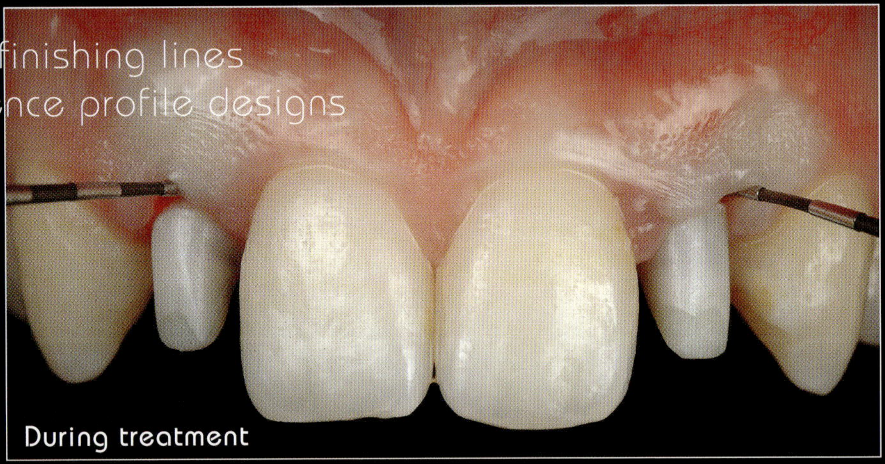

During treatment

Final

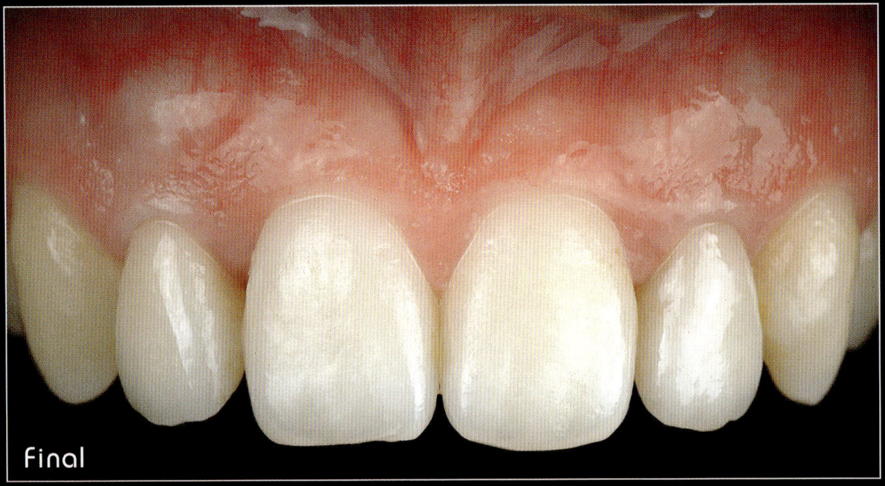

Final

Dentogingival angle and emergence profile

The ideal dentogingival angle of the emergence profile should mimic that of the natural tooth as closely as possible. Any greater angulation in the anterior region may lead to potential problems, especially at the interproximal bone level. One of the best ways to visualize the ideal angle and emergence profile for an implant is to evaluate the ridge area by inspecting and critically assessing any fixed or removable provisional restoration, which can serve as an excellent diagnostic tool to determine treatment objectives. An ideal emergence profile of an implant restoration should provide uniform support of the soft tissue topography 360 degrees around, with an overall angle between 10 and 20 degrees. In such an ideal implant position, the prosthetic abutment should support 90% of the soft tissue and the crown restoration the remaining 10%.

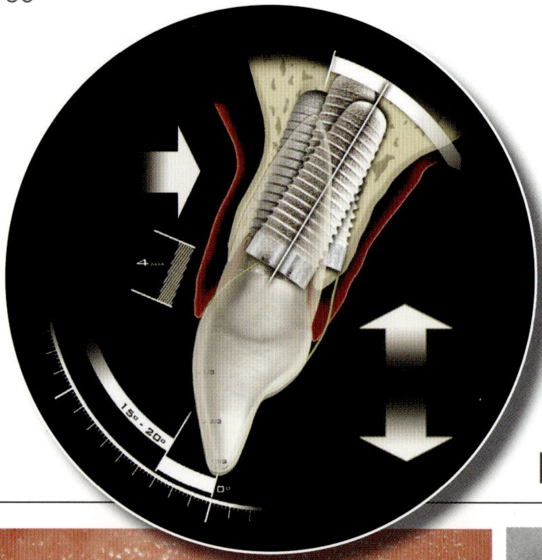

Ideal contour: Flat

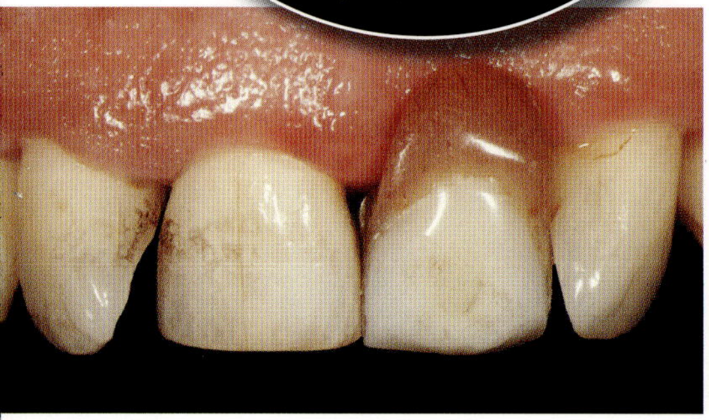

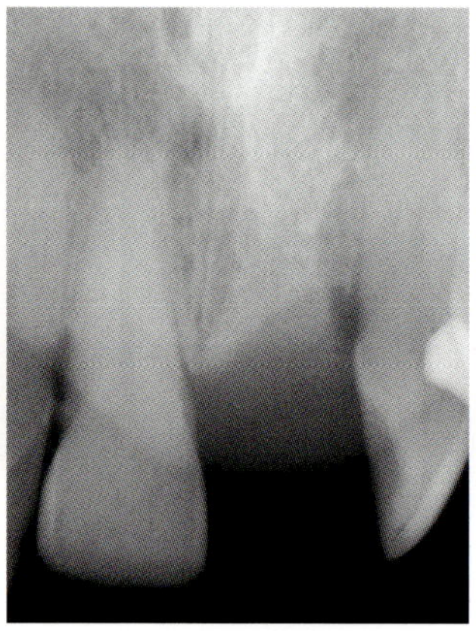

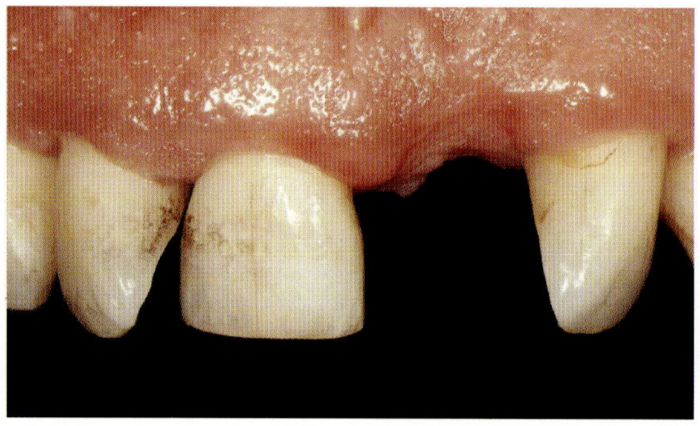

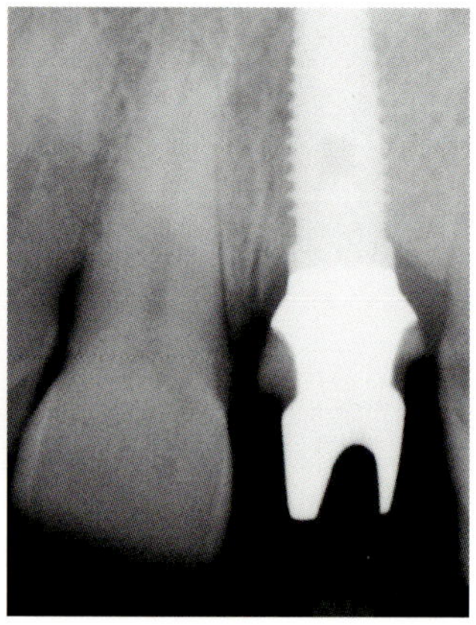

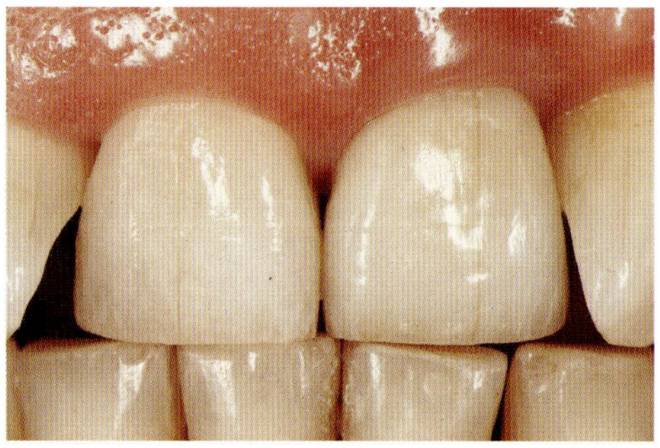

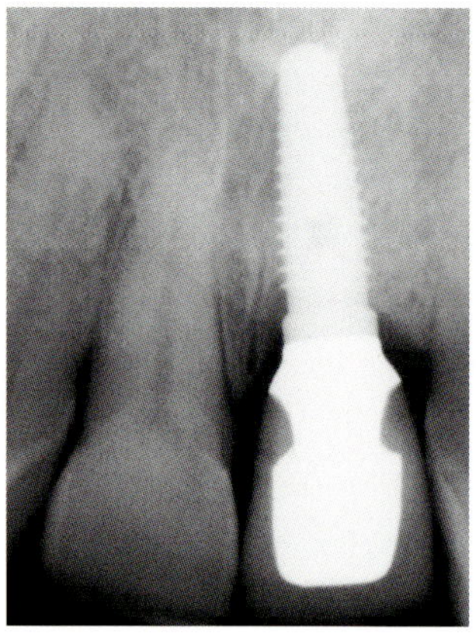

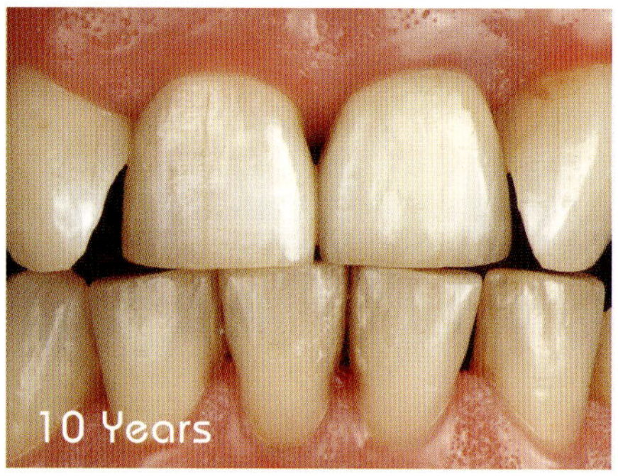

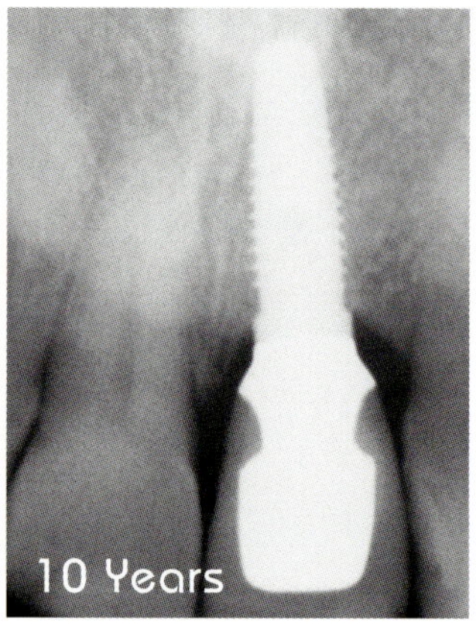

The 10-year results demonstrate the long-term stability of this approach. The major variation was at the tissue level, especially at the interproximal area between the central incisors. The radiograph reveals the same pattern of resorption at the mesial aspect of the implant.

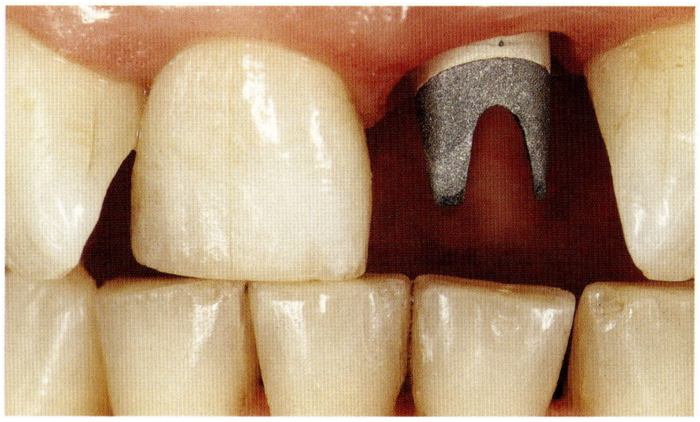

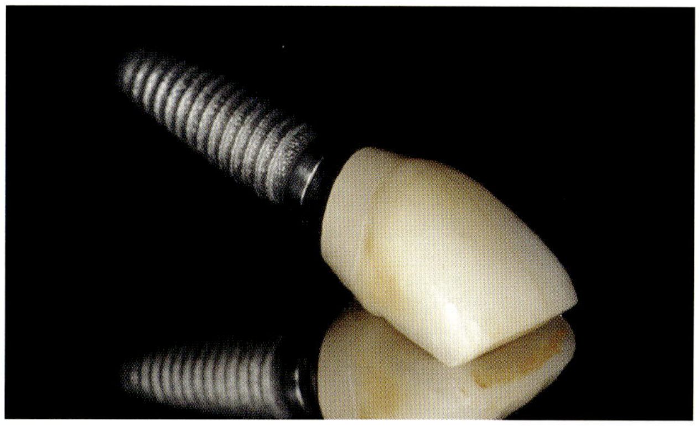

This clinical situation illustrates the long-term stability of a flat emergence profile. The patient presented with a provisional restoration on the left central incisor. A NobelReplace implant (4.3 × 13 mm with an external connection) was placed with a CTG to compensate for lost tissue volume.

The path of the screw access hole should be evaluated because it reveals the perfect orientation of the implant toward the incisal edge, providing a flat support to the buccal soft tissues. It provides a progressive and smooth transition from the implant head to the abutment to the definitive crown restoration.

This clinical scenario illustrates that flat emergence profiles allow for more stability in the long term than concave or ridge lap emergence profiles. Today's trends suggest the creation of emergence profiles with more concave areas below the soft tissue crest. These circumferential concavities allow for a thicker band of soft tissue and create a "ring effect" that provides a thicker biotype at the abutment level, which ultimately results in a more stable peri-implant tissue collar.

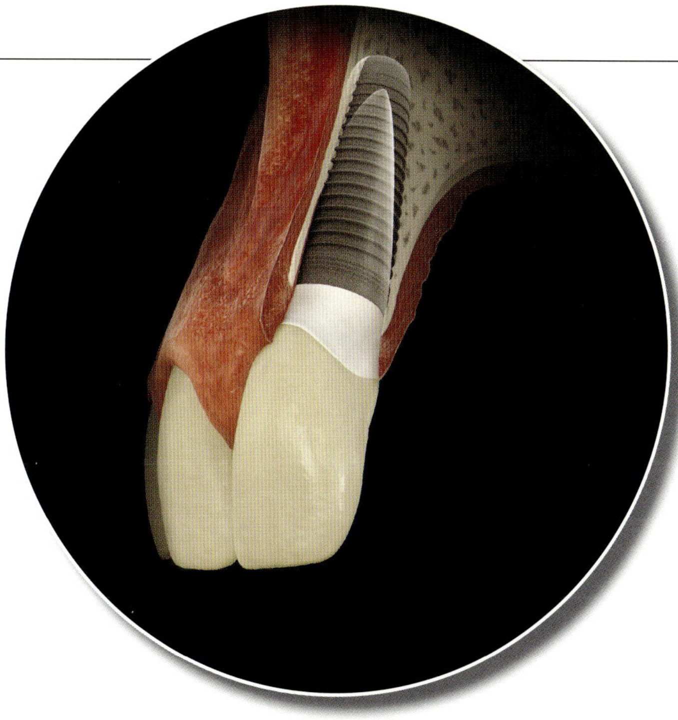

Finish line and crown contour

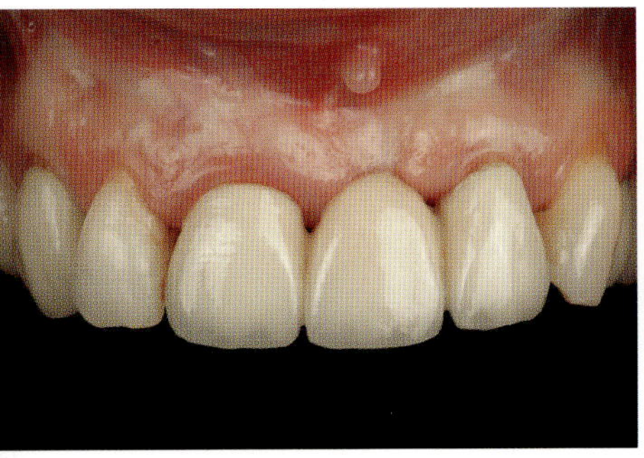
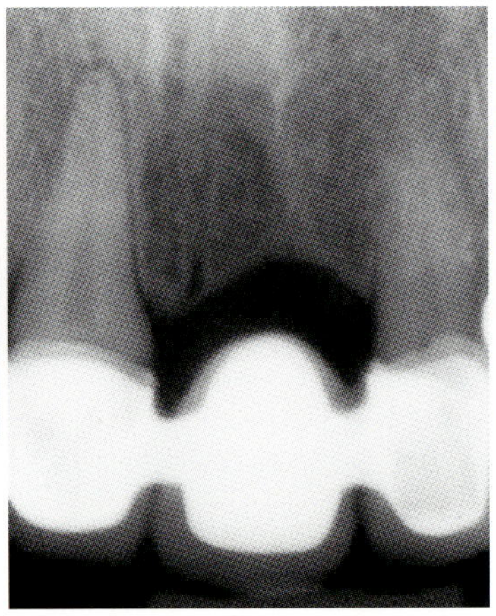
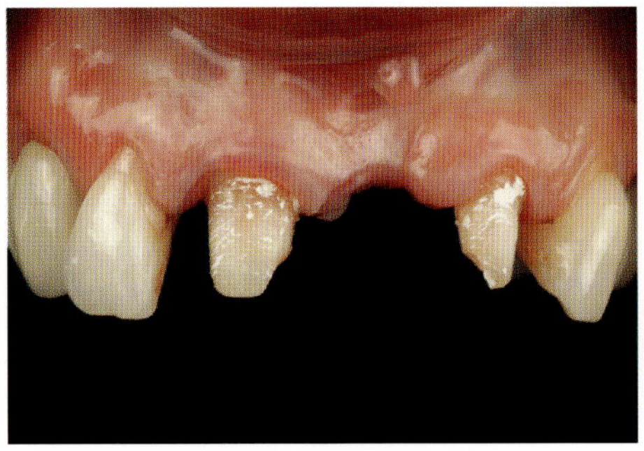
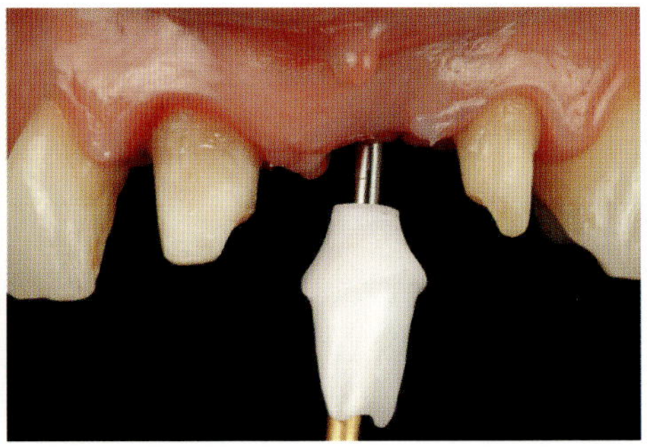

This clinical situation illustrates a current trend in implant dentistry, which suggests that the definitive abutment should be inserted on the first day of the prosthetic phase, and demonstrates its clinical consequences. The implant was positioned and angulated correctly, as indicated by the path of the screw access hole. The ideal angulation provides a smooth transition from the implant to the prosthetic components. A NobelReplace Tapered implant (4.3 × 13 mm) was placed with a PS adapter and CTG.

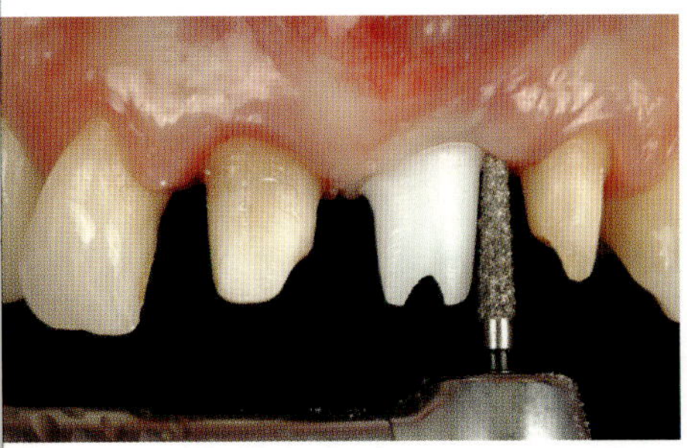
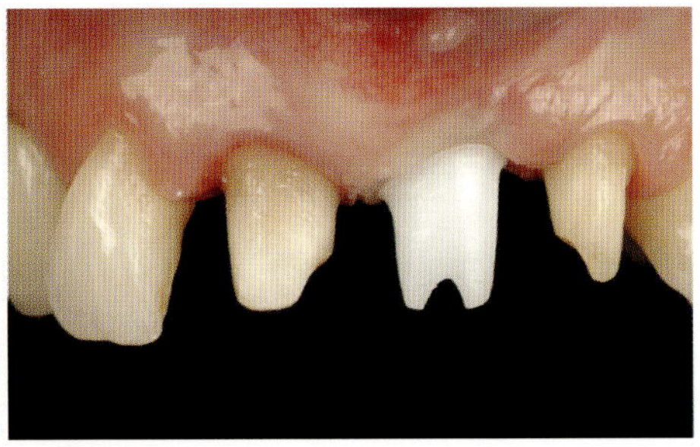

The margin of the abutment was placed slightly supragingivally compared with the adjacent tooth margin. However, the margin should be placed further apically to be level with the adjacent tooth margin to support and emerge from the peri-implant soft tissue in the same manner as the adjacent natural tooth. When the margin is placed more apically, the diameter is reduced because of the concave design of the abutment, leaving the support of the gingival third to the crown.

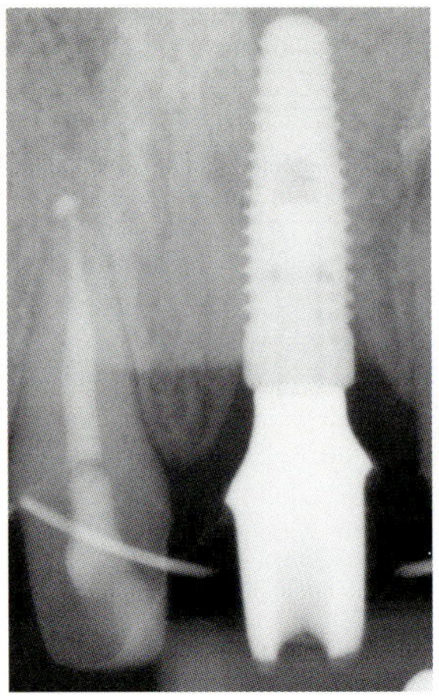
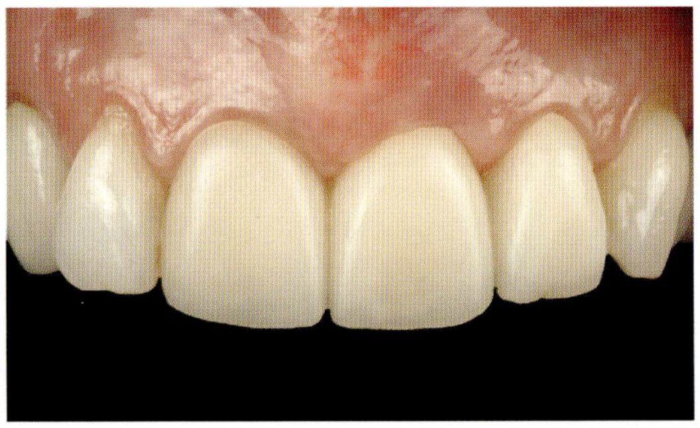

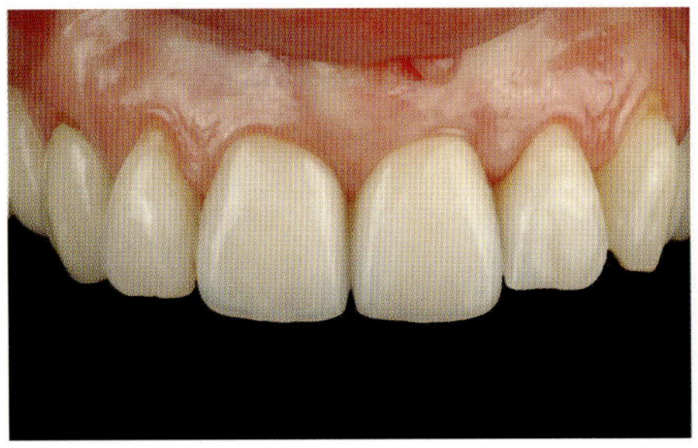
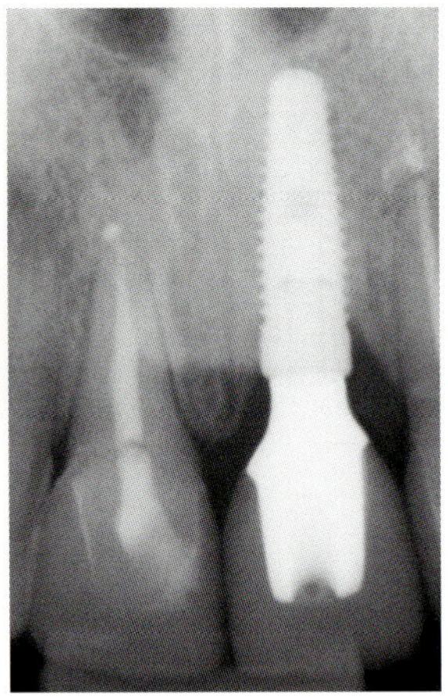
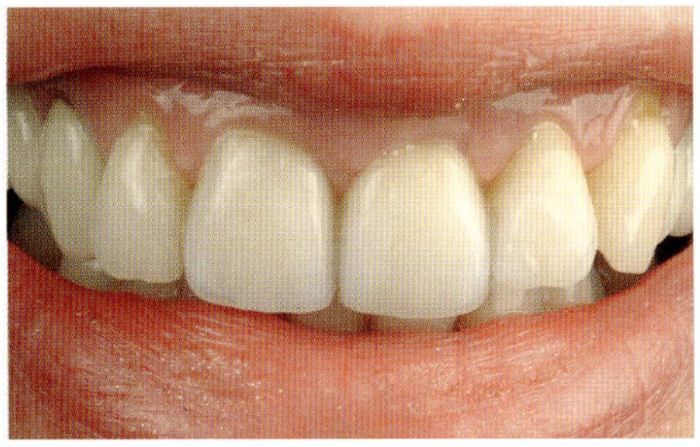

Five years after cementation, tissue maturation and stability are evident. A thicker band of connective tissue around the concave-designed abutment provided greater stability for the peri-implant soft tissue.

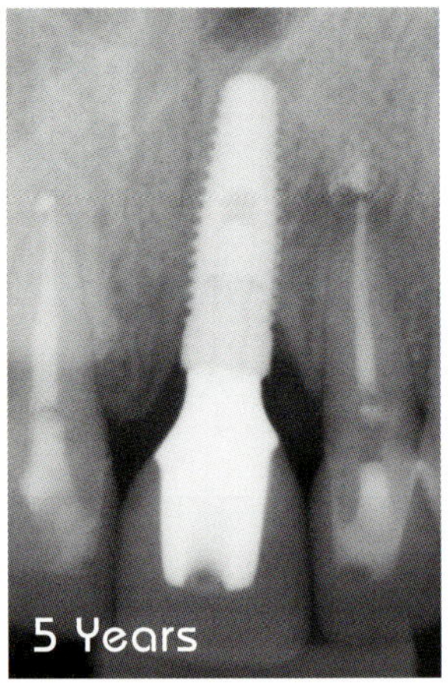

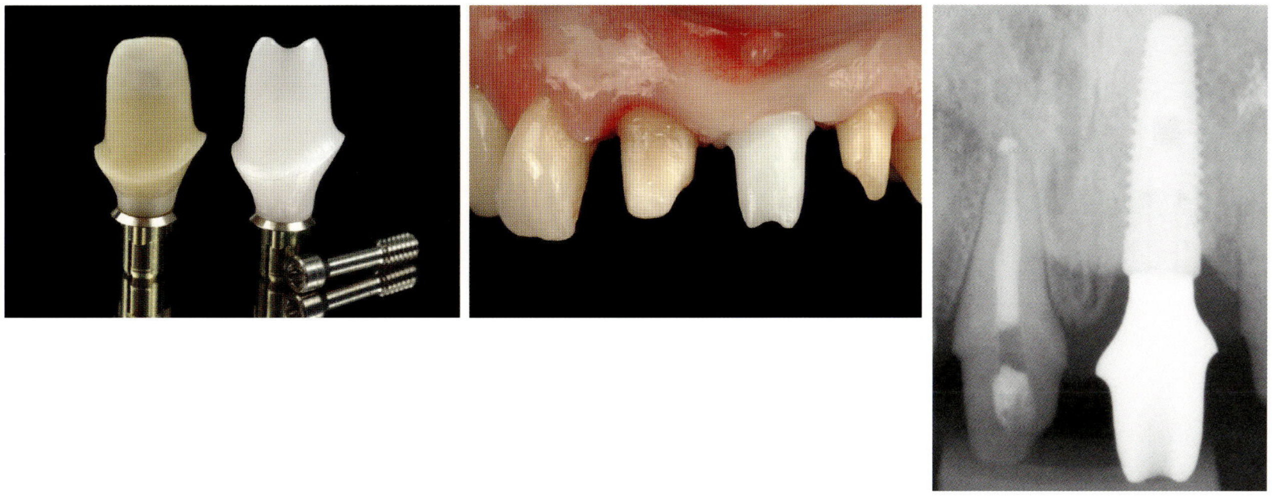

The definitive zirconia abutment was fabricated from a composite replica created on the master cast. The abutment was designed with a circumferential concavity below the finishing line. The diameter of the abutment should be as close as possible to that of the missing tooth in the area of soft tissue penetration to support the tissue in the same manner.

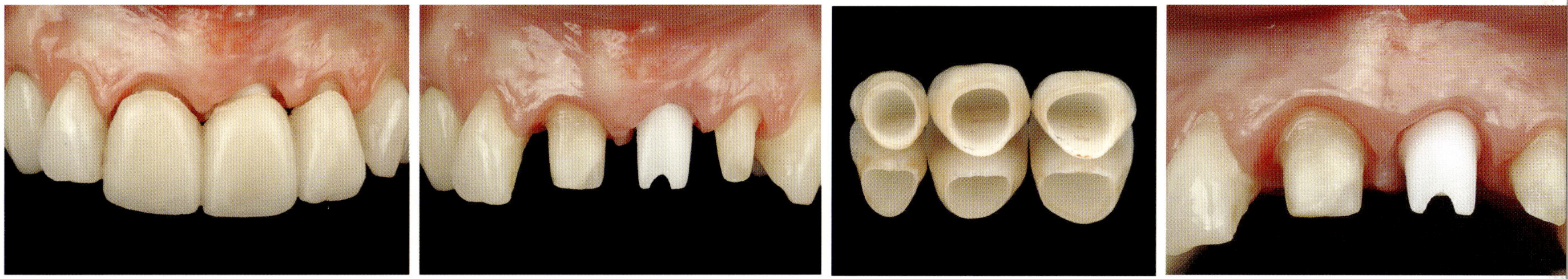

The provisional restoration was relined and reshaped to provide tissue support in the same manner as the natural tooth. Despite the effort during the provisional stage to establish identical profiles on the tooth and the implant through margin location and crown contours, the margin was deeper than desired.

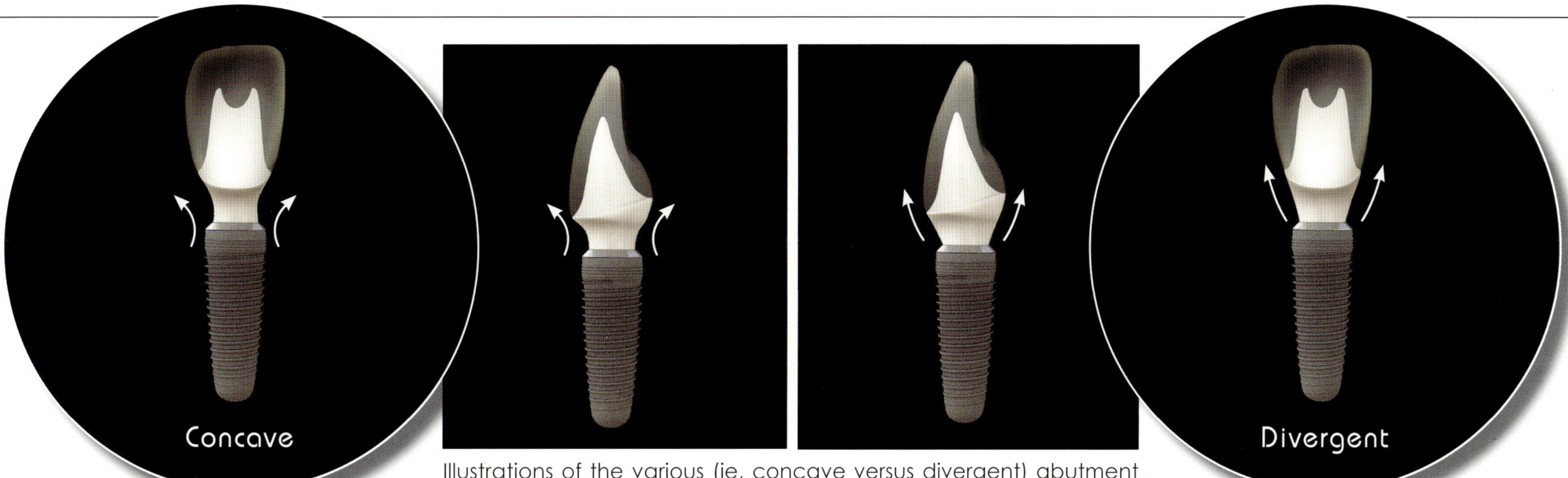

Illustrations of the various (ie, concave versus divergent) abutment designs show the potential of each design to maintain stability. The concave design has greater stability, like a "donut effect," with thicker tissue around the peri-implant soft tissue, especially when grafting has been performed. The divergent design will promote more recession under function because it creates a thinning of the tissues.

Emergence profile with lack of soft tissue

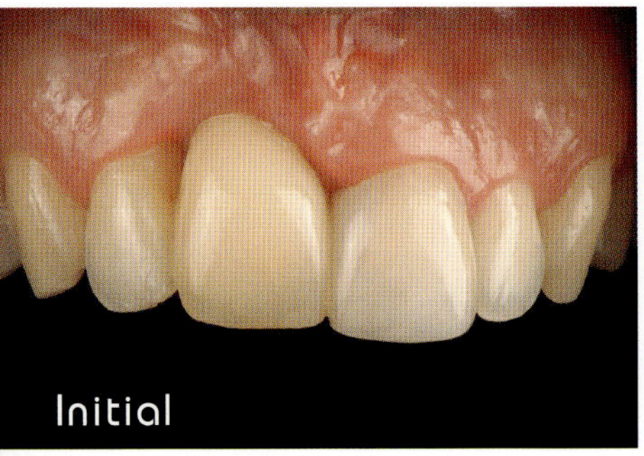

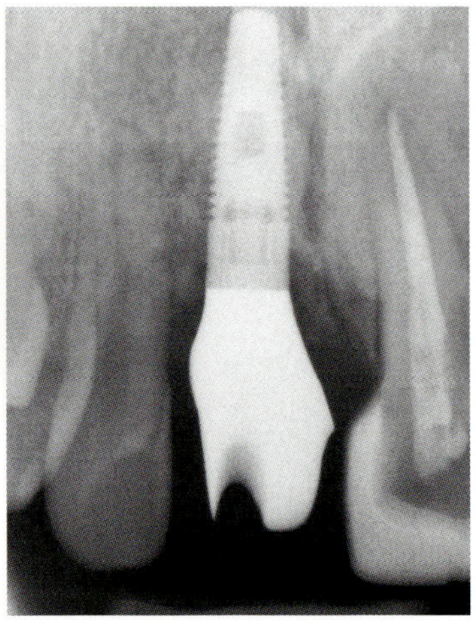

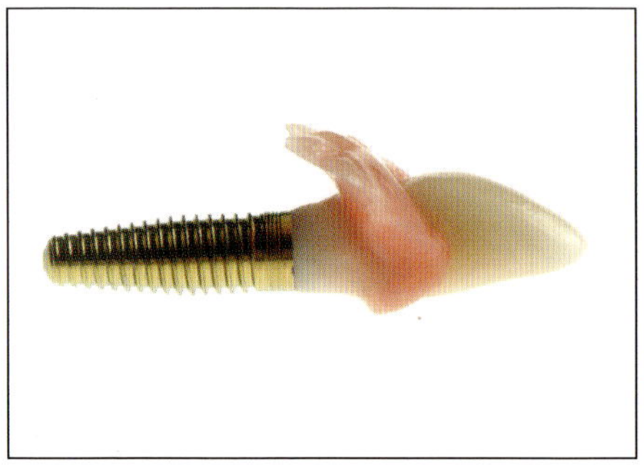

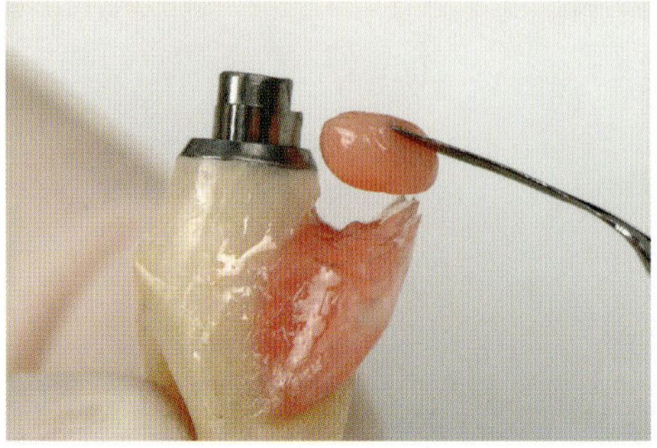

It is difficult to create a proper emergence profile without sufficient soft tissue. Some important aspects to take into consideration before planning a hybrid screw-retained restoration are the screw access hole of the implant (eg, angulation), the implant depth necessary for generating the ideal emergence profile, and the ability to support the remaining buccal tissue. First, an ideal ridge lap provisional restoration with pink composite was fabricated to re-create the soft tissue volume and to compensate for the morphologic deficiencies.

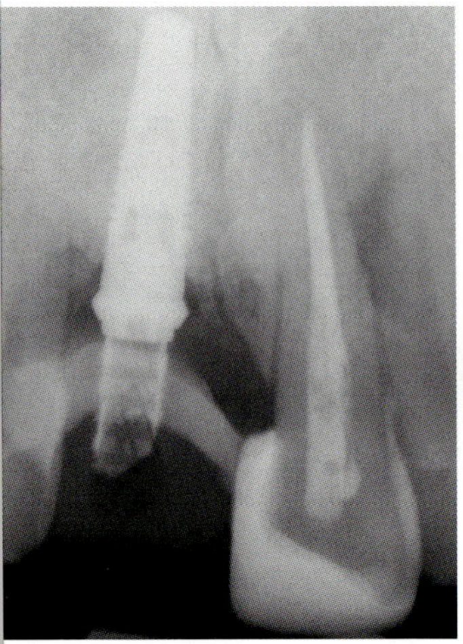

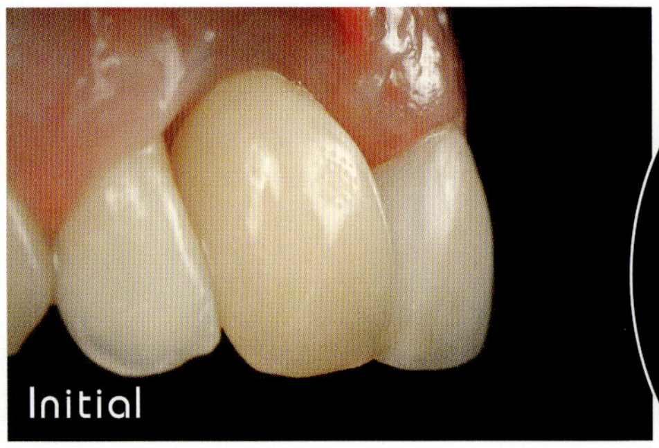

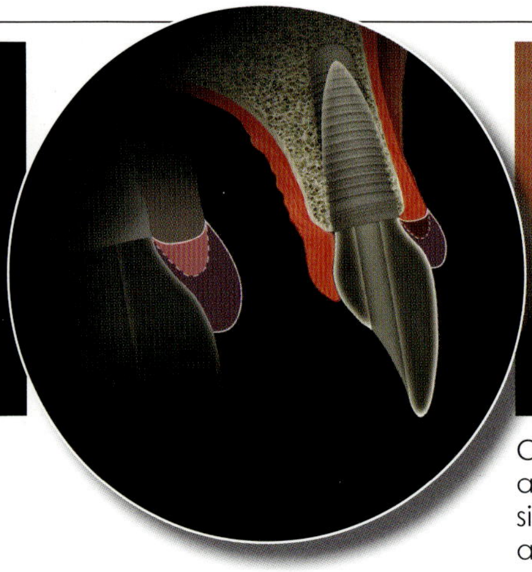

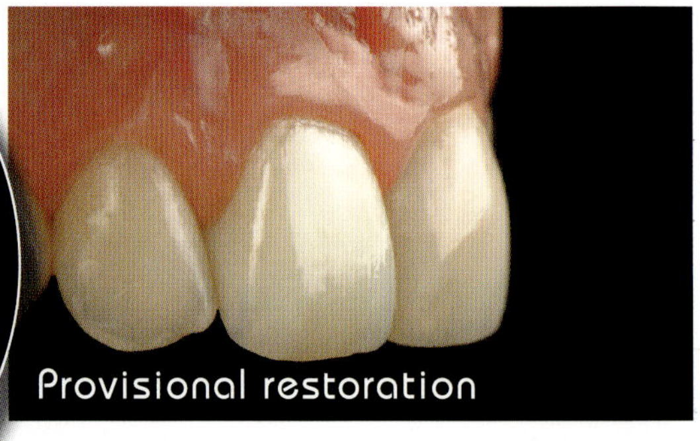

Composite was added at the ridge lap level and relined several times until the ideal transition was created. Note the tissue support achieved through the pink composite.

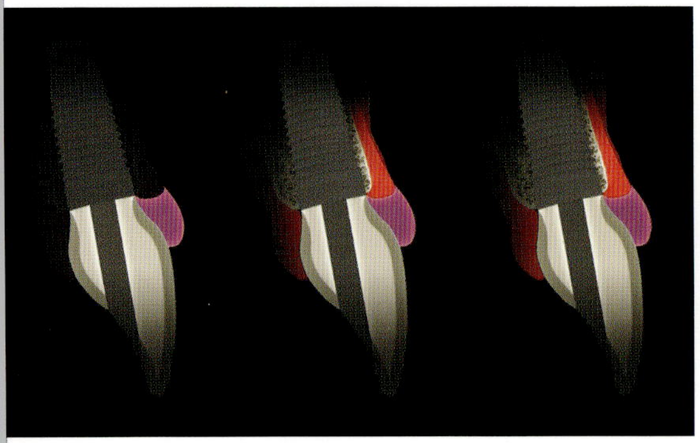

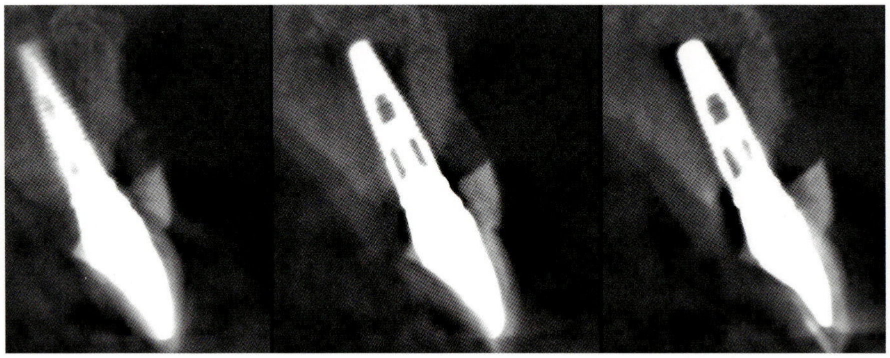

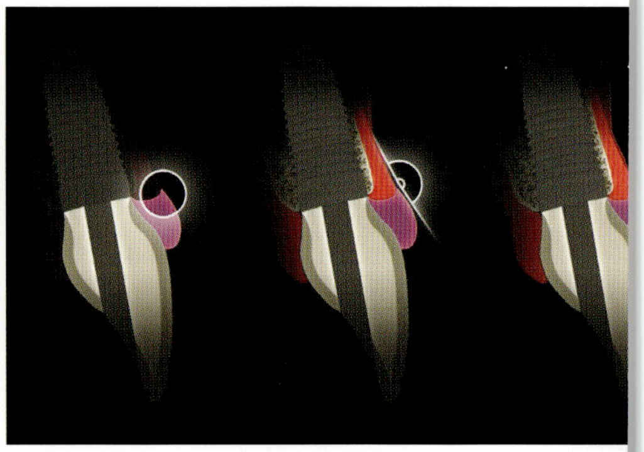

CT scans were taken to visually perceive the amount of soft tissue volume lost and replaced with pink composite. Note the precise tissue support from the pink buccal semi-pontic, which supports the entire soft tissue volume vertically in order to blend the hybrid implant prosthesis to the peri-implant soft tissue. The visual perception is thereby achieved without a grayish transition due to the flat pontic design into the surrounding soft tissue.

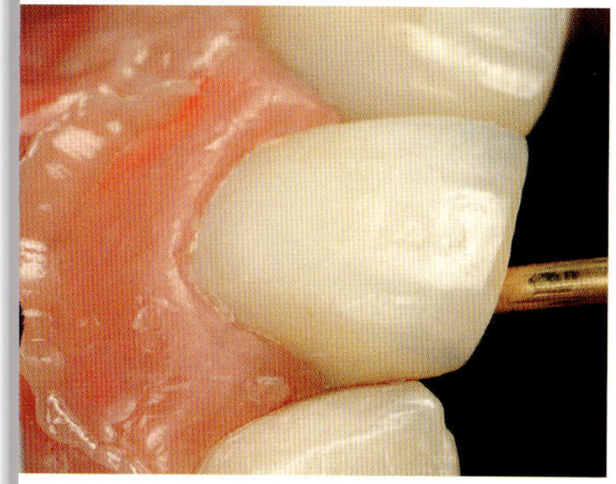

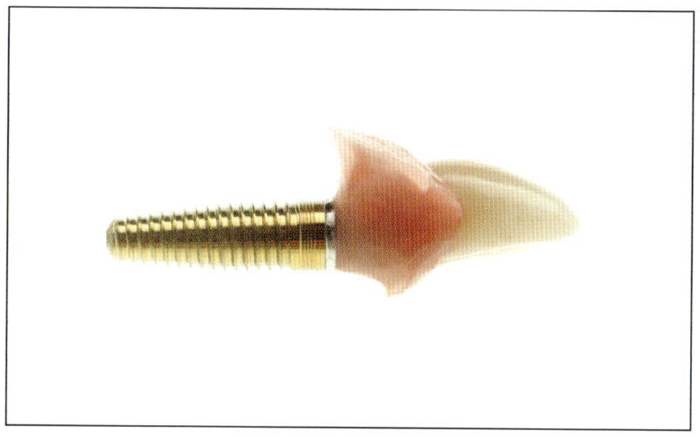

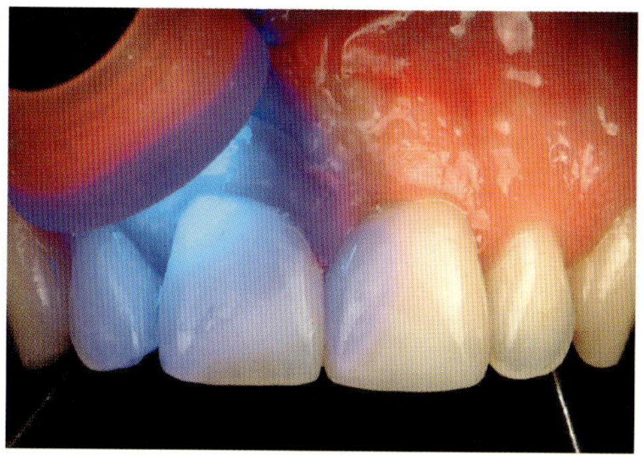

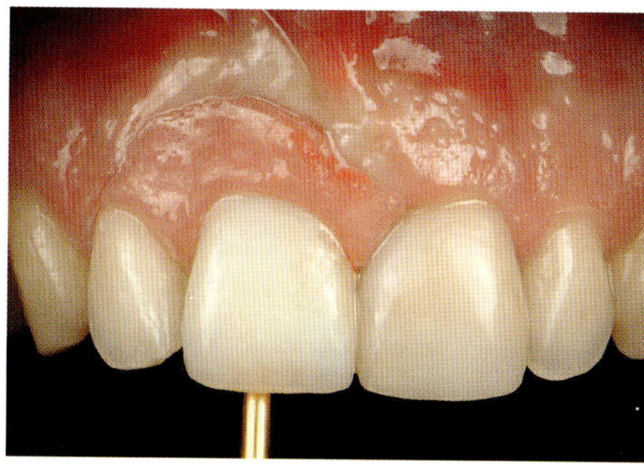

During a second stage, an ideal emergence profile from the implant shoulder to the tissue emergence is created. Ideally, the tissue emergence should be at least level with or coronal to the implant shoulder to create a smooth transition.

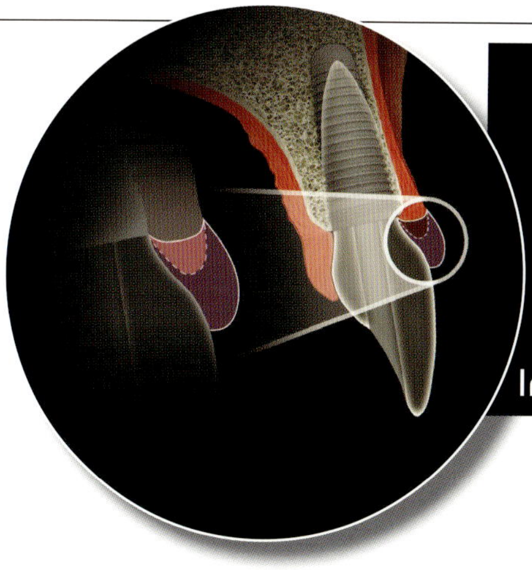

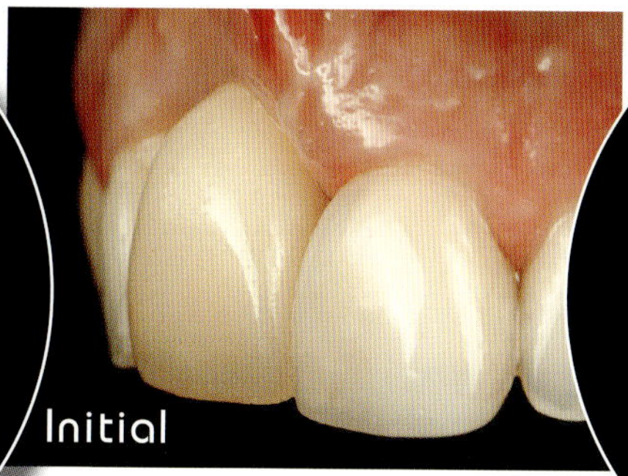

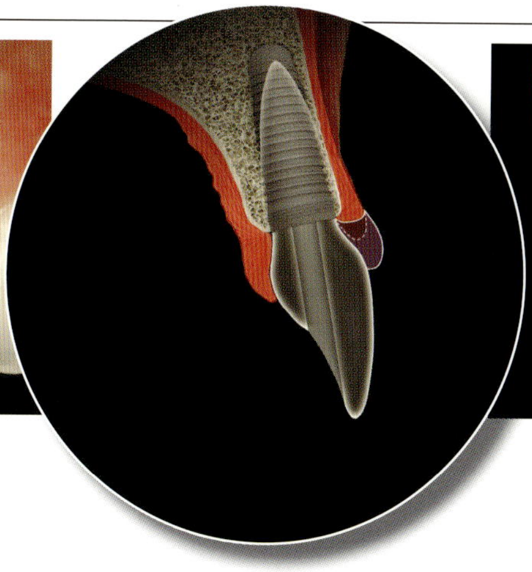

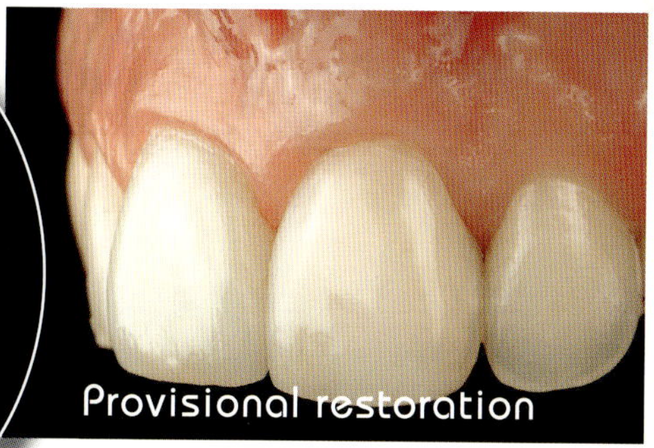

Once the provisional restoration is placed, the definitive restoration can be fabricated in a predictable manner. The ideal emergence profile should provide an inconspicuous transition from the natural tissue profile of the patient to the pink composite.

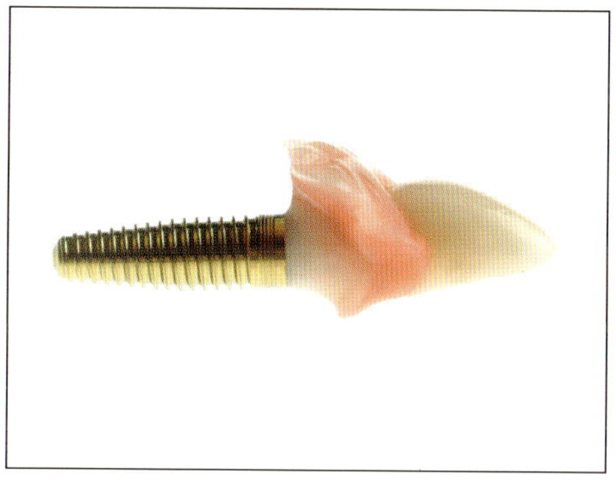

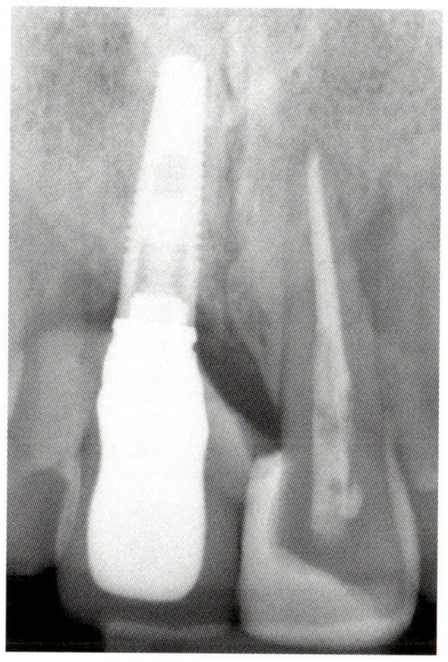

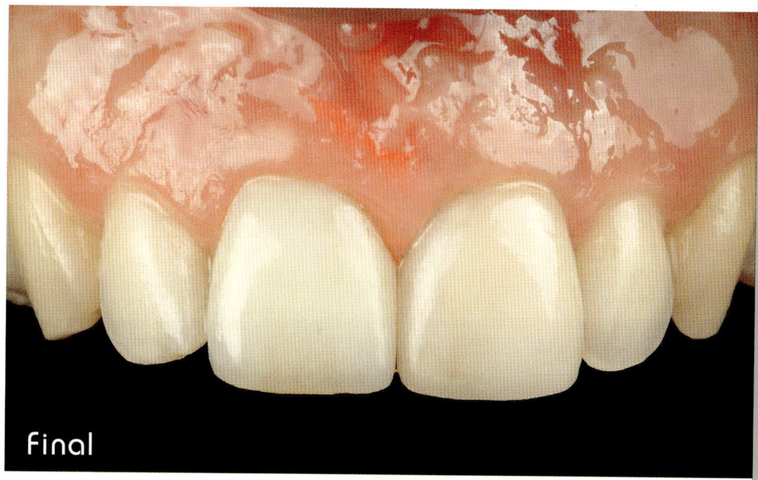

Crown contour and tissue support

This patient presented with bilateral agenesis of the maxillary lateral incisors. Two NobelActive NP implants (3.5 × 13 mm) were placed in the lateral incisor positions. Slim temporary healing abutments maximized CTG volume around the implants and the possibility of using stable provisional restorations during the healing phase.

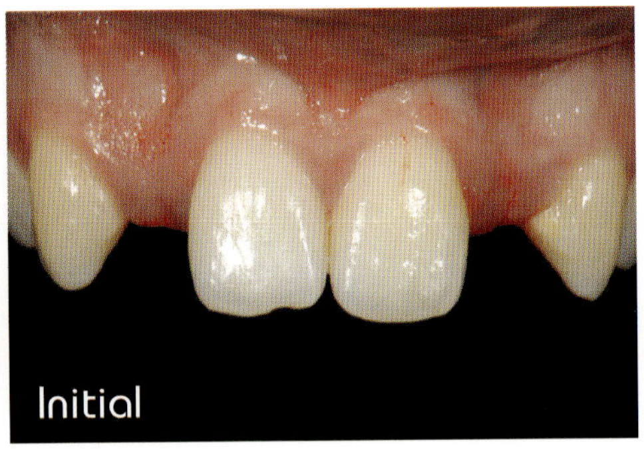
Initial

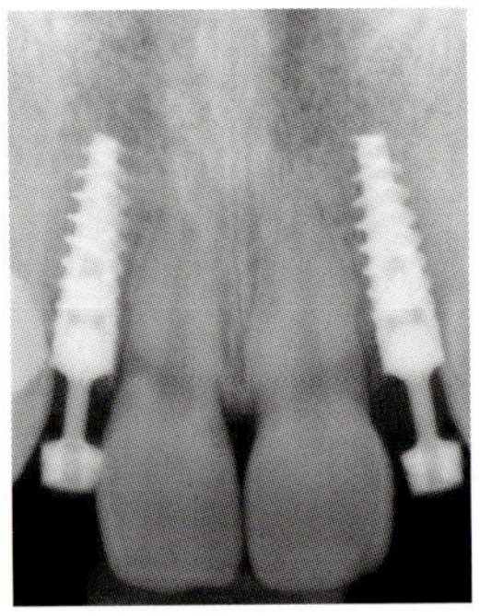

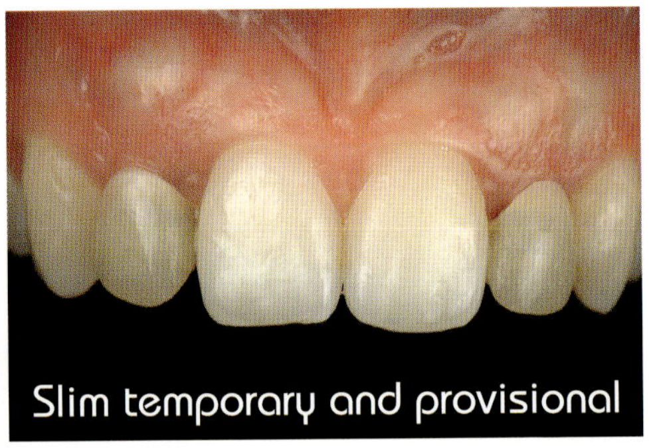
Slim temporary and provisional

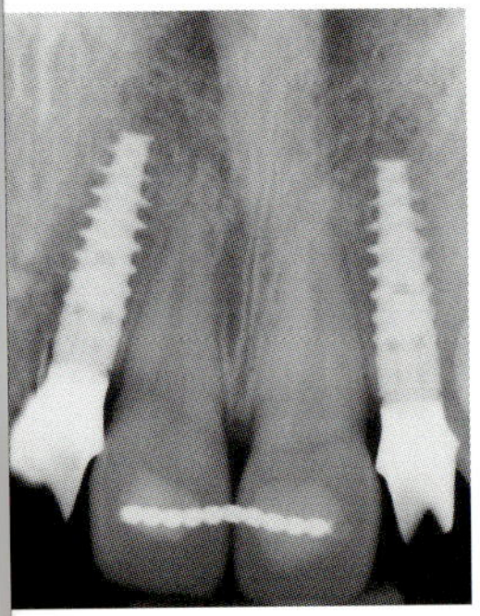

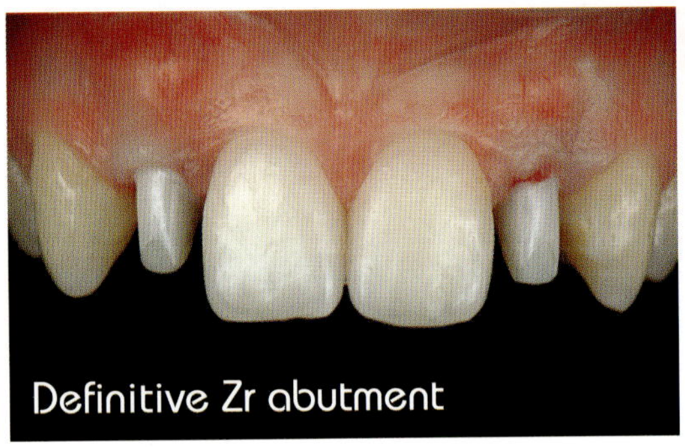
Definitive Zr abutment

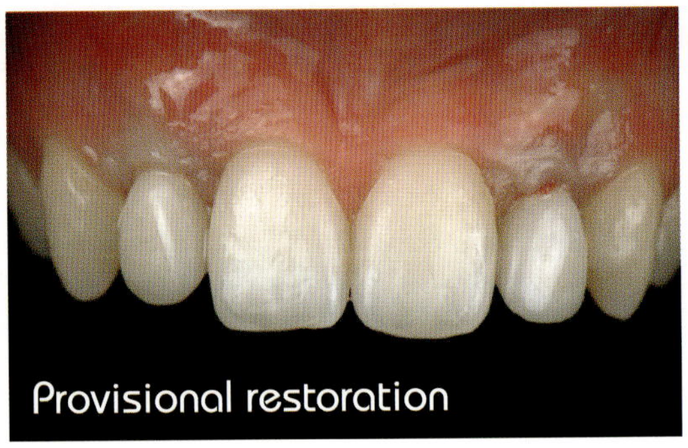
Provisional restoration

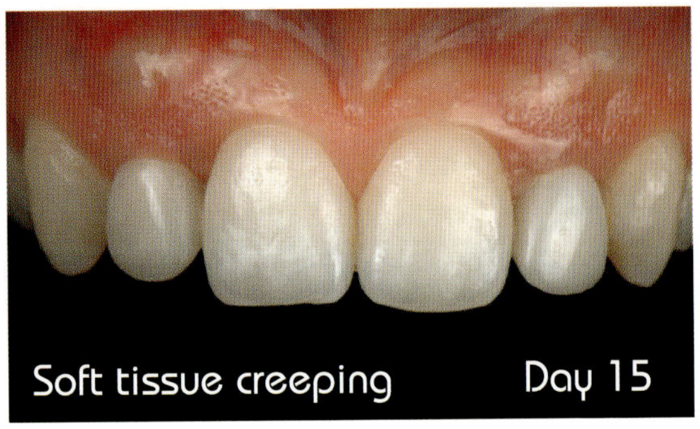
Soft tissue creeping Day 15

Note the blanching of the tissues and the re-formation after 15 days due to excess tissue and the lack of volume contour from the abutment and crown.

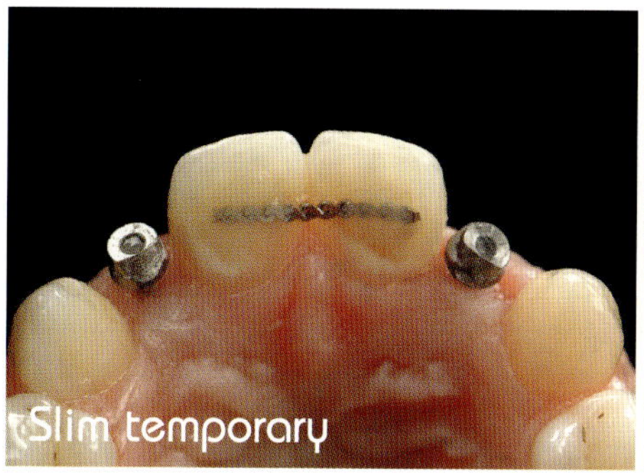

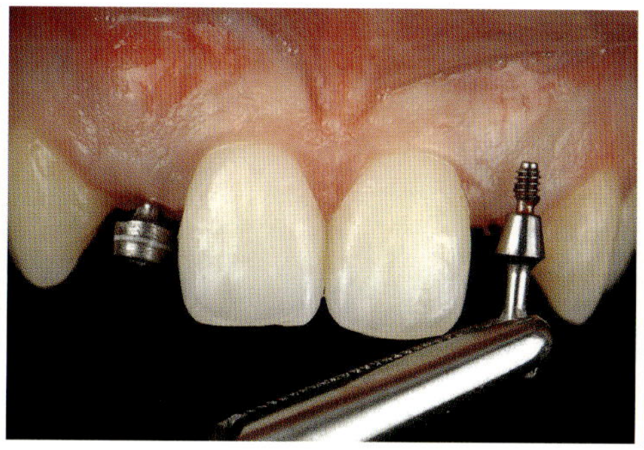
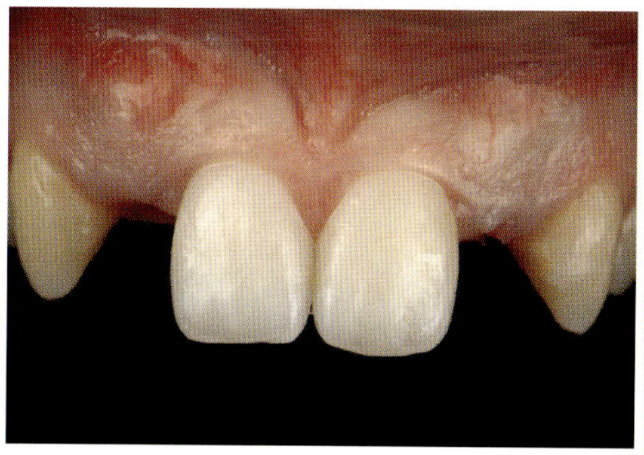
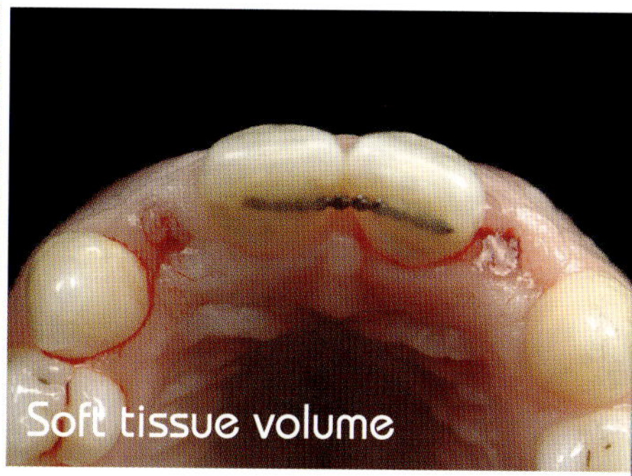

The temporary healing abutments were removed for implant impressions. Note the amount of coronal soft tissue volume available for modification.

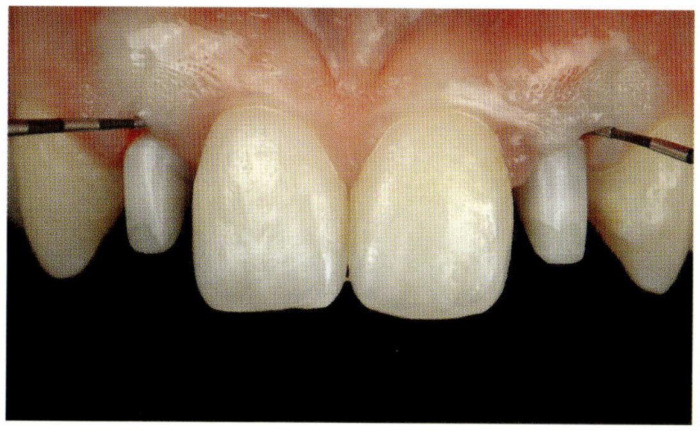
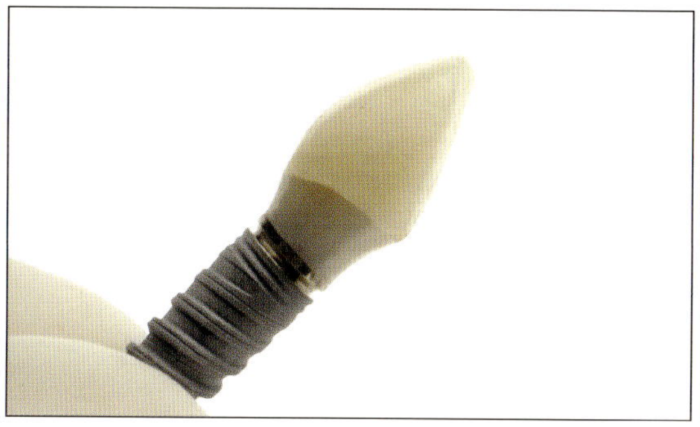
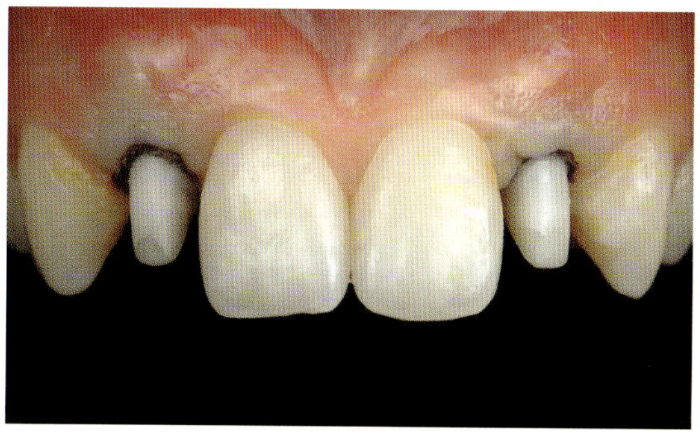

Vertical pressure needs to be applied through the crown contour as the "one-abutment-one-time" concept with the definitive zirconia abutment chosen. A repositioned margin and possible overcontouring of the crown need to be assessed to create the desired soft tissue scalloping and gingival levels.

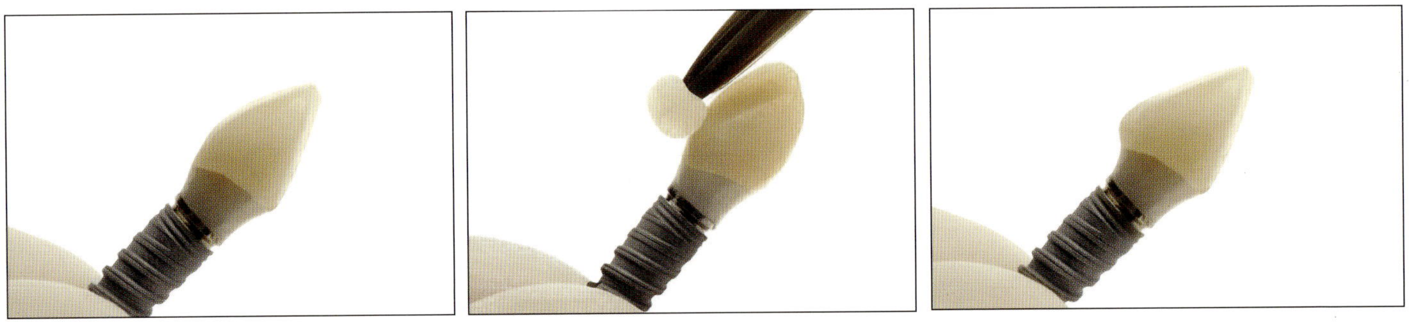

After verifying level vertical positions of the preparation finish lines with periodontal probes, the definitive abutments were disconnected and attached to the implant analogs chairside. The provisional crowns were placed on the abutments, and acrylic was added cervically to shape the desired tissue contour.

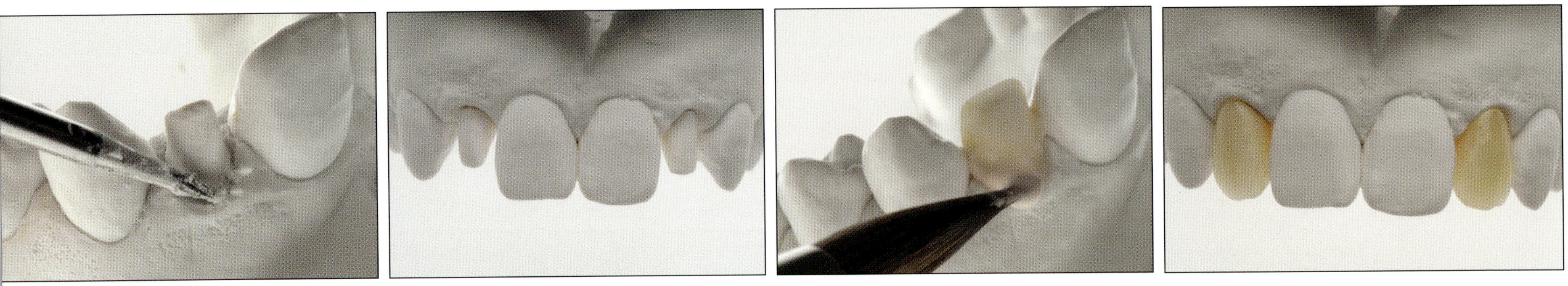

The final PVS impression was poured in stone. An idealized tissue contour was carved into the stone to create the emergence profile, which must be communicated with the laboratory technician.

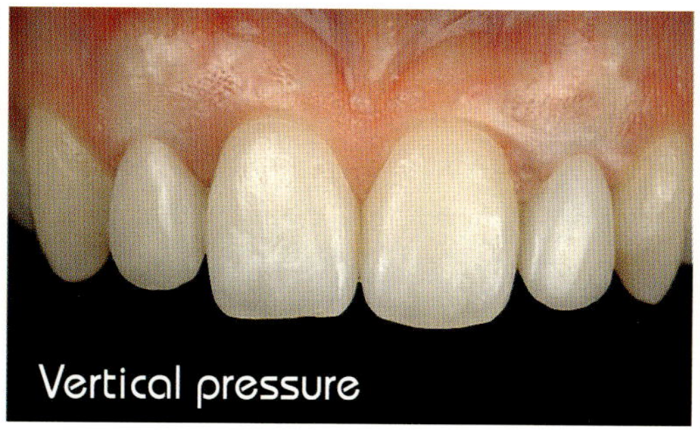

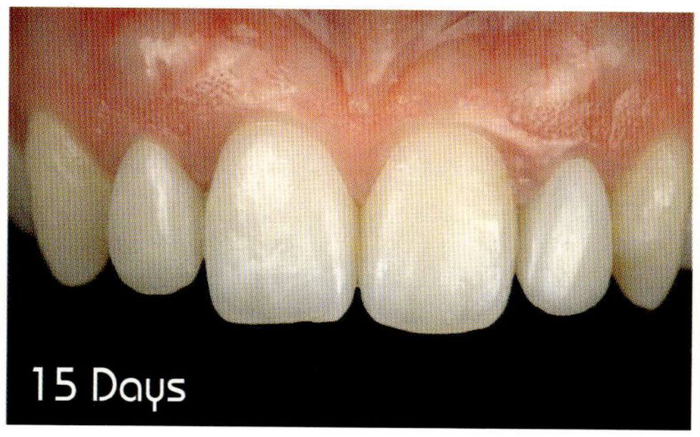

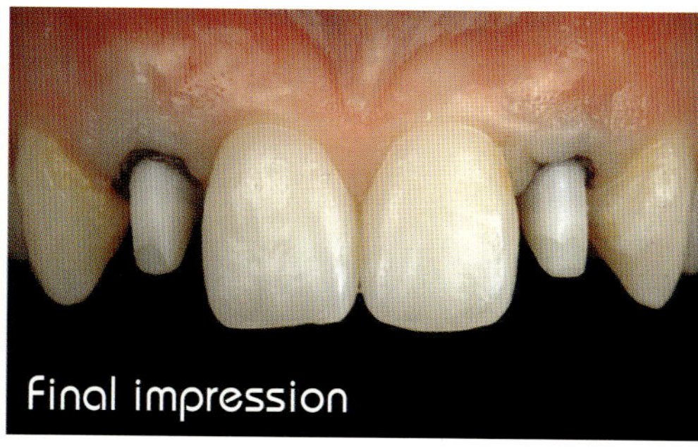

Provisional crowns were polished and provisionally cemented onto the abutments. The blanching of the tissues is an obvious indicator of the amount of pressure applied. After 15 days, the tissue contour seemed acceptable, and a final impression was made in a conventional manner with a retraction cord.

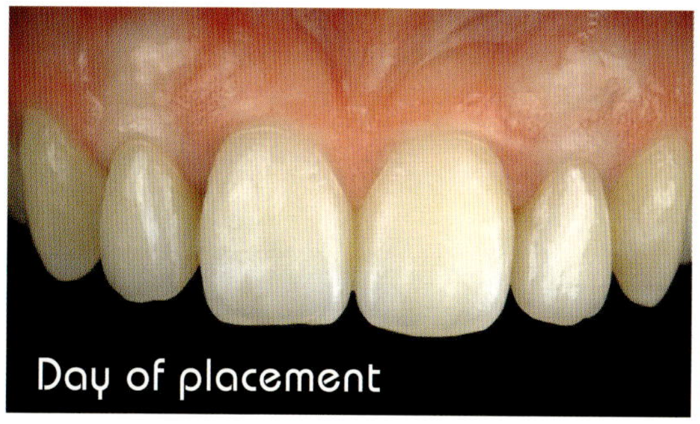

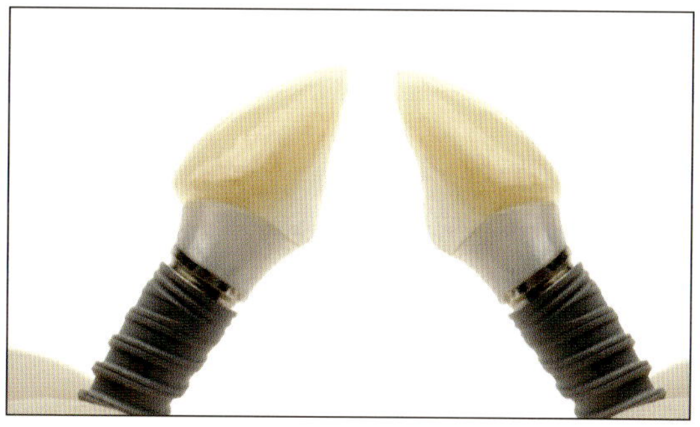

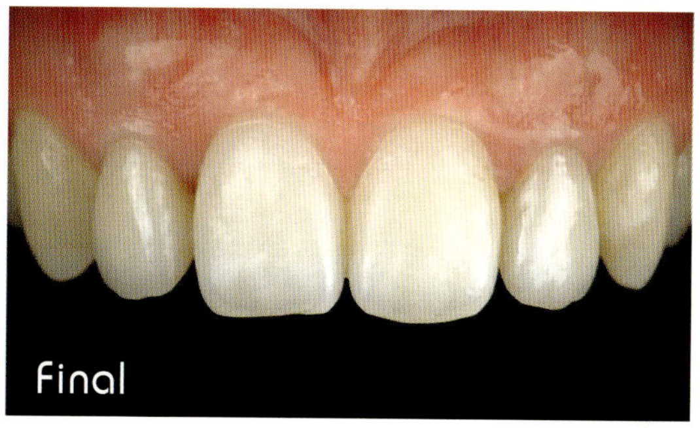

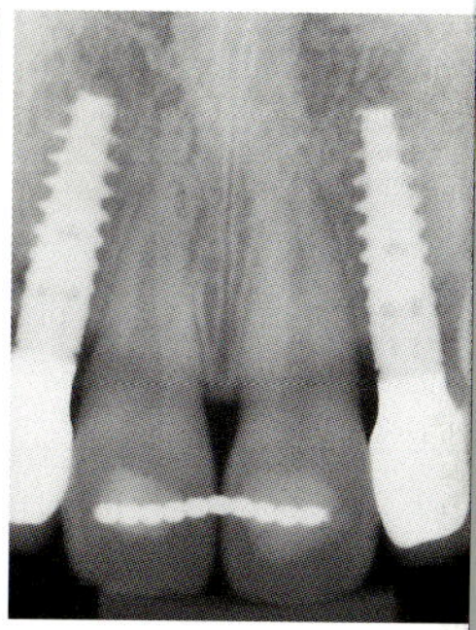

A recontoured definitive crown always causes at least a slight blanching of the buccal tissues. The buccal aspect of the crown was bulkier and overcontoured to compensate for the lack of support by the abutment. Yet tissues and bone support remained stable 1 year postoperatively.

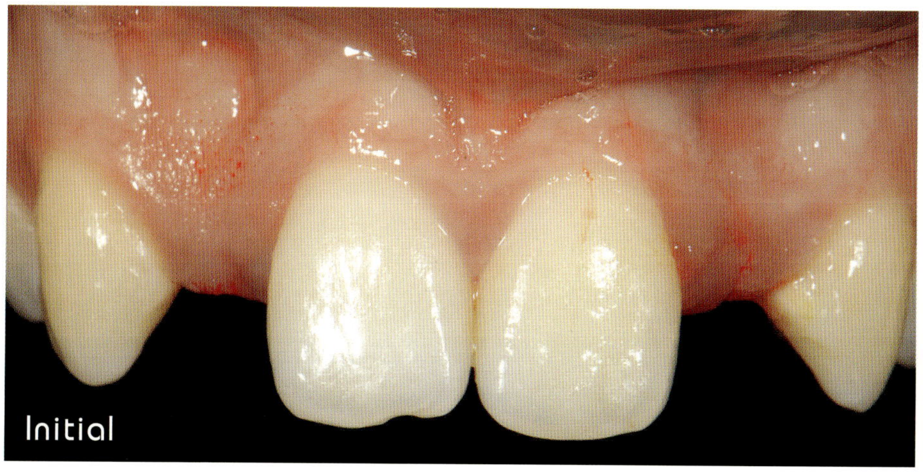

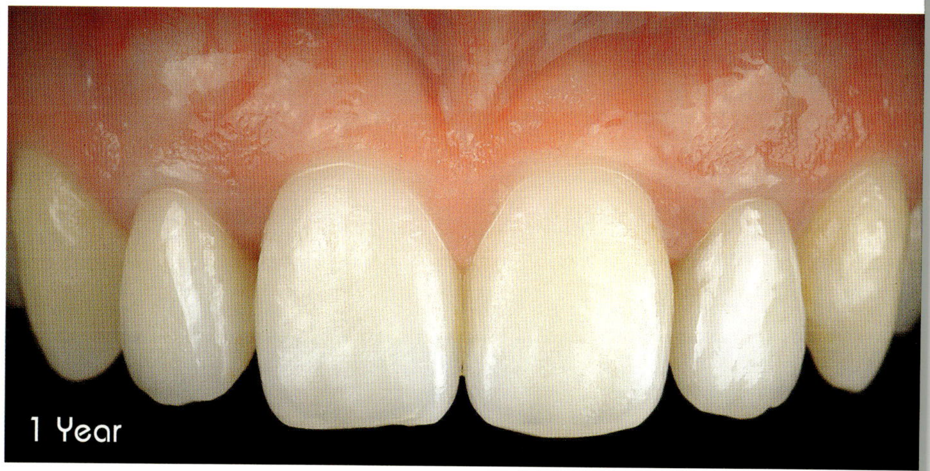

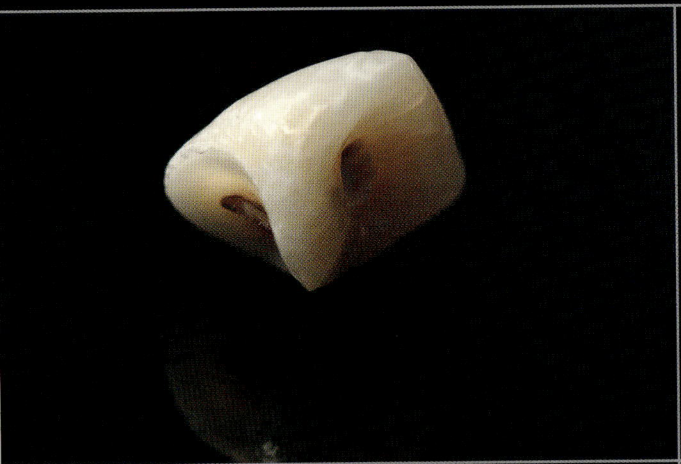

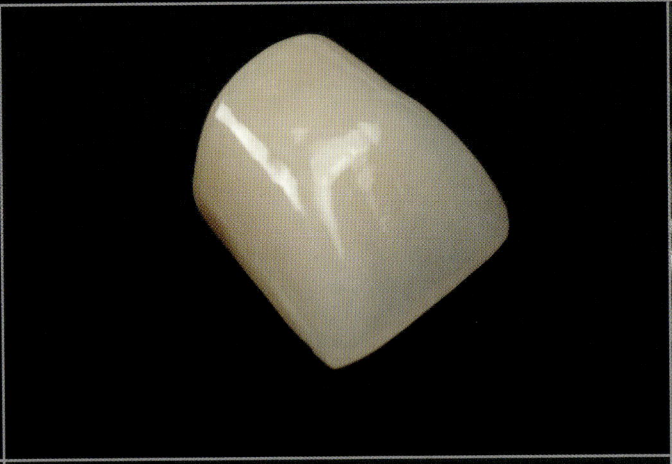

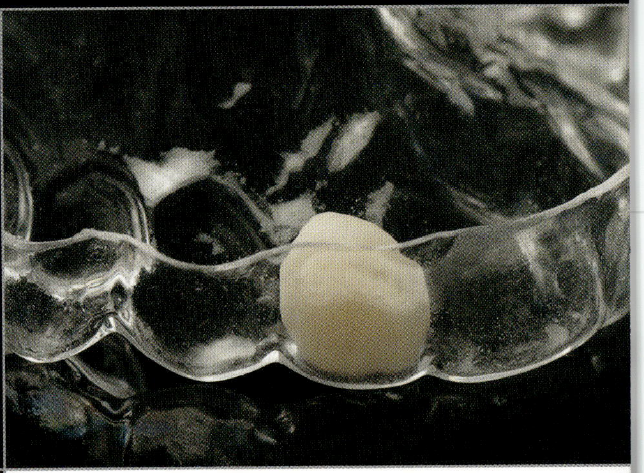

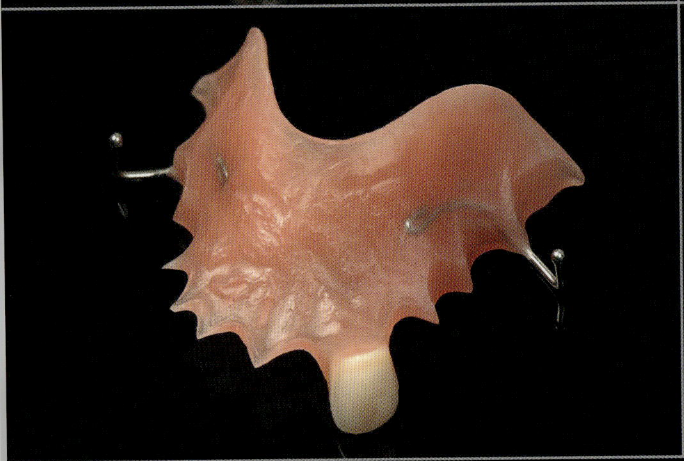

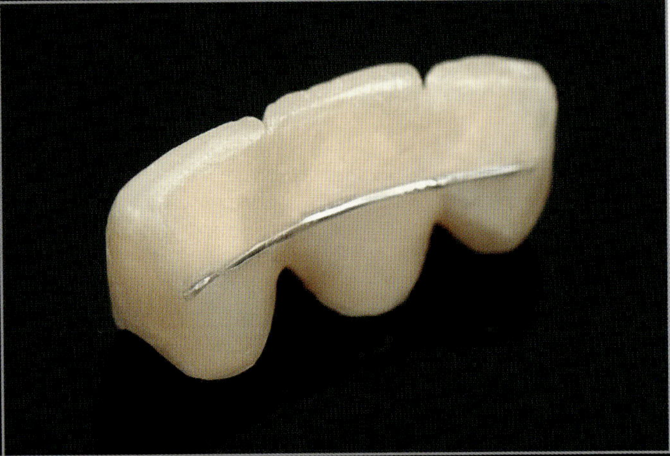

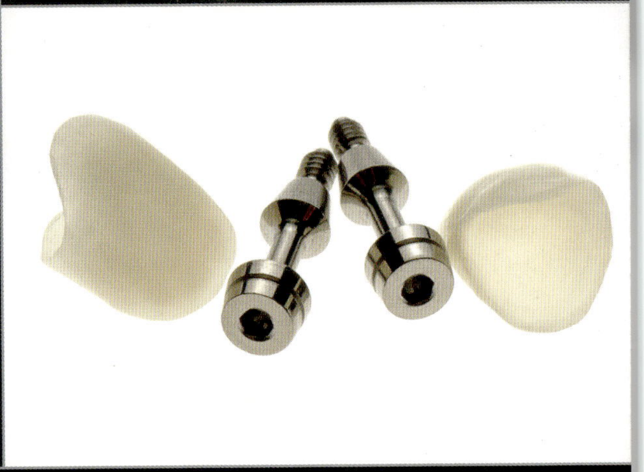

Interim restorations

Interim restorations, whether fixed or removable, need to provide satisfactory esthetics to the patient during the multiple phases of restorative implant therapy. They are also key diagnostic tools and provide invaluable guidance in the decision-making process for the design and material selection of the definitive restoration. Many different options are available, as outlined in the following clinical examples. Certain key factors need to be taken into consideration to prevent deleterious effects on the edentulous ridge.

The interim restorations must:
- Eliminate vertical pressure on the ridge
- Have a ridge lap or flat pontic design during the healing phase
- Maintain good interproximal contacts to maintain the original mesiodistal space
- Protect tooth contours and soft tissue topography
- Provide satisfactory esthetics to the patient
- Be durable and easy to fabricate and maintain
- Provide some diagnostic value

Interim restorations can include any of the following: bonded tooth, vacuform retainer, removable partial denture (RPD), provisional FPD, or immediately loaded restorations.

Composite tooth

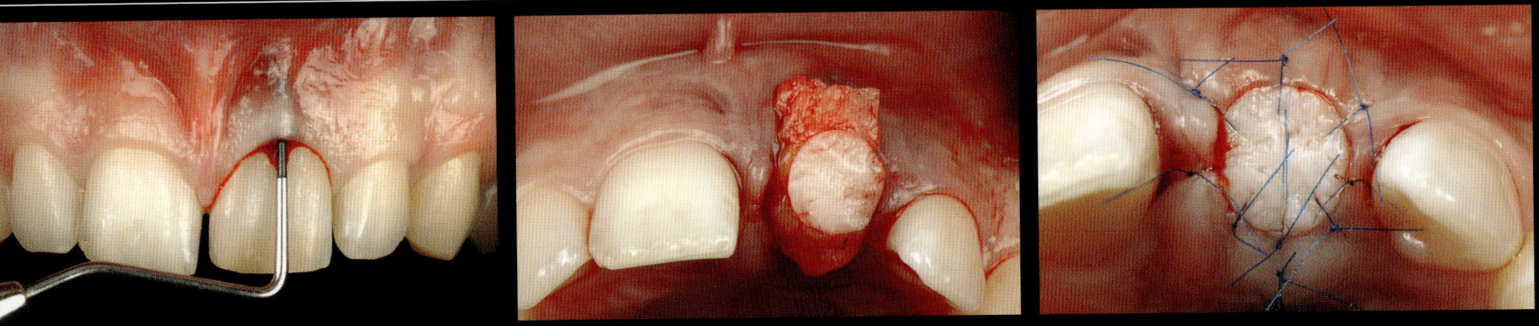

A bonded composite tooth is fabricated prior to tooth extraction and provides several benefits, including fixed esthetics, the elimination of vertical pressure, and protection of the CTG. Fabricating the provisional tooth from the same composite material as the one used for bonding it to the adjacent teeth has the benefit of increased bond strength and, therefore, a longer-lasting restoration.

Own natural tooth

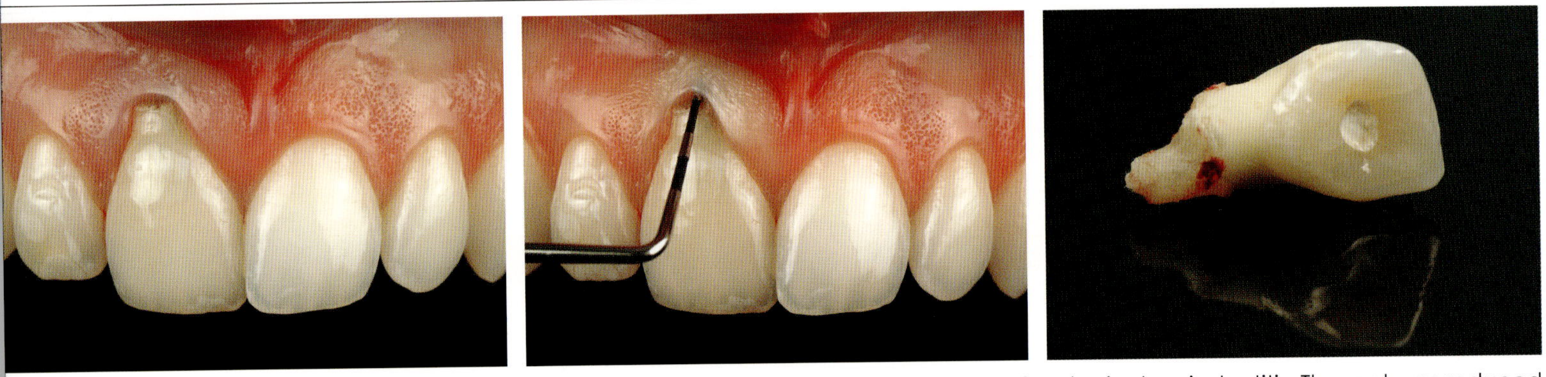

A tooth with root resorption had to be extracted because of periapical periodontitis. The root was reduced carefully, and a ridge lap pontic design was created to avoid vertical pressure and protect the soft tissue graft.

Orthodontics and vacuform retainer

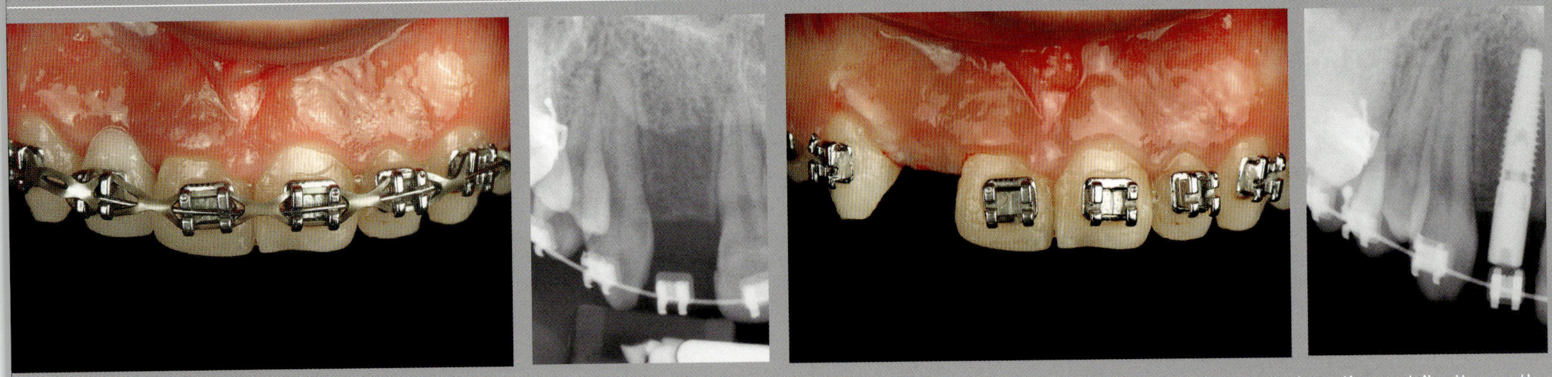

The aim of this multidisciplinary approach is to place the implant and provisional restoration while the orthodontic treatment is being performed, thereby reducing the overall duration of treatment.

Orthodontist: Dr Domingo Martín

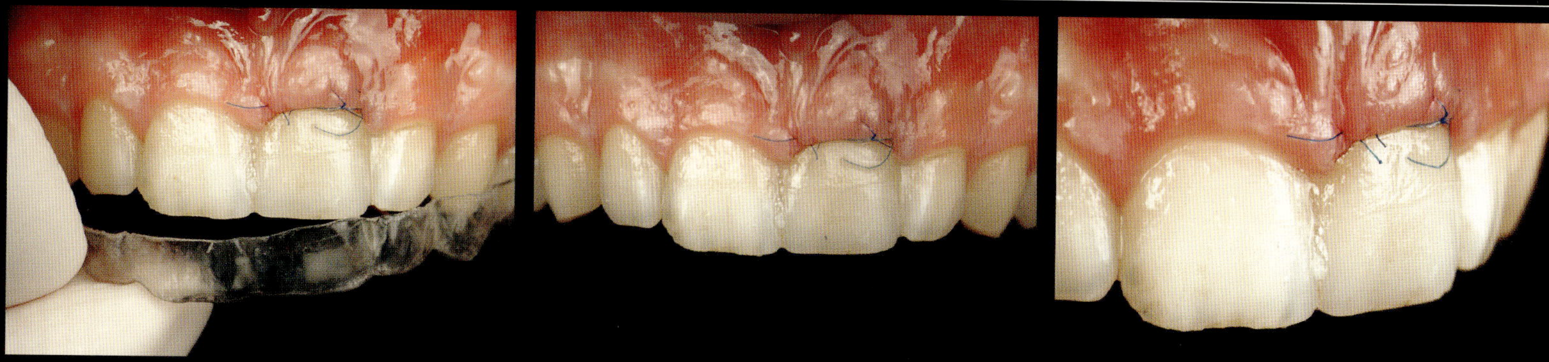

A diastema was present, and a bonded composite restoration was placed for increased strength because the natural tooth was fractured.

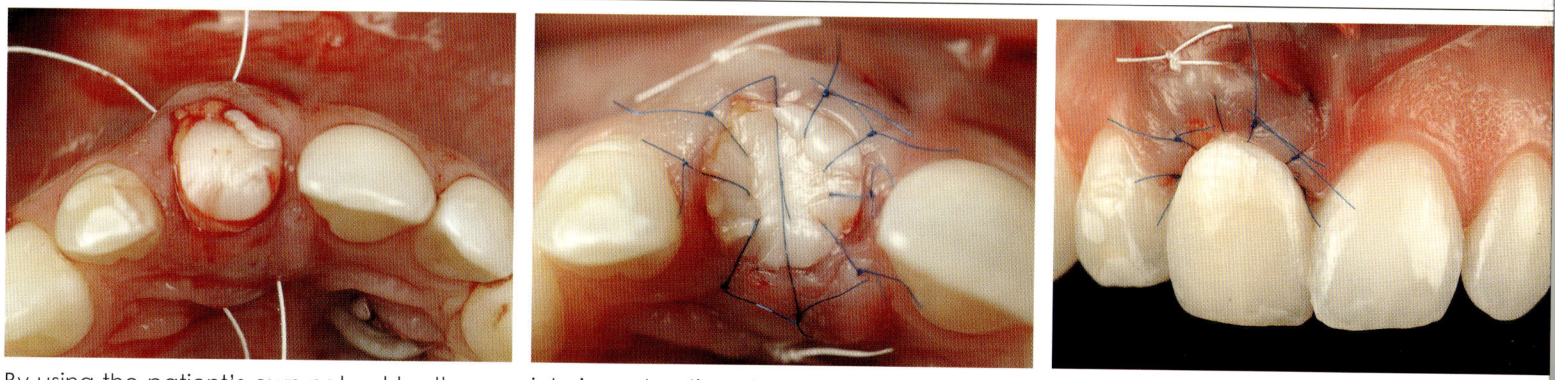

By using the patient's own natural tooth as an interim restoration, the original esthetics are maintained. The tooth is resin bonded with composite to the interproximal enamel of the adjacent teeth. Besides providing a simple, easy-to-make, and durable solution, it may serve as an excellent indicator and diagnostic tool for identifying and evaluating future soft tissue changes and resorption.

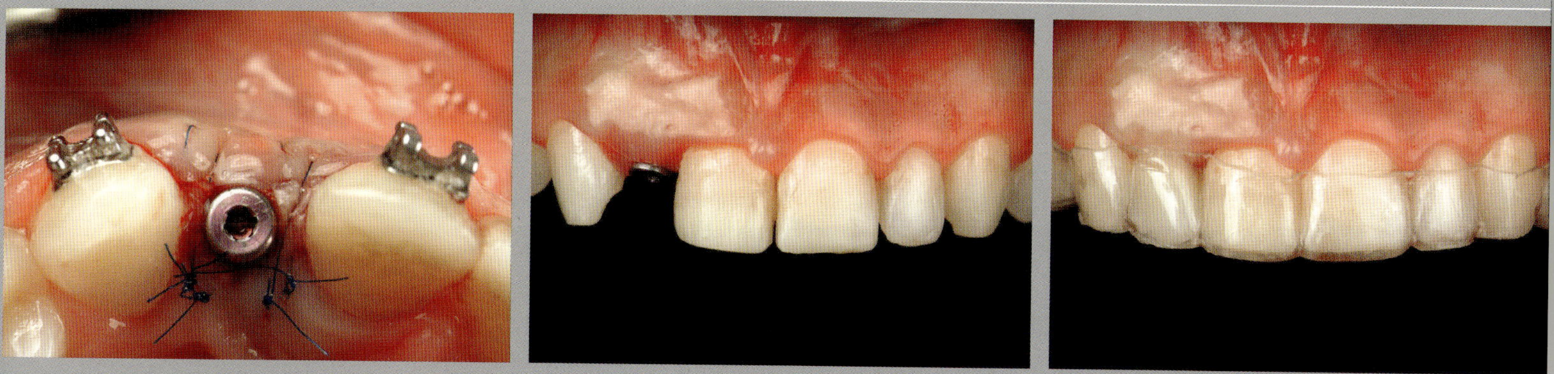

In this patient, orthodontic treatment was completed before complete healing from the implant surgery. A clear vacuform retainer, typically used by the orthodontist as a retainer and space maintainer after orthodontic treatment and during implant therapy, was used as an interim restoration. These retainers are easy to fabricate but are not recommended for extended use because of wear and possible fractures. A natural, denture, or composite tooth is integrated into the retainer as a pontic. When shaped appropriately, it eliminates vertical forces and protects the soft tissues in the pontic area during the healing phase without impinging on them.

Removable partial denture

The biggest disadvantage of RPDs as interim restorations is the possible vertical pressure to the edentulous ridge during the healing phase. Therefore, RPDs are only recommended when the patient presents with one and when it can be adjusted appropriately. Fixed interim solutions should be provided whenever possible. Vertical support can be provided by the teeth through wrought-wire ball-type interproximal clasps and by the palatal tissues through fabrication of a stable and well-fitting acrylic base. The acrylic base should be extended into the embrasure spaces of the posterior teeth for increased stability and retention as well as distribution of influencing forces. Even if relieved in the pontic area, RPDs are not recommended if bone grafting is planned because of the potential for intermittent pressure on the grafted site and consequential resorption.

This patient presented with an RPD that fulfilled all the requirements to avoid pressure on the ridge in the implant site. The RPD was helpful to assess tissue volume loss and to determine the surgical approach necessary to regain that volume.

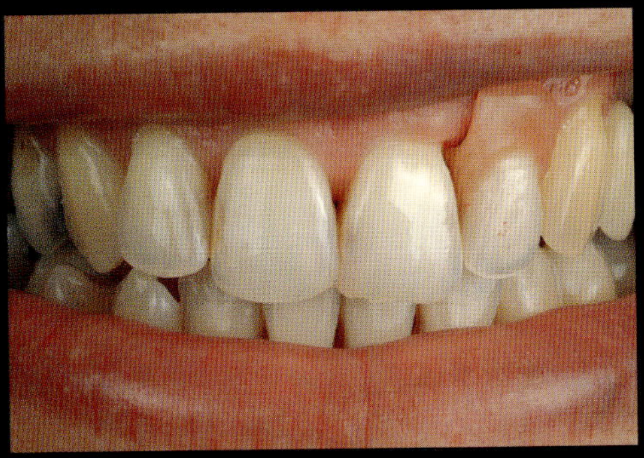

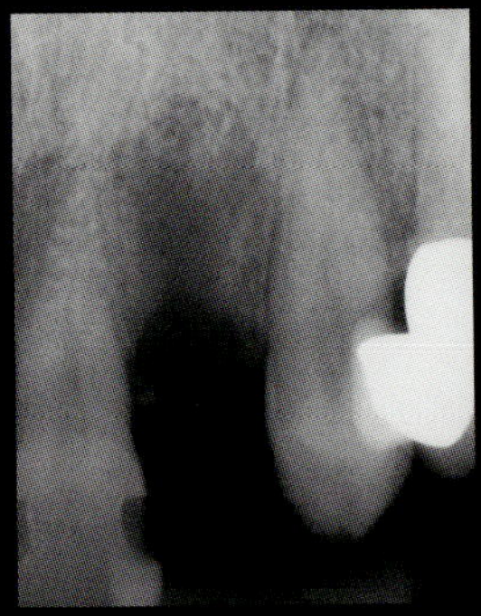

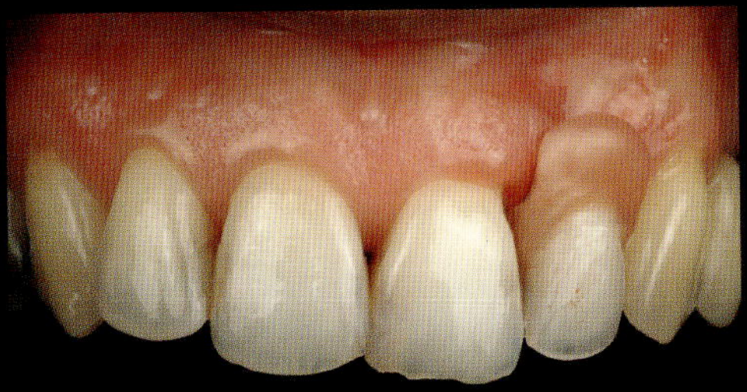

Provisional fixed partial denture

If teeth adjacent to the implant site have crowns or will receive full-coverage restorations, an FPD interim restoration provides the best solution for ideal esthetics and function while the implant site is healing.

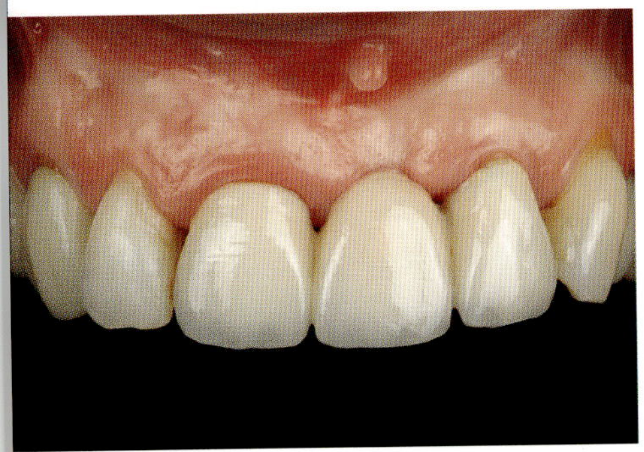

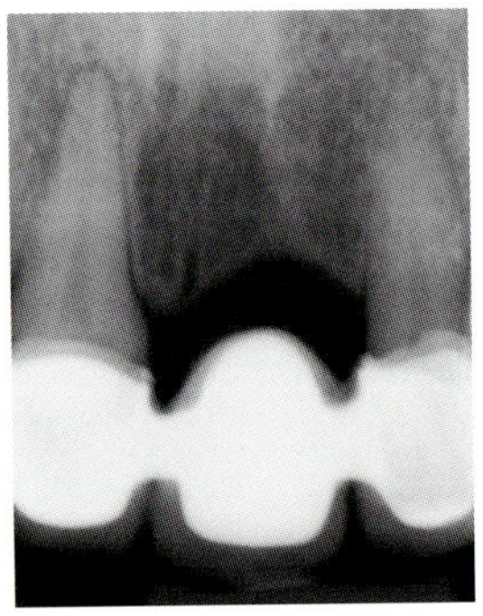

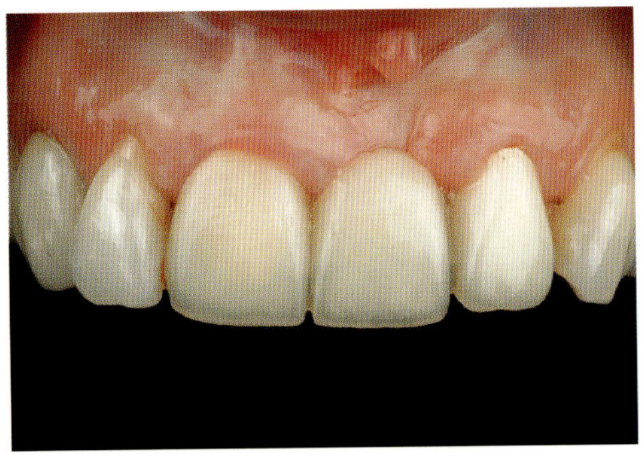

In this clinical situation, a three-unit provisional FPD was fabricated from a provisional acrylic material (Caulk/Dentsply) before the surgical implant phase. A NobelReplace Groovy implant (4.3 × 13 mm) was inserted with a 5-mm-high NP healing abutment, a PS adapter, and a CTG during a one-stage surgery. The provisional FPD was relined to accommodate the new tissue topography at the surgical site as the tissues matured.

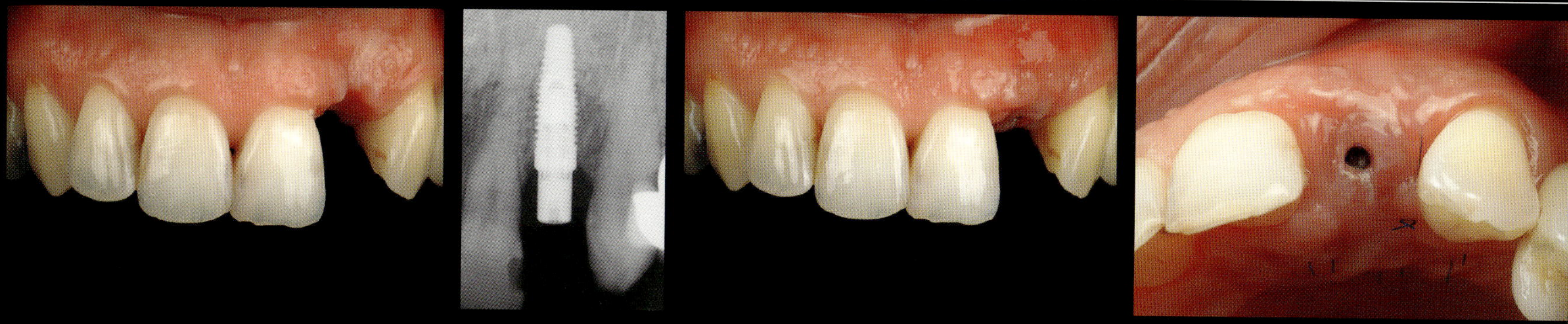

Different phases of the healing process are shown. The RPD was designed so that neither the flange nor the pontic came in contact with the soft tissue or the healing abutment.

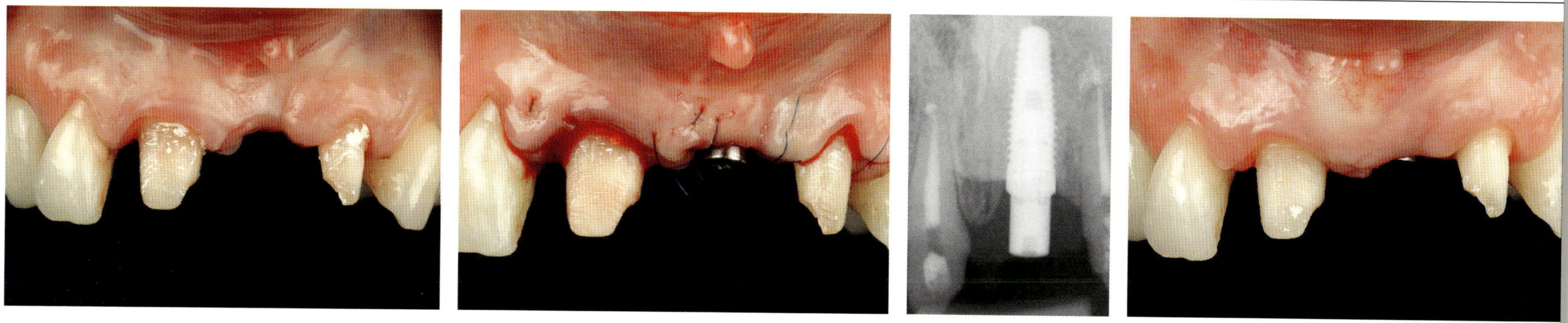

Immediate loading: Temporary healing abutment

Slim temporary abutments allow for a totally different approach whenever the surgeon is able to ideally place the implants with a minimum torque of 35 Ncm. This type of healing abutment allows for an immediate interim restoration with the possibility to place a CTG around the implant (a major asset for ideal esthetics during implant treatment) and excellent primary closure due to its 1-mm narrow transmucosal part. An abutment is placed on top (prosthetic part) of the healing abutment for the retentive part of the crown restoration. Care must be taken when relining the shell provisional restoration because of the undercut of the design. To avoid locking the provisional crown in place, it is recommended to never let the acrylic material polymerize completely on the healing abutment.

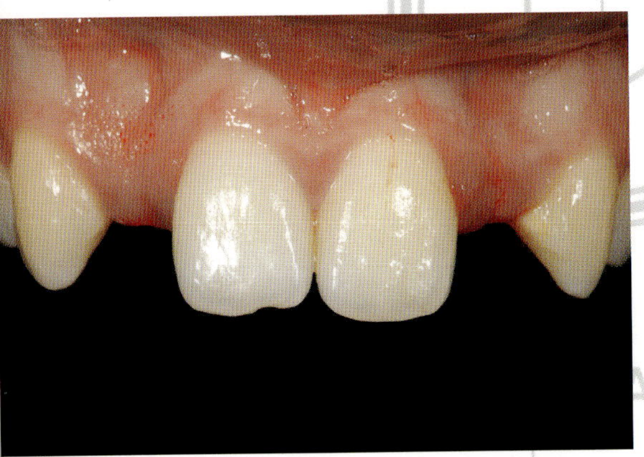

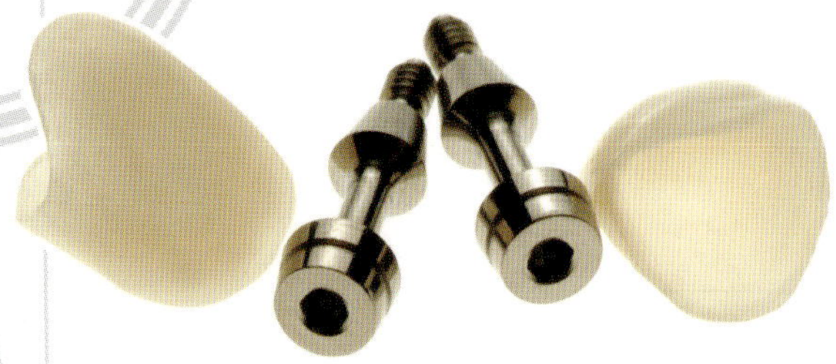

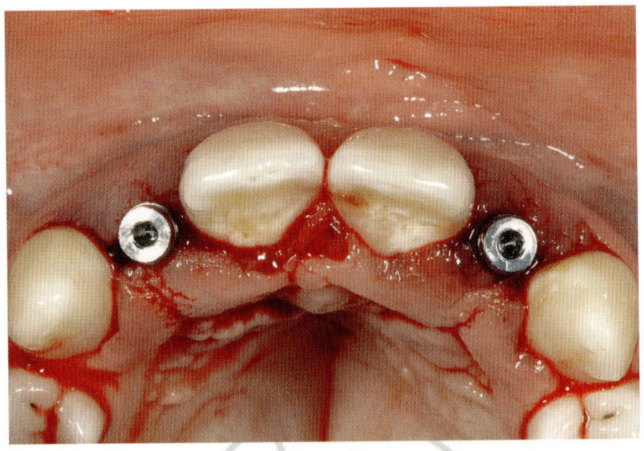

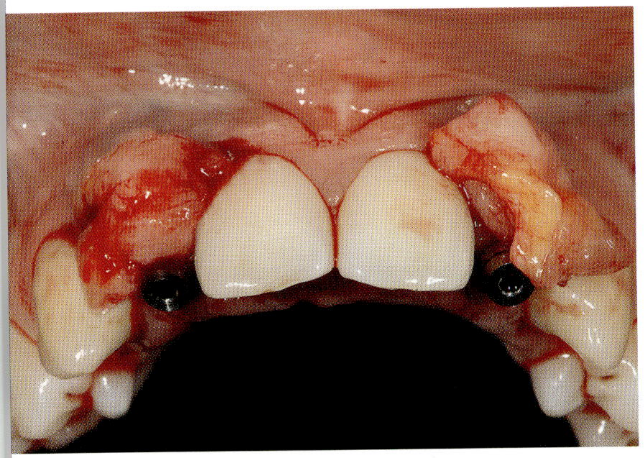

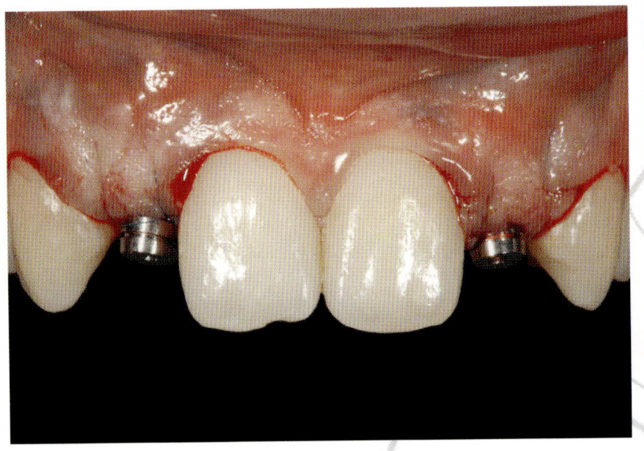

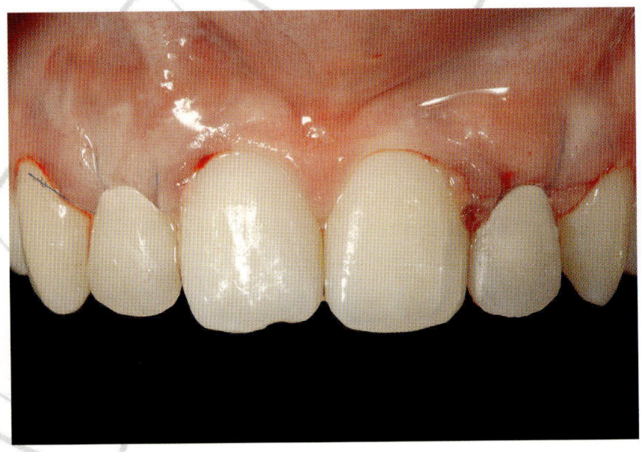

Silicone matrices from a previous diagnostic wax-up can be fabricated for visualization of the abutment and implant placement in reference to the overall crown contour and interocclusal space. It may become necessary to customize the abutment in the event of limited occlusal space to allow thicker walls of the provisional crown restoration.

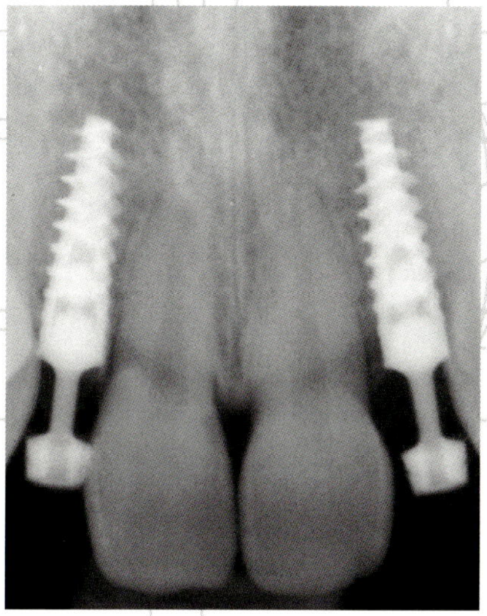

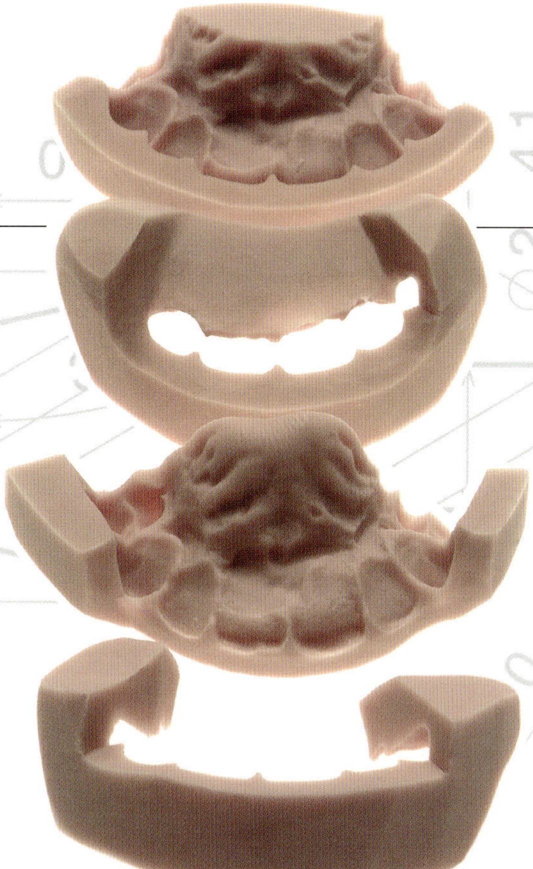

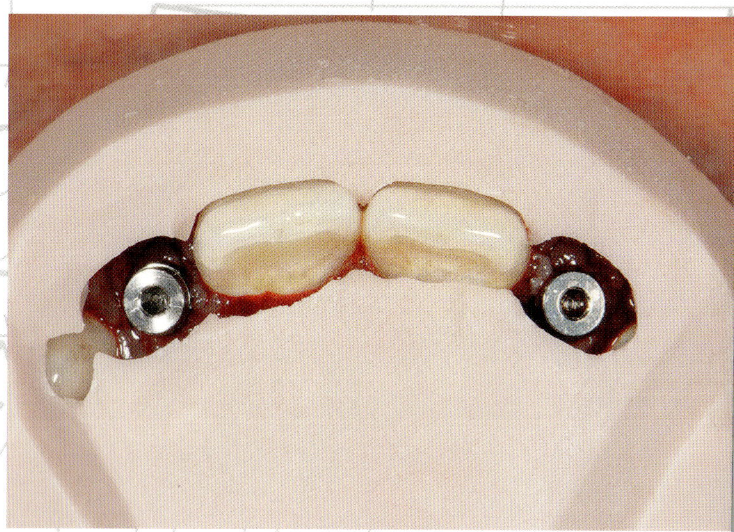

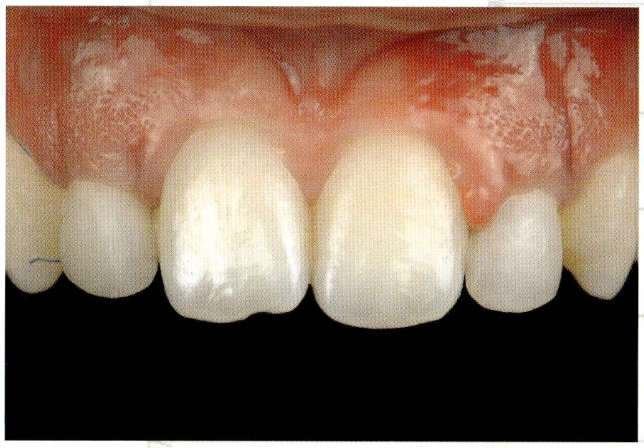

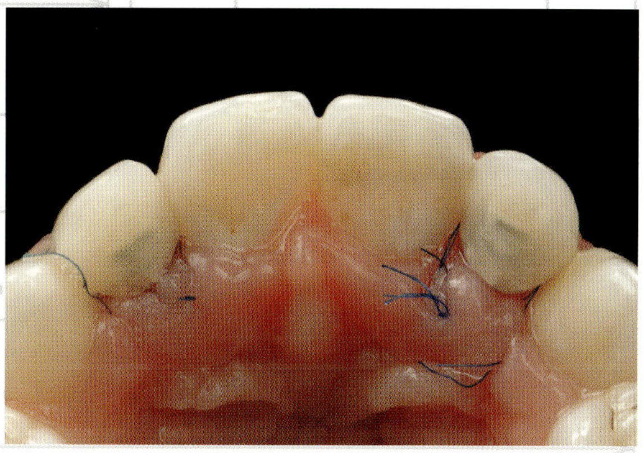

CTGs from the tuberosity were placed on both sites for long-term tissue stability and esthetic results. The voluminous soft tissue grafts were positioned at the most coronal and central areas of the implant long axes and allowed for ideal suturing and primary wound closure.

The 2-week postsurgery view depicts the soft tissue integration from the buccal and palatal aspects and the space required for the CTG and the interim crown restoration. Another benefit of this type of interim restoration is that it eliminates the need for resin bonding to the adjacent teeth, which always causes trauma to the enamel of these teeth and negatively influences overall contour of the original crown.

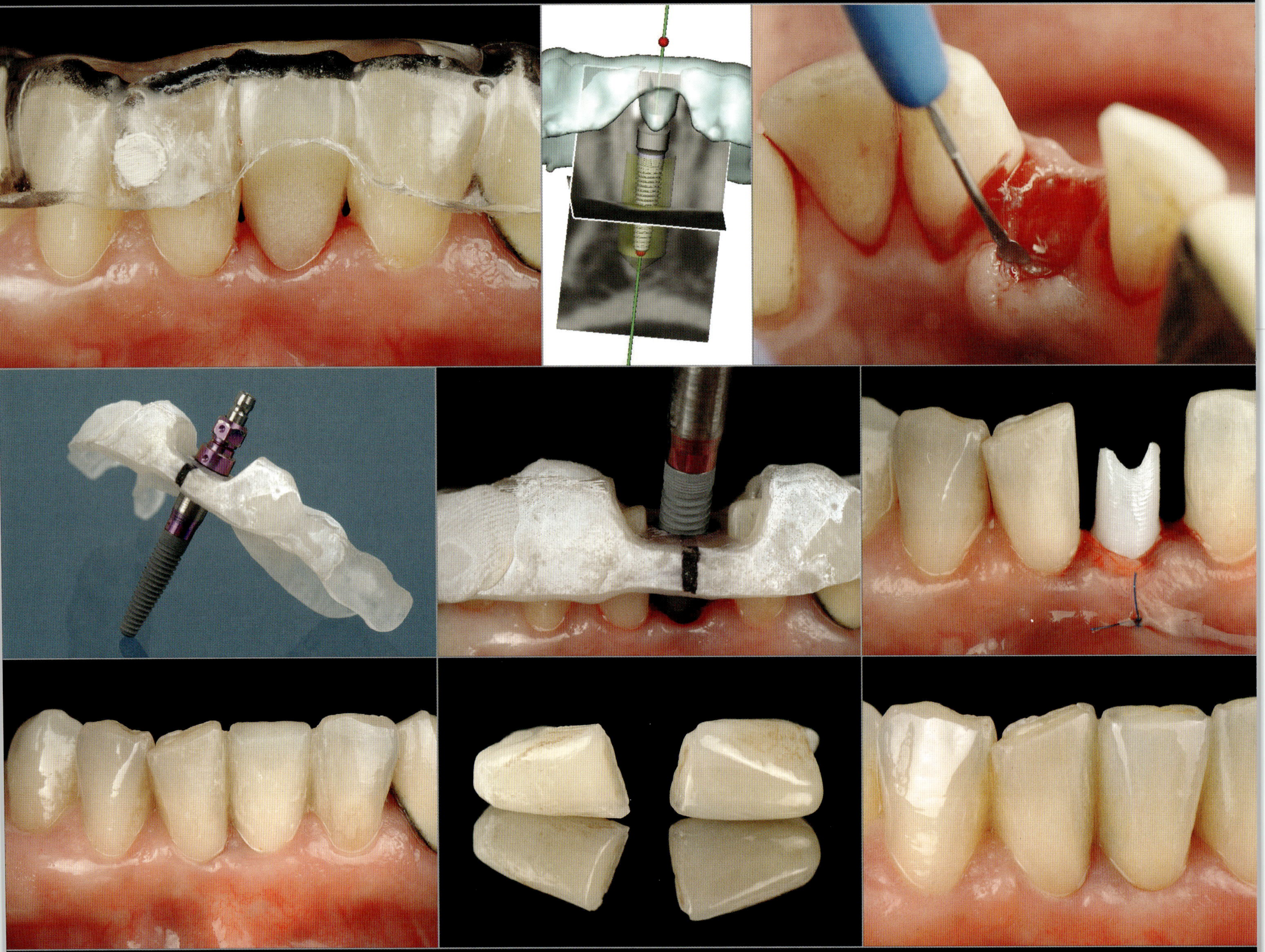

Guided Surgery

Initial situation

It is difficult to justify the use of guided surgery for a single-tooth implant placement. However, in a situation like the one presented here, where anatomical limitations such as angulation of adjacent root tips provide a great challenge and high risk for compromising the outcome, guided surgery adds a level of precision and accuracy that is simply not possible by pure "eyeballing" and tactile sensation even of the most skilled surgeon.

Therefore, guided surgery adds precision, predictability, and safety to the surgical procedure. The most important aspects of this technique are the adaptation, fit, and design of the radiographic template to ensure precise implant placement with a well-fitted and well-designed surgical stent.

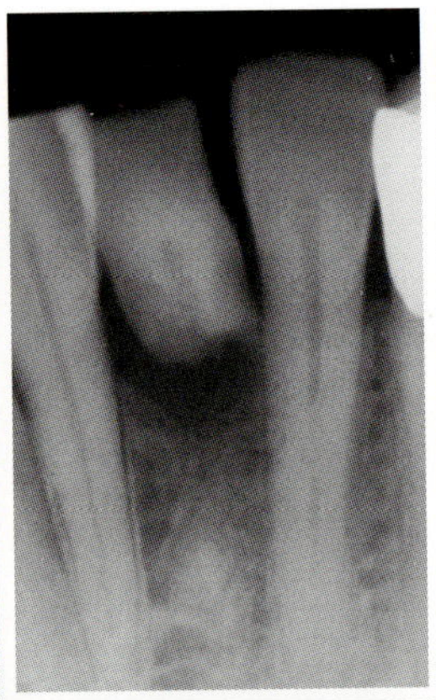

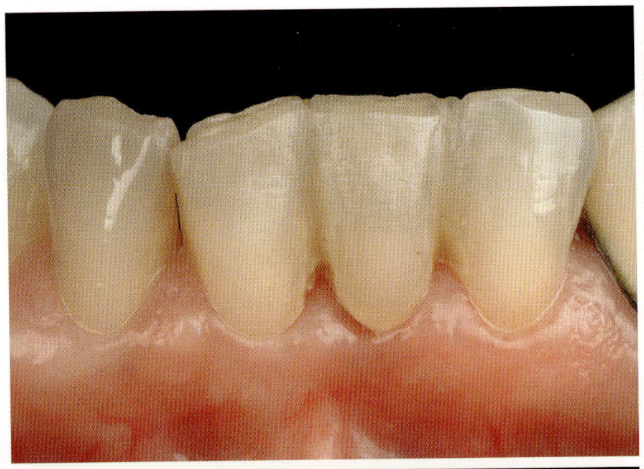

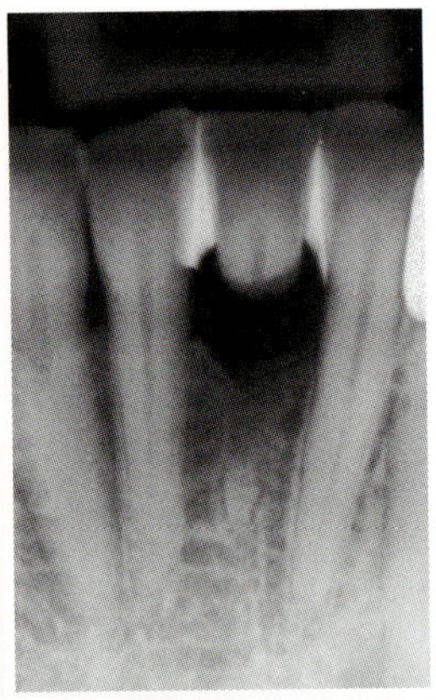

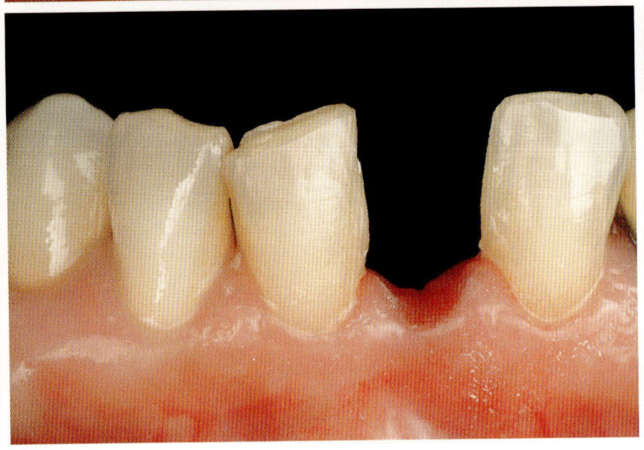

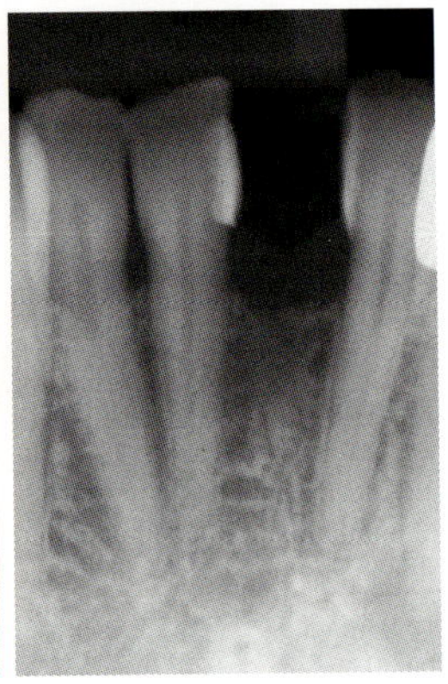

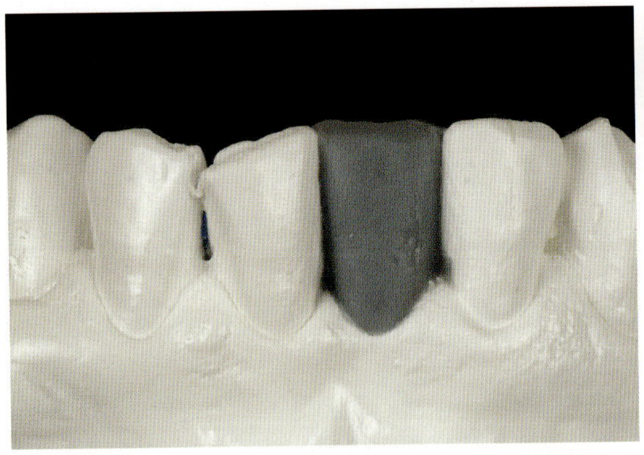

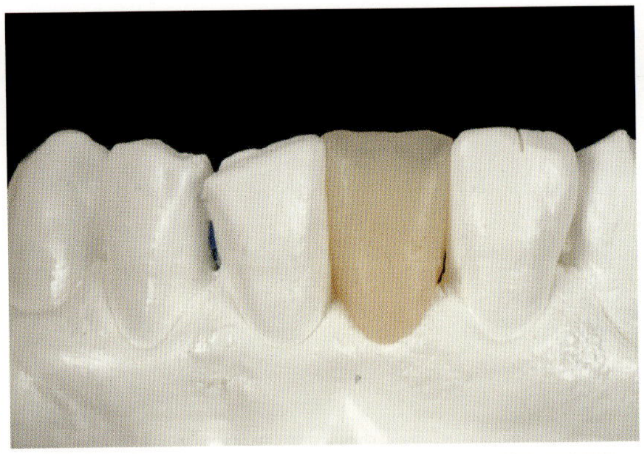

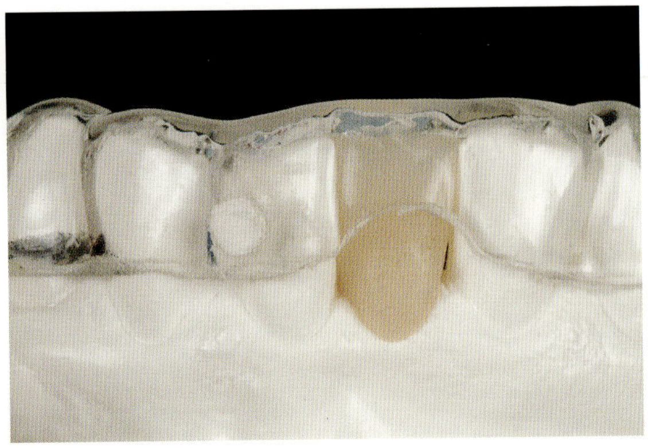

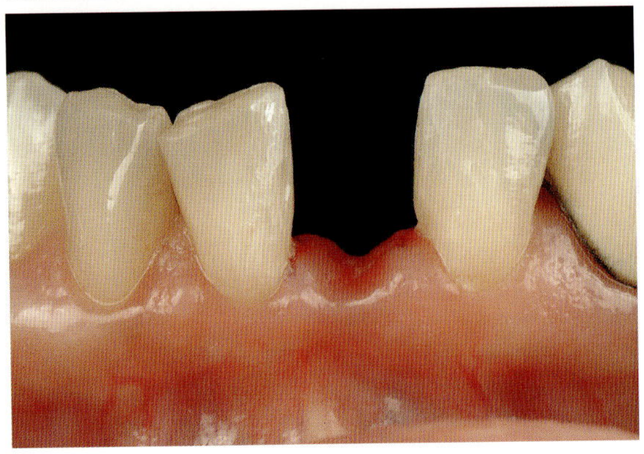

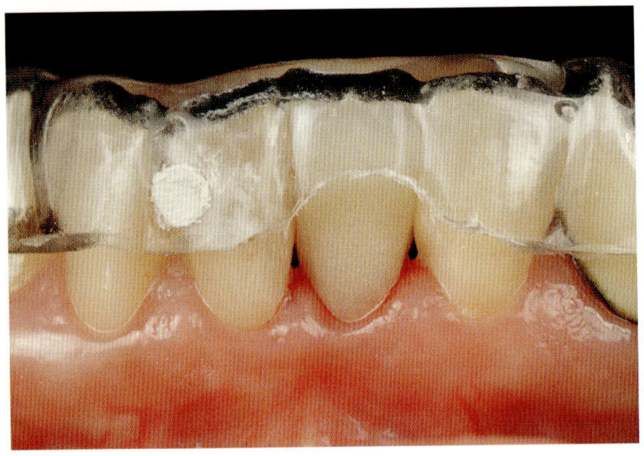

Diagnostic

A diagnostic wax-up that restored the contour and characteristics of the missing tooth was fabricated on a precise master cast. The master cast with the diagnostic wax-up was then duplicated to fabricate a clear thermoplastic splint with a 1-mm-thick polyvinyl chloride (PVC) material. An acrylic tooth was fabricated from the wax-up and integrated into the clear splint.

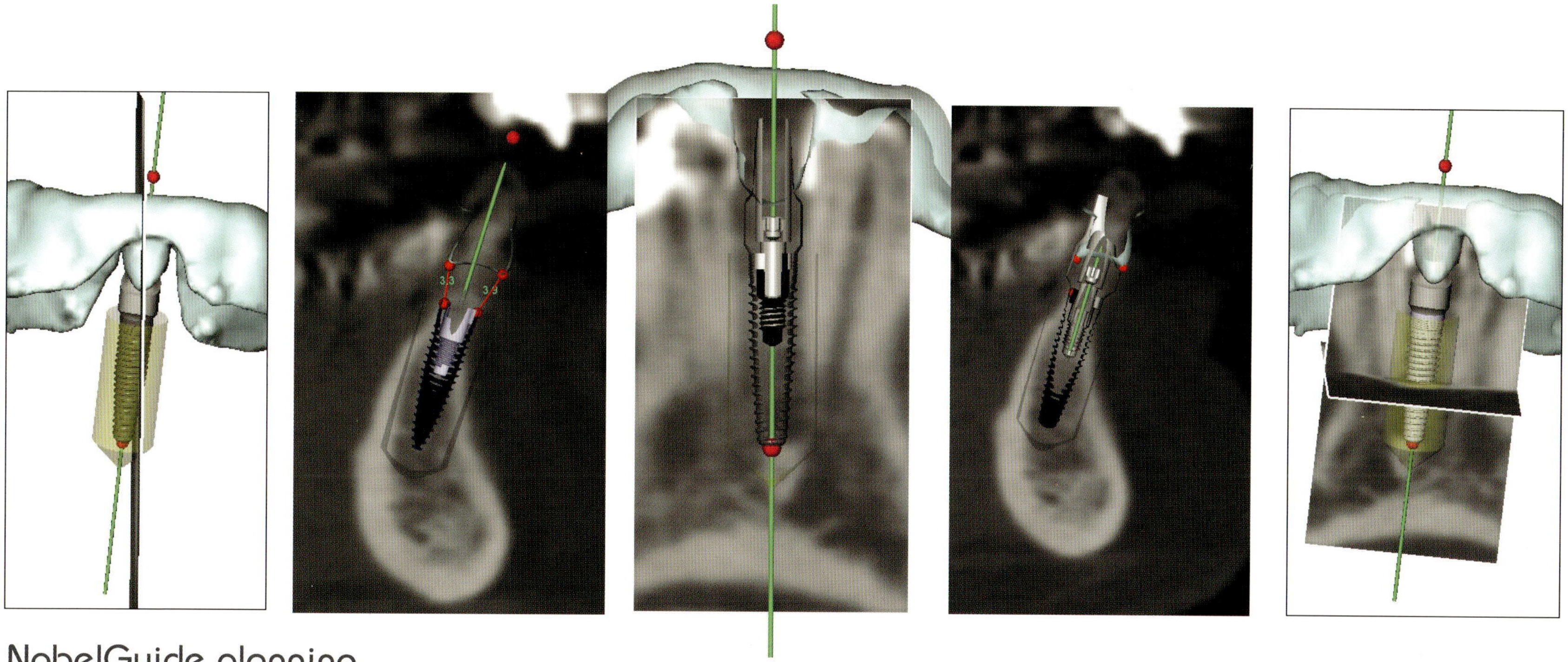

NobelGuide planning

Gutta-percha dots 1 mm in diameter were placed throughout the stent to superimpose the scan of the patient and the radiographic stent into the NobelGuide software. Care was taken to try in the radiographic stent intraorally to verify its perfect adaptation. The patient was scanned (computer tomography) with the stent in place, and, in addition, the stent was scanned by itself. The digital information was processed with the NobelGuide software, allowing for 3D implant placement while the ideal tooth position for the implant treatment was visually assessed. The different views and the ability to evaluate the abutment together with the implant placement and the tooth reference make this method ideal for treatment planning. A two-piece NobelActive 3.0 implant would have been ideal but was not available at the time of surgery. Therefore, a 3.5 NobelReplace Groovy NP was chosen over the NobelActive NP because of its smaller tip.

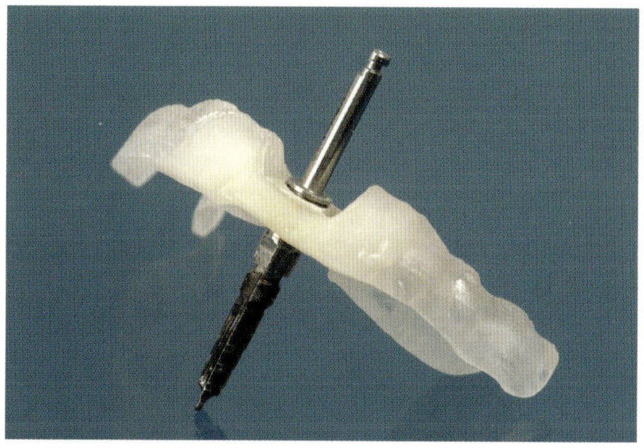

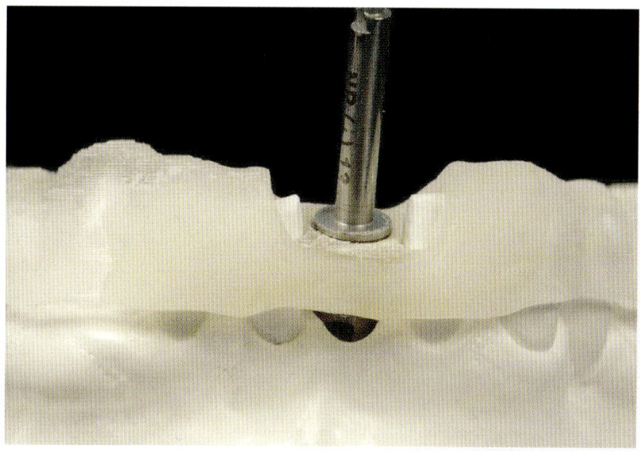

Stent adaptation

Once the surgical stent was fabricated, it was sent to the clinician. Great care was taken to adapt the surgical stent into position on the master cast and to accurately embed the laboratory analog through the modified guide cylinder inserted in the surgical template. Orientation of the laboratory analog is a crucial element for the positioning. One of the trichannel lobes of the internal implant connection must be directed toward the buccal aspect, which was marked with a black line for optimal transfer and accurate delivery of the immediate definitive zirconia abutment.

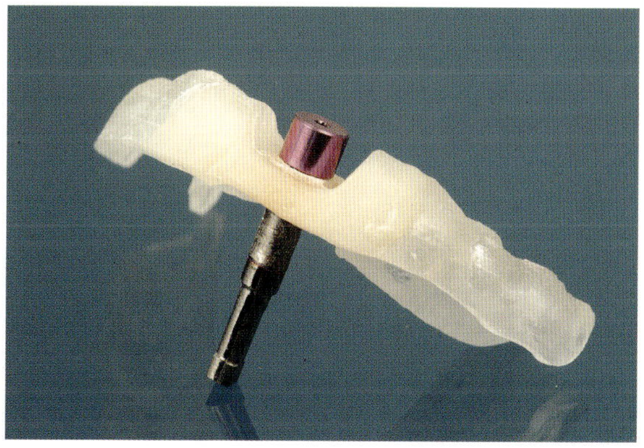

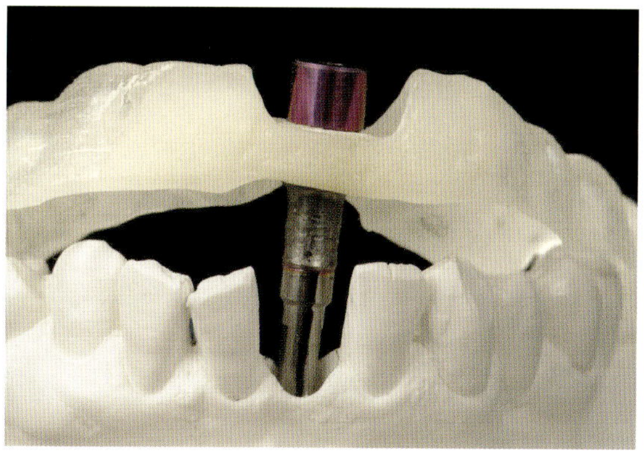

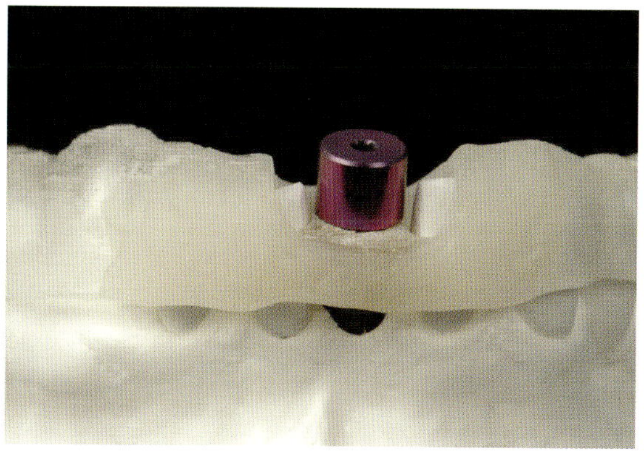

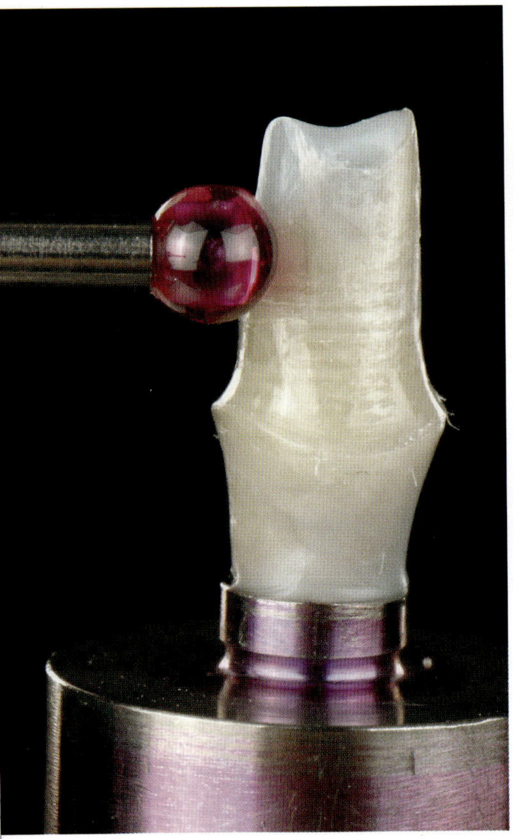

Abutment fabrication

A provisional plastic abutment was modified with composite resin to achieve the ideal shape and contour according to the provisional and diagnostic wax-up. Polyvinyl siloxane matrices were then made from the diagnostic wax-up to design and scan the zirconia abutment. The abutment was disinfected with 2% glutaraldehyde for 5 minutes before final insertion.

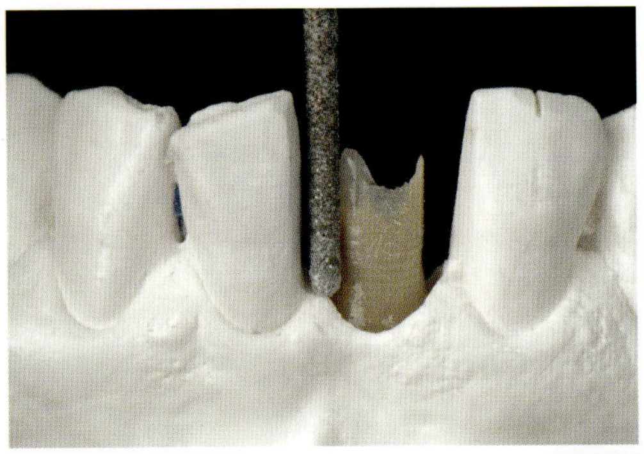

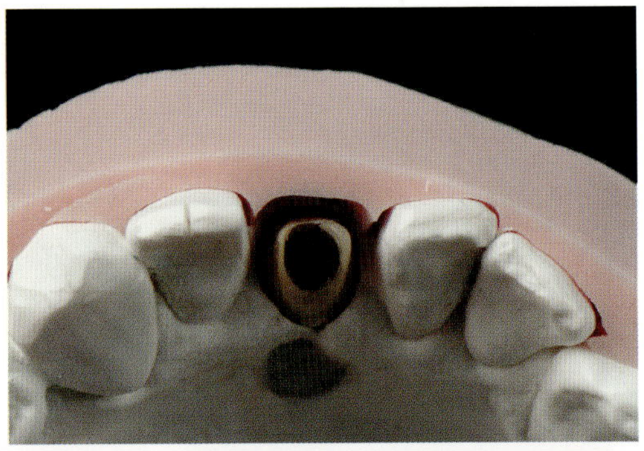

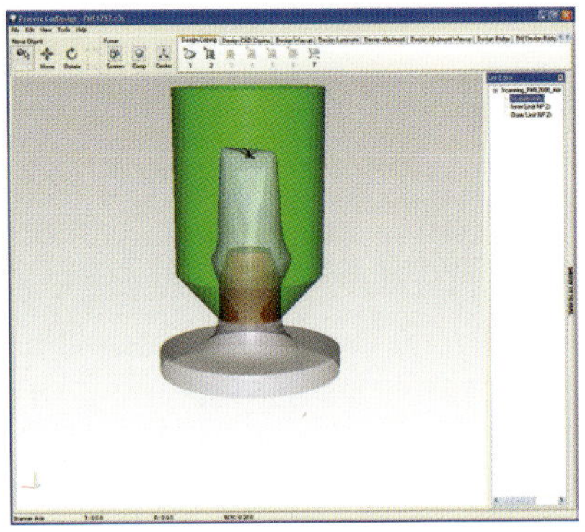

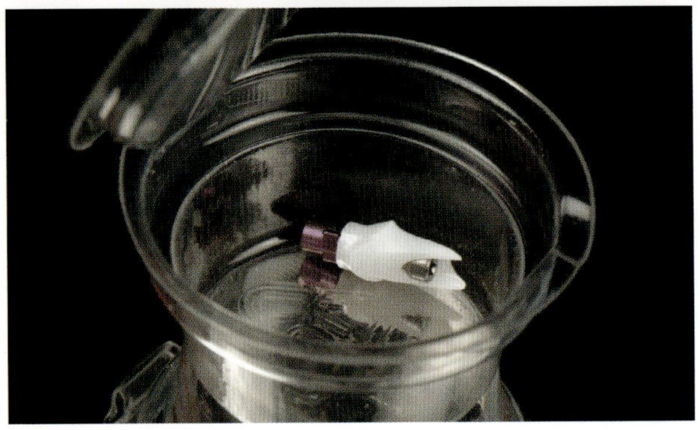

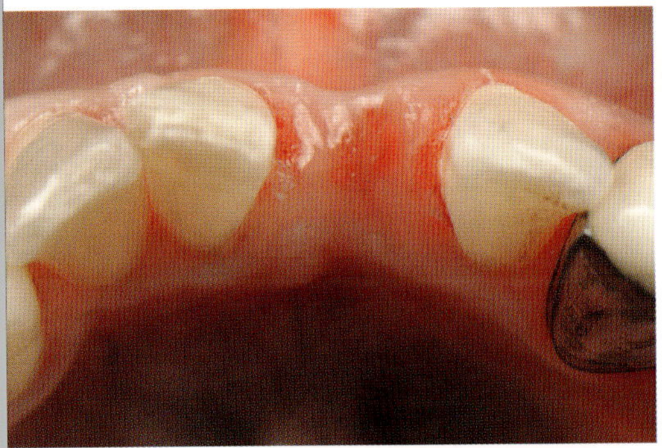

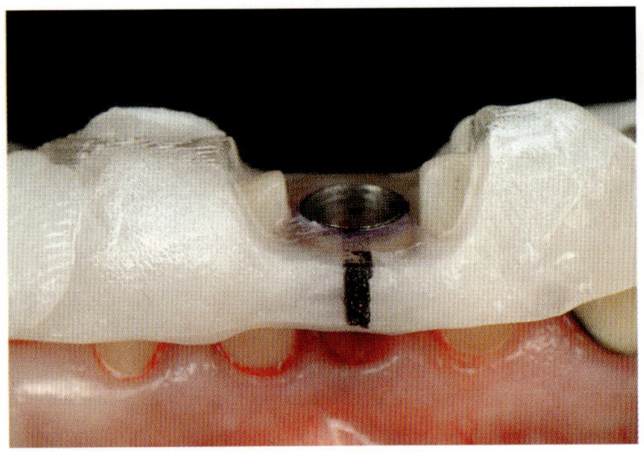

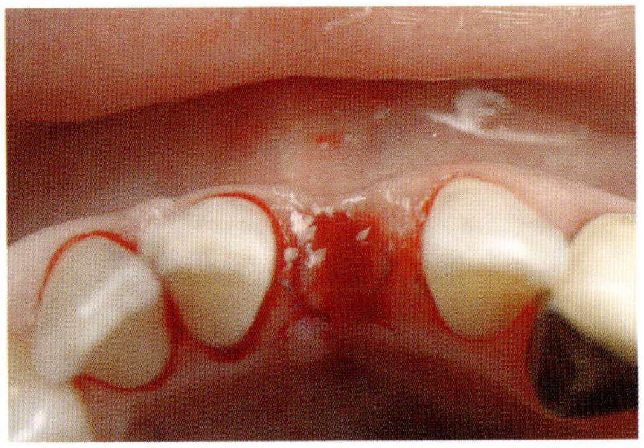

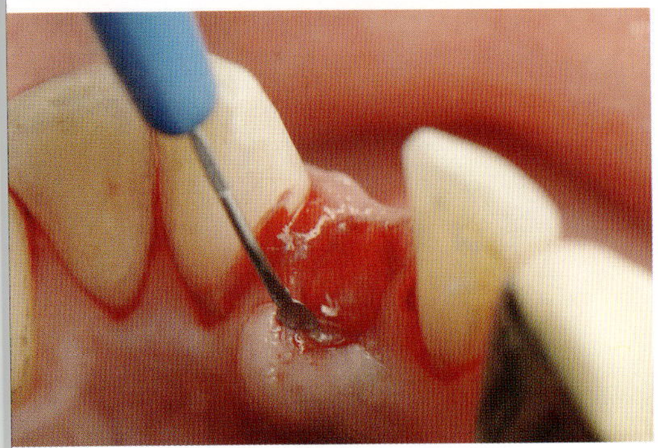

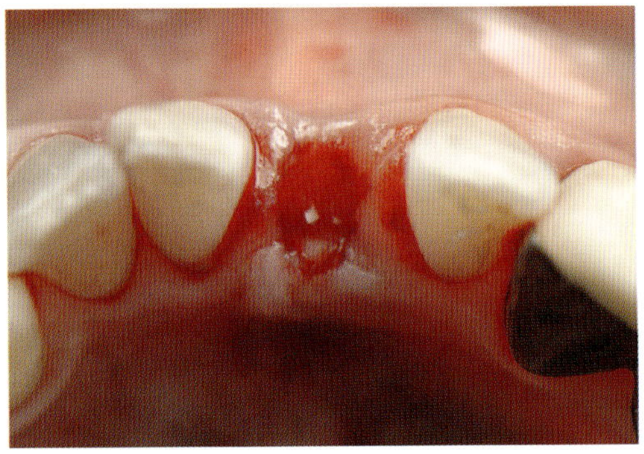

Guided soft tissue management

Soft tissue manipulation of the edentulous site through the Nobel-Guide stent is possible and predictable. Because the exact implant placement location and angulation were known, a circular incision with split-thickness flaps was made through the stent 1 mm into the tissue. Then, a microsurgical blade was used to prepare a tunnel incision on the palatal aspect of the edentulous ridge to rotate the coronal tissue lingually, allowing the drilling for the implant without damaging the valued surrounding soft tissue (usually the pedicle of tissue is sutured to avoid trauma or tearing during implant placement).

Guided implant placement

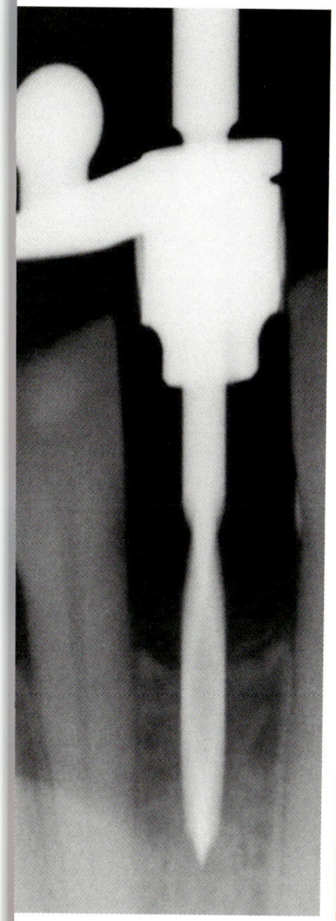

The surgical template was reinforced with acrylic resin. A periapical radiographic sequence was taken during the drilling to ensure the accurate positioning of the implant. The black line on the stent transferred the information from the master cast, including the trilobe position of the implant. Depth is crucial and was assessed with conventional carriers to place the implant exactly 3 mm from the desired gingival margin emergence. Note the correct orientation of the trilobe with the desired depth and volume shift to compensate for the lingual defect.

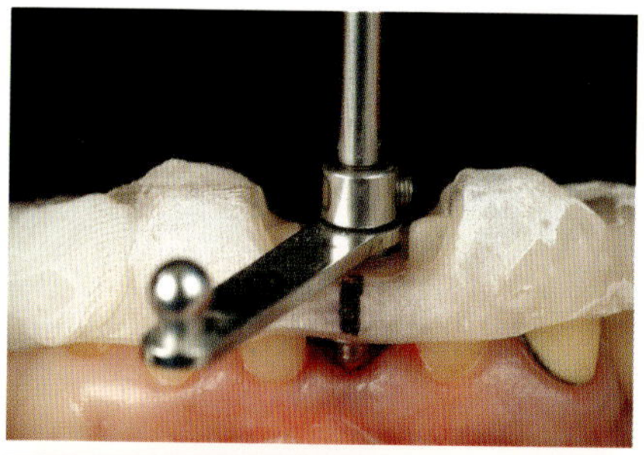
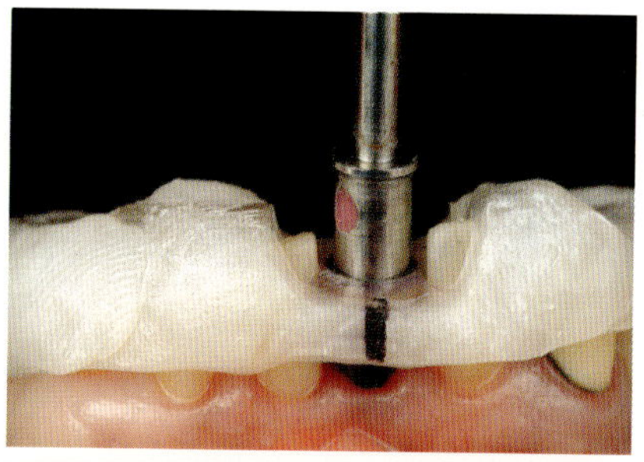
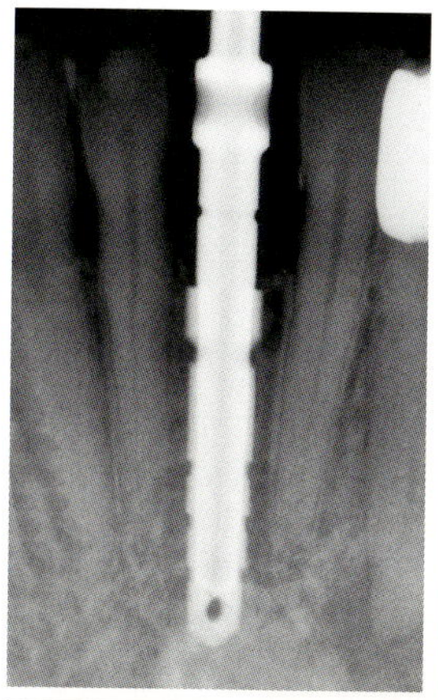
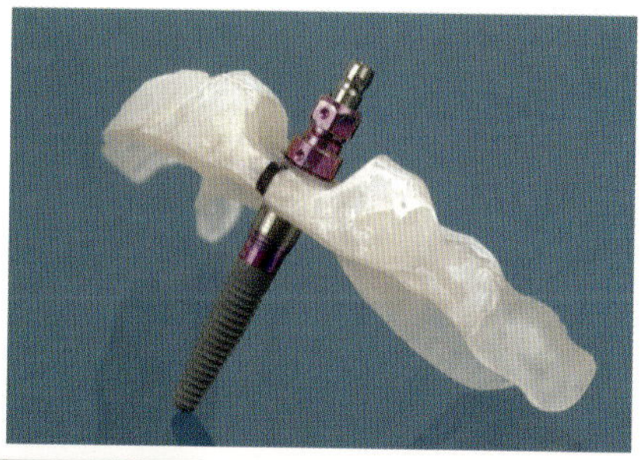

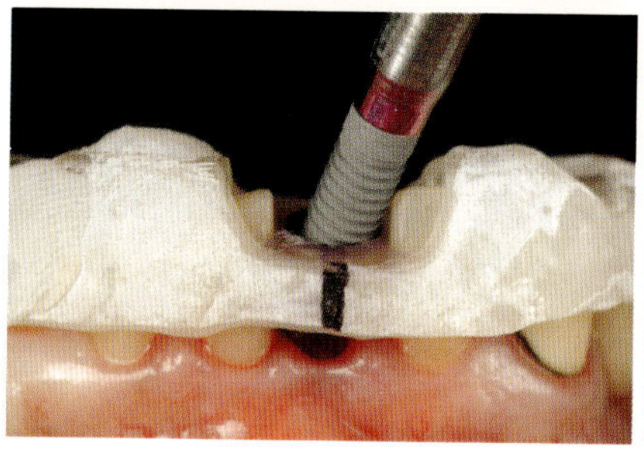
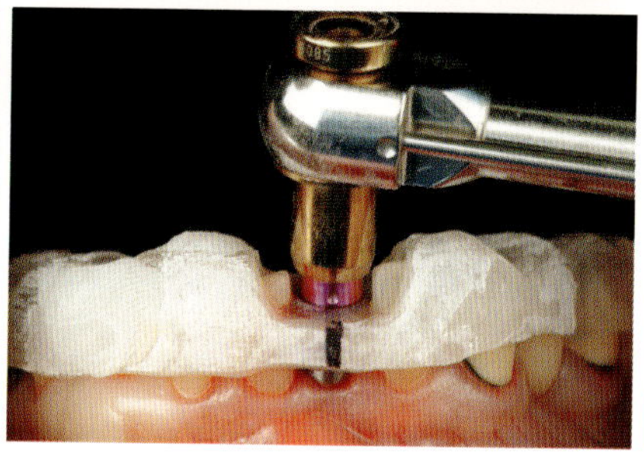
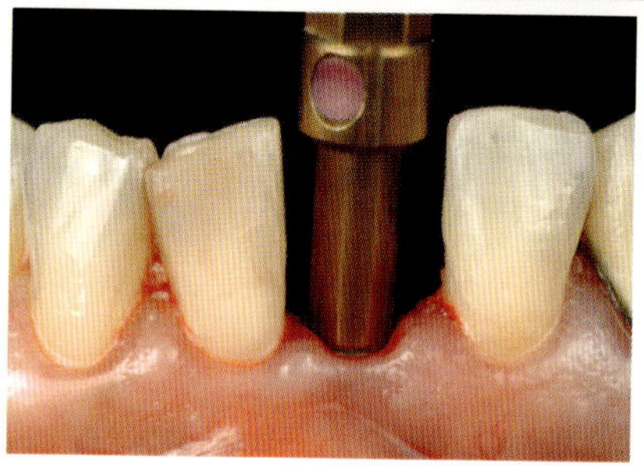
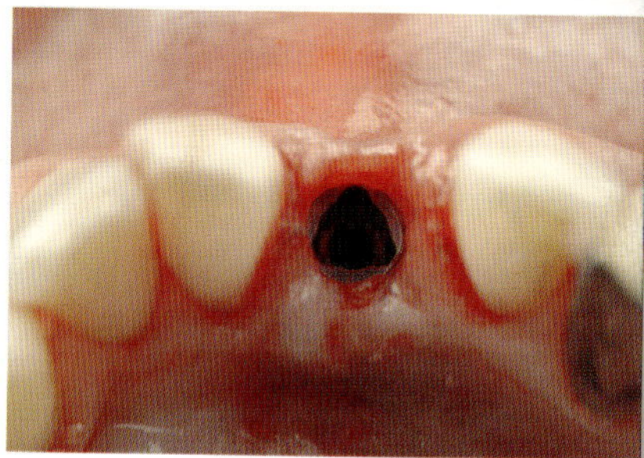

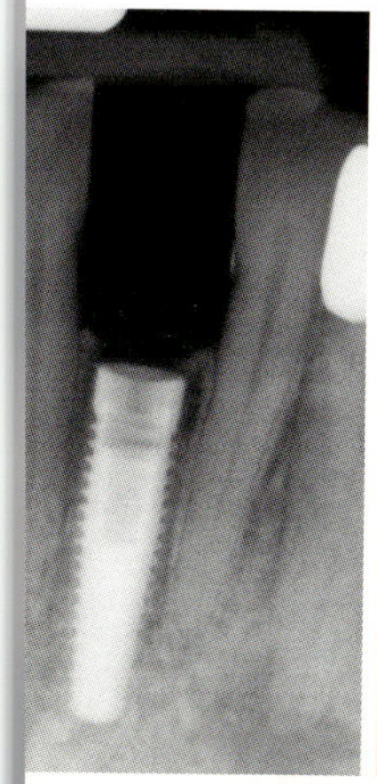

Abutment and CTG management

Once the implant was placed, the buccal defect and interproximal space were tunneled and elevated to be filled with a CTG harvested from the tuberosity to thicken the biotype. Because of space concerns with the CTG, the zirconia abutment was reduced, and a concavity was created to allow as much space as possible for maximizing tissue thickness. Once the balance was achieved between the tissue thickness volume and the available prosthetic space, the CTG was sutured in place, and the abutment was connected. The provisional restoration was then relined, adapted, and cemented with provisional cement (TempBond, Kerr).

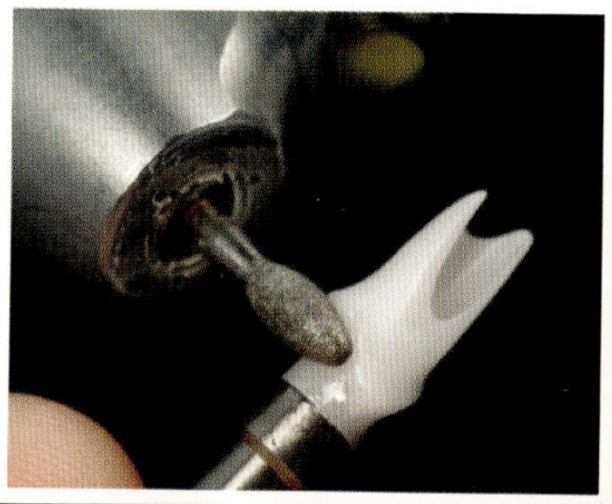
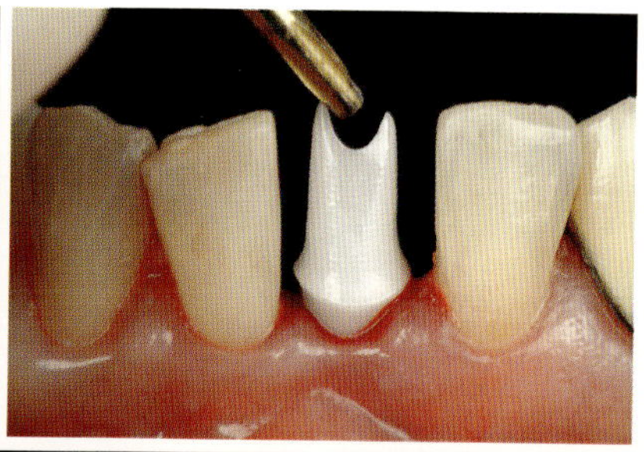
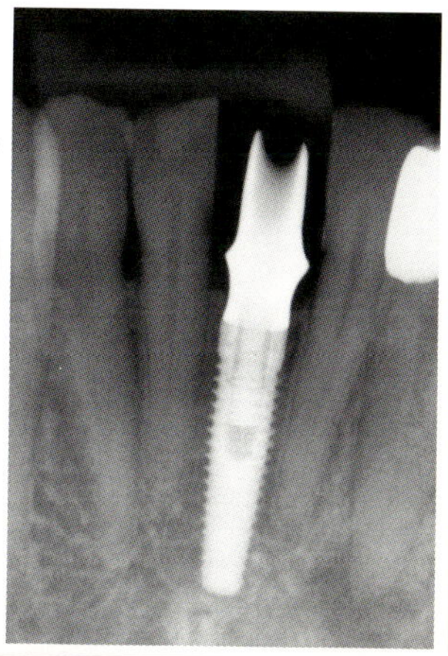
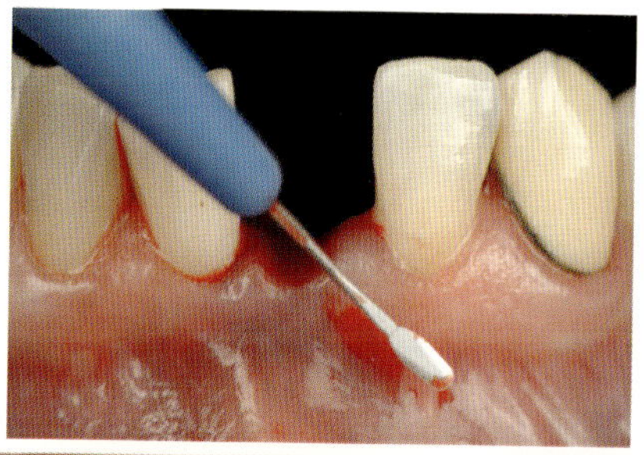
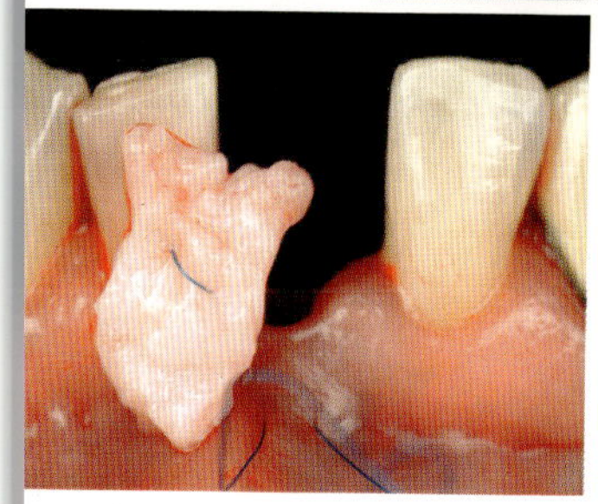
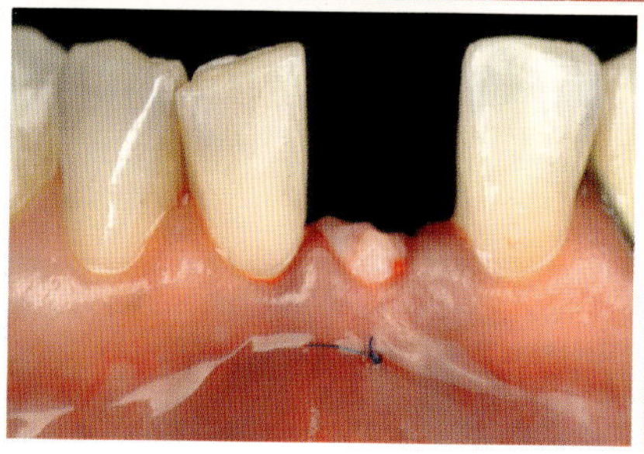
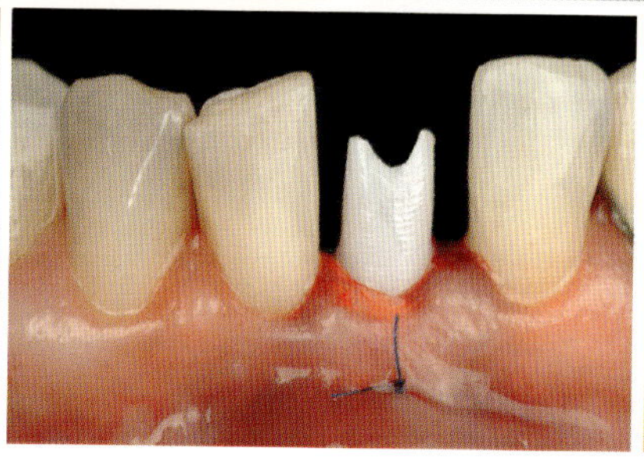
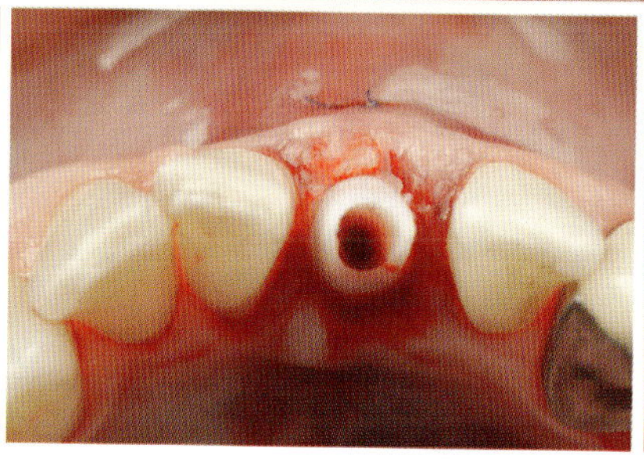
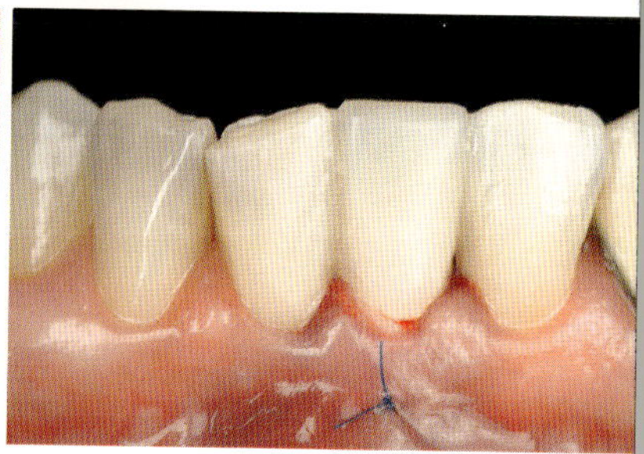

Soft tissue healing

The intraoral situation of the healing process after implant placement, definitive zirconia abutment placement, provisional restoration, and CTG delivery is shown. Note the balance and adaptation between the prosthetic contours and the space left for the grafting volume.

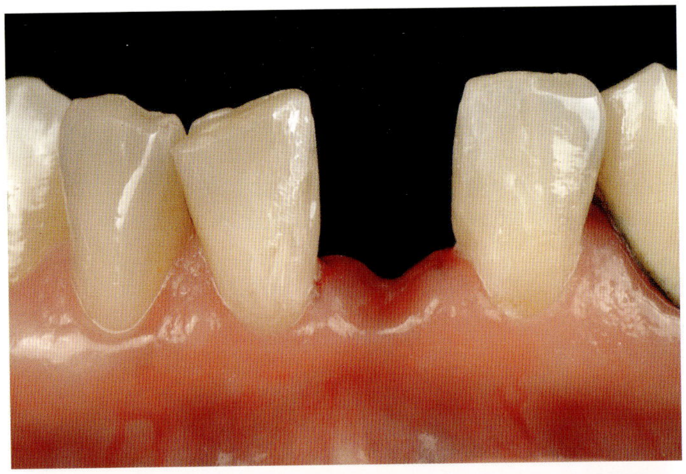

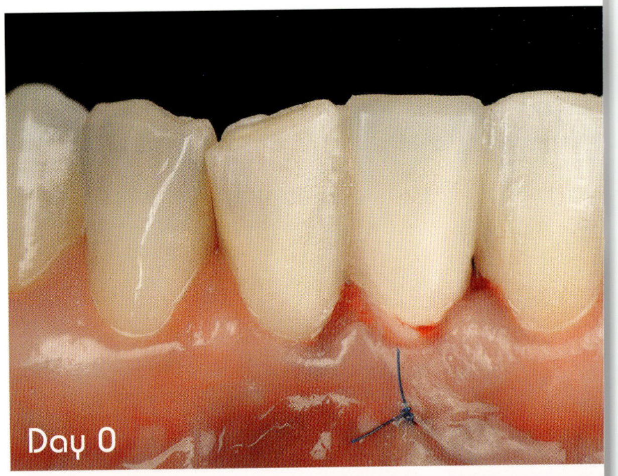

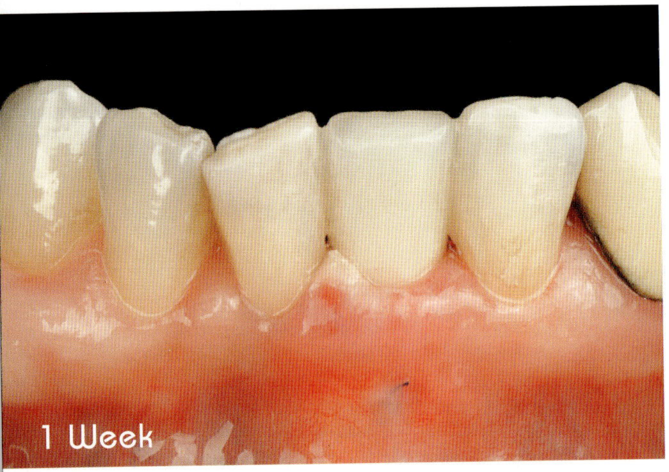

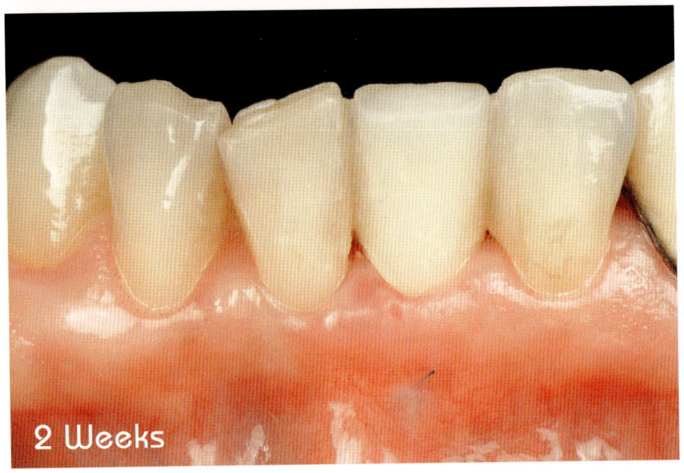

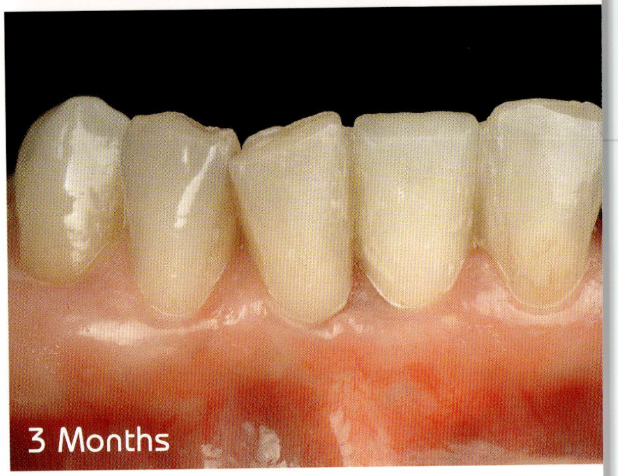

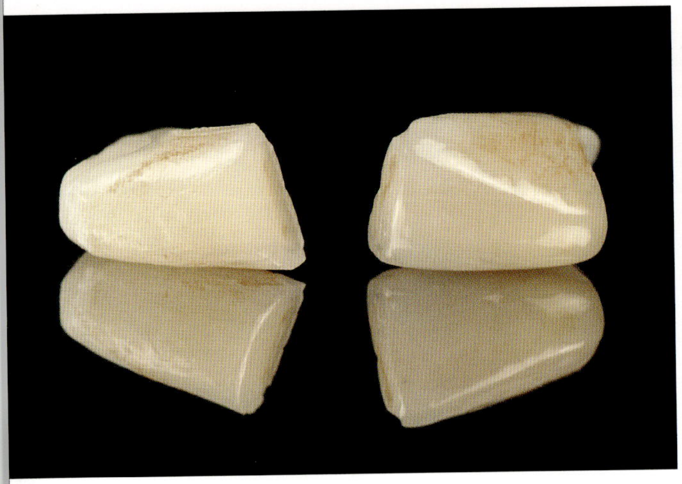

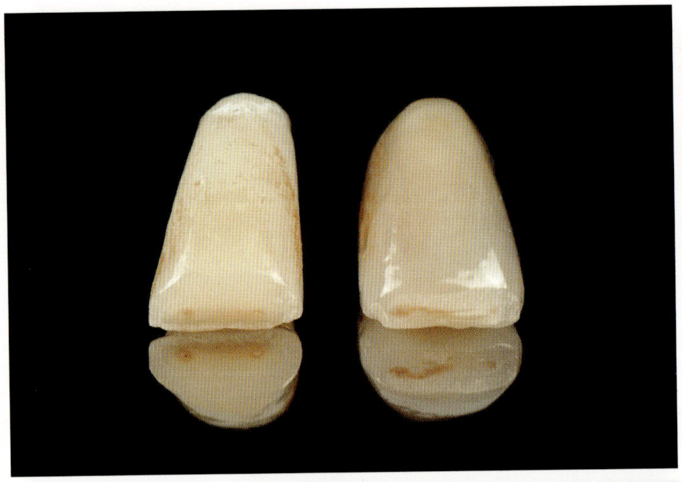

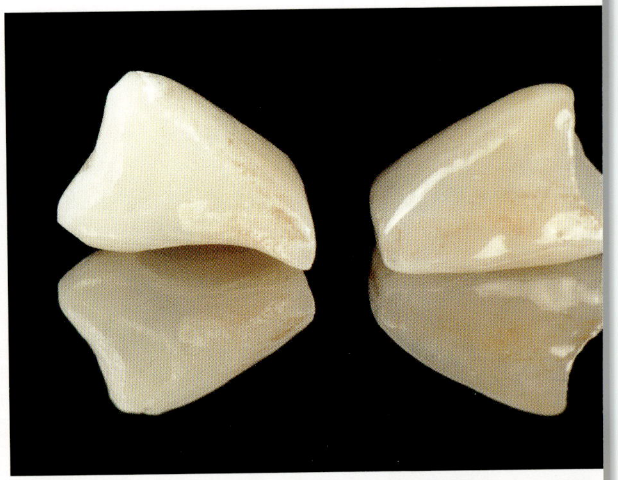

Crown adaptation

The alumina crown restoration on the left central incisor mimics the characteristics of the natural right central incisor.

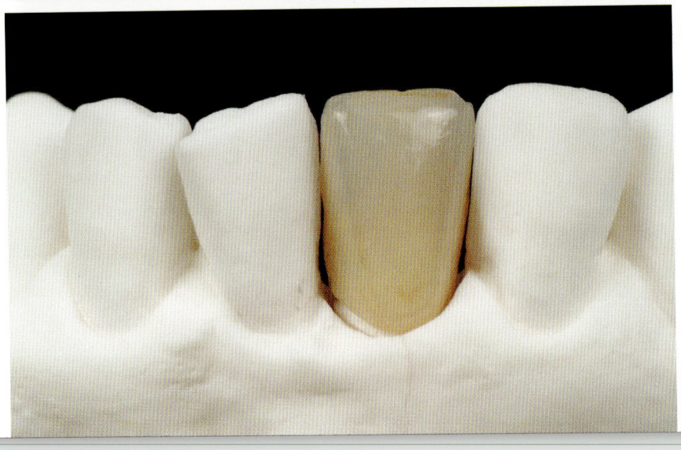

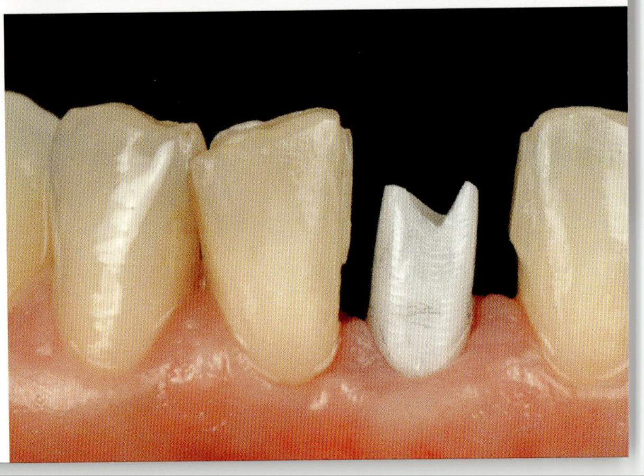

Final result

Clinical and radiographic views of the definitive mandibular left central incisor with an alumina crown restoration on a NobelReplace Groovy 3.5 × 13–mm implant are shown at 1 year and 3 years posttreatment.

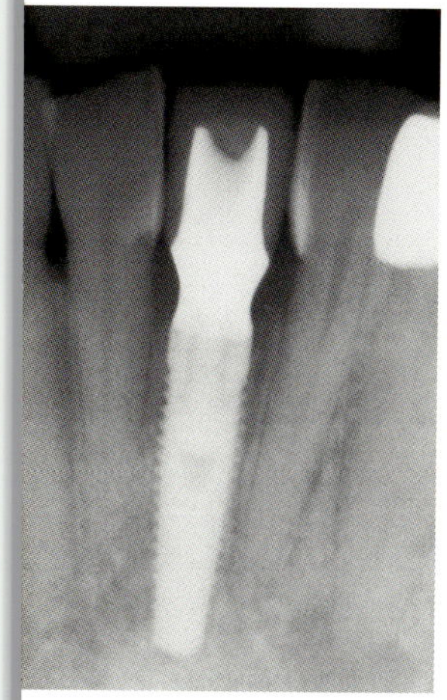

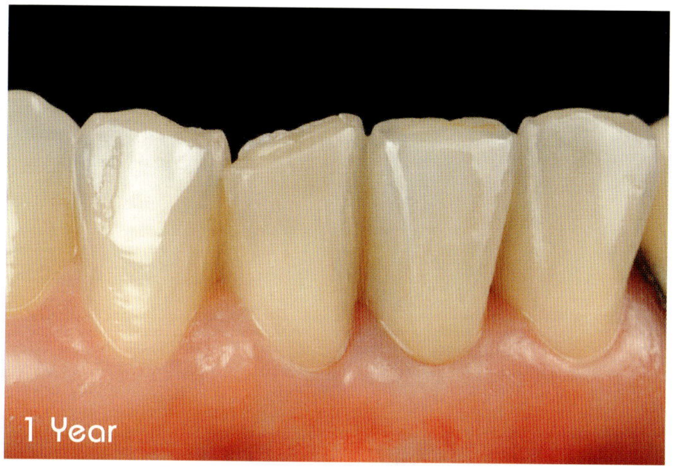

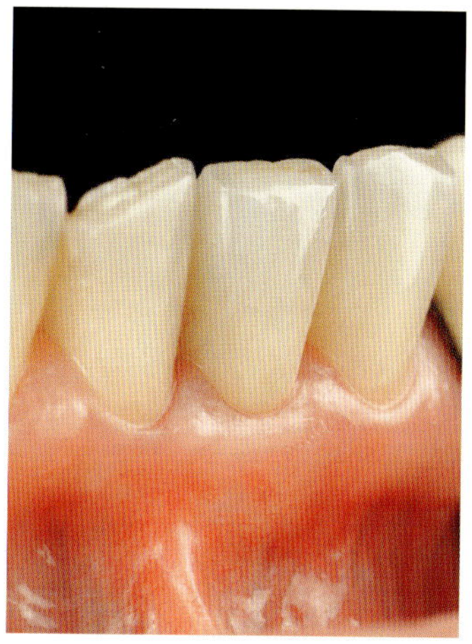

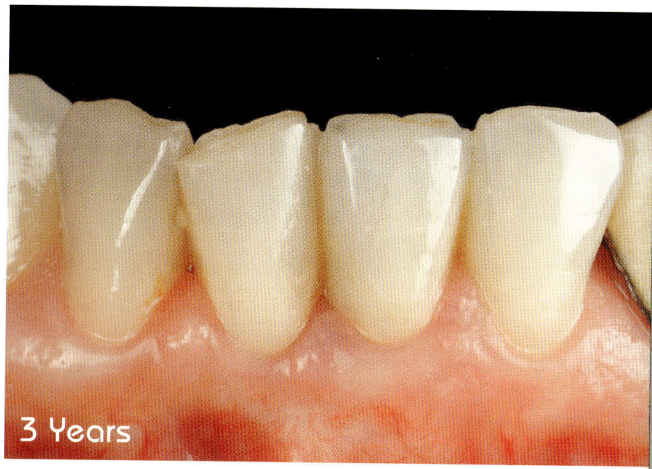

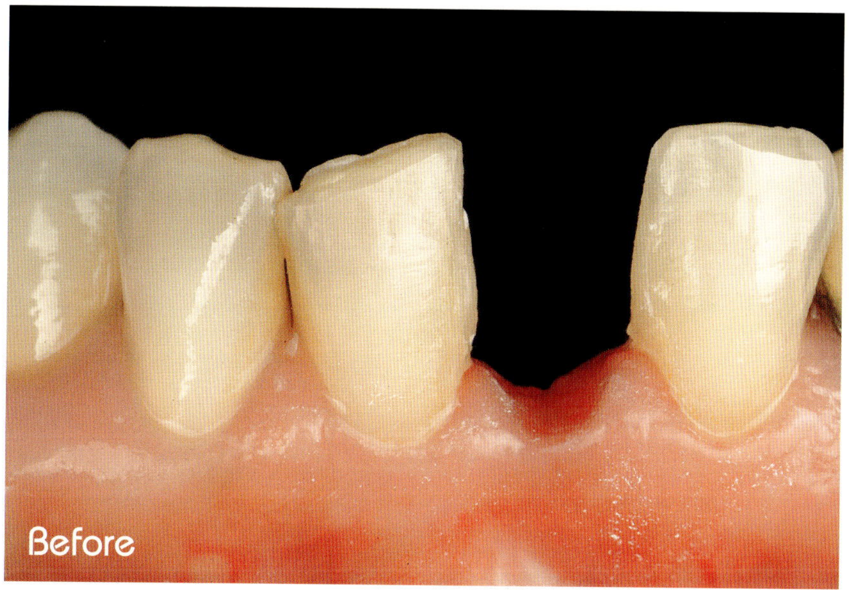

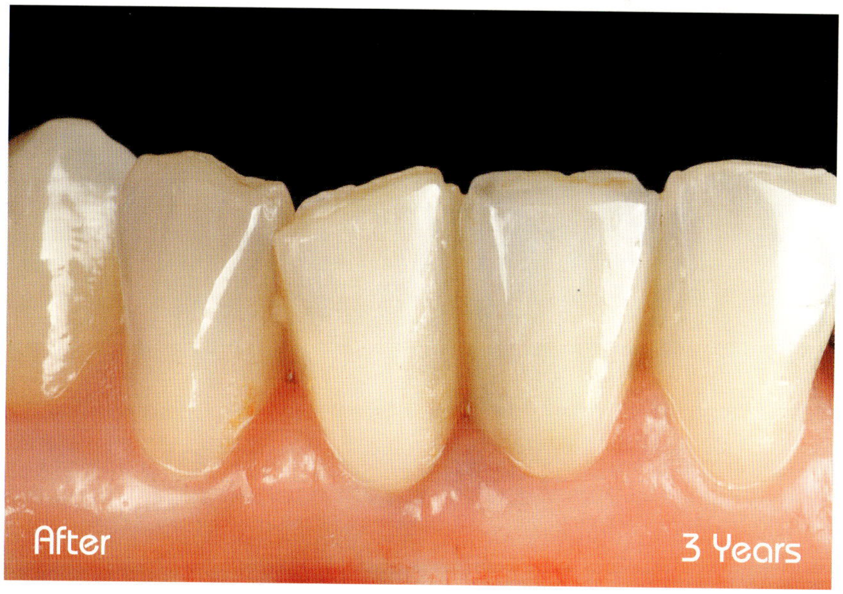

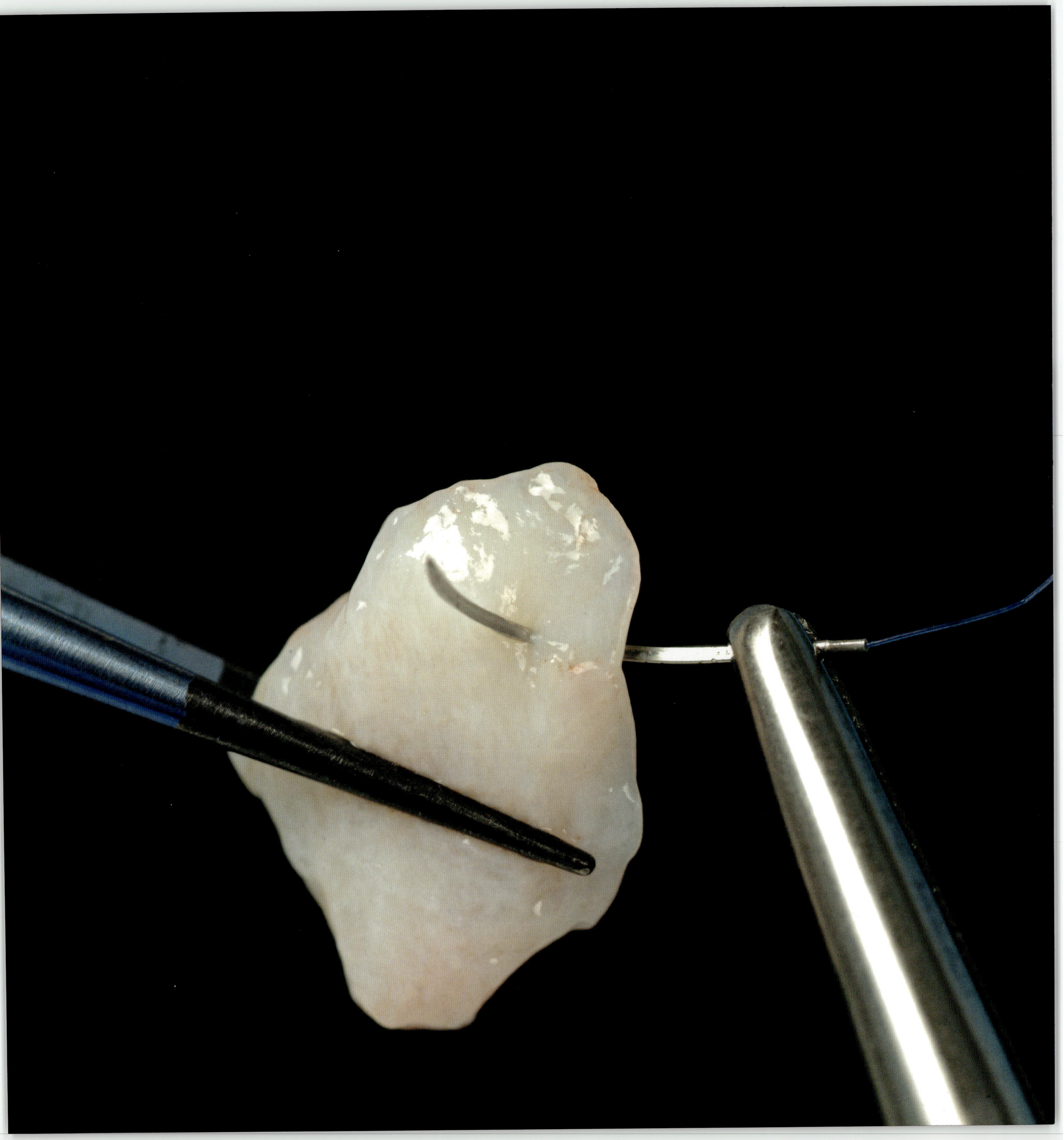

Creating a Natural Soft Tissue Contour

- Bone Grafting
- Soft Tissue Grafting Procedures
  - – Donor site manipulation
  - → Research: Soft tissue graft donor site
  - → Research: Tissue graft clinical outcomes
  - – Recipient site manipulation
  - → Research: Socket grafting
- Creating a Soft Tissue Contour Prosthetically Through Provisional Restoration
  - – Abutment design and provisional fabrication
  - – Implant abutment selection
  - → Research: Implant abutments
- Orthodontics to Maximize Soft Tissue Esthetics
  - → Research: Orthodontics
  - – Orthodontic extrusion
  - – Intrusion and torque

Chapter 4

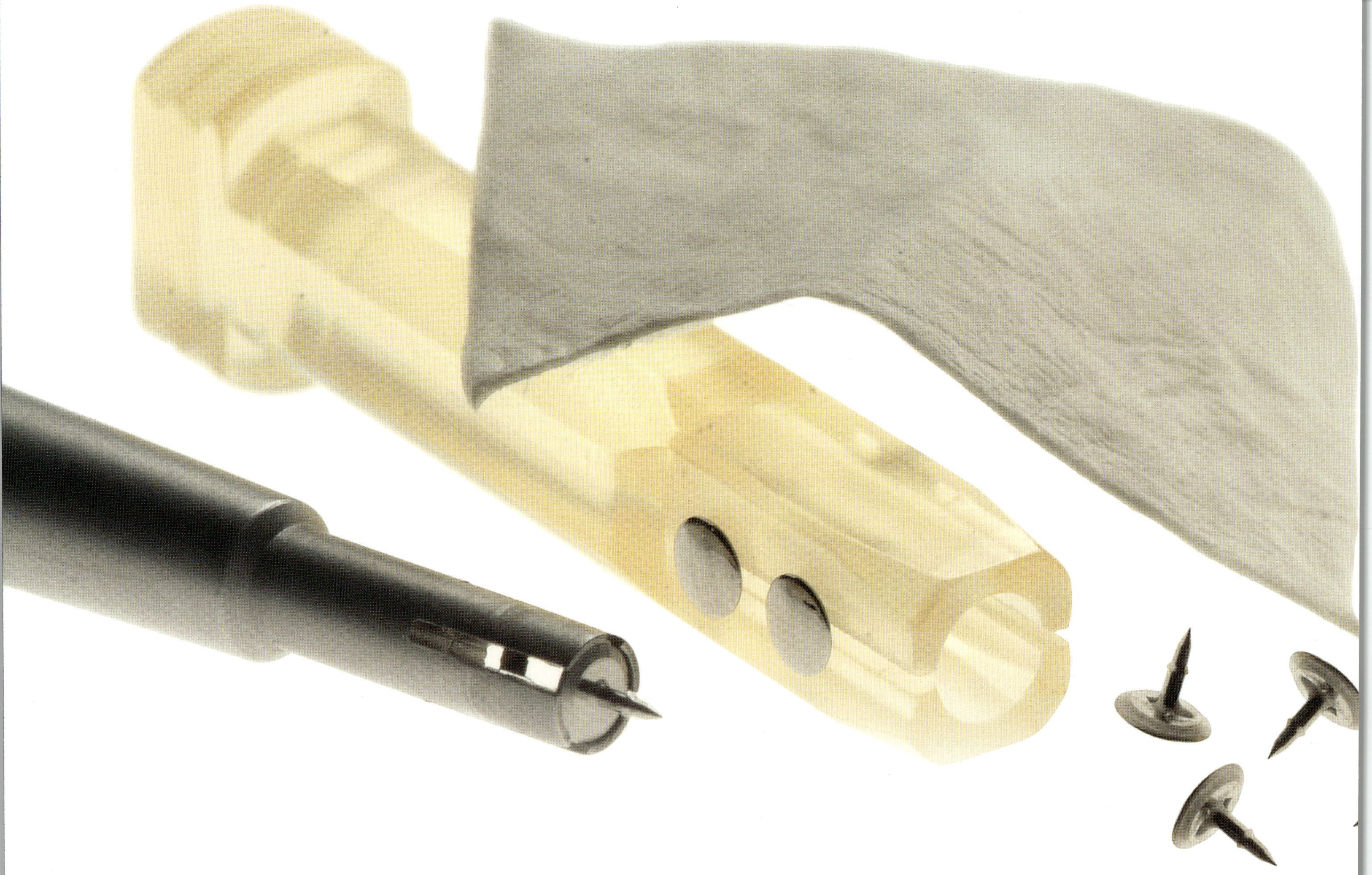

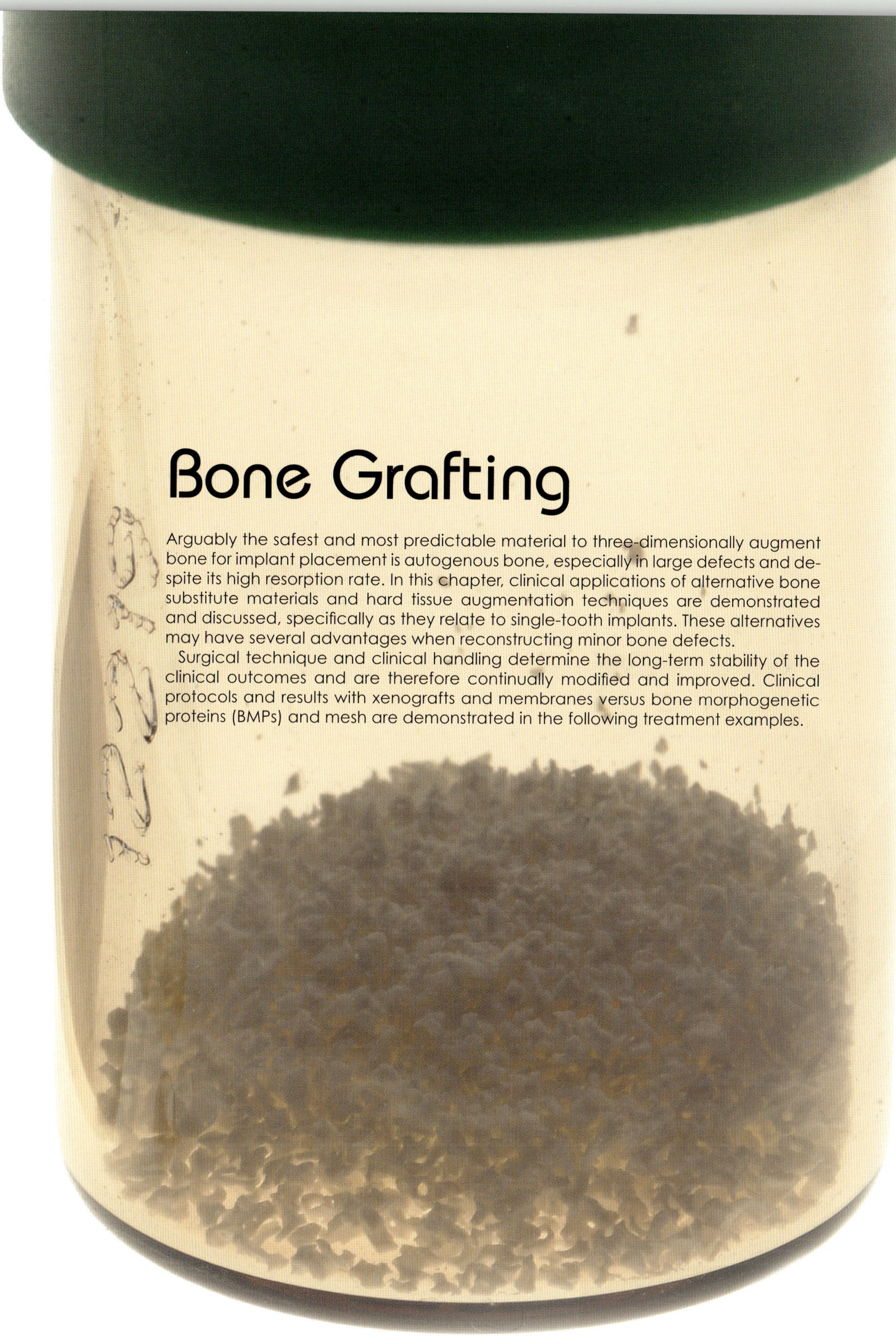

Bone Grafting

Arguably the safest and most predictable material to three-dimensionally augment bone for implant placement is autogenous bone, especially in large defects and despite its high resorption rate. In this chapter, clinical applications of alternative bone substitute materials and hard tissue augmentation techniques are demonstrated and discussed, specifically as they relate to single-tooth implants. These alternatives may have several advantages when reconstructing minor bone defects.

Surgical technique and clinical handling determine the long-term stability of the clinical outcomes and are therefore continually modified and improved. Clinical protocols and results with xenografts and membranes versus bone morphogenetic proteins (BMPs) and mesh are demonstrated in the following treatment examples.

Xenografts with membranes

The patient presented with an implant placed in the area of the right central incisor. The implant was placed in contact with the lateral incisor, causing the patient numbness and discomfort and necessitating extraction of the implant. In addition, the severe angulation and close proximity to the adjacent tooth made it impossible to restore the implant and to achieve a natural-looking outcome. The patient had high esthetic demands, and orthodontic treatment was suggested to control the diastemata and proportions as well as the interproximal bone height.

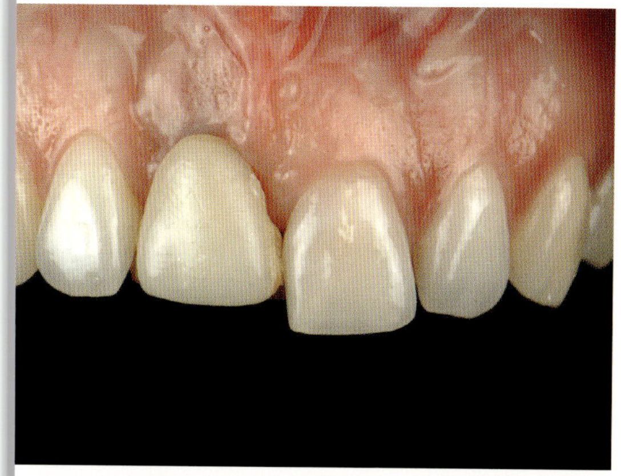

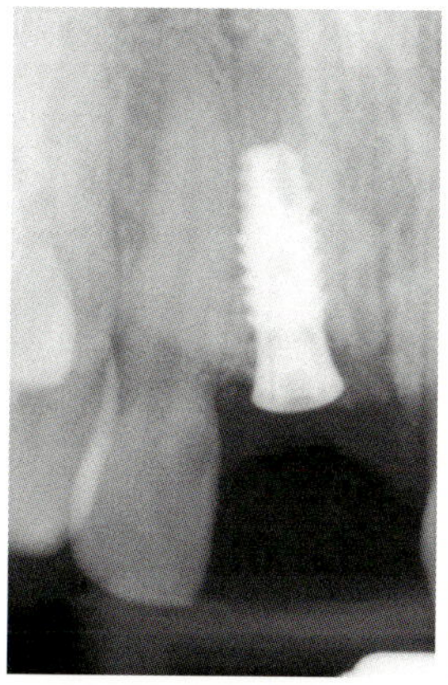

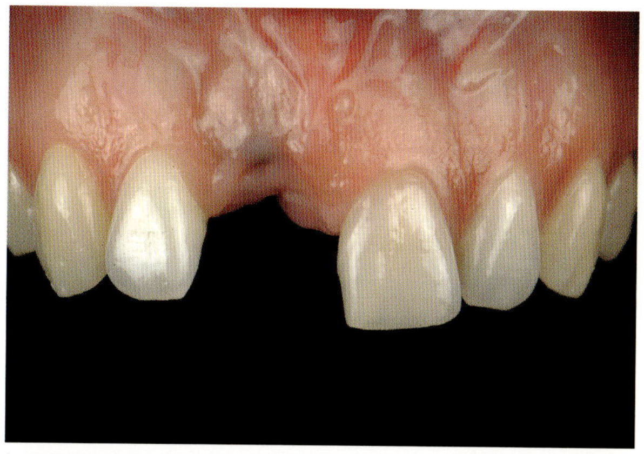

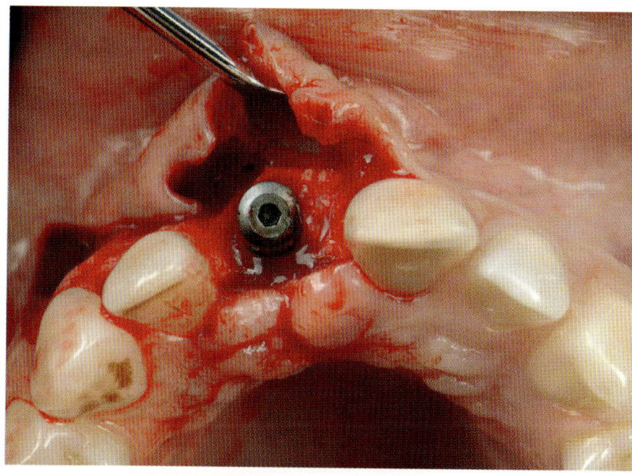

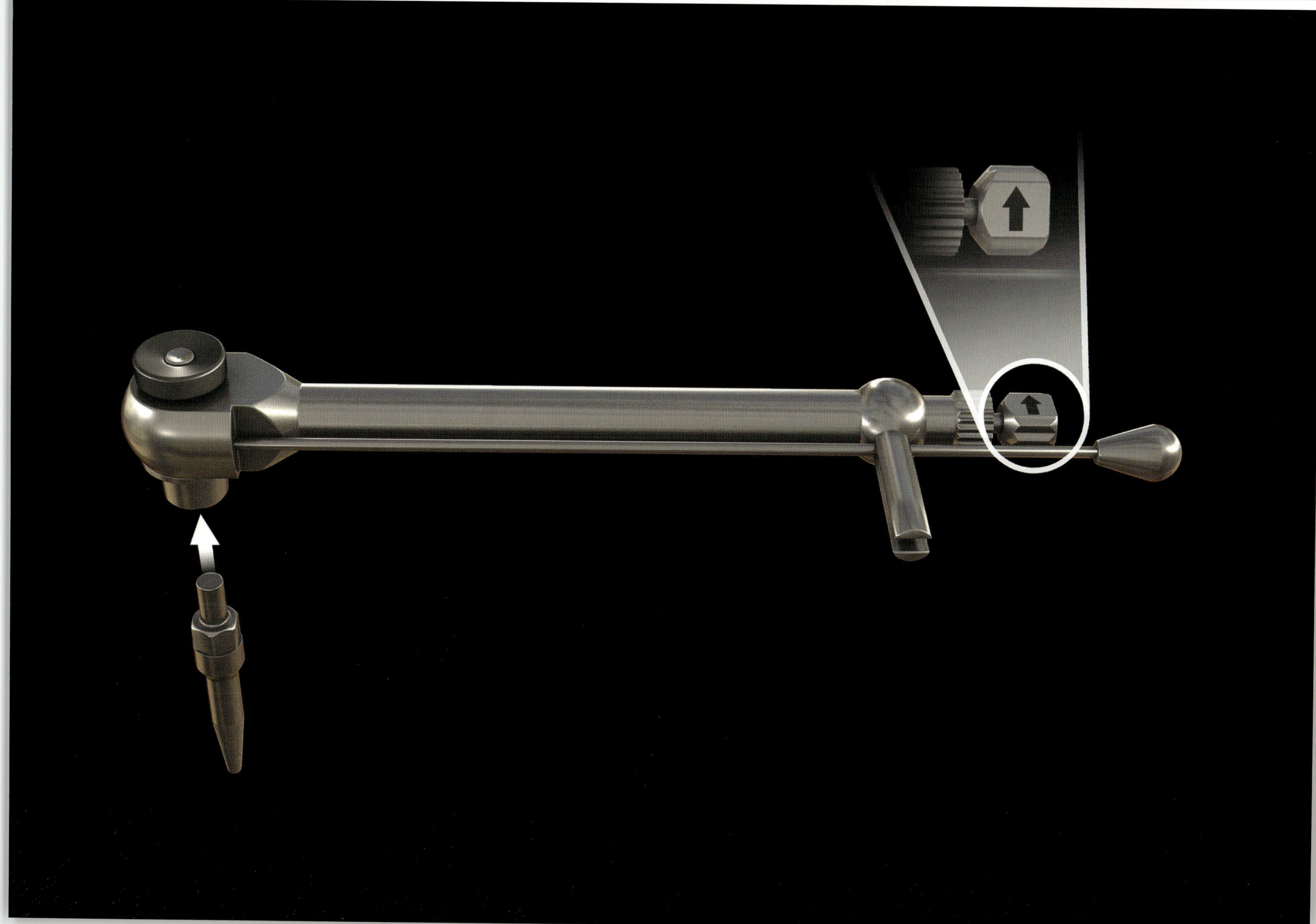

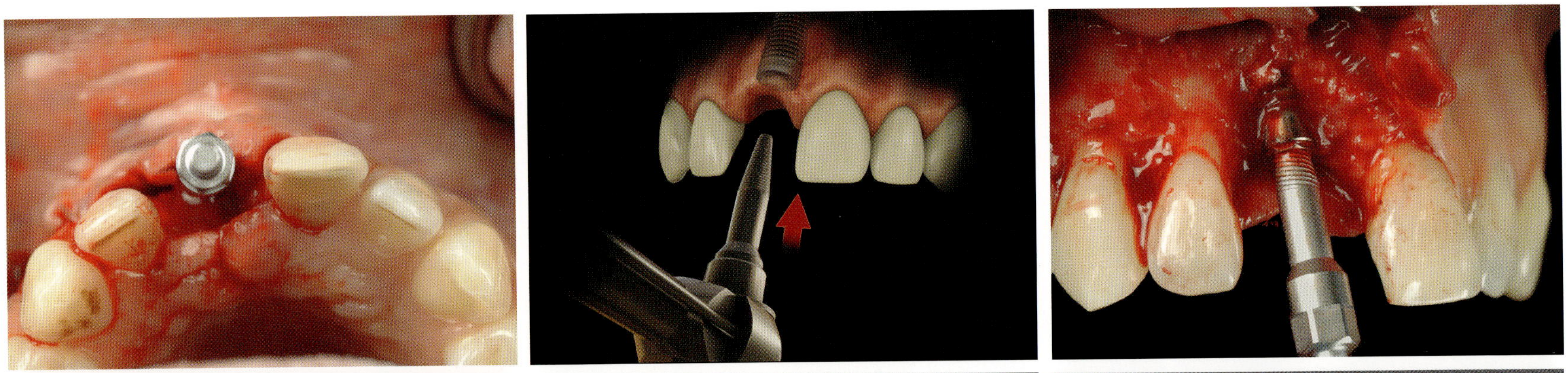

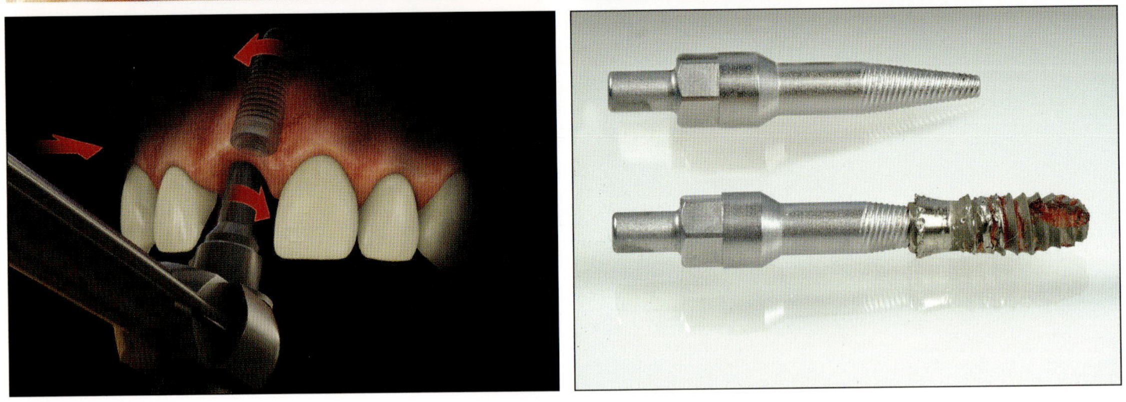

Newly available implant-retrieval tools simplify the removal procedure of osseointegrated dental implants. The implant-retrieval instrument rotates in a clockwise direction while the insert on the internal connection of the implant rotates counterclockwise, thereby breaking the implant-bone interfacial connection and allowing for nontraumatic implant removal. Trephines should not be used for implant extraction because they cause significant destruction and bone loss.

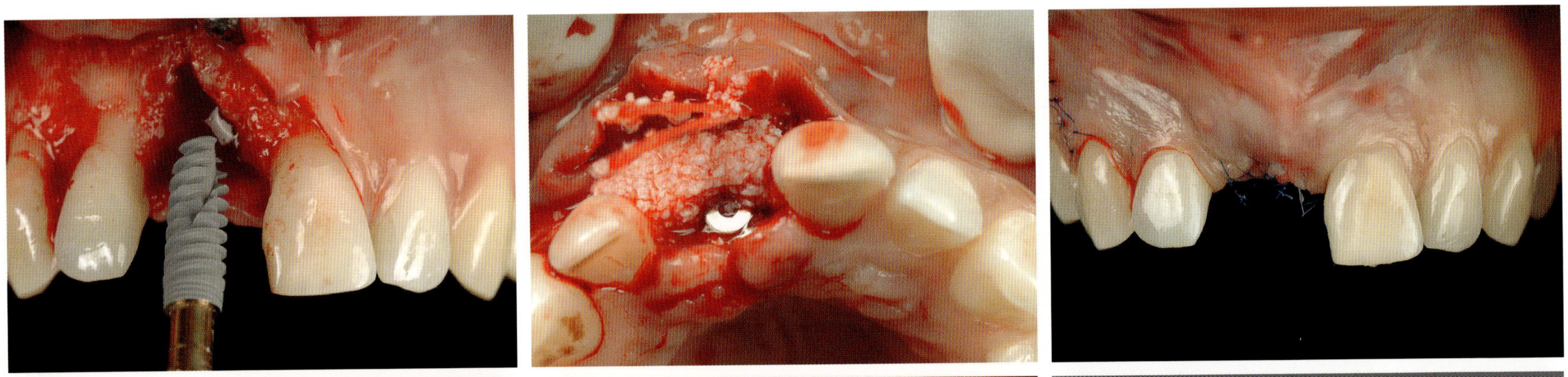

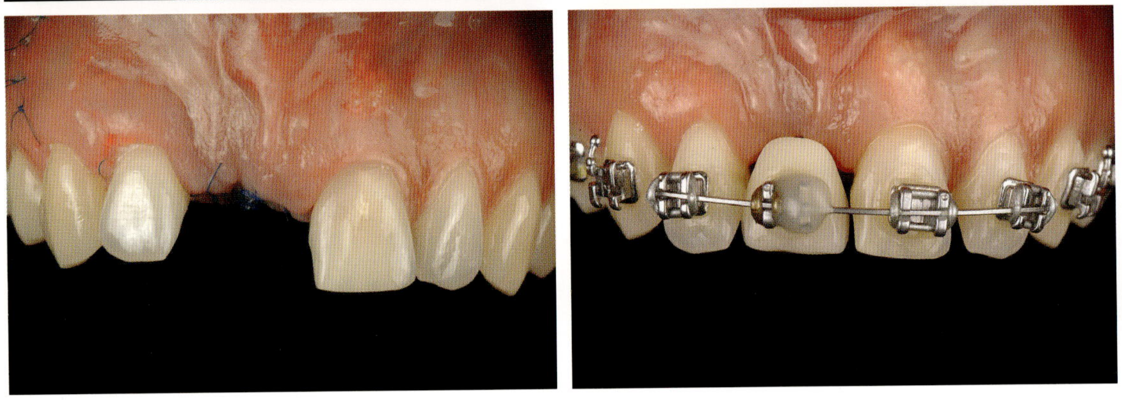

After implant retrieval, a 4.3 × 13–mm NobelActive implant (Nobel Biocare) was placed and redirected to maximize the esthetic potential of the implant restoration. A single releasing incision was prepared in the premolar area to avoid scarring of the soft tissue. Two Bio-Oss membranes (Geistlich) were then placed to cover the few exposed implant threads, limit bone resorption, and preserve bone maturation. Meanwhile, orthodontic treatment was carried out to properly align the teeth and redistribute spaces.

Orthodontist: Dr Domingo Martín

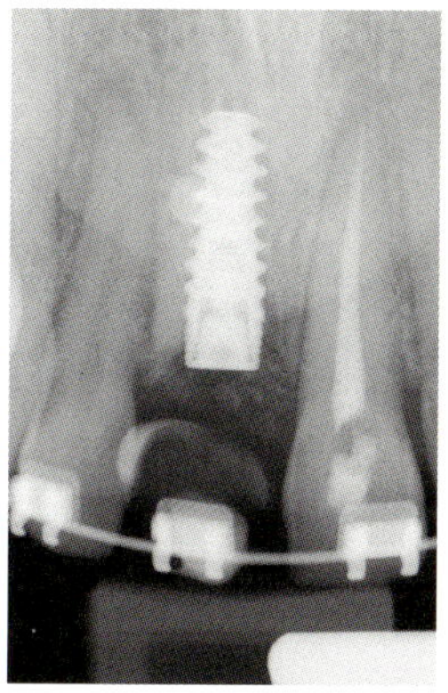

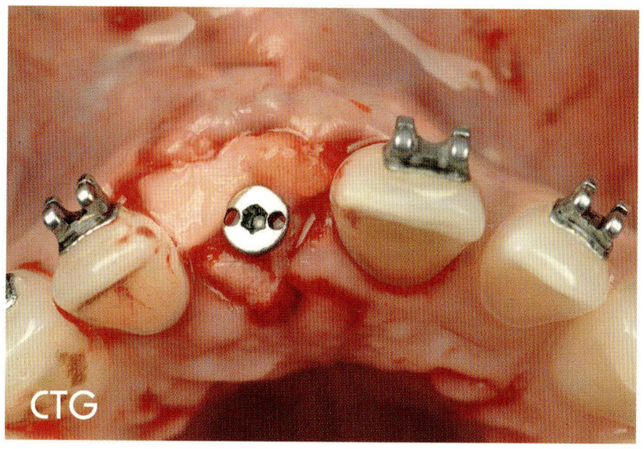

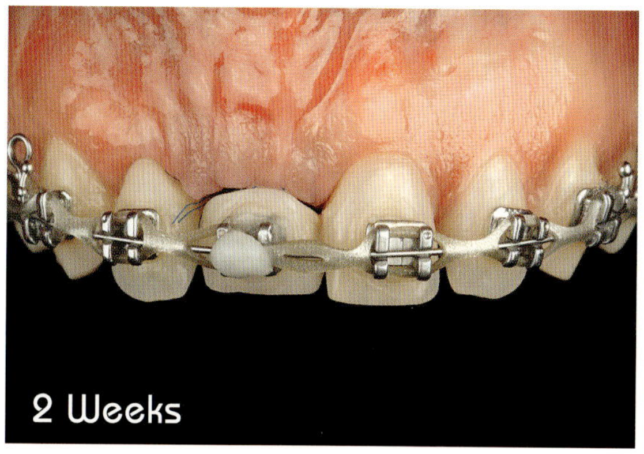

Stage-two surgery was performed with a connective tissue graft (CTG) from the tuberosity after 8 months of bone healing. A concave healing abutment with holes was inserted to allow more space for the CTG and thereby thicken the peri-implant soft tissue at the most coronal part of the healing abutment with the help of the suturing holes.

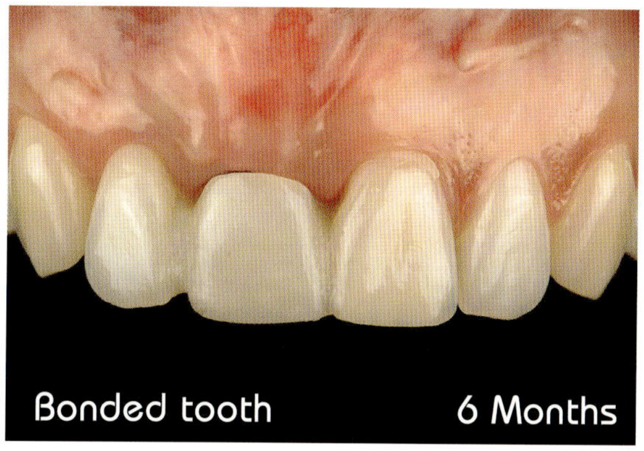

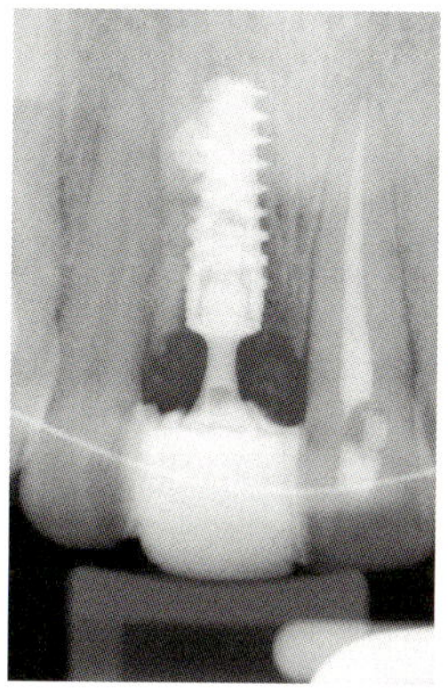

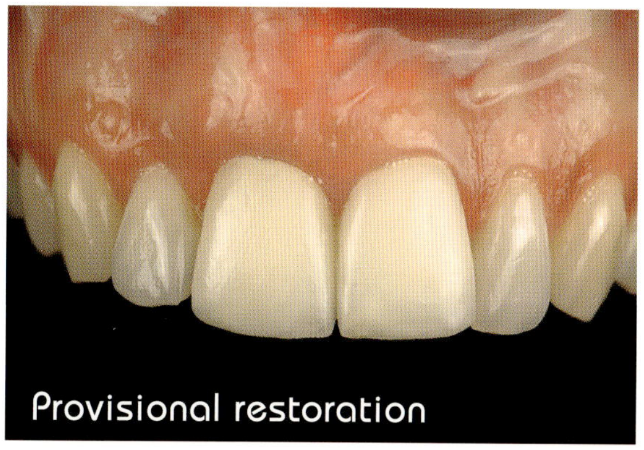

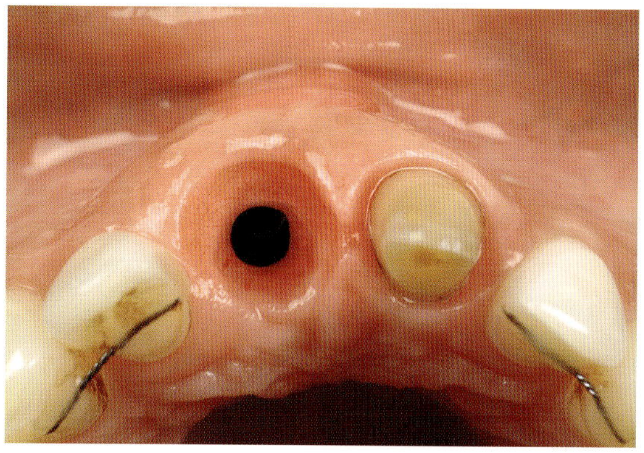

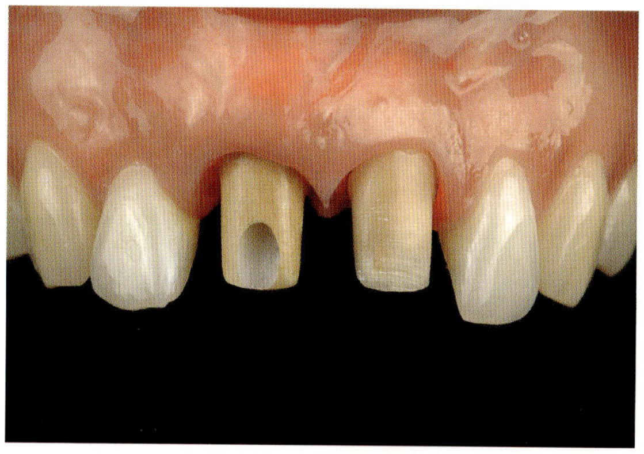

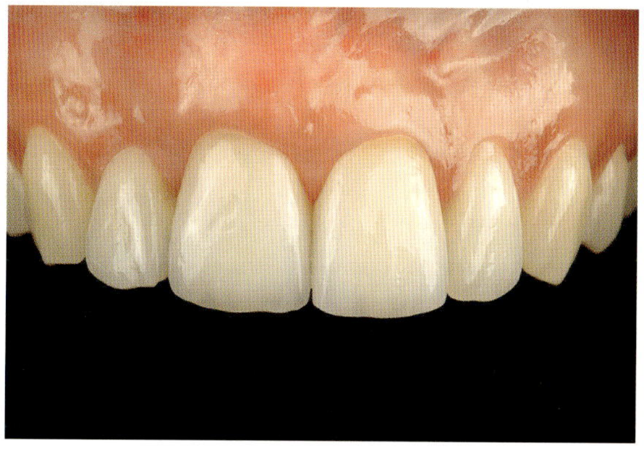

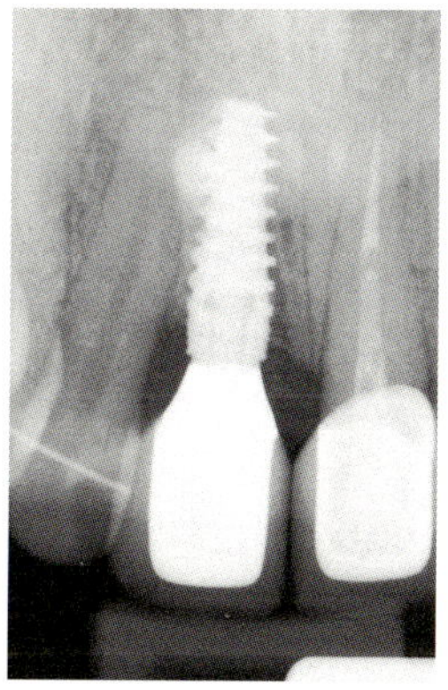

A provisional restoration was placed on the adjacent central incisor to improve the contour and tissue support. The definitive zirconia abutment was colored to match the shade of the adjacent natural abutment central incisor, which was impossible to bleach. Having the same stump shade for both the natural abutment and the implant abutment simplifies fabrication of the zirconia crowns in the laboratory, as both need the same opacity and shade.

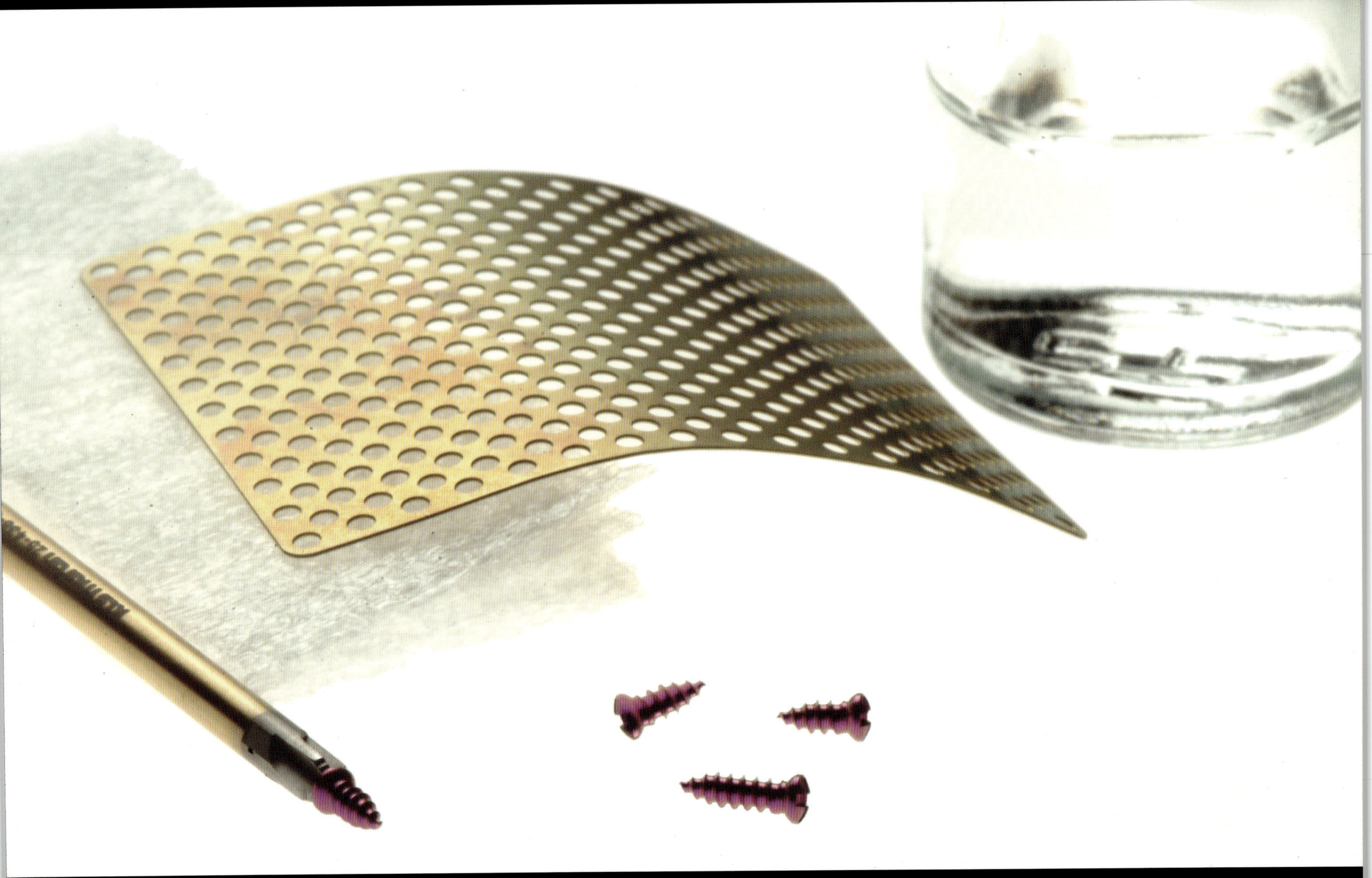

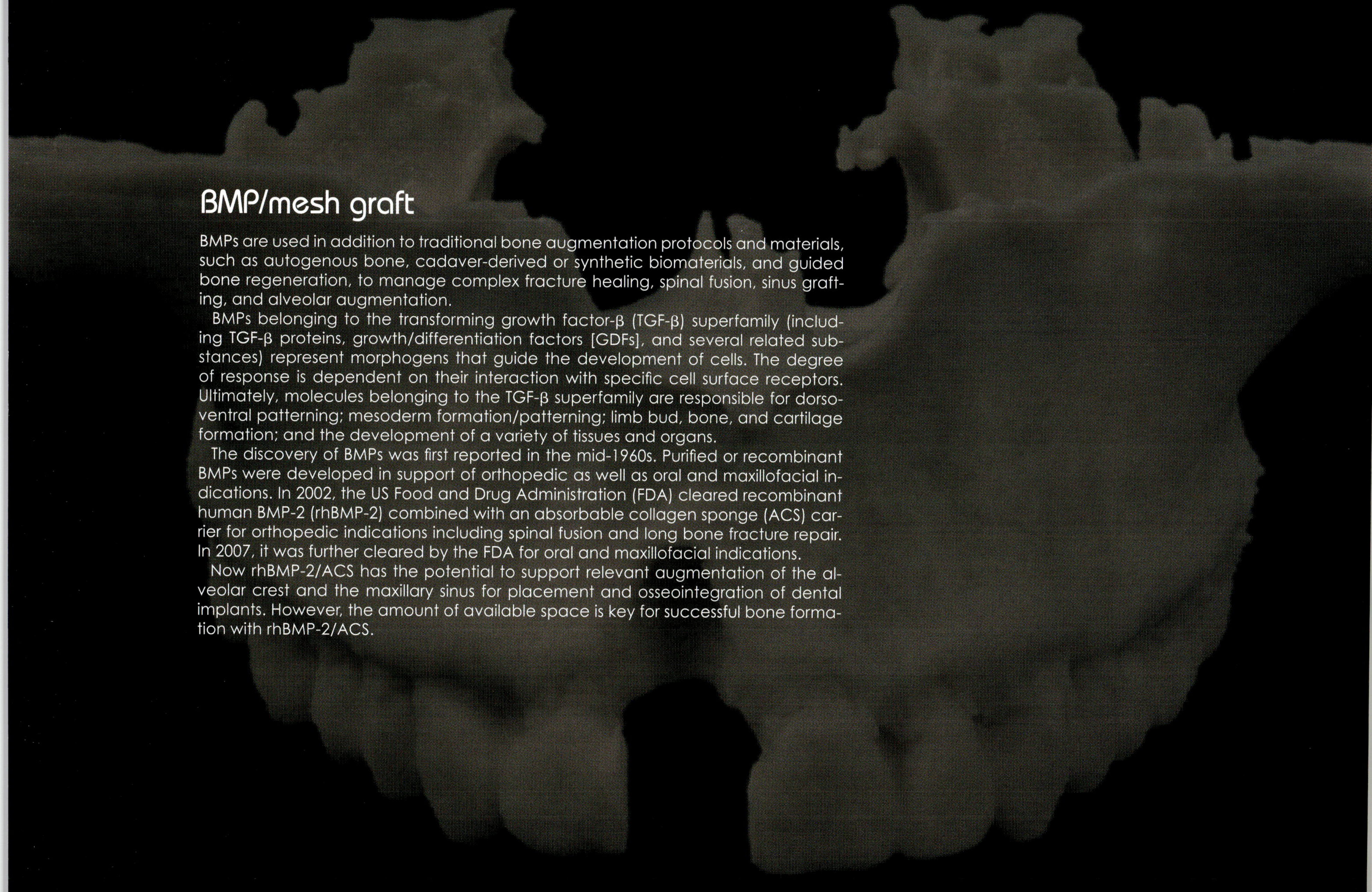

BMP/mesh graft

BMPs are used in addition to traditional bone augmentation protocols and materials, such as autogenous bone, cadaver-derived or synthetic biomaterials, and guided bone regeneration, to manage complex fracture healing, spinal fusion, sinus grafting, and alveolar augmentation.

BMPs belonging to the transforming growth factor-β (TGF-β) superfamily (including TGF-β proteins, growth/differentiation factors [GDFs], and several related substances) represent morphogens that guide the development of cells. The degree of response is dependent on their interaction with specific cell surface receptors. Ultimately, molecules belonging to the TGF-β superfamily are responsible for dorsoventral patterning; mesoderm formation/patterning; limb bud, bone, and cartilage formation; and the development of a variety of tissues and organs.

The discovery of BMPs was first reported in the mid-1960s. Purified or recombinant BMPs were developed in support of orthopedic as well as oral and maxillofacial indications. In 2002, the US Food and Drug Administration (FDA) cleared recombinant human BMP-2 (rhBMP-2) combined with an absorbable collagen sponge (ACS) carrier for orthopedic indications including spinal fusion and long bone fracture repair. In 2007, it was further cleared by the FDA for oral and maxillofacial indications.

Now rhBMP-2/ACS has the potential to support relevant augmentation of the alveolar crest and the maxillary sinus for placement and osseointegration of dental implants. However, the amount of available space is key for successful bone formation with rhBMP-2/ACS.

The patient presented with significant external root resorption, a cavernous periradicular bone defect, and fistulation on the maxillary right central incisor. The tooth was extracted, and the site was cleaned of infected material and granulation tissue. A three-dimensional (3D) scan of the teeth was made, and a composite resin master model was fabricated from the scan to visualize the magnitude of the defect. Care was taken to meticulously customize the ACS mesh to the intended site.

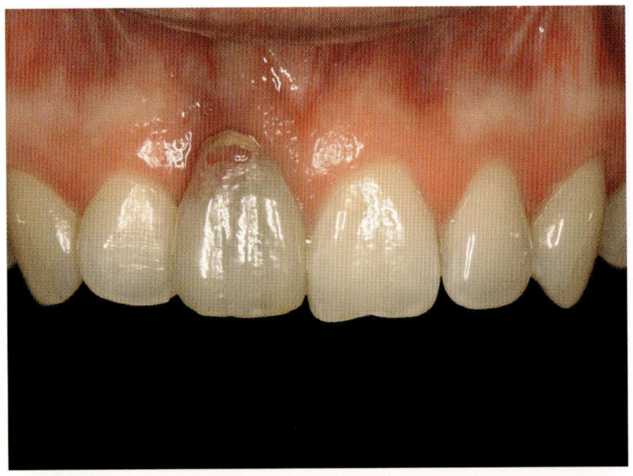

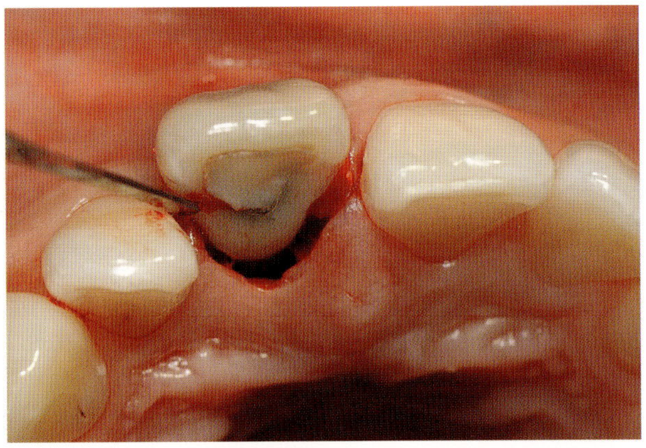

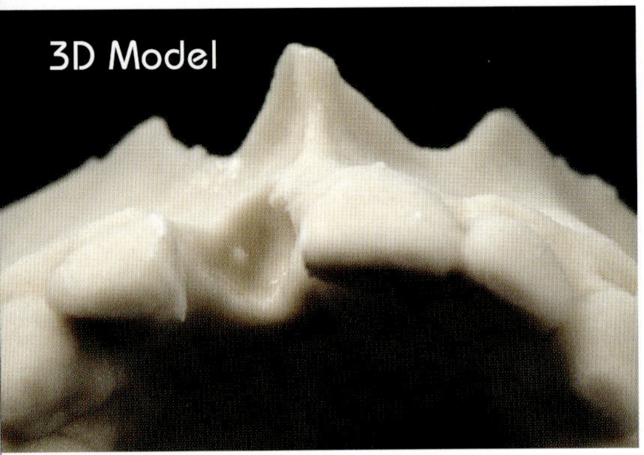

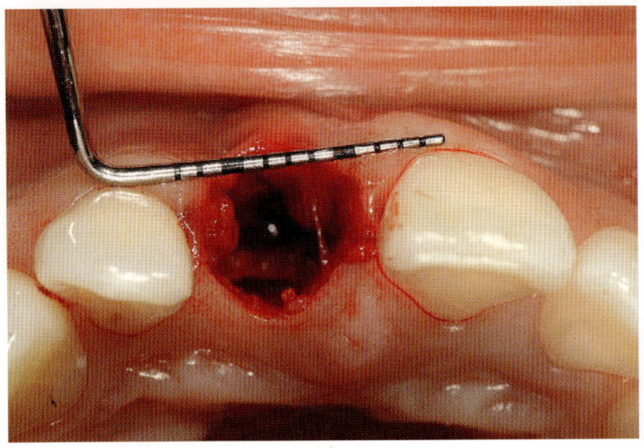

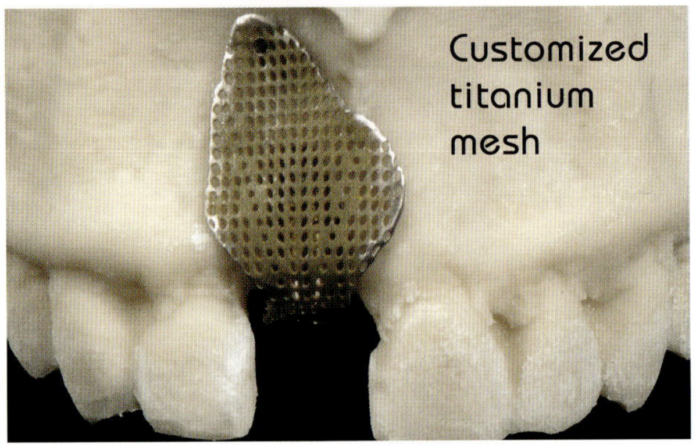

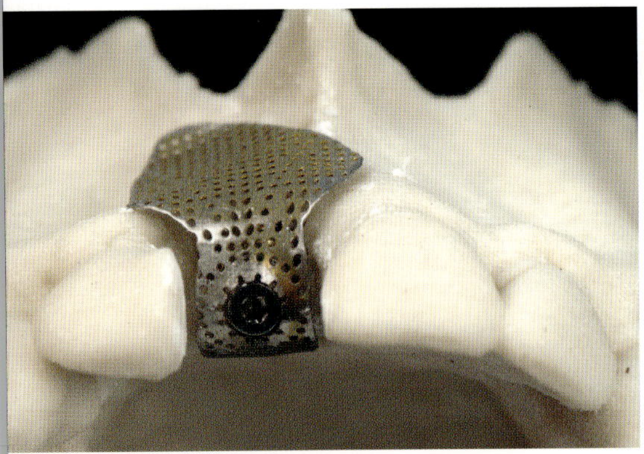

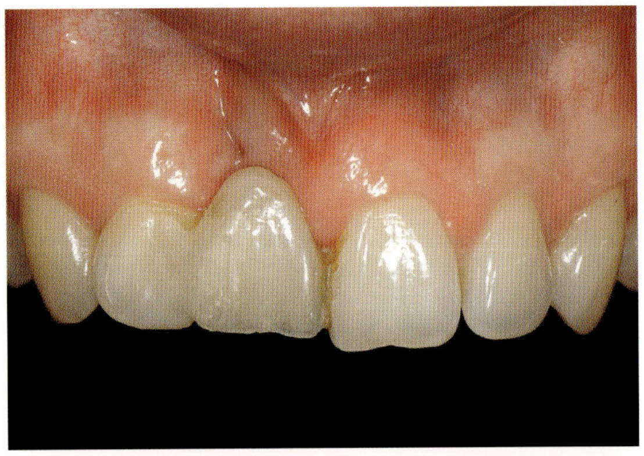

After 3 months, a full-thickness flap was reflected on the central incisor site. The flap extension was deflected laterally to the first premolar and across to the lateral incisor without a vertical releasing incision. The defect was well exposed, and the custom mesh was held in place apically with a horizontal screw. The absorbable sponges were then impregnated with rhBMP-2 and covered with the titanium mesh, which was fixed in place with a palatal bone screw.

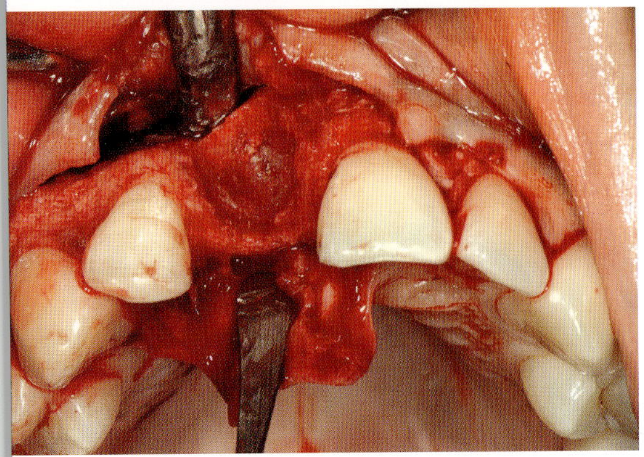

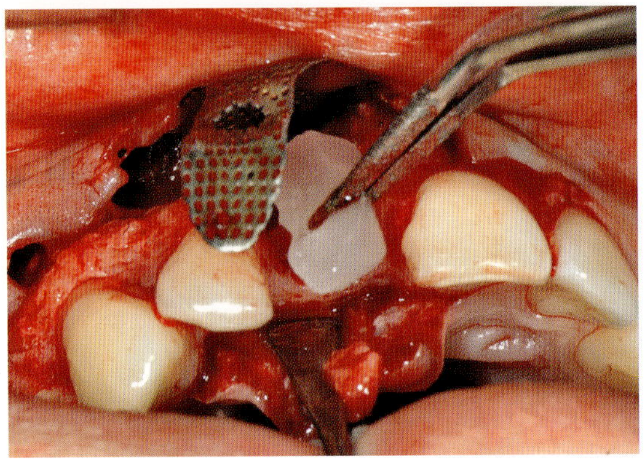

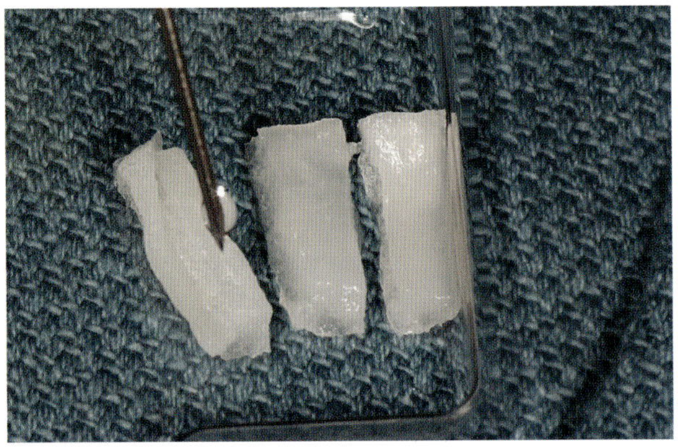

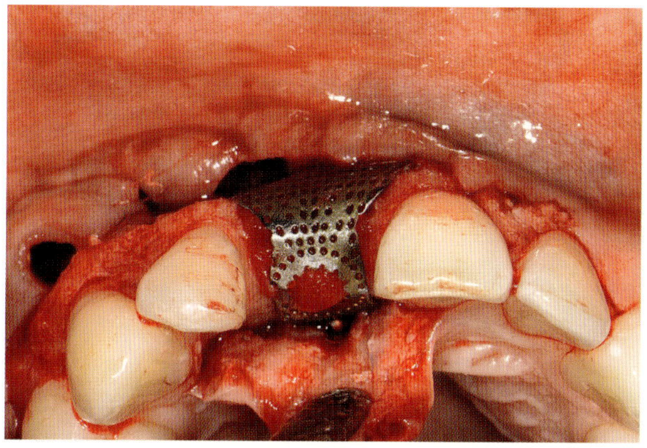

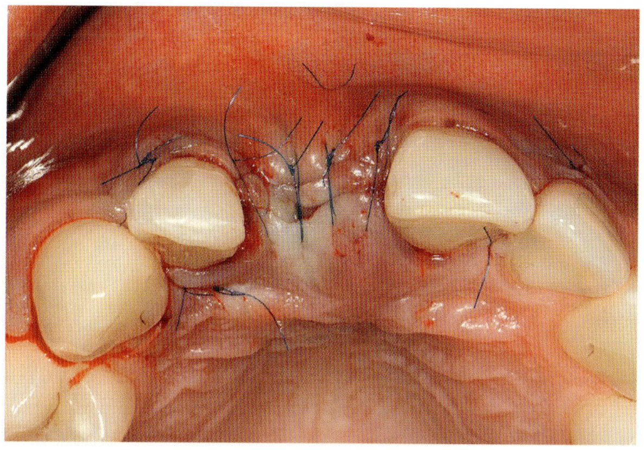

Care was taken to close and suture the wound to the exact position of the original incisions. The cone beam computed tomography (CBCT) image shows the bone healing and volume as well as soft tissue maturation after 4 months.

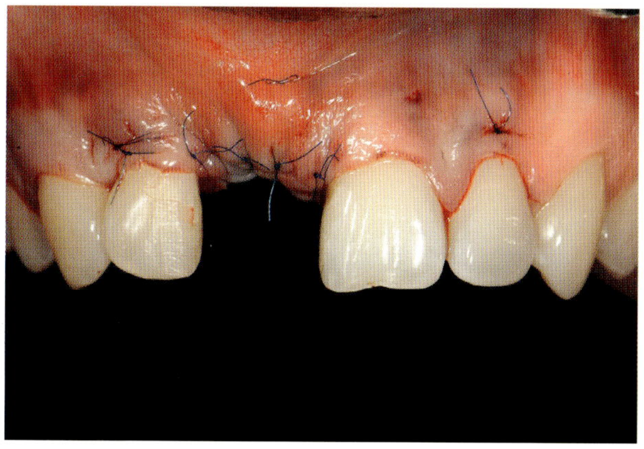

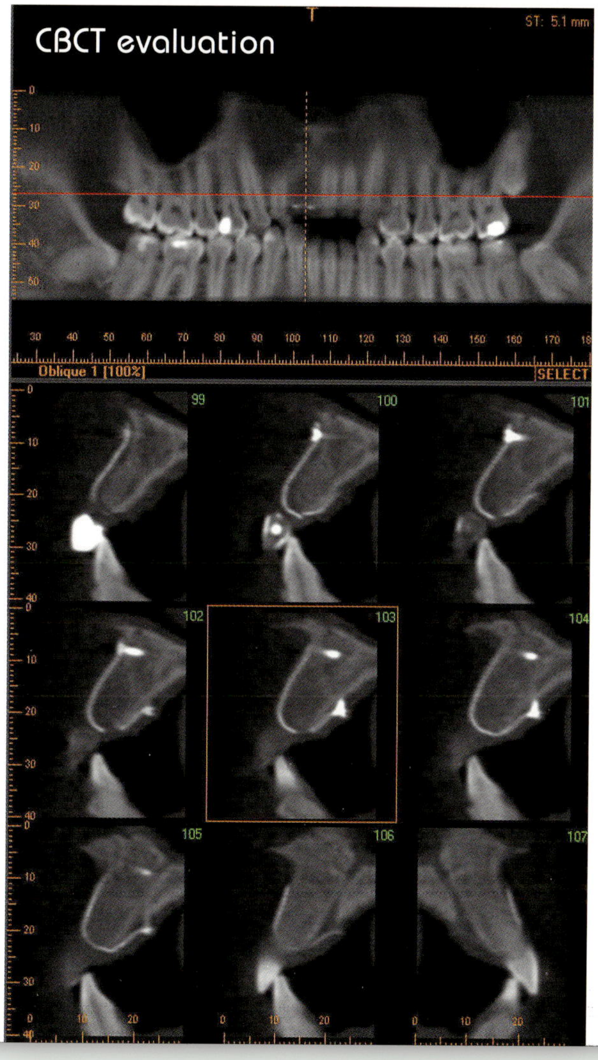

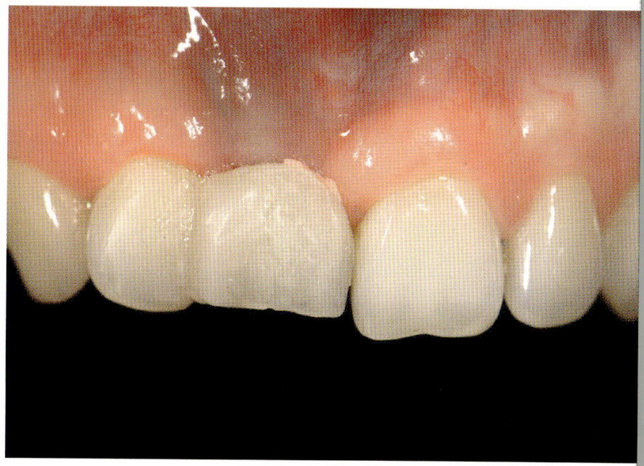

Bone surgery performed at the Medical College of Georgia, Department of Periodontics, under the supervision of Dr U.M. Wikesjö and team (Dr J. Lee and Dr C. Susin).

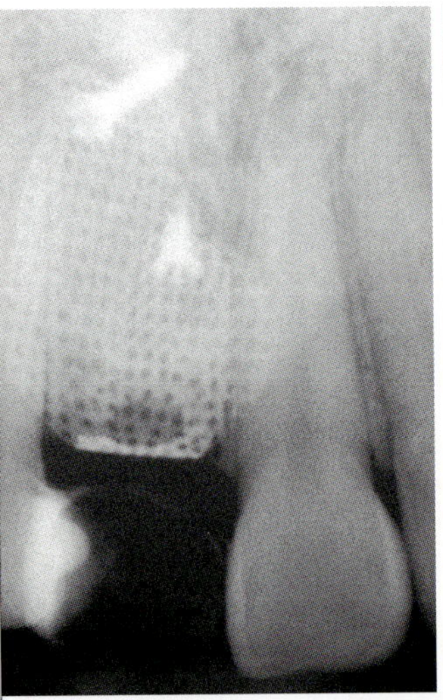

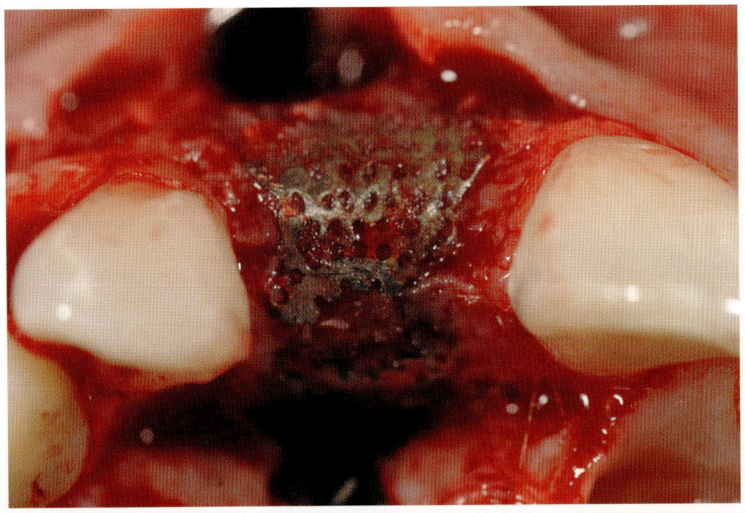

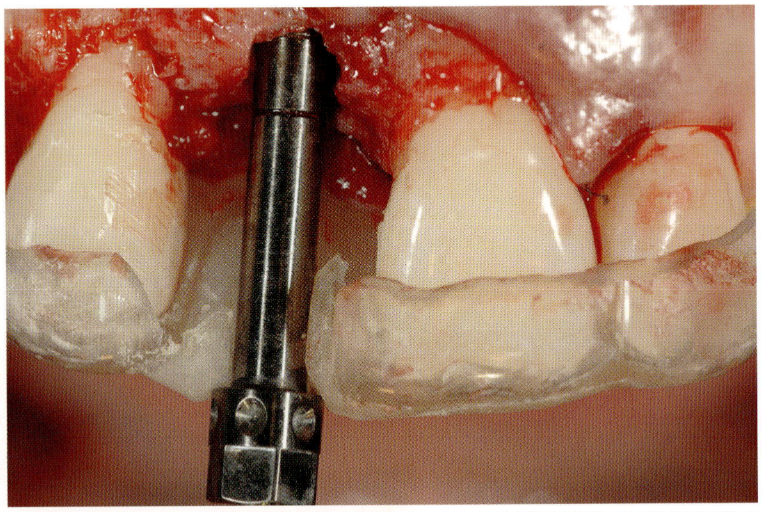

After 6 months, a crestal partial-thickness flap was prepared, and the mesh and screws were removed. A 4.3 × 15–mm NobelActive implant was placed with a straight healing abutment and a CTG.

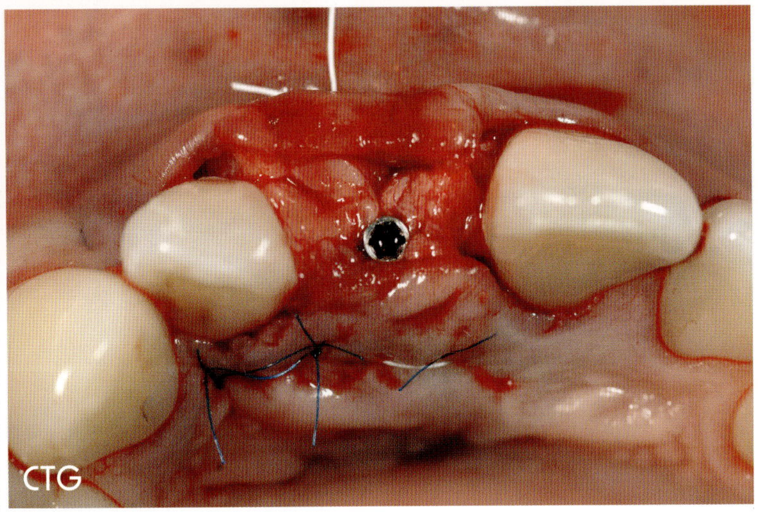

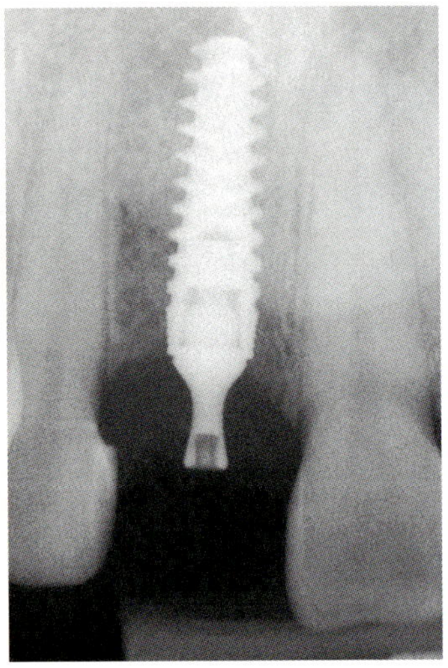

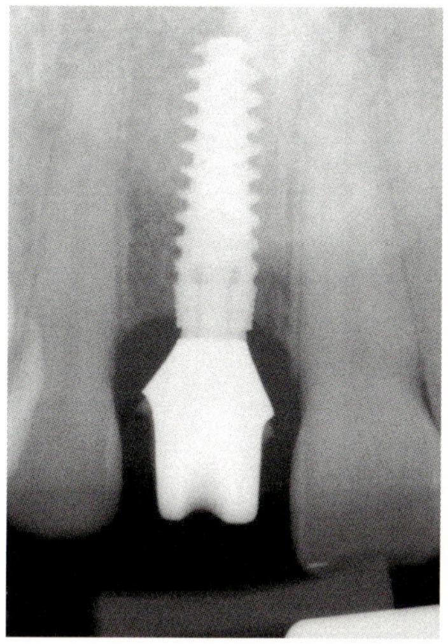

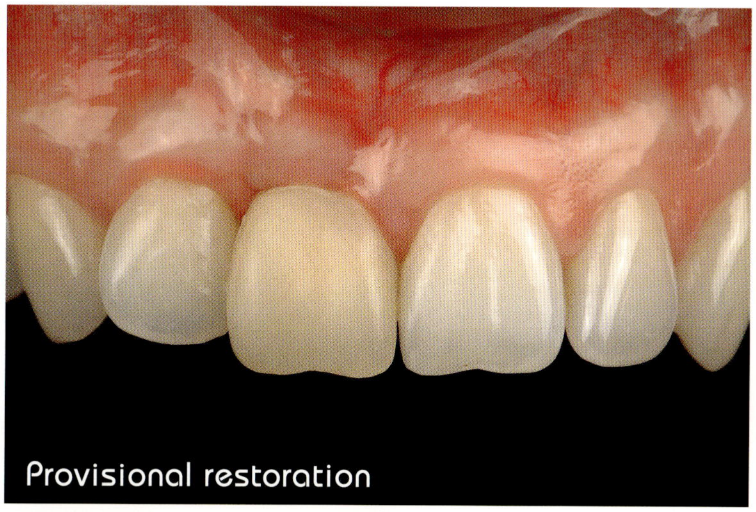

Provisional restoration

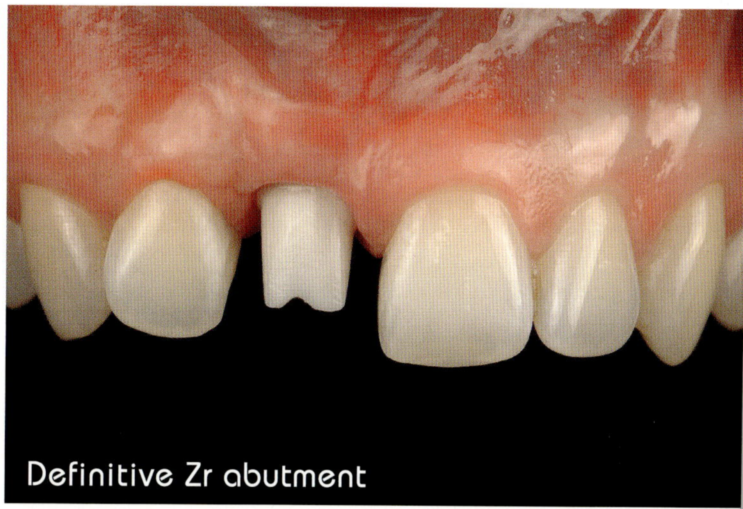

Definitive Zr abutment

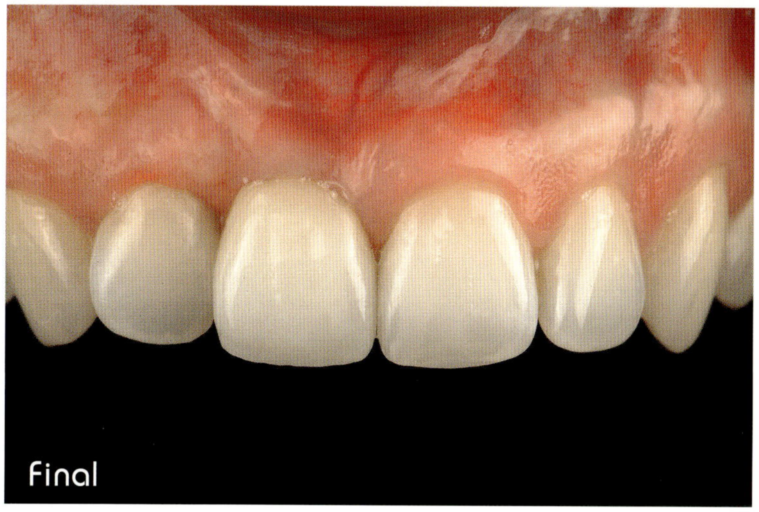

Final

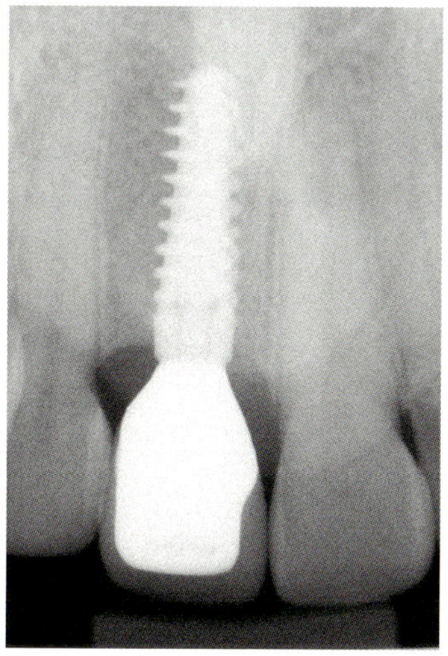

Six months after surgery, a definitive zirconia abutment and provisional restorations were placed for prosthetically guided soft tissue manipulation. After 3 months of soft tissue stability, the definitive zirconia crown restoration was inserted. Additional soft tissue grafting was necessary to achieve the desired result. However, the patient did not agree to another CTG.

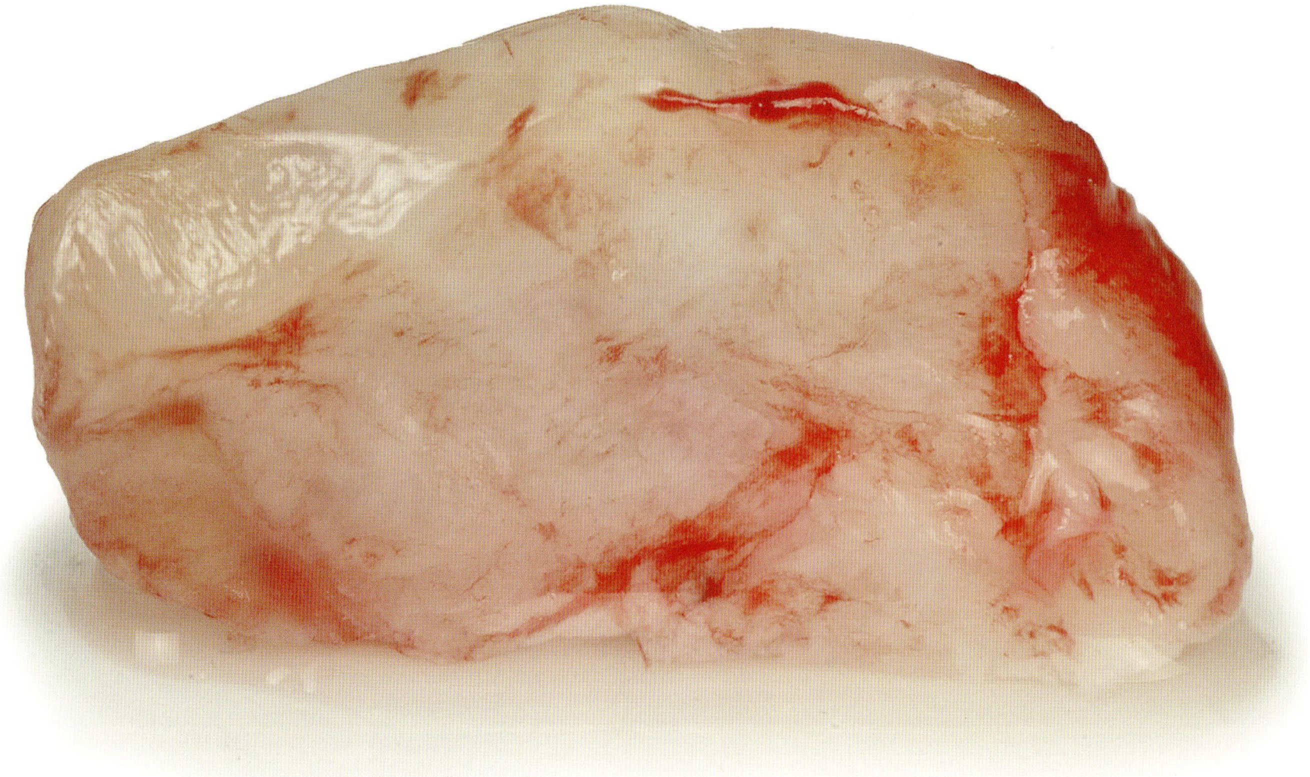

Soft Tissue Grafting Procedures

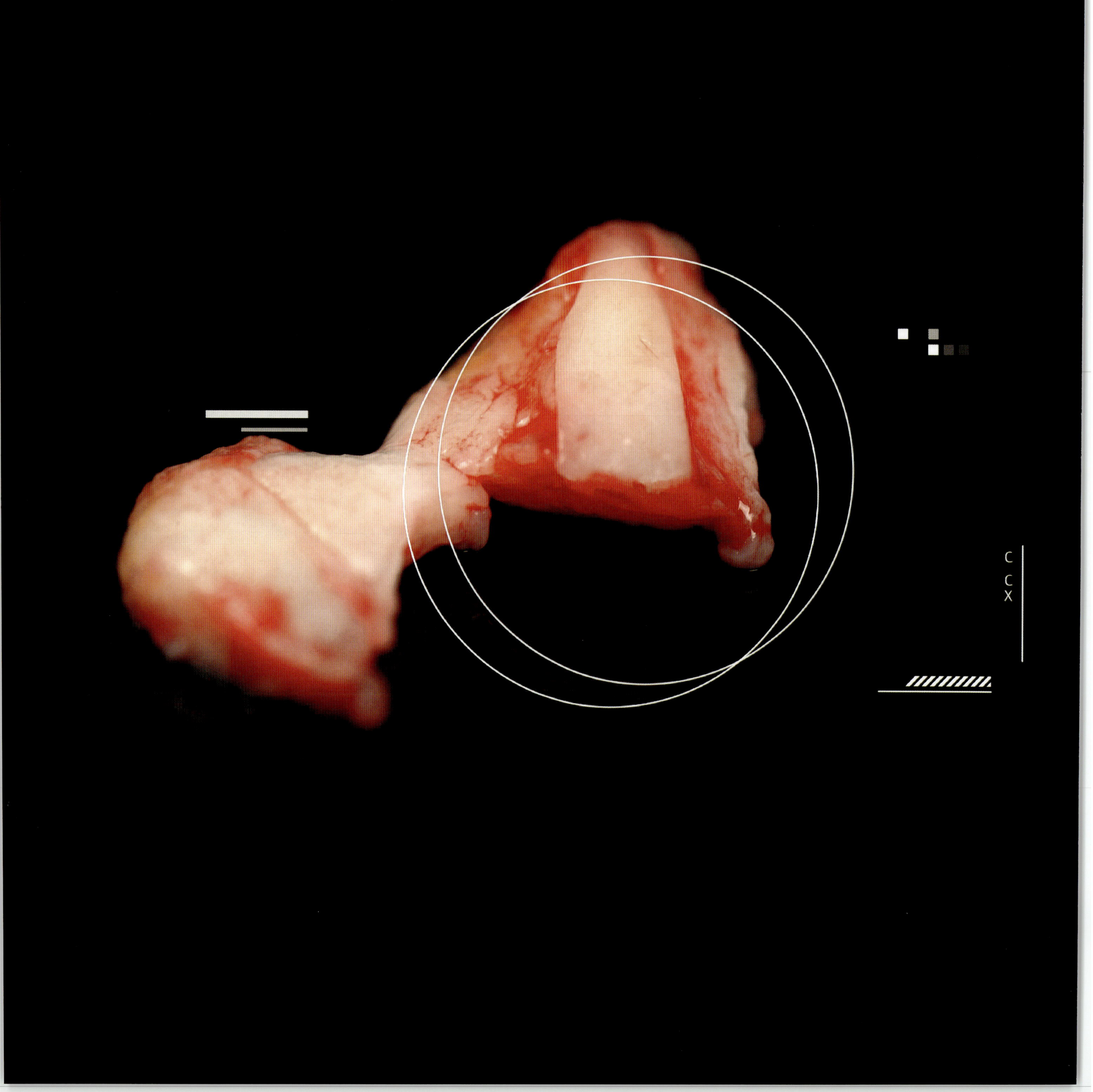
CCX

Donor site manipulation

Research

Soft tissue graft donor site

Systematic reviews on the benefits of soft tissue augmentation procedures around dental implants in the esthetic zone could not identify conclusive evidence on any such interventions, due to lack of long-term clinical studies with sufficient sample size and absence of clear outcome measures and quantitative data analyses.[1] The goal to create a harmonious esthetic outcome that mimics the surrounding dentition and soft tissue condition and morphology is indeed difficult to assess in a quantifiable manner.

Nevertheless, the subepithelial CTG is a preferred technique to treat and prevent gingival and peri-implant soft tissue recessions.[2–5] It is usually placed in combination with a coronally advanced flap[6,7] or with an envelope flap or pouch.[8–10] Traditionally, the palatal mucosa has served as the favored connective tissue donor site.[11] Its thickness, however, varies significantly among patients and is limited by anatomical structures such as the greater palatine artery.[12–15] Healing is associated with significant discomfort, especially when vertical releasing incisions are prepared and areas are left uncovered postsurgically. Procedures that are less traumatic have been proposed but are clinically demanding.[16] Hirsch et al[17] first described the area of the maxillary tuberosity as a donor site for subepithelial CTGs with greater and more consistent tissue thickness. A histologic and clinical description was later provided by Jung et al,[18] who found successful recession coverage associated with a change from a thin to a thick soft tissue biotype and gain in keratinized tissue. Surgical procedures and postoperative hemostasis seemed simpler as compared with the palatal donor site. This approach was then applied around dental implants with excellent clinical success in respect to the amount of recession coverage and esthetic outcomes.[19]

The decision on donor site and surgical technique selection is mainly a clinical one, based on the intended application of the CTG and the tissue morphology at the prospective donor site.[7,20] Endodontic files and rubber stops have been recommended to clinically assess the individual mucosal thickness and tissue density.[20] Subepithelial connective tissue from the tuberosity has a higher density than that from the palate, which usually contains more fat.[18,20] Therefore, it may be less prone to postoperative shrinkage but more difficult to vascularize.[20] A split-thickness flap pouch technique[8] where the periosteum remains on the bone is preferred for CTGs from the tuberosity to ensure maximum vascularization.

Dellavia et al[21] conducted histologic and molecular analyses of tuberosity and palatal mucosa. At microscopic evaluation, the palatal mucosa showed a loose connective tissue containing several blood vessels, while the connective tissue from the tuberosity was dense and poorly vascularized. Histologic and cell-culture studies indicate additional dissimilarities, which support the different clinical outcomes when CTGs from the maxillary tuberosity are used for tissue augmentation. The high cross-linking of tuber collagen seems to maintain the graft stability over time, but in some patients it could induce hypertrophic reactions when used for large soft tissue augmentation procedures.[21]

References

1. Levine RA, Huynh-Ba G, Cochran DL. Soft tissue augmentation procedures for mucogingival defects in esthetic sites. Int J Oral Maxillofac Implants 2014;29(suppl):155–185.

2. Langer B, Calagna L. The subepithelial connective tissue graft. J Prosthet Dent 1980;44:363–367.

3. Langer B, Langer L. Subepithelial connective tissue graft technique for root coverage. J Periodontol 1985;56:715–720.

4. Rosetti EP, Marcantonio RA, Rossa C Jr, Chaves ES, Goissis G, Marcantonio E Jr. Treatment of gingival recession: Comparative study between subepithelial connective tissue graft and guided tissue regeneration. J Periodontol 2000;71:1441–1447.

5. Paolantonio M, di Murro C, Cattabriga A, Cattabriga M. Subpedicle connective tissue graft versus free gingival graft in the coverage of exposed root surfaces. A 5-year clinical study. J Clin Periodontol 1997;24:51–56.

6. Burkhardt R, Joss A, Lang NP. Soft tissue dehiscence coverage around endosseous implants: A prospective cohort study. Clin Oral Implants Res 2008;19:451–457.

7. Zucchelli G, Mazzotti C, Mounssif I, Mele M, Stefanini M, Montebugnoli L. A novel surgical-prosthetic approach for soft tissue dehiscence coverage around single implant. Clin Oral Implants Res 2013;24:957–962.

8. Silverstein L, Lefkove M. The use of the subepithelial connective tissue graft to enhance both the aesthetics and periodontal contours surrounding dental implants. J Oral Implantol 1994;20:135–138.

9. Hsu YT, Shieh CH, Wang HL. Using soft tissue graft to prevent mid-facial mucosal recession following immediate implant placement. J Int Acad Periodontol 2012;14:76–82.

10. Cosyn J, DeBruyn H, Cleymaet R. Soft tissue preservation and pink aesthetics around single immediate implant restorations: A 1-year prospective study. Clin Implant Dent Relat Res 2013;15:847–857.

11. Reiser GM, Bruno JF, Mahan PE, Larkin LH. The subepithelial connective tissue graft palatal donor site: Anatomic considerations for surgeons. Int J Periodontics Restorative Dent 1996;16:130–137.

12. Studer SP, Allen EP, Rees TC, Kouba A. The thickness of masticatory mucosa in the human hard palate and tuberosity as potential donor sites for ridge augmentation procedures. J Periodontol 1997;68:145–151.

13. Müller HP, Schaller N, Eger T, Heinecke A. Thickness of masticatory mucosa. J Clin Periodontol 2000;27:431–436.

14. Stipetić J, Hrala Z, Celebić A. Thickness of masticatory mucosa in the human hard palate and tuberosity dependent on gender and body mass index. Coll Antropol 2005;29:243–247.

15. Song JE, Um YJ, Kim CS, et al. Thickness of posterior palatal masticatory mucosa: The use of computerized tomography. J Periodontol 2008;79:406–412.

16. Hürzeler M, Weng D. A single incision technique to harvest subepithelial connective tissue from the palate. Int J Periodontics Restorative Dent 1999;19:279–287.

17. Hirsch A, Attal U, Chai E, Goultschin J, Boyan BD, Schwartz Z. Root coverage and pocket reduction as combined surgical procedures. J Periodontol 2001;72:1572–1579.

18. Jung UW, Um YJ, Choi SH. Histologic observation of soft tissue acquired from maxillary tuberosity area for root coverage. J Periodontol 2008;79:934–940.

19. Roccuzzo M, Gaudioso L, Bunino M, Dalmasso P. Surgical treatment of buccal soft tissue recessions around single implants: 1-year results from a prospective pilot study. Clin Oral Implants Res 2014;25:641–646.

20. Zuhr O, Baumer D, Hürzeler M. The addition of soft tissue replacement grafts in plastic periodontal and implant surgery: Critical elements in design and execution. J Clin Periodontol 2014;41(suppl):123–142.

21. Dellavia C, Ricci G, Pettinari L, Allievi C, Grizzi F, Gagliano N. Human palatal and tuberosity mucosa as donor sites for ridge augmentation. Int J Periodontics Restorative Dent 2014;34:179–186.

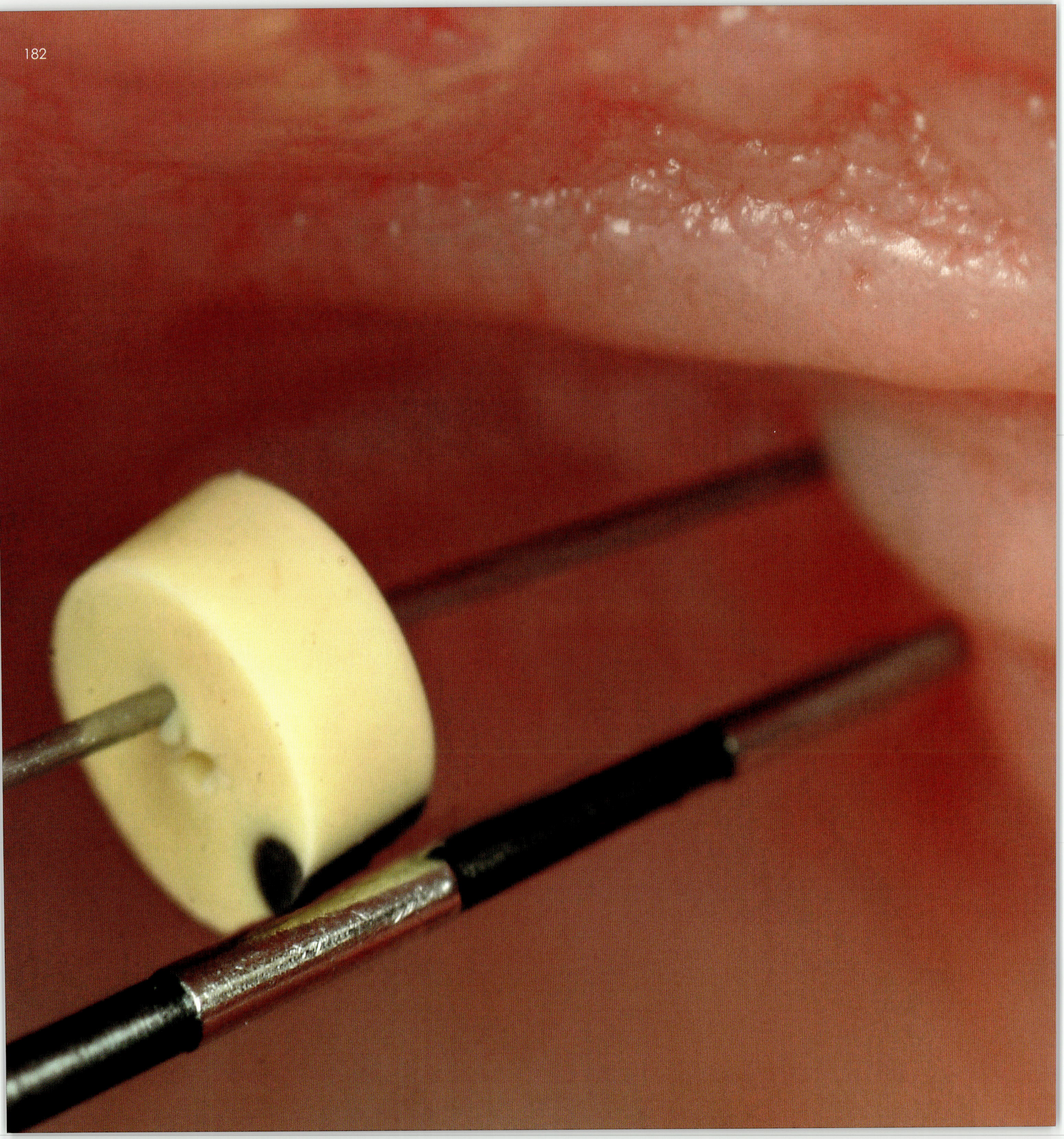

Thickness evaluation

To avoid multiple entries or excessive interventions and to get an estimation of the maximum dimensions of a subepithelial CTG that can be harvested, it is helpful to know the tissue thickness at the prospective donor sites. Average tissue thickness values at various donor sites have been published in the literature and are summarized in the following.

This information serves the surgeon but also the restorative dentist as a guide to select the proper donor site. Today's advanced radiologic technologies and computed tomography allow for better treatment planning and a more predictable surgical approach, because the available tissue can be quantified more easily before surgically entering the site for the CTG.

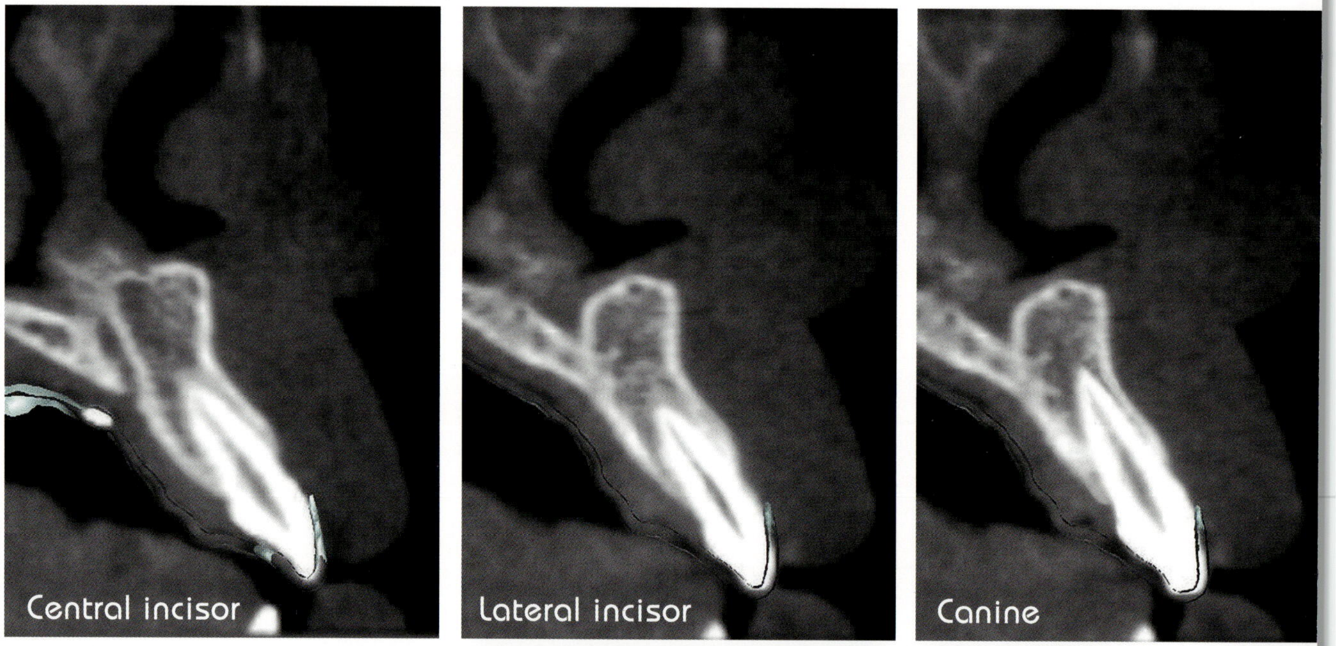

Palatal tissue thickness

Average tissue thickness values of the palatal mucosa are shown in different areas. Palatal anatomy, patient phenotype, sex, and arch configuration are limiting factors. The thickest tissue is typically found in the area of the second premolar. The area of the first molar is usually the thinnest due to the voluptuous palatal root. Greater tissue thicknesses can be found anteriorly and posteriorly to the first molar.

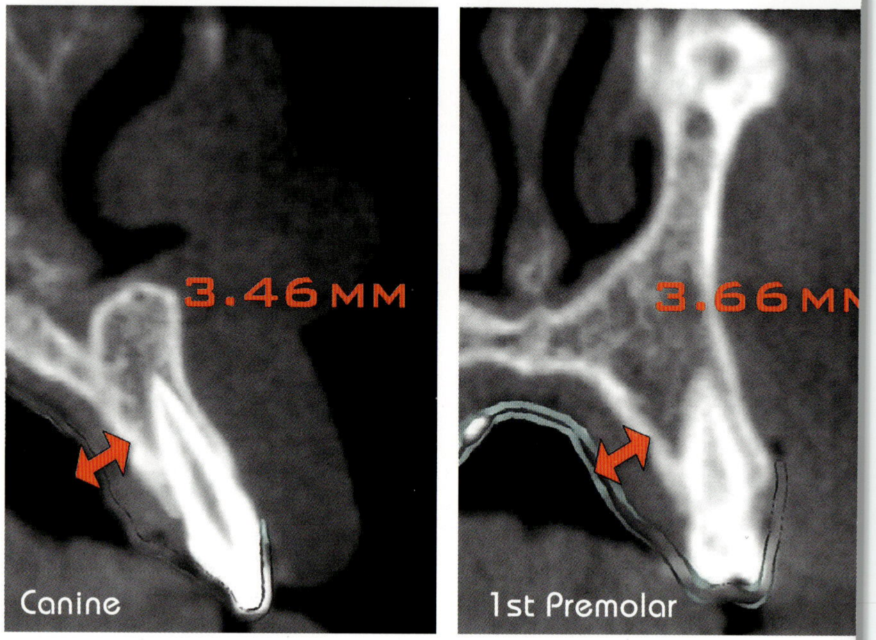

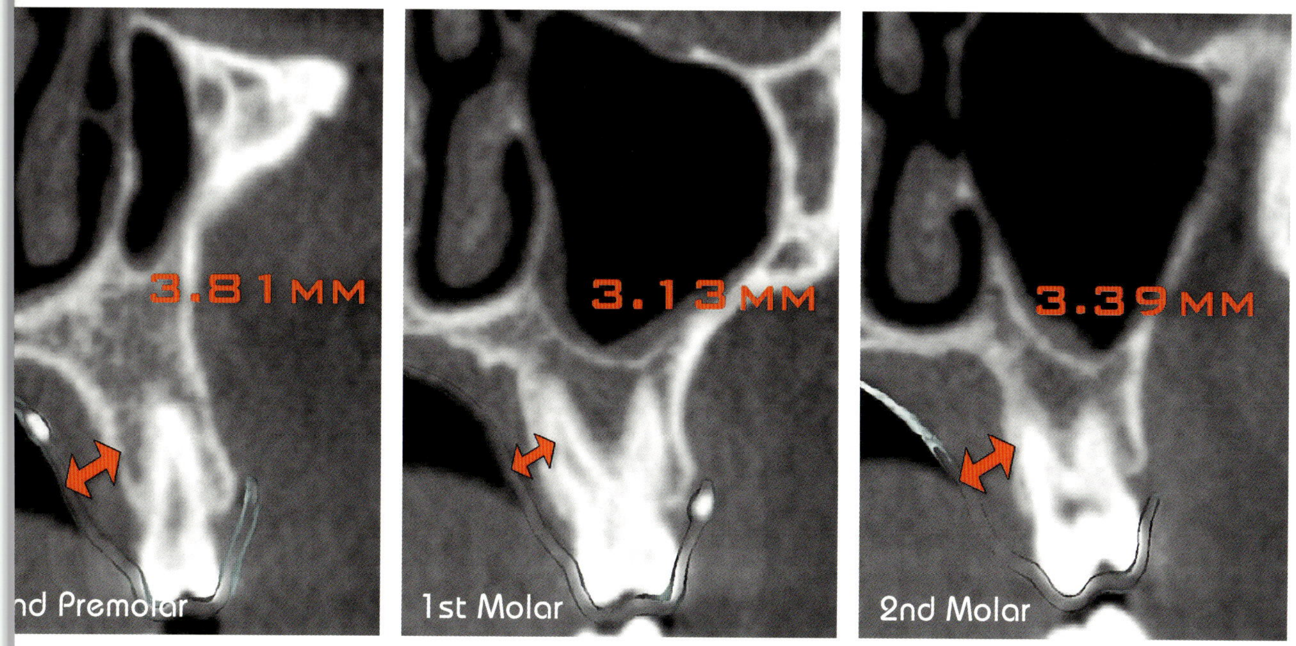

The greater palatine artery presents a significant anatomical landmark and surgical limitation when harvesting tissue from the palate. It is typically located between the second and third molars about 14 mm palatally to their cementoenamel junctions (CEJs). This number, however, is not absolute, and the distance shows great individual variation.

Tuberosity tissue thickness

A subepithelial CTG from the maxillary tuberosity has several advantages, such as higher density. Because the quality and not just the quantity of connective tissue is important for long-term augmentation success, the maxillary tuberosity and retomolar pad areas have become increasingly popular donor sites. These sites are specifically attractive after third molar extraction and can be considered about 6 months thereafter. Patient discomfort and tissue morbidity is significantly less than with the palate. In fact, the CTG harvested from the tuberosity may be too large to handle and difficult to suture in place. One of the challenges of harvesting a CTG from the maxillary tuberosity, however, is surgical access due to the posterior location and the coronoid apophysis.

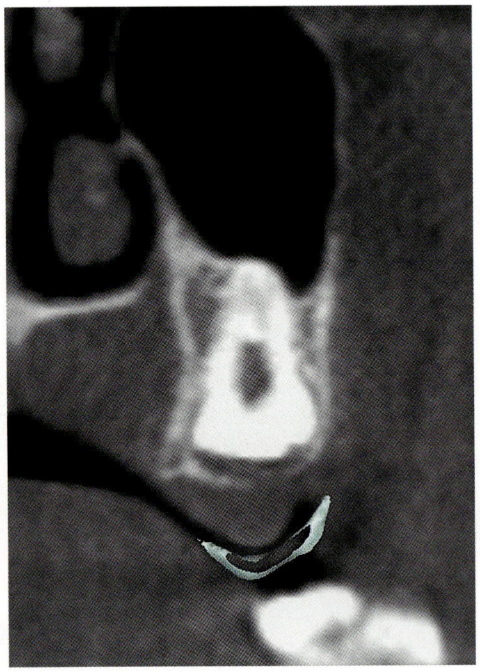

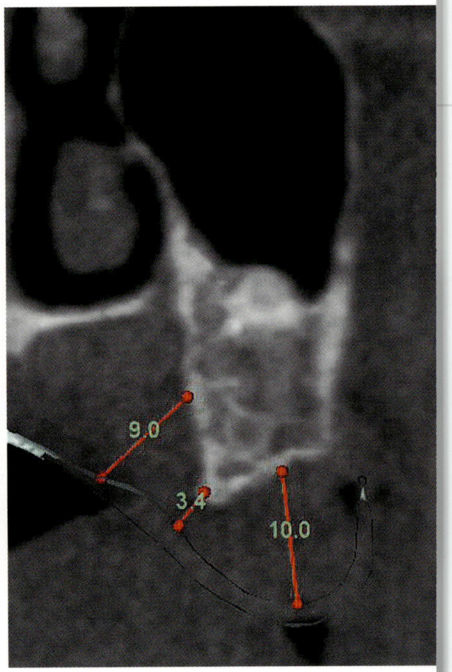

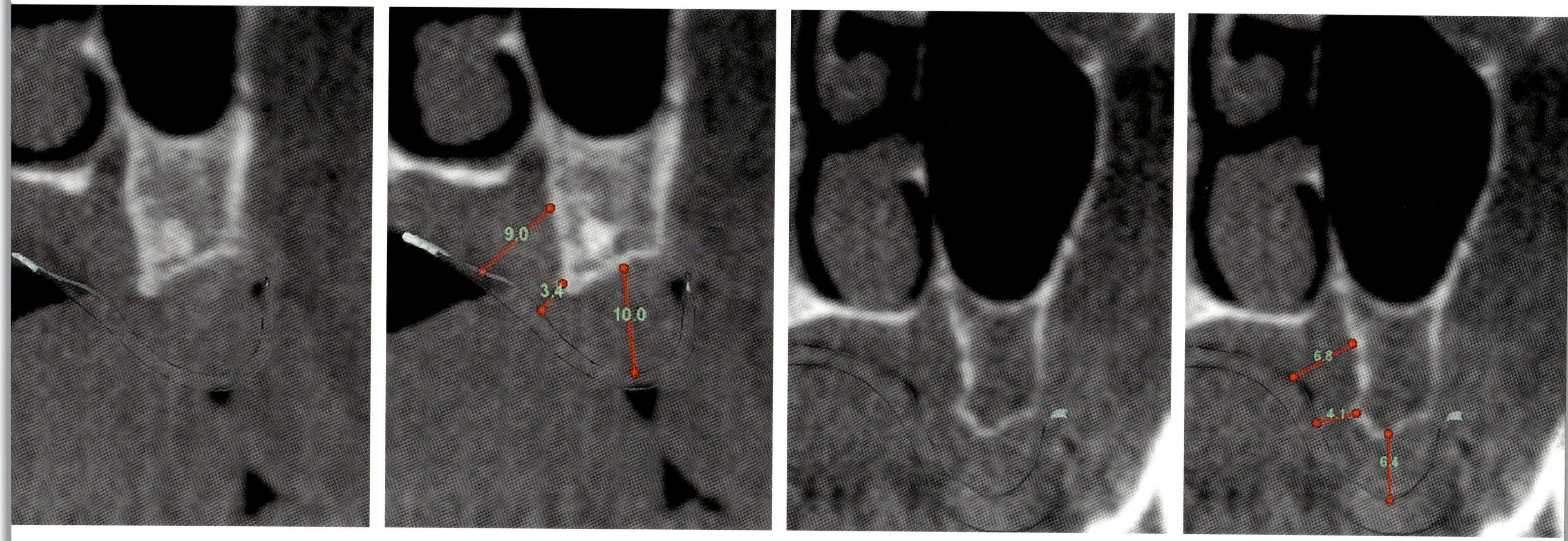
9.0
3.4
10.0
6.8
4.1
6.4

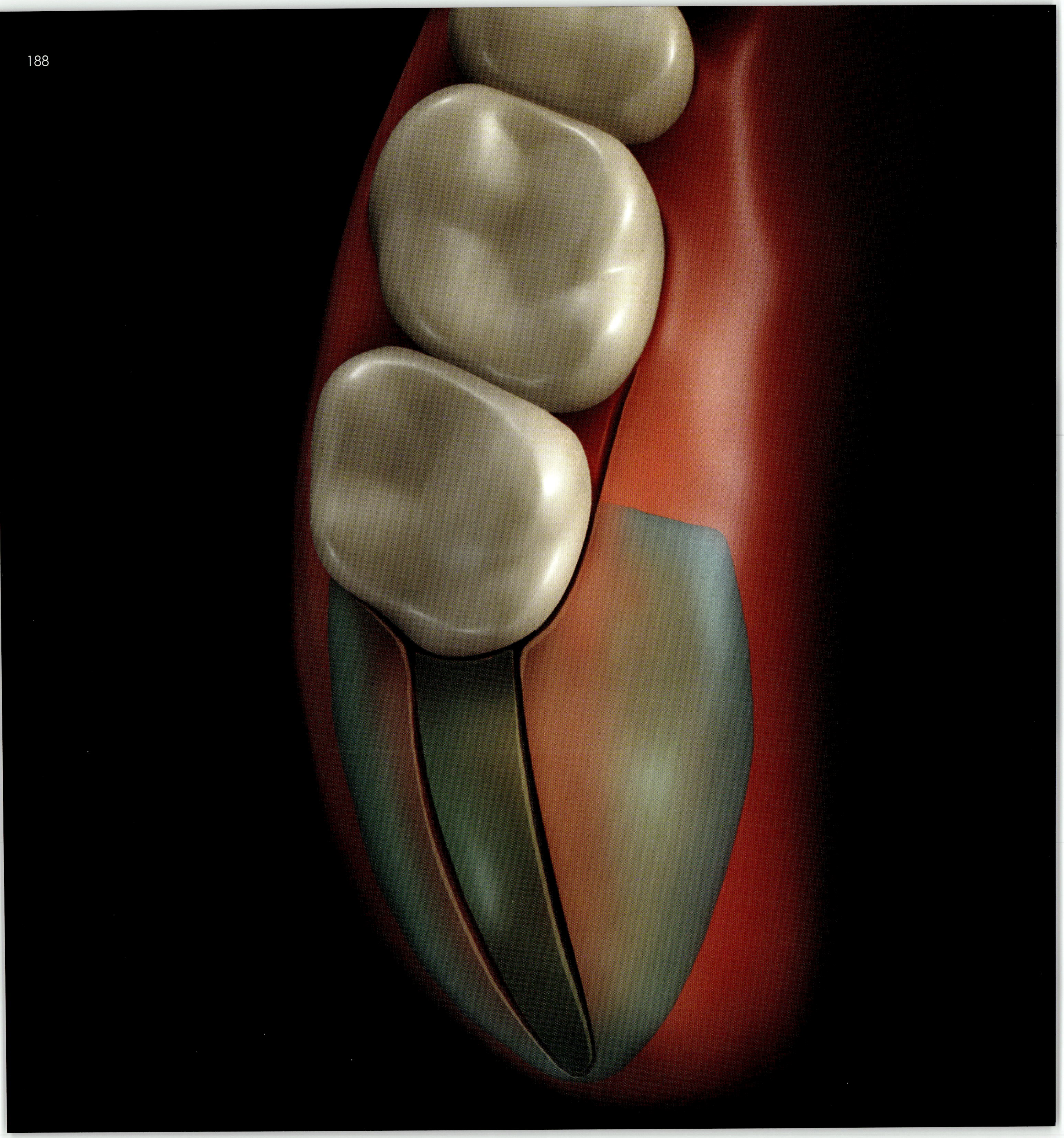

Surgical technique

The retromolar pad in the mandible and the maxillary tuberosity present unique challenges to the clinician. They generally involve hyperplastic tissues, unusual underlying osseous topography, and in the case of the retromolar area, a fatty, glandular, mucosal-type tissue. Historically, while periodontal surgery techniques were constantly developed and improved, progress in surgical techniques for these areas remained stagnant. Gingivectomy was the treatment of choice for various pathologic conditions and hyperplastic tissues. The distal wedge procedure overcame the shortcomings of a simple gingivectomy, which, due to its limited access and visibility, did not allow treatment of irregular osseous deformities or access to the distal furcation areas of maxillary molars. As a technique to harvest a subepithelial CTG, the wedge procedure offers multiple advantages in addition to the histologic and morphologic benefits of tissues from the retromolar pad and maxillary tuberosity.

Advantages of the distal wedge technique

- Minimal trauma, fast healing, limited pain for the patient (unlike palatal CTGs)
- Maintenance of attached tissue, simple primary wound closure (limits postoperative discomfort)
- Closure with mature thin tissue especially important in the retromolar pad area

The few limitations include access and anatomical restrictions (eg, ascending ramus, coronoid apophyses, or external oblique ridge); increased illumination (eg, surgical head light) is recommended to improve vision.

Wedge designs

- Triangular
- Square, parallel, or H-design
- Linear or pedicle

Triangular design

The triangular wedge requires an adequate zone of keratinized tissue and can be applied in a very short or small maxillary tuberosity. A triangular incision is made distal to the last molar with a no. 12 or no. 15 scalpel blade. The resulting triangular tissue wedge is removed with scalers, hoes, or knives. The walls of the wedge are thinned or undermined with scalpel blades to allow proper adaptation of the proximal tissues to the underlying bone. Note the outline of the incisions, removal of the secondary wedges, and reflection of the flap for bone exposure, which is typically achieved with periosteal elevators. It may be necessary to prepare small releasing incisions at the apex of the primary incision to relieve tissue tension. Primary closure is accomplished with interrupted sutures.

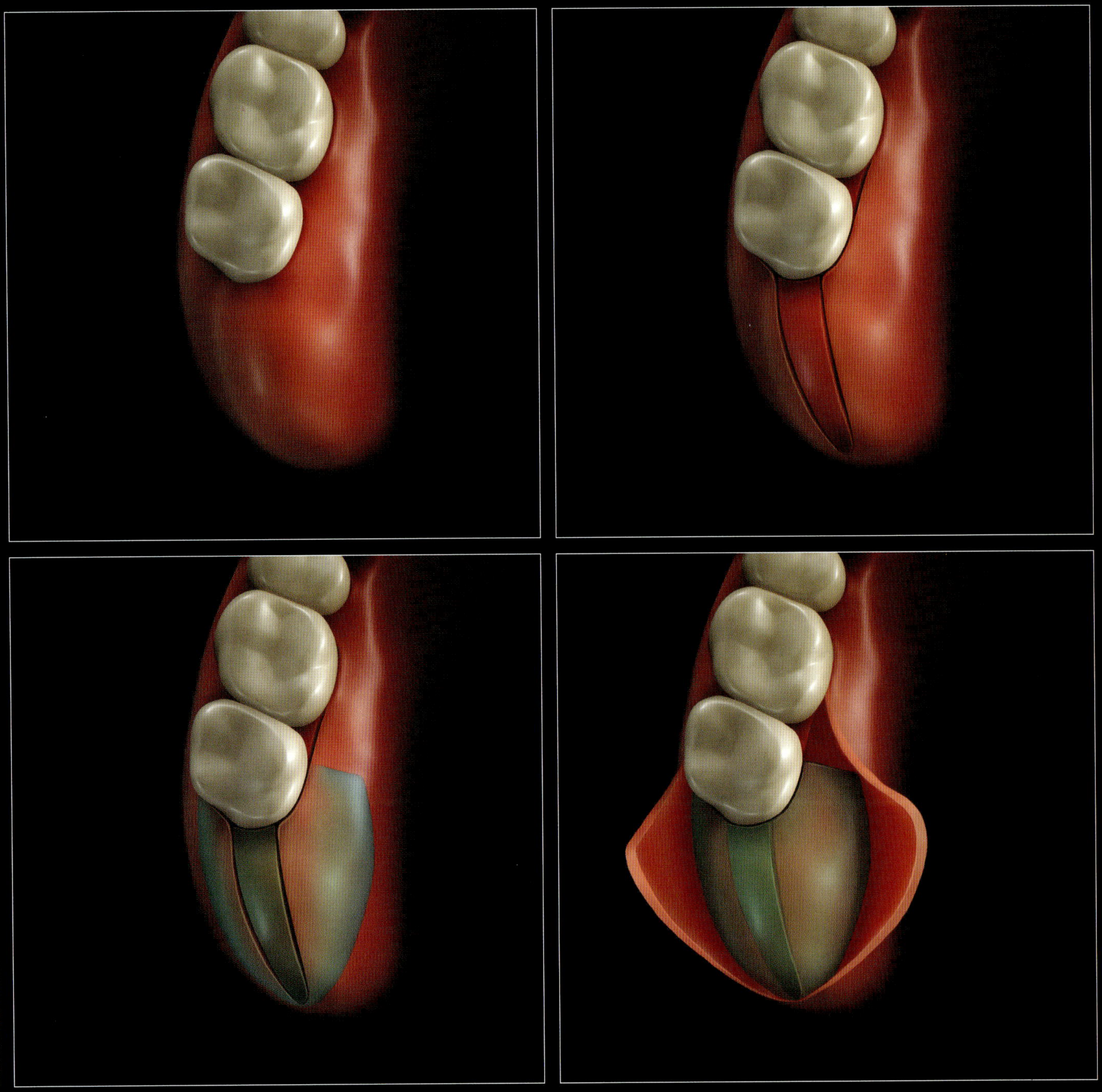

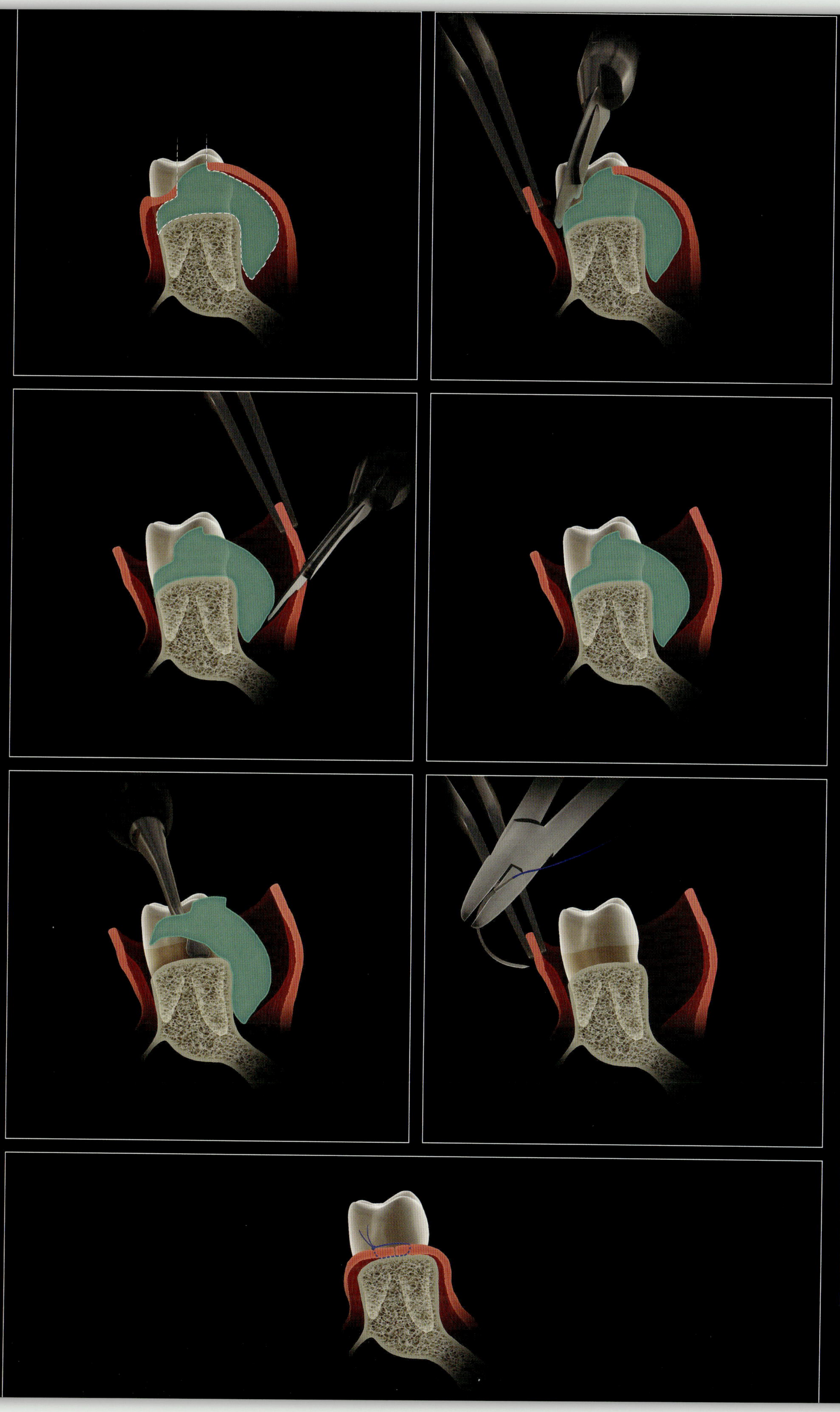

Square or parallel

This technique allows for harvesting large amounts of keratinized tissue and maximum closure. It also provides greater access to the underlying bony topography and the distal furcation of the most posterior molar if necessary. It is indicated when the maxillary tuberosity is long or large.

As a first step, two parallel inversely beveled thinning incisions are made with a no. 12 blade. They start at the hamular notch at the mucosal part on the distal end of the edentulous area and are continued to the tooth. Two more incisions are made to release the flaps, one directed toward the buccal and the other toward the palatal aspect of the edentulous ridge.

The flaps are raised buccally and lingually or palatally with periosteal elevators. Kirkland or Orban knives may be used to remove the wedge of tissue from the bone. After the bone is exposed, the tissue is thinned and manipulated as necessary to provide primary closure with interrupted sutures.

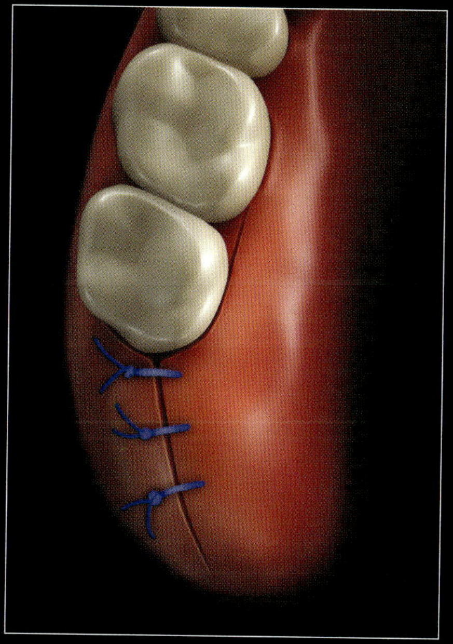

Tuberosity surgical technique

Modified parallel

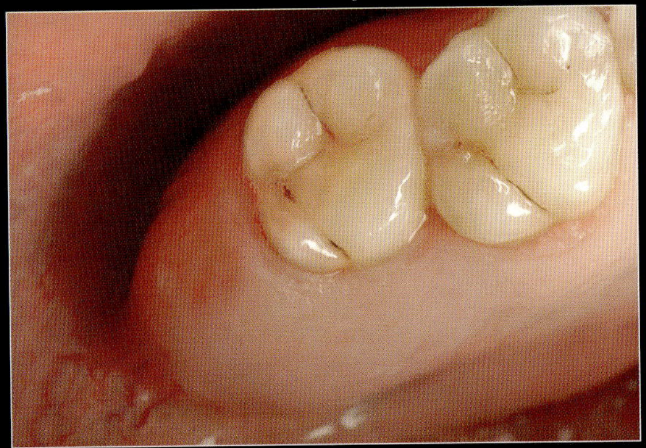

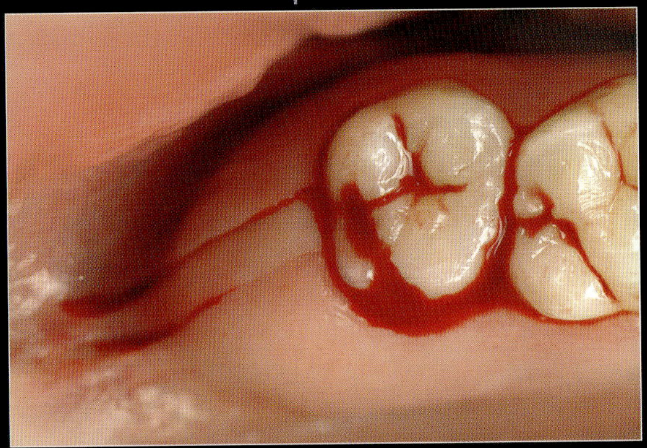

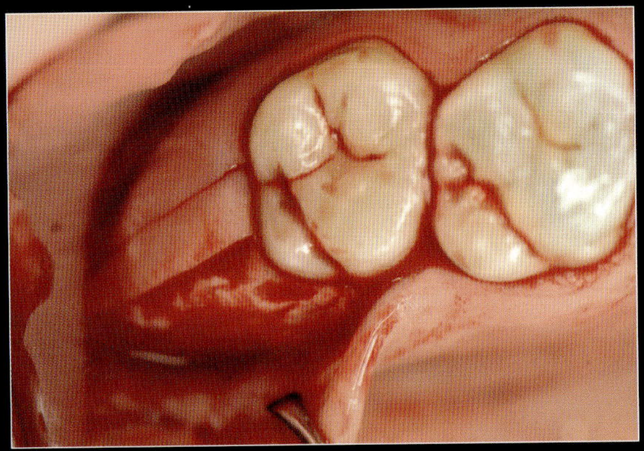

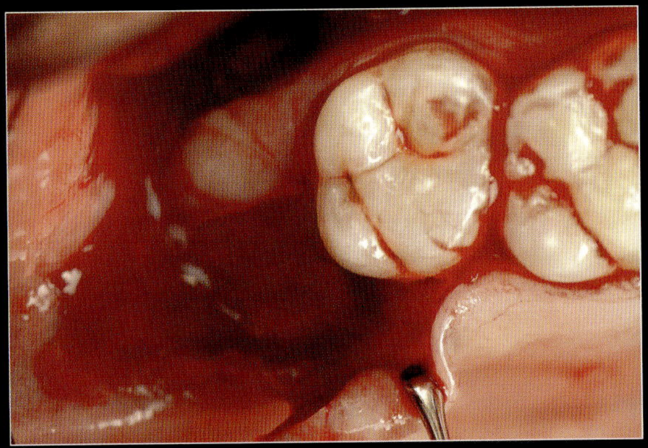

This technique allows for the maximum amount of tissue that can be harvested from the maxillary tuberosity area. The maximum quantity of tissue is located on the ridge and on the palatal aspect of the tuberosity. This technique is indicated when large quantities of connective tissue are required and, obviously, in the presence of large tuberosities.

Two parallel incisions are made with a no. 12 blade from the distal part of the tuberosity (hamular notch at the mucosal aspect of the tuberosity) to the distal aspect of the second molar. The buccal incision can be inversely beveled or parallel to the bone and extend all the way to the bone. The palatal incision runs parallel to the buccal incision but is only 1 to 2 mm in depth and continues around the distal and palatal aspects. A sulcular incision is made to release the inner flap before removal of the connective tissue all the way to the second molar and straight to the first molar, whenever large CTGs are necessary.

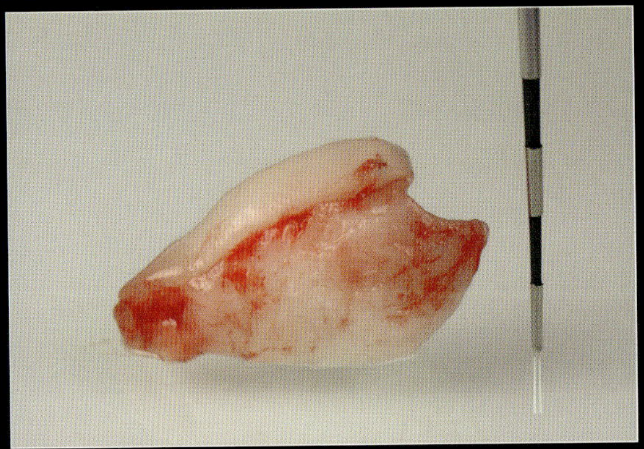

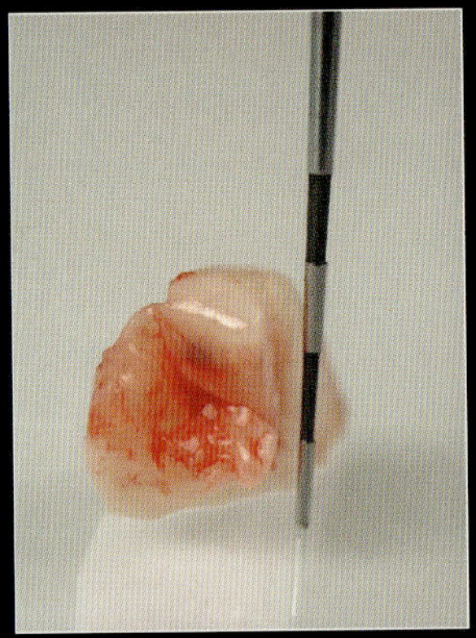

The palatal epithelium is carefully dissected with a no. 15 scalpel, starting at the palatal incision and following the anatomy of the palate. This should leave a 2-mm-thick flap from the posterior to the anterior aspect, which could extend to the first molar. Curved cotton pliers are recommended to reflect the palatal flap and prepare a vertical incision around the mesial aspect of the second molar and straight to the bone. Then periosteal elevators are used to lift and loosen the inner flap until the bone is exposed. This is best achieved by using the second molar as a fulcrum to apply leverage on the elevators and, starting from the parallel buccal incision, move the instruments toward the center of the palate. Subsequently, a horizontal or parallel incision is made to sever the inner second flap or CTG at the base, which is then pulled out, leaving the bone exposed. The flap is adapted and sutured with interrupted sutures.

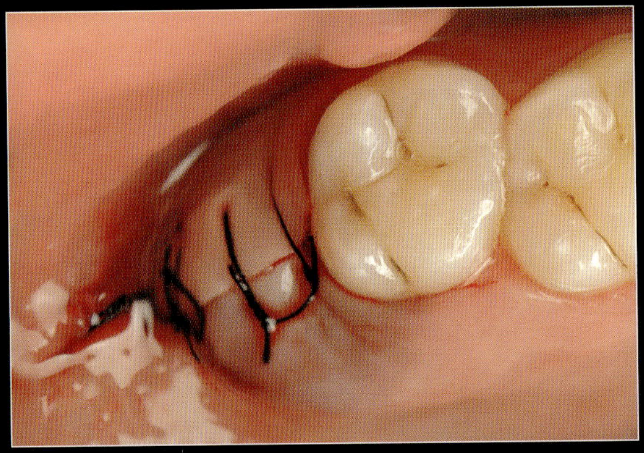

Retromolar pad surgical technique

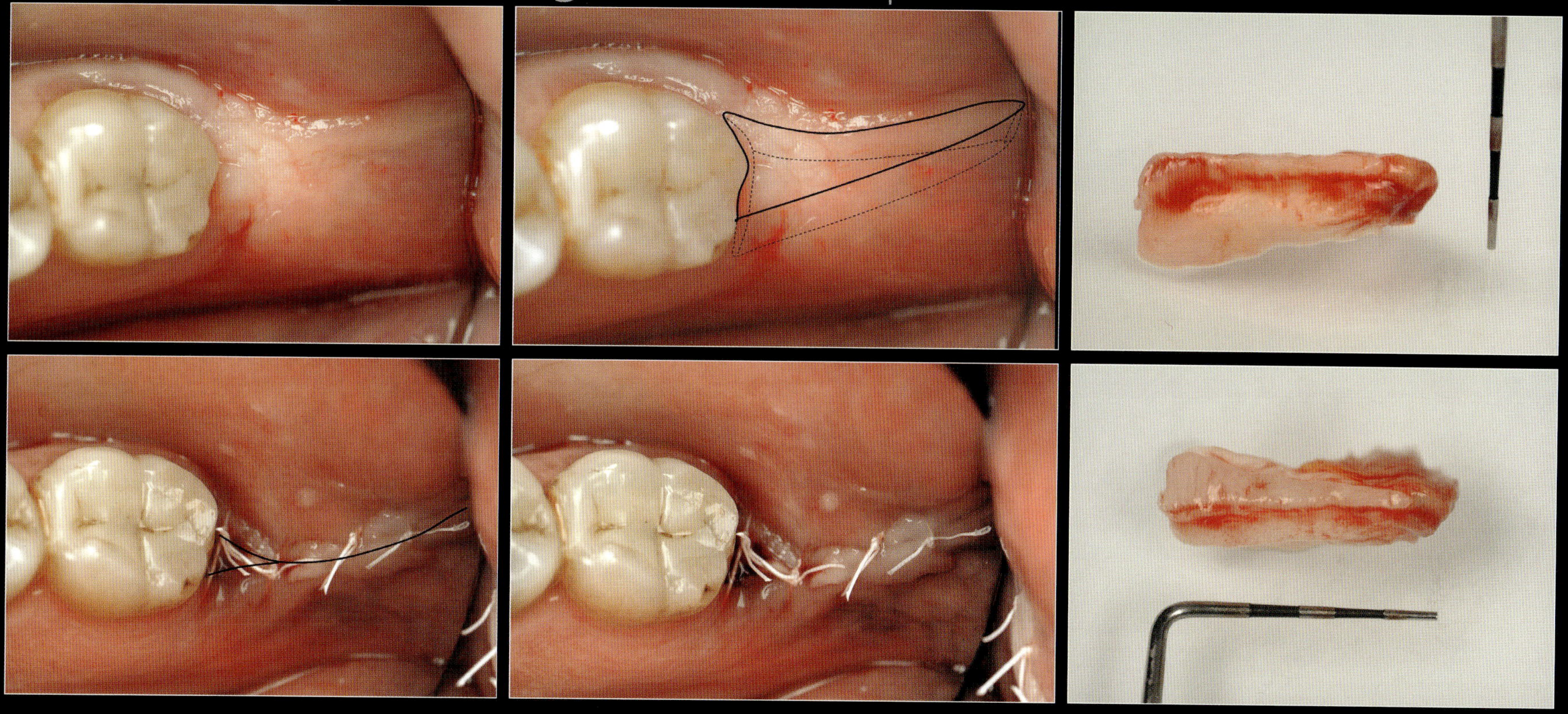

The retromolar area often has minimal keratinized tissue that is primarily mucosal glandular. A simple wedge technique is the only possible method to thin and reduce the tissue in this area. Typically, only limited amounts of tissue can be harvested, which may be sufficient to provide volume and stability for small teeth like mandibular anterior or maxillary lateral incisors. No information could be found in the literature that refers to the use of this site for grafting. This area and its importance for removable prosthodontics requires further study.

The distal wedge technique was applied in the retromolar area of the mandible. Probing revealed a 9-mm-deep pocket with a wide band of gingiva, which made it a viable option for connective tissue grafting. This area is not always ideal, but it should be considered as an alternative donor site, for example when third molars are to be extracted. Two vertical parallel incisions are made to the bone and joined at the distal end of the retromolar pad. The wedge incision should allow at least 1 mm of gingiva on each side lingually and buccally from the incision to the mucogingival line. A wedge is then elevated, dissected with a perpendicular incision, and removed. A large amount of tissue was harvested in this situation.

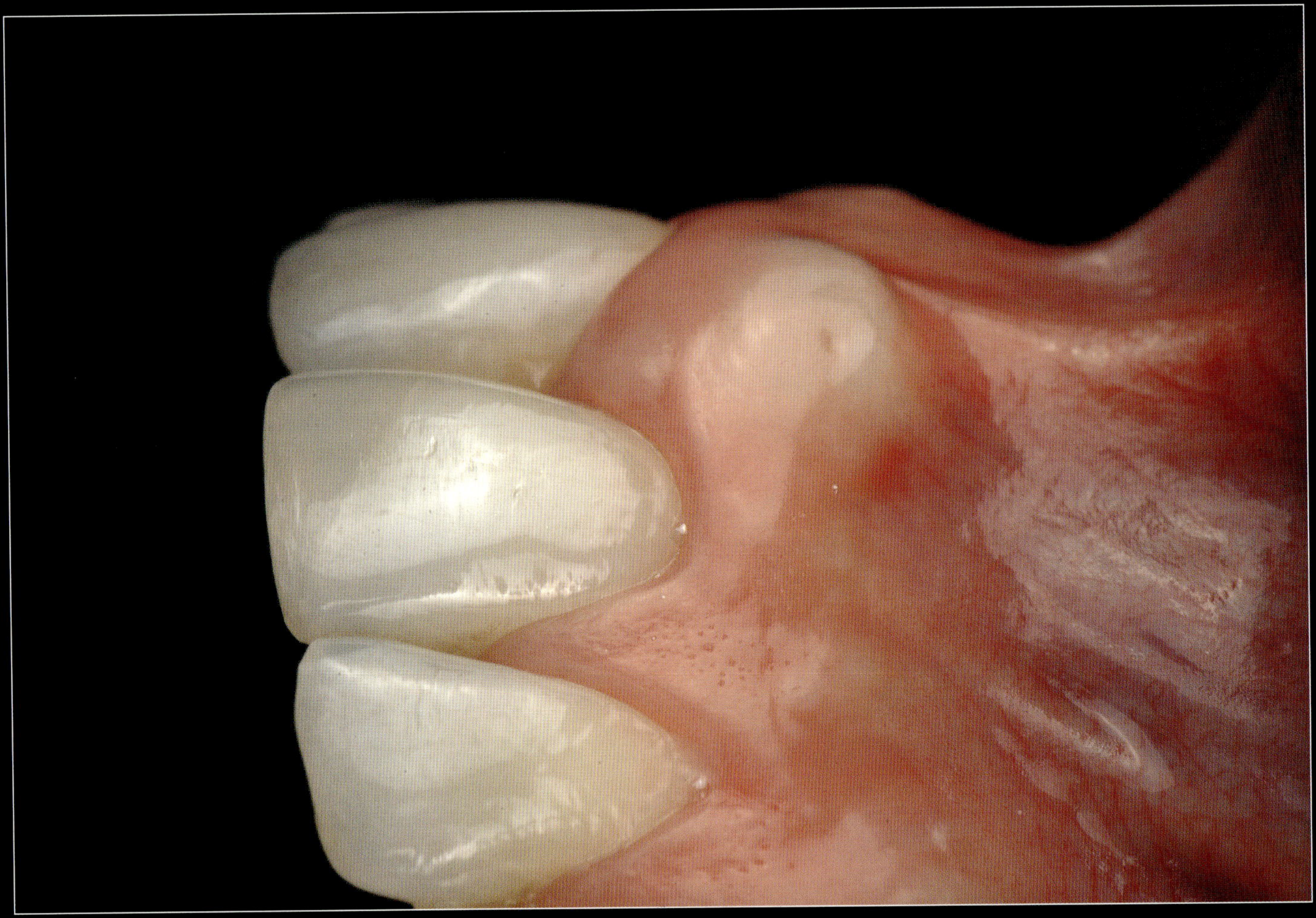

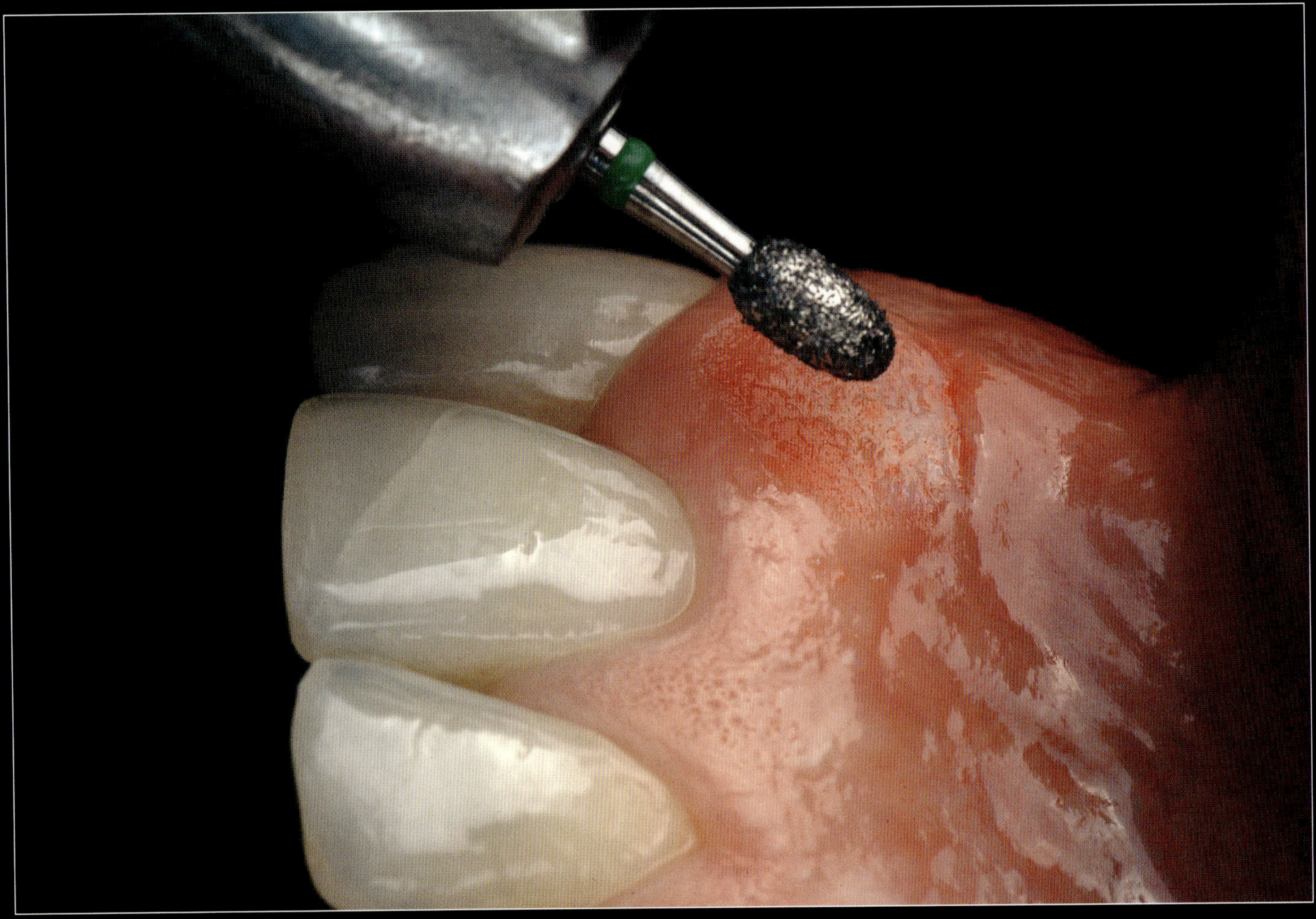

Long-term grafting results

In the esthetic zone, every implant should receive a CTG. It seems that long-term outcomes with CTGs from the tuberosity or retromolar area are far superior than those without a CTG or with a CTG from the palate. Five patient scenarios are presented to illustrate outcomes and possibilities with such novel approaches in implant therapy:

1. Hypertrophic reaction
2. Restoring lost volume with only a CTG from the tuberosity, with 5-year recall
3. The consequences of 10 years of implant function without a CTG, as well as the contemporary line of treatment
4. Comparison of treatment with a CTG on one site versus treatment without a CTG on another site and problems that occur in the long term, as well as the solution for long-term stability
5. Retromolar area as the donor site and long-term results

Research

Tissue graft clinical outcomes

The current scientific evidence on clinical outcomes of soft tissue augmentation procedures of peri-implant mucogingival defects remains inconclusive.[1] It is even less clear on bone augmentation techniques, bone graft materials, and their respective timing.[2] Existing clinical studies focus more on implant survival and success rates than on esthetic outcomes, which are difficult to standardize, quantify, and analyze. With advanced soft tissue augmentation techniques, however, the need for bone grafting procedures in single-tooth edentulous sites has diminished.[3]

In a clinical study, peri-implant recessions were treated with CTGs from the palate and coronally advanced partial thickness flaps.[3] While early success rates were excellent, recurring recessions could not be avoided 6 months postoperatively. Zucchelli et al[4] used a similar approach but achieved significantly better late success. They attributed this to the fact that in their study, the implant abutments were removed, reshaped, and repolished before the surgery to create more space for the CTG and better tissue adaptation.

A CTG placed in a pouch or envelope is probably the most popular technique to treat peri-implant soft tissue deficiencies. In a 1-year prospective study of 22 immediately placed implants, two cases demonstrated advanced midfacial recession of 1.5 and 2.0 mm after 3 months.[5] CTGs were placed, and the recessions were limited to 0.5 mm for both cases at the 1-year follow-up.

Grunder[6] demonstrated the effectiveness and volumetric soft tissue gain when placing a CTG at the time of immediate implant insertion. The benefits are not limited to morphologic and biologic success but also improved soft tissue esthetics.[7] Subepithelial CTGs can be placed at any stage of treatment and are especially effective and stable in patients with a thin soft tissue biotype.[8]

The initial soft tissue thickness at the crest seems to have a significant influence on marginal bone stability around implants.[9] A thin peri-implant soft tissue of 2.0 mm or less may lead to greater crestal bone loss.[9] Clinical studies indicate that soft tissue recession around implants is an ongoing process that does not halt after 1 year.[10,11] Sites with a thick tissue biotype showed significantly less changes at the facial gingival level than sites with a thin tissue biotype, both at 1-year (–0.25 mm versus –0.75 mm) and 4-year (–0.56 mm versus –1.50 mm) follow-ups after implant placement. In general, thin gingival biotypes seem more prone to tissue recessions, but even thick biotypes can be susceptible.[12] Thin peri-implant tissues are more friable and less vascularized than thick biotypes.[11,13] Postoperative tissue recession is especially common in immediate tooth replacement situations.[14–16]

Therefore, biotype enhancement and soft tissue augmentation with subepithelial CTGs[17–20] should be considered for all implant procedures, especially immediate implant placement, and even with thick tissue biotypes. The graft should ideally be placed at the time of implant placement.[17–20]

References

1. Levine RA, Huynh-Ba G, Cochran DL. Soft tissue augmentation procedures for mucogingival defects in esthetic sites. Int J Oral Maxillofac Implants 2014;29(suppl):155–185.

2. Kuchler U, von Arx T. Horizontal ridge augmentation in conjunction with or prior to implant placement in the anterior maxilla: A systematic review. Int J Oral Maxillofac Implants 2014;29(suppl):14–24.

3. Burkhardt R, Joss A, Lang NP. Soft tissue dehiscence coverage around endosseous implants: A prospective cohort study. Clin Oral Implants Res 2008;19:451–457.

4. Zucchelli G, Mazzotti C, Mounssif I, Mele M, Stefanini M, Montebugnoli L. A novel surgical-prosthetic approach for soft tissue dehiscence coverage around single implant. Clin Oral Implants Res 2013;24:957–962.

5. Cosyn J, DeBruyn H, Cleymaet R. Soft tissue preservation and pink aesthetics around single immediate implant restorations: A 1-year prospective study. Clin Implant Dent Relat Res 2013;15:847–857.

6. Grunder U. Crestal ridge width changes when placing implants at the time of tooth extraction with and without soft tissue augmentation after a healing period of 6 months: Report of 24 consecutive cases. Int J Periodontics Restorative Dent 2011;31:9–17.

7. Speroni S, Cicciu M, Maridati P, Grossi GB, Maiorana C. Clinical investigation of mucosal thickness stability after soft tissue grafting around implants: A 3-year retrospective study. Indian J Dent Res 2010;21:474–479.

8. Linkevicius T, Apse P, Grybauskas S, Puisys A. The influence of soft tissue thickness on crestal bone changes around implants: A 1-year prospective controlled clinical trial. Int J Oral Maxillofac Implants 2009;24:712–719.

9. Wiesner G, Esposito M, Worthington H, Schlee M. Connective tissue grafts for thickening peri-implant tissues at implant placement. One-year results from an explanatory split-mouth randomised controlled clinical trial. Eur J Oral Implantol 2010;3:27–35.

10. Kan JYK, Rungcharassaeng K, Cosyn J. Immediate placement and provisionalization of maxillary anterior single implants: A 1-year prospective study. Int J Oral Maxillofac Implants 2003;18:31–39.

11. Kan JYK, Rungcharassaeng K, Lozada JL, Zimmerman G. Facial gingival tissue stability following immediate placement and provisionalization of maxillary anterior single implants: A 2- to 8-year follow-up. Int J Oral Maxillofac Implants 2011;26:179–187.

12. Evans CDJ, Chen ST. Esthetic outcomes of immediate implant placements. Clin Oral Implants Res 2008;19:73–80.

13. Lee A, Fu JH, Wang HL. Soft tissue biotype affects implant success. Implant Dent 2011;20:e38–e47.

14. Kan JYK, Rungcharassaeng K, Morimoto T, Lozada J. Facial gingival tissue stability after connective tissue graft with single immediate tooth replacement in the esthetic zone: Consecutive case report. J Oral Maxillofac Surg 2009;67:40–48.

15. Kan JYK, Rungcharassaeng K, Umezu K, Kois JC. Dimensions of peri-implant mucosa: An evaluation of maxillary anterior single implants in humans. J Periodontol 2003;74:557–562.

16. De Rouck T, Collys K, Cosyn J. Immediate single-tooth implants in the anterior maxilla: A 1-year case cohort study on hard and soft tissue response. J Clin Periodontol 2008;35:649–657.

17. Cornellini R, Brone A, Covani U. Connective tissue grafts in postextraction implants with immediate restoration: A prospective controlled clinical study. Pract Proced Aesthet Dent 2008;20:337–343.

18. Bianchi AE, Sanfilippo F. Single-tooth replacement by immediate implant and CT graft: A 1 to 9-year clinical evaluation. Clin Oral Implants Res 2004;15:269–277.

19. Redemagni M, Cremonesi S, Garlini G, Maiorna C. Soft tissue stability with immediate implants and concave abutments. Eur J Esthet Dent 2009;4:328–337.

20. Chung S, Rungcharassaeng K, Kan JY, Roe P, Lozada JL. Immediate single tooth replacement with subepithelial connective tissue graft using platform switching implants: A case series. J Oral Implantol 2011;37:559–569.

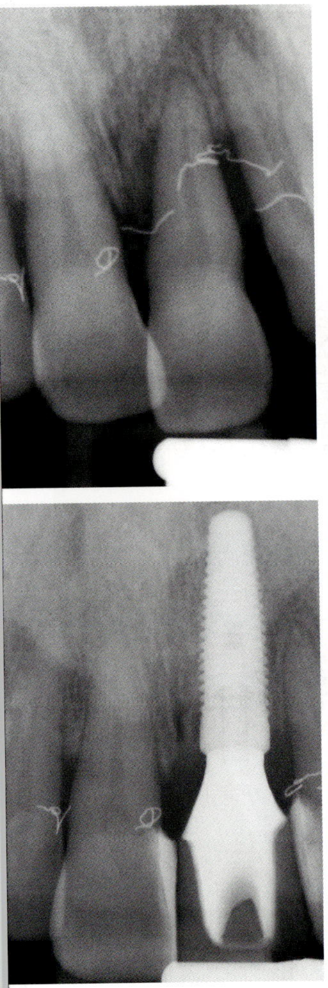

Long-term grafting results

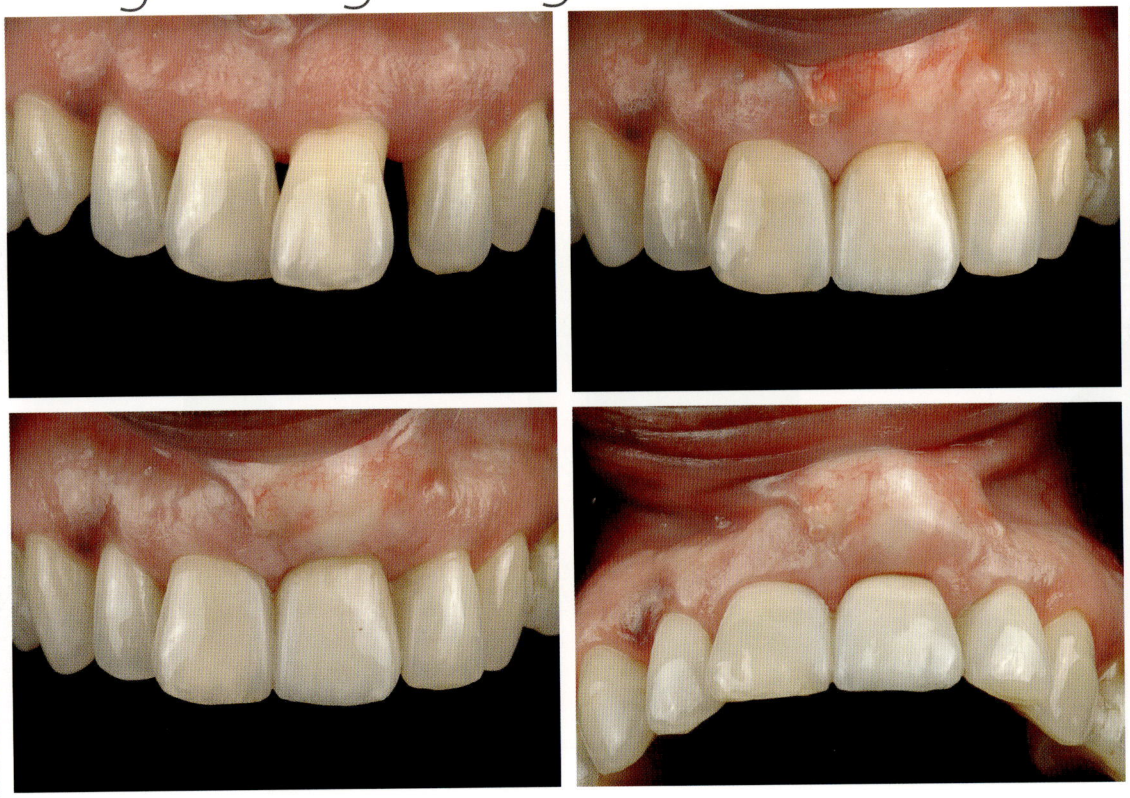

Patient scenario 1

This patient had suffered from periodontitis, and the maxillary left central incisor had to be extracted. After 3 months of bone healing, a 4.3 × 15-mm implant (NobelReplace Groovy) was placed with a PS adapter from regular platform (RP) to narrow platform (NP), along with an NP 5-mm healing abutment and a CTG from the tuberosity. Six months later, the definitive zirconia abutment and the provisional restoration were placed to idealize the soft tissue contours. The definitive alumina crown was ultimately cemented to complete the treatment. At the 1-year recall appointment, the patient presented with a swelling that was not present on the day of crown delivery. This scenario demonstrates a hypertrophic reaction, which may occur in certain patients. Gingivoplasties are recommended to blend the tissues, but the patient refused further surgery.

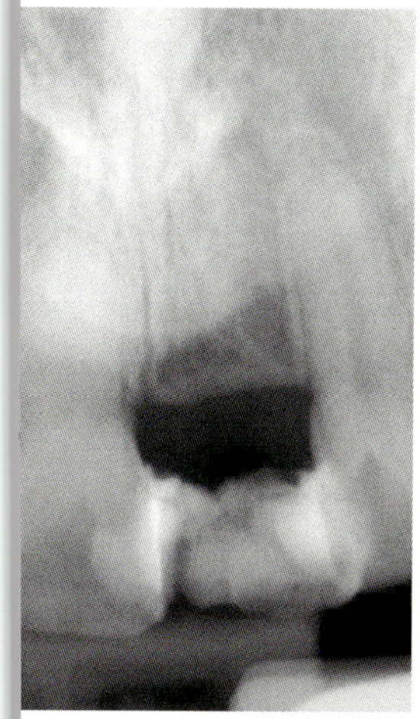

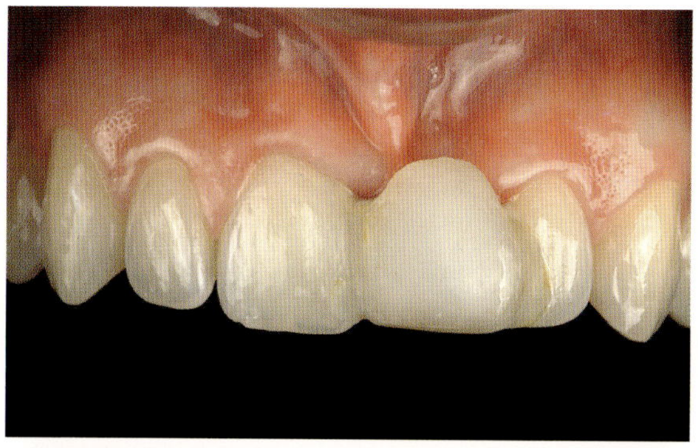

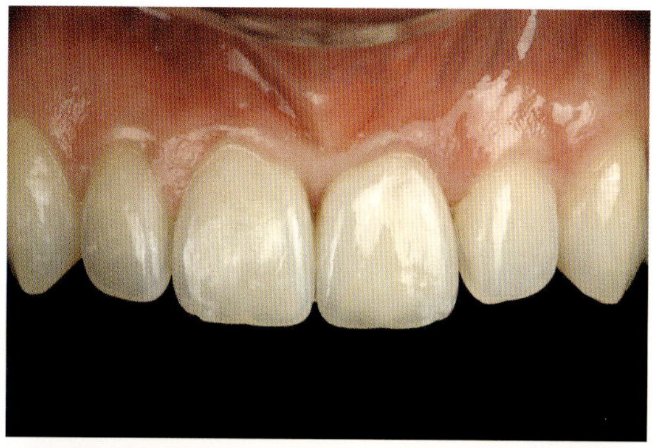

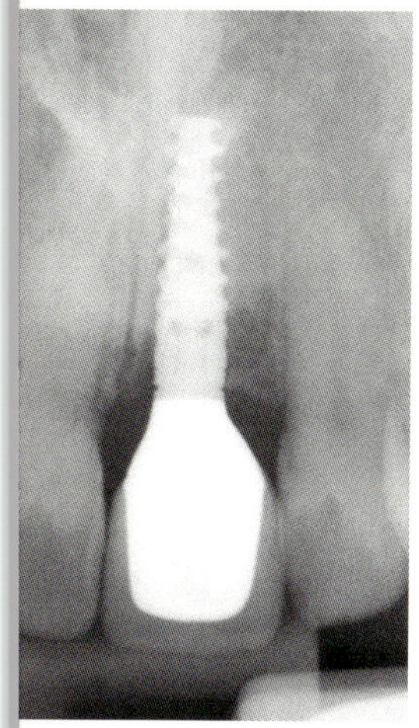

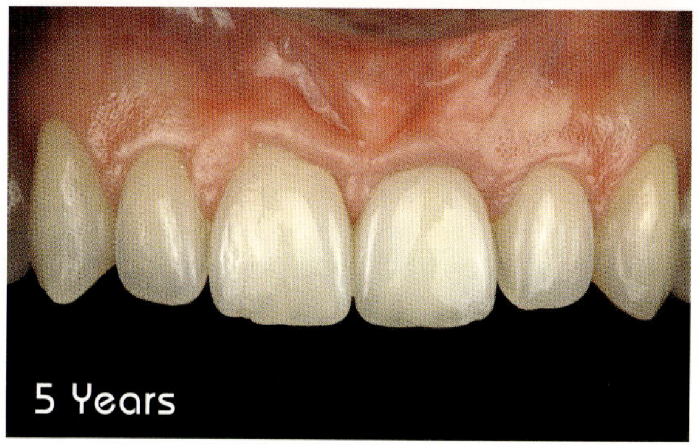

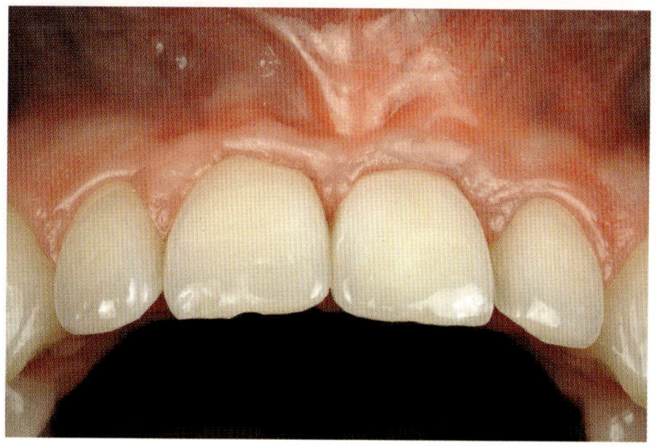

Patient scenario 2

CTGs from the tuberosity provide consistent and predictable results. CTGs are preferred for one- and two-tooth defects with moderate severity. It is critical to avoid bone exposure and limit bone resorption.

Therefore, partial-thickness flaps without vertical releasing incisions are recommended. The differences in tissue levels between the day of final delivery and the 5-year postcementation visit, where the tissue has grown over the original emergence profile, are obvious. This growth is the result of either: *(1)* the growth factor genetics of the patient leading to excessive growth or *(2)* the amount of grafted tissue being bigger than the defect.

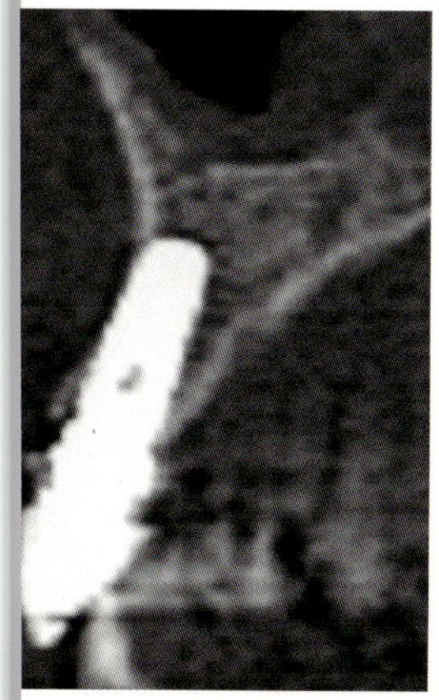

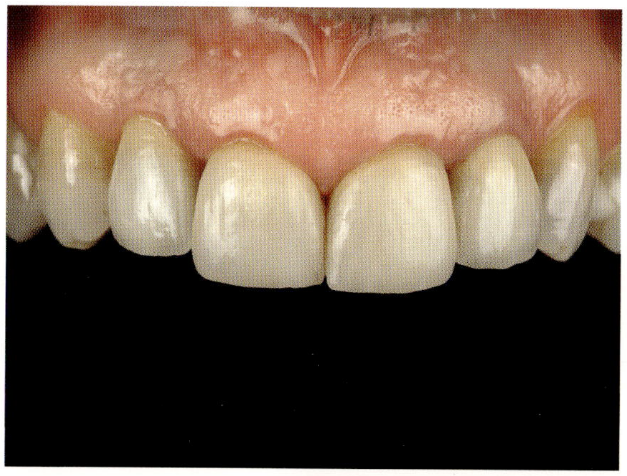

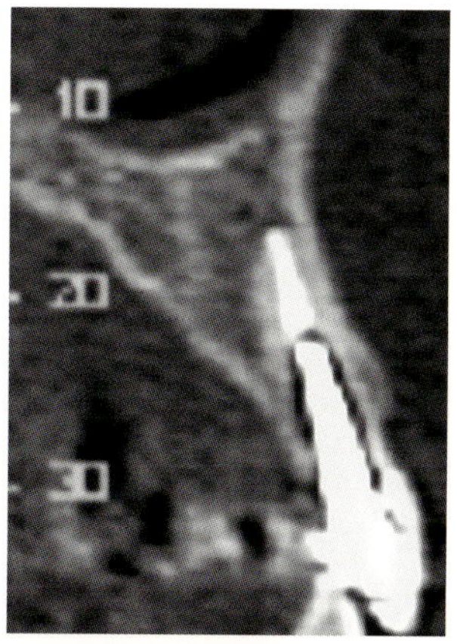

Patient scenario 3

This patient was restored 10 years prior with a NobelReplace external 5 × 13–mm implant in the maxillary right lateral incisor site. The consequences of not grafting are obvious. Later, the contralateral lateral incisor required extraction and implant therapy.

The implant was placed in the left lateral incisor site, and the right lateral incisor site was augmented with a CTG to improve the buccal support and create similar emergence profiles for both implants. The results after 2 years of treatment are shown.

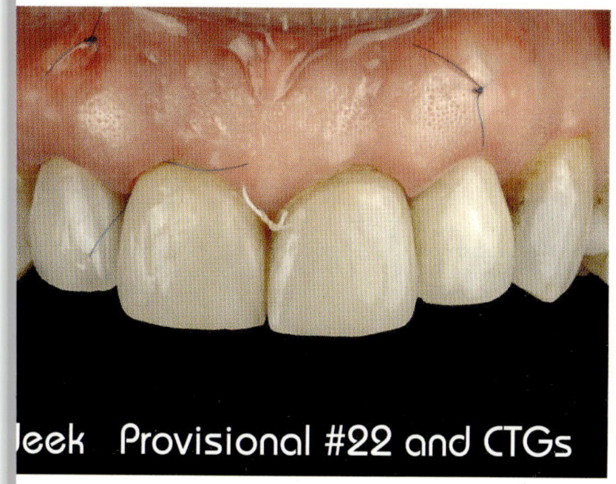

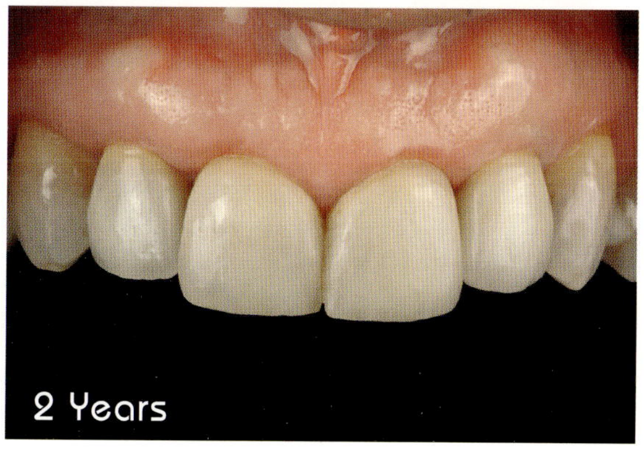

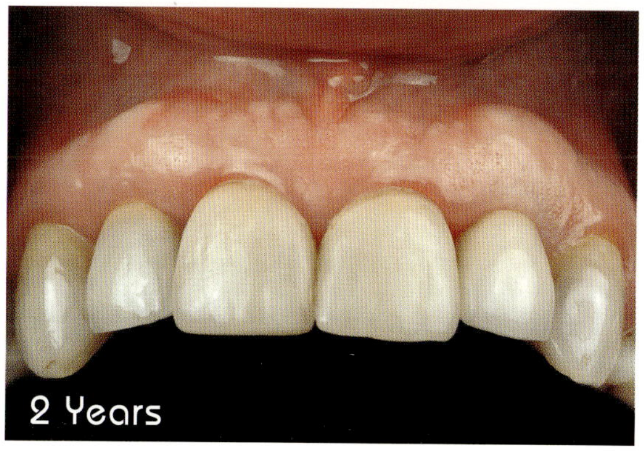

Patient scenario 4

In a patient with bilateral agenesis of the maxillary lateral incisors, the canines were orthodontically repositioned anteriorly and altered into lateral incisors through coronoplasty and a direct composite resin restoration. NobelReplace Groovy 4.3 × 13–mm implants were placed in the canine sites. The implant placed in the maxillary right canine site received no CTG, but the implant placed in the contralateral canine site received a CTG from the tuberosity. The difference is noticeable. At the 1-year recall visit, the patient presented with an extensive hypertrophic reaction.

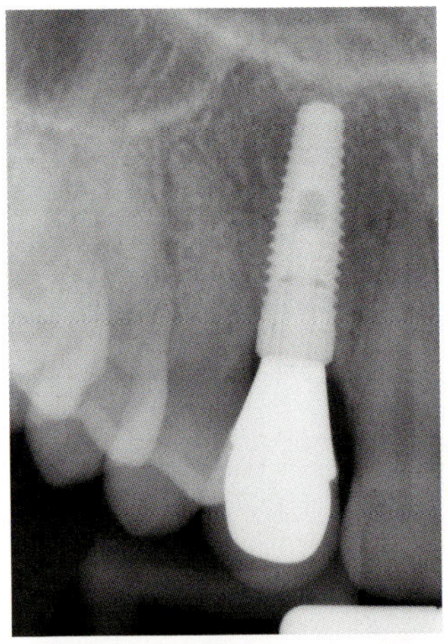

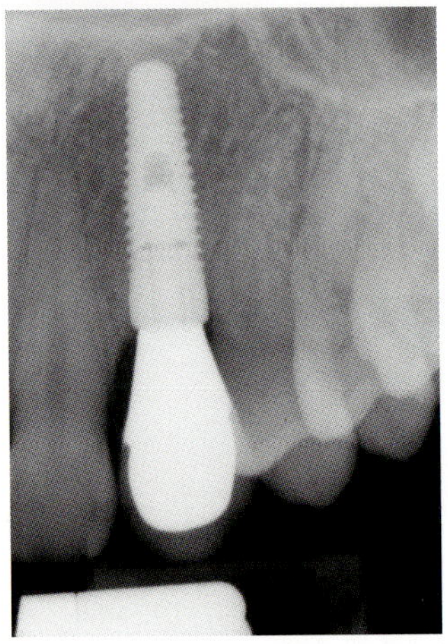

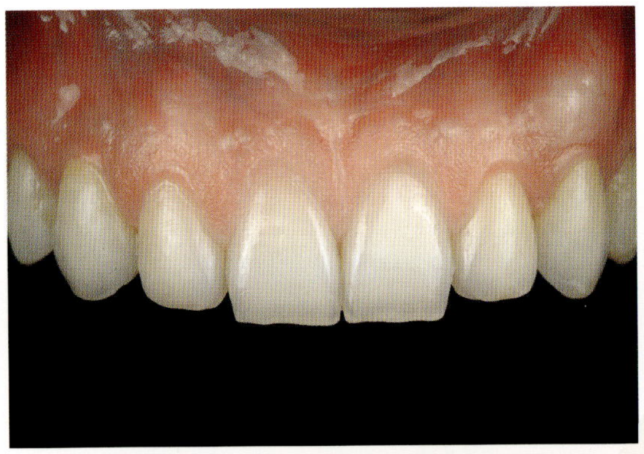

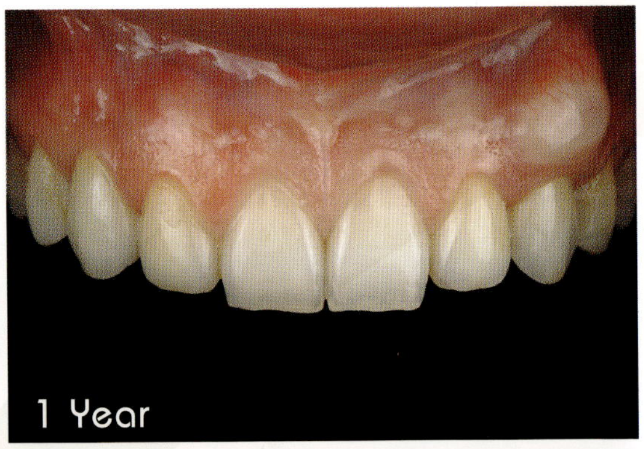

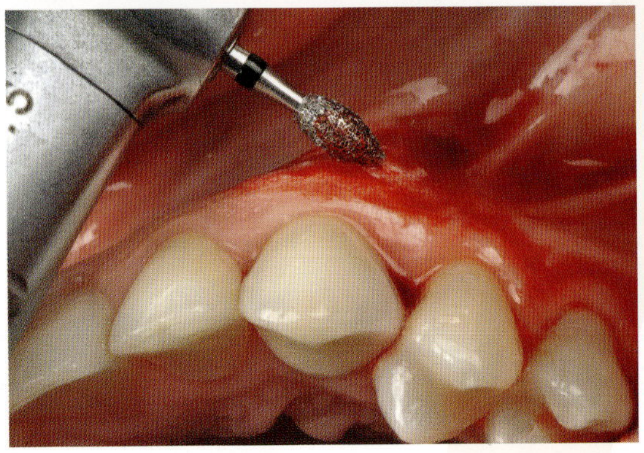

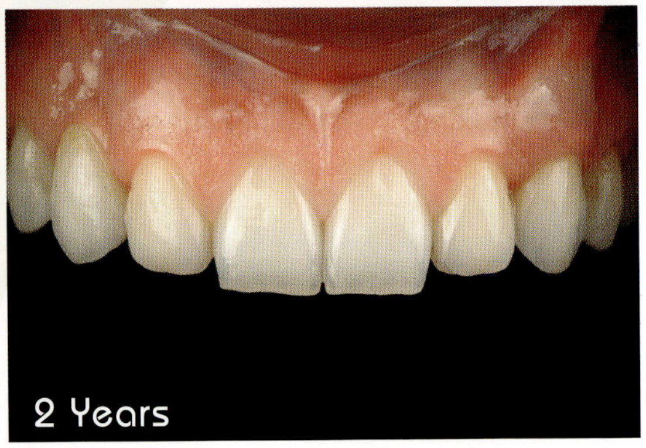

Four gingivoplasties were performed with a coarse diamond bur every 3 months. The outcome after 2 years is shown.

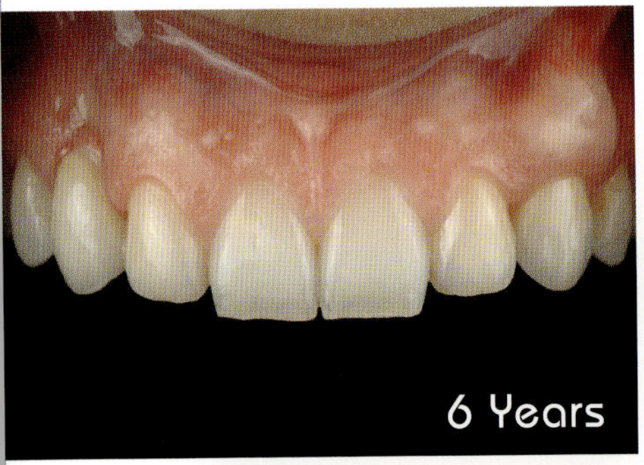

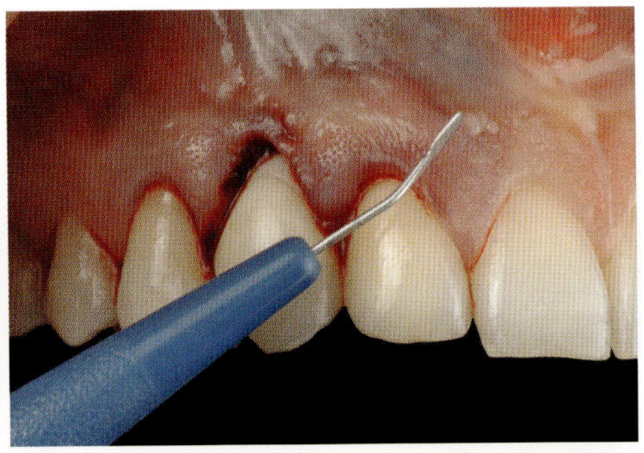

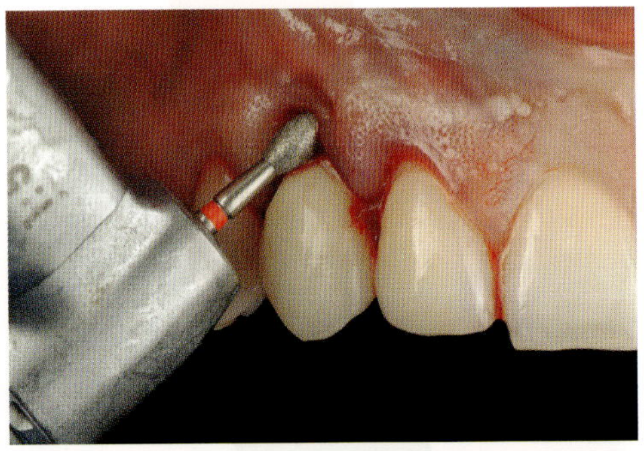

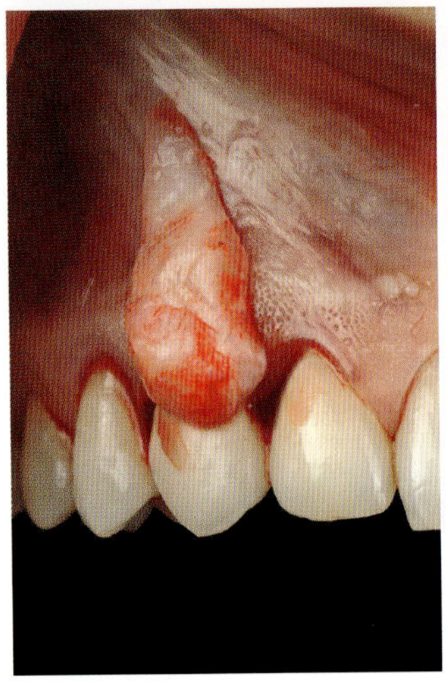

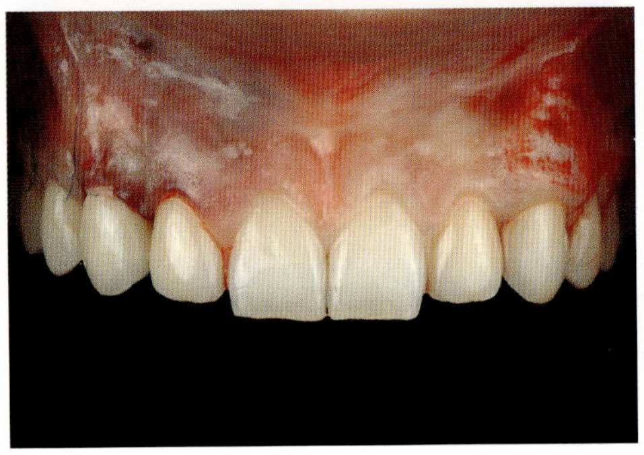

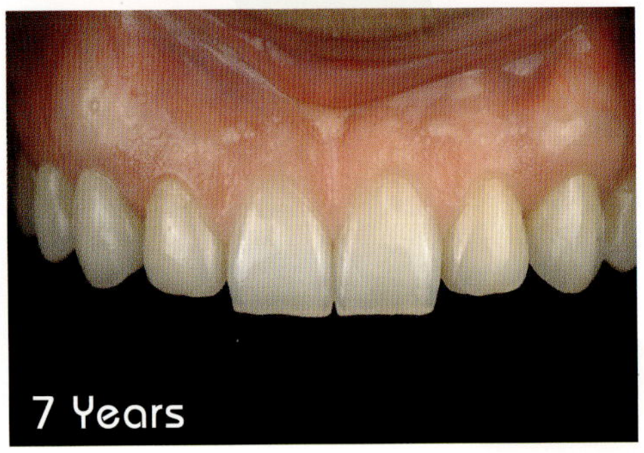

One year postsurgically, the tissue on the left canine receded again. The patient was also complaining about discomfort in the tissue around the right canine. A CTG was placed at the right canine site, while the left canine site was leveled surgically. A sulcular incision was made to the implant site, both adjacent teeth, and apically above the mucogingival line to create a tunnel for placement of the CTG in the most coronal and buccal aspect of the implant crown. To create a smooth surface and more space for the CTG, the crown and the abutment were modified with a fine diamond bur. The graft from the tuberosity was then inserted to provide the necessary volume in a coronal position and sutured in place, and the flap was sutured coronally to cover the graft. The situation 4 years after the last surgery and 7 years after cementation are shown.

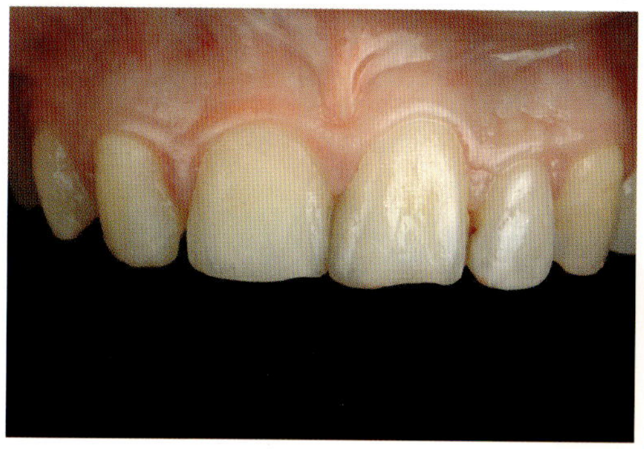

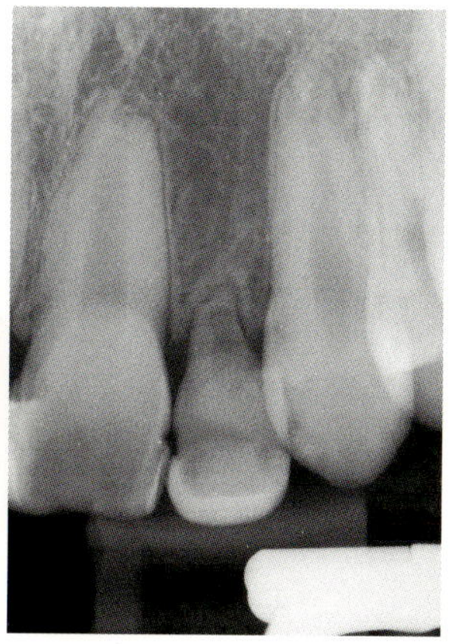

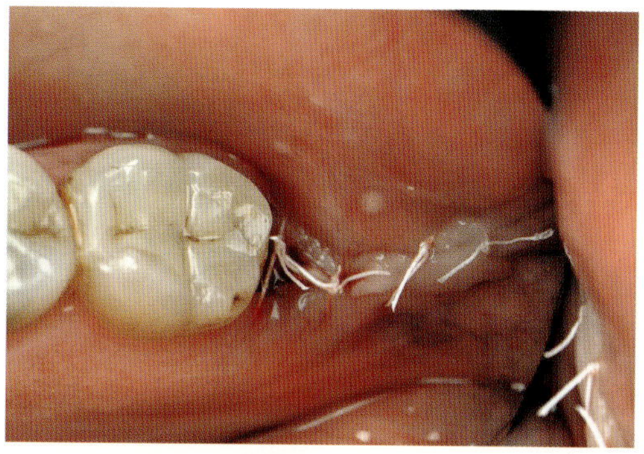

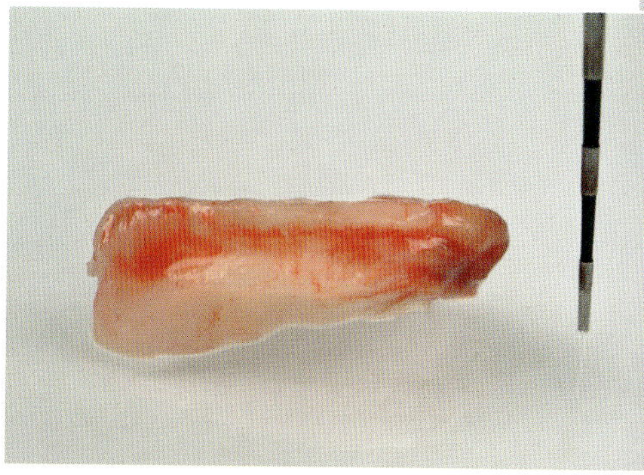

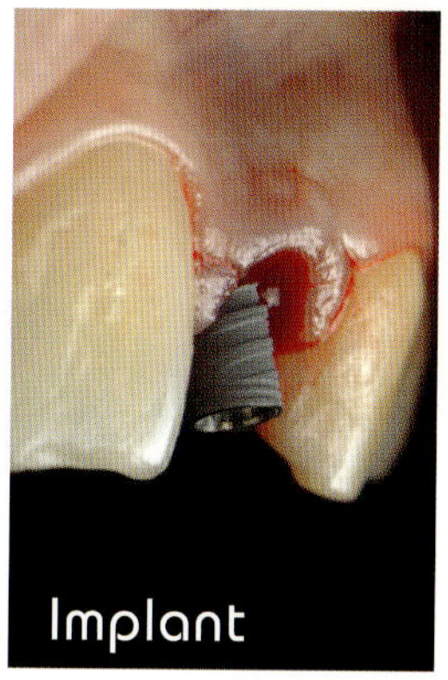

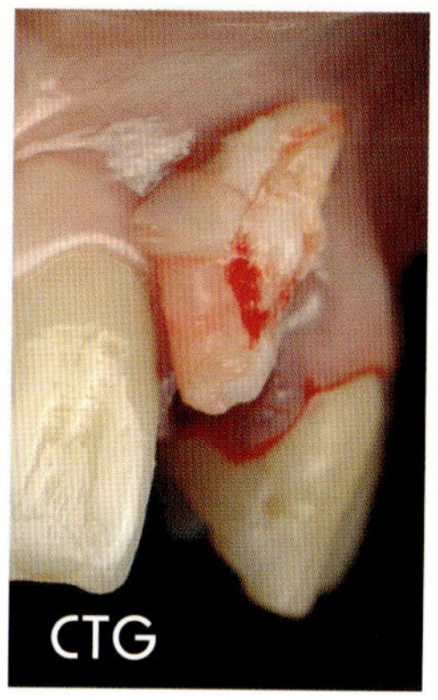

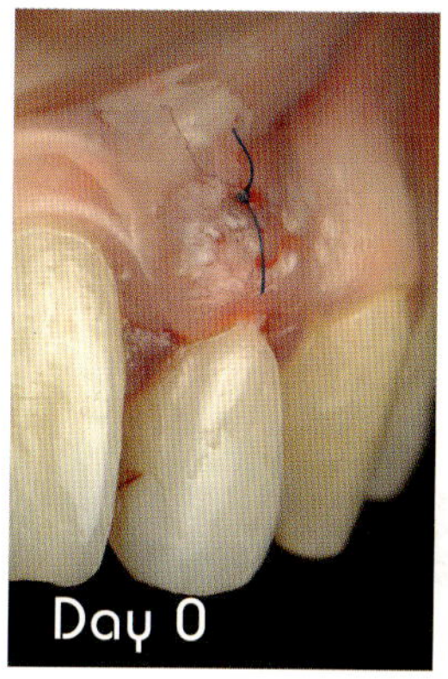

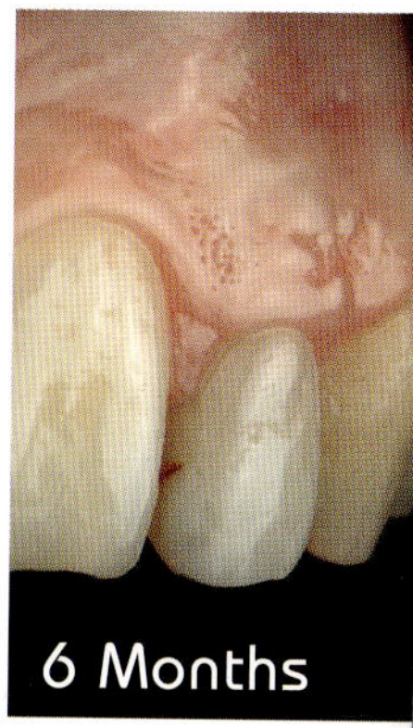

Patient scenario 5

A primary lateral incisor required extraction and was replaced with a NobelActive NP 3.5 × 13–mm implant. A CTG was harvested from the retromolar area due to the limited tissues available after various periodontal surgeries done before the implant treatment. A distal wedge design was performed on the distal aspect of the second molar, and the entire retromolar area was harvested. The buccal aspect of the implant site was tunneled, and the CTG was inserted and sutured into position.

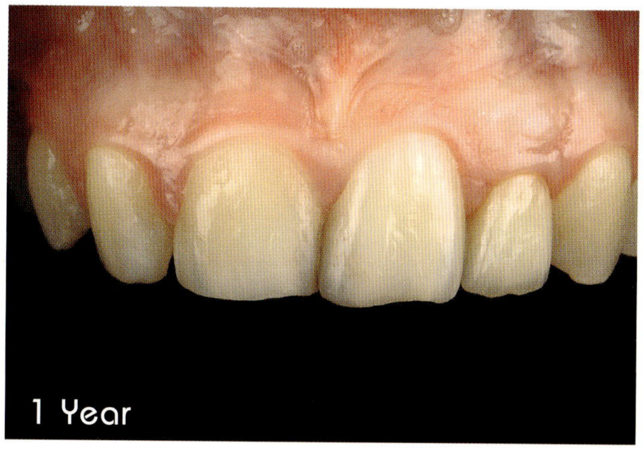

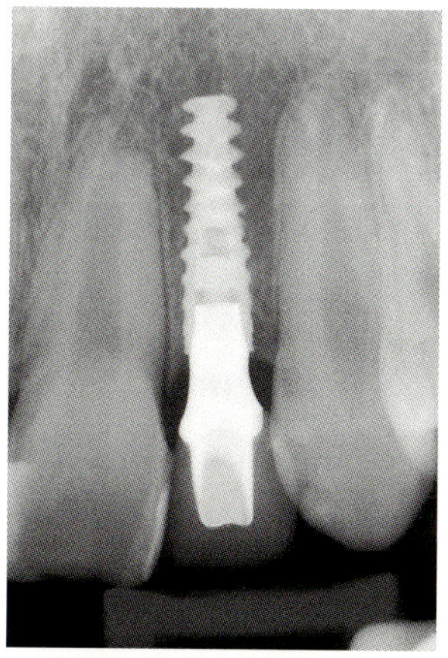

Evaluation of the tissue response at 1 year and 3 years posttreatment shows the tissue stability compared with that of CTGs from tuberosity donor sites.

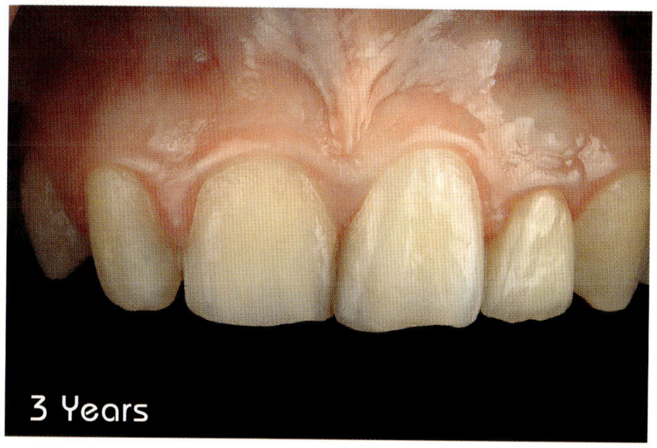

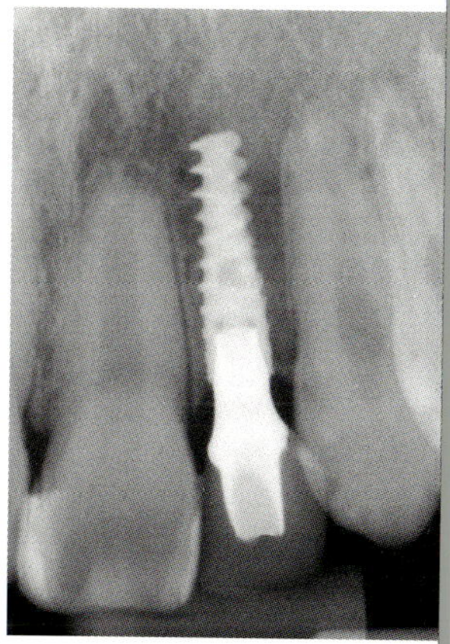

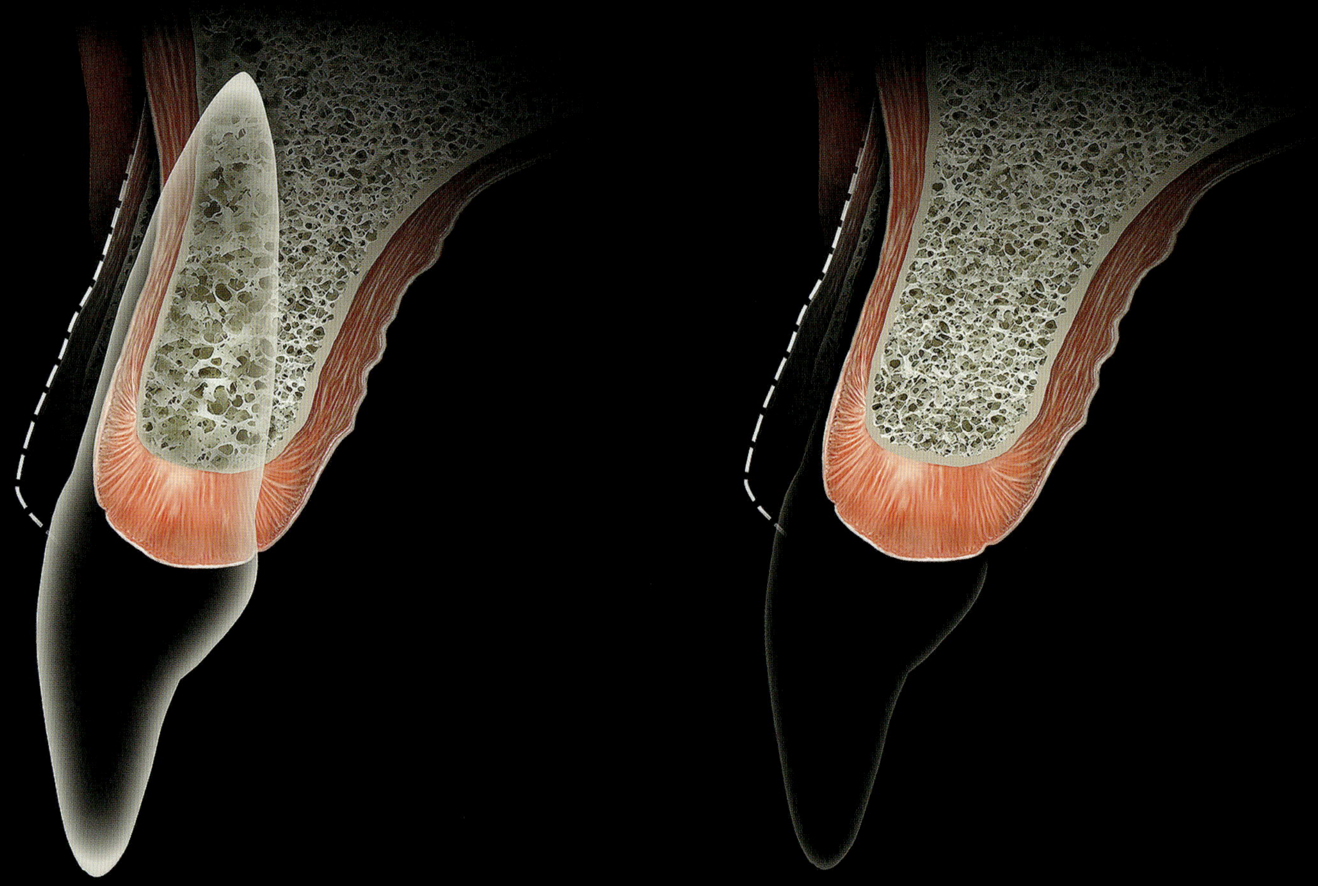

Recipient site manipulation

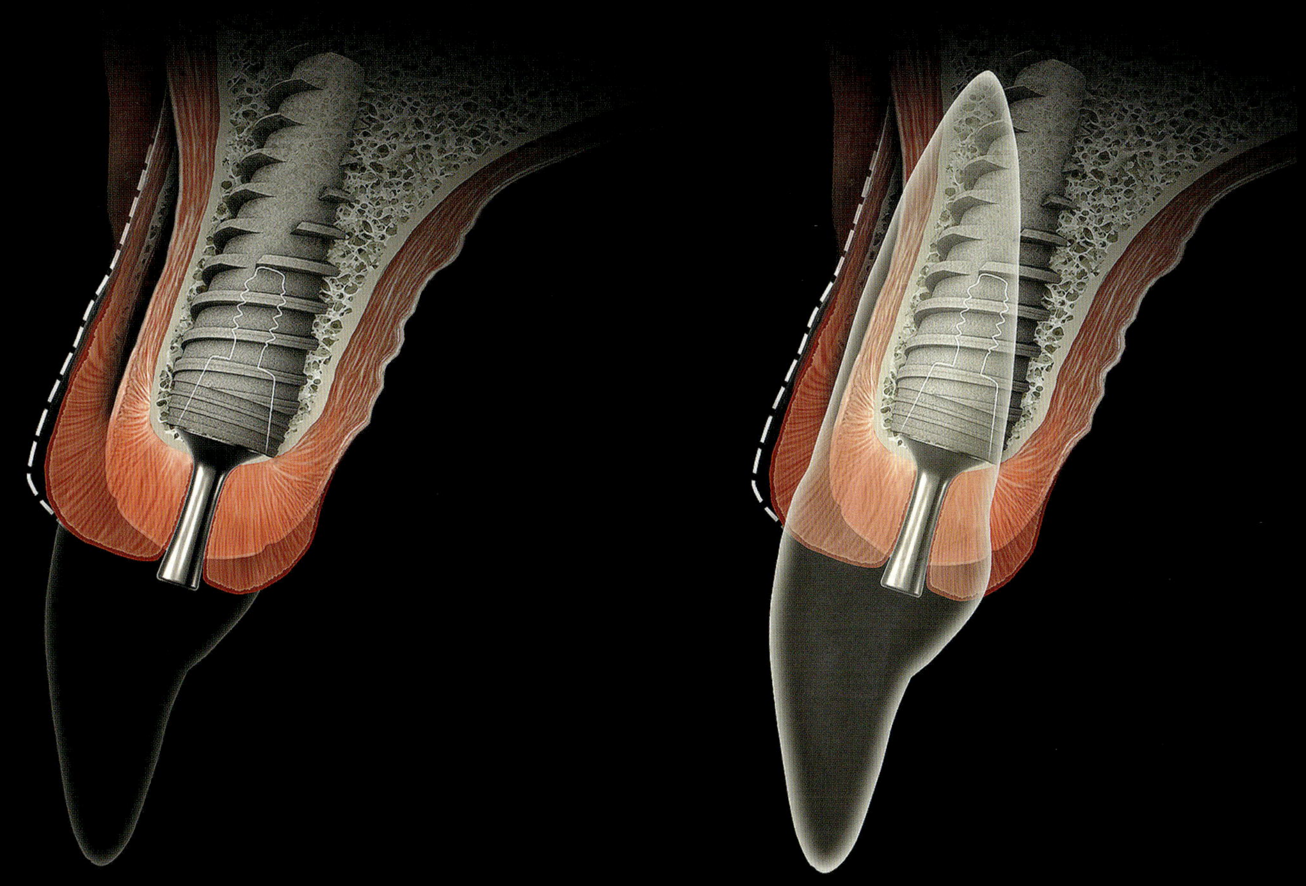

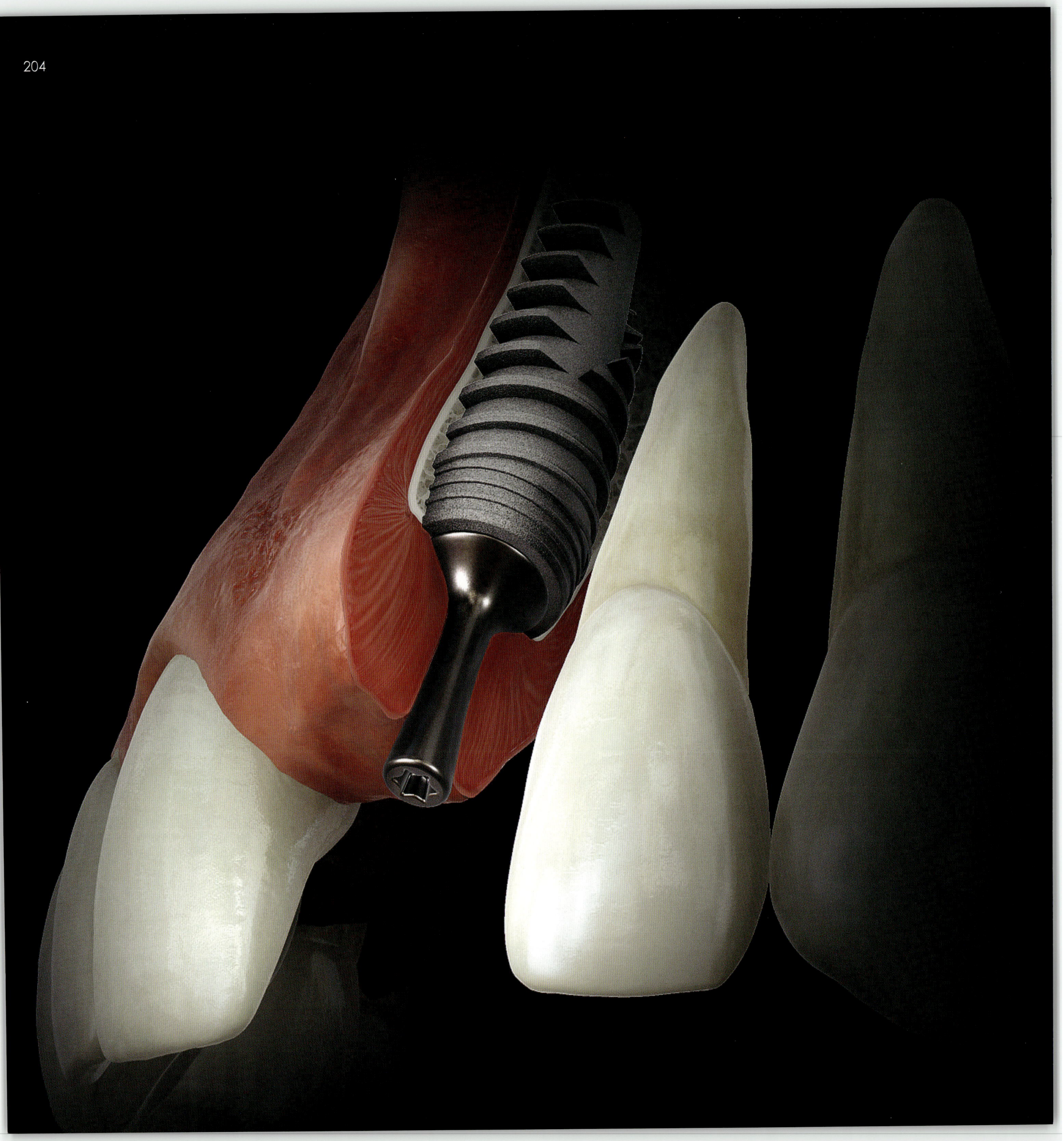

Surgical objectives and criteria

A comprehensive surgical approach is needed once an implant is planned. Five factors are crucial to the final outcome of any implant treatment:

1. Incision and flap design
2. Healing abutment choice
3. Connective tissue graft donor site selection
4. Tissue graft manipulation
5. Suturing technique

Incision and flap design

The benefits of minimally invasive surgical interventions are explained and emphasized throughout this book. In general, less trauma means faster healing, less pain, greater predictability, and increased longevity. Minimally invasive surgery starts with an atraumatic incision technique and clean cuts. Consequently, the choice of surgical instruments is crucial. Only the sharpest knives and scalpel blades, preferably microsurgical instruments, provide clean and less invasive cuts, as they minimize tear and distortion of the tissues. Bleeding is significantly reduced, which often comes as a great surprise to clinicians who apply these principles for the first time. The use of microsurgical instruments requires magnification through surgical loupes or microscopes.

Incision outlines and flap designs have also changed dramatically over the last few years, especially with the increasing use of partial-thickness flaps. For example, vertical releasing incisions are not necessary in modern, less invasive implant dentistry. They may provide easy access, but other than that they must be considered harmful, cutting lateral blood supply to the reflected flap, reducing its mobility, and potentially creating unnecessary scars. Today's minimally invasive surgical philosophy recommends exposing bone as little as possible and only when bone grafting is necessary, in which case only the specific grafted site is exposed. Partial-thickness flaps should be prepared in every other situation, leaving the periosteum attached to the bone and thereby ensuring continuous blood supply and decreasing the likelihood of tissue flap necrosis. Extension of the flap beyond the adjacent teeth is crucial when no vertical releasing incisions are performed to sufficiently elevate the flap and provide primary wound closure and tissue adaptation. Once the flap has been sufficiently mobilized, the implant can be placed without causing excessive bleeding while giving the surgeon ample visual access to the site for tissue adaptation and closure.

Healing abutment choice

The healing abutment design, height, and diameter are key factors for peri-implant soft tissue manipulation and CTG positioning, especially with thick and dense grafts from the maxillary tuberosity. The minimum height of the healing abutment should be 5 mm for it to serve as a reference for the necessary flap elevation when the implant is placed 3 mm below the prospective gingival margin or flush to the adjacent bone. The diameter of the healing abutment is directly related to the amount of tissue and space needed between the adjacent teeth and the healing abutment. Narrow healing abutments provide the unique advantage of allowing space for thick CTGs and primary wound closure without harmful tension.

Connective tissue graft donor site selection

A subepithelial CTG from the maxillary tuberosity offers excellent outcomes but is more difficult to handle surgically. Similar to membranes used for guided tissue regeneration, a CTG from the tuberosity should not be exposed to the oral cavity due to its high concentration of collagen fibers and poor blood supply, which increases the chance of necrosis. Palatal CTGs are less ideal for implant sites because they are less stable and unpredictable in the long term. They do not contain enough collagen but rather too much fat. In addition, palatal CTG harvesting and postoperative healing of the donor site are very painful for the patient.

Graft manipulation

Narrow healing abutments offer more space for graft manipulation, especially when thick and dense tissue is used. Because of the available space, the graft and adaptation can be tailored to the specific site and needs. The graft is always sutured first to avoid mobility and to ensure close adaptation to the underlying bone or periosteum while the flap is adapted over it. Final suturing is key for consistent primary wound closure and healing.

Suturing technique

Good suturing technique limits patient discomfort and provides faster healing with less scarring. However, it is an acquired skill that needs to be learned and constantly practiced. This is especially true for small-diameter sutures, which must be handled with adequate magnification of at least × 3.5 through surgical loupes or microscopes. Suturing under high magnification differs substantially from macroscopic techniques, since most of the handling occurs in a confined area (limited field of vision) and with two hand instruments. It must therefore be practiced to gain proficiency and avoid frustration.

The general rule for suture materials is as follows: smaller diameter means less trauma. Of course, they still have to be suitable for the type and thickness of tissue being sutured and the tension that needs to be applied to the flap. In that respect, suture sizes of 7-0 and 6-0 provide an excellent compromise, given that the flaps were prepared properly and can be adapted passively without much tension. Suture sizes are commonly defined by the United States Pharmacopeia (USP). A 6-0 USP designation suture translates to a 0.07-mm diameter for nonresorbable materials, while a 7-0 suture has a diameter of 0.05 mm. The authors prefer monofilament polypropylene sutures (eg, Prolene [Ethicon]), which are nonresorbable and hydrophobic and accumulate less plaque than other materials while still providing sufficient strength. If greater tension must be applied, suture materials made from polytetrafluoroethylene (PTFE), which became popular under the registered trademark GORE-TEX (W. L. Gore), provide excellent biocompatible properties, flexibility, and tear strength (eg, Cytoplast PTFE suture [Osteogenics Biomedical]). The needle size and configuration should match the specific needs and tissue thickness. For example, larger needles are required to adapt both buccal and palatal papillae, while smaller needles are better suited for thin tissue flaps. Triangular needles of 12 to 15 mm in length are the authors' preference.

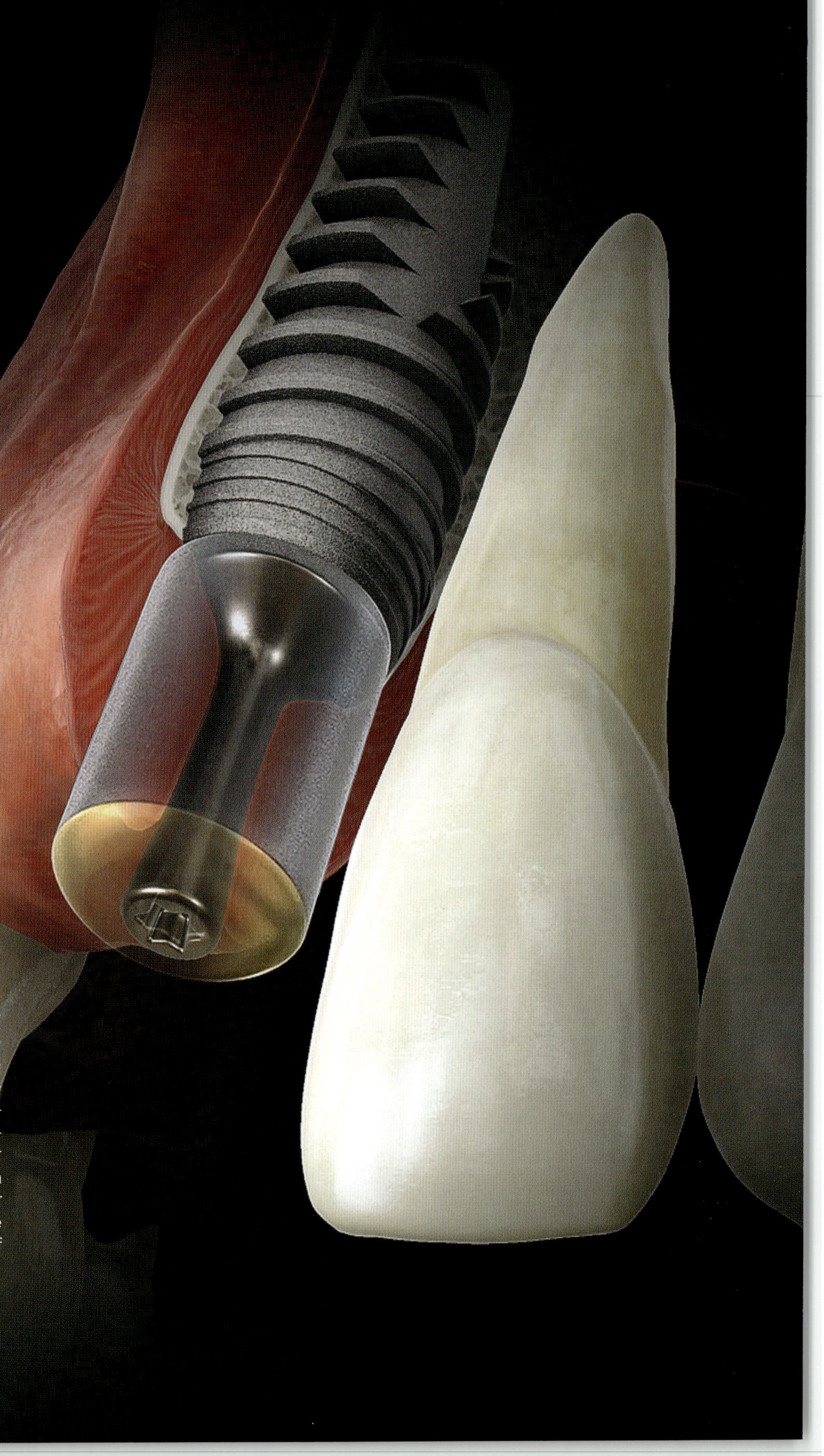

Surgical criteria

Successful implant treatment requires close communication between the surgeon and the restorative dentist. It is essential to identify and implement common goals and objectives. These three key aspects must be considered in respect to the peri-implant soft tissue:

1. Interproximal tissue height
2. Free gingival margin height location
3. Buccal tissue volume

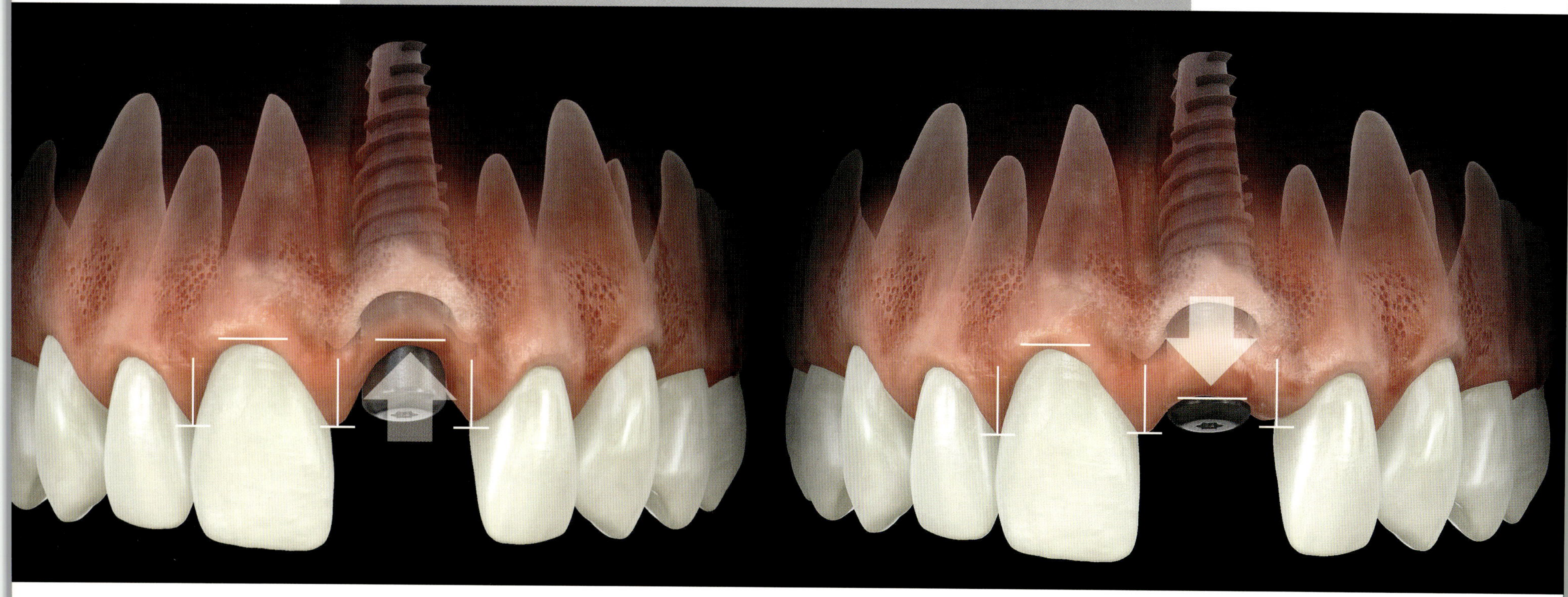

Interproximal tissue height

The interproximal papilla height determines the difficulty of a specific case: greater papilla deficiency means greater difficulty. In a healthy situation, the interproximal papilla occupies the space between two teeth up to the interproximal contact point. It is therefore determined by the supporting bone crest and the location, size, and shape of the interproximal contact area. The gingival margin is typically located about 2 mm coronal to the CEJ of a tooth, following the crest of the bone. According to the location of the interproximal contact area, the largest papilla is the one between the two central incisors. Because the interproximal contact areas are located increasingly more apically from anterior to posterior regions, the papillae are progressively shorter and smaller toward the posterior. The interproximal papilla has two peaks, vestibularly and lingually, with a crest, the so-called col, in between. The width and depth of the col are determined by the size and location of the contact area and increase from anterior to posterior regions.

Once a site is evaluated for placement or restoration of an implant, the papillary heights are evaluated for adequacy in relation to the adjacent teeth and symmetry between contralateral teeth on both sides of the oral cavity. Tooth loss, trauma, and inflammation often cause loss of bone and papillary height, creating deficient and asymmetric soft tissue conditions. They are common shortcomings in edentulous sites and therefore most challenging in implant dentistry. The greater the mismatch between papillary heights of the implant site and the natural teeth, the more difficult the clinical situation becomes. Consequently, preservation of bone through careful selection and application of atraumatic surgical techniques is key to maintaining papillary height and providing an inconspicuous implant restoration and soft tissue framework that perfectly blends with the natural teeth.

Buccal tissue volume

The largest amount of buccal tissue volume should be located at the most coronal aspect of the implant site, which is why healing abutment selection is so crucial. Tissue volume is probably the single most important indicator for success in implant dentistry. Surgical incision and flap management, healing abutment selection, CTG donor site selection, graft manipulation, and suturing are essential to maximize and ideally position buccal tissue volume.

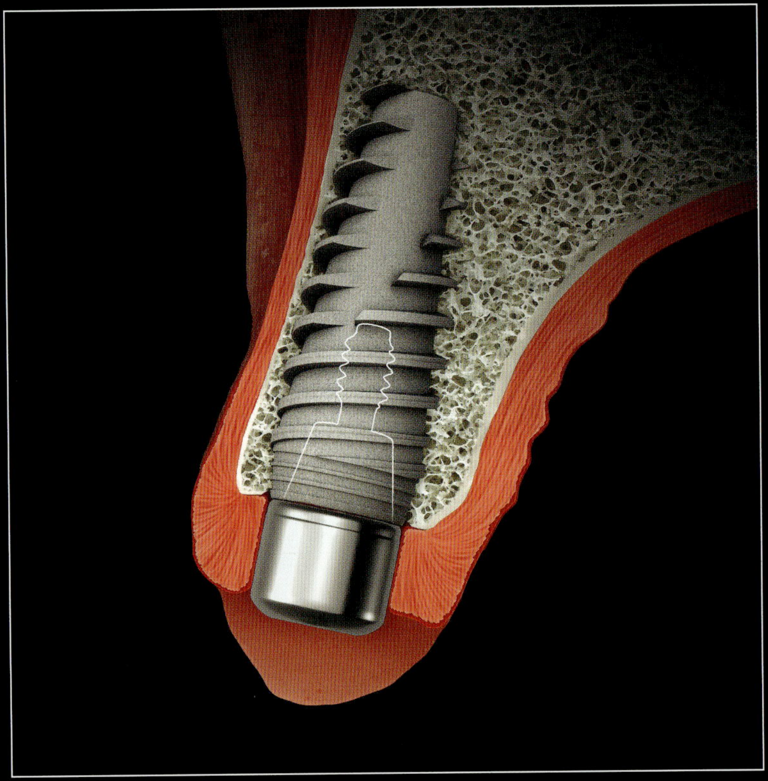

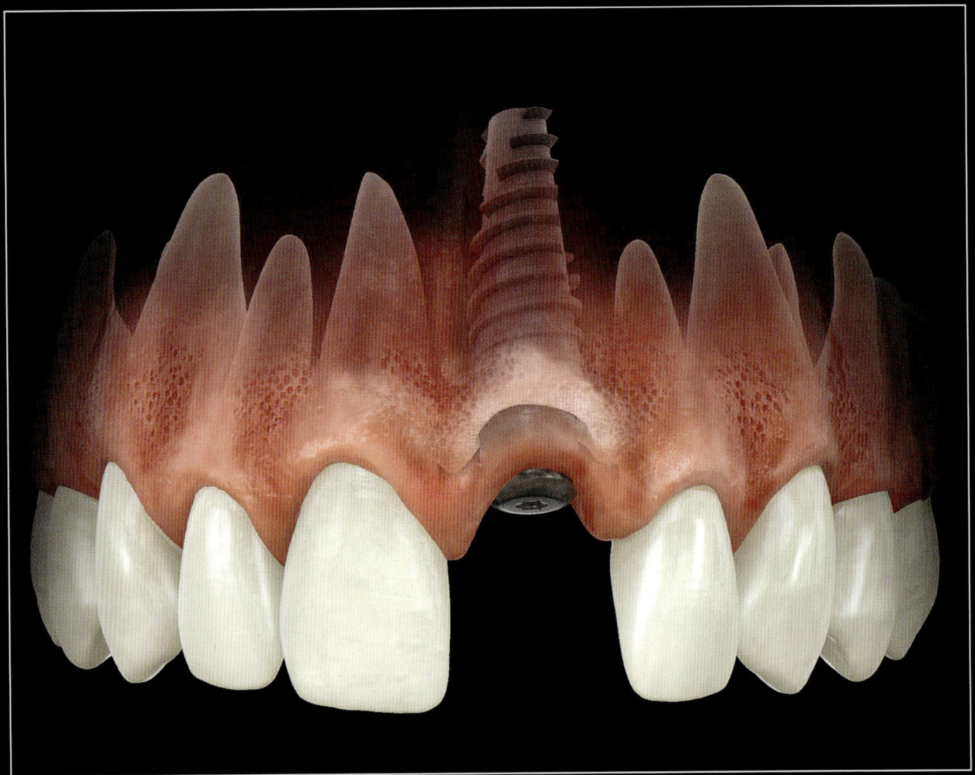

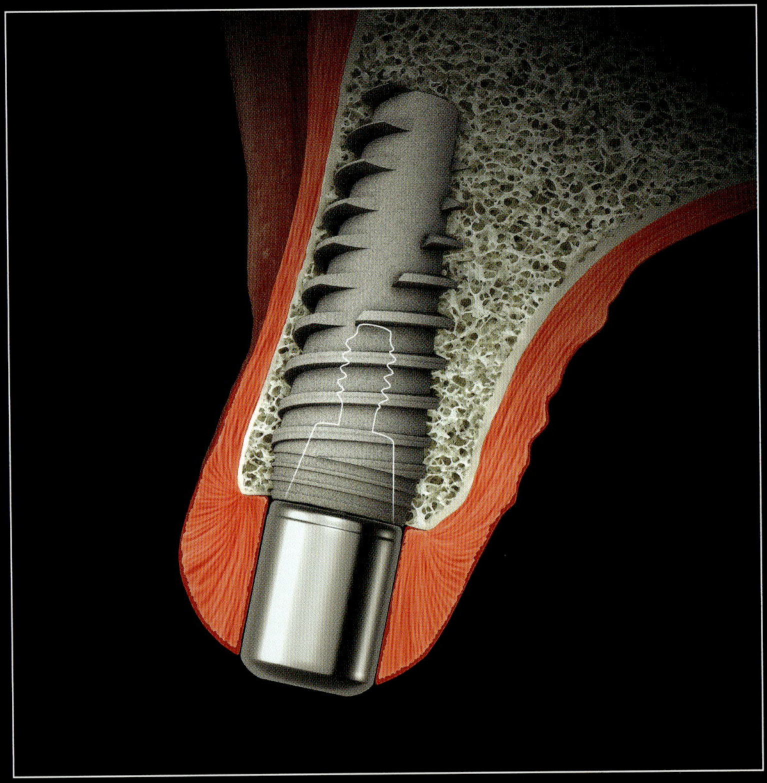

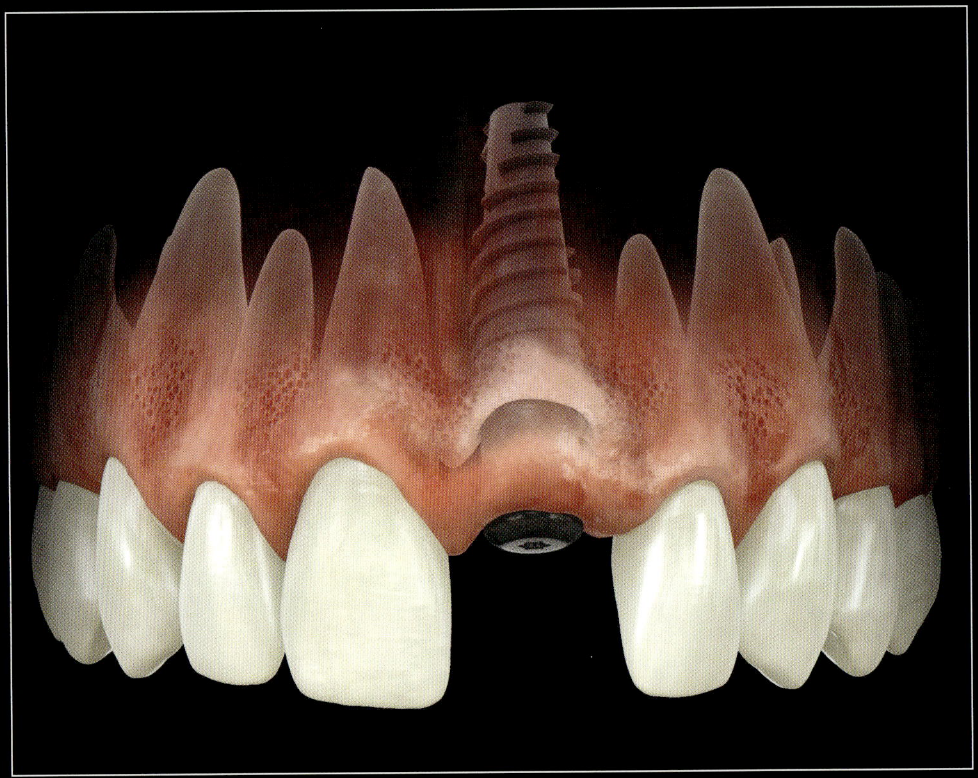

Drawing healing abutment heights

Healing abutments are critical for soft tissue management. Short healing abutments (eg, 3 mm) facilitate sufficient coronal tissue displacement. A 5-mm-tall healing abutment used with an implant of the same depth increases the chances of having to coronally advance the flap. When the surgical phase is complete, the gingival margin on the healing abutment should be at least 2 mm coronal to the one on the adjacent or reference tooth.

Because height is important for coronal tissue displacement, diameter becomes a key factor for a predictable final outcome. The narrowest healing abutment (eg, 1 mm diameter) provides the largest space for the thickest CTG, ensuring a consistent long-term result with the simplest flap closure technique.

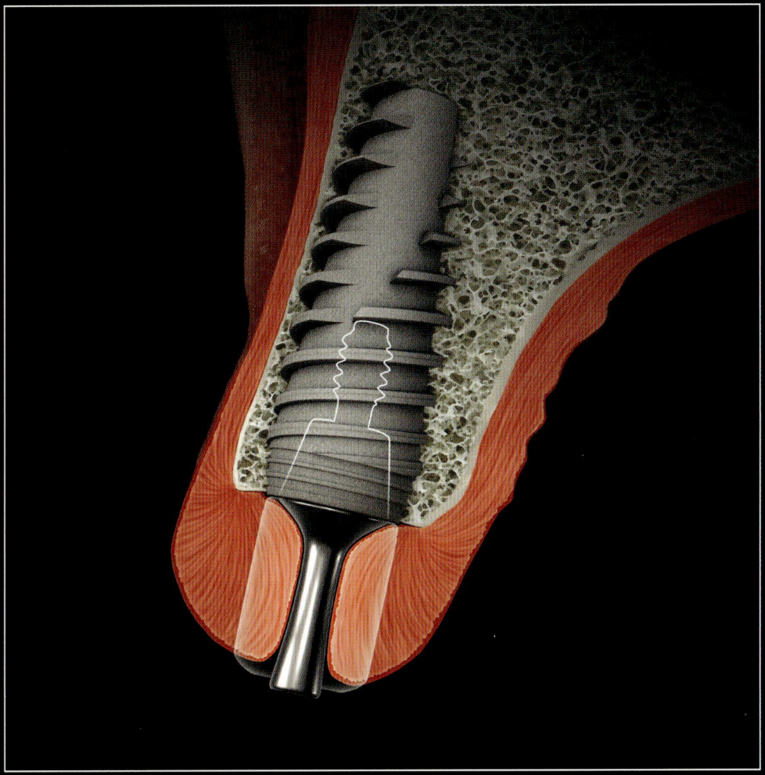

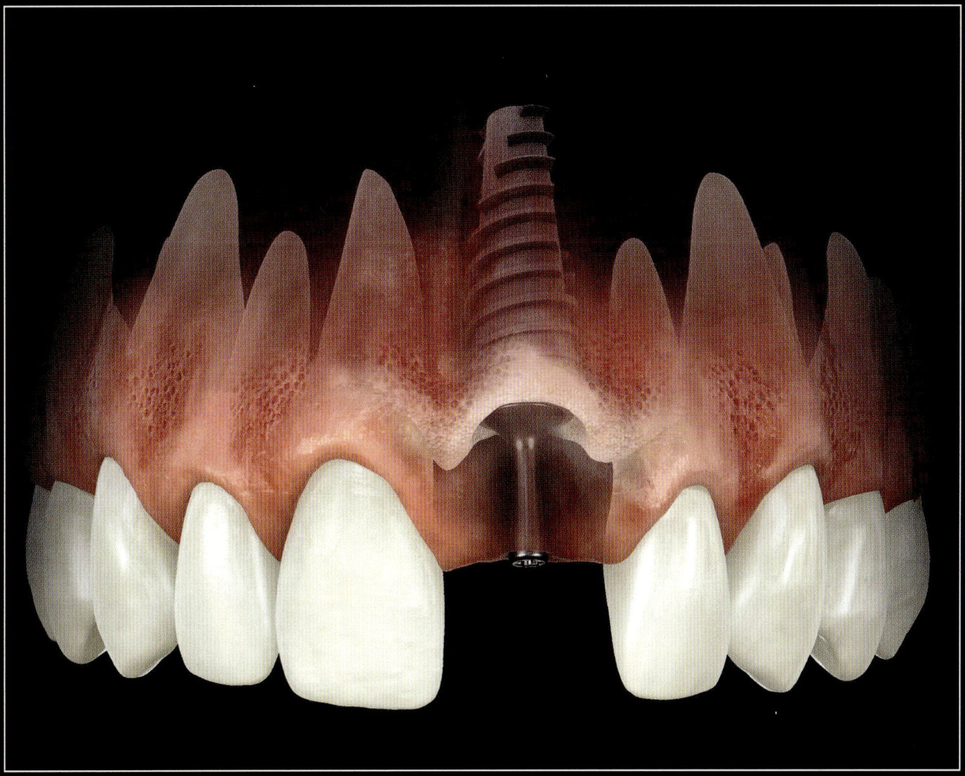

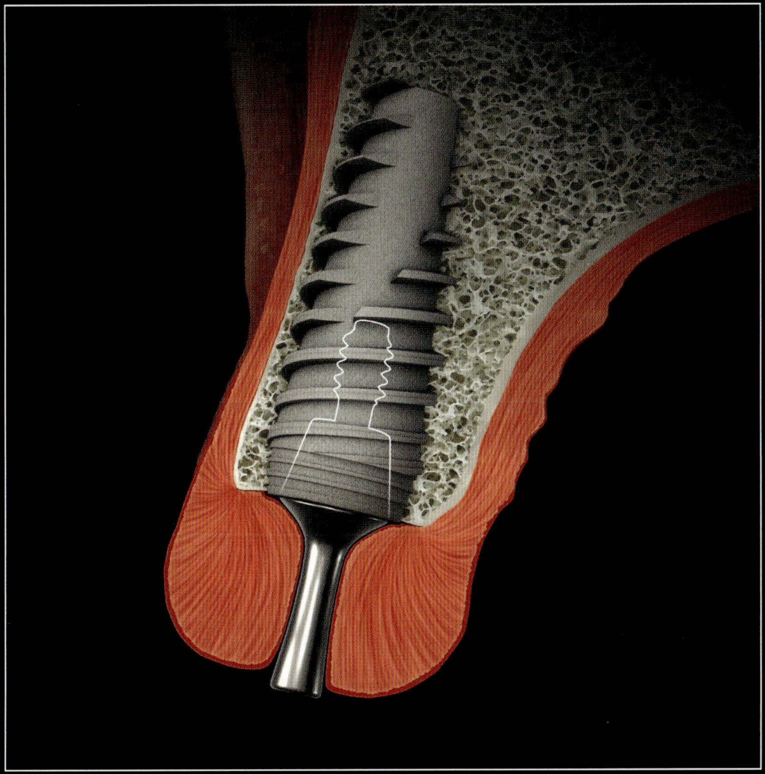

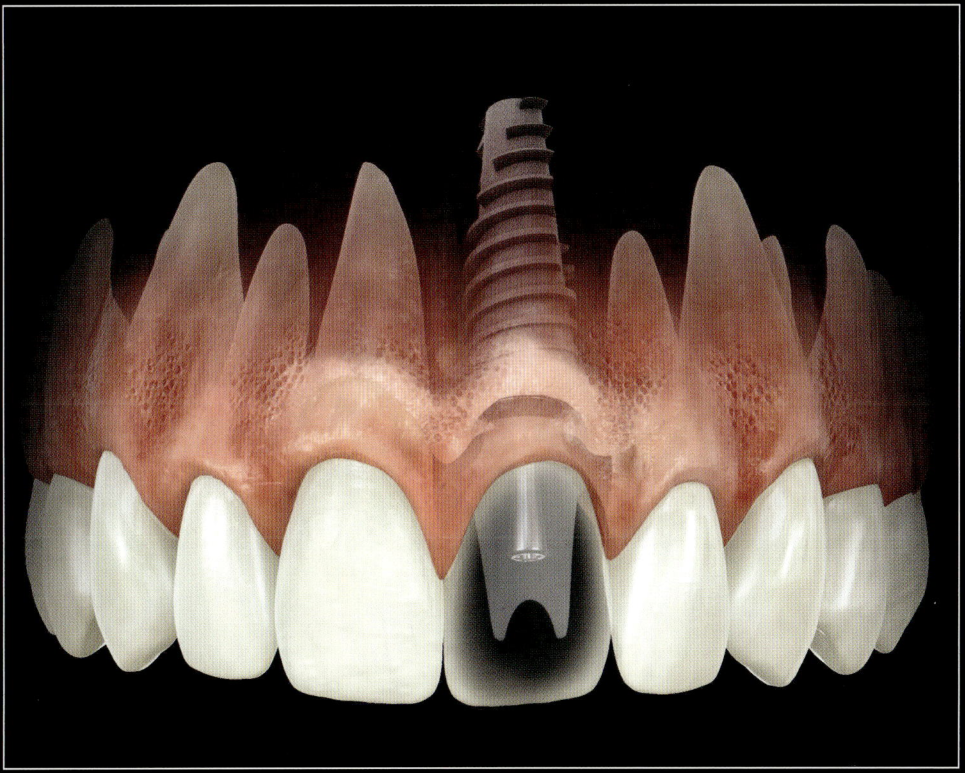

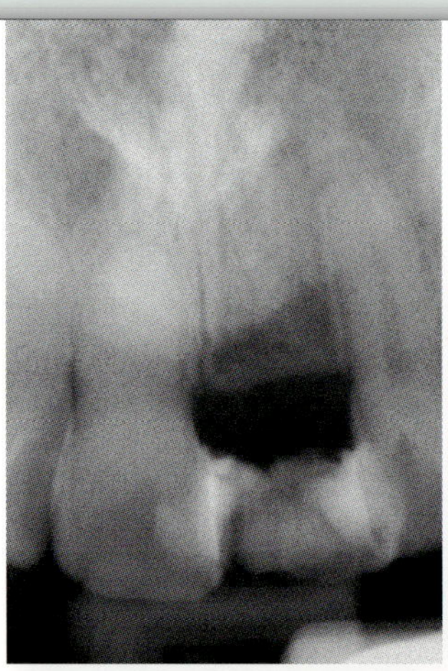

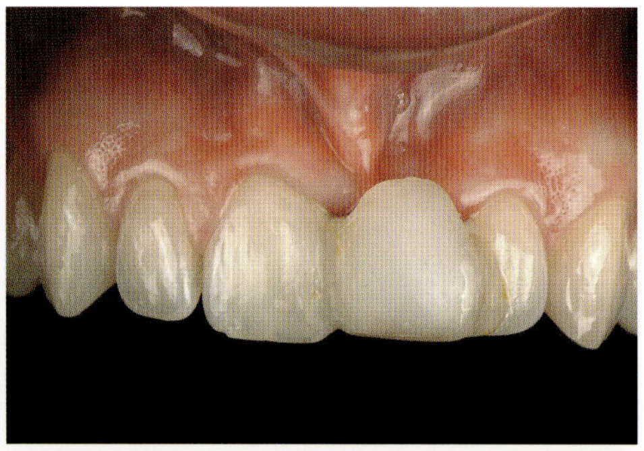

Clinical case

The left central incisor was lost during a bike accident when the patient was 16 years old. Implant treatment was postponed until skeletal growth was complete, in his case at the age of 20 years. The periapical radiograph and CBCT scan revealed the magnitude of the bone loss, especially when compared with the adjacent central incisor. The interproximal papilla height was almost ideal, but the mesial papillae of the lateral incisors showed signs of inflammation. The large buccal defect caused a drift of the frenum. A frenectomy was contraindicated, as it may have caused additional volume loss.

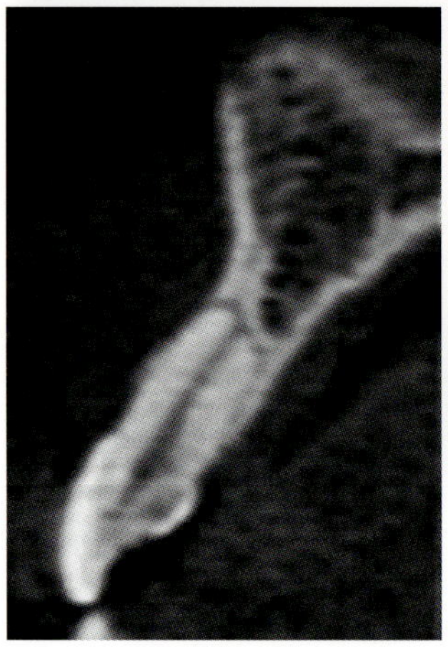

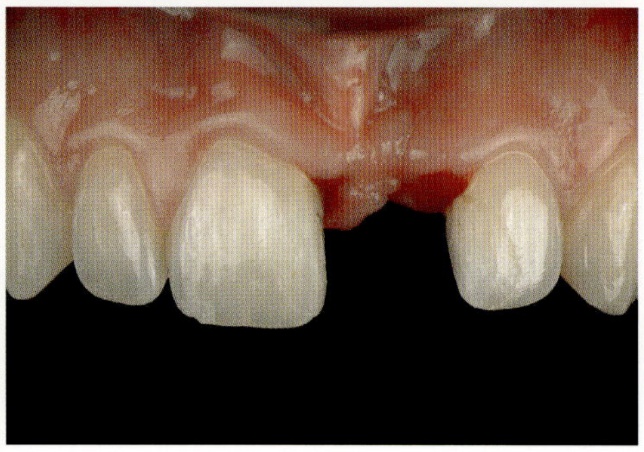

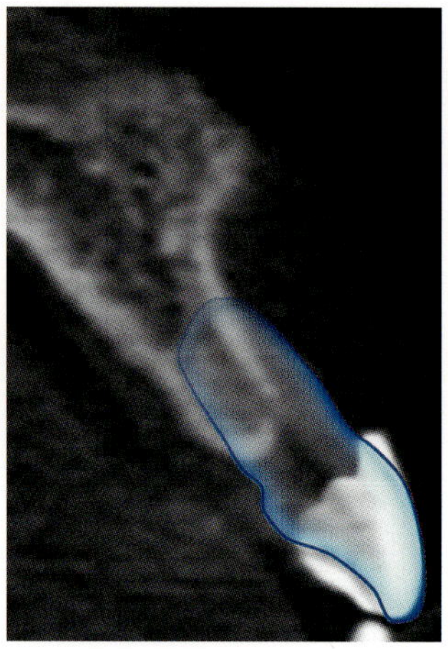

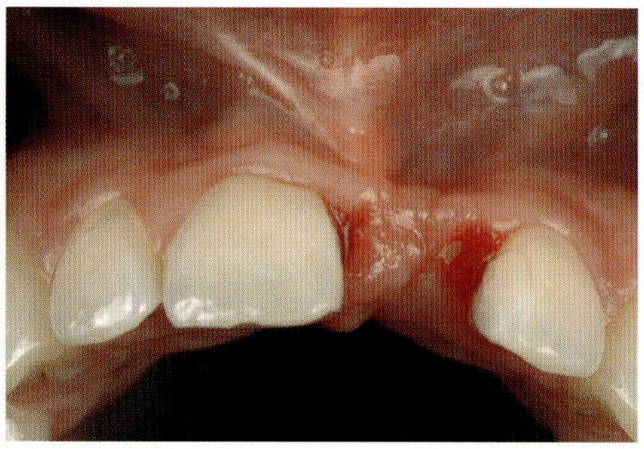

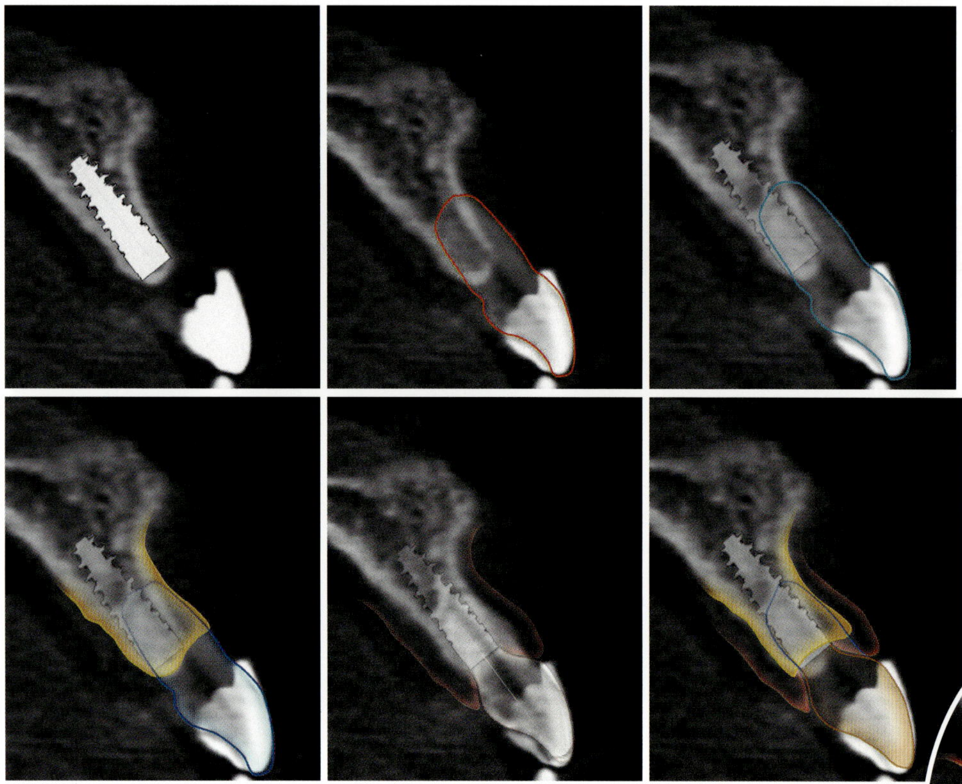

Digital implant planning software was used to assess existing bone morphology and the feasibility of placing an implant. Virtual implant selection and placement suggested a NobelActive implant (3.5 × 13 mm). Due to its unique shape and thread design, this type of implant offers various advantages in questionable bone in the anterior region. It condenses the bone and provides high primary stability but also allows reorientation of the implant during insertion to accommodate challenging anatomical conditions. The next question is whether to graft the obviously deficient bone with bone or only with soft tissue, which always depends on multiple factors. If the implant was placed exactly as planned and without damaging buccal bone, grafting with bone or bone substitute would provide little additional support for the implant itself while increasing the surgical complexity of the case.

Implant placement planning

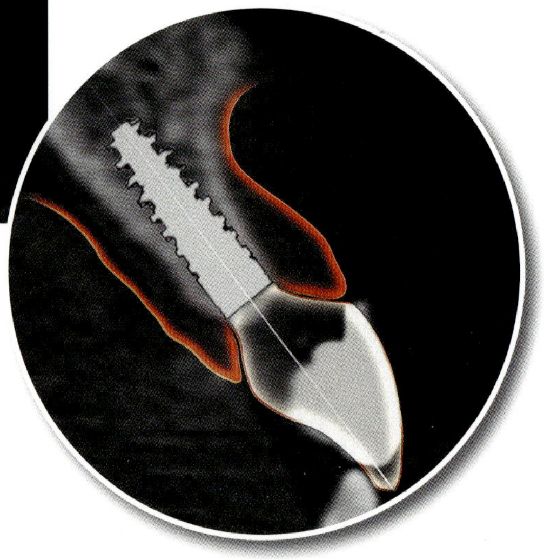

Implant placement and straight healing abutment

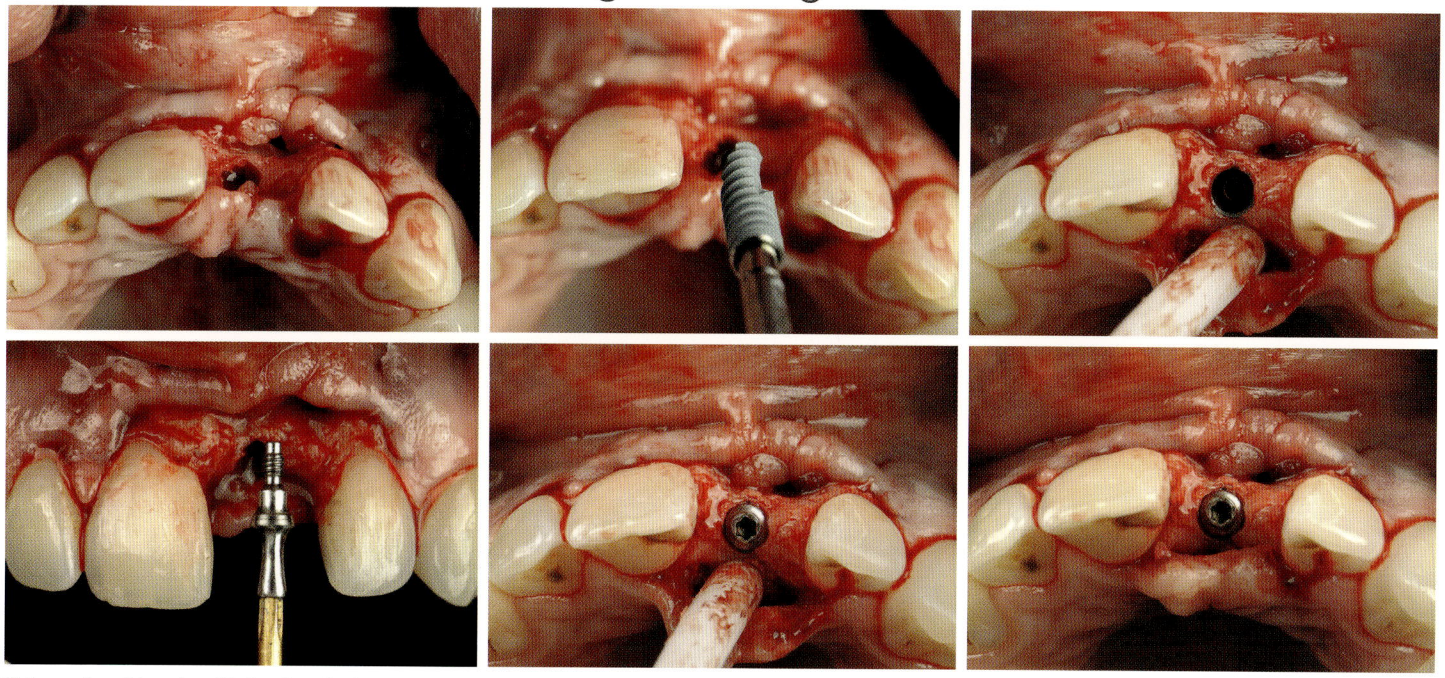

This patient had sufficient soft tissue thickness in the areas of the maxillary tuberosities to serve as excellent donor sites for CTGs. For all the above reasons, it was decided to graft the deficient buccal bone with a CTG. A crestal incision was performed at the edentulous ridge, and a partial-thickness flap was elevated. A sulcular incision was made around the mesial and distal aspects of the teeth, and the papillae adjacent to the defect were elevated. Finally, the partial-thickness flap was prepared and raised above the mucogingival junction (MGJ) until it reached the desired coronal position. No vertical releasing incisions were performed, and the periosteum was left attached to the bone. The implant was inserted, and the narrowest (5-mm) straight healing abutment was attached.

CTG from tuberosity

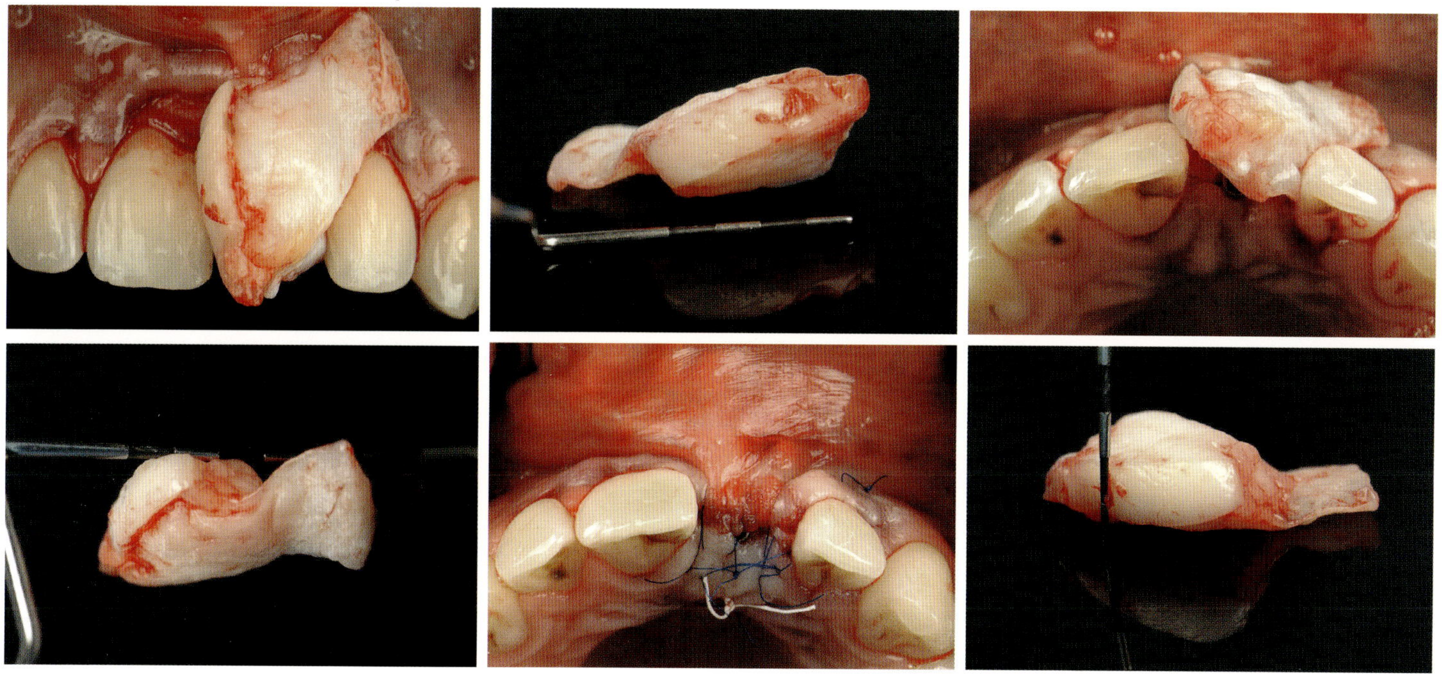

To maximize the graft tissue amount, a large free tissue graft was harvested from the maxillary tuberosity and carefully de-epithelialized. The graft measured approximately 21 × 9 mm, which was large enough to compensate for the volume lost at the implant site. The CTG was sutured in position to the palatal aspect of the flap. The buccal flap was then sutured exactly to the initial incision to close the wound. A 2-0 PTFE monofilament suture material was necessary to secure the tissues in place, while 6-0 monopropylene suture was used for precise flap closure. The intention should always be to perform this type of surgery in one stage.

Healing progression from the initial situation to 6 months post-surgery: The goals of coronally displacing the tissue and creating sufficient volume compared with the adjacent gingival margin were achieved. Palatal bone and tissue support are crucial to re-create buccal esthetics and provide stability. Rotating flaps or pedicle grafts from the palatal aspect are not recommended. These techniques thin the palatal tissue, thereby eliminating the palatal support that the buccal tissues need for long-term stability and success. The bone stability around the implant is verified radiographically.

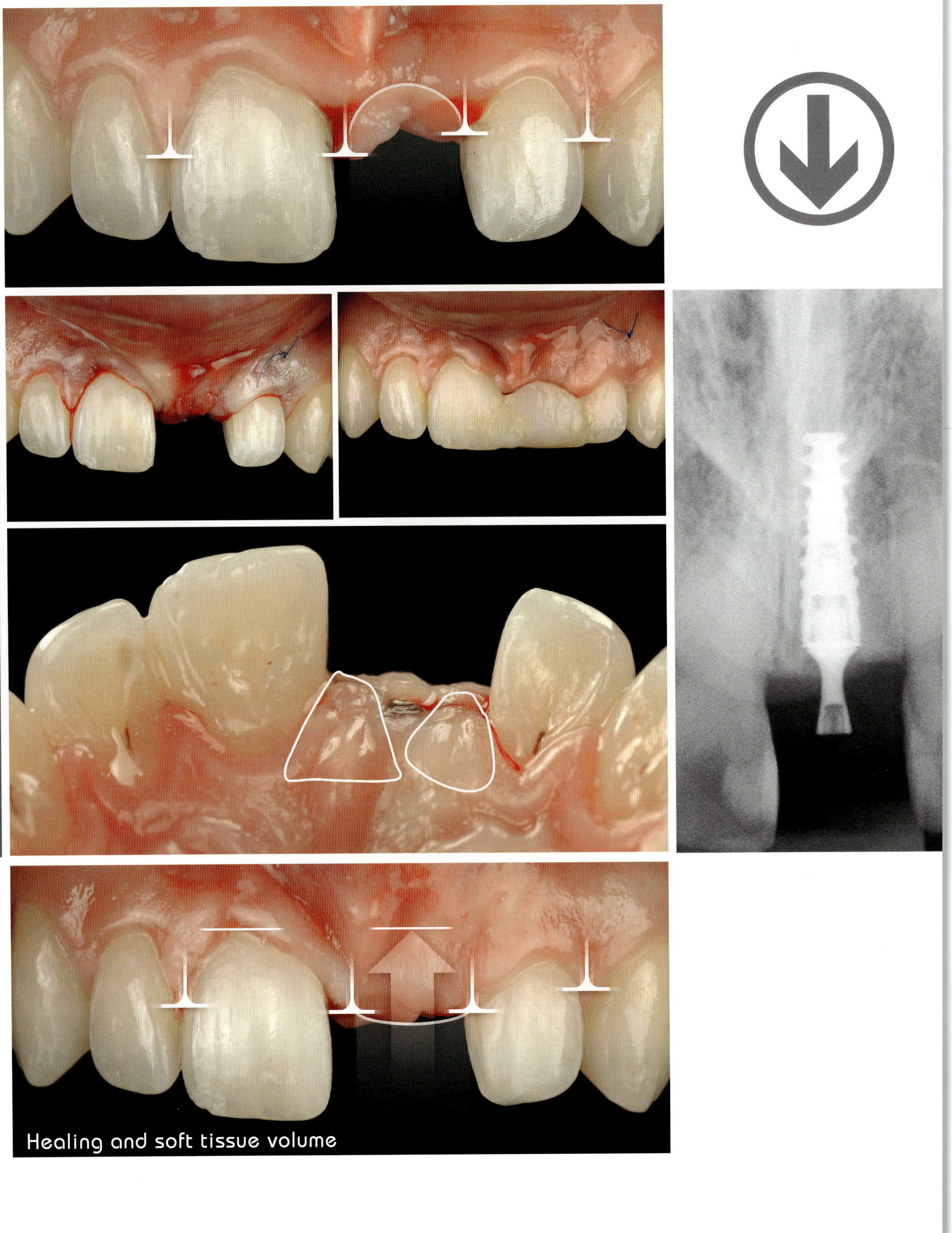

Prosthetic phase

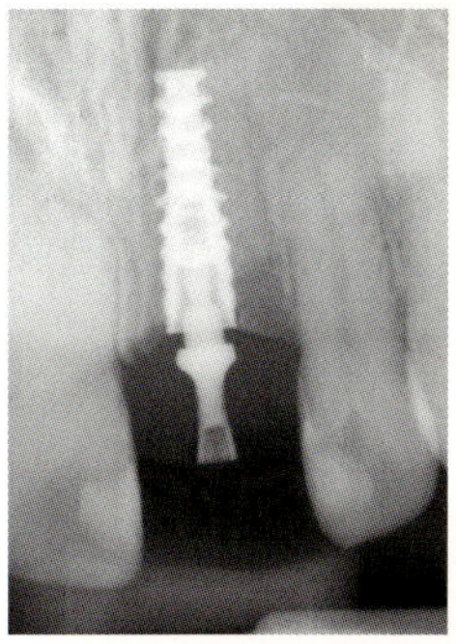
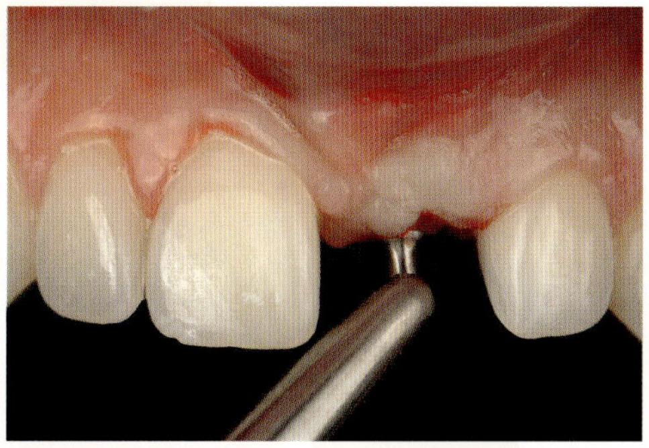
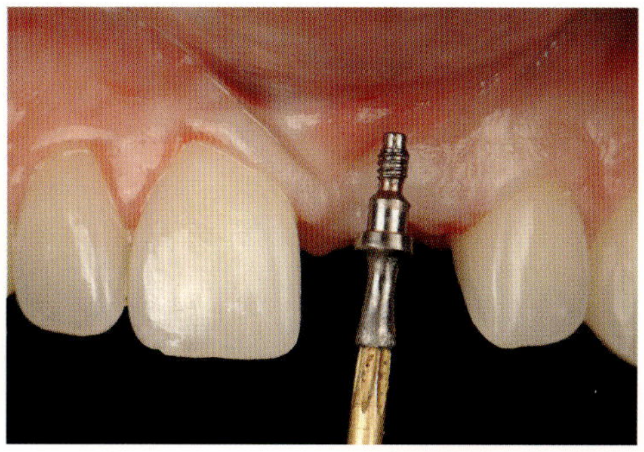

Six months after the surgery, an impression of the implant was made. Removal of the healing abutment and connection of the impression coping require a careful approach due to the large amount of tissue and the diameter of the impression coping. The definitive zirconia abutment was inserted together with a provisional crown, which was relined chairside.

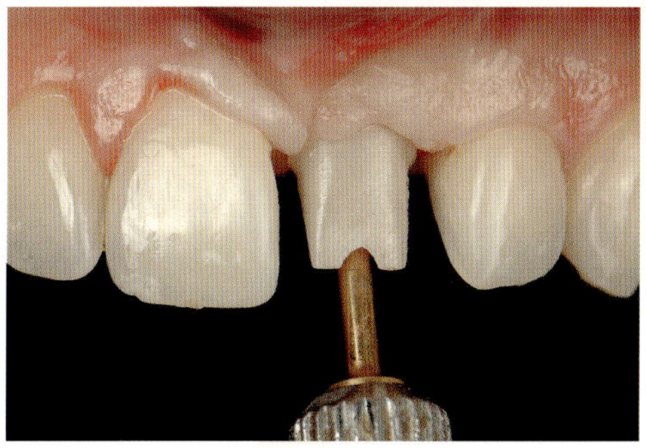
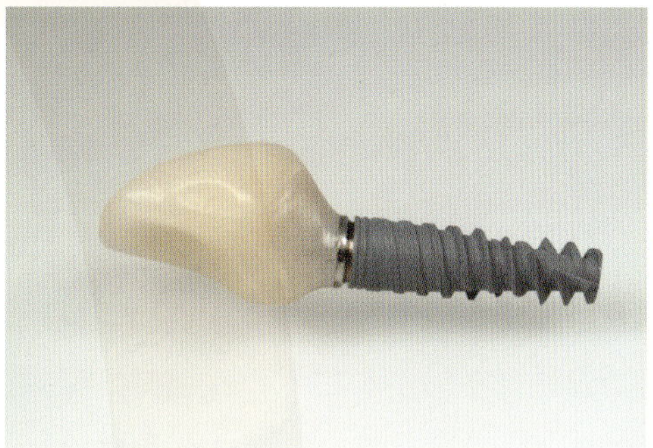
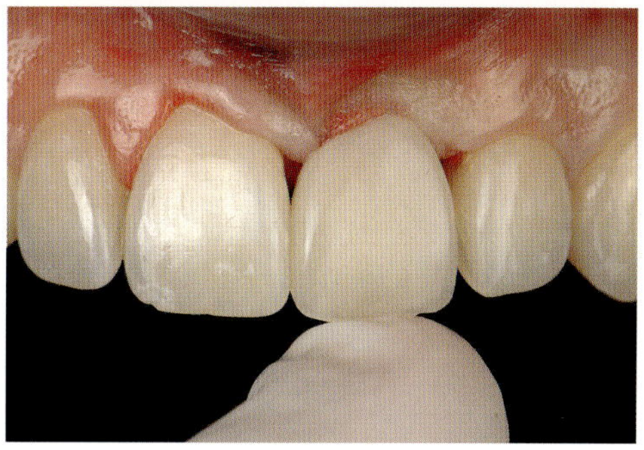

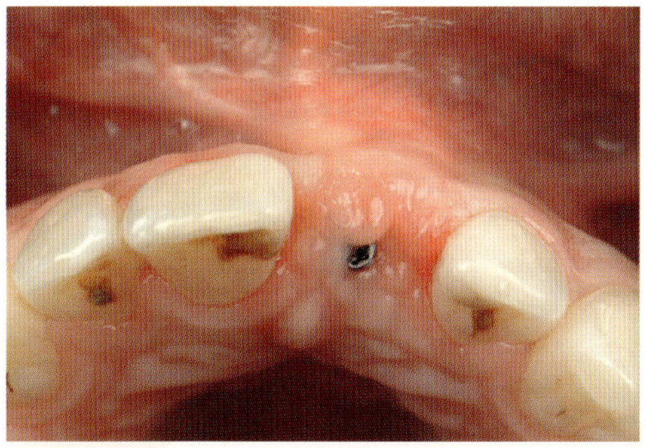
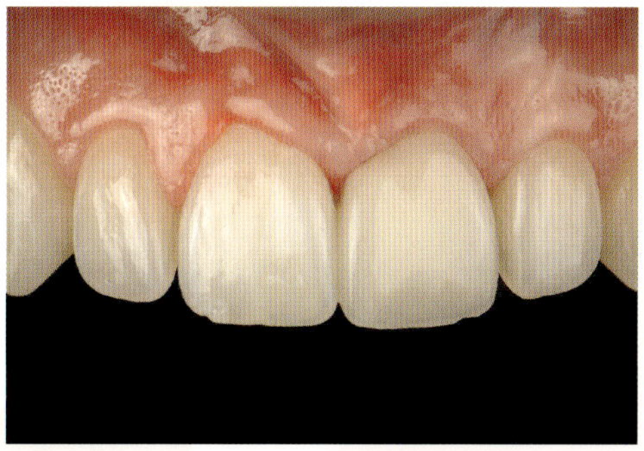
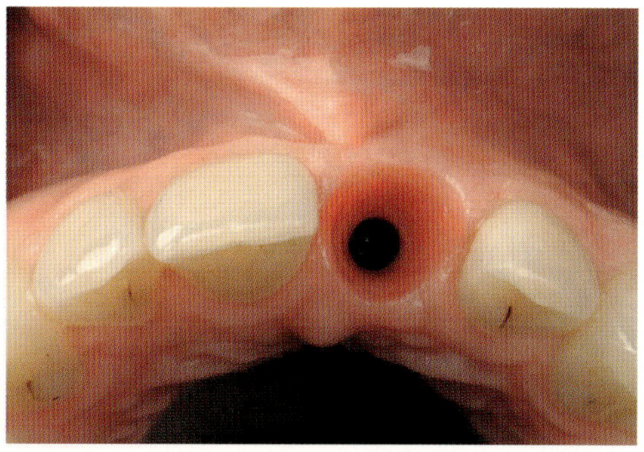

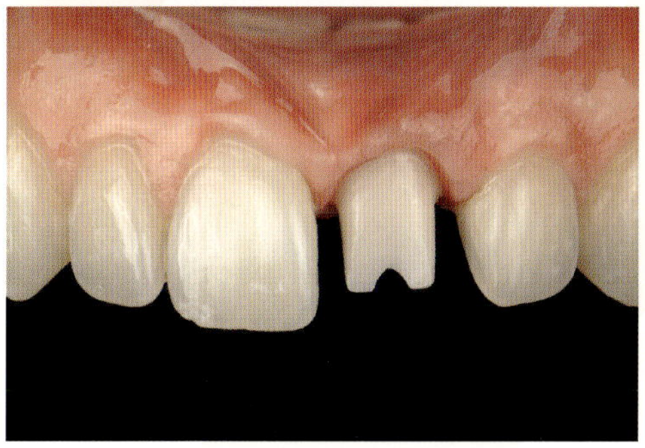
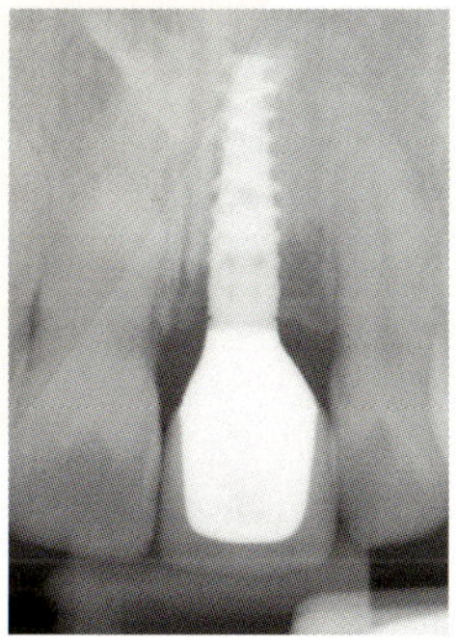
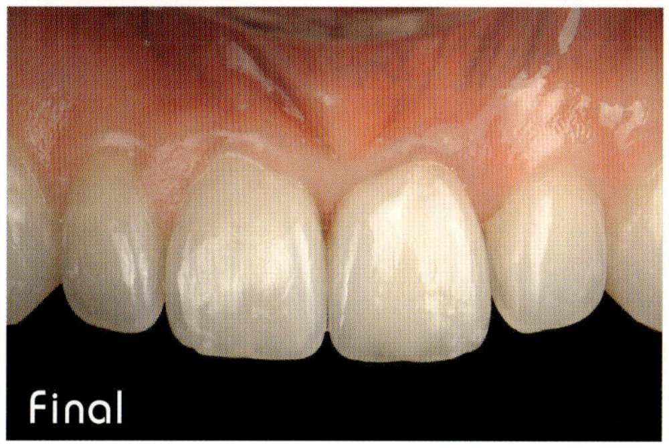

Three months after insertion of the provisional restoration, the soft tissue situation around the restoration and the outcome of the comprehensive approach were re-evaluated. The definitive zirconia crown was placed, and the frenum was repositioned in a more central location.

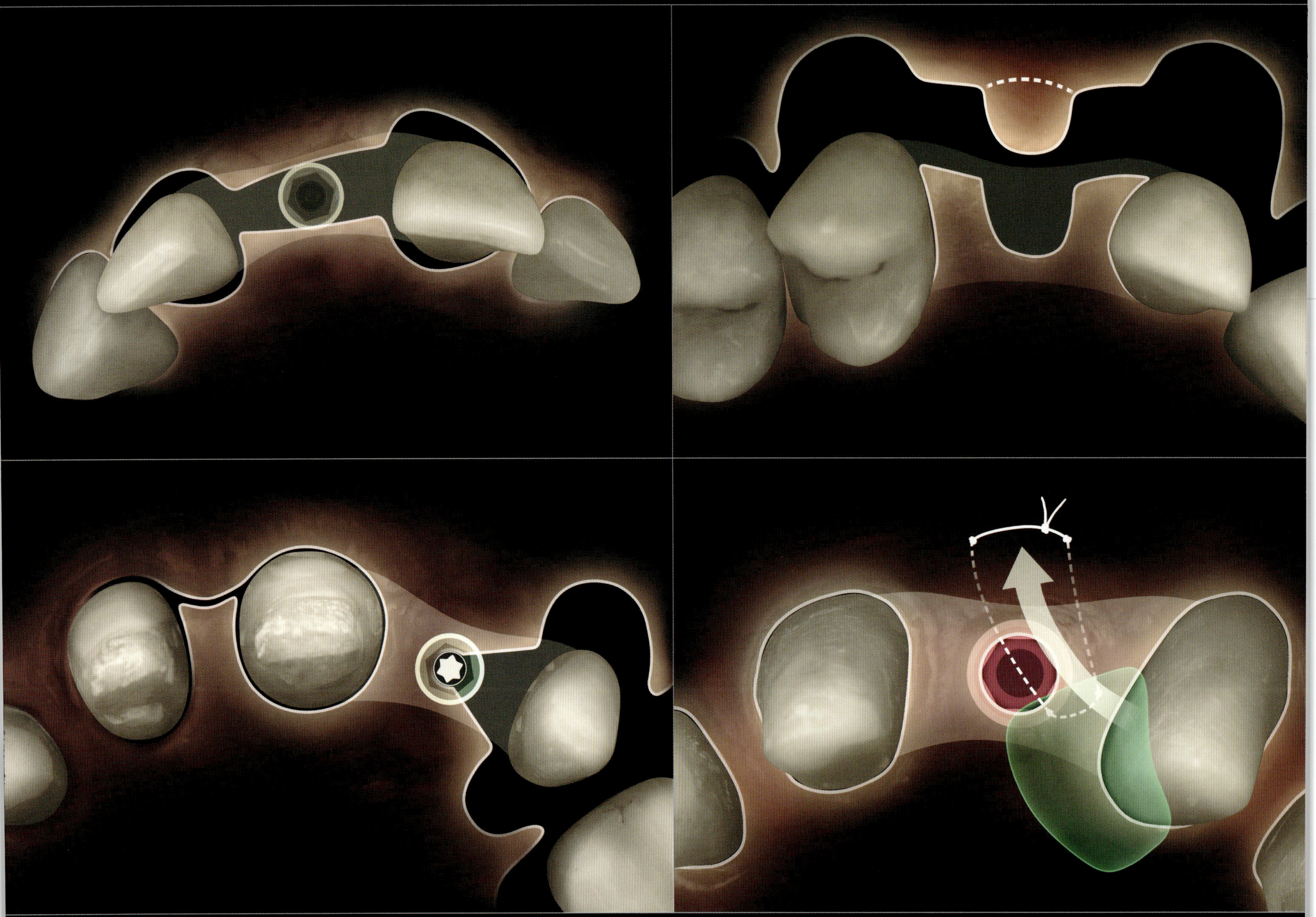

Updated surgical techniques

The overriding philosophy is to complete all procedures in one stage and avoid any vertical releasing incisions or bone exposure, which will limit trauma and postoperative resorption.

The type of incision should be individually selected based on the present situation and the defect size. The interproximal tissue or papillary height is crucial for the incision preparation design. It may either be modified and included in the incision (eg, when not level with the adjacent papillae) or, even better, simply preserved. It should be noted that the proximity of the implant to the adjacent root will influence the ultimate papillary height.

Another goal is to locate the free gingival margin more coronally than the one on the reference tooth to allow for prosthetic soft tissue management and compensate for the likely postoperative and postinsertion recessions. This, however, requires specific soft tissue flap preparation design and elevation techniques.

The buccal tissue volume is the most important surgical parameter for optimal and long-term esthetic outcomes of implant-supported restorations. Almost every implant site requires additional soft tissue volume, and specific surgical techniques are constantly updated for predictable outcomes, limited trauma, and long-term success.

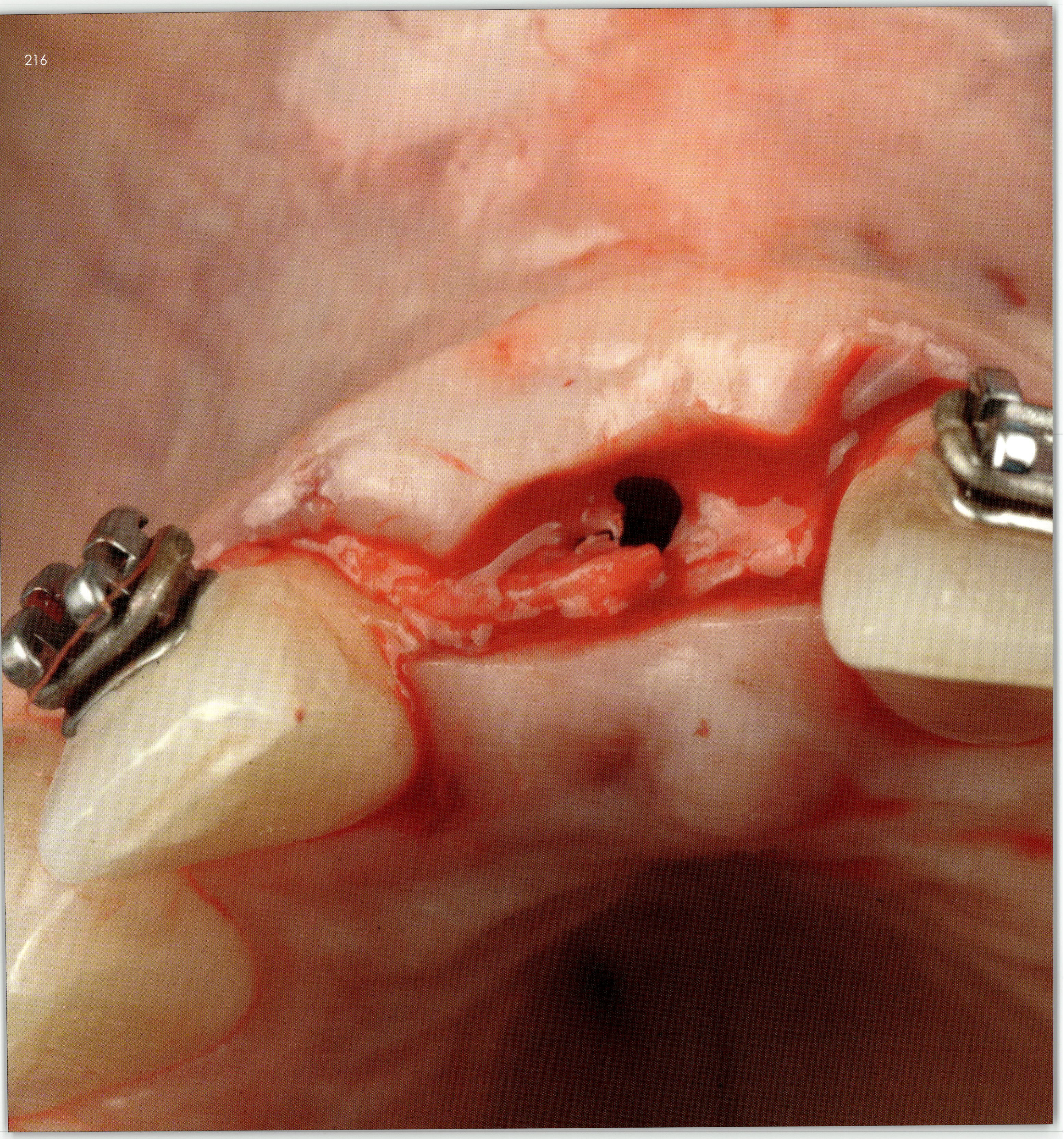

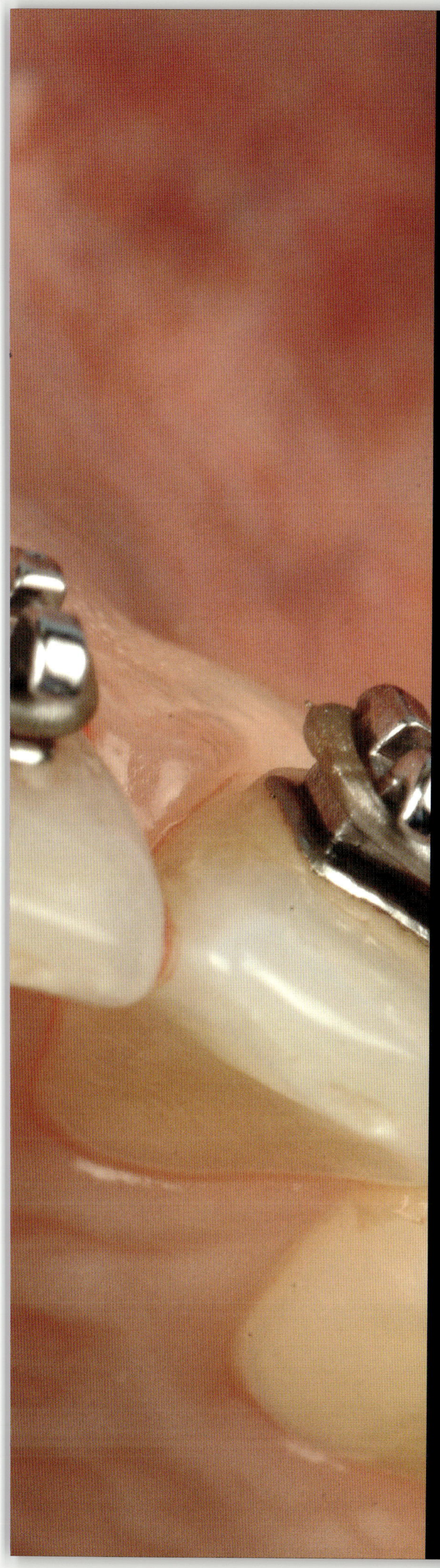

Straight incision

A straight incision is a crestal incision involving the interproximal papilla and a split-thickness flap with sulcular incisions extending over half of the tooth on either side, mesial and distal to the implant site. The straight incision allows elevation of the papilla and creation of space for a CTG without excessive tension. A partial-thickness flap is carefully dissected and elevated off the ridge while leaving the periosteum attached to the bone for better vascularization and integration of the graft. The flap extends vertically above the MGJ to allow sufficient elevation and primary wound closure over a graft. Wide-diameter healing abutments may add difficulties to achieving passive wound closure and adaptation.

Indications:

- When visual assessment of the supporting bone and possible defect is necessary for implant placement
- To augment the ridge volume and papillae vertically and/or horizontally

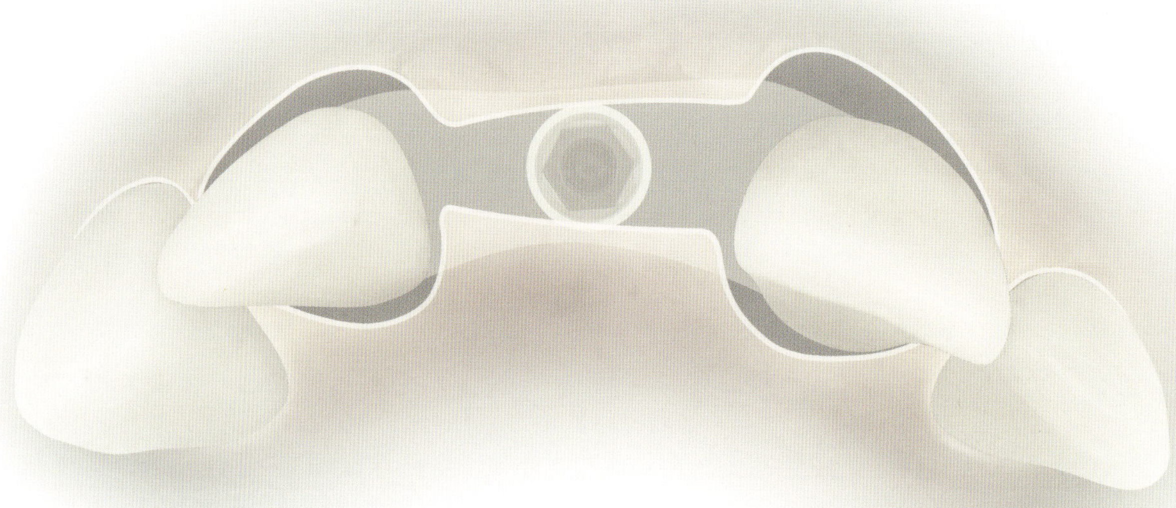

Orthodontist: Dr Domingo Martín

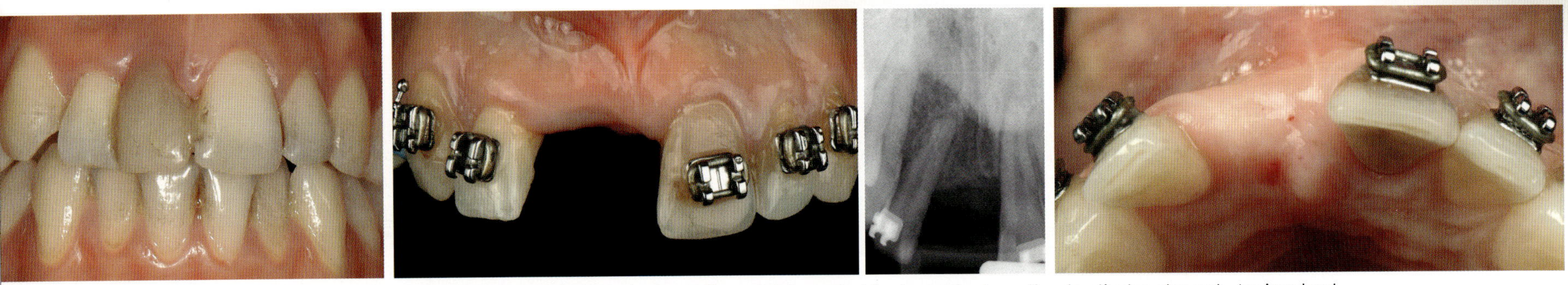

The patient presented with a resin-bonded maxillary right central incisor prior to orthodontic treatment. An implant was planned to assist orthodontic straightening of the root toward the distal aspect. A straight incision design was made to visualize the supporting bone and maximize the soft tissue volume coronally and interproximally.

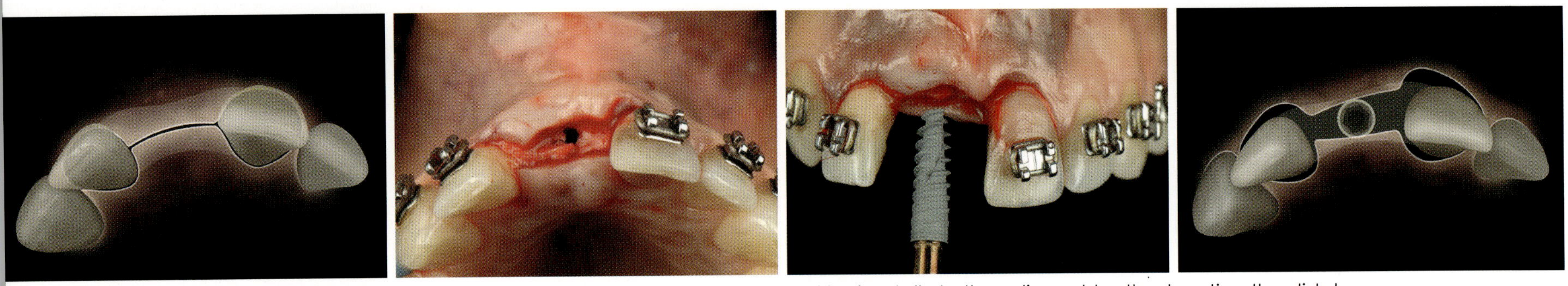

A partial-thickness flap was raised vertically to the MGJ and horizontally to the adjacent teeth, elevating the distal papillae to allow sufficient vertical flap displacement and achieve primary wound closure.

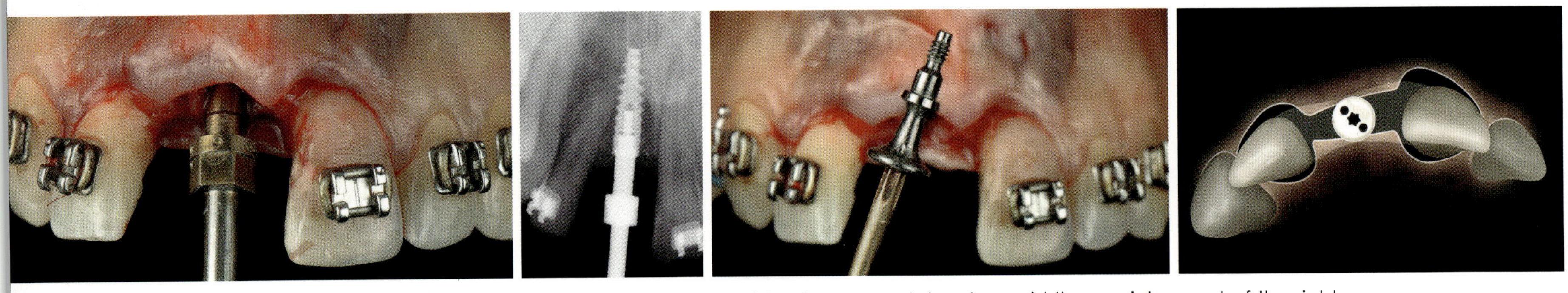

A NobelActive NP 3.5 × 13–mm implant was placed, and care was taken to avoid the mesial aspect of the right lateral incisor root. Then a concave healing abutment with holes was placed to secure the CTG.

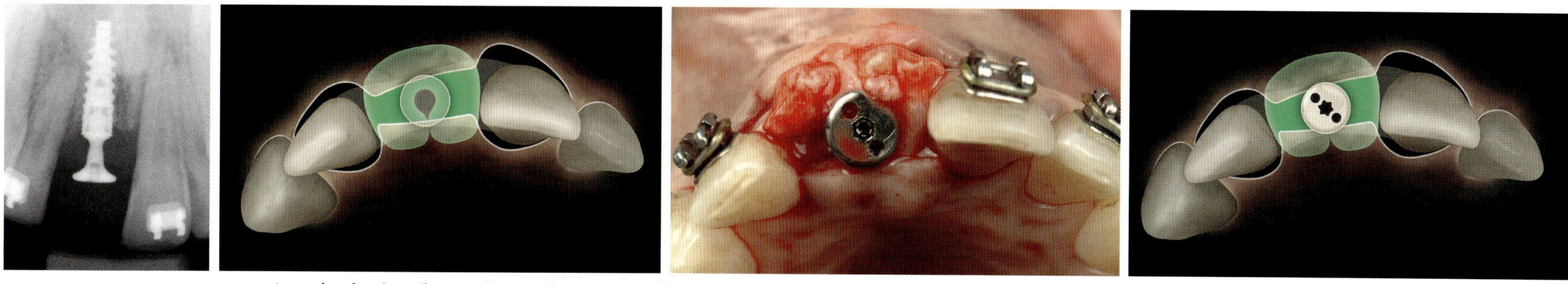

A periapical radiograph was taken to verify complete seating of the healing abutment. A CTG was harvested from the maxillary tuberosity and trimmed to fit the recipient site.

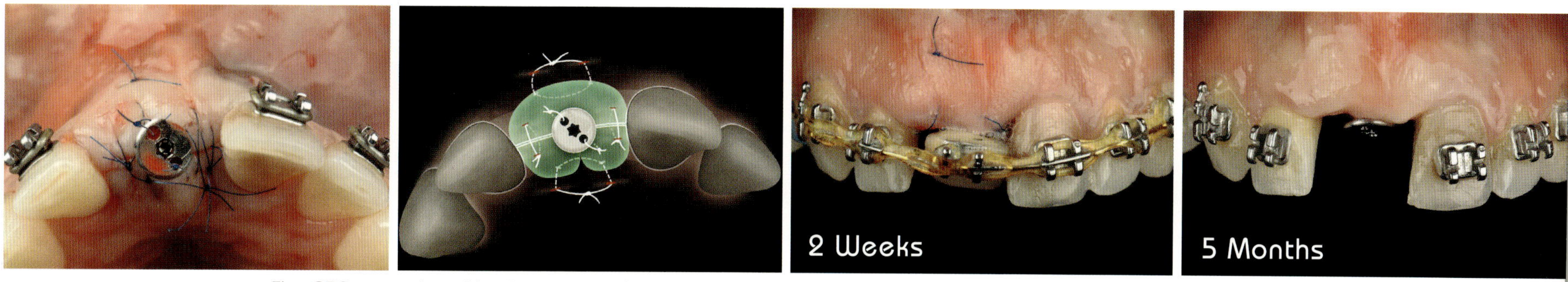

The CTG was sutured in place and, with the help of the holes of the healing abutment, secured in position. The flap was then sutured over the grafted area.

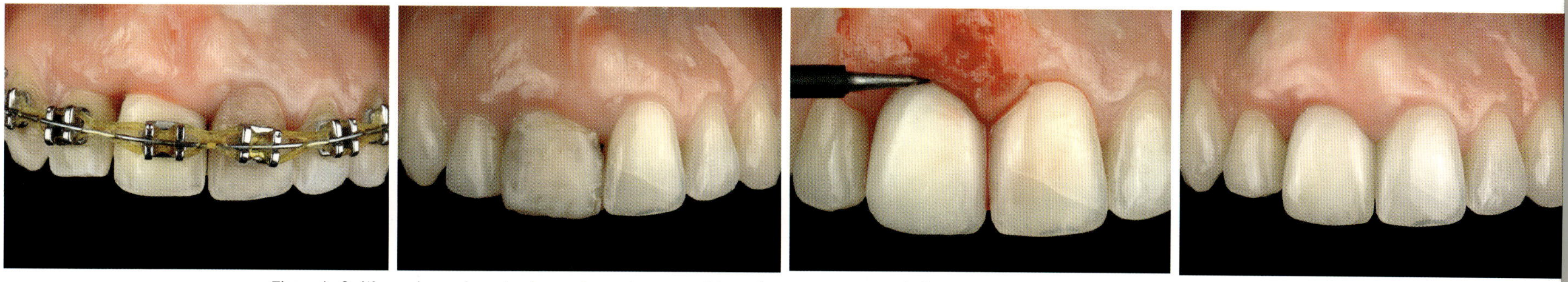

The definitive zirconia abutment and a provisional crown were delivered 4 months postoperatively. Once the orthodontic treatment was completed, a new provisional restoration was inserted to restore the proportions of the right central incisor.

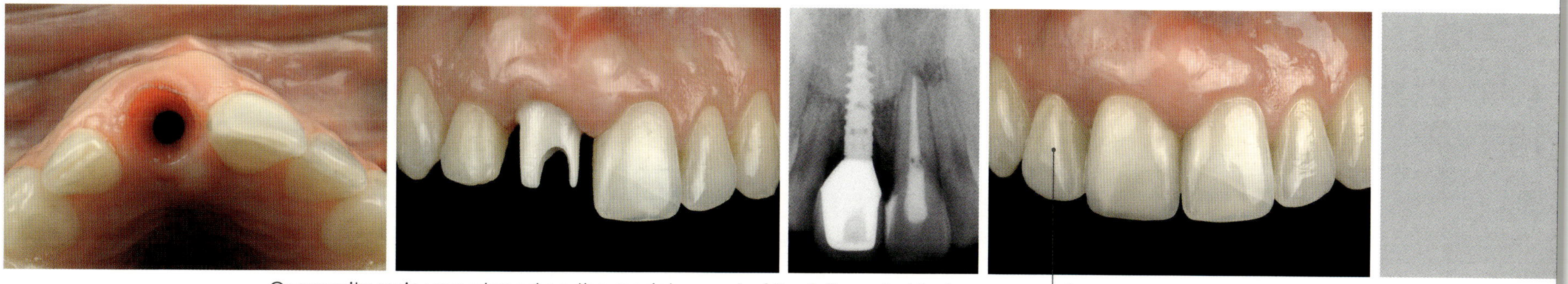

Composite resin was placed on the mesial aspect of the left central incisor to restore the interproximal contact and papillary height. The peri-implant soft tissue architecture was reshaped through gingivoplasty, and the treatment was completed with a veneered zirconia crown.

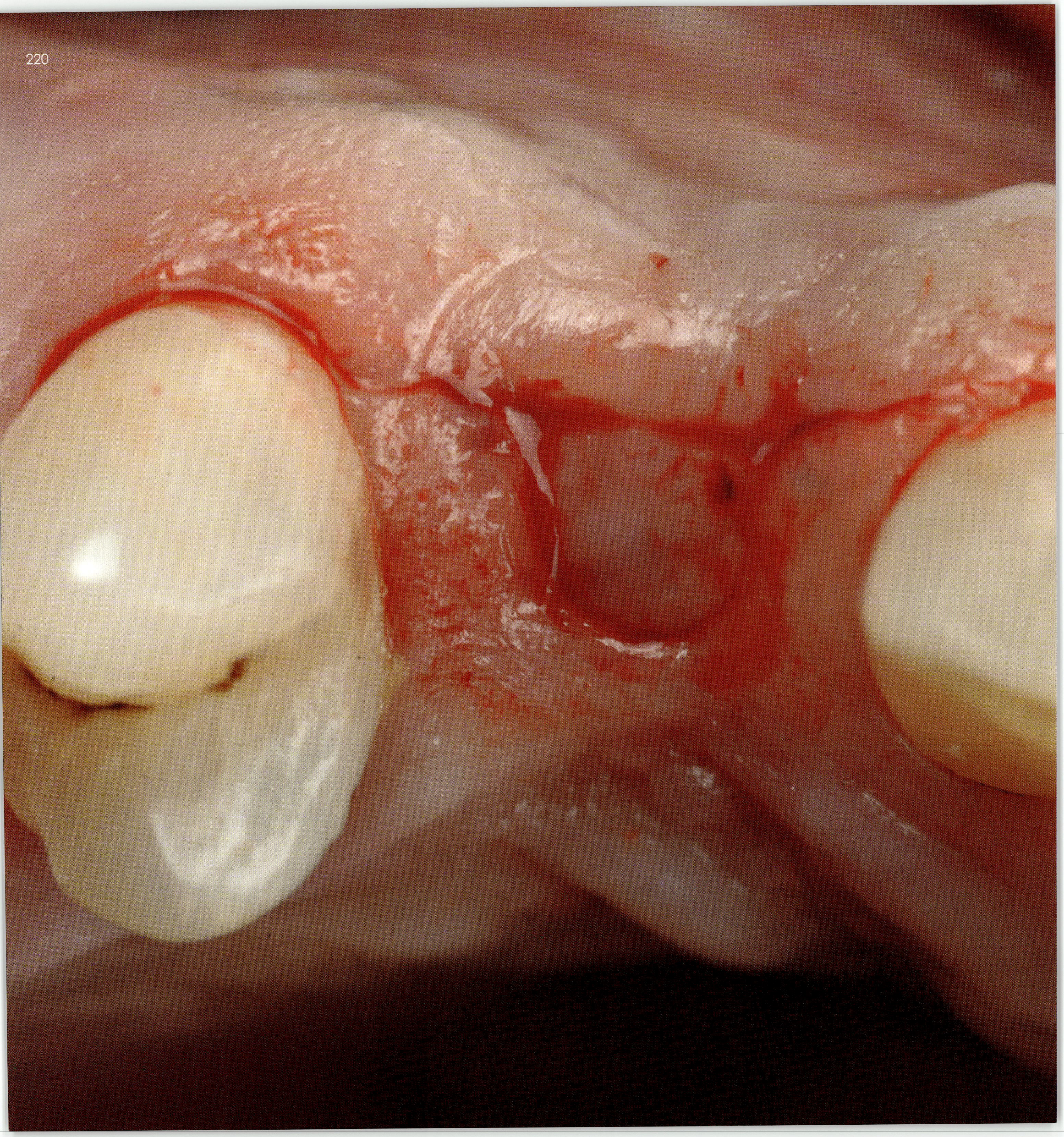

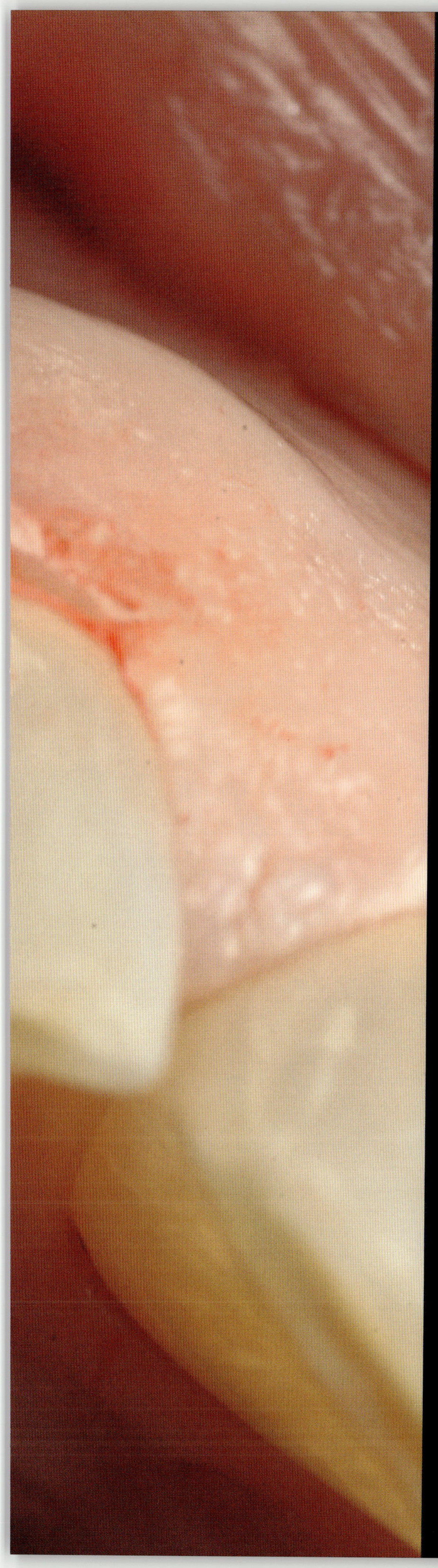

Anatomical incision

The anatomical incision is a 2-mm-deep, crestal circular incision performed with a circular blade or tissue punch in the exact location where the implant will be placed. The small half-circular tissue flap above the prospective implant is then de-epithelialized with a coarse diamond to be folded in with an envelope technique to gain additional volume on the buccal aspect. CBCT scanning is helpful to identify the ideal position and extent of the incision. The diameter of the circular incision should match that of the healing abutment for best possible tissue adaptation. This incision is indicated for defects where only small amounts of tissue grafting are necessary in the buccal and/or interproximal areas. Then a straight incision is prepared to the bone from the interproximal contact area through the papilla and connected to the circular incision. This crestal incision has two possible locations: buccal or centered on the buccolingual ridge. The buccal incision is indicated in situations of ideal papillae that do not require augmentation. Conversely, the centered incision is preferred when the papillae need grafting.

The next step includes sulcular incisions on the adjacent teeth that are one and a half tooth widths distal to the implant site on either side. The distal papillae on the adjacent teeth are typically elevated to allow better mobilization of the flap. A buccal partial-thickness flap is raised, and the half-circular de-epithelialized tissue flap is folded into the envelope between the flap and the buccal ridge to graft the site. If needed, additional connective tissue may be placed on the buccal and interproximal aspects and sutured to the palatal flap.

Indications:

- When visual assessment of the supporting bone and possible defect is necessary for implant placement
- To augment smaller bone defects when tissue grafting is necessary in the buccal/interproximal areas

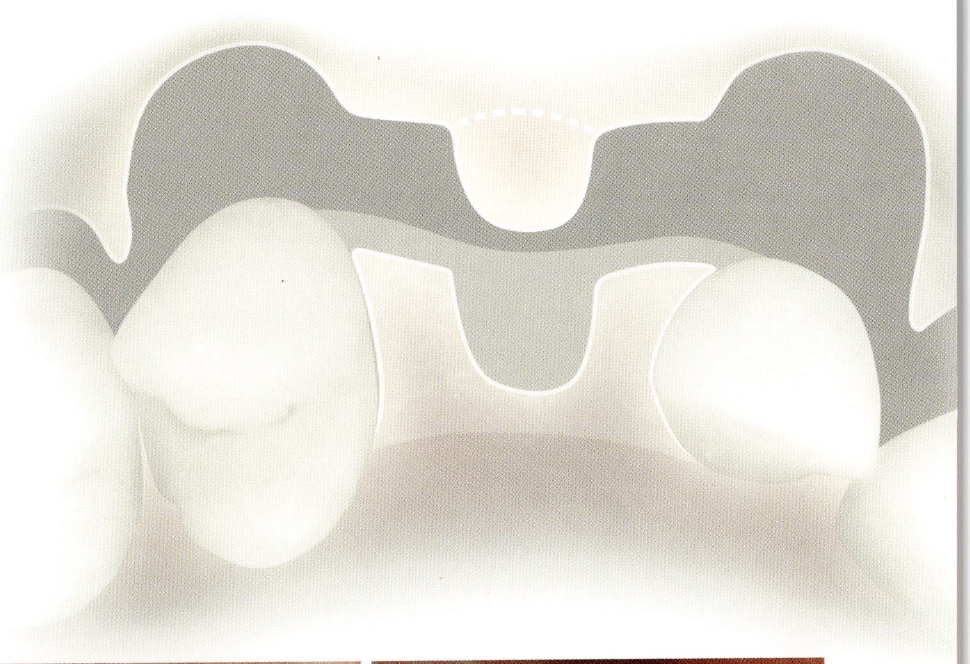

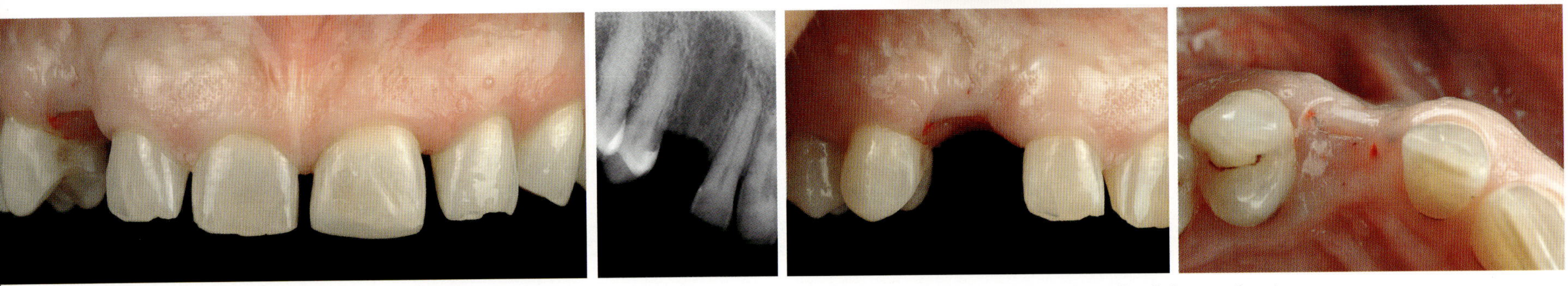

An implant-supported restoration was planned in the area of the missing maxillary right canine. The interproximal tissue was level, but the buccal volume and location of the margin needed improvement.

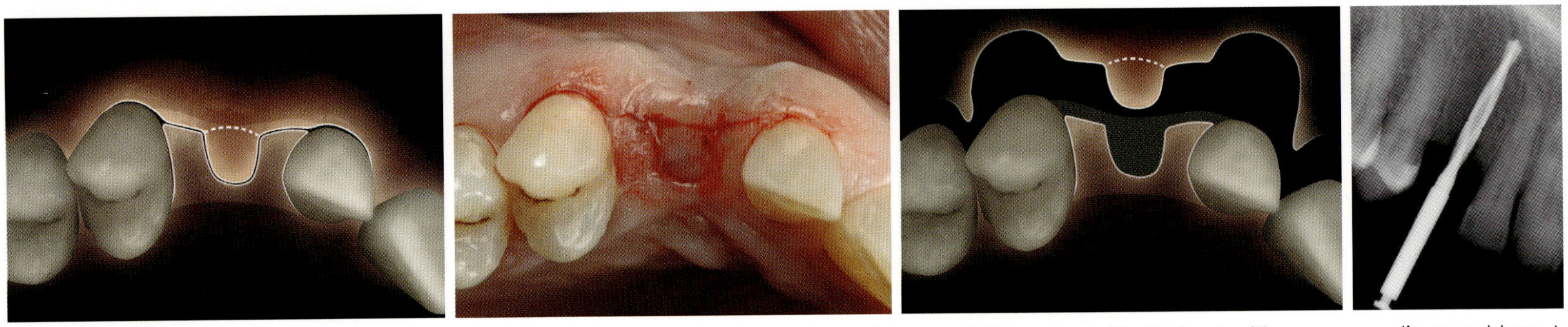

A circular incision was performed about 1 to 2 mm deep in the middle of the ridge and then de-epithelialized with a coarse diamond bur. A straight incision was prepared on the buccal aspect from the mesial to the distal line angles of the adjacent teeth. The straight mesial incision was connected to the circular one and followed into the straight distal incision. The distal papillae of the adjacent teeth were not completely excised but rather elevated to reduce tension on the flap during suturing.

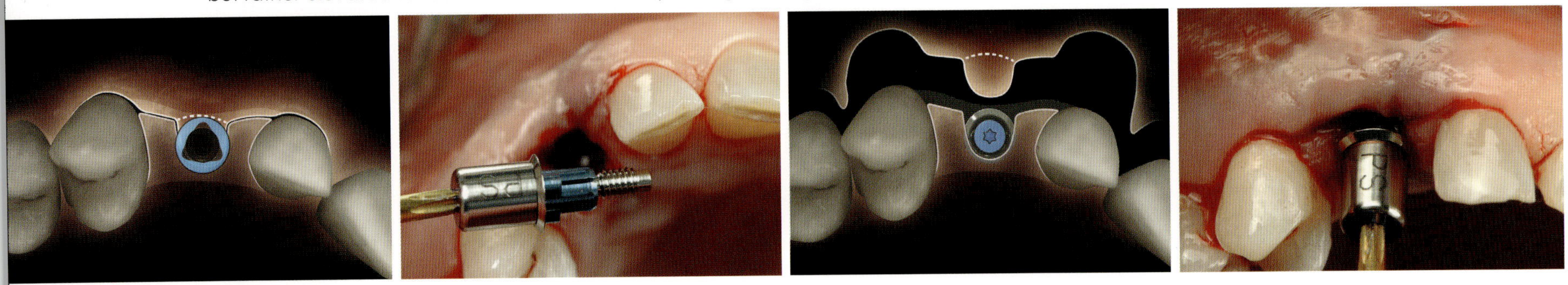

A NobelReplace Groovy 5 × 13–mm implant with PS adapter from NP to wide platform and a 4.3 × 5–mm healing abutment were placed exactly in the planned position.

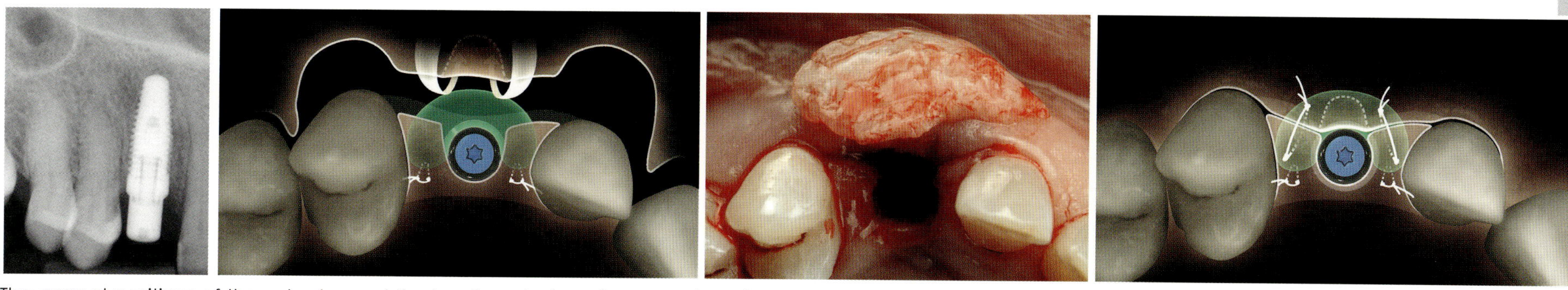

The correct positions of the adapter and the healing abutment were verified with a periapical radiograph. A CTG was sutured in place on the buccal aspect, and the half-circular de-epithelialized tissue flap was folded in to gain additional soft tissue volume. The flap was then sutured to the interproximal tissue, which may be elevated for better adaptation by preparing a partial-thickness flap.

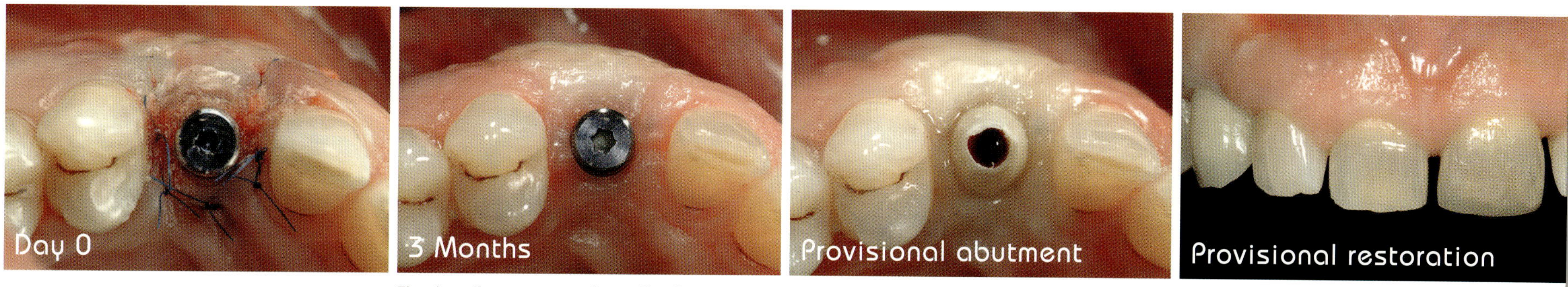

The healing process from the implant placement to the provisional restoration and the creation of the emergence profile.

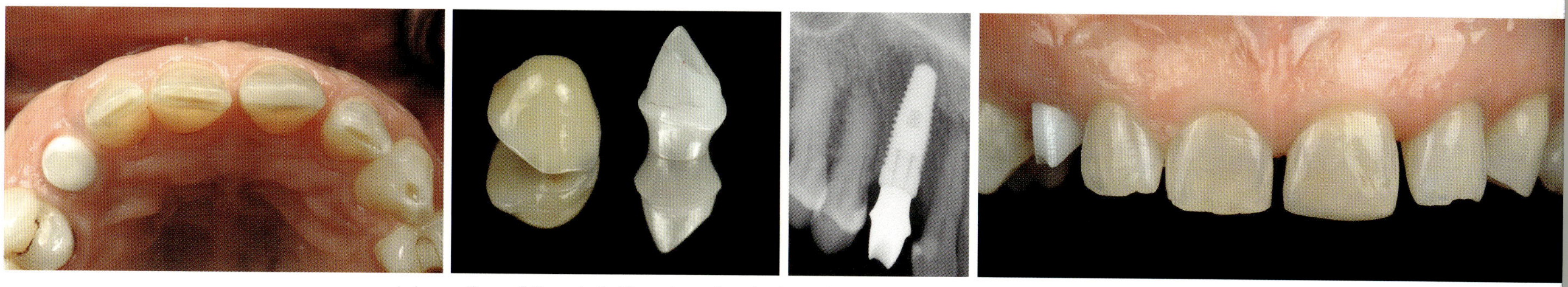

Integration of the definitive zirconia abutment and support of the peri-implant tissue. The periapical radiograph demonstrates accurate precision of fit.

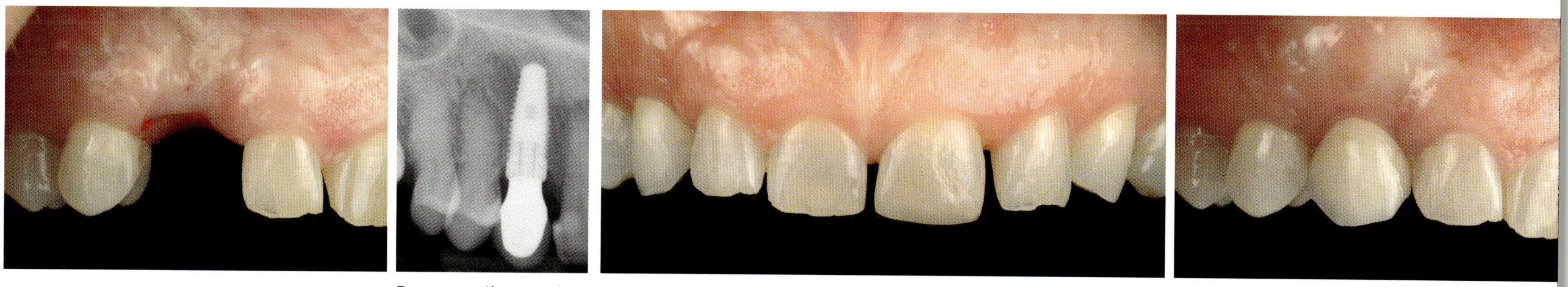

Preoperative and postoperative views of the single-tooth implant-supported restoration in the maxillary right canine area.

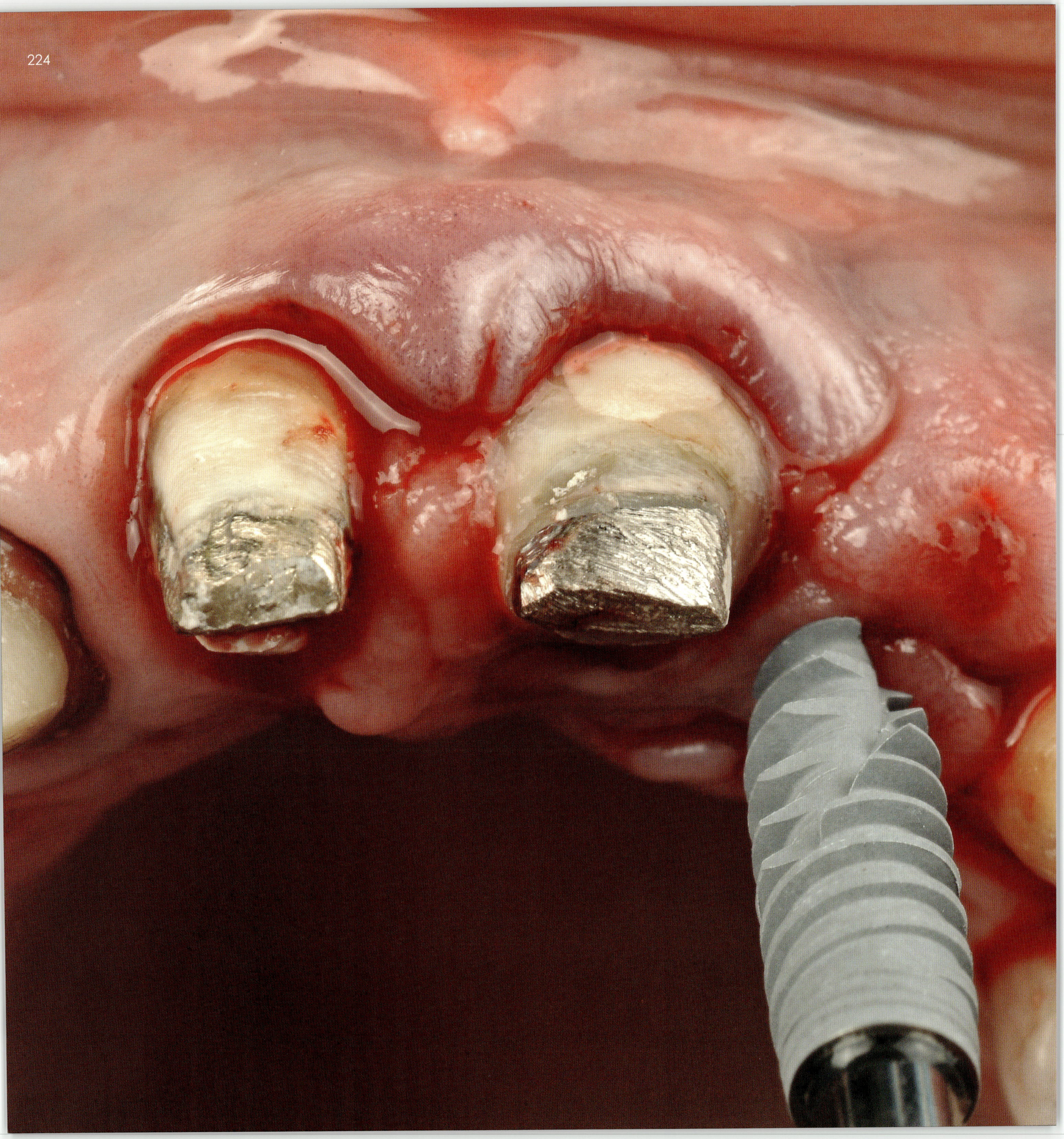

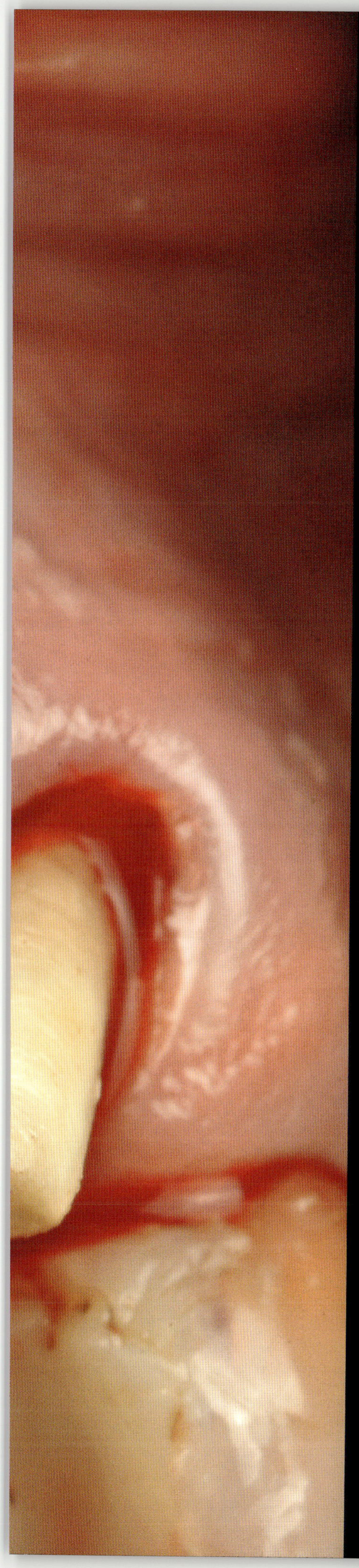

Half conservative incision

In situations where one of the two papillae adjacent to the edentulous area was restored through orthodontic extrusion or other means, the new supporting bone may still be fragile and prone to rapid resorption when exposed. A half conservative incision is indicated to preserve this papilla and not interfere with the newly created bone. It starts with a crestal incision centered on the edentulous ridge that extends about half the distance from one tooth to the next, starting in the area of the planned implant and sparing the newly restored papilla. All incisions are prepared as partial-thickness flaps, and only one papilla is raised for visual access to assess the bone morphology and defect type. The newly restored papilla is not cut and only undermined with a split-thickness tunnel technique, leaving the periosteum on the bone. A graft can be placed into the prepared tunnel to increase the soft tissue volume without exposing bone. Similarly, partial-thickness flaps are elevated around the adjacent teeth to form a tunnel and provide space for a CTG, which is placed through a palatal incision on the distal aspect of the adjacent tooth.

Indications:

- When partial visual assessment of the supporting bone and possible defect is necessary for implant placement
- To decrease trauma to fragile or new bone and prevent resorption
- To minimize resorption and maximize tissue volume through a tunnel technique

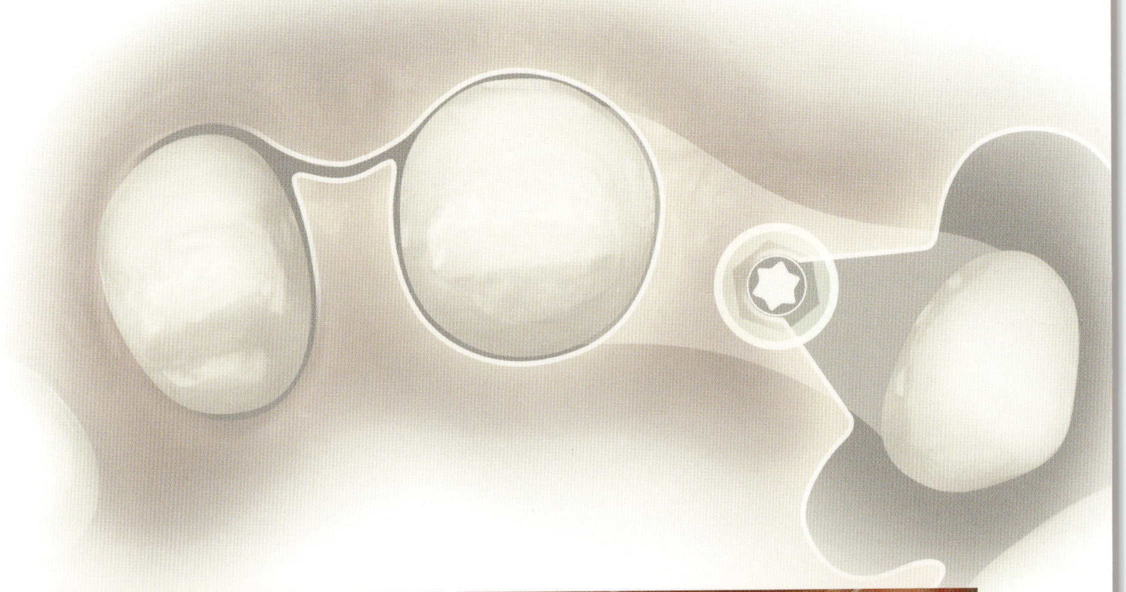

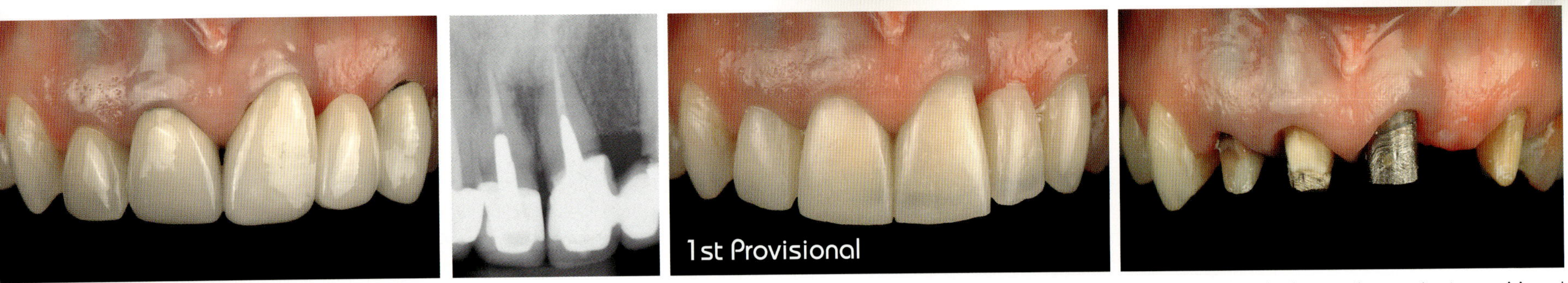

The five anterior porcelain-fused-to-metal (PFM) crown restorations were defective. An extensive bone defect in the area of the maxillary left central incisor and canine as well as a vertical and horizontal defect around the maxillary left lateral incisor were visible in the radiograph. A provisional restoration was inserted to evaluate newly established tooth proportions and the smile line.

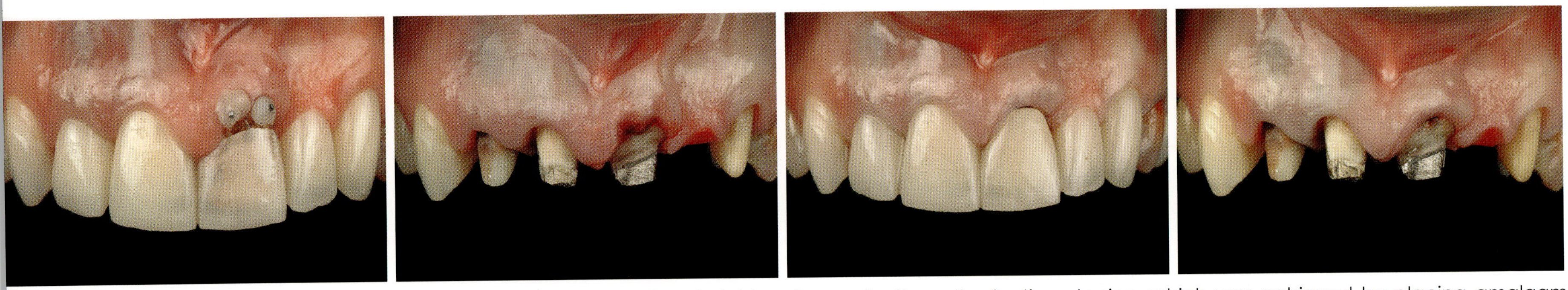

Orthodontic extrusion was planned to improve the papillary height on the distal of the left central incisor for later implant placement in the area of the left lateral incisor. The provisional restoration functioned as anchorage for the orthodontic extrusion, which was achieved by placing amalgam pins into the root and elastic bands to force tooth eruption.

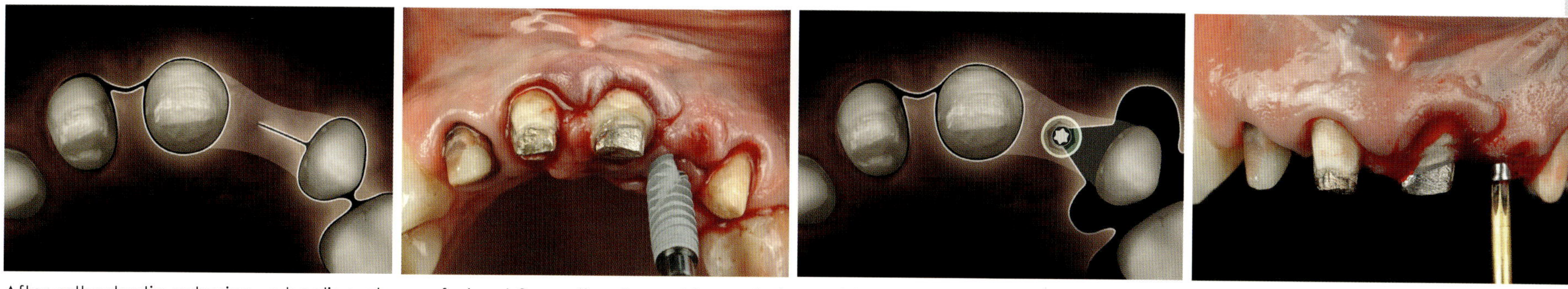

After orthodontic extrusion, a healing phase of about 8 months allowed for bone remineralization and tooth stability before the implant was placed. A half conservative incision was performed to prevent exposure of the newly formed bone. Sulcular and partial-thickness flaps were elevated to gain sufficient visual access to place the implant (NobelActive 4.3 × 13 mm). A straight healing abutment was attached to maximize the space for grafting.

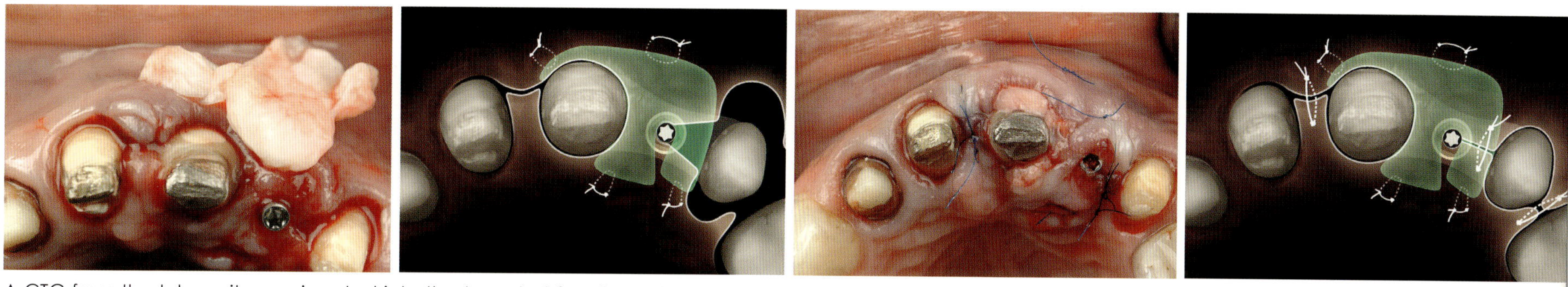

A CTG from the tuberosity was inserted into the tunneled flap through two access points: one between the central incisors and the other on the palatal aspect between the left canine and the first premolar. This allowed for grafting underneath the tunneled flap without tearing it as well as better graft adaptation and suturing around the straight healing abutment.

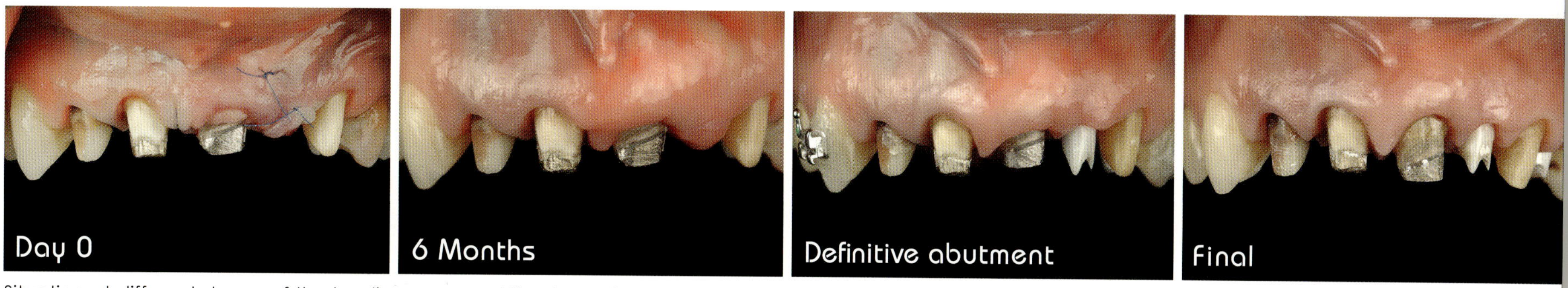

Situation at different stages of the healing process. After 6 months, the left central incisor had relapsed. Another phase of orthodontic extrusion was performed after placement of the definitive zirconia abutment to increase the papillary height on the mesial aspect of the implant. The situation was stable after another 6 months.

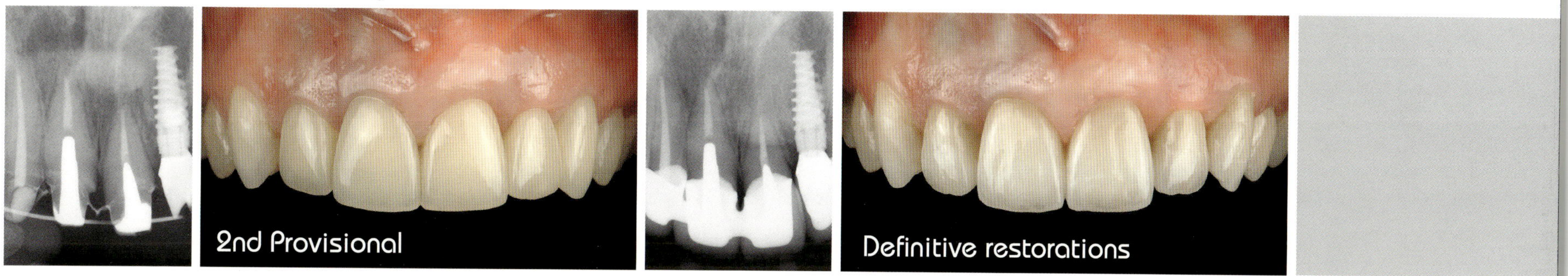

A second provisional restoration and the subsequently placed definitive restorations restored esthetic tooth proportions and supported the buccal and interproximal soft tissue architecture. The definitive zirconia restorations were splinted from the right lateral incisor to the left central incisor to avoid future tooth movement. The implant restoration remained separated.

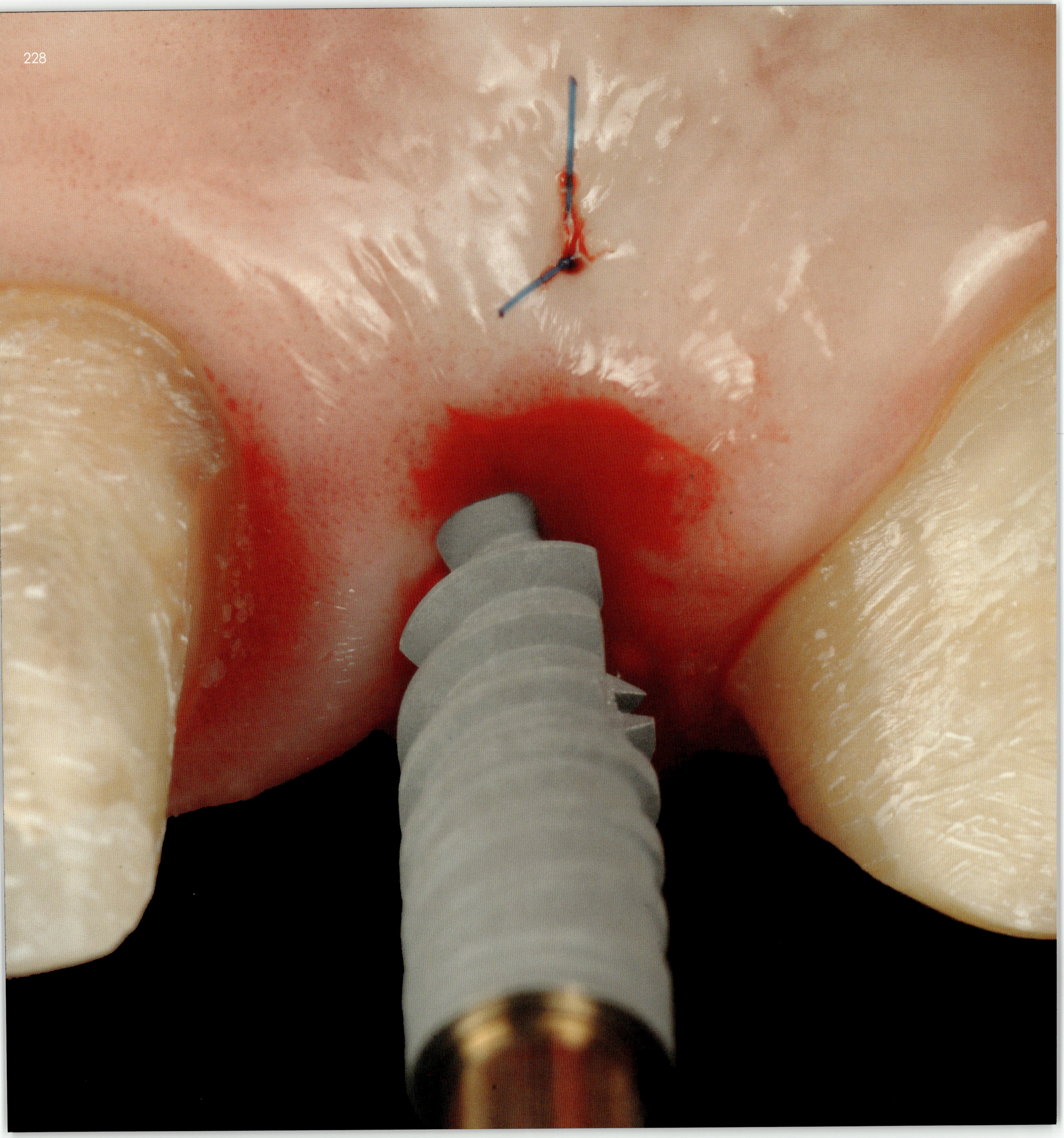

Total conservative incision

A total conservative incision is a circular incision in the center of the edentulous ridge, usually performed with the smallest-diameter circular blade or tissue punch (eg, 3 mm) and in the prospective location of the planned implant. The diameter of the circular blade should match the diameter of the healing abutment to ensure precise tissue adaptation. A CBCT scan is necessary for precise preoperative implant planning and optimal incision placement. Then a sulcular incision is made on the teeth adjacent to the site of the prospective implant, followed by a partial-thickness flap and tunneling of the soft tissue on the ridge all the way to the MGJ to displace the tissue vertically and horizontally. The flap can be mobilized for at least partial visualization of the ridge during implant placement. To place the CTG in the desired position underneath the flap, a crestal incision is made in the area of the adjacent papillae, preferably on the distal aspect of the implant to conceal it.

Indications:

- When direct visual access to the bone is not necessary (CBCT scan advised)
- To create ideal morphology only through vertical and horizontal soft tissue grafting
- To avoid trauma to fragile or new bone
- To minimize resorption through the tunnel technique

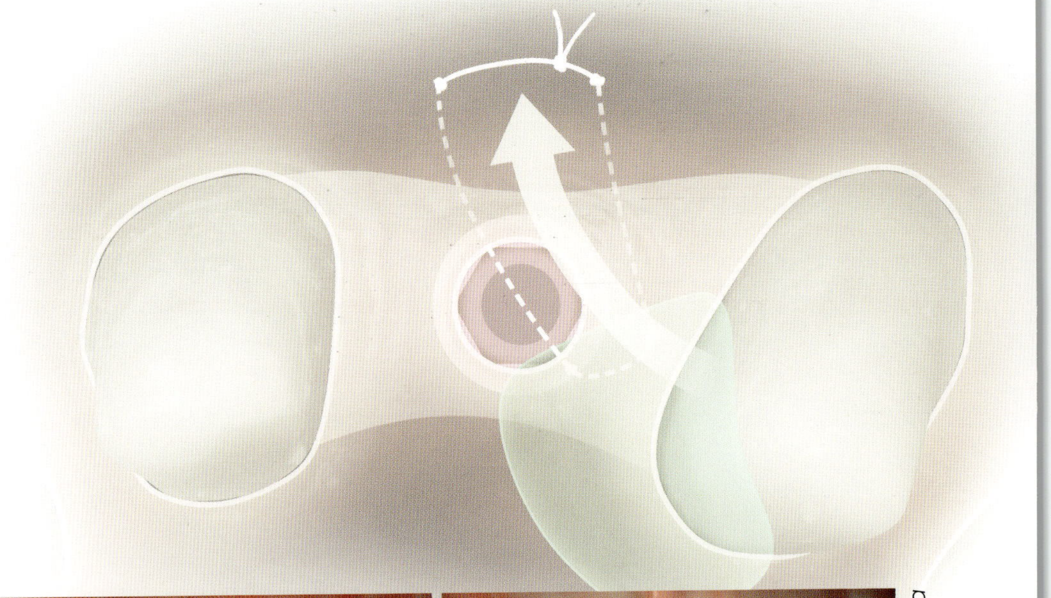

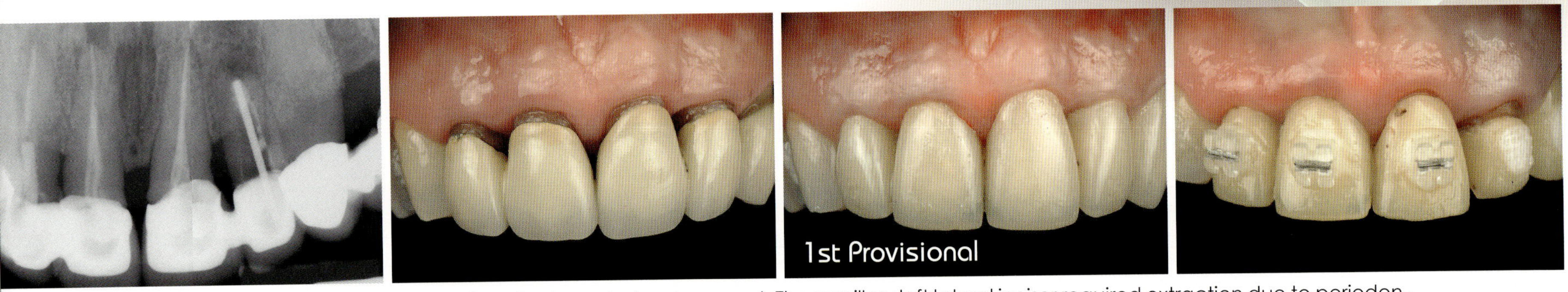

Orthodontist: Dr Vincente Sada

The defective PFM restorations in this patient needed replacement. The maxillary left lateral incisor required extraction due to periodontal and endodontic failure. A provisional restoration was placed to restore the abutment teeth. During the second phase, orthodontic treatment was performed to level the interproximal bone and tissue.

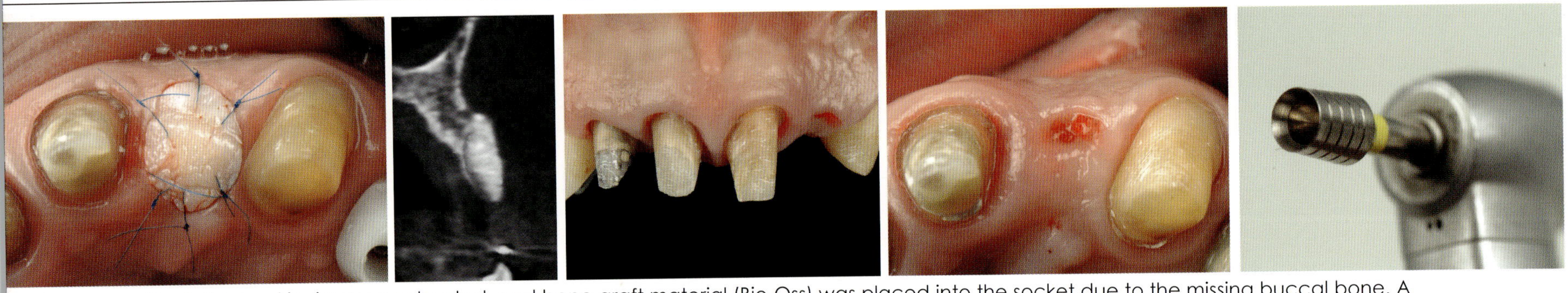

The left lateral incisor was extracted, and bone graft material (Bio-Oss) was placed into the socket due to the missing buccal bone. A round free tissue graft was sutured in place to seal the socket. A CT scan was performed 8 months after bone healing, and the implant was placed.

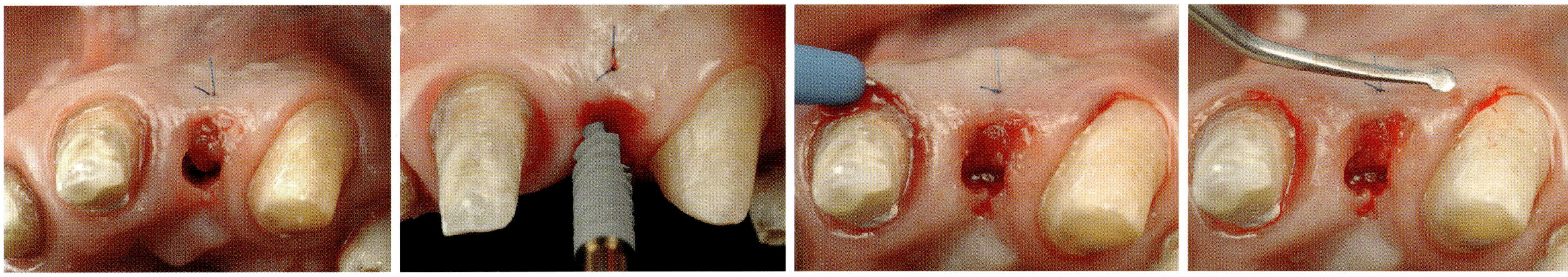

A total conservative approach was applied to avoid any exposure of the underlying grafted bone and prevent resorption. A 3-mm circular blade was used to make a 2-mm-deep initial circular incision. The top of the circular tissue was de-epithelialized with a coarse diamond bur before the site was undermined with a partial-thickness flap.

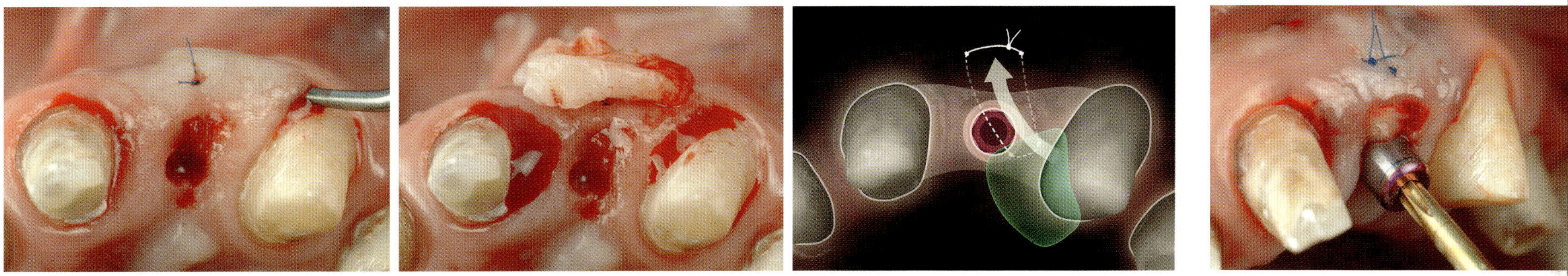

A sulcular incision was performed on the adjacent teeth, and a partial-thickness flap was elevated to connect this incision to the circular incision, thereby creating a tunnel in all directions. The previously excised circular tissue was sutured to the buccal aspect to avoid surgical trauma during the perforation for the implant (NobelActive 3.5 × 13 mm). A CTG from the tuberosity was then inserted from the lateral aspect and positioned with rounded hand instruments and specific suture techniques.

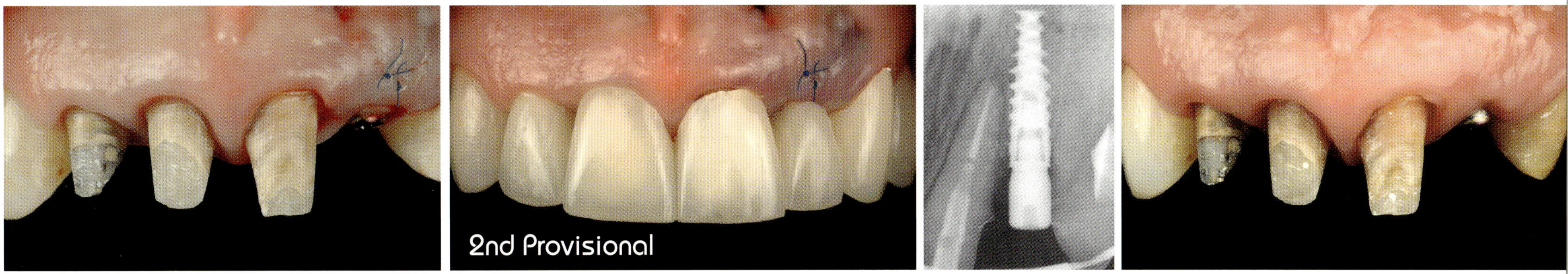

The suture entered the created tunnel and exited at the adjacent tooth, suturing the graft into position. A conventional healing abutment was placed, and a provisional restoration was relined without creating any pressure at the grafted site. A 3-month healing period followed, which is the minimum for such surgical procedures.

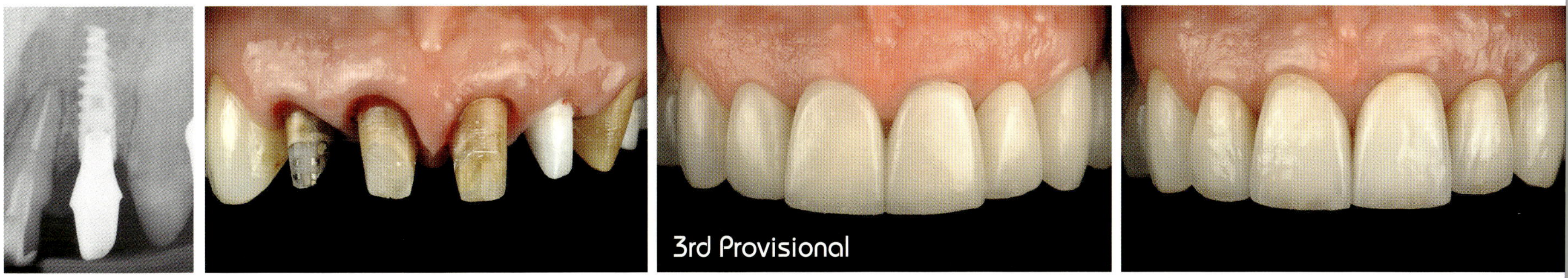

After an implant impression was made, the definitive zirconia abutment was inserted, and the provisional restoration was relined. The definitive zirconia crown was then finalized. Despite the difficult initial situation and bone defect, the minimally invasive approach was able to gain and maintain adequate tissue volumes.

Surgical blades

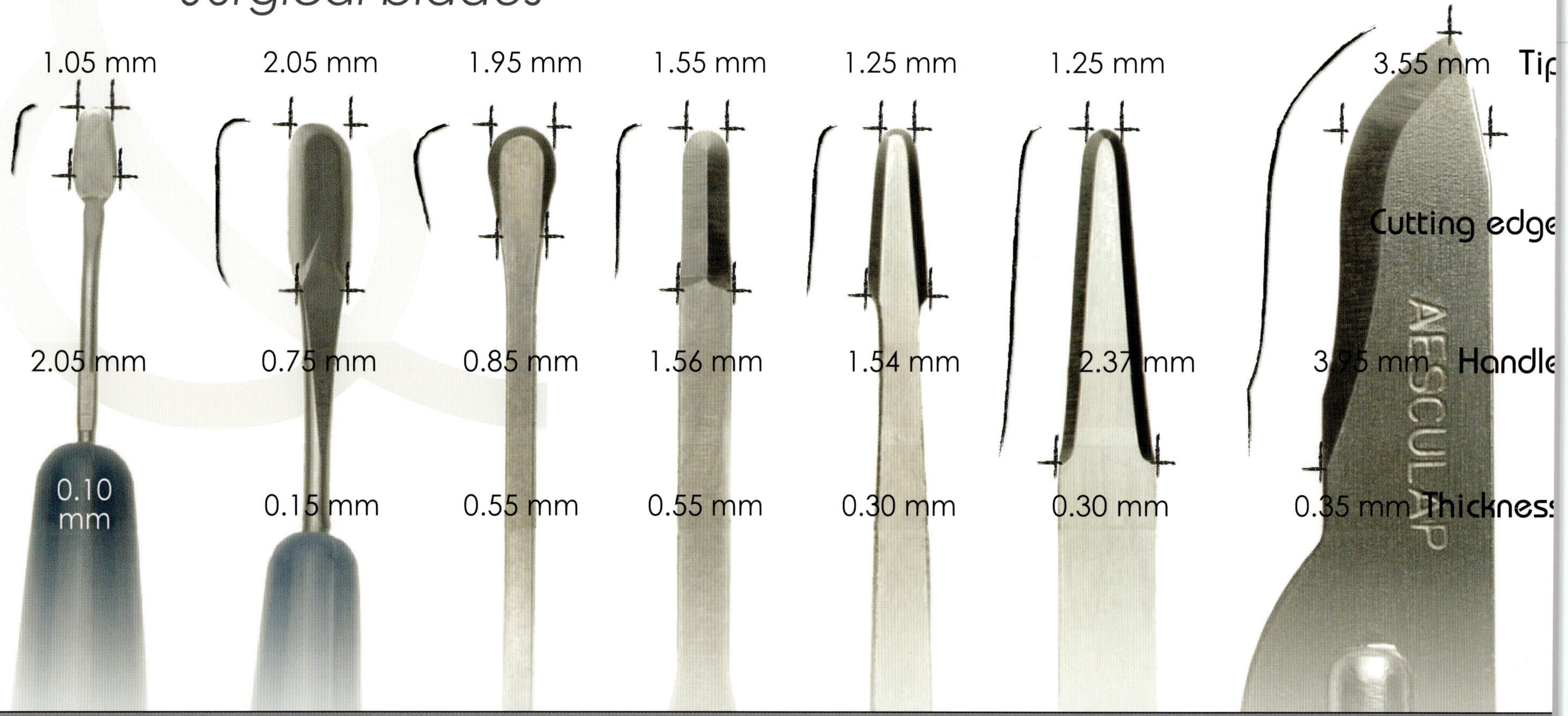

Surgical instruments

Minimally invasive peri-implant surgical procedures cannot be performed with conventional surgical instruments. The complexity of the delicate techniques, variety of movements in restricted areas, and limited tissue thicknesses require very small and specially shaped instruments. Micro instruments and blades are only rarely used in dentistry, but they are slowly being introduced to the market. The preferred resource for such instruments is the field of surgical ophthalmology. The microblades are significantly smaller and require sufficient magnification. They are also considerably sharper, which provides a clean cut and eliminates tissue drag and distortion.

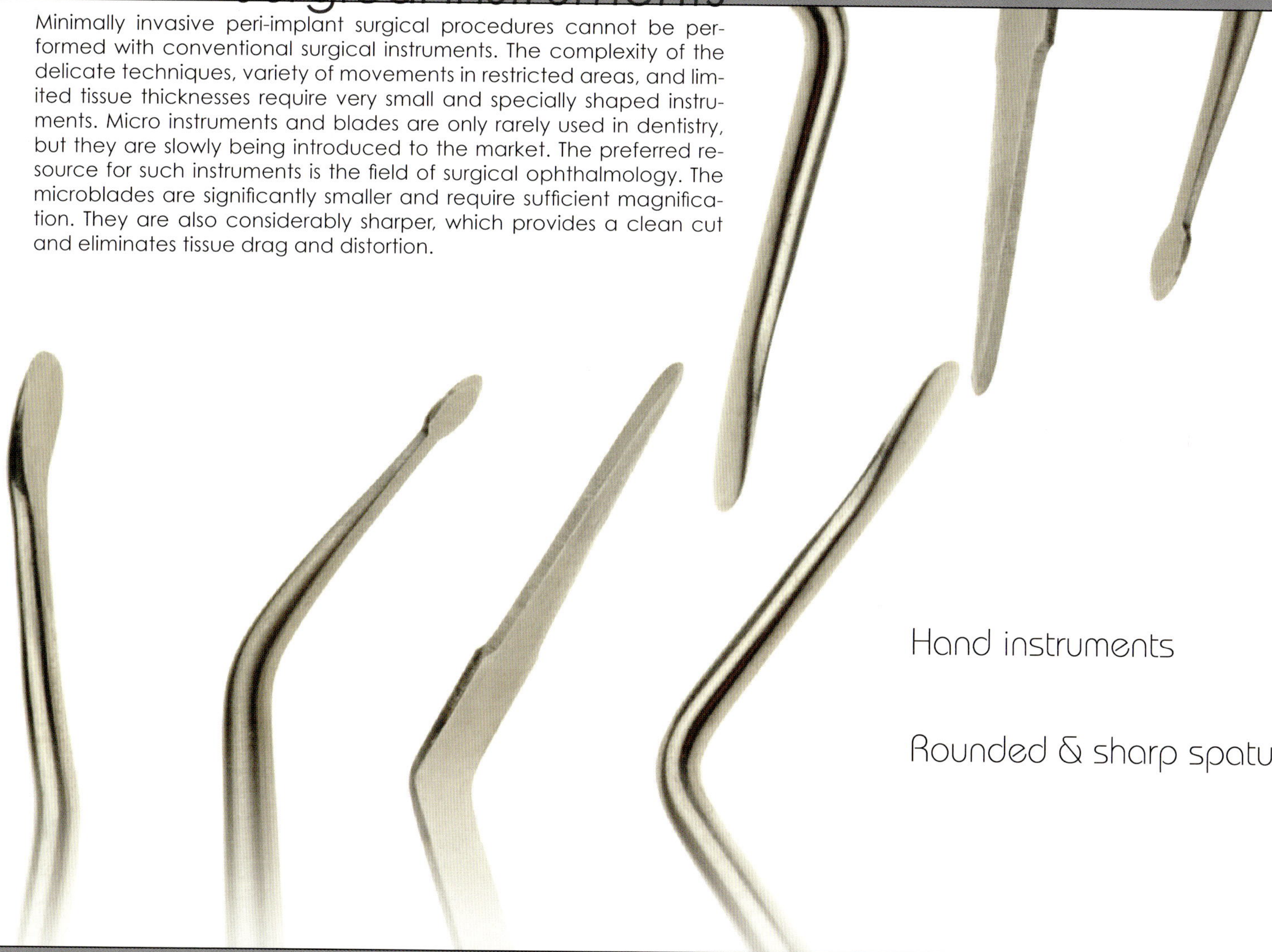

Hand instruments

Rounded & sharp spatulas

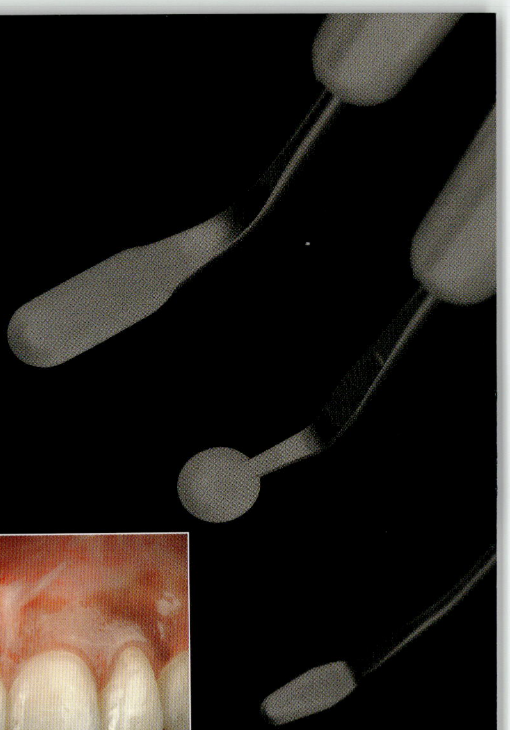

The authors' preferred rounded blades are the following: a 2.0-mm angled crescent knife available with various bevels (Sharpoint Sharptome, Angiotech), a 1.25-mm angled double-bevel mini-crescent knife (Sharpoint), and a 2.2-mm angled double-bevel spoon knife (Sharpoint). These disposable blades can be bent to a certain limit to create different angles and allow almost limitless possibilities and versatility. They are used for fine and delicate cuts for papillae elevation, partial-thickness incisions for tunneling purposes, fibrotomies after horizontal gingivectomy procedures, or dissection of the periodontal ligament for noninvasive extractions. Because these instruments are originally designed for ophthalmic surgeries, some may find the handle not rigid enough for all periodontal surgery purposes. Rounded knives are recommended over pointed ones because they provide greater control, especially for tunneling techniques.

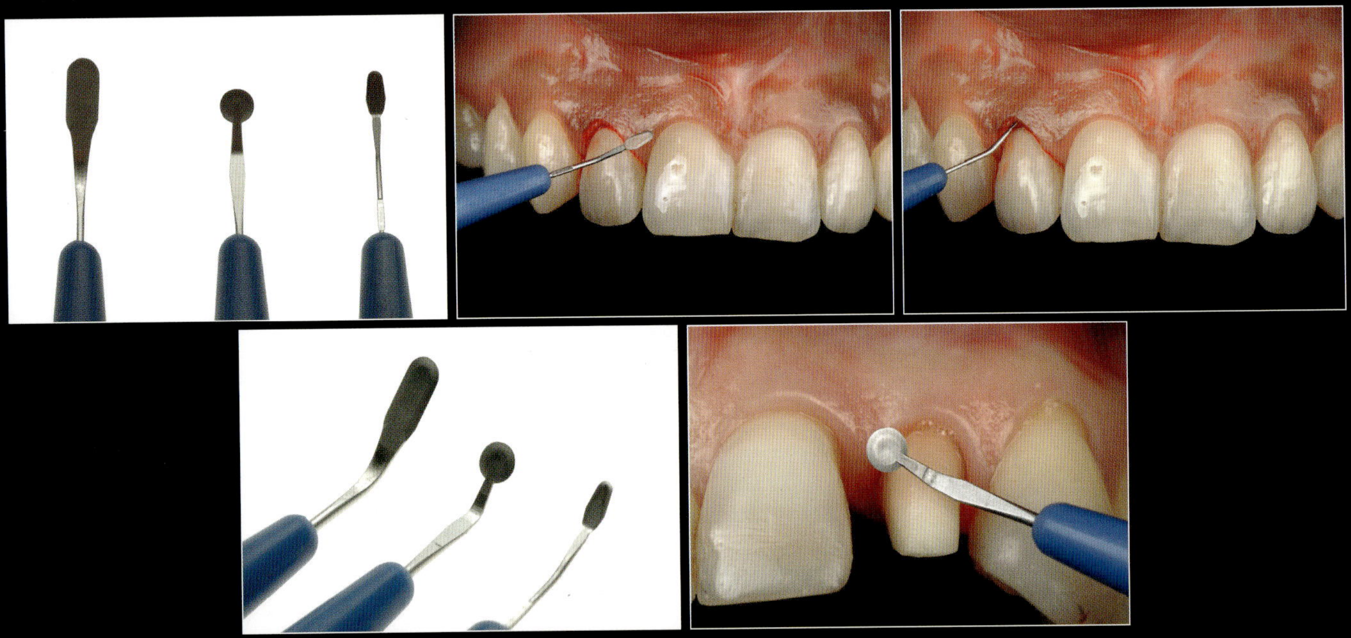

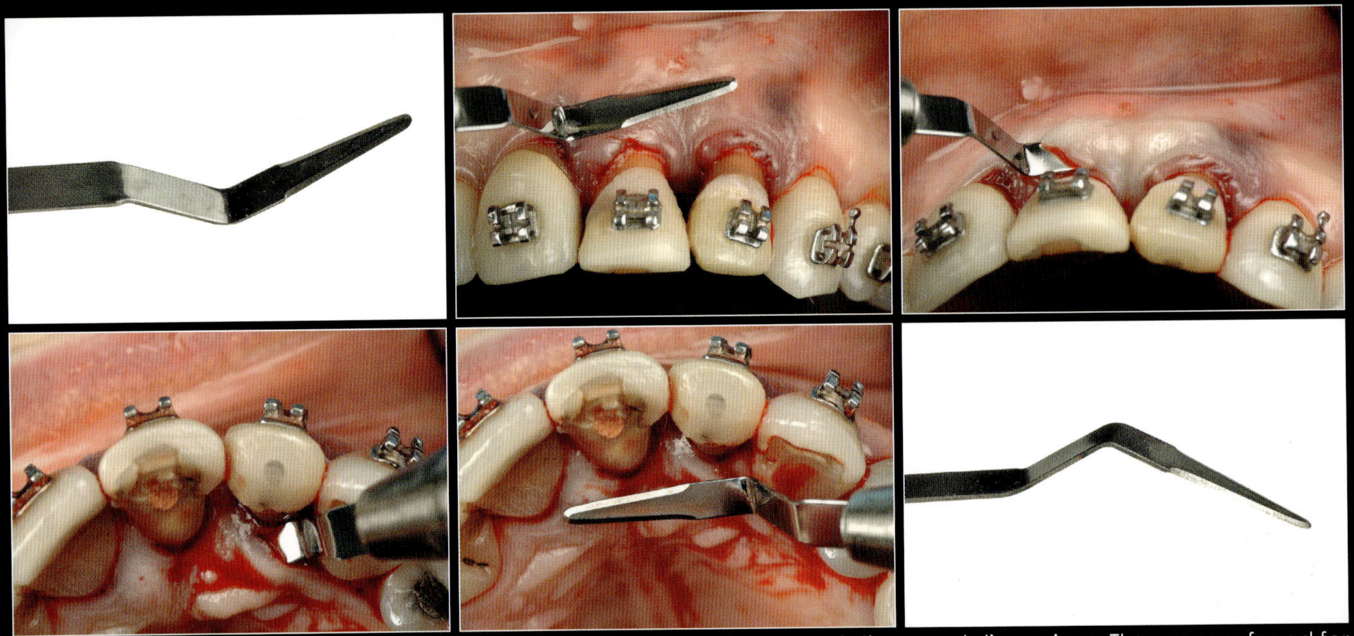

Angulated pointed blades are available in a variety of configurations, angulations, and dimensions. They are preferred for slightly more forceful cuts, such as elevating papillae from the palatal aspect. A shortcoming of this particular knife is the long cutting edge, which easily perforates the tissues during rotational movements. It is quite simple, however, to customize and modify the length of the cutting edges chairside with rotating instruments. The incorporated angulation makes this the preferred knife for palatal CTG harvesting.

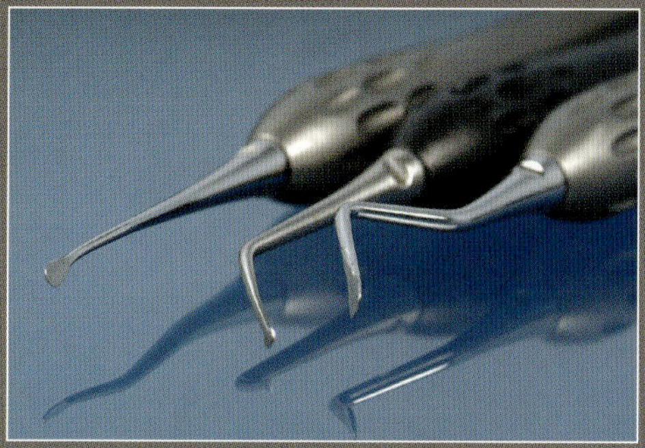

These hand instruments (mamadent Macro tunneling instruments Nos. 1, 2, and 3; American Dental Systems) are ideal as spatulas or elevators for creating pressure for tissue elevation after dissection of the partial-thickness flaps. They have two different degrees of angulation and a relatively straight design. Their cutting ability, however, is limited, unless they are sharpened before the surgery.

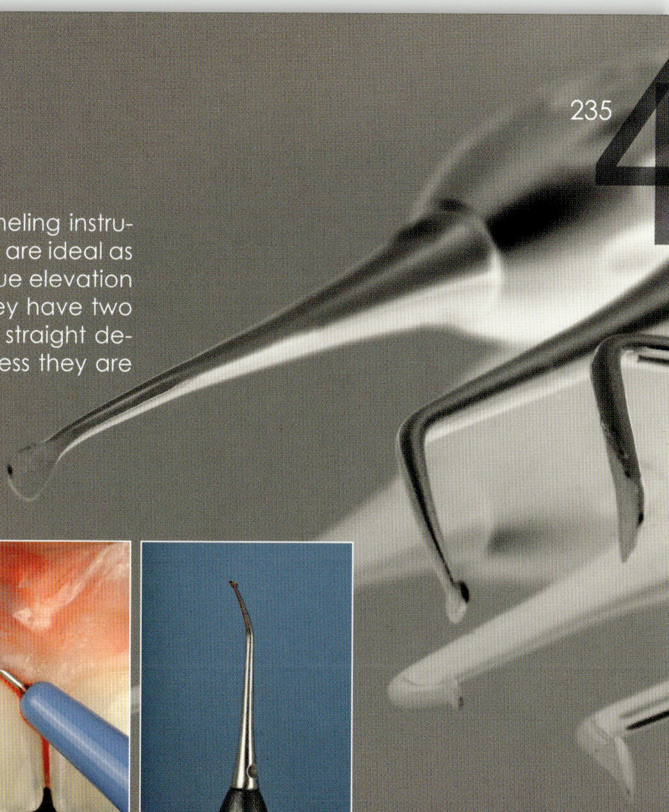

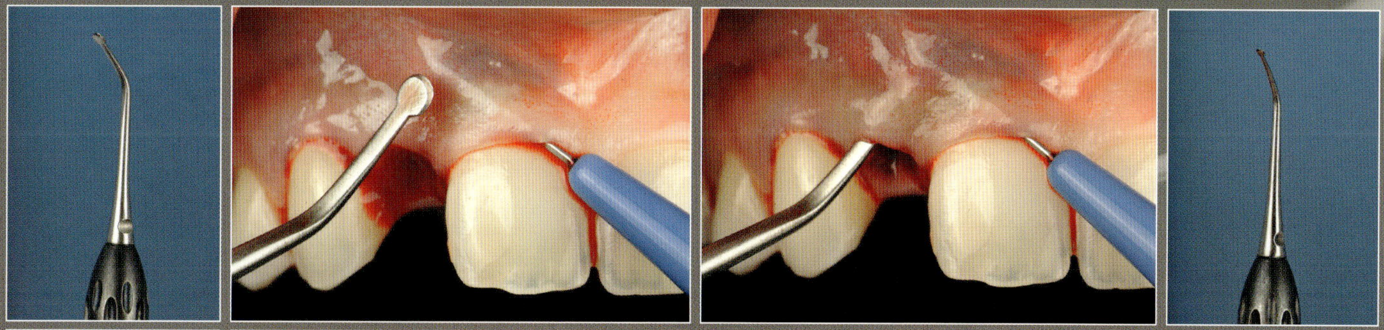

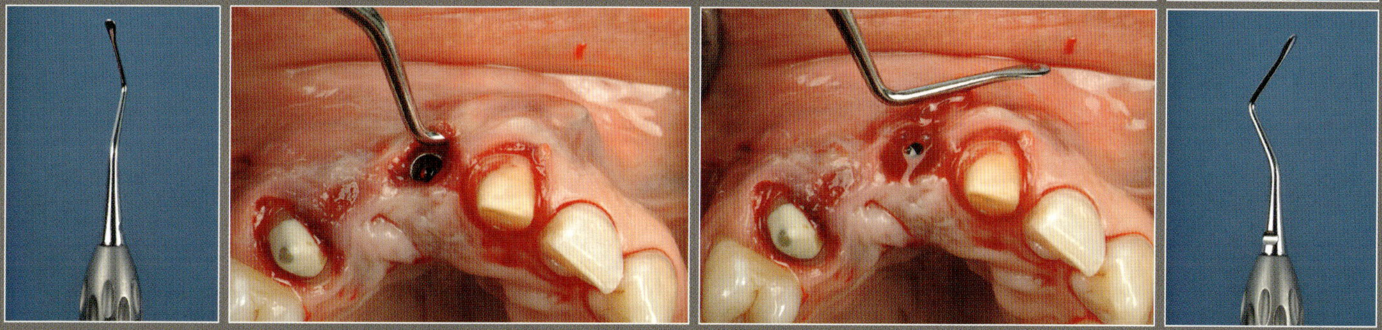

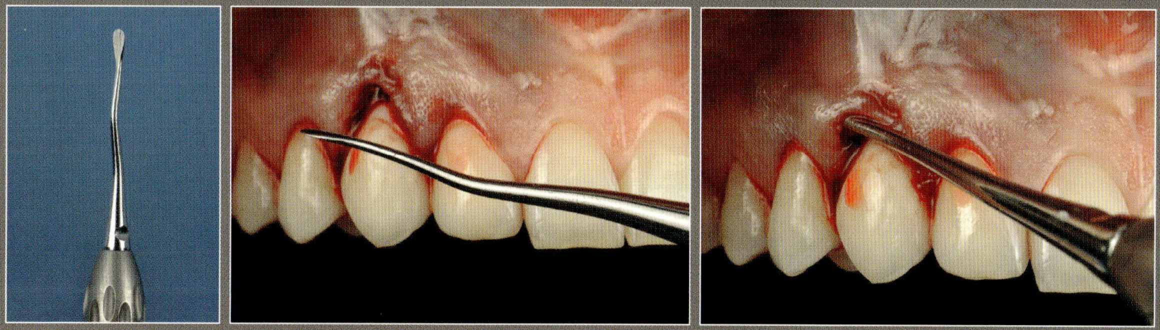

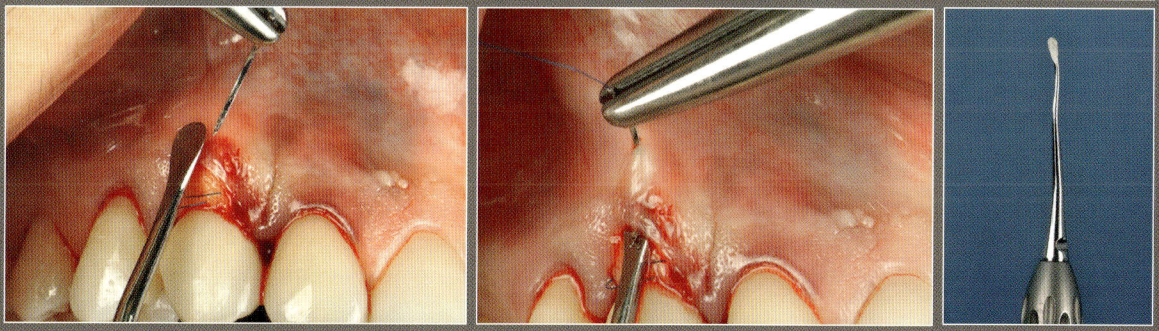

The initial incision and preparation should be made with a microblade while these elevators are used as tunneling instruments. They are also useful to protect the base of the CTG during suturing. The straight No. 3 instrument penetrates deep into partial-thickness flaps and, due to its limited angulation, provides control even in the presence of buccal concavities in the maxillary bone.

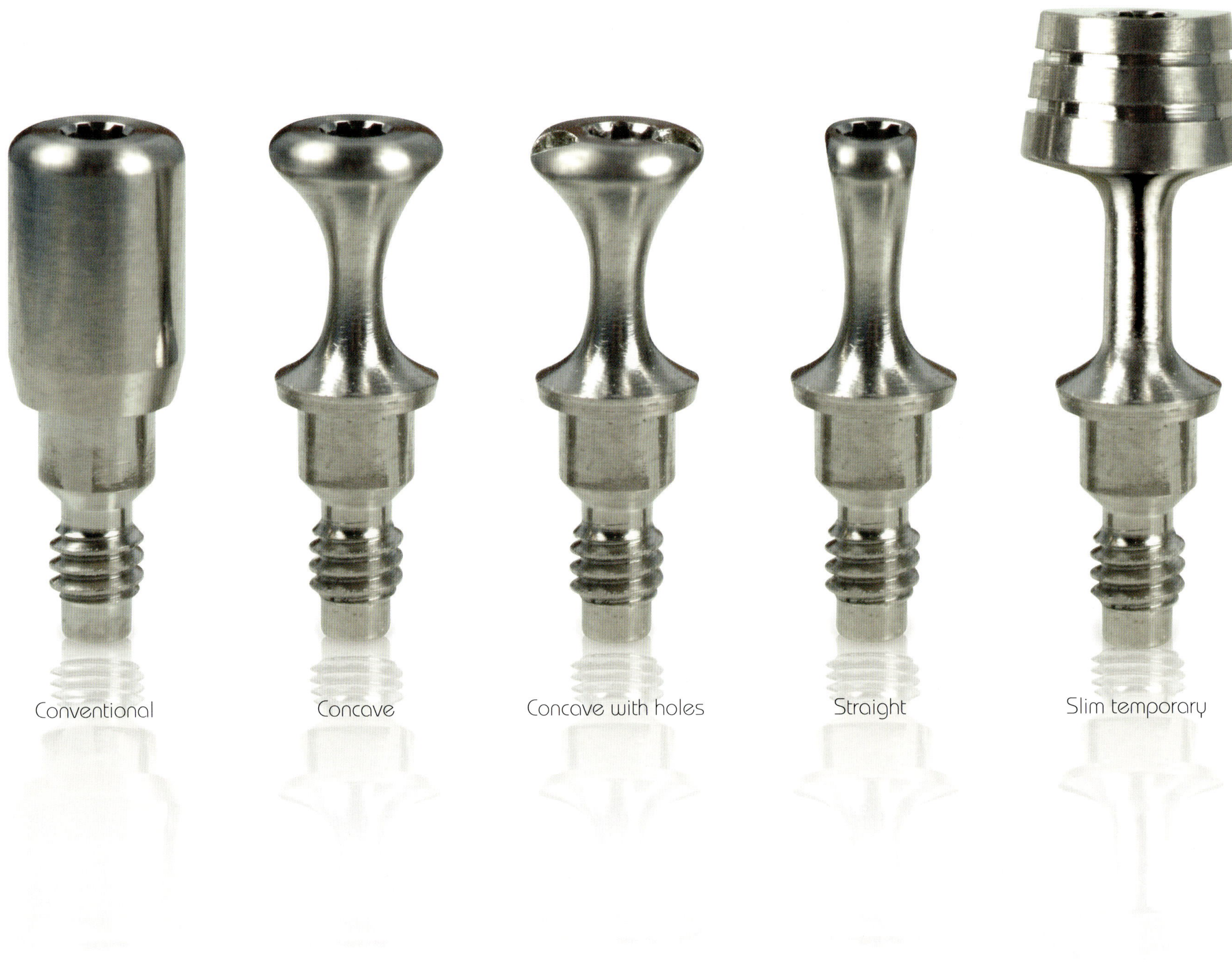

Conventional Concave Concave with holes Straight Slim temporary

Healing abutment design

The healing abutment is a critical component for peri-implant soft tissue manipulation. Today, two important design aspects must be considered: *(1)* Healing abutment height should serve as a reference for coronal displacement of the soft tissue flap, and *(2)* the diameter of the healing abutment should provide extra space for a CTG. In the early 1990s, wider-diameter healing abutments were recommended to shape the desired emergence profile from day 1, with the theory to create an ideal tissue topography for the definitive crowns and effortless results immediately after implant placement. In the meantime, it was learned that, while possibly successful in select patients with a thick soft tissue biotype, this concept does not provide the desired outcomes in the majority of patients and certainly not in the esthetic zone. Wide-diameter healing abutments do not allow coronal positioning of a CTG. However, this is the area where a graft is usually needed the most to hide the implant-abutment-crown interface and create the required tissue volume.

The two main problems with wide-diameter healing abutments are: *(1)* They create a recession from the day of the surgery even with a CTG, and *(2)* the thickness of tissue created is usually level to or below the implant head. It is very difficult for the surgeon to place a thick CTG in a most coronal position and passively reposition the soft tissue flap over the graft and the wide-diameter healing abutment. Therefore, it is recommended to always select a healing abutment that has the same or a smaller diameter than the respective implant or modify it through grinding. Current knowledge and trends suggest placement of a CTG for any implant treatment, especially in the anterior maxilla and regardless of the patient's soft tissue biotype. The goal is to place a thick and dense CTG, harvested preferably from the maxillary tuberosity at the time of implant insertion. A small-diameter healing abutment provides the necessary 3D space for the CTG and passive wound closure.

The healing abutment must be tall enough, at least 5 mm, depending on the location and depth of the implant shoulder, which is usually placed about 3 mm below the free gingival margin of the prospective tooth. It is key to create a soft tissue level that is coronal to the gingival margin of the adjacent tooth to counteract future soft tissue recessions, which usually occur after prosthetic connection of the abutment and crown. The diameter of the healing abutment should be as small as possible.

These considerations paired with the quest for clinical simplicity led to the development and experimental use of four prototypes of small-diameter healing abutments with the following designs and features:

1. Concave
2. Concave with holes
3. Straight
4. Slim temporary

Concave

While many clinicians have discussed and recommended concave healing abutments, manufacturers have shown only limited interest. In those discussions, the importance of the height of the healing abutment as a surgical reference has been largely ignored but was implemented by the authors in the design of this prototype abutment. Another key aspect is the diameter of the concave healing abutment at its most coronal aspect in relation to the diameter of the pre-existing tooth. The idea was to create a wider platform with a toothlike diameter at the top of the abutment to protect, like an umbrella, the soft tissue flap and CTG underneath. A shortcoming of this design is that when the implant shoulder is positioned deeper than 3 mm below the free gingival margin of the prospective tooth, the coronal part of the concave healing abutment may be located too deep and has to be covered with the flap, which may present a challenge due to its width.

This patient presented with agenesis of the maxillary right lateral incisor. Orthodontic treatment was performed to widen the space for implant placement. An anatomical incision was selected due to the leveled papilla. A circular incision was made with the smallest circular blade available at that time (2 mm). A partial-thickness flap was then elevated with a sulcular incision to visualize the bone defect and the tissue volume to be recreated.

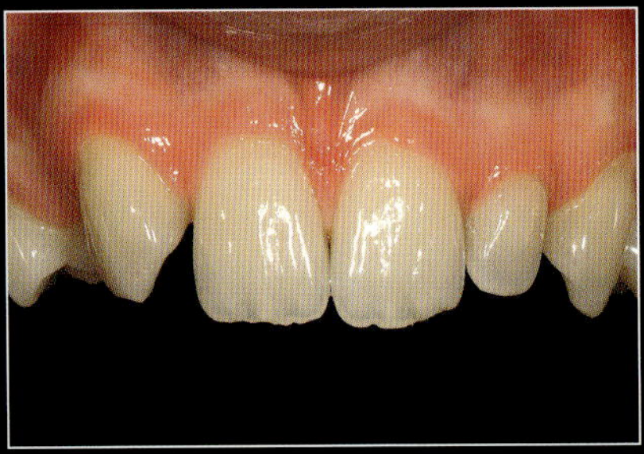
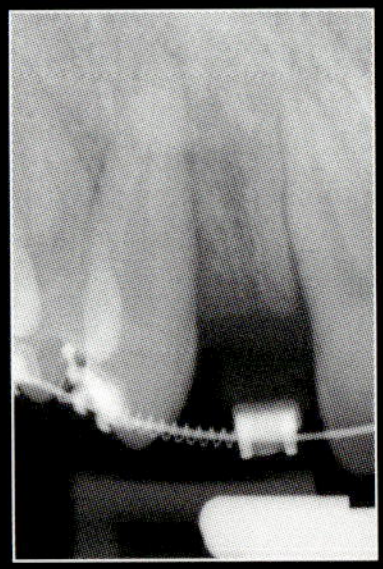
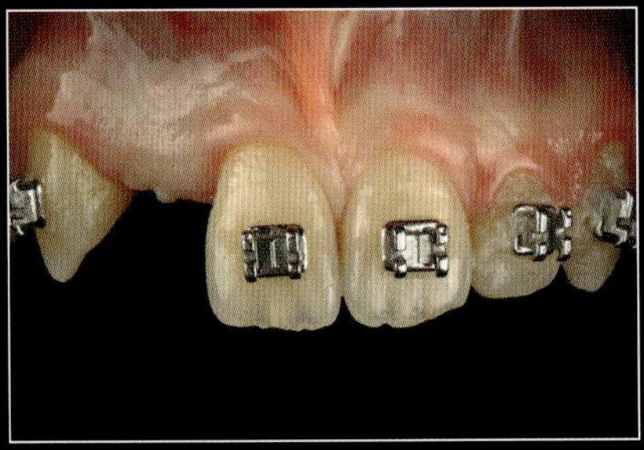
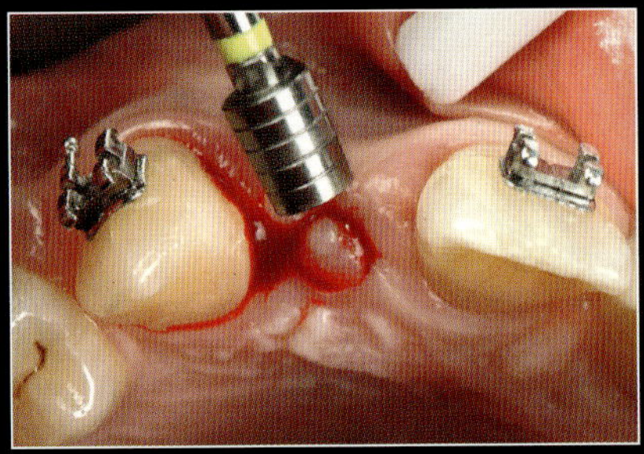
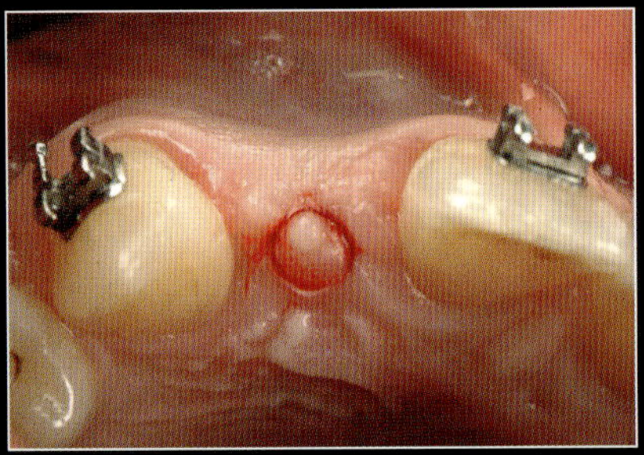
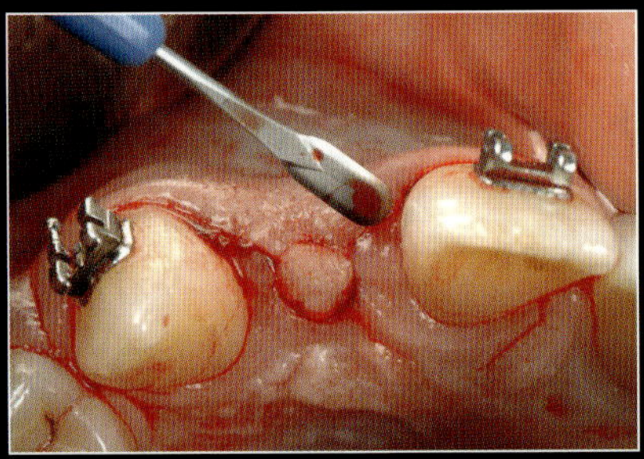

Orthodontist: Dr Domingo Martín

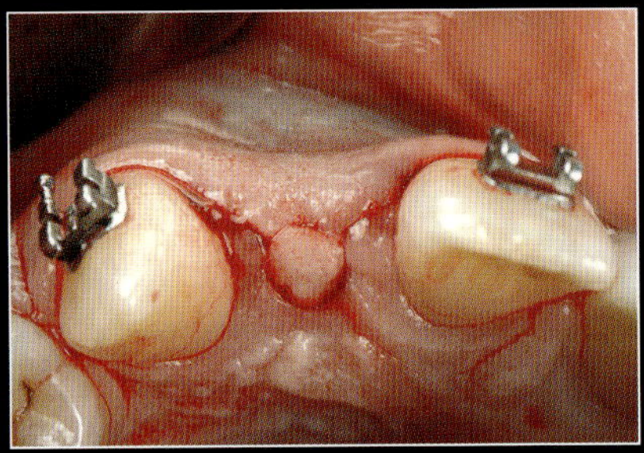
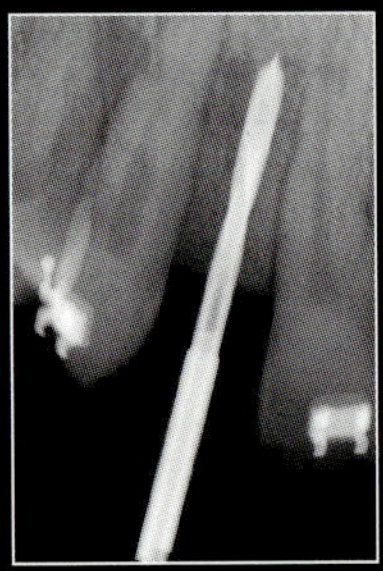
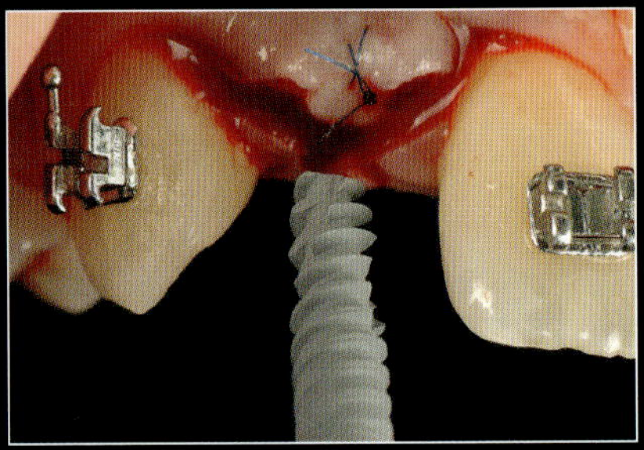
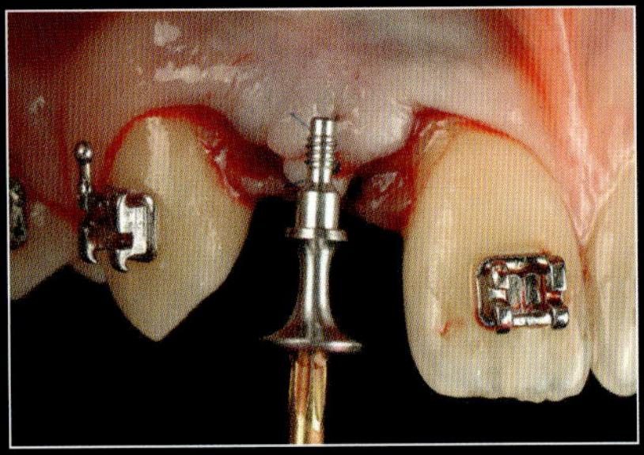
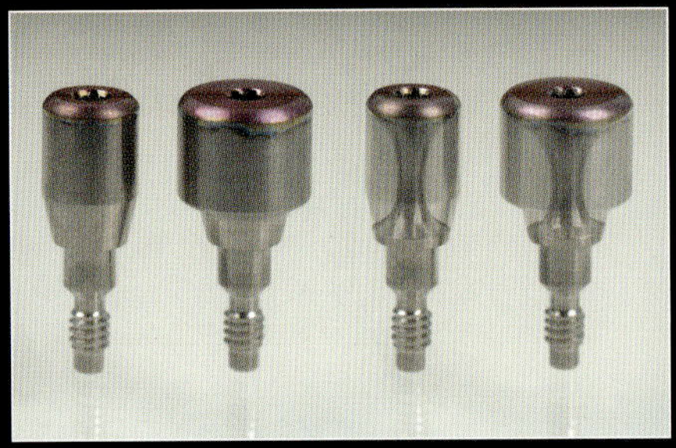
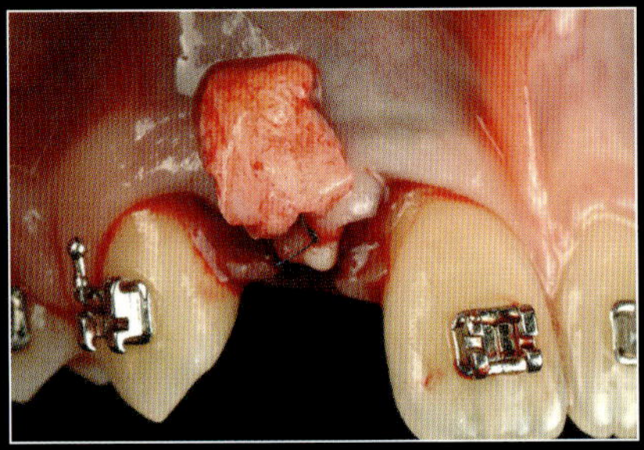

Once the flap was elevated coronally above the mucogingival line and laterally one tooth's width on either side of the edentulous site, a NobelActive NP 3.5 × 13–mm implant was placed. A radiograph was taken during the ostectomy to verify the correct positioning of the implant. A CTG was harvested from the tuberosity and tried into place to increase the buccal as well as the interproximal volume. A concave healing abutment with a wider coronal platform was selected to match the diameter of the tooth to be replaced and to protect the underlying CTG.

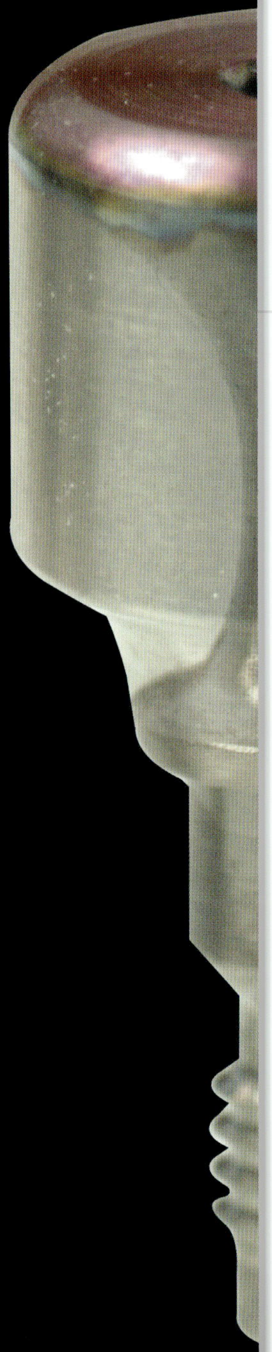

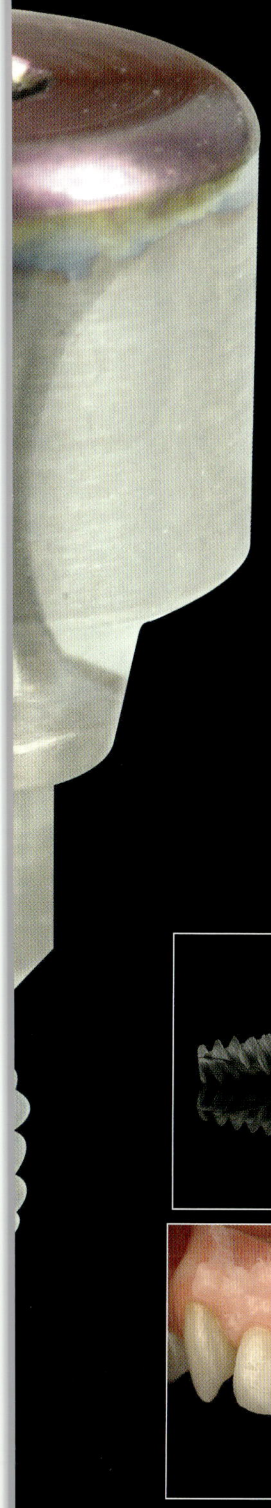

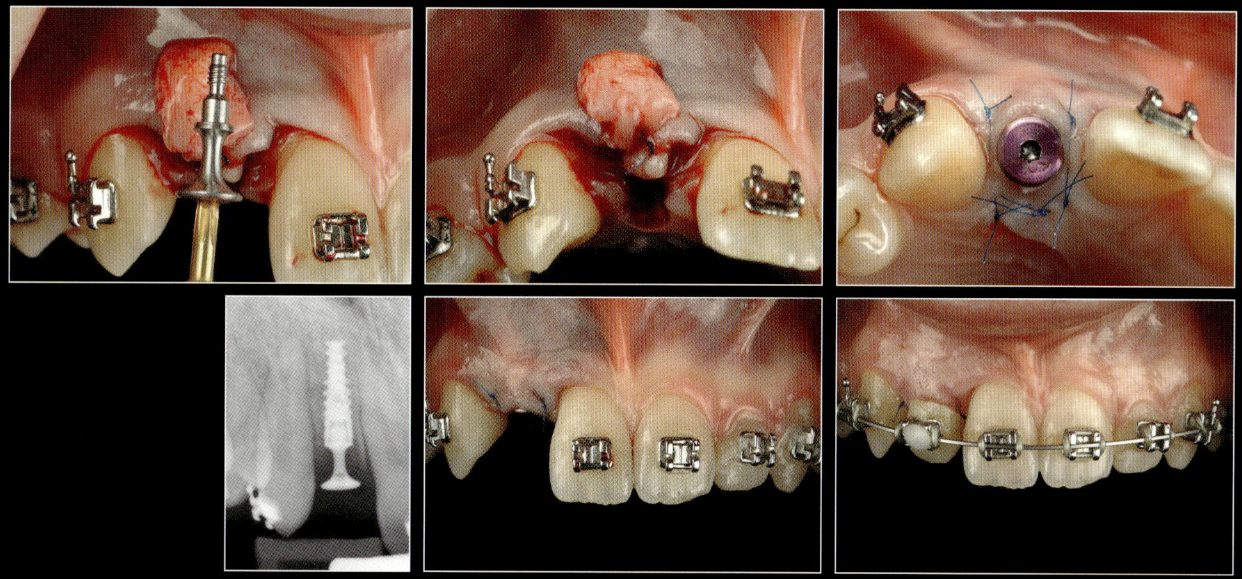

To ensure adequate flap closure, the interproximal papillae were elevated with a partial-thickness flap. This also created the space for the desired interproximal graft and the best transition from the buccal flap to the elevated interproximal palatal tissue. An incision in the middle of the CTG allowed its winglike placement at the narrow part of the concave healing abutment and positioning underneath the elevated papillae to increase their volume. First, the CTG was sutured to the palatal flap and secured into the desired position. Then, the flap was sutured over it and adapted. A periapical radiograph was taken to verify the correct connection of the healing abutment. Care was taken to avoid any contact of the provisional restoration with the grafted site. The gained volume is noticeable 6 months postoperatively. An impression was made to fabricate the definitive zirconia abutment and provisional crown restoration. Another radiograph confirmed the correct position of the zirconia abutment and successful excess cement removal.

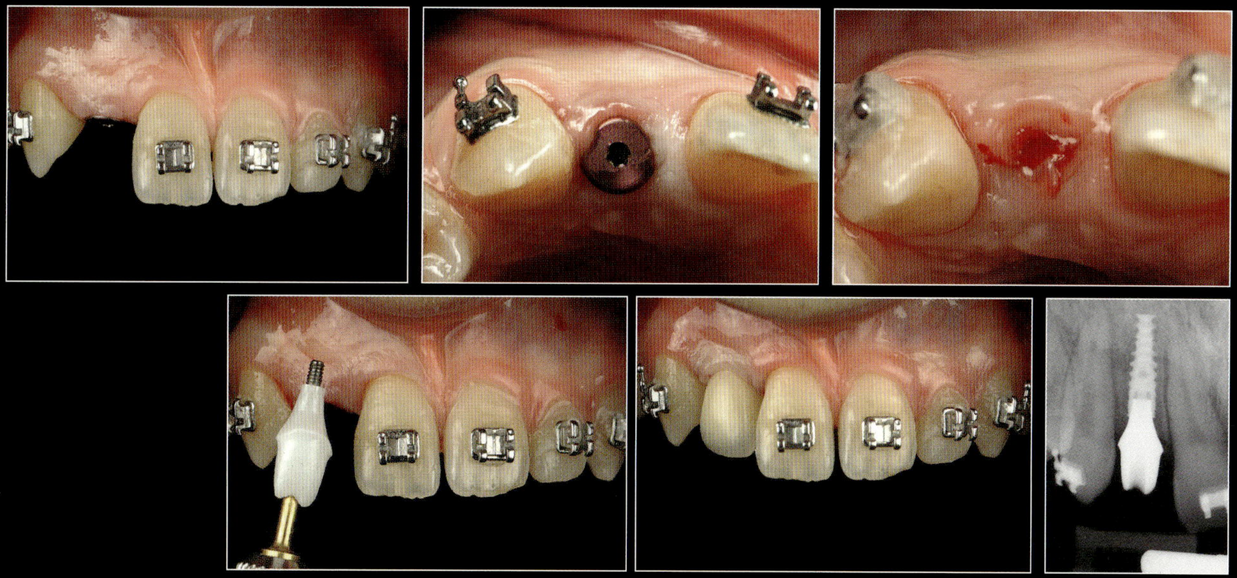

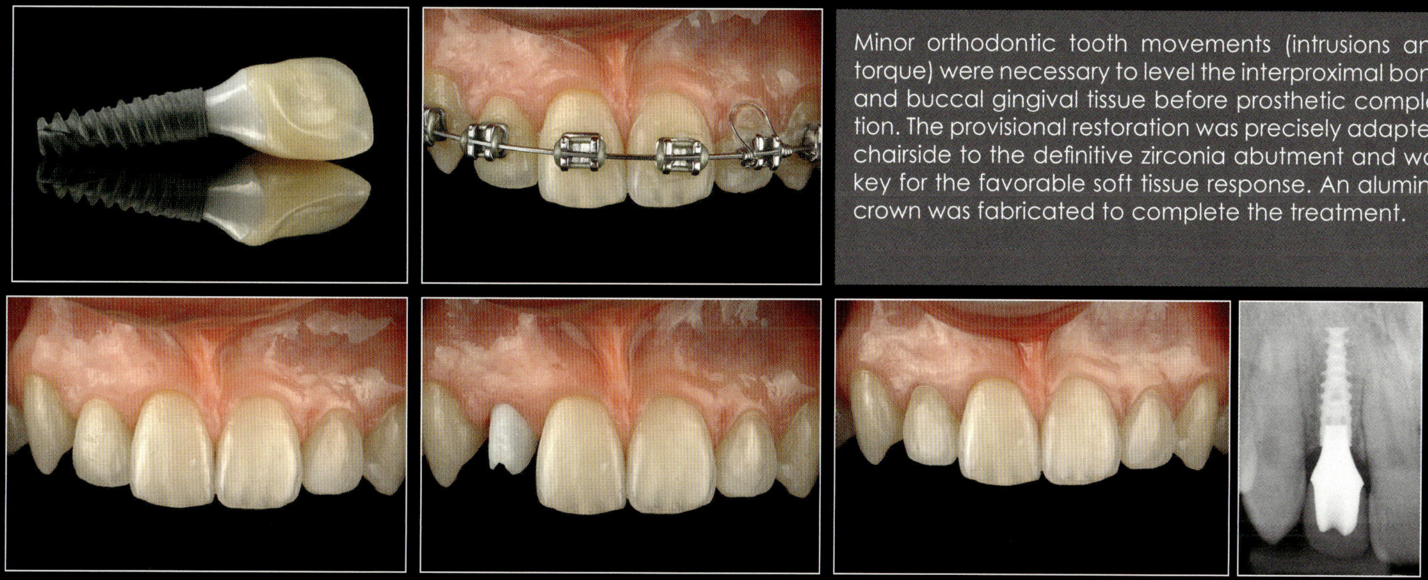

Minor orthodontic tooth movements (intrusions and torque) were necessary to level the interproximal bone and buccal gingival tissue before prosthetic completion. The provisional restoration was precisely adapted chairside to the definitive zirconia abutment and was key for the favorable soft tissue response. An alumina crown was fabricated to complete the treatment.

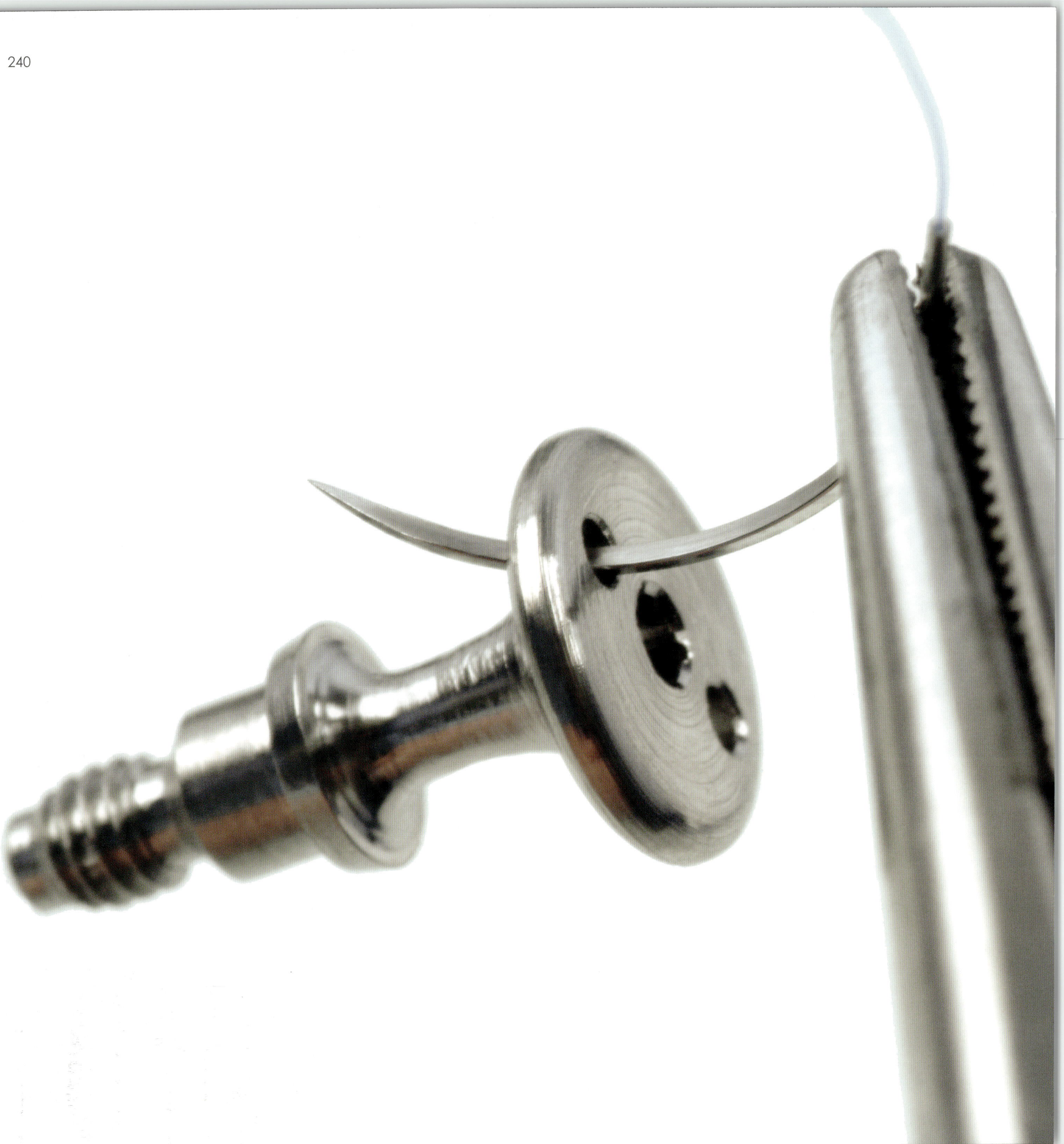

Concave with holes

This novel abutment features small holes to suture the CTG to the coronal abutment platform and secure it into position. The reflected flap must be released horizontally and vertically to allow coverage without tension. The main goal is to create an abundance of soft tissue with greater 3D volume than ultimately needed in the desired location. Different coronal diameters have been fabricated to address the different tooth diameters to be restored. As with the concave healing abutment, the coronal platform provides protection for the CTG while the holes offer stable anchorage for the sutures to secure the CTG in position. Clinical outcomes with this abutment are similar to those with the concave healing abutment. However, threading the sutures through those holes may be challenging. The needle size must be small enough to rotate in a small area with a maximum length of 7 mm and a suture size of 6-0 or smaller. This becomes increasingly difficult when the implant is placed deeper than ideal.

While this concept makes a lot of sense, it is difficult to use in a clinical setting with limited space.

This patient presented with a maxillary left lateral incisor requiring extraction due to periapical and periodontal pathologies. No additional surgery was performed on the day of the extraction. A composite restoration was bonded to the adjacent teeth for the duration of the healing period. Note the different diameters of the holes in the coronal platforms of the healing abutments.

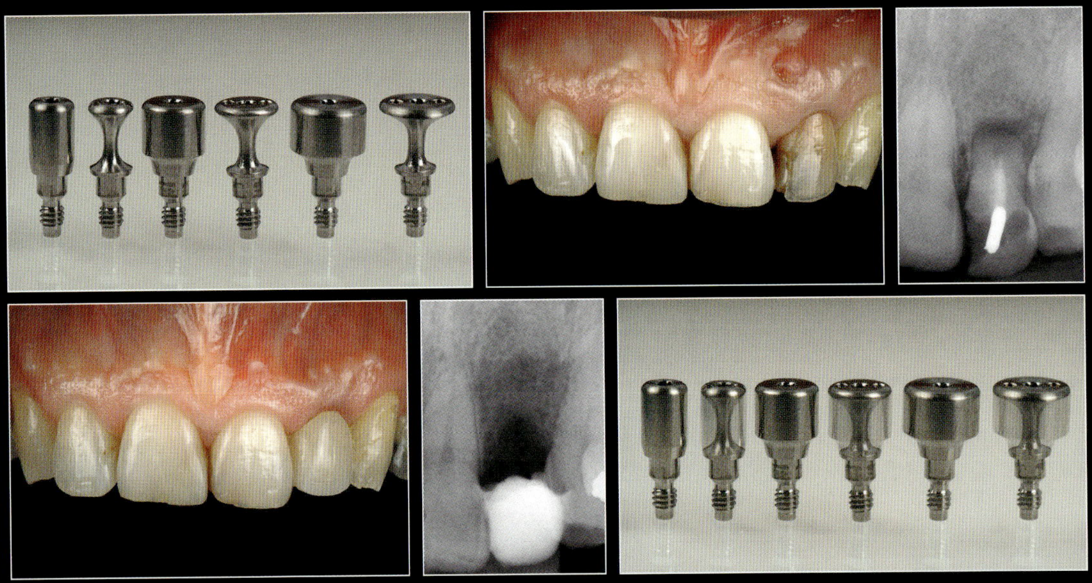

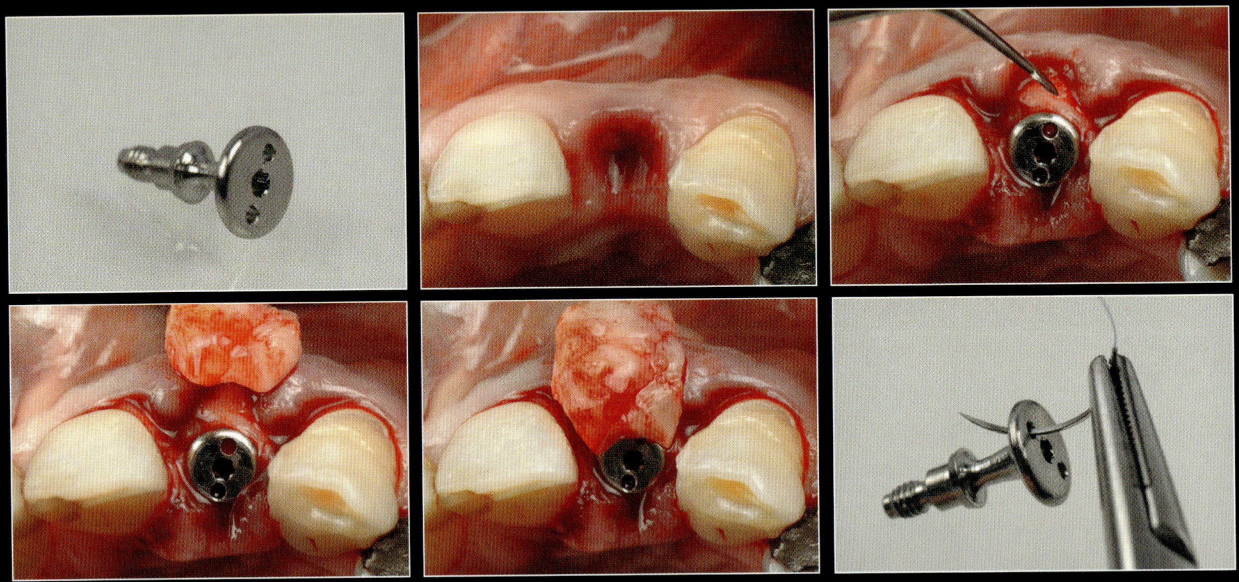

An implant (NobelActive NP 3.5 × 13 mm) was placed together with a concave healing abutment with holes 3 months after the extraction. A straight incision was prepared for visual access to the interproximal and labial defect. A CTG was harvested from the tuberosity and adapted to the site to increase the 3D soft tissue volume. An incision was made in the center of the CTG to position the created wings in a manner to gain as much interproximal volume as possible. Once in the desired position, the graft was secured in place by suturing it to the abutment holes.

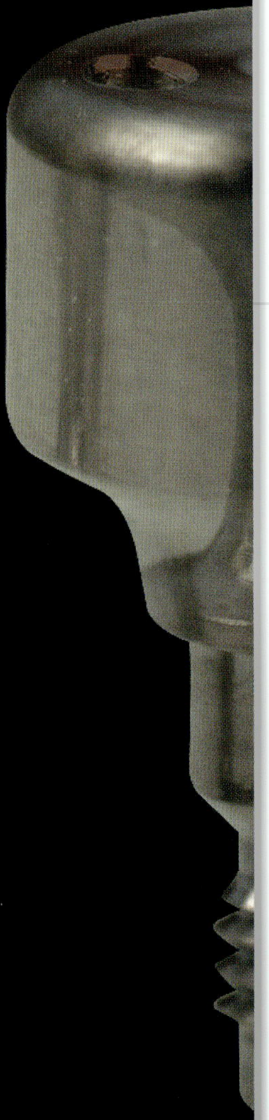

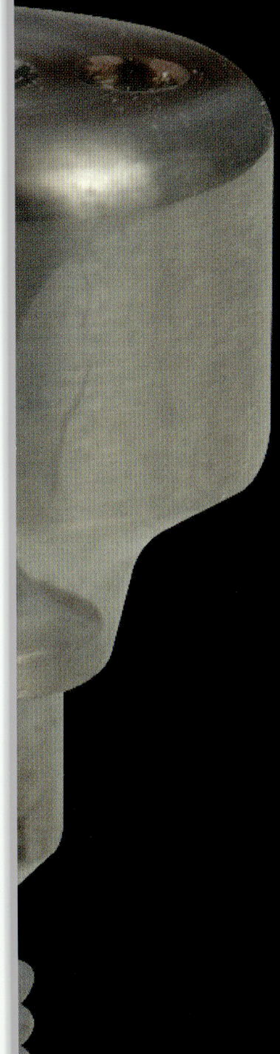

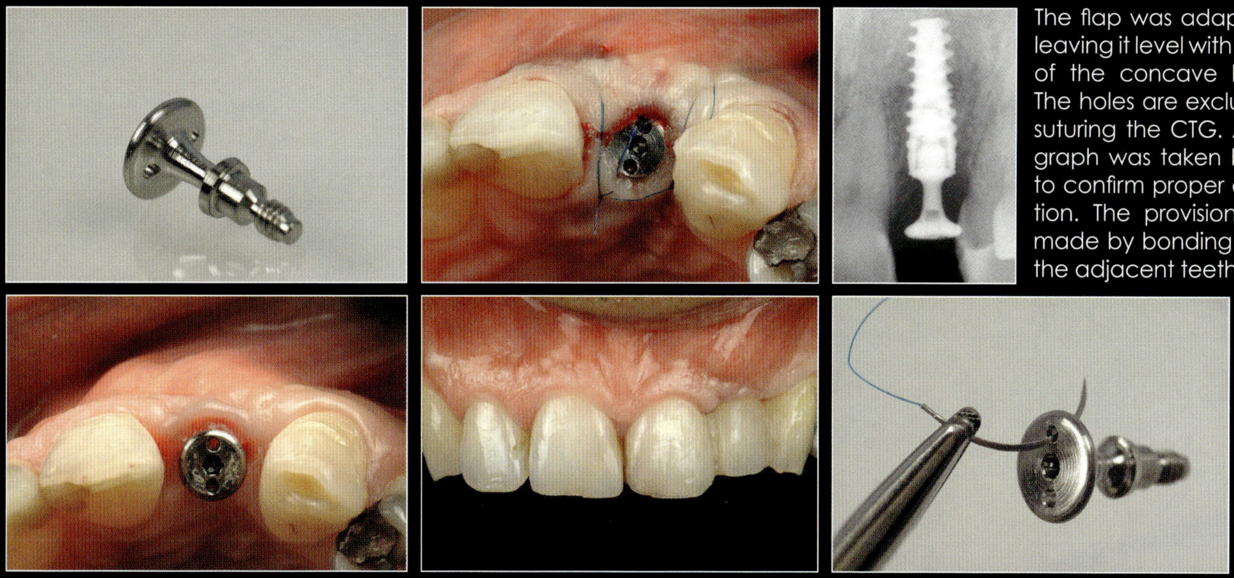

The flap was adapted over the CTG, leaving it level with the coronal aspect of the concave healing abutment. The holes are exclusively intended for suturing the CTG. A periapical radiograph was taken before the suturing to confirm proper abutment connection. The provisional restoration was made by bonding composite resin to the adjacent teeth.

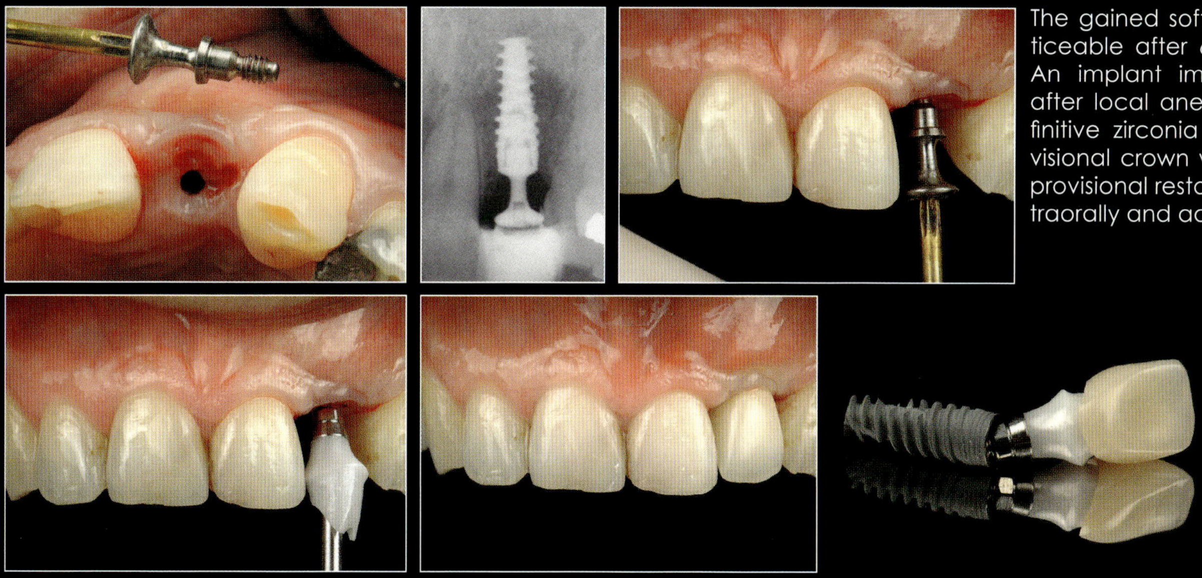

The gained soft tissue volume is noticeable after 6 months of healing. An implant impression was made after local anesthesia, and the definitive zirconia abutment and provisional crown were fabricated. The provisional restoration was relined intraorally and adjusted chairside.

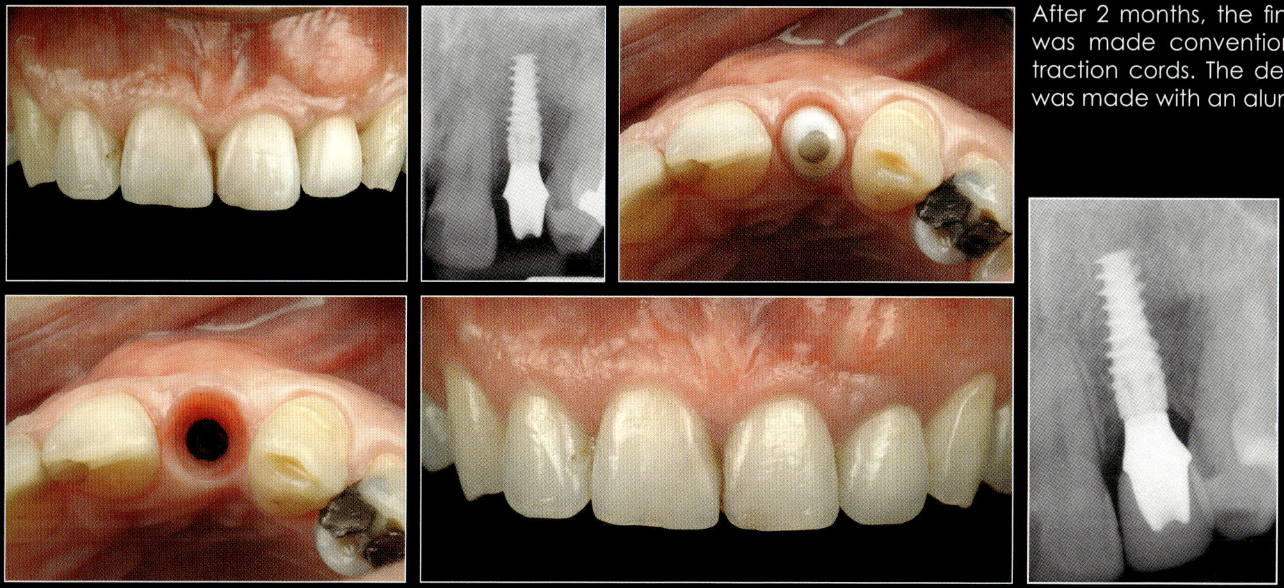

After 2 months, the final impression was made conventionally with retraction cords. The definitive crown was made with an alumina coping.

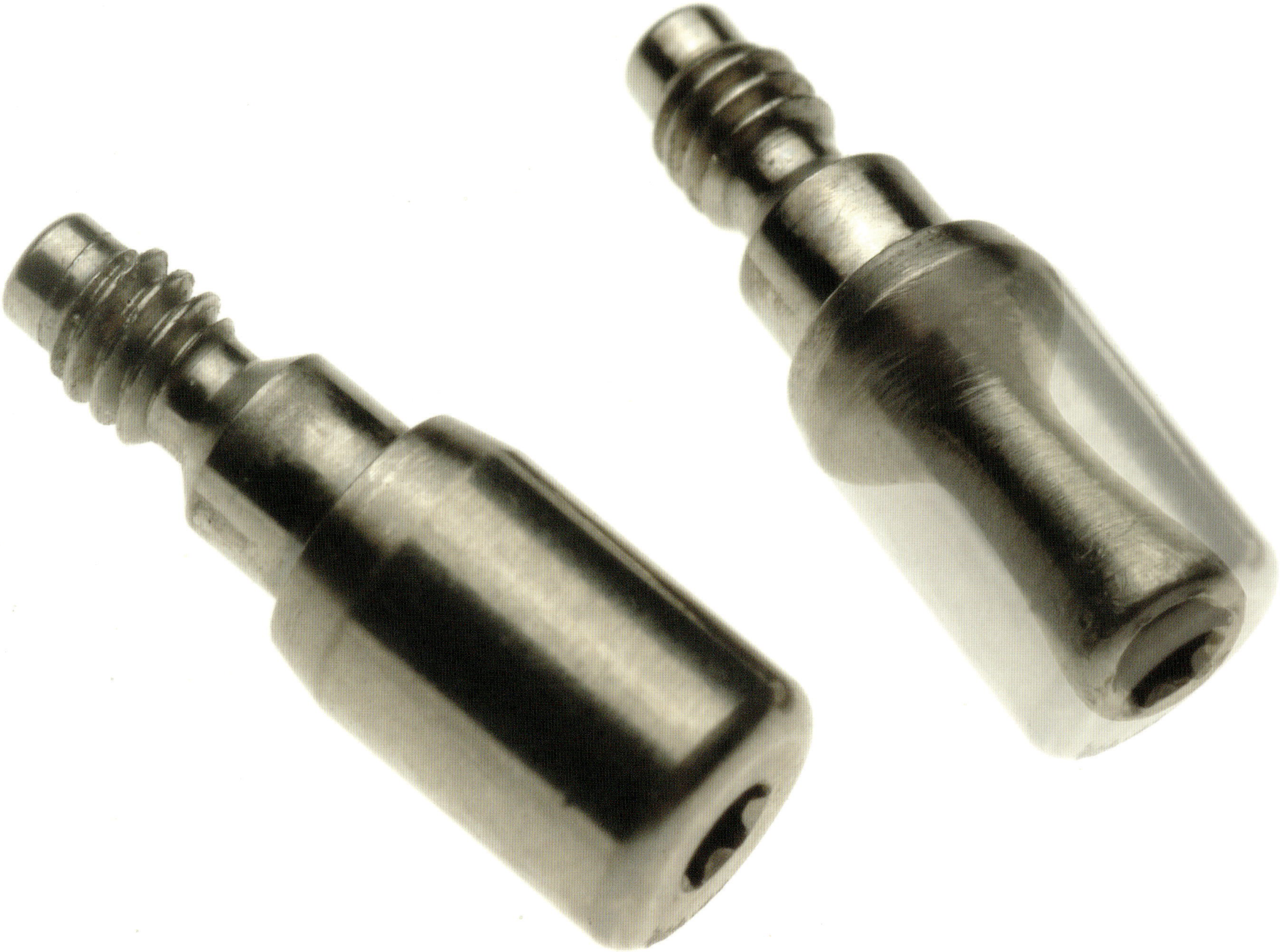

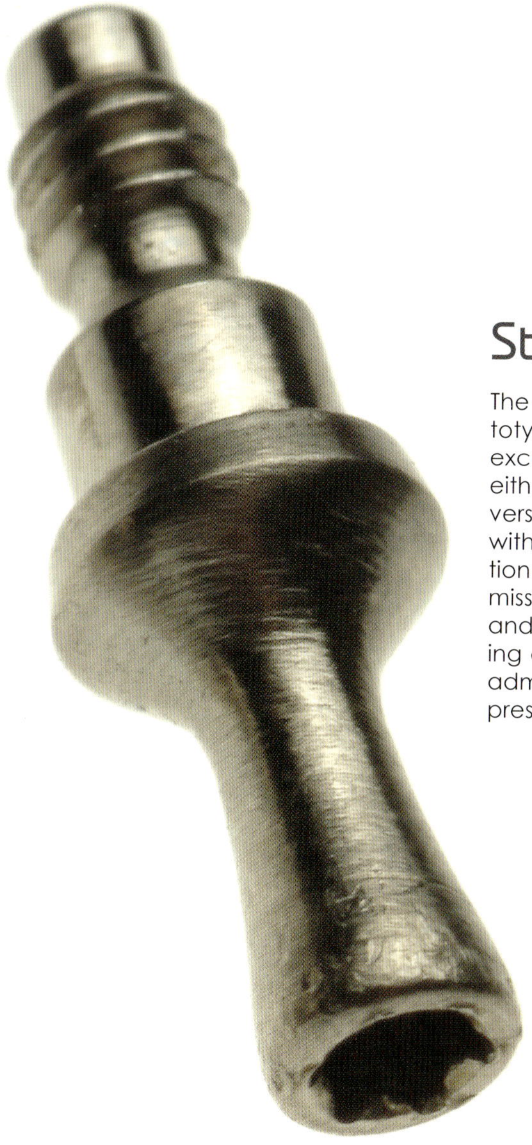

Straight

The straight healing abutment is perhaps the most attractive of the prototypes. It is the most versatile, easy to use, and allows for large CTGs and excellent flap closure. This simplistic healing abutment is 1.2 mm wide and either 5 or 7 mm long, depending on the depth of the implant. It can be universally applied and allows the clinician to easily close any flap with a CTG without the healing abutment being an obstacle and with direct visualization of the initial incision. If there is enough bone to place an implant, any missing soft tissue volume is compensated with a CTG from the tuberosity, and a straight healing abutment is placed for ideal and simple positioning of the CTG. The only shortcoming of this design is the possible need to administer local anesthesia whenever wider-diameter components (eg, impression copings or abutments) that may exert painful pressure are inserted.

This patient underwent extraction of the mandibular left lateral incisor. The procedure caused a substantial bone defect as demonstrated in the periapical radiographs taken 1 week and 3 months postoperatively. Note the large cleft-type bone defect in the middle of the ridge buccally and palatally as well as the excellent interproximal volume and height. CBCT revealed adequate bony support for implant placement without the need for bone grafting. The objective was to restore the defective buccal and palatal ridge volume with a CTG from the tuberosity and a properly positioned flap with the help of a straight healing abutment.

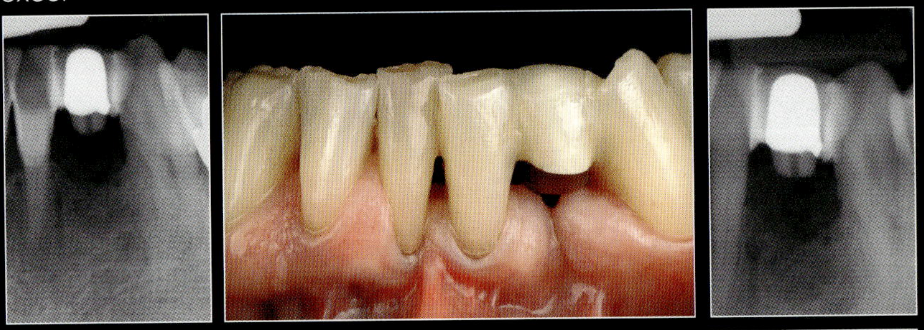

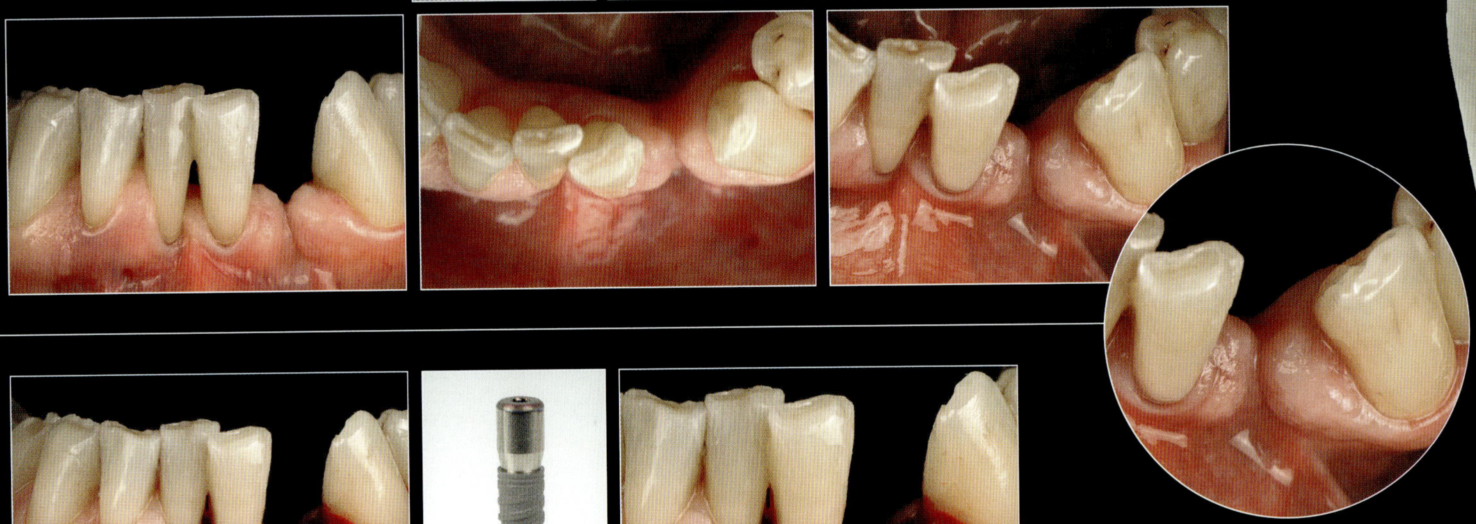

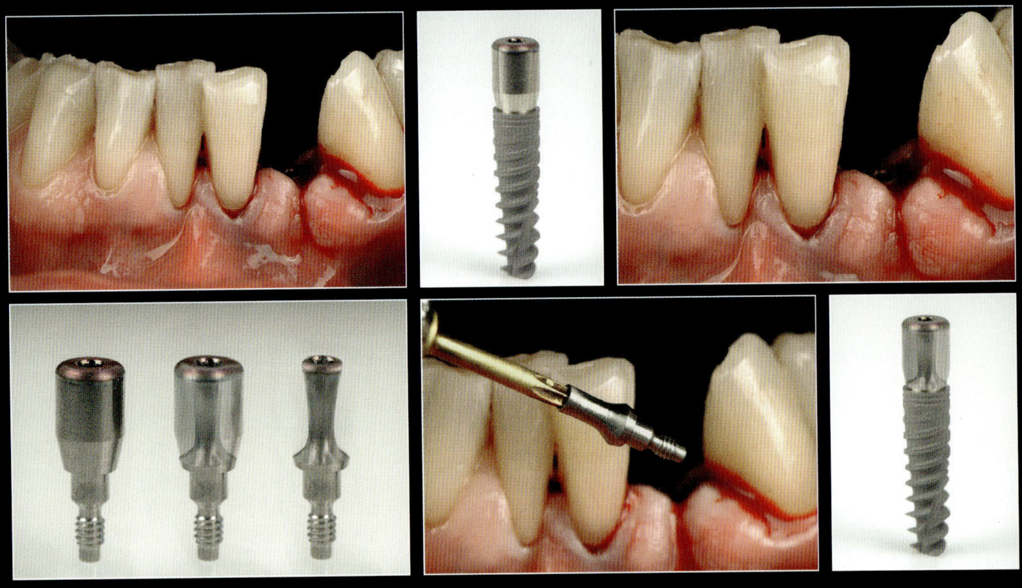

A straight crestal incision was made at ridge level, followed by a sulcular incision up to the distal aspect of the canine and mesially to the central incisor. A partial-thickness flap was elevated to expose the defect for optimal implant placement. The contralateral papillae adjacent to the defect were elevated to allow horizontal mobility of the flap above the MGJ and vertical elevation to allow flap closure over the CTG. A NobelActive NP 3.5 × 13–mm implant was placed together with a straight healing abutment.

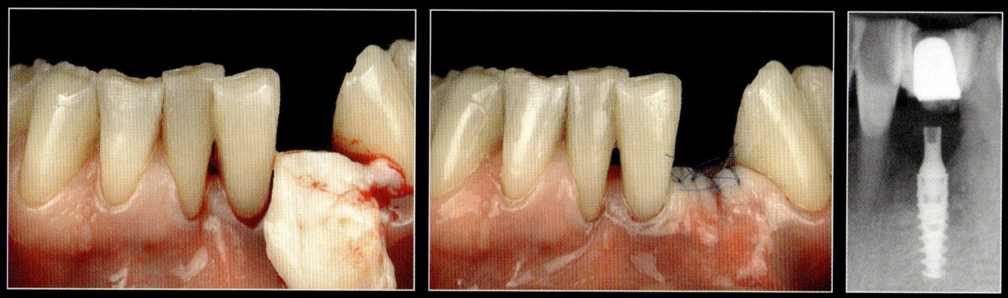

The CTG from the tuberosity was tried on top of the defect and adjusted as needed. An incision was made at the center of the graft at the position of the straight healing abutment. The graft was sutured in place with a buccal and palatal suture placed as apically as possible, and the flap was sutured over the CTG, leaving the small screw access hole of the healing abutment exposed to the oral cavity. Note the tissue volume 6 months later.

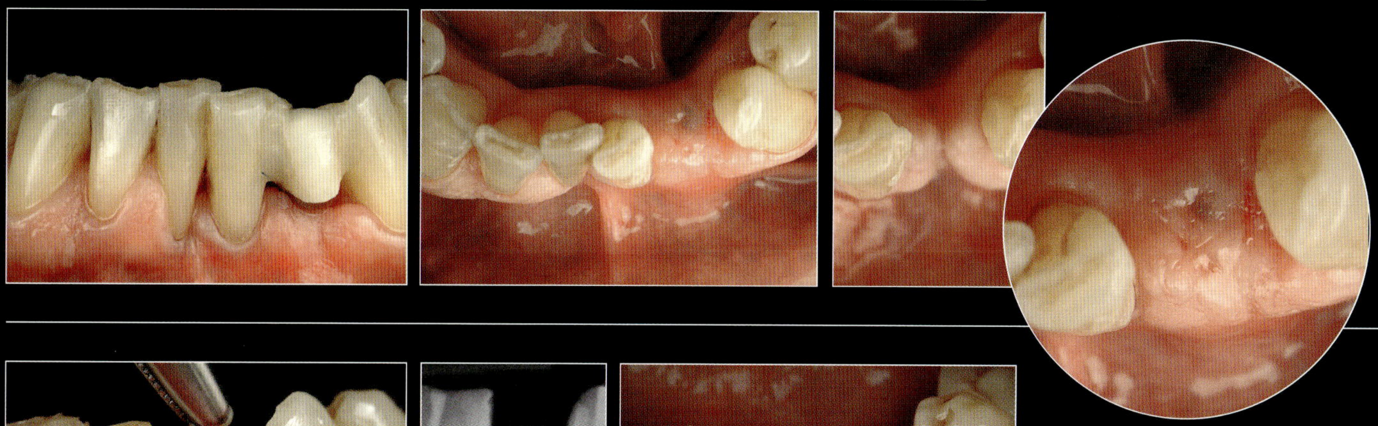

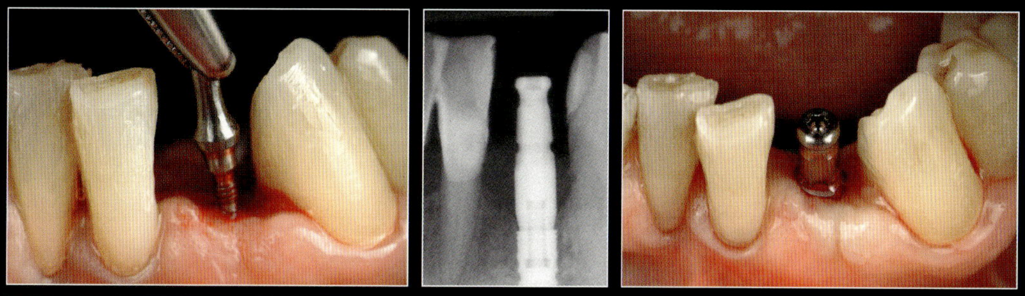

A small incision was necessary to reach the top of the healing abutment. An impression was made to fabricate the definitive zirconia abutment and provisional crown. The zirconia abutment was designed with the exact diameter of the adjacent tooth based on the diagnostic wax-up. It had a concave shape below the finishing line to accommodate the increased soft tissue. Blanching and even slight tissue resorption are not concerning due to the volume and quality of the graft.

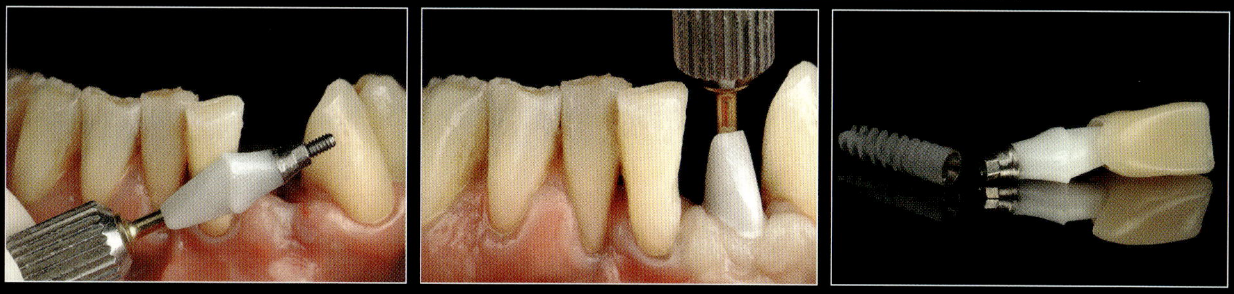

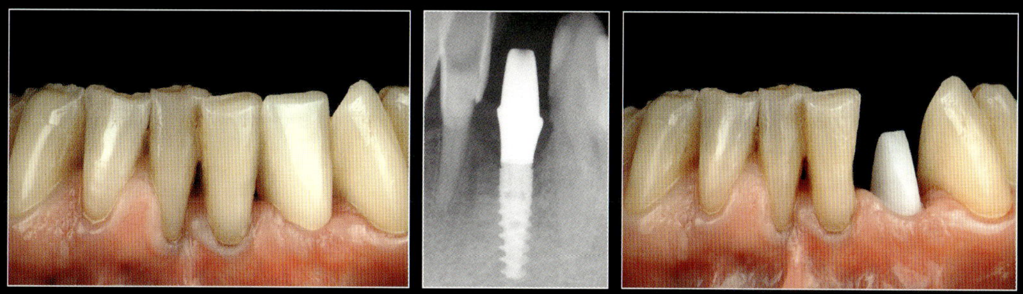

Situation 3 months postoperatively. Proper seating of the definitive alumina crown was verified with a periapical radiograph.

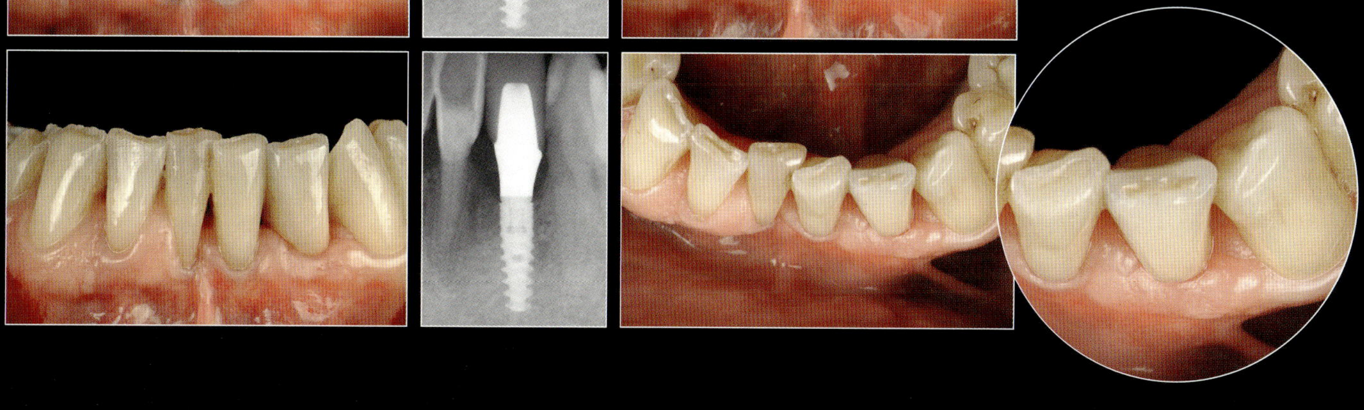

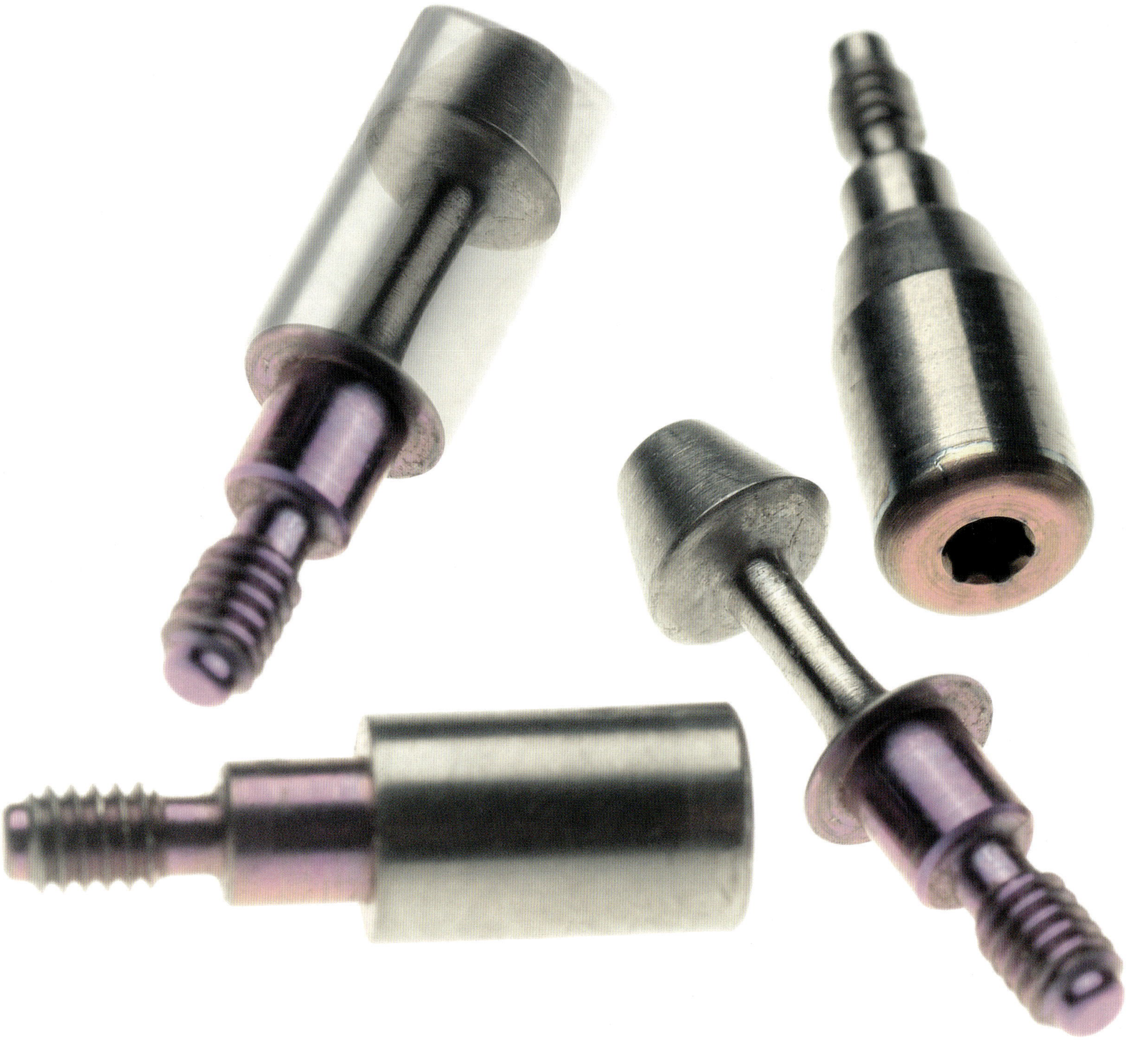

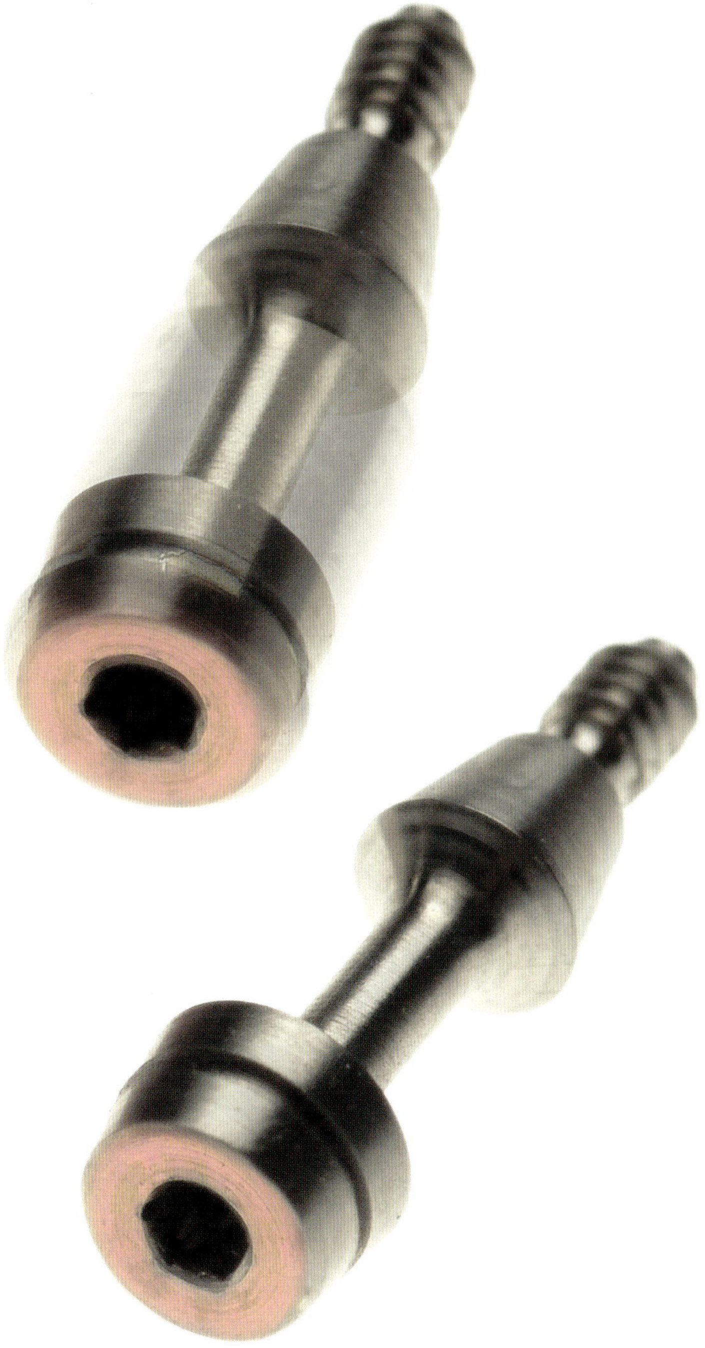

Slim temporary

The slim temporary healing abutment is an evolution of the straight healing abutment. It offers the ability to place a tissue graft around the implant in a coronal position and primary flap closure. In addition, it provides support for an immediate fixed provisional restoration or accommodates a restoration bonded to the adjacent teeth. The option of a fixed immediate prosthetic solution is a great advantage for the patient but also means that vertical loading of the grafted tissue during the healing phase can be avoided.

The prerequisites for the slim temporary healing abutment include: *(1)* ideal implant placement in respect to depth and angulation, which may affect the position of the abutment and the interocclusal space for crown relining, and *(2)* high primary implant stability with a minimum torque of 35 Ncm to allow for immediate provisionalization. One of the shortcomings of the slim temporary abutment, mainly used in single-tooth situations, is that its angulation may complicate the path of insertion and subsequent provisional crown relining. The inexperienced clinician may find it challenging to avoid locking the provisional crown in place during relining, due to the abutment's steep undercut. Proper implant placement is needed to support the crown in an ideal manner. However, if needed, the slim healing abutment can be customized with a bur to best accommodate the provisional crown.

This type of healing abutment is recommended for implants with self-tapping features, which allows the surgeon to reorient the implant exactly based on prosthetic needs without losing torque. A specially designed implant carrier with the abutment embedded into it allows the surgeon to have a better perspective during the implant surgery in respect to the interocclusal space and crown position.

The slim healing abutments consist of two parts: *(1)* the surgical component, only 1.2 mm in diameter, and *(2)* the prosthetic component, comprised of the abutment with a cone for provisional crown restoration cementation. They were developed with two different surgical component heights, based on the implant design and implant depth. The prosthetic component was designed in two different heights, one for lateral incisors and another one for central incisors, canines, and premolars.

This patient had a root-fractured mandibular left lateral incisor with an alumina crown fabricated a few years earlier. The crown to the mesial made it difficult to provide a bonded fixed provisional restoration for the implant healing period. A slim temporary healing abutment allowed placement of a provisional restoration on the day of implant placement. A NobelReplace Groovy NP implant (3.5 × 13 mm) was placed, and a straight incision was performed to maximize the tissue volume around the implant. The drawings illustrate partial-thickness flap preparation around the implant site in the interproximal area and its vertical elevation buccally and lingually.

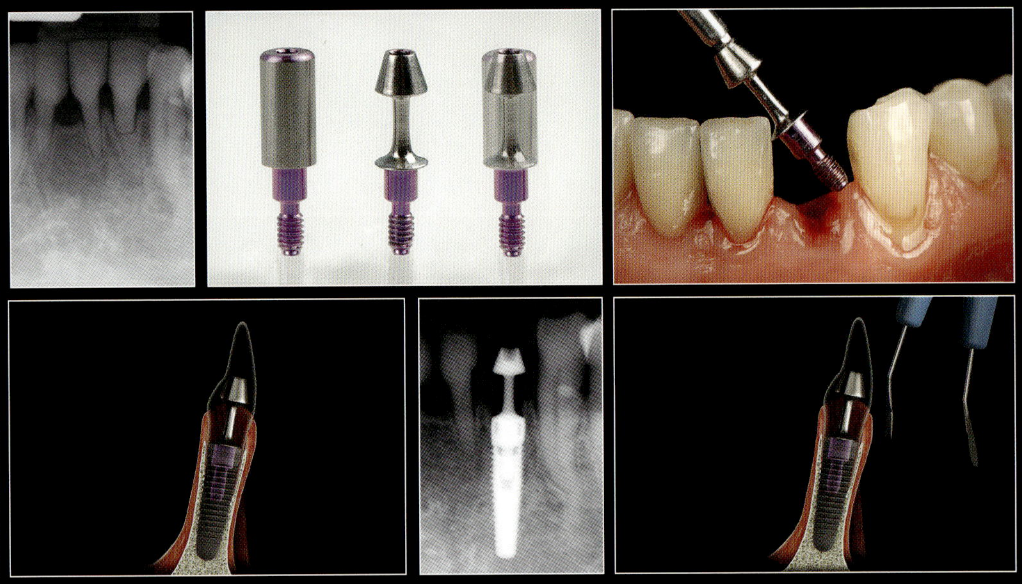

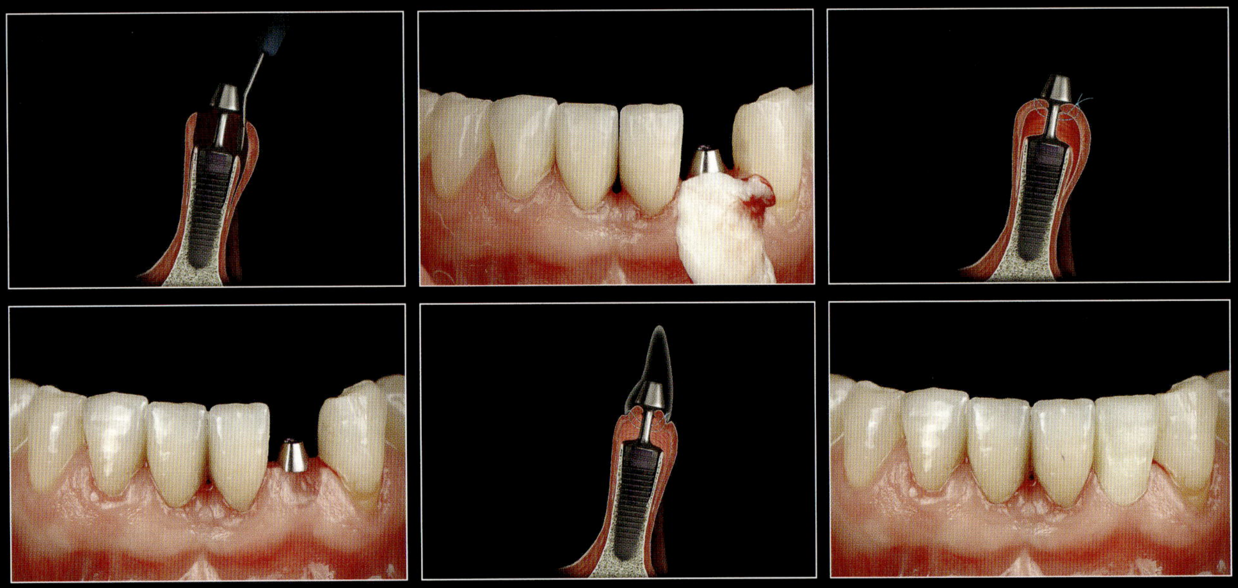

Once the partial-thickness flap was released, the CTG was adapted and trimmed to create an ideal ridge. A small incision was made at the center of the CTG to slide it over the slim temporary healing abutment for best possible anchorage. The partial-thickness flap was then elevated above the CTG and secured with a 6-0 suture, flush to the base of the prosthetic component. The shell provisional was relined and cemented on top of the prosthetic cone without exerting any pressure onto the graft.

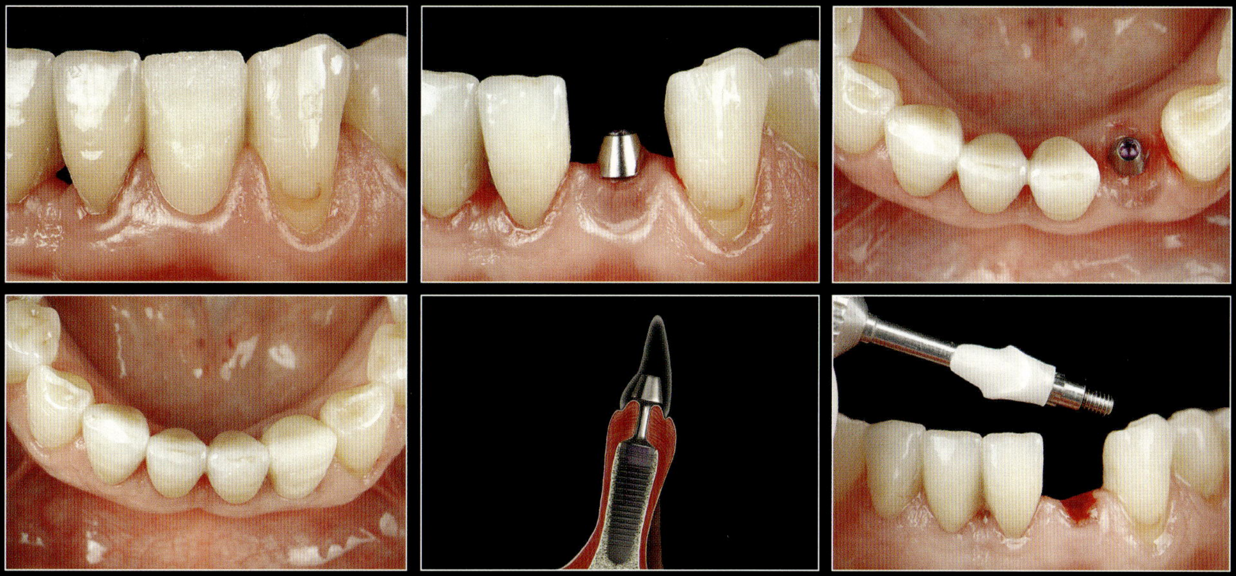

The 6-month follow-up situation reveals the gain in soft tissue volume on the lingual and buccal aspects as well as an ideal emergence profile without loss of tissue height. The amount of lingual volume provides a predictable ridge situation for an optimal result on the buccal aspect. Impressions were made of the implant and the provisional restoration to provide a reference and transfer the emergence profile to the definitive zirconia abutment. The same provisional restoration was then relined on the definitive abutment and cemented.

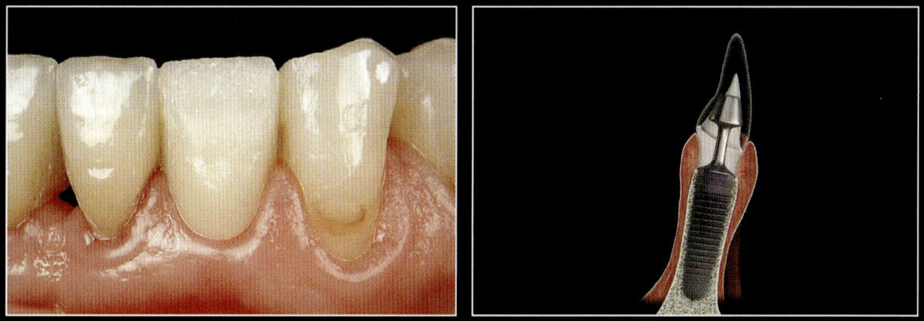

The narrowest healing abutment was used to maximize 3D soft tissue volume coronal to the implant. The provisional crown was cemented onto the conical prosthetic component of the slim healing abutment, reconstructing the contour of the lost tooth, which becomes the reference for the necessary soft tissue volume. Compare the situation 3 months after the definitive abutment and provisional crown were delivered *(bottom right)* to the transitional situation *(top left)*. The soft tissue was maintained through the different phases of the prosthetic treatment.

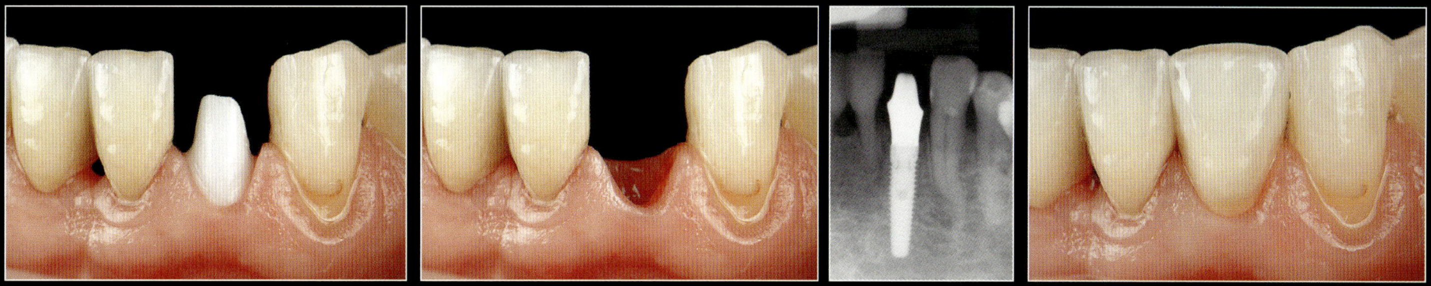

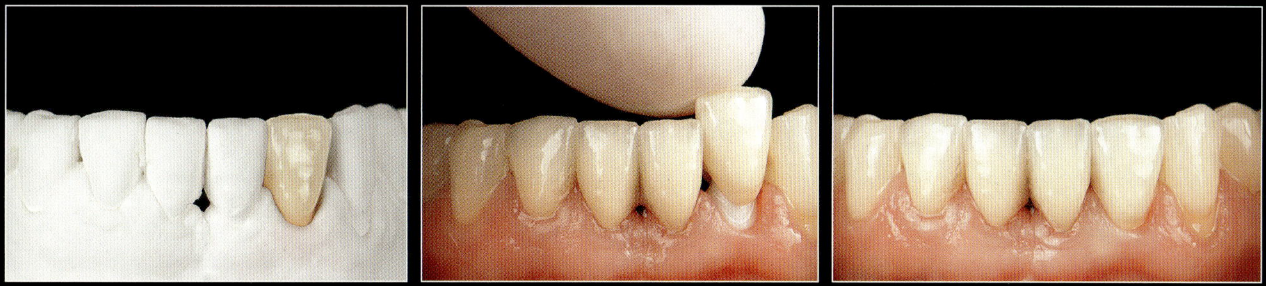

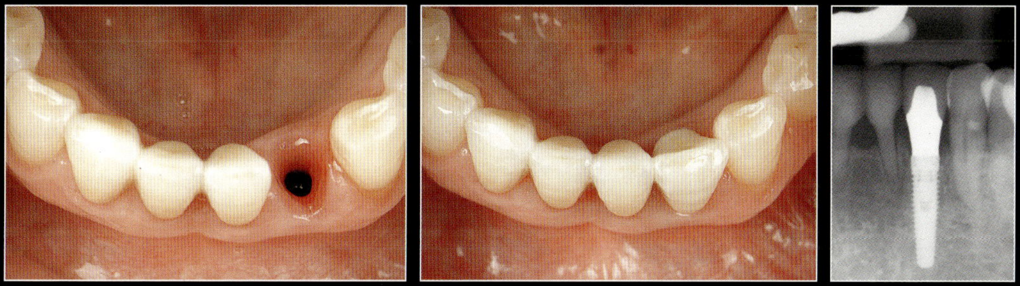

The final impression was made with one retraction cord (size #0) and treated in the same manner as done for conventional crown restorations on natural teeth. An alumina crown was fabricated to blend with the other three pre-existing mandibular anterior incisor crowns. The definitive restoration was tried in before final cementation to verify functional aspects, interproximal contacts, and fit. The definitive zirconia abutment was unscrewed to demonstrate the amount of tissue volume. The final radiograph reveals the bone response to the treatment.

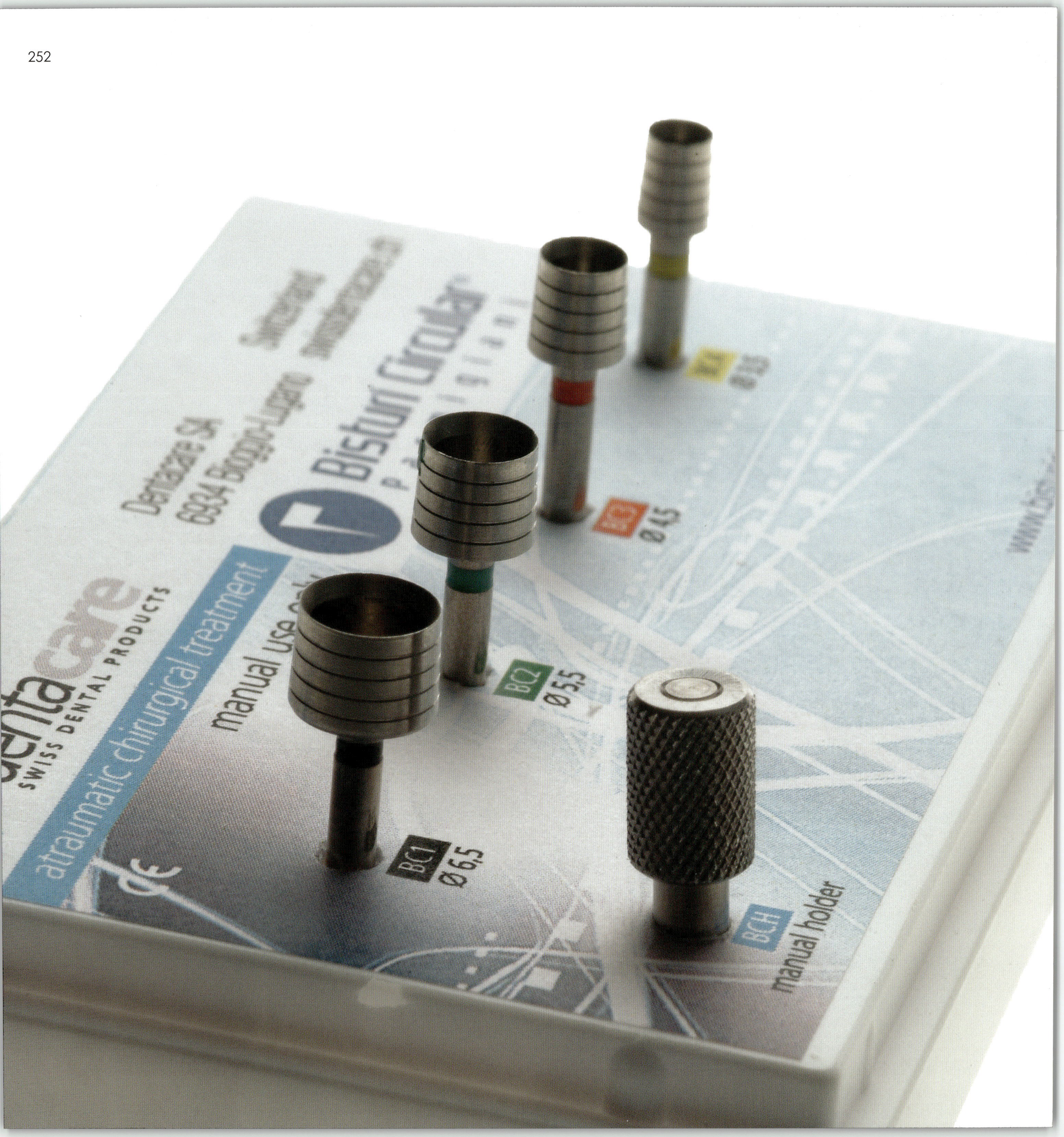
SWISS DENTAL PRODUCTS
atraumatic chirurgical treatment
Bisturi Circular
BC1
Ø 6,5
BC2
Ø 5,5
BC3
Ø 4,5
BCH
manual holder

Socket grafting

After tooth extraction, physiologic and pathologic wound-healing events cause resorption of the alveolar ridge and a 3D reduction of the surrounding bone both in height and thickness, especially within the first 6 months. Various ridge preservation techniques have been developed over the years to limit the amount of bone resorption and subsequent bone graft procedures after tooth extraction. The techniques illustrated and described here follow the latest recommendations based on the scientific evidence as well as long-term personal experience with socket grafting techniques in the esthetic zone, where bone resorption has the most devastating impact, especially from an esthetic standpoint.

Socket grafting is usually not necessary when the entire buccal bone is still intact after extraction. The first and most important step is therefore nontraumatic tooth extraction.

A proper socket grafting technique is one of the most difficult surgical procedures. It should ideally be performed with a flapless tunnel or a full-thickness buccal flap to affix a separating membrane against the bone to prevent the periosteum from migrating into the grafted extraction site. Then a bone substitute is placed into the socket and covered with the membrane. Once the membrane is attached to the palatal bone or sutured to the palatal soft tissue flap, a circular free gingival autograft is harvested from the palate to seal the socket and facilitate guided bone regeneration.

The last step of sealing the extraction socket with a free gingival graft is very important. Without that, the wound will be closed by secondary intention healing and granulation of the blood clot, leading to a thin and fragile soft tissue covering that is difficult to handle during implant placement.

Primary wound closure with a free tissue graft allows faster healing and provides a preferred soft tissue thickness and density. The free gingival tissue graft is easily harvested with a tissue punch. However, the diameter of the graft is important: The incidence of necrosis is rather high when the tissue graft is too small in respect to the diameter of the extraction socket. In addition, it should be at least 4.5 mm thick.

Research

Socket grafting

The alveolar process undergoes varying degrees of atrophy and resorption after removal of a tooth.[1] The physiologic and pathologic events, dimensional changes, dynamics, and resorptive patterns are well documented.[1–3] The buccal plate typically undergoes greater resorption than the lingual plate, and loss of bone width is reportedly three times greater than the loss of height: The mean horizontal reduction of the alveolar ridge measures 3.8 mm and the vertical reduction 1.24 mm 6 months after tooth extraction.[1,4] According to studies with a 12-month follow-up, the rapid and substantial bone volume reductions in the first 3 to 6 months are followed by a continuous but more gradual resorption thereafter.[5]

The loss of bone complicates subsequent implant placement and compromises functional and esthetic outcomes. Various techniques have been suggested to preserve the alveolar ridge, generally following established guided bone regeneration (GBR) concepts.[6] These socket grafting techniques typically include placement of autogenous bone, allograft, xenograft, or synthetic materials, which are also categorized into slow- and fast-resorbing materials.[1] The addition of growth factors (eg, platelet-derived growth factor, transforming growth factor β) and proteins (eg, bone morphogenetic protein) has also been discussed, but the current evidence is still inconclusive.[7]

Numerous clinical studies and systematic reviews conclude that ridge preservation techniques are effective in minimizing ridge resorption after tooth extraction.[1,7–14] These techniques seem to be less effective, however, when all four bone walls of the extraction socket are still intact.[15] In addition, the direct effects of ridge preservation on the outcomes of implant therapy need further validation,[1,7–10] especially since they may not be able to entirely eliminate additional grafting procedures at the time of implant placement or thereafter.[1]

The large number of techniques, bone graft materials, and membranes available for GBR and ridge preservation as well as the vast heterogeneity of clinical parameters and investigative tools make it difficult to identify one technique or material as superior based on scientific evidence.[16] The use of a bovine bone mineral material in combination with a collagen membrane has been demonstrated to be one of the most successful ridge preservation techniques and has been shown to significantly limit bone resorption after tooth extraction.[17–19]

Sealing the extraction wound and covering the bone graft material placed into the socket with a soft tissue graft harvested with a biopsy punch seems to further improve clinical outcomes and limit resorption.[20] This technique allows for primary would closure and provides better soft tissue conditions than the ones achieved when the socket opening is left open to heal by secondary intention. Colorimetry revealed that, after healing, the color of the grafted tissue matches that of the adjacent tissue quite closely and below the detectable threshold.[20]

A modification of this technique with a combination epithelialized-subepithelial connective tissue graft may provide an even greater degree of vascularization, limiting the risk of necrosis.[21,22]

References

1. Kassim B, Ivanovski S, Mattheos N. Current perspectives on the role of ridge (socket) preservation procedures in dental implant treatment in the aesthetic zone. Aust Dent J 2014;59:48–56.
2. Cardaropoli G, Araujo M, Lindhe J. Dynamics of bone tissue formation in tooth extraction sites. An experimental study in dogs. J Clin Periodontol 2003;30:809–818.
3. Schropp L, Wenzel A, Kostopoulos L, Karring T. Bone healing and soft tissue contour changes following single-tooth extraction: A clinical and radiographic 12-month prospective study. Int J Periodontics Restorative Dent 2003;23:313–323.
4. Hämmerle CH, Araujo MG, Simion M. Evidence-based knowledge on the biology and treatment of extraction sockets. Clin Oral Implants Res 2012;23(suppl 5):80–82.
5. Tan WL, Wong TL, Wong MC, Lang NP. A systematic review of post-extractional alveolar hard and soft tissue dimensional changes in humans. Clin Oral Implants Res 2012;23(suppl 5):1–21.
6. Block MS, Jackson WC. Techniques for grafting the extraction site in preparation for dental implant placement. Atlas Oral Maxillofac Surg Clin North Am 2006;14:1–25.
7. Darby I, Chen ST, Buser D. Ridge preservation techniques for implant therapy. Int J Oral Maxillofac Implants 2009;24(suppl):260–271.
8. Horowitz R, Holtzclaw D, Rosen PS. A review on alveolar ridge preservation following tooth extraction. J Evid Based Dent Pract 2012;12(3 suppl):149–160.
9. Ten Heggeler JM, Slot DE, Van der Weijden GA. Effect of socket preservation therapies following tooth extraction in non-molar regions in humans: A systematic review. Clin Oral Implants Res 2011;22:779–788.
10. Vignoletti F, Matesanz P, Rodrigo D, Figuero E, Martin C, Sanz M. Surgical protocols for ridge preservation after tooth extraction. A systematic review. Clin Oral Implants Res 2012;23(suppl 5):22–38.
11. Felice P, Soardi E, Piattelli M, Pistilli R, Jacotti M, Esposito M. Immediate non-occlusal loading of immediate post-extractive versus delayed placement of single implants in preserved sockets of the anterior maxilla: 4-month post-loading results from a pragmatic multicentre randomised controlled trial. Eur J Oral Implantol 2011;4:329–344.
12. Norton MR, Wilson J. Dental implants placed in extraction sites implanted with bioactive glass: Human histology and clinical outcome. Int J Oral Maxillofac Implants 2002;17:249–257.
13. Patel K, Mardas N, Donos N. Radiographic and clinical outcomes of implants placed in ridge preserved sites: A 12-month post-loading follow-up. Clin Oral Implants Res 2013;24:599–605.
14. Sandor GK, Kainulainen VT, Queiroz JO, Carmichael RP, Oikarinen KS. Preservation of ridge dimensions following grafting with coral granules of 48 post-traumatic and post-extraction dento-alveolar defects. Dent Traumatol 2003;19:221–227.
15. Heberer S, Al-Chawaf B, Jablonski C, Nelson JJ, Lage H, Nelson K. Healing of ungrafted and grafted extraction sockets after 12 weeks: A prospective clinical study. Int J Oral Maxillofac Implants 2011;26:385–392.
16. Jensen SS, Terheyden H. Bone augmentation procedures in localized defects in the alveolar ridge: Clinical results with different bone grafts and bone-substitute materials. Int J Oral Maxillofac Implants 2009;24:218–236.
17. Cardaropoli D, Tamagnone L, Roffredo A, Gaveglio L. Relationship between the buccal bone plate thickness and the healing of postextraction sockets with/without ridge preservation. Int J Periodontics Restorative Dent 2014;34:211–217.
18. Cardaropoli D, Tamagnone L, Roffredo A, Gaveglio L, Cardaropoli G. Socket preservation using bovine bone mineral and collagen membrane: A randomized controlled clinical trial with histologic analysis. Int J Periodontics Restorative Dent 2012;32:421–430.
19. Barone A, Aldini NN, Fini M, Giardino R, Calvo Guirado JL, Covani U. Xenograft versus extraction alone for ridge preservation after tooth removal: A clinical and histomorphometric study. J Periodontol 2008;79:1370–1377.
20. Jung RE, Siegenthaler DW, Hämmerle CH. Postextraction tissue management: A soft tissue punch technique. Int J Periodontics Restorative Dent 2004;24:545–553.
21. Stimmelmayr M, Allen EP, Reichert TE, Iglhaut G. Use of a combination epithelized-subepithelial connective tissue graft for closure and soft tissue augmentation of an extraction site following ridge preservation or implant placement: Description of a technique. Int J Periodontics Restorative Dent 2010;30:375–381.
22. Stimmelmayr M, Güth JF, Iglhaut G, Beuer F. Preservation of the ridge and sealing of the socket with a combination epithelialised and subepithelial connective tissue graft for management of defects in the buccal bone before insertion of implants: A case series. Br J Oral Maxillofac Surg 2012;50:550–555.

Punch technique failure

The socket grafting technique is ideally combined with a free gingival graft, harvested from the palate with a biopsy tissue punch (ie, punch technique) to cover the membrane and bone graft material and close the extraction socket opening. Since blood supply to the graft is severely compromised and predominantly provided through the surrounding soft tissue, the diameter and thickness of the graft are crucial to prevent necrosis. A graft that is too small and too thin will not have sufficient blood supply and likely necrotize. In addition, tight adaptation through proper suturing is important for adequate vascularization.

A necrotic free gingival tissue graft does not necessarily affect the bone graft, but it usually requires a CTG before or at the time of implant placement.

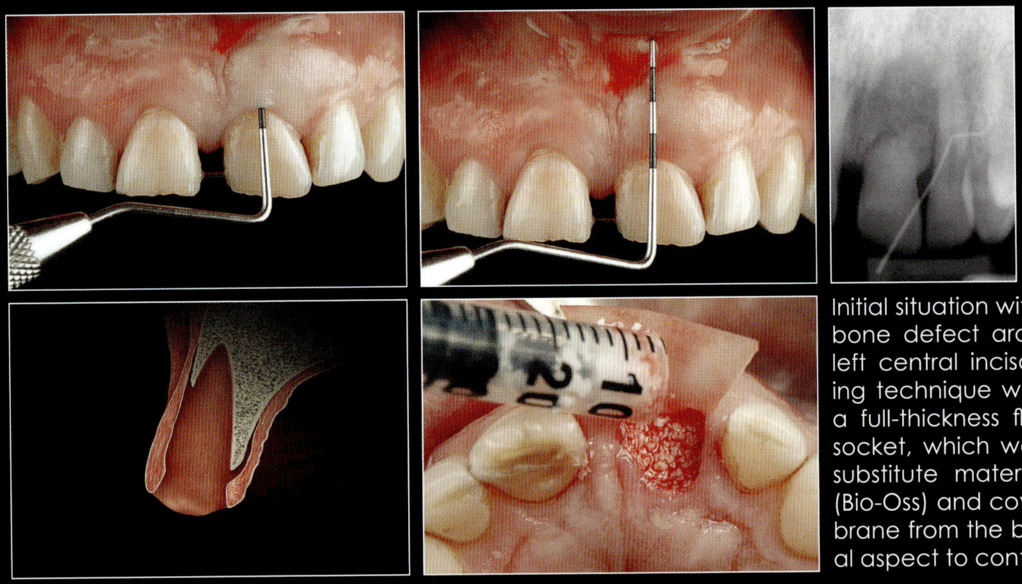

Initial situation with a severe buccal bone defect around the maxillary left central incisor. A socket grafting technique was performed with a full-thickness flap buccal to the socket, which was filled with bone substitute material with a syringe (Bio-Oss) and covered with a membrane from the buccal to the crestal aspect to contain the particles.

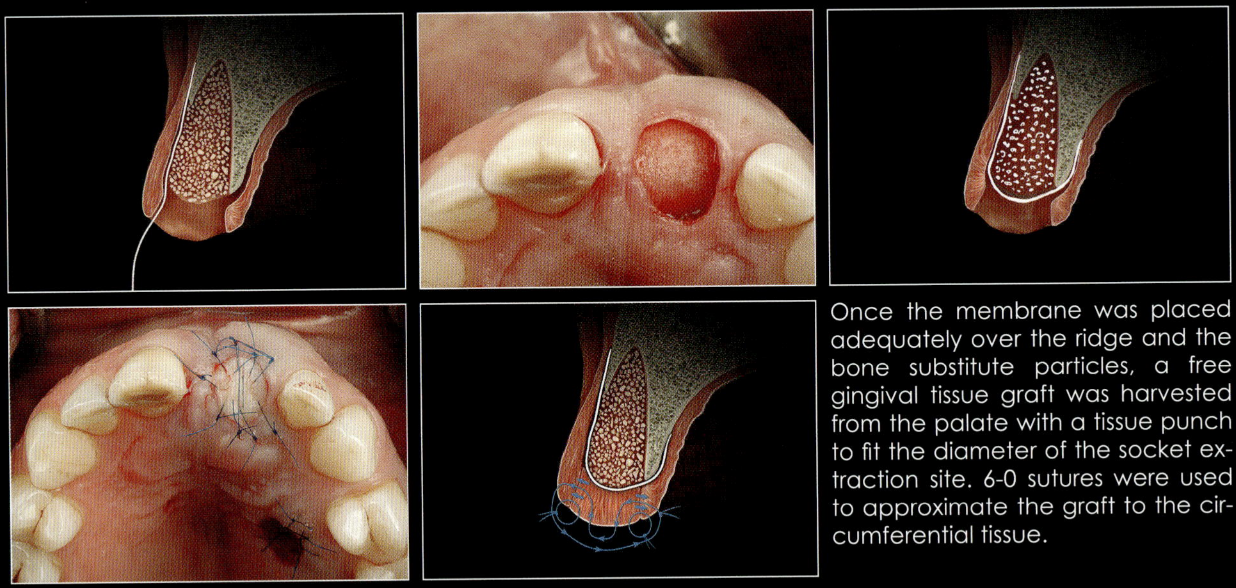

Once the membrane was placed adequately over the ridge and the bone substitute particles, a free gingival tissue graft was harvested from the palate with a tissue punch to fit the diameter of the socket extraction site. 6-0 sutures were used to approximate the graft to the circumferential tissue.

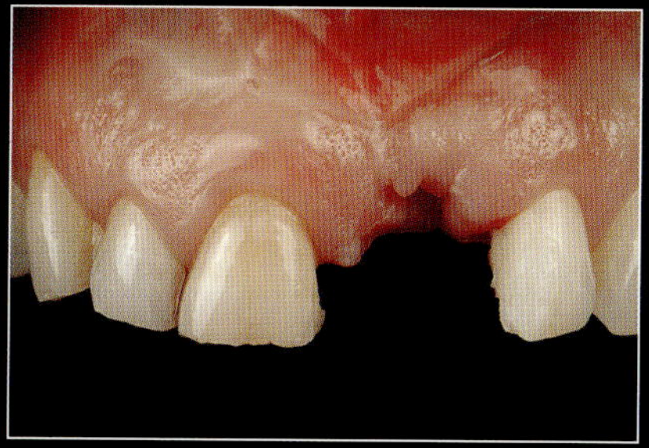
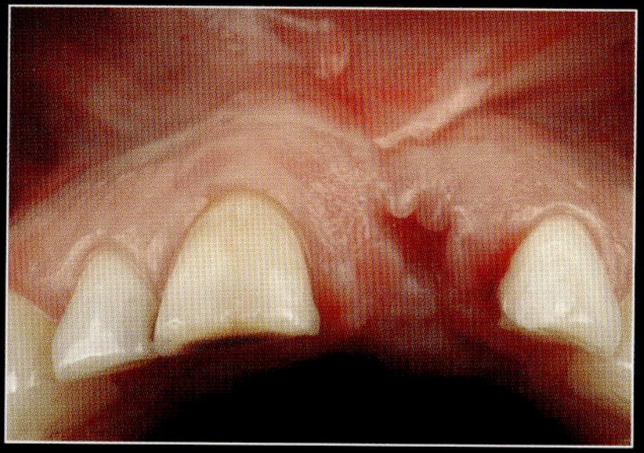
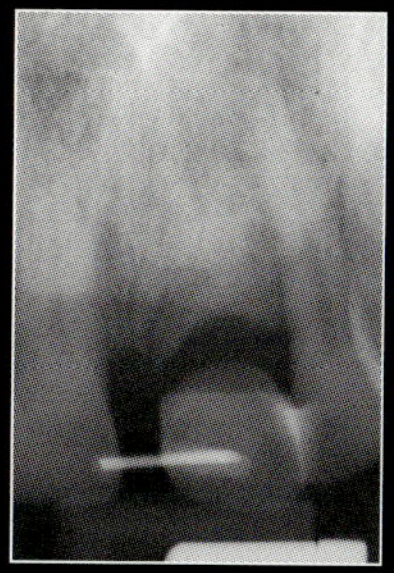
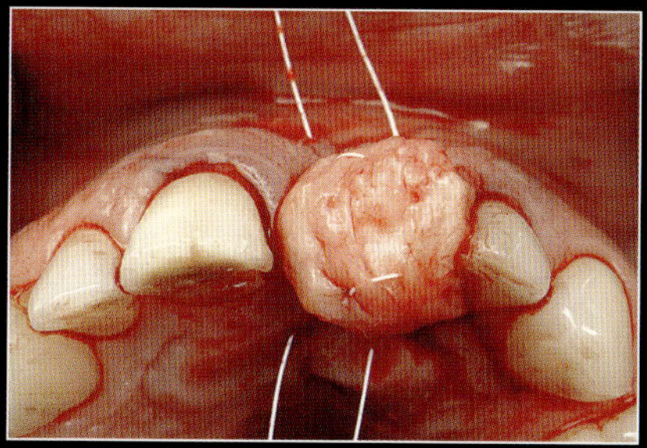
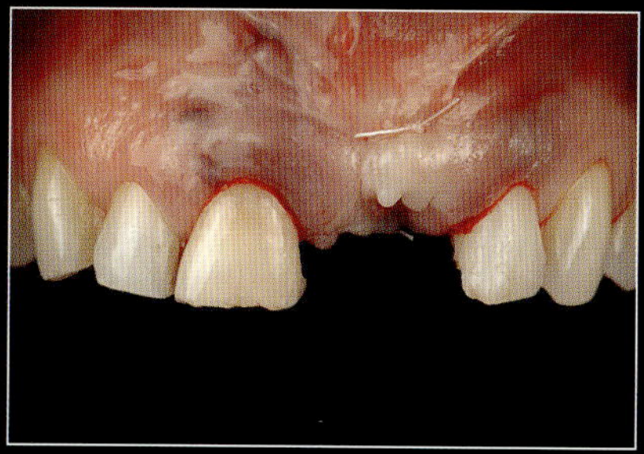

The free tissue graft necrotized during the healing phase. The extent of the resulting defect became most obvious at the 6-month follow-up. The site was then grafted with a CTG to replace the lost tissue volume without elevating flaps via tunneling incisions. A healing period of 8 to 10 months was necessary before implant placement.

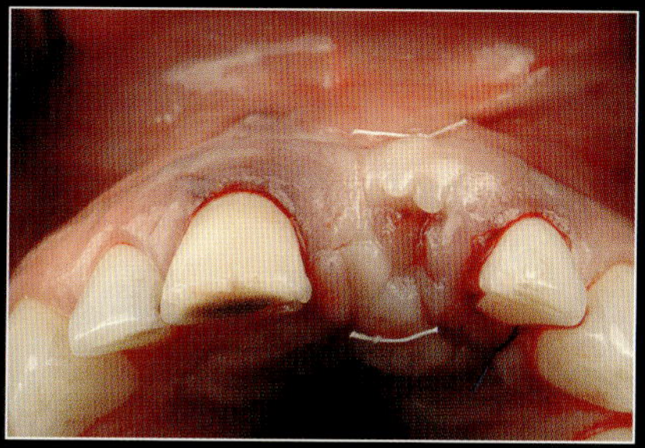
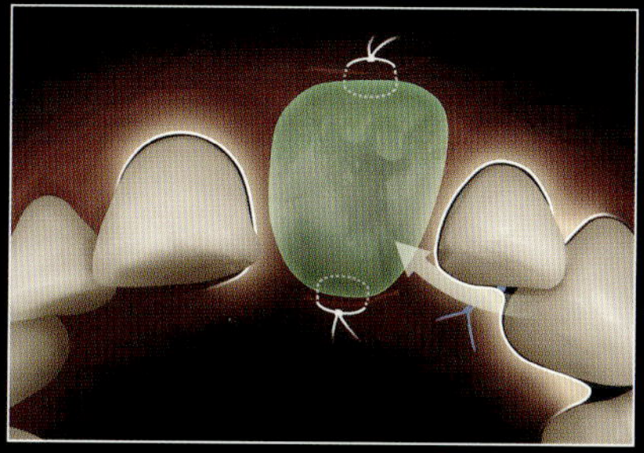
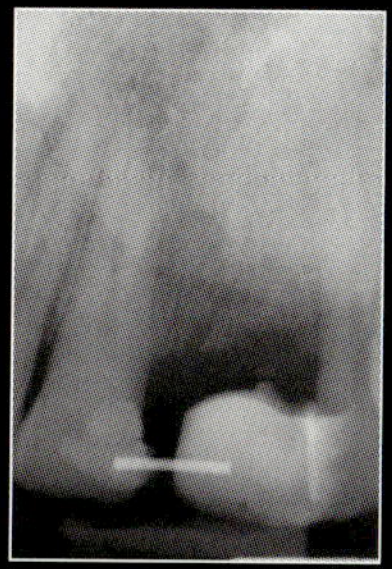
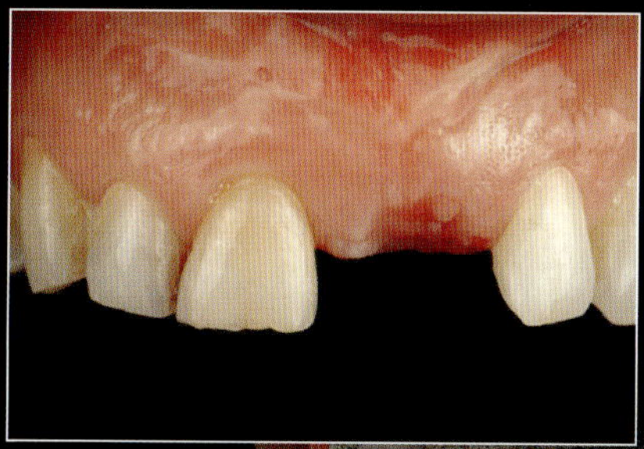
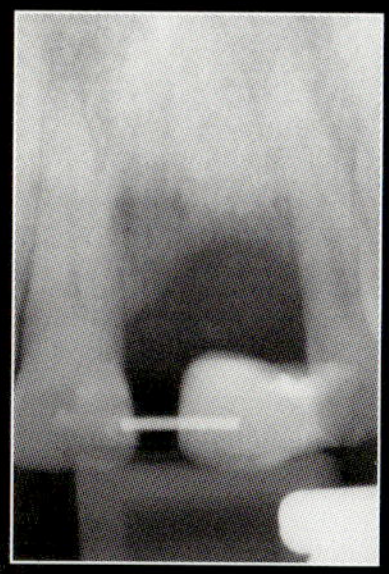

The illustration depicts the surgical procedure and incisions to elevate the tissue with a tunnel technique and without elevating a full soft tissue flap as well as proper placement of the CTG. Clinical and radiographic situation 1 year after ridge preservation.

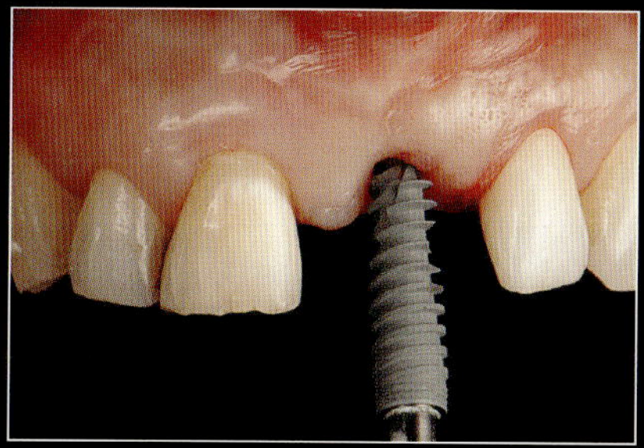
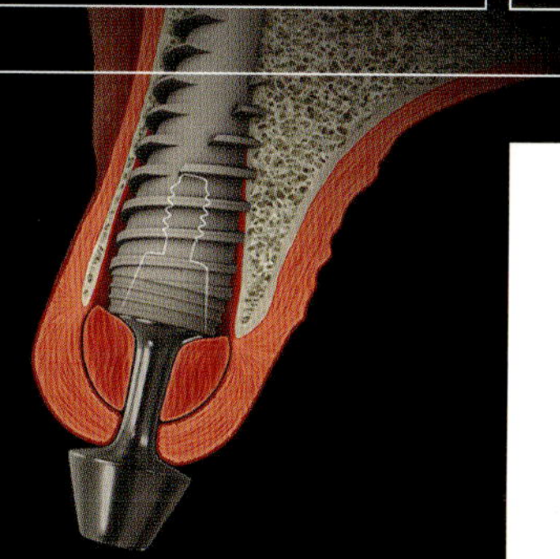
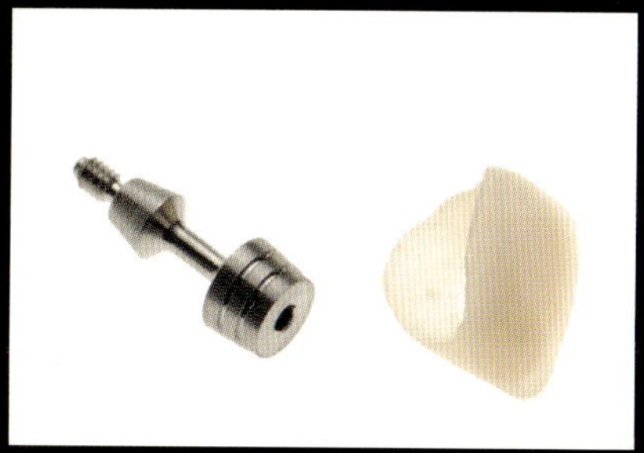
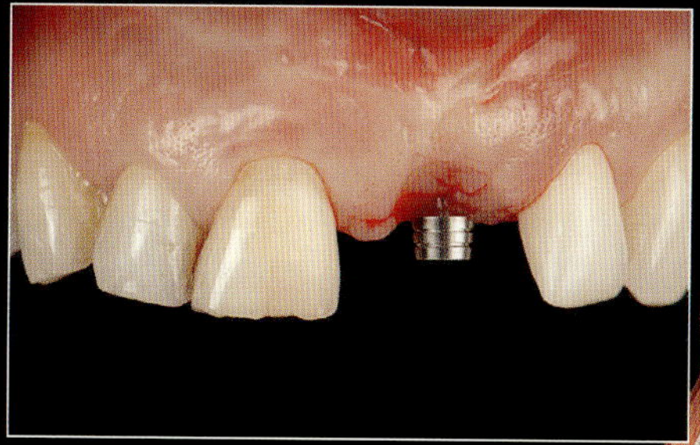
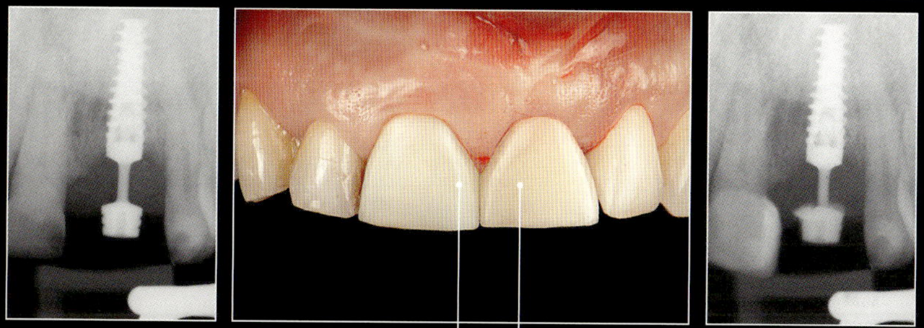

Composite — Provisional restoration

A NobelActive implant (4.3 × 15 mm) was placed with a flapless technique to preserve as much of the underlying bone and soft tissue as possible. Due to the primary stability, a slim healing abutment was inserted together with a provisional crown to provide immediate esthetics. Composite resin was placed on the maxillary right central incisor to facilitate closure of the diastema.

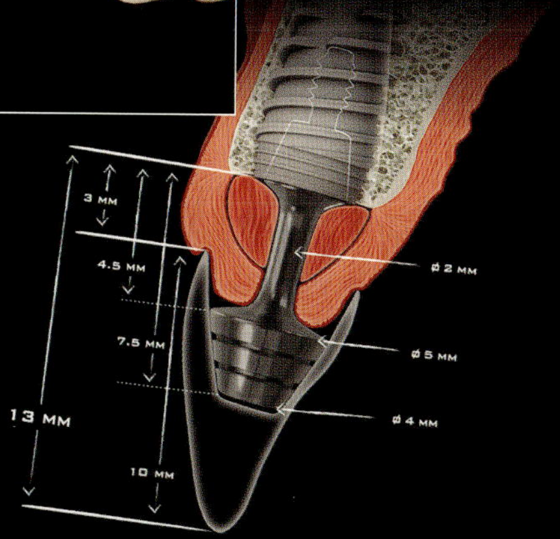

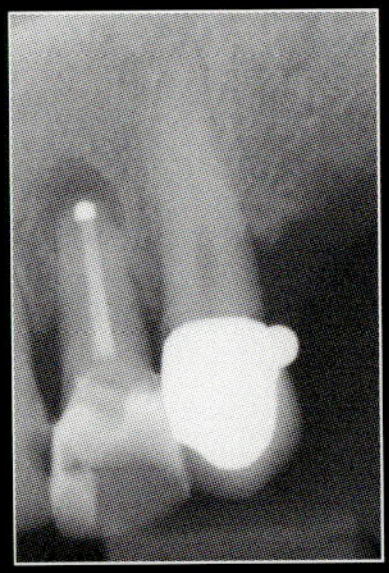

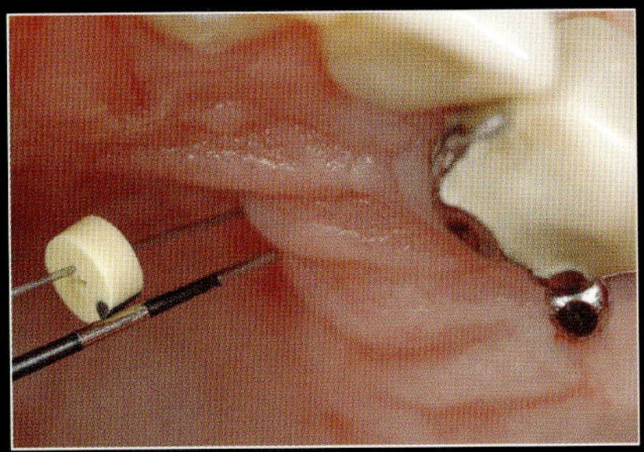

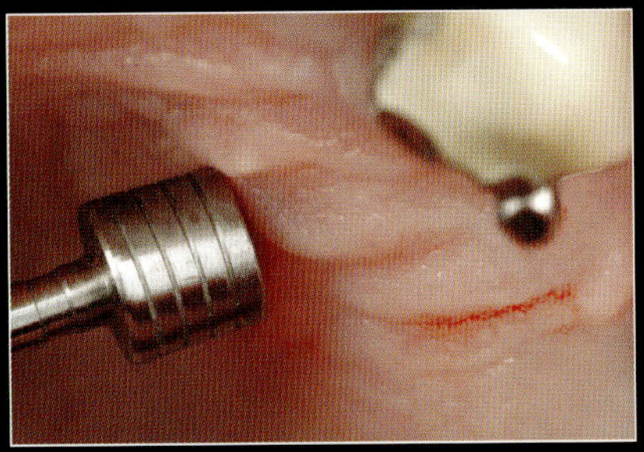

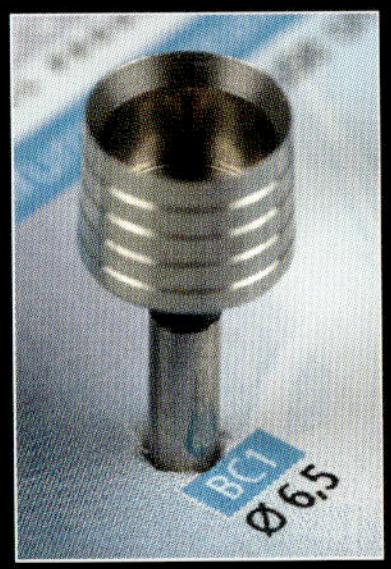

Punch technique success

A detailed sounding of the palate is necessary to identify the optimal donor site and harvest a free gingival graft at least 4.5 mm thick. Different diameters of circular biopsy tissue punches are available to harvest a graft that properly fits the tissue opening left by the tooth extraction. In fact, the diameter of the graft should be approximately 1 mm larger than the opening to ensure intimate contact between the graft and the surrounding soft tissue to optimize vascularization and prevent necrosis of the graft.

The buccal plate of the extraction socket was completely intact, so a bone substitute was not necessary. It was decided, however, to seal the socket opening with a free gingival punch graft due to the periapical bone defect. After tooth extraction and thorough cleaning of the socket by removing the periapical granuloma, the graft was placed and secured with 7-0 sutures.

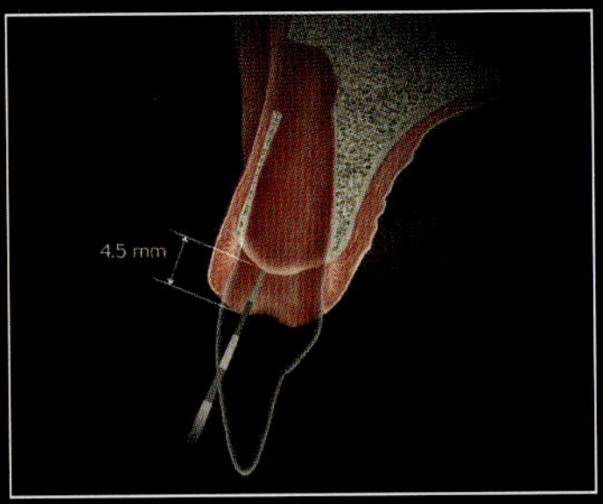

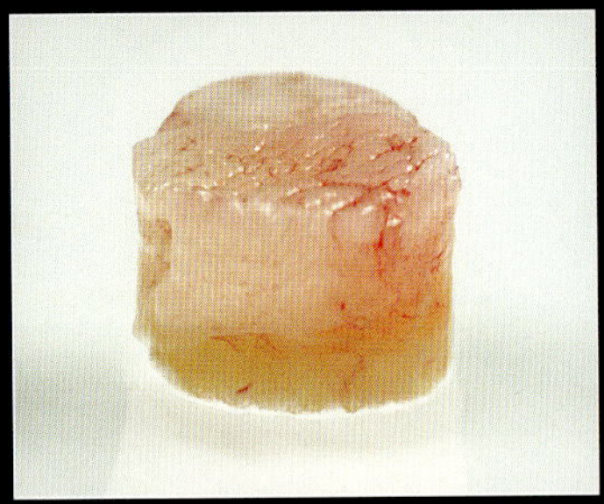

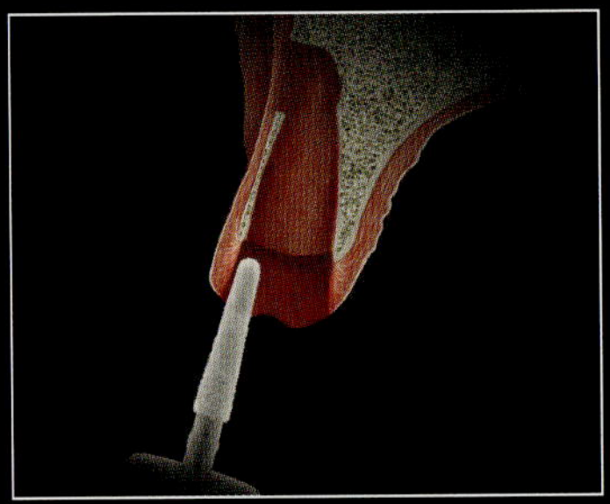

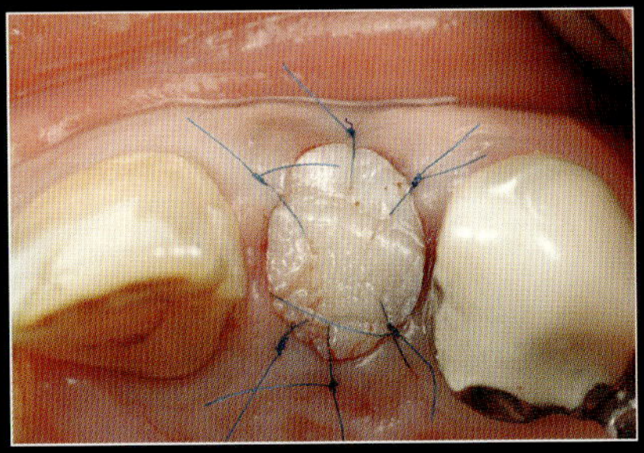

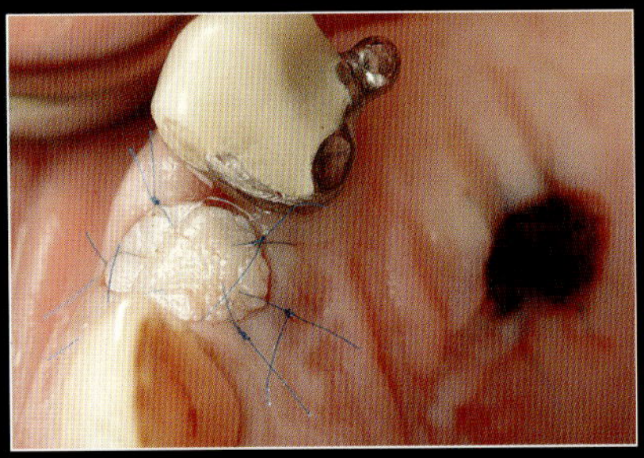

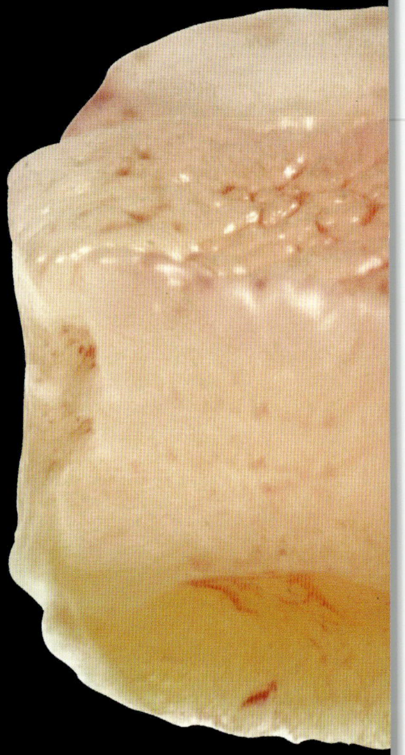

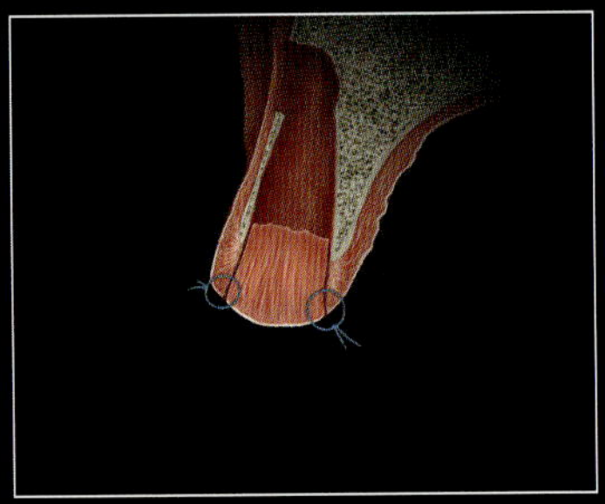

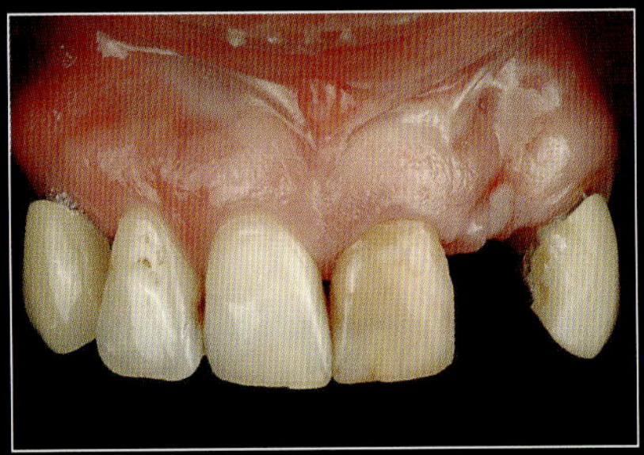

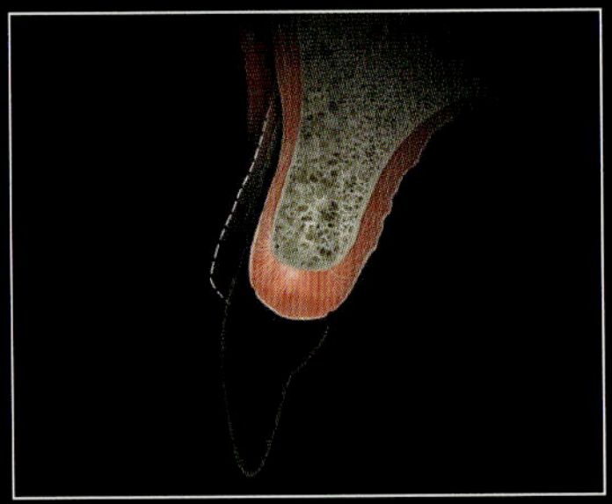

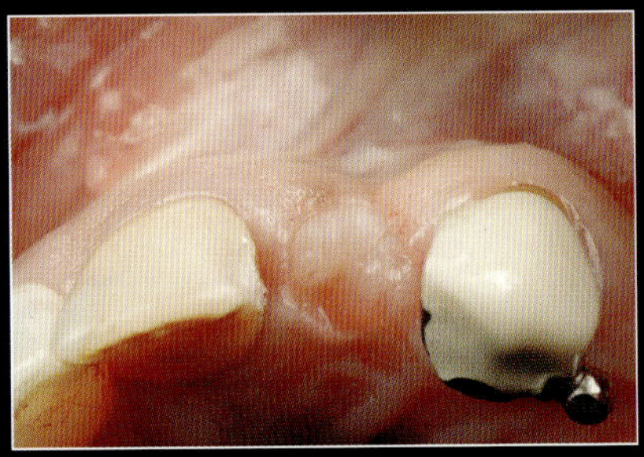

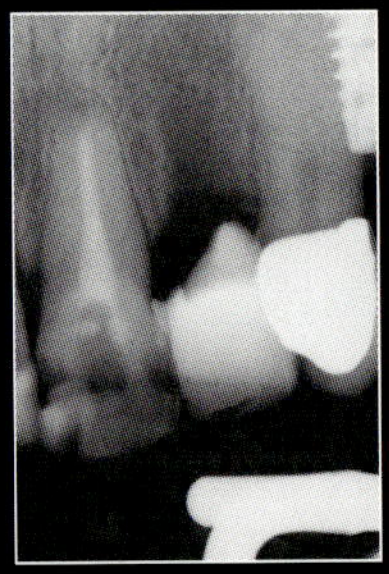

Three months after the socket was sealed, the tissue volume collapsed as the graft was fully integrated. Despite the collapse, placement of a narrow implant and grafting with a CTG from the tuberosity were still an option.

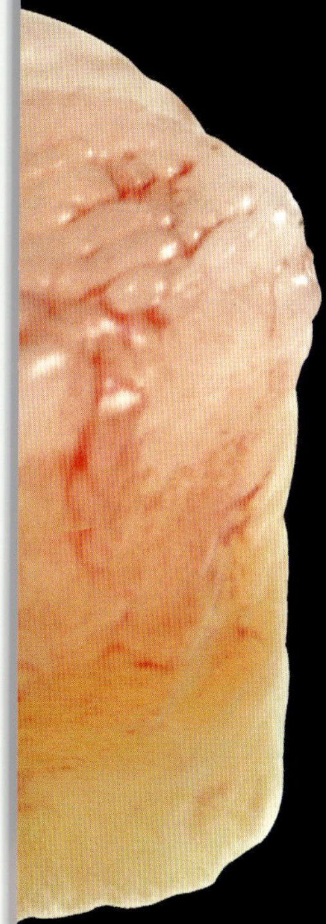

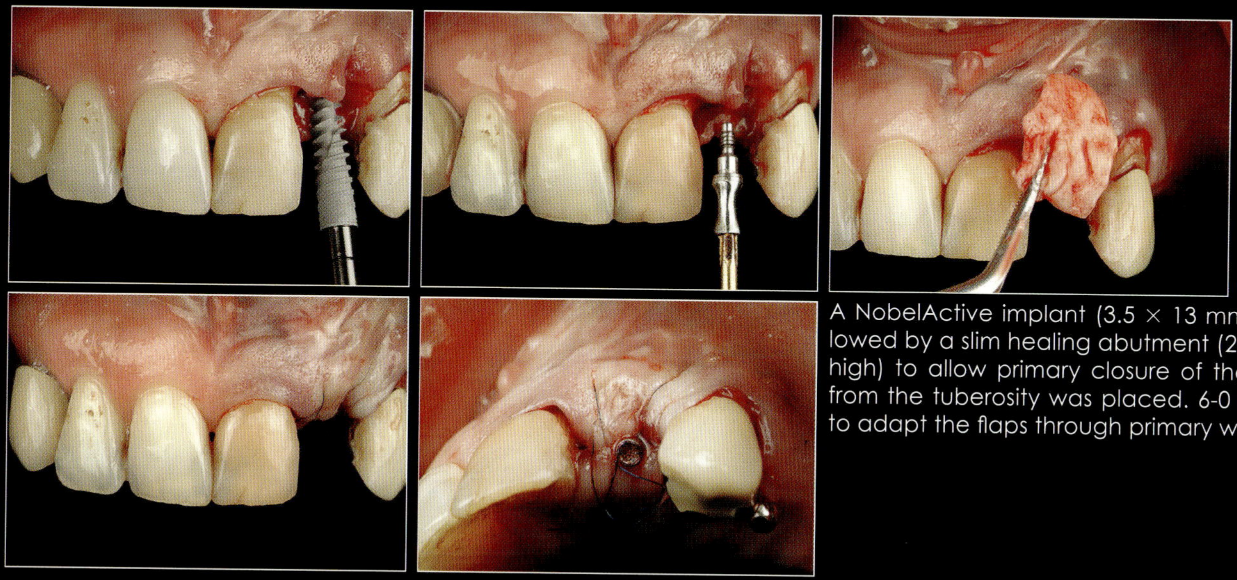

A NobelActive implant (3.5 × 13 mm) was placed followed by a slim healing abutment (2 mm wide × 5 mm high) to allow primary closure of the flap as the CTG from the tuberosity was placed. 6-0 sutures were used to adapt the flaps through primary wound closure.

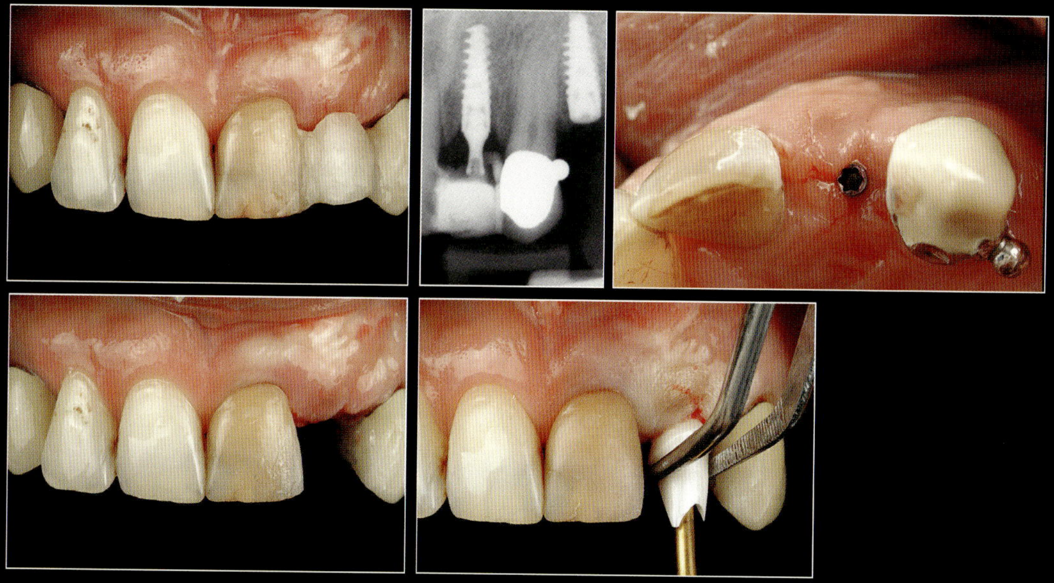

After a 6-month healing period, the tissue volume achieved with the CTG was obvious. An implant impression was made after local anesthesia. The definitive zirconia abutment was fabricated in the laboratory together with a provisional crown. The abutment was screwed onto the implant while secured in place with cotton pliers for proper abutment orientation and tissue displacement.

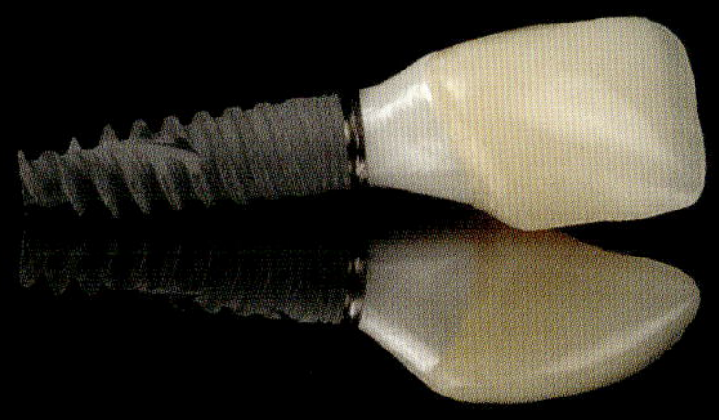

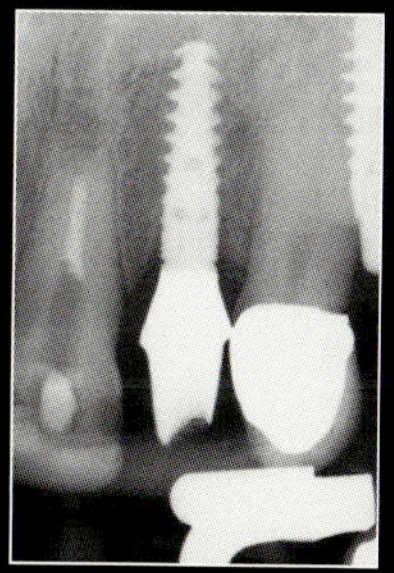

Radiographic evaluation was necessary to verify proper fit and placement of the zirconia abutment on the implant before the provisional crown restoration was relined. The soft tissue contour was shaped through the emergence profile of the provisional restoration, which was transferred to the definitive crown 1 year later.

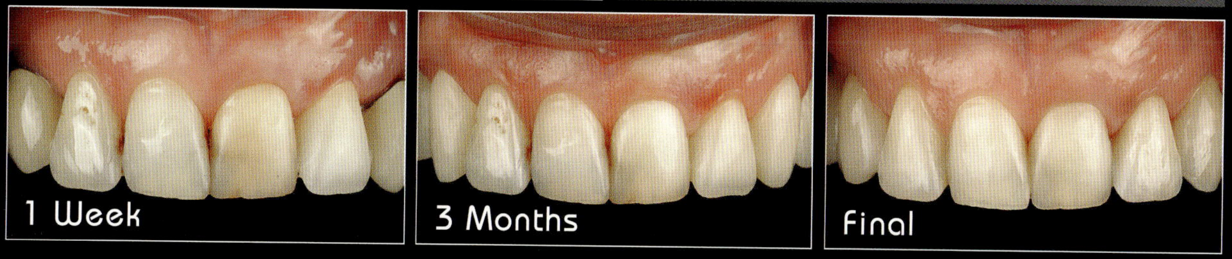

Modified punch technique

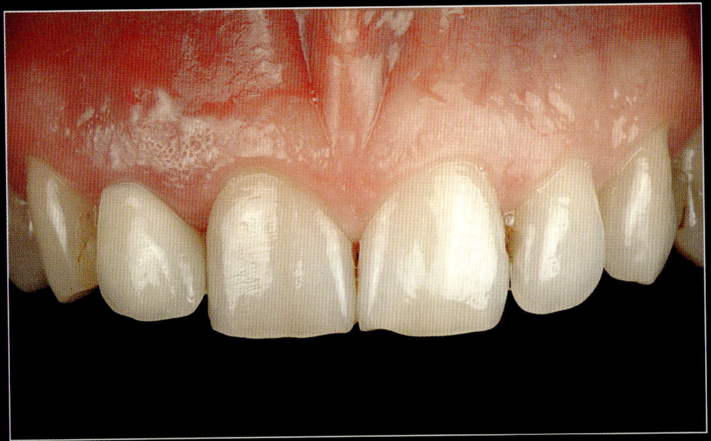

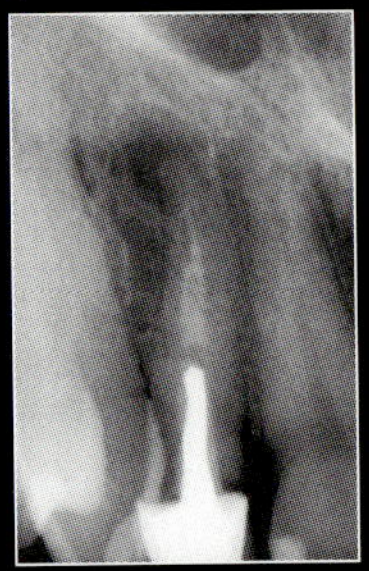

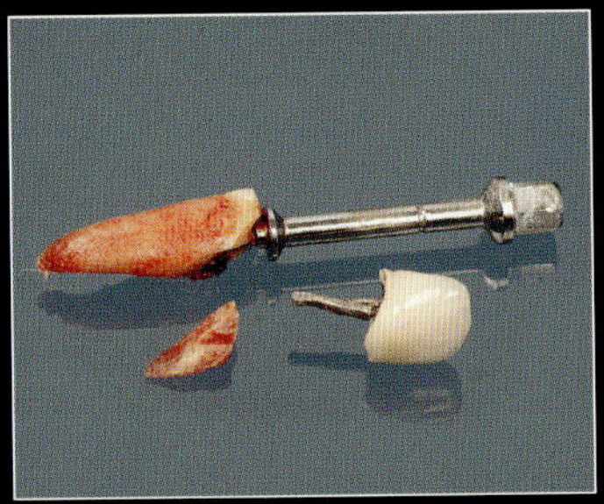

The patient presented with a root fracture of the maxillary right lateral incisor, associated with a bone defect on the buccal aspect and an active periapical granuloma. The tooth was extracted, and a ridge preservation technique was performed. A tunnel technique was applied to avoid releasing incisions and elevation of a full-thickness flap. The membrane was slid in the buccal pouch, and the socket was filled with bone substitute material through a syringe.

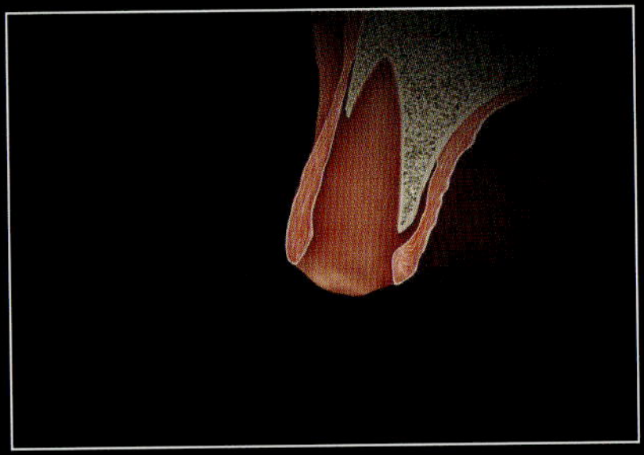

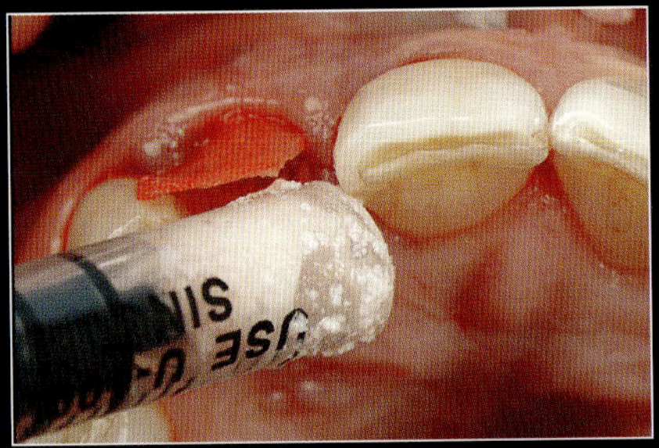

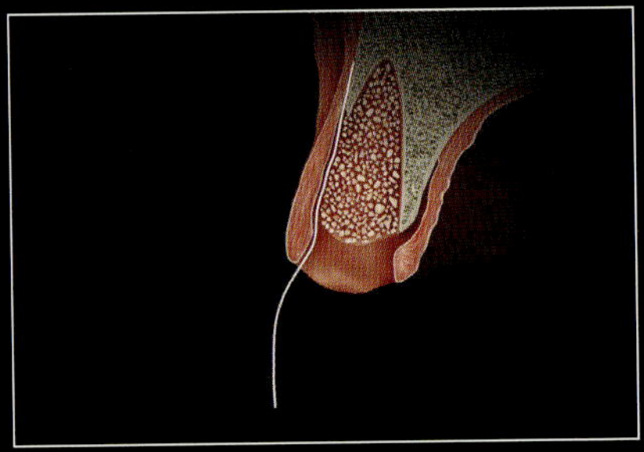

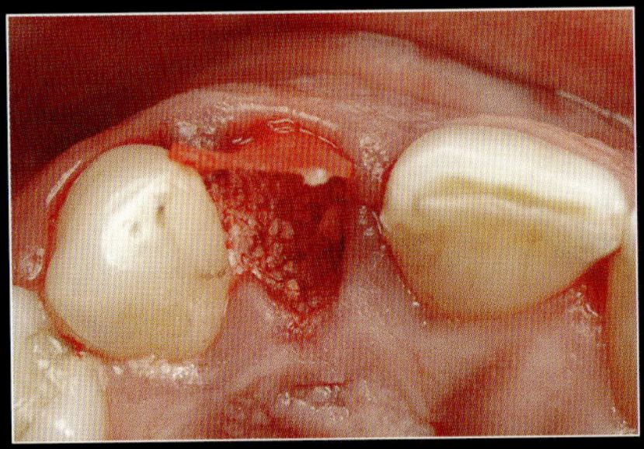

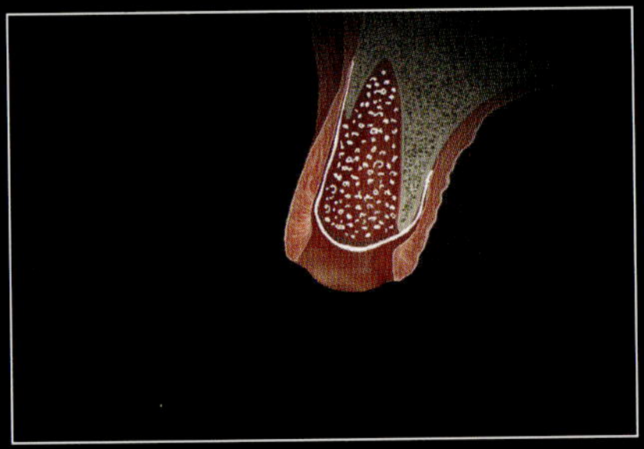

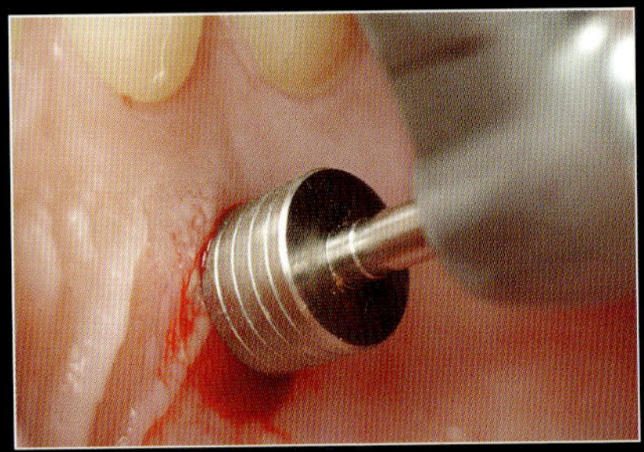

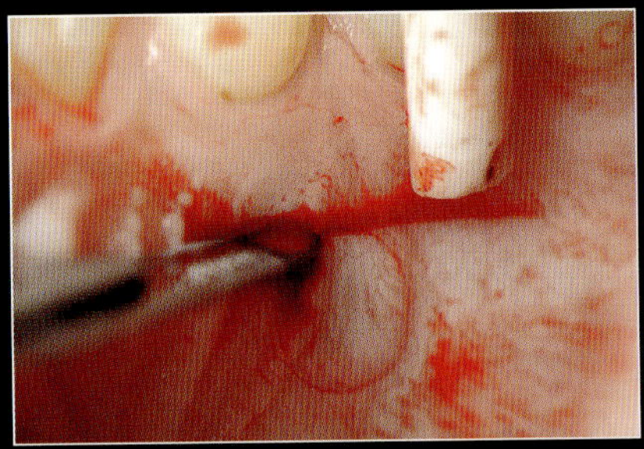

After the membrane was placed over the socket and covered the entire ridge from the buccal to the palatal aspect, a combined epithelial-subepithelial CTG was harvested from the palate to seal the socket. A circular tissue punch blade was selected based on the diameter of the tooth socket, and a circular incision was performed on the palate about 2 mm deep. Subsequently, another 2-mm-deep incision was placed parallel to the gingival margins. The epithelium mesial and distal to the circular incision was then delicately deflected with a split-thickness flap technique, leaving about 1.5 mm of epithelium mesial and distal to the initial circular punch incision.

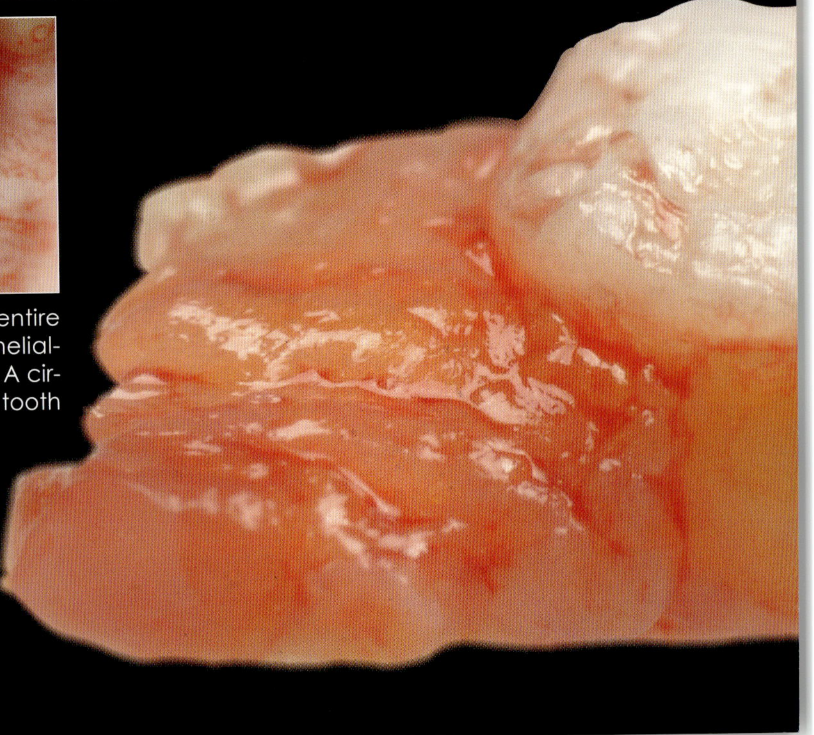

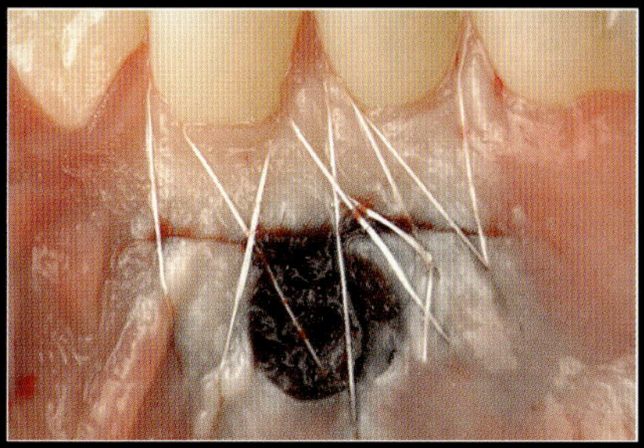

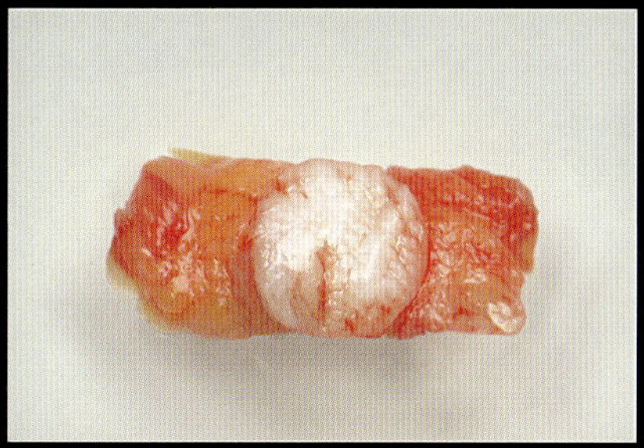

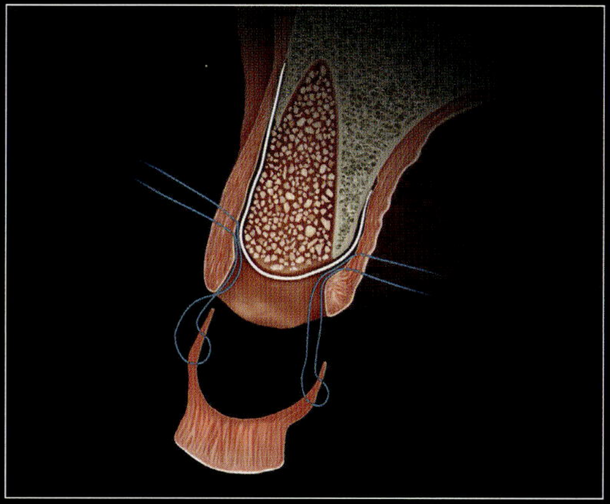

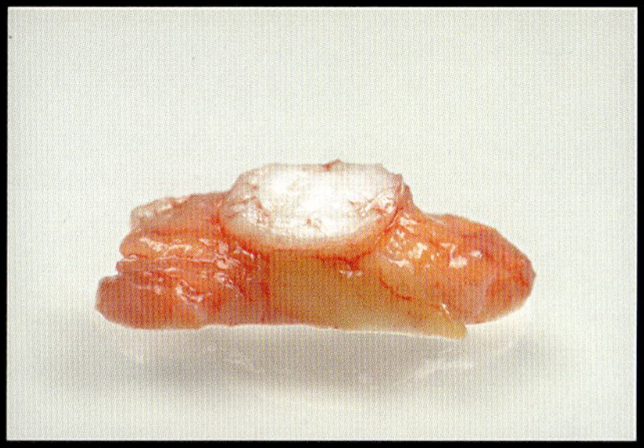

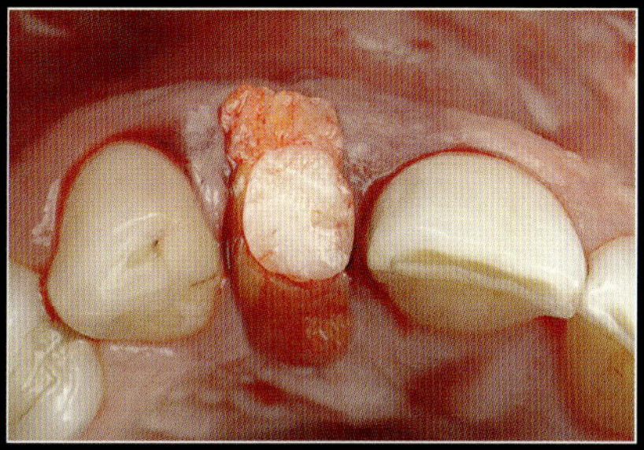

The epithelium was deflected around the circular incision in the center. A vertical incision on the mesial and distal of the subepithelial connective tissue was performed. Then a horizontal incision was placed parallel to the first horizontal incision occlusally to shape a rectangular subepithelial CTG with a circular "island" of epithelium the same size as the socket diameter. Once the graft was harvested from the palate, a pouch was prepared on the palatal and buccal aspects of the socket to suture it in place, centering the epithelialized aspect of the graft to the gingival margins of the socket. With this technique, the central graft is provided additional blood supply from the buccal and palatal subepithelial connective tissue extensions.

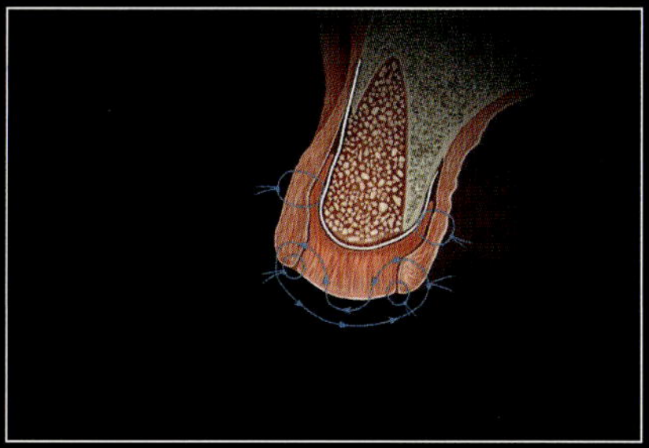

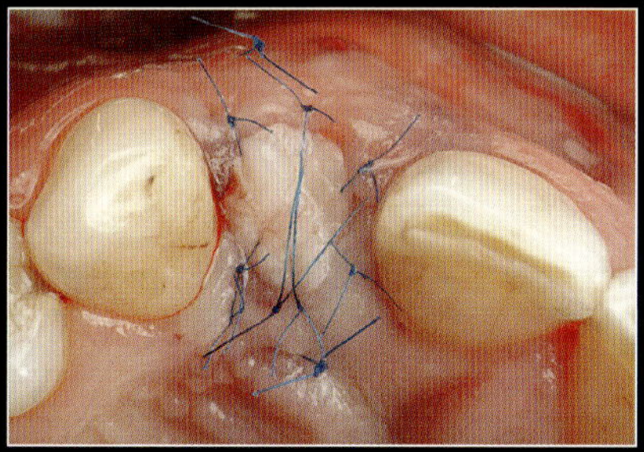

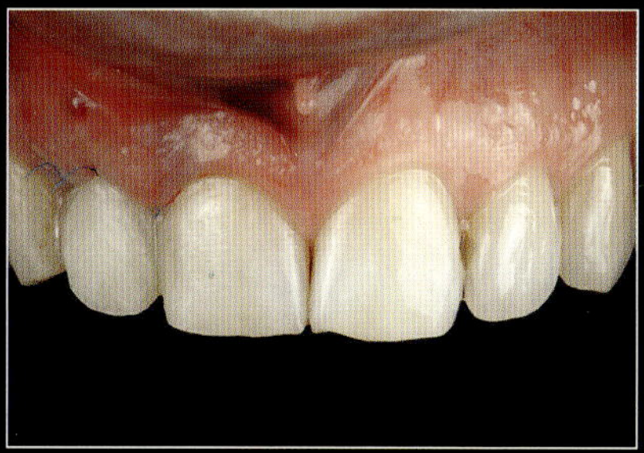

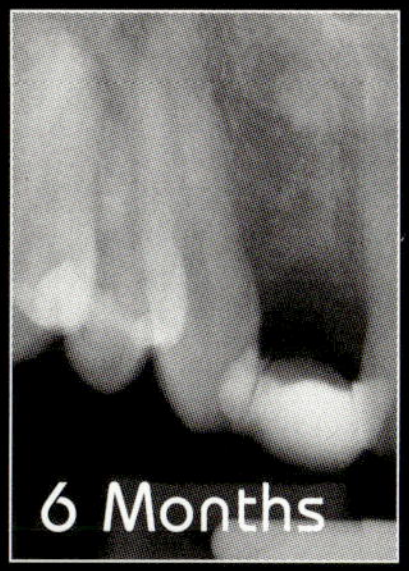

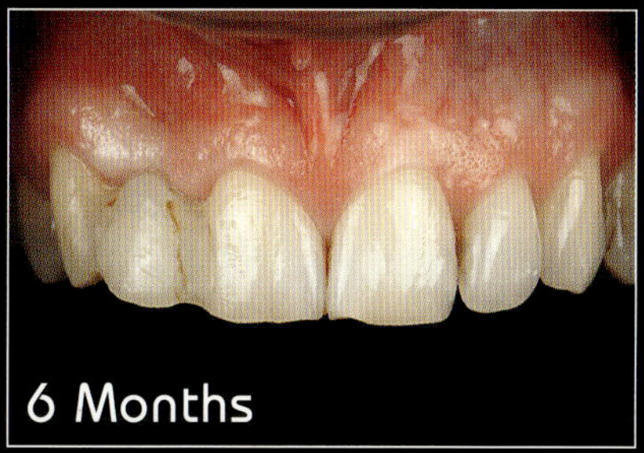

The buccal and palatal subepithelial connective tissue extensions were secured in place with horizontal mattress sutures to center the graft. Then a centered vertical mattress suture was tied through the palatal flap, graft, and buccal flap to approximate the edges of the socket to the epithelialized area of the tissue graft. Once the graft was centered and placed into position, single interrupted sutures were used to achieve an intimate seal. A composite tooth was adhesively bonded to the adjacent teeth as an immediate provisional restoration. The clinical situation after 1 year indicates a slight tissue collapse but favorable soft tissue appearance.

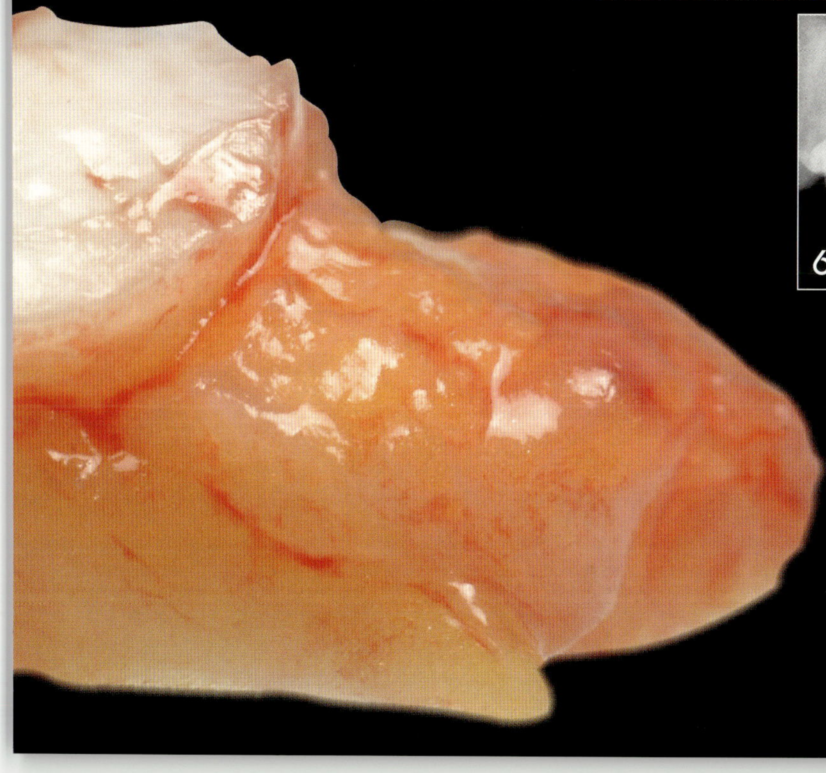

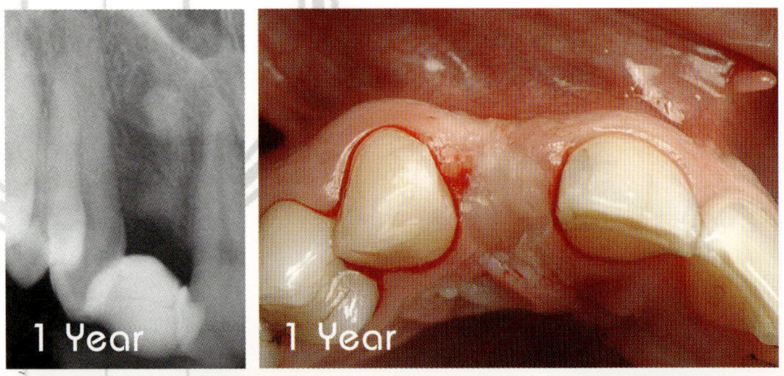

The 1-year postoperative periapical radiograph and occlusal view depict the integration of the grafted tissue. Through a crestal partial-thickness flap, a NobelActive 3.5 × 13–mm implant was inserted with a slim temporary abutment to provide adequate space for the CTG and insertion of an immediate provisional restoration.

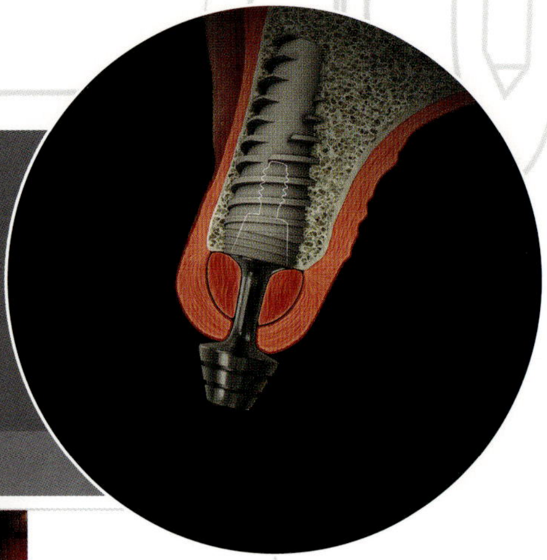

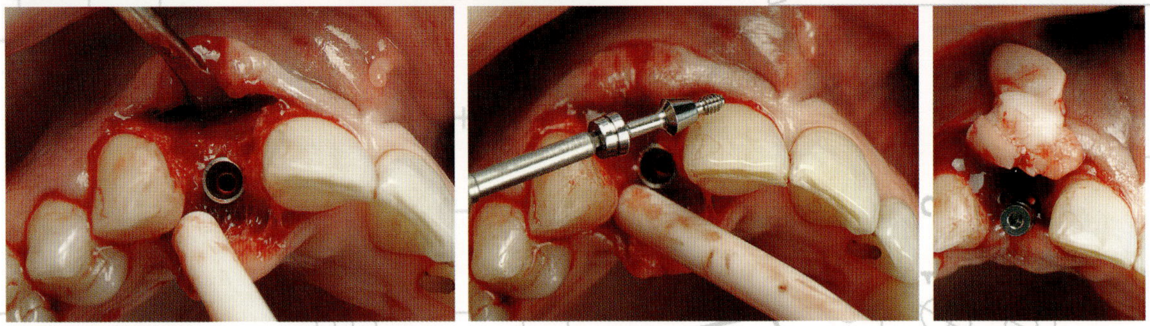

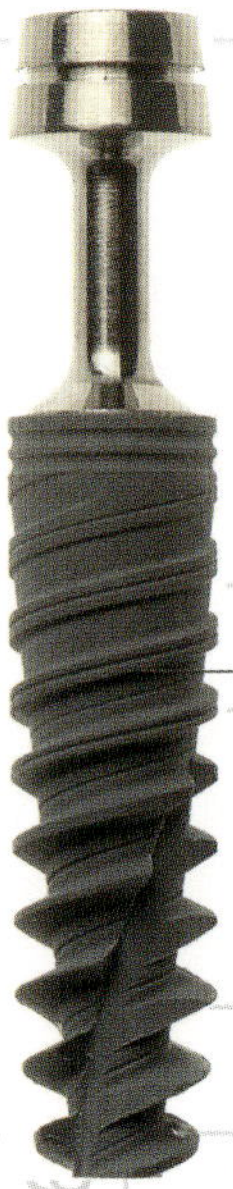

Periapical radiograph verifying correct adaptation of the healing abutment and proper positioning of the implant. The CTG was again sutured in layers, first the CTG and then the flap over it, to achieve primary wound closure. After 6 months of healing, the volume achieved with the CTG confirms the efficacy of this technique.

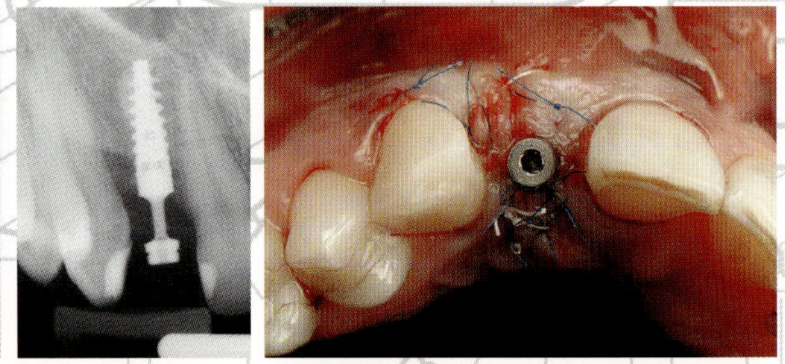

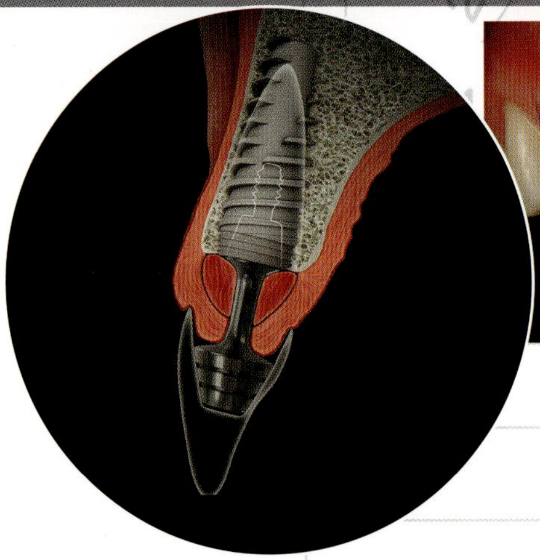

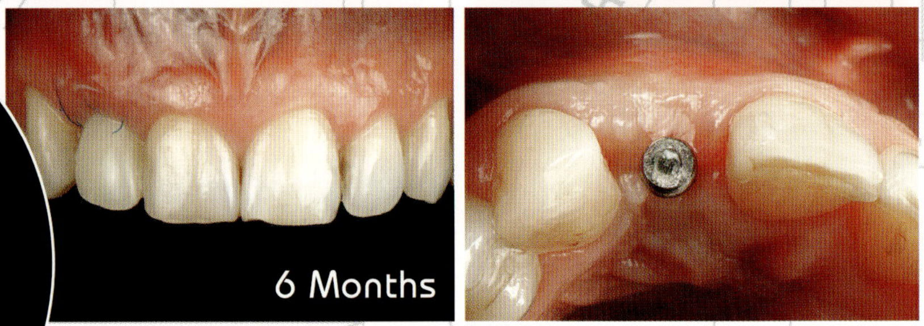

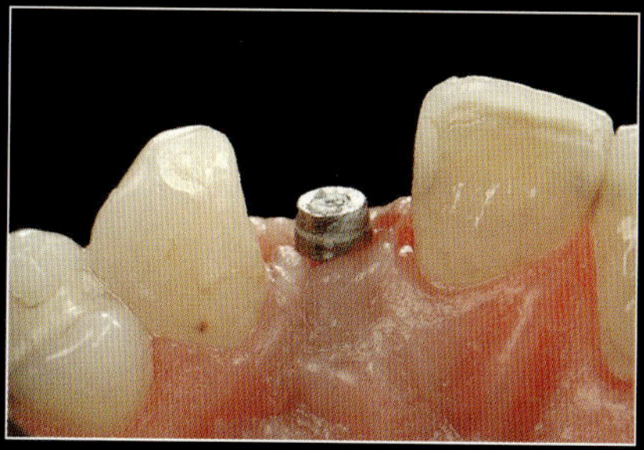
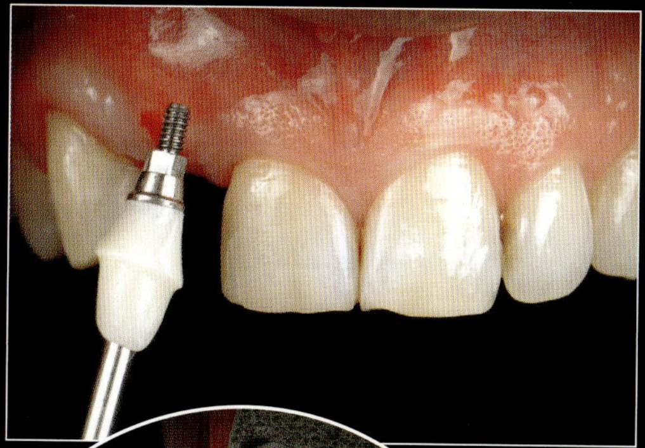
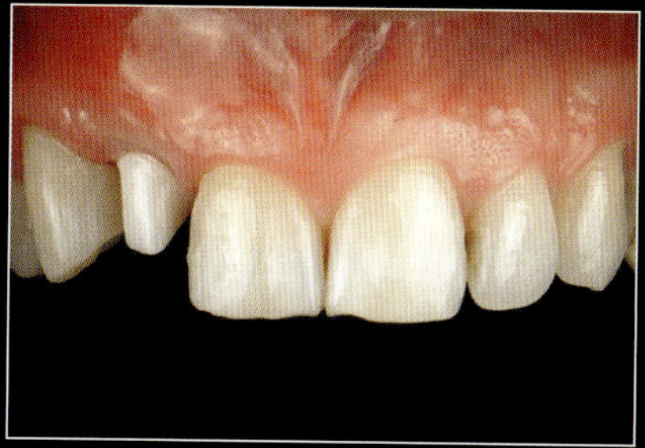
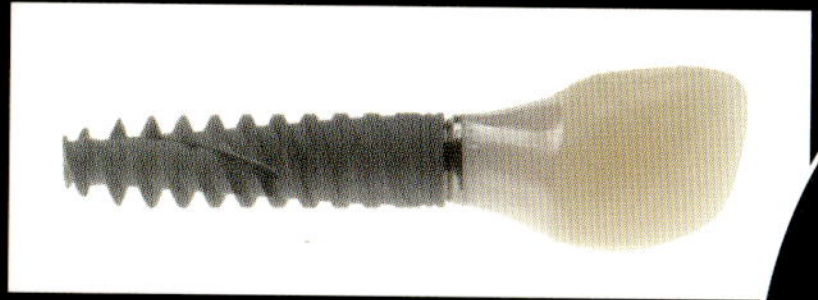
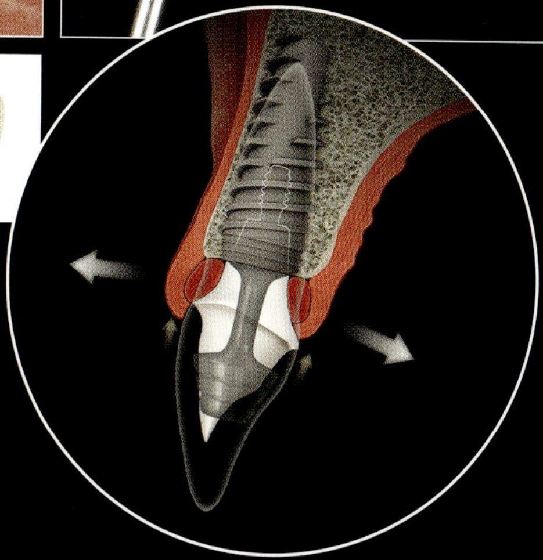

The provisional restoration was removed for the final implant impression. A definitive zirconia abutment and provisional crown were fabricated. The provisional crown was positioned and relined with acrylic intraorally and then finalized for optimal fit and proper soft tissue response. The illustration depicts the definitive abutment concept from day 1 of the prosthetic phase to minimize bone resorption and remodeling. It also illustrates the concept to create ideal pressure for tissue modification and emergence profile, which is carefully designed through a diagnostic wax-up and carving of the stone cast.

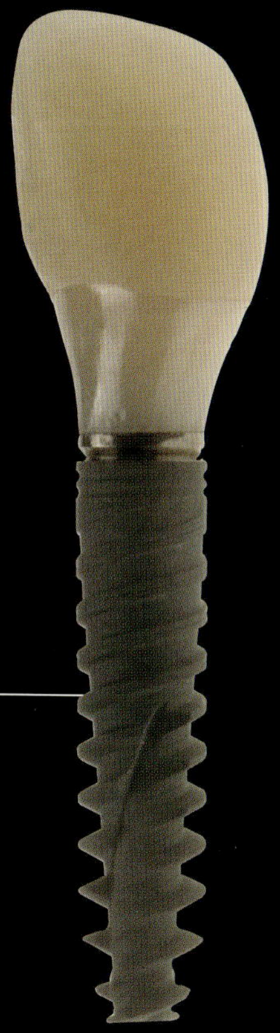

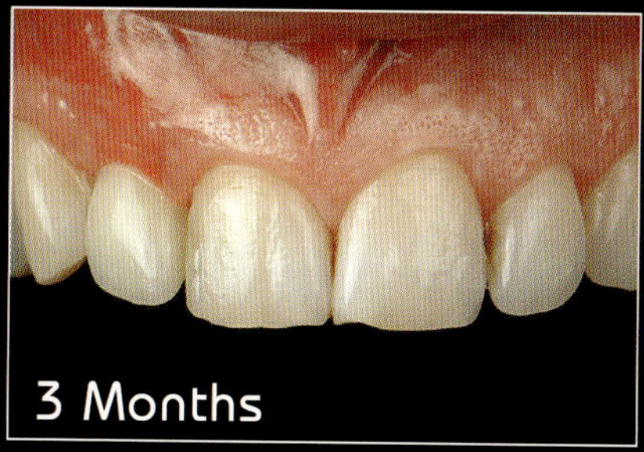

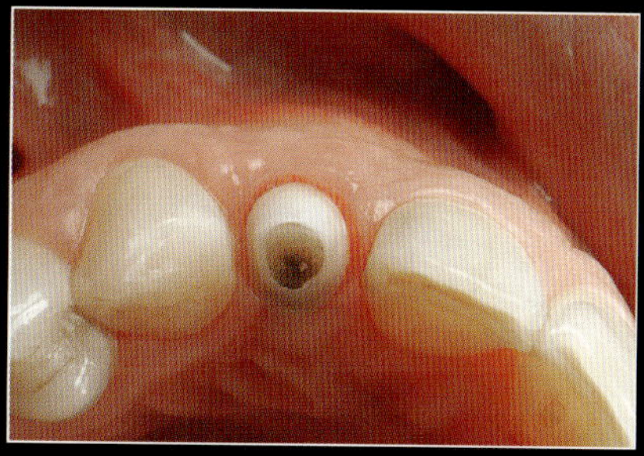

The tissue response around the definitive zirconia abutment and provisional restoration was re-evaluated 3 months after their insertion. The occlusal view indicates the tissue volume gained with the CTG. A veneered zirconia crown served as the definitive restoration.

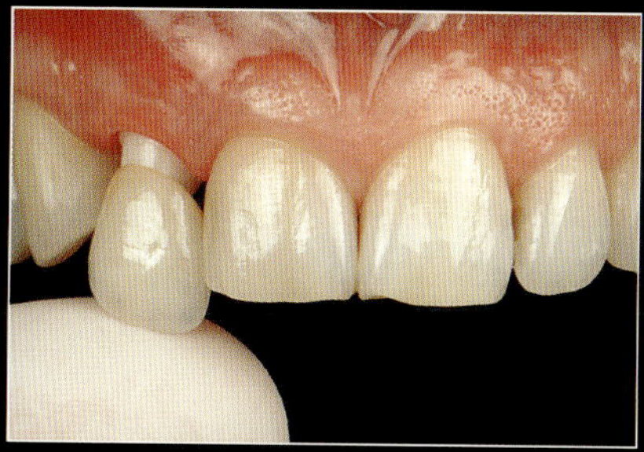
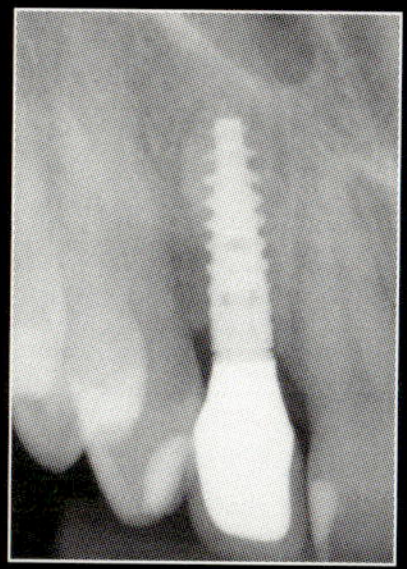
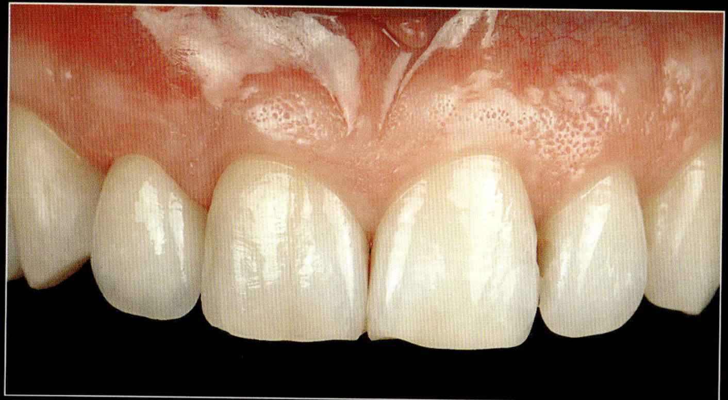

Biomaterials

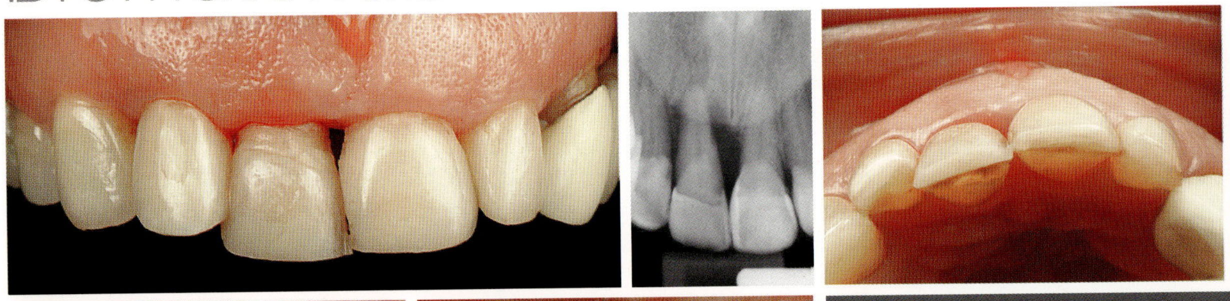

The maxillary right central incisor required extraction because of severe periodontitis. Due to the severely resorbed bone and increased mobility of the six anterior teeth, a multi-unit fixed partial denture (FPD) was planned as the preferred prosthetic solution after periodontal pretreatment. It was planned to augment the pontic site to improve the esthetic and functional outcome. The tissue thickness in the area of the maxillary tuberosity was also compromised, suggesting a ridge preservation technique with GBR as a first step and a CTG at a later stage. A membrane made of porcine collagen and specifically designed as an alternative for autologous soft tissue grafts (Mucograft, Geistlich) was selected in combination with bovine bone substitute material (Bio-Oss).

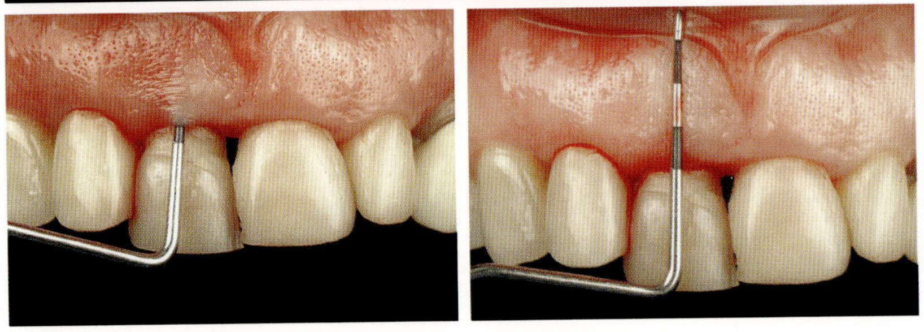

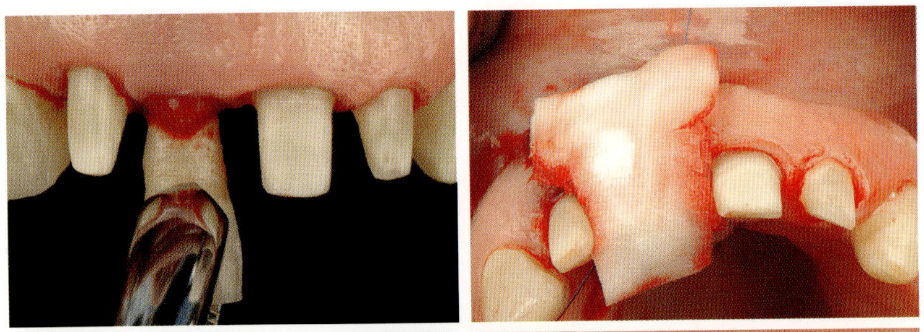

The adjacent teeth were prepared for full-coverage FPDs. The maxillary right central incisor was extracted, and the membrane was slid between the buccal bone and the tissue flap to protect the bone substitute particles. The membrane was folded twice to increase its thickness.

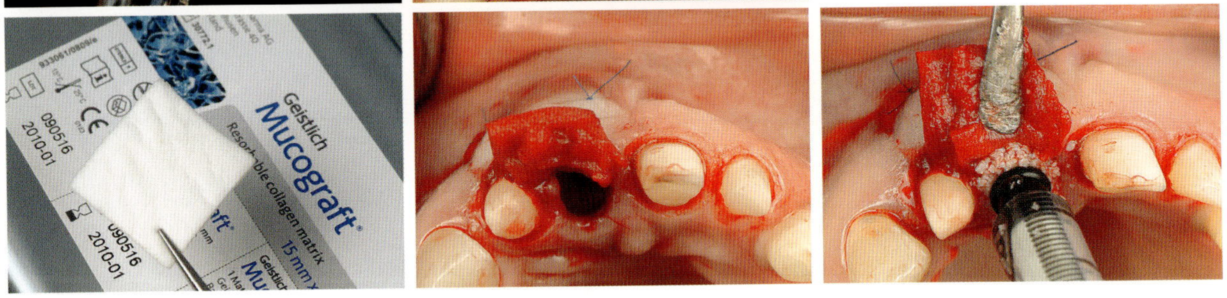

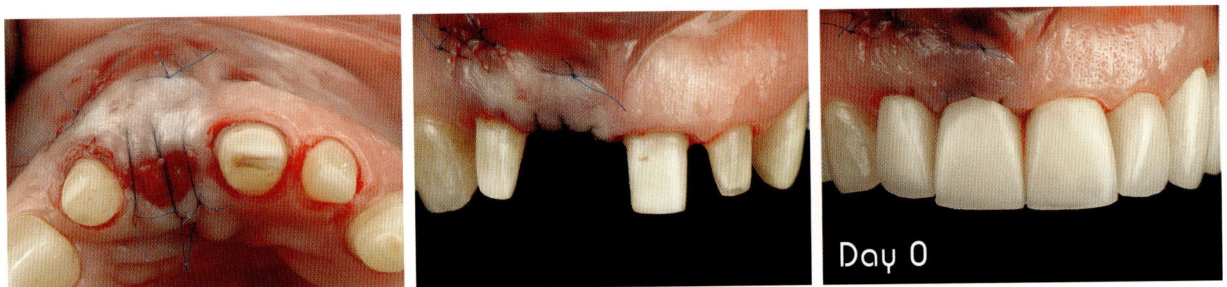

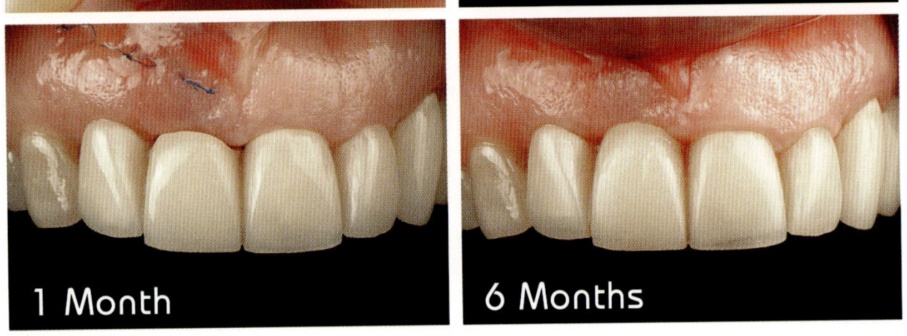

6-0 sutures were used to seal the socket in the crestal area and the fistula on the buccal aspect. The provisional restoration was relined with acrylic on the abutment teeth, adjusted, and polished. The typical resorption and difference in tissue volume is noticeable between the 1- and 6-month re-evaluation visits.

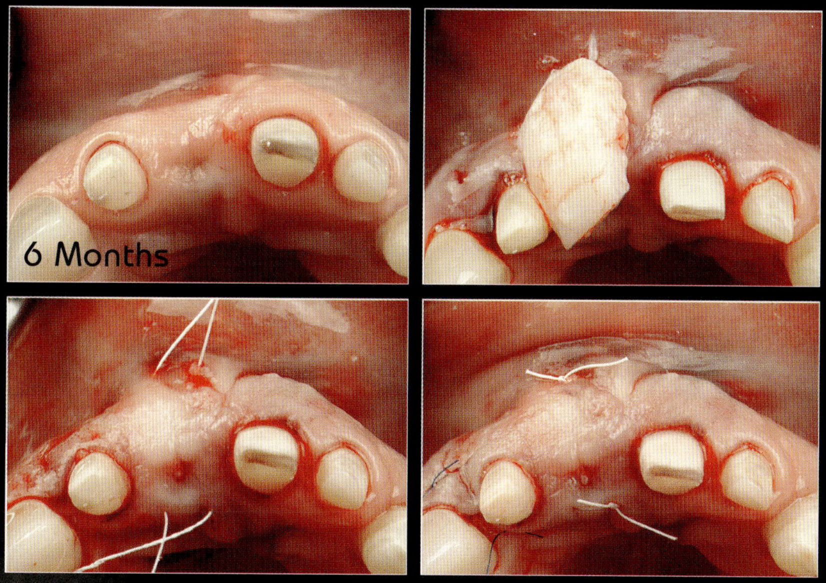

Six months after surgery, the pontic site was grafted with the entire tissue of the tuberosity. A tunnel incision was prepared on the ridge from the buccal aspect to the MGJ and toward the palatal aspect to create space for the dense CTG. An entrance to the tunnel was prepared between the maxillary right lateral incisor and the canine to insert the graft onto the ridge and create an improved pontic site. The graft was sutured in place, and the tissue flap was secured with vertical mattress sutures to conceal the graft.

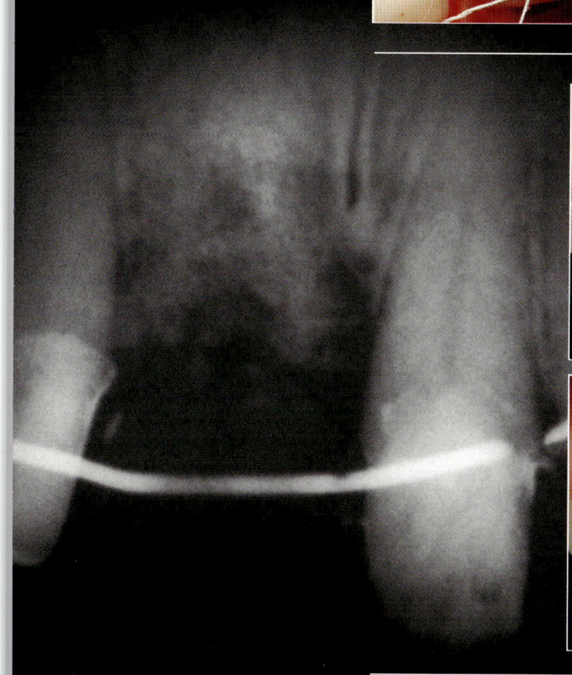

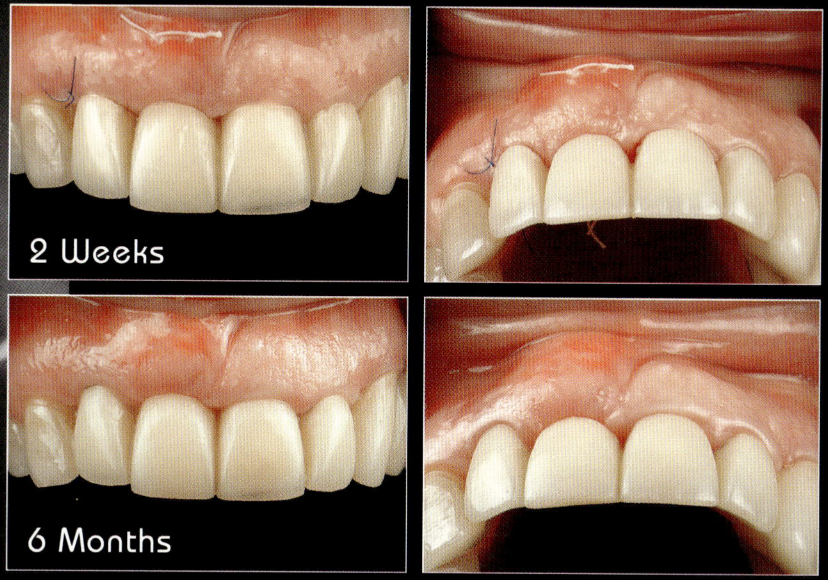

Different views to assess the tissue volume at 2 weeks and 6 months post-surgery, indicating stability of the soft tissue condition. Therefore, the final impression was made 1 year after the grafting procedure.

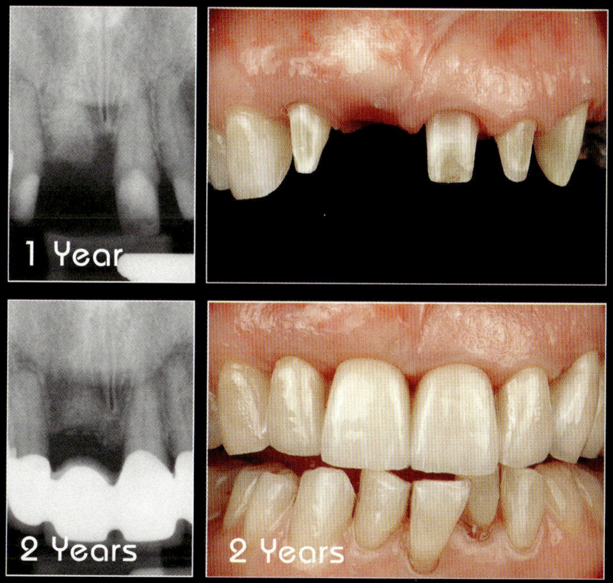

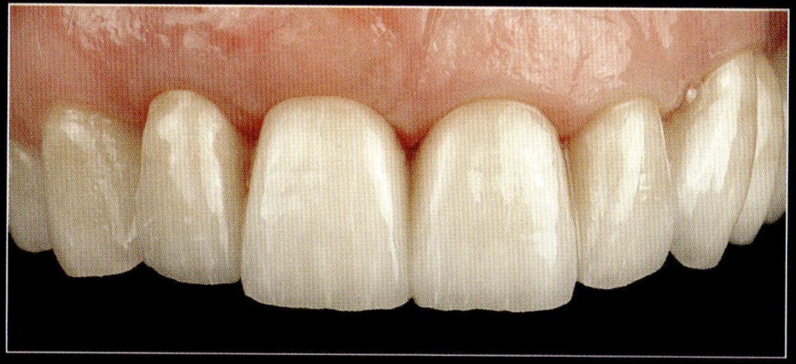

Definitive preparations of the abutment teeth. The soft tissue pontic site was conditioned with the provisional restoration.

Situation after cementation of the definitive zirconia-based FPD and corresponding periapical radiograph 2 years later.

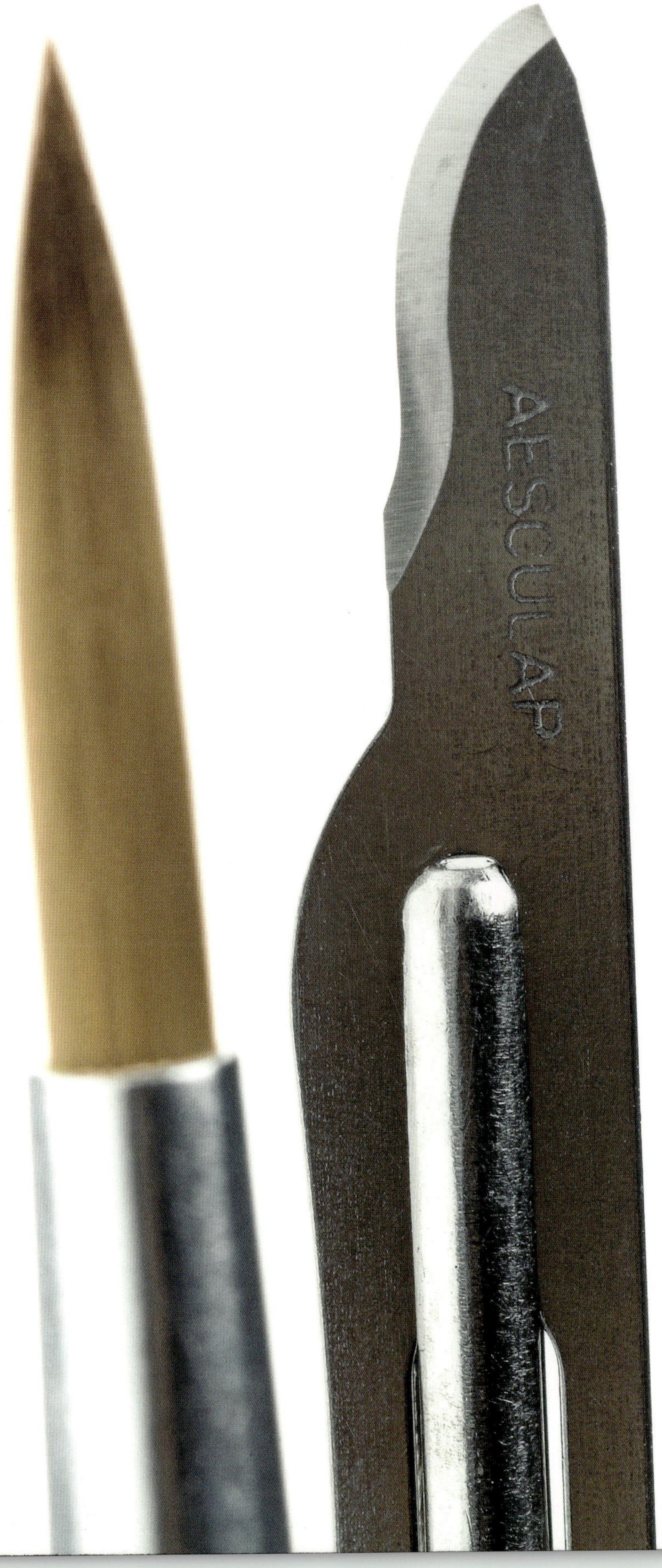
AESCULAP

Creating a Soft Tissue Contour Prosthetically Through Provisional Restoration

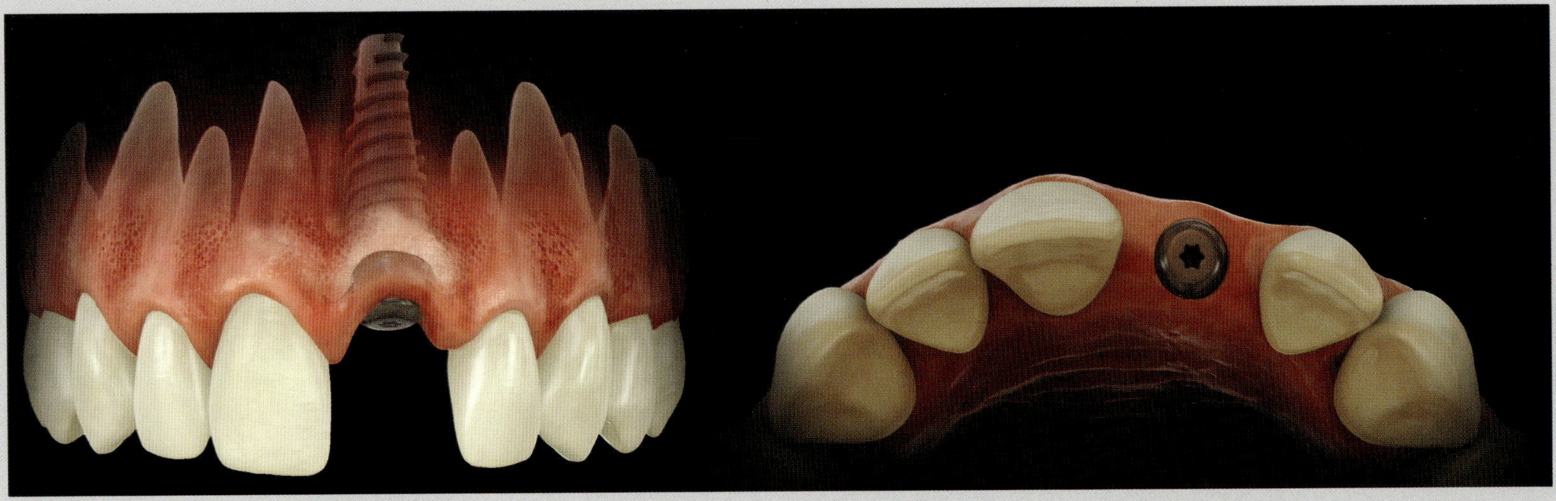

Interproximal tissue height

Interproximal tissue height refers to the papillary position adjacent to the implant site and the other papillae in the esthetic zone, which greatly affects the difficulty level of a patient situation. Even and symmetric interproximal soft tissue heights provide better predictability of the final outcome. The complexity and need for multidisciplinary intervention, such as orthodontic extrusion, increases with dissimilar tissue heights, often caused by lack of bone support on the adjacent teeth. Such deficiencies are often caused by periodontal inflammation, trauma, or surgical iatrogenic manipulation and may provide a major challenge to the goal of creating balance and symmetry.

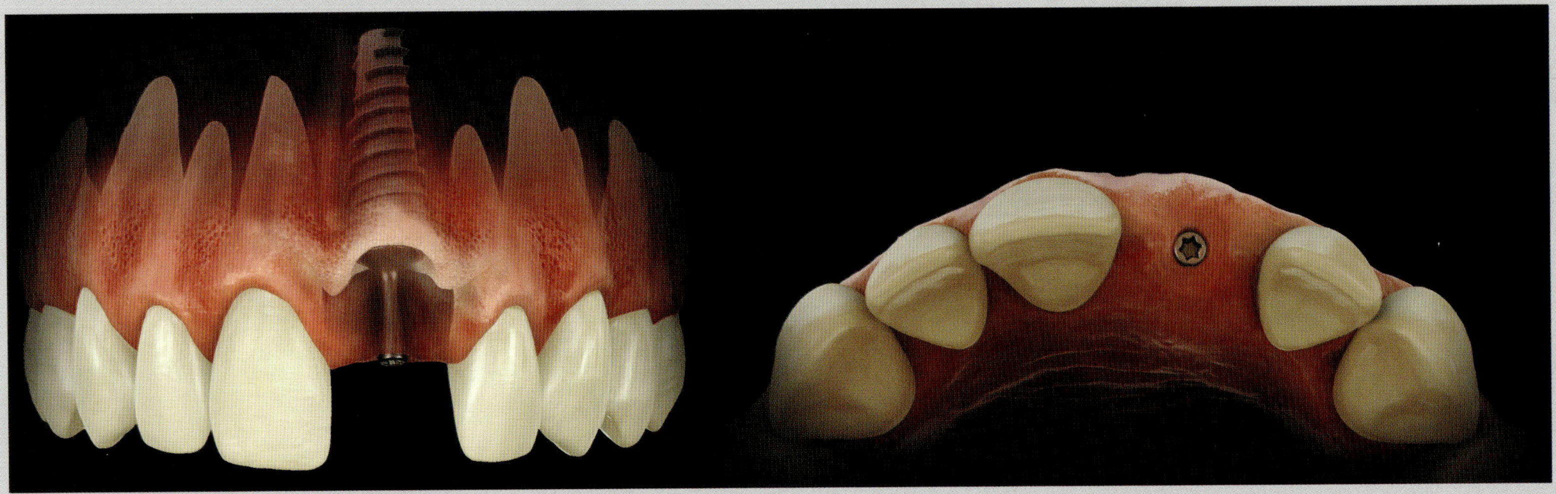

Free gingival height

Free gingival height location describes the vertical height of the free gingival margin on the buccal aspect of the implant site in comparison with the gingival margin on the reference tooth (the tooth to be copied, including its gingival scallop). This parameter is a decisive factor for the amount of pressure that needs to be applied to the soft tissue through the implant abutment and the respective crown restoration to achieve a height of the free gingival margin that is level with the site to be copied.

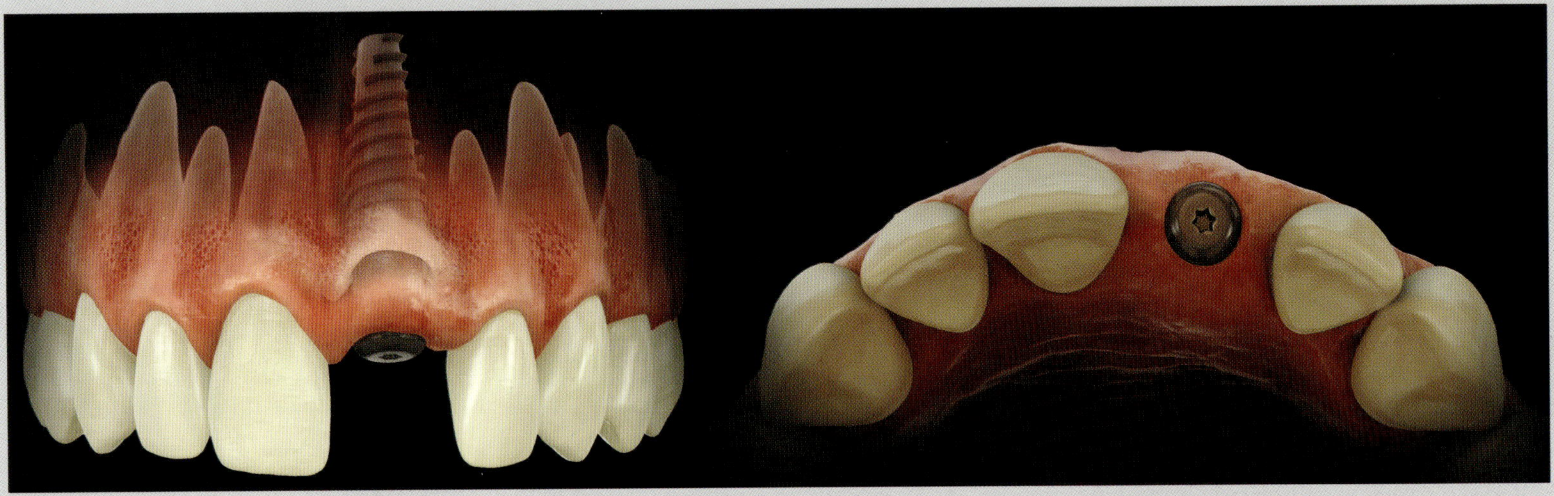

Buccal volume

Buccal soft tissue volume relates to the horizontal relationship or "thickness" of the tissue around the implant site in comparison with the site to be copied. It is important for the restorative dentist to know if a CTG was placed around the implant and, if so, which donor site it was harvested from to determine the appropriate prosthetic treatment.

Criteria for soft tissue evaluation

When facing the restorative phase of implant treatment, the correct treatment plan depends on accurate diagnosis and criteria established during the re-evaluation phase. The symbiosis between surgeon and restorative dentist has never been so interdependent as it is today. The surgeon must know the restorative prerequisites of ideal implant placement and conservative, minimally invasive incision approaches to be able to create various soft tissue volumes—thick, dense, centered, and coronal to the implant. Conversely, the restorative dentist must adequately assess the soft tissue situation to identify the type of necessary surgery and grafting procedure associated with the donor site selection and determine the anticipated time of wound healing. Before starting the prosthetic phase, it is essential to recognize the potential of the implant site that needs to be restored. The level and volume of tissue are key to an inconspicuous implant restoration. For long-term esthetic results, an abundance of tissues around the implants is critical, which, in most cases, cannot be accomplished without soft tissue grafting and thickening of the biotype. The three main points of reference discussed in the surgical objectives must be confirmed.

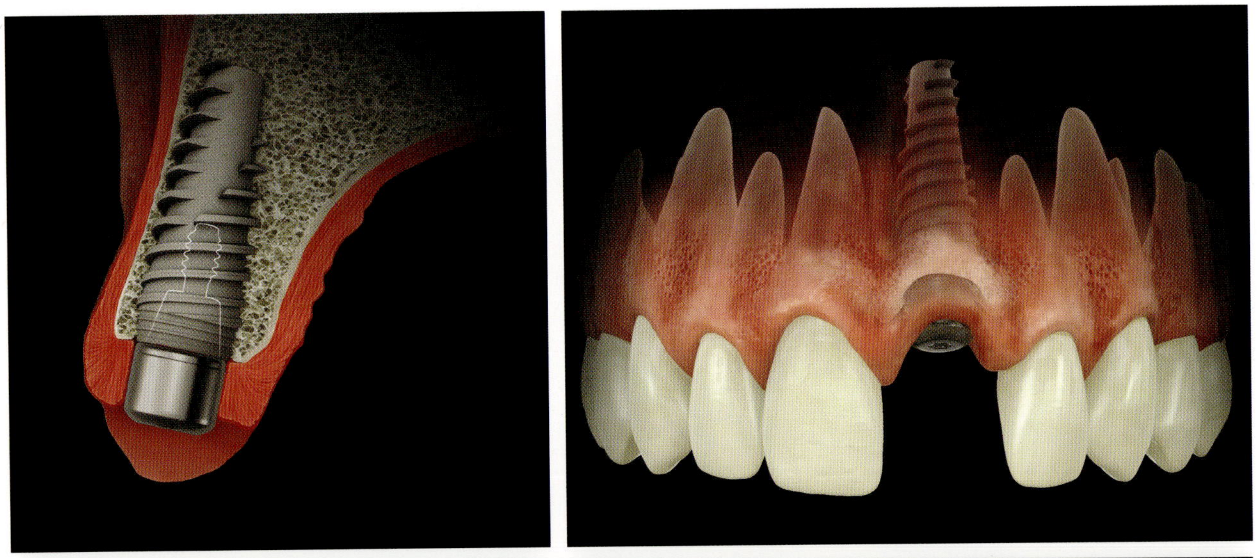

Short (3-mm) healing abutments limit the surgeon's ability to develop the desired soft tissue height, unless a flap is raised above the healing abutment. Short healing abutments often cause insufficient soft tissue height and, in case a CTG was placed, an apically displaced graft. The initial prosthetic situation is therefore compromised.

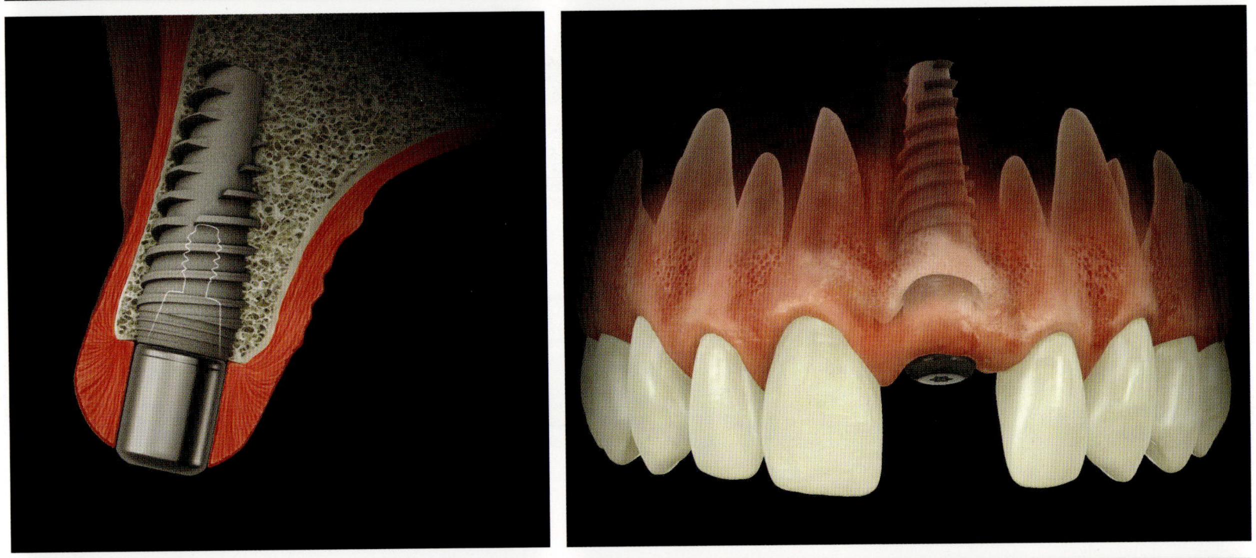

5-mm healing abutments provide a greater reference to how much the flap and graft should be coronally advanced for an ideal restorative result. The taller healing abutment provides greater visibility for the surgeon when placing the implant at the same depth. The free gingival margin on the implant site should be at least 2 mm above the margin of the reference tooth. The diameter of a standard healing abutment does not provide sufficient space for the graft to be sutured in the most coronal aspect.

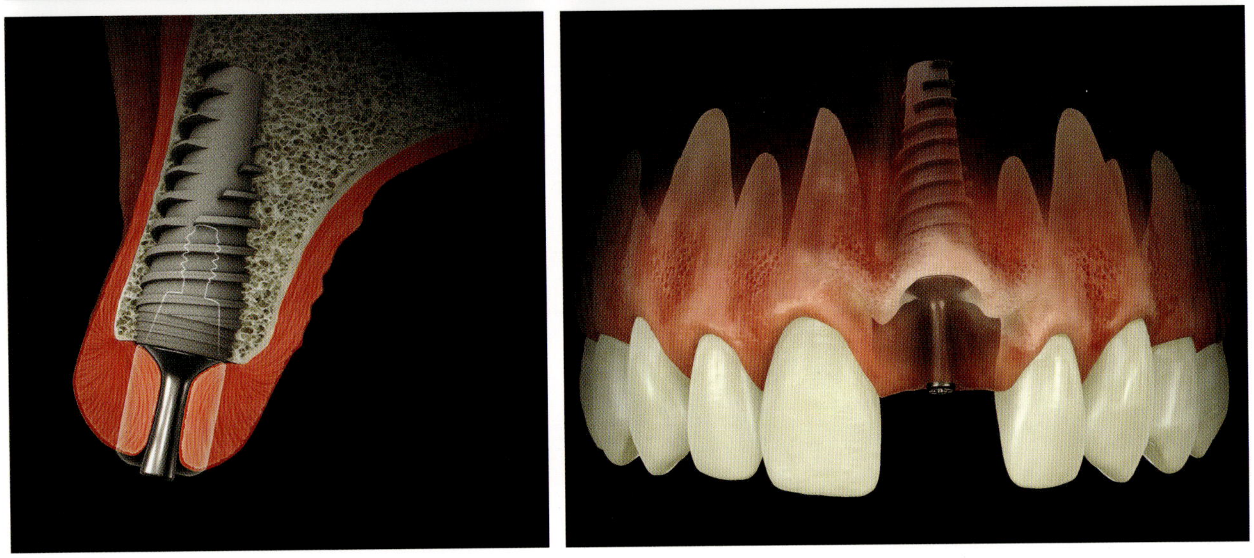

5-mm straight healing abutments provide the best alternative in controlling the vertical and horizontal dimensions and a great advantage for flap closure and adaptation in a most coronal position. The narrow diameter of the straight healing abutment allows the surgeon to create the desired tissue volume for the restorative dentist and preferred wound closure.

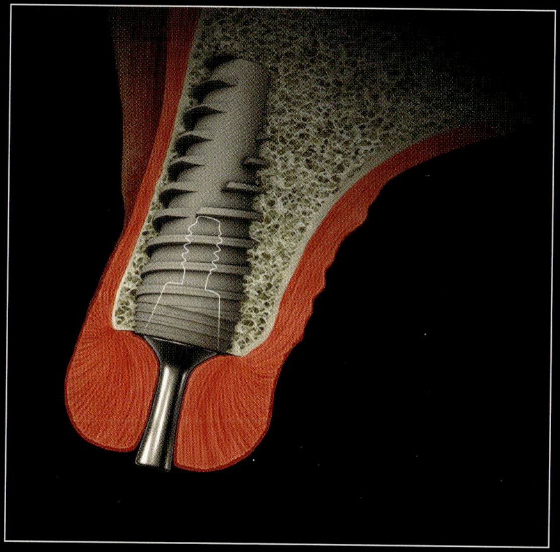

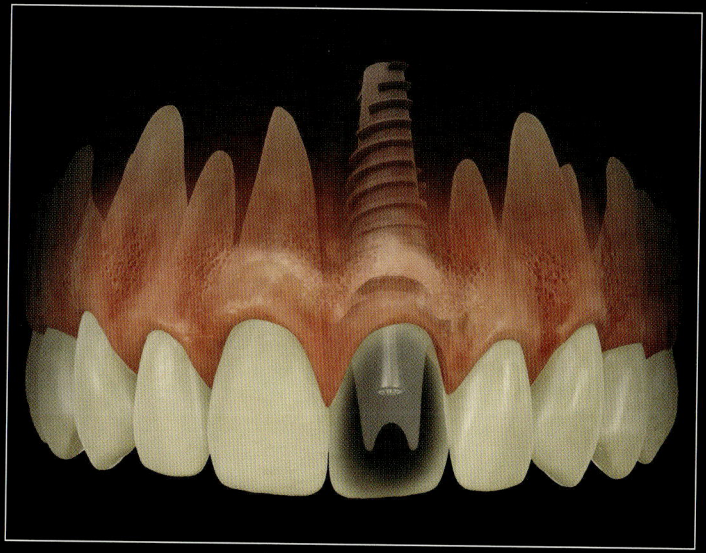

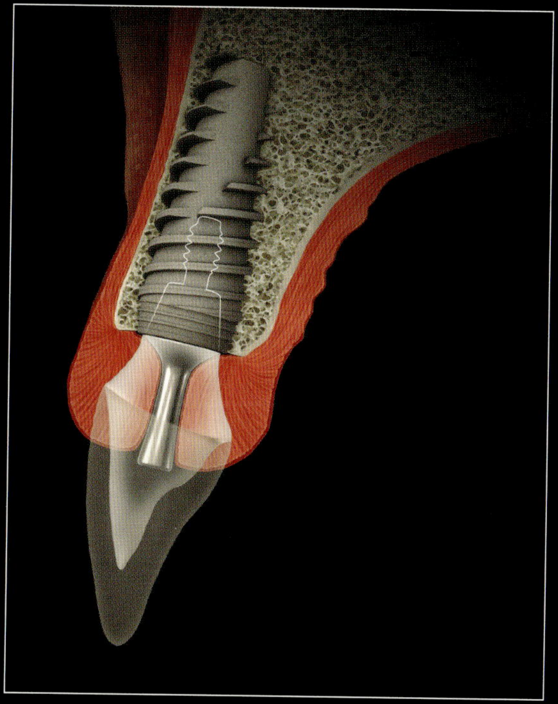

The amount of pressure from the abutment-crown complex is directly related to the implant position, but, more importantly, it is directly related to the peri-implant soft tissue quantity (volume) and quality (density of donor site) both vertically and horizontally. Prosthetic connection inevitably creates soft tissue recession, regardless of the emergence profile design.

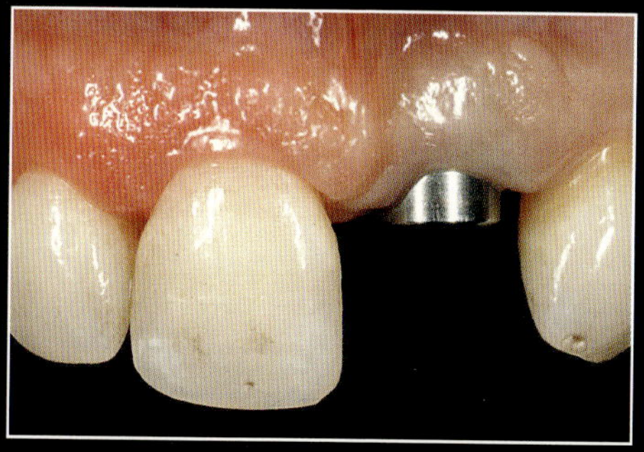

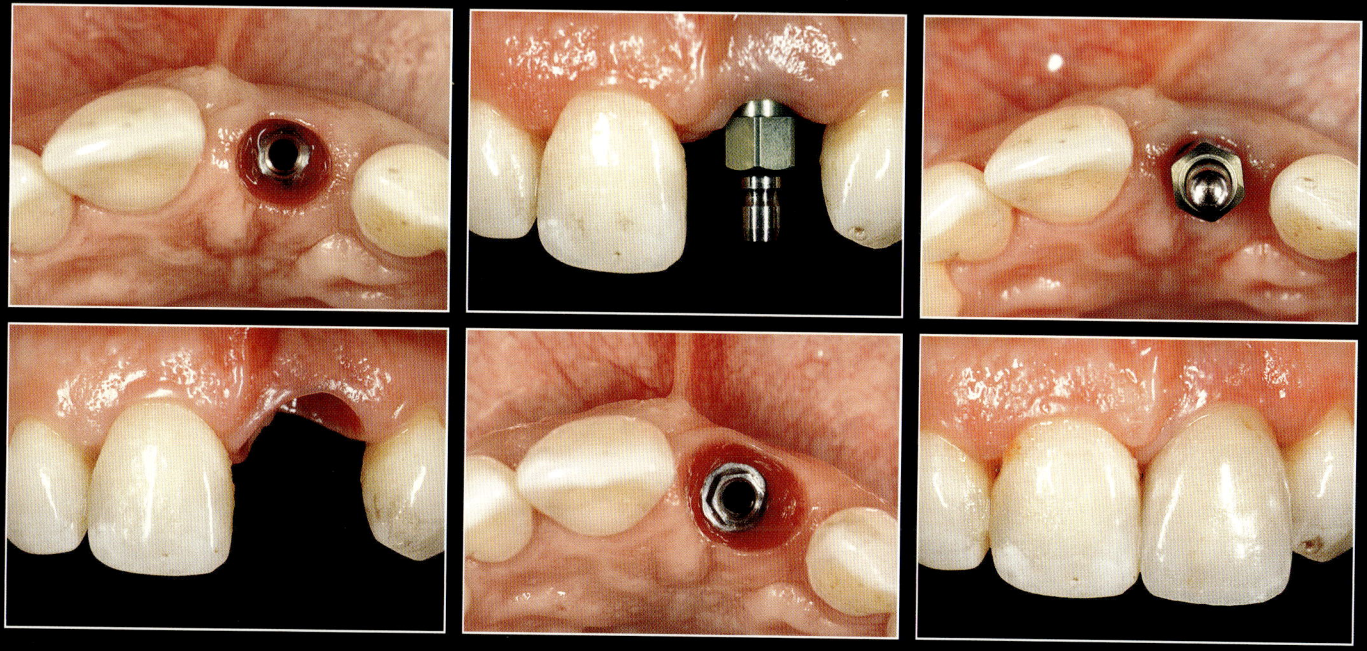

The clinical situation reflects the above discussion. A conventional 3-mm healing abutment (with a diameter wider than the implant) was placed without CTGs in a patient with a moderately thick gingival biotype. The interproximal height was lost to a certain degree, the free gingival margin was leveled, and the buccal volume was nonexistent. The definitive restoration demonstrates the treatment deficiencies.

Independent of the emergence profile, whether flat or concave, connecting the restoration to the implant always creates a soft tissue recession. Coined as "the arc width concept" in 1994 by Phillips and Kois, height will always be lost. It is therefore of utmost importance to increase the height of the tissue by at least 2 mm coronal to the ideal final free gingival margin. The implant surgeon should concentrate not only on raising the tissue coronally as much as possible but also on thickening it. To compensate for the recession created by the connection of the prosthetic restoration, the peri-implant soft tissue should be grafted with thick and dense CTGs harvested from the tuberosity.

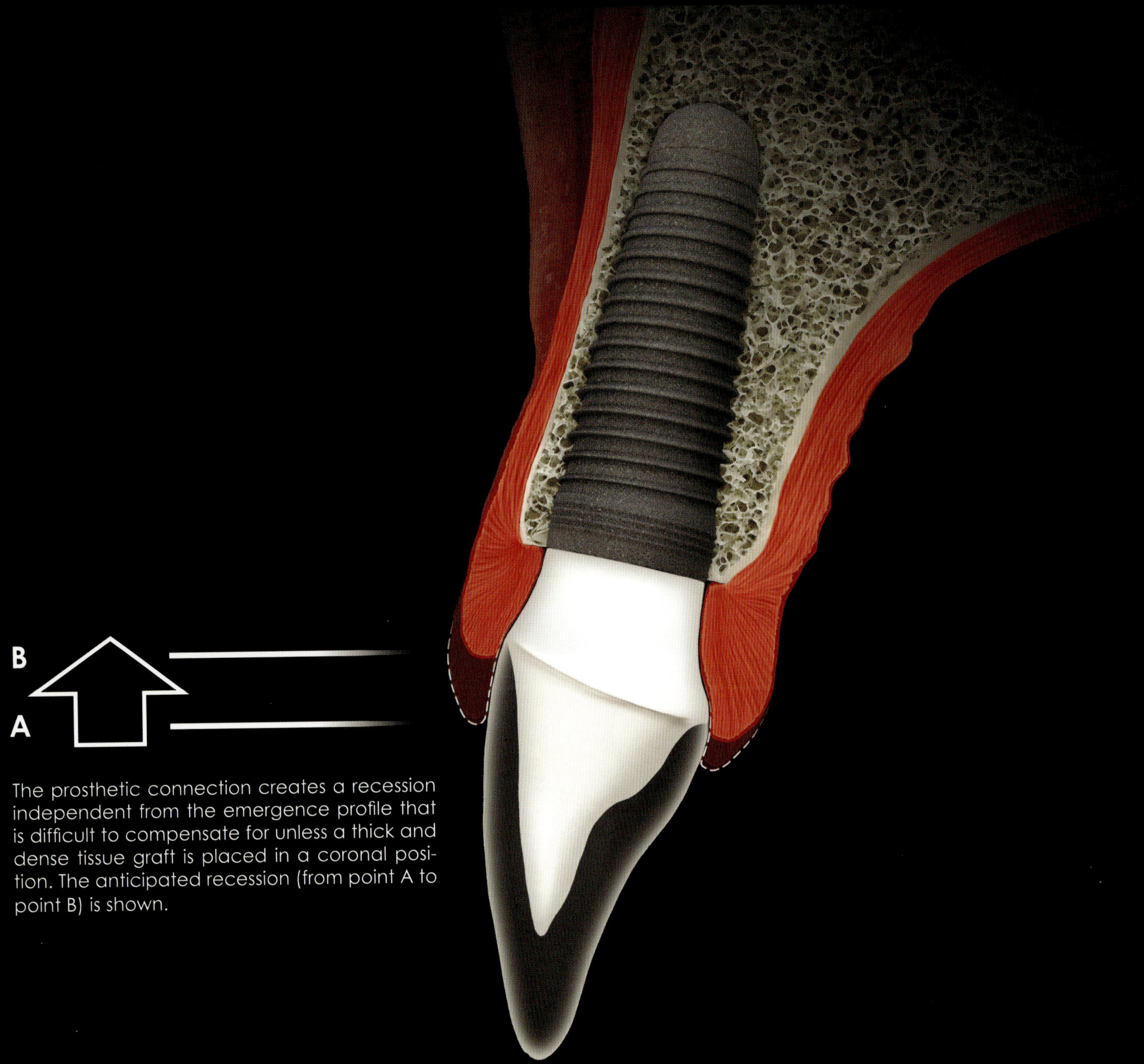

The prosthetic connection creates a recession independent from the emergence profile that is difficult to compensate for unless a thick and dense tissue graft is placed in a coronal position. The anticipated recession (from point A to point B) is shown.

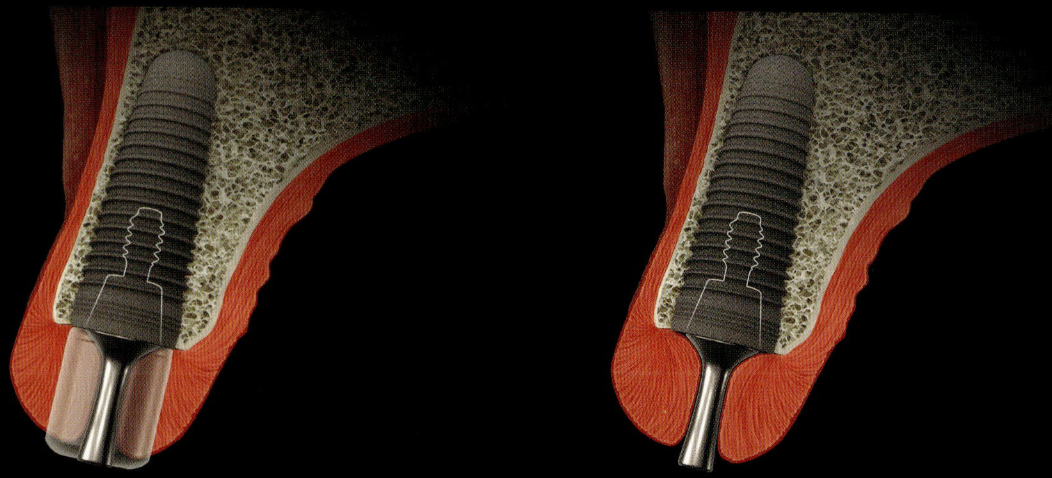

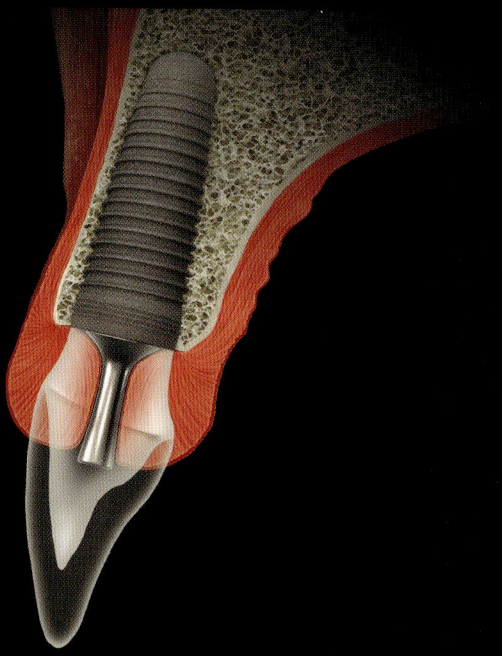

With thick and dense soft tissue, the prosthetic phase becomes simplified with increasing chances to achieve the desired restorative pressure and ultimate outcome. Ischemia is related in the prosthetic field to pressure blanching of the tissues, reducing the amount of blood supply and eventually resulting in necrosis of the surrounding tissues. The patient scenarios discussed in this book predominantly include prosthetic pressure applied to soft tissue augmented with grafts harvested from the tuberosity.

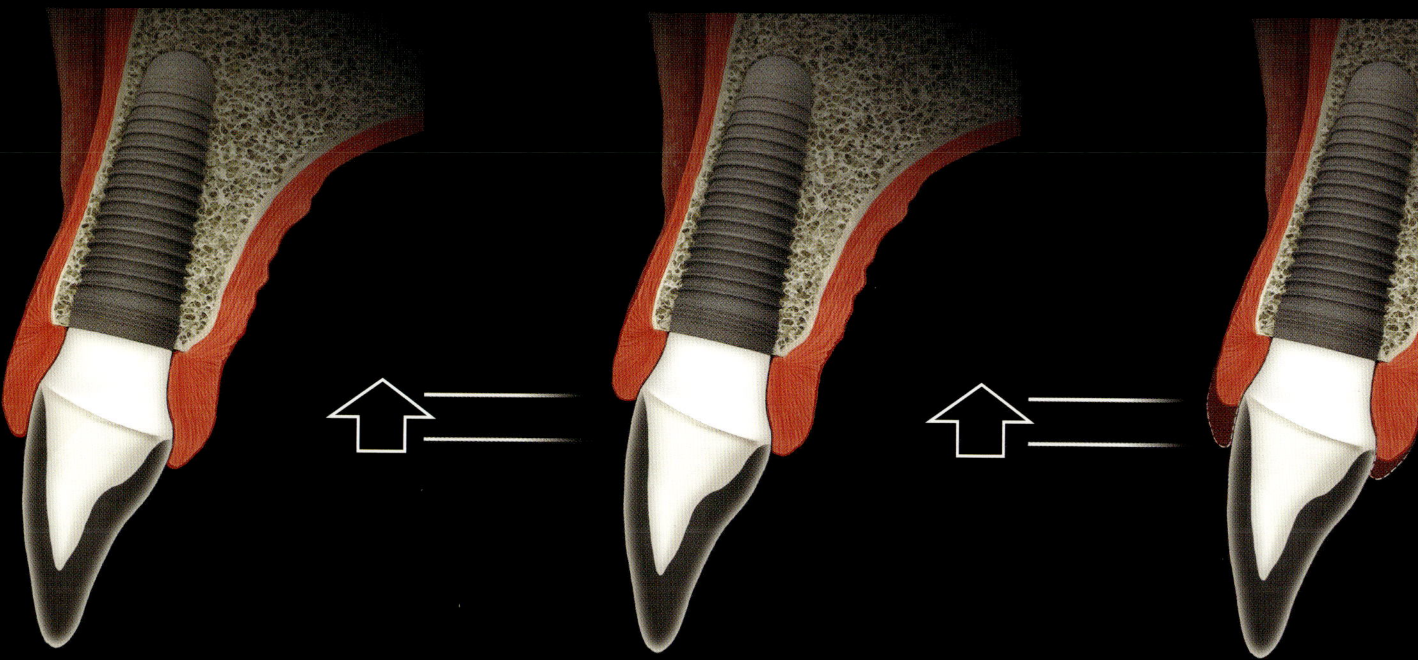

The amount of pressure from the implant abutment–crown restoration is directly related to the diameter of the original tooth. This pressure is first designed from a diagnostic wax-up, which provides information about the desired contour of the crown. The stone master cast is then carved to create the emergence profile needed to meet the contour designed in the wax-up. The subgingival abutment aspect follows a concave design to create the so-called "O-ring" or "doughnut" effect, which thickens the peri-implant soft tissue and provides long-lasting esthetic results.

Patient situations

Four patient situations are presented, demonstrating different treatment philosophies based on the clinical situation and the necessary treatment.

- Patient situation 1 revealed insufficient soft tissue for immediate restoration. The patient was unwilling to undergo further treatment, so an ideal provisional restoration was inserted. After a 3-month healing period for soft tissue maturation and stability, the definitive crown restoration was inserted.
- Patient situation 2 included an abundance of soft tissue. The soft tissue contour could be managed through staged provisional manipulation. The donor site for a CTG was then selected to decide the sequence of the prosthetic phase. The amount of pressure from the abutment-crown complex is directly related to the quantity (volume) and quality (density of the donor site) of the CTG both vertically and horizontally.
- Excessive pressure was applied during fabrication of the provisional restoration in patient situation 3, which was a direct result of a poor-quality tissue graft donor site. This led to an extensive recession defect that was difficult to correct.
- In patient situation 4, placement of a definitive zirconia abutment and provisional crown restoration with soft tissue management provided predictable results.

Patient situation 1: Insufficient soft tissue

This particular clinical situation is especially difficult to treat. The lack of a CTG means insufficient soft tissue, and the existing soft tissue is located apical to the implant head. In situations like these, the soft tissue may be deficient on the interproximal aspect, the buccal aspect, or both, which presents the greatest challenge. When a CTG was not placed and a lack of soft tissue is evident, the only recommendation for the restorative dentist (when the patient refuses further surgery) is to insert a provisional restoration and observe the tissue reaction. The provisional restoration is designed to the same contours and interproximal contact areas as the missing tooth. After a 3-month healing period, the soft tissue topography is re-evaluated before the definitive crown is fabricated and placed. In any case, once the provisional restoration is inserted, the soft tissue situation should be re-evaluated every 10 days for the first month. Sometimes, especially in patients with high lip lines, esthetic failure may convince the patient of the need for a CTG augmentation.

Surgeon: Dr José Antonio Arruti

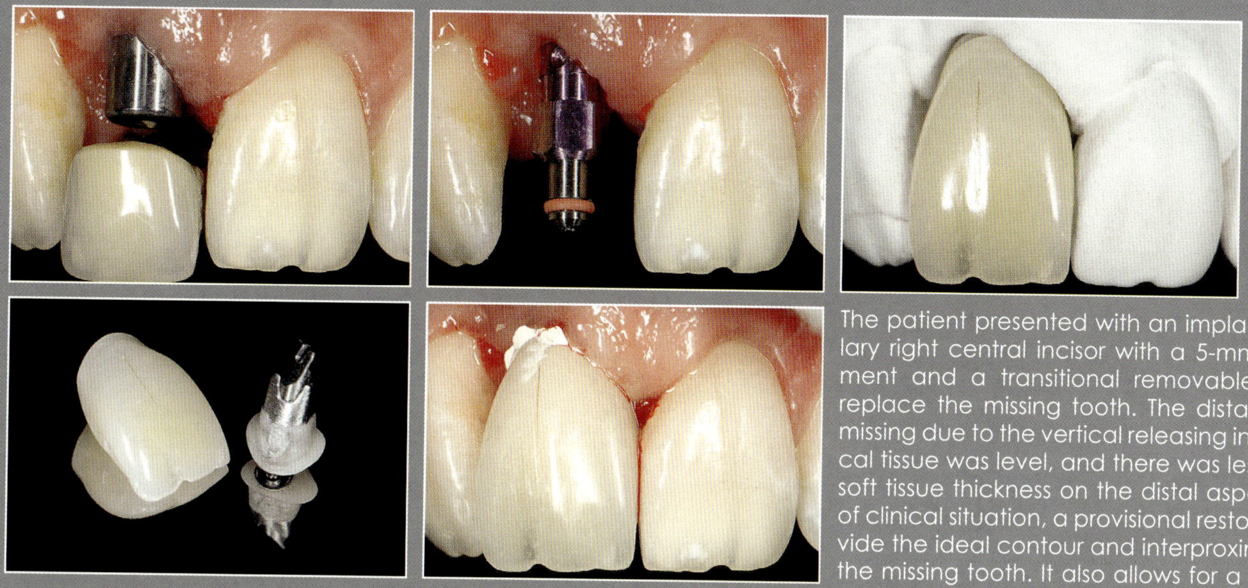

The patient presented with an implant on the maxillary right central incisor with a 5-mm healing abutment and a transitional removable appliance to replace the missing tooth. The distal papillae were missing due to the vertical releasing incision. The buccal tissue was level, and there was less than 1 mm of soft tissue thickness on the distal aspect. In this type of clinical situation, a provisional restoration may provide the ideal contour and interproximal contacts of the missing tooth. It also allows for a 3-month observation period of the soft tissue reaction.

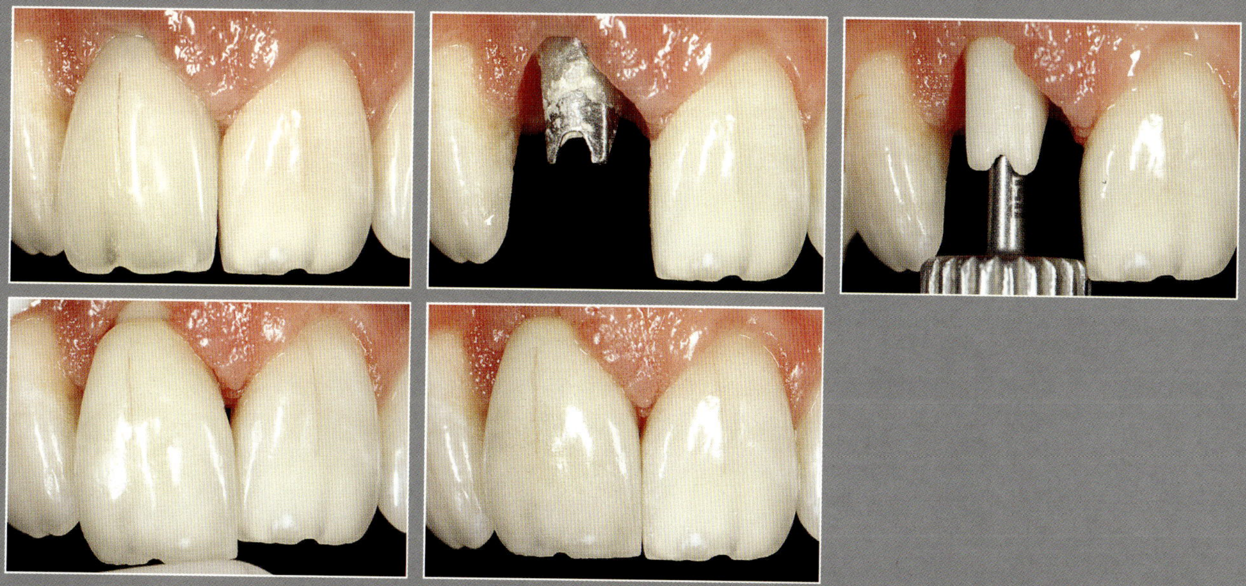

Three months after provisional restoration, the soft tissue had responded to the provisional contour and regenerated by secondary intention. Then the implant restoration was finalized. Note the longer implant restoration and the asymmetric emergence profile after 1 year. Having visualized and understood this outcome, the patient was satisfied with the final results.

Patient situation 2: Ideal situation with an abundance of soft tissue

The patient presented with an ideal implant situation on the maxillary left central incisor, with a CTG from the palate. Interproximal tissues were level, the free gingival margin on the implant site was coronal to the adjacent central incisor, and the buccal volume was coronally displaced, though scarce on the buccodistal aspect. In clinical situations in which the CTG was harvested from the palate, the prosthetic phase should be performed sequentially (staged approach) to guide the soft tissue, which has a low density and is prone to recession under provisional pressure. A triangular tooth with a concave or straight emergence profile is designed so that the pressure of the buccal recession can be controlled. The patient is then seen every 10 days for re-evaluation, and chairside modifications are performed with composite or acrylic resin until an ideal scallop has been achieved. It is always recommended in these types of cases to start with an acrylic or composite abutment or screw-retained type of restoration (if implant placement allows it) to have more control over the emergence profile during the provisional stage. It is recommended in most cases to provide the definitive abutment and provisional crown restoration at the beginning of the prosthetic treatment. The poor quality of the palatal CTG, however, requires a more careful approach to avoid soft tissue recessions and costly prosthetic remakes as well as to ensure long-term stability.

Surgeon: Dr José Antonio Arruti

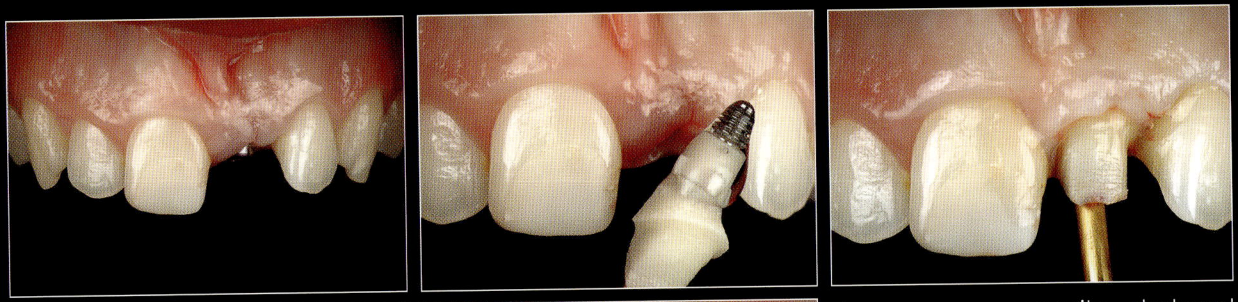

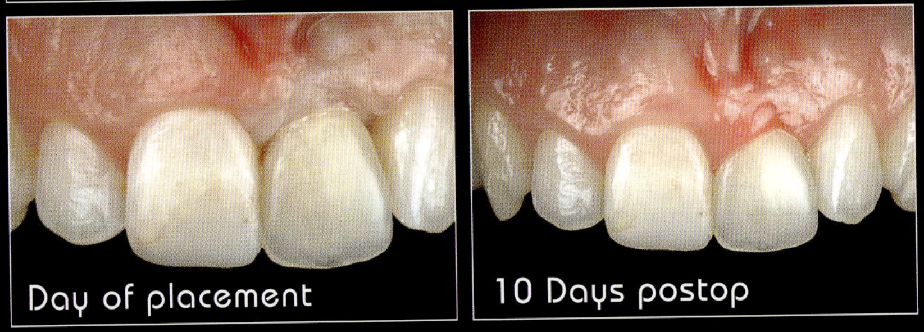

A concave composite abutment was designed to allow controlled pressure on the soft tissue with a triangular provisional crown and scalloping of the soft tissue in the interproximal area. The patient was then seen every 10 days to control the soft tissue management and make additional modifications chairside. The coronal growth of the tissue is obvious 10 days after implant insertion.

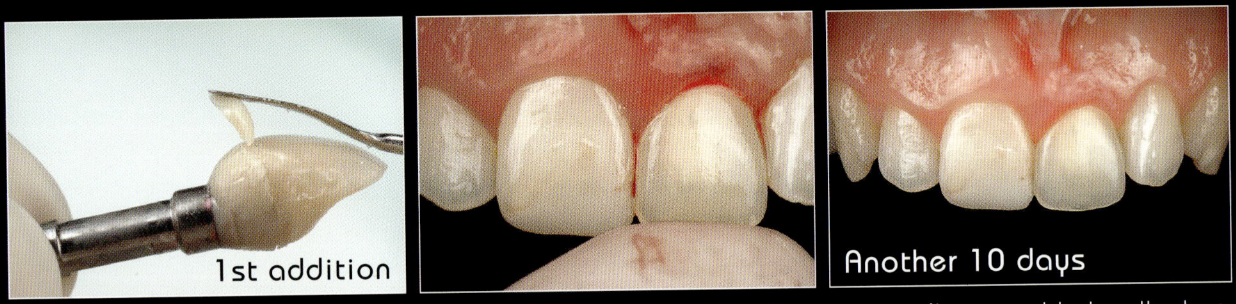

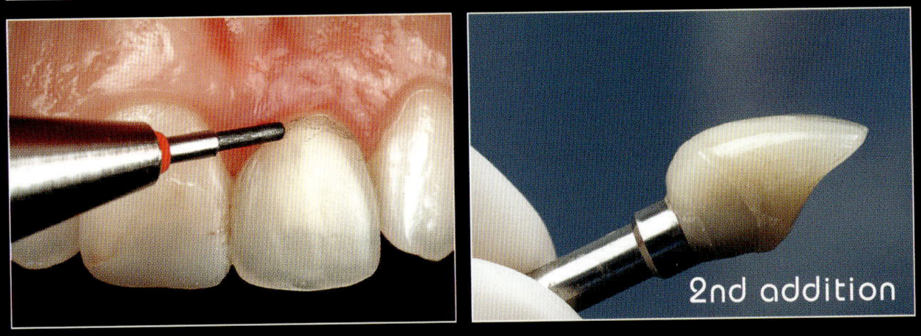

Composite was added on the buccal aspect of the abutment to create a greater buccal recession. After 10 more days, a flatter gingival scallop on the adjacent central incisor was observed. The gingival scallop that was achieved was marked with a pencil to visualize it once the abutment-crown complex was unscrewed. Additional modifications were made chairside to closely imitate the adjacent soft tissue morphology.

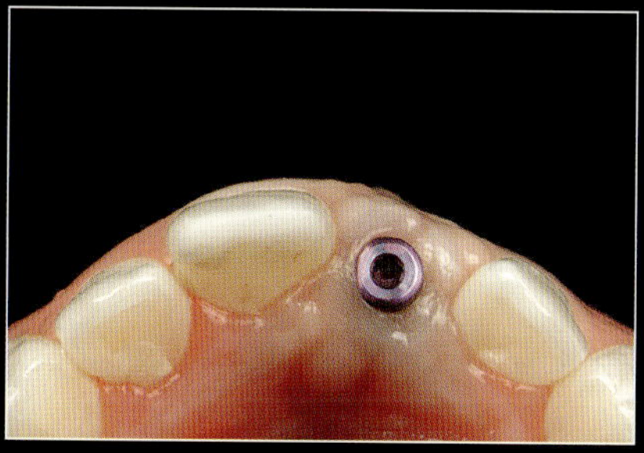
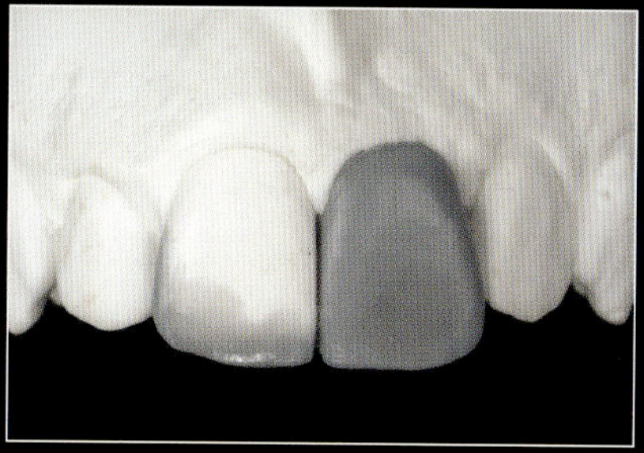
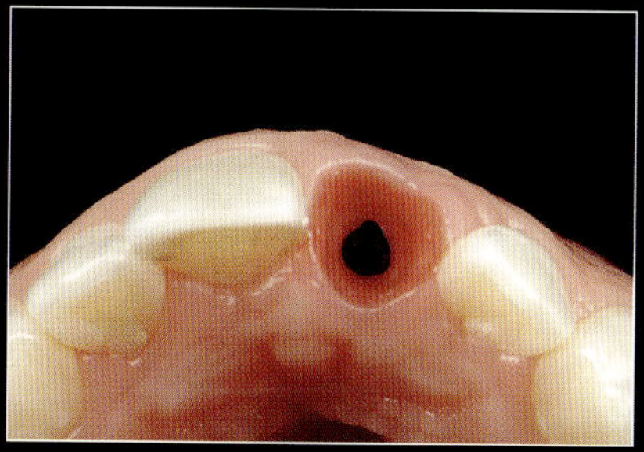
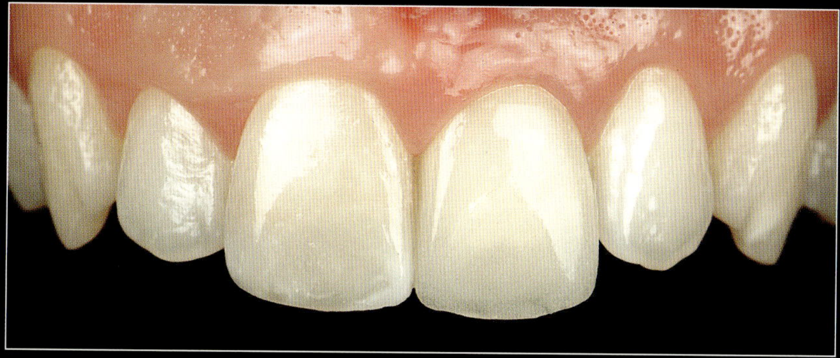

After a month of soft tissue manipulation, which achieved the ideal gingival contour, new provisional restorations were fabricated to create more dominant central incisors. A wax-up was made on a preliminary impression cast. A composite veneer and provisional crown restoration were fabricated and designed to support the soft tissue in an ideal manner. The occlusal view depicts the gradually established soft tissue morphology.

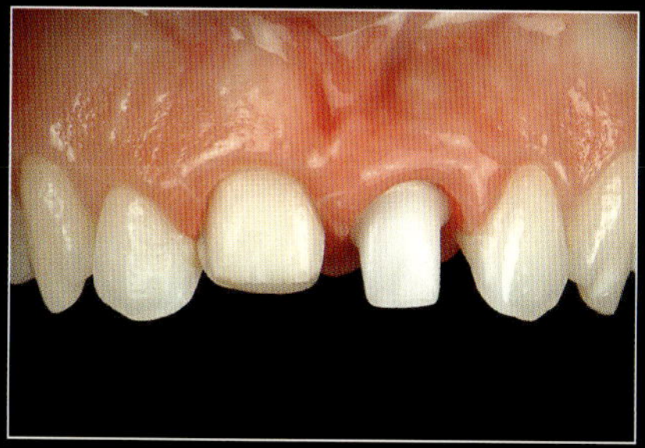
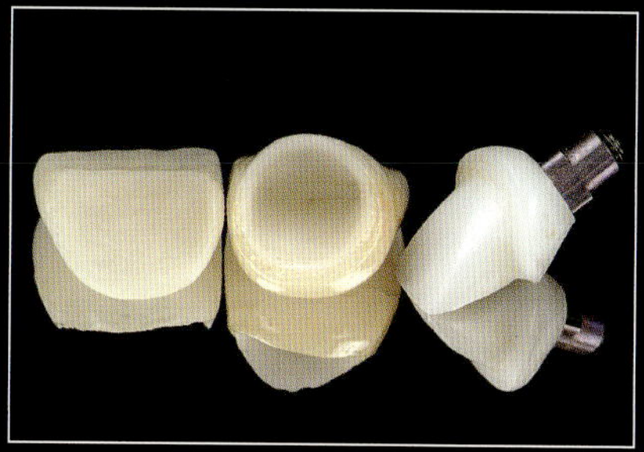
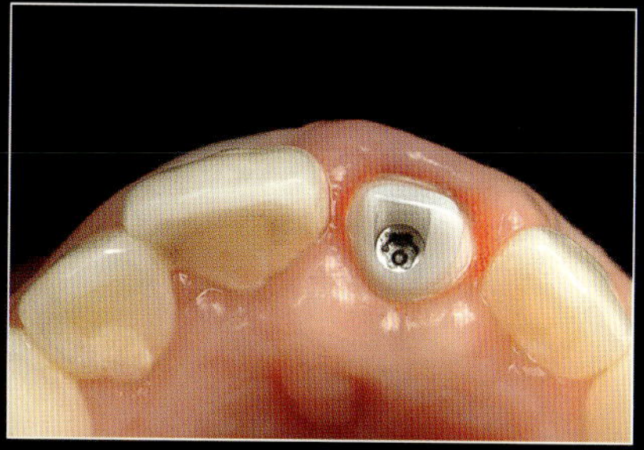
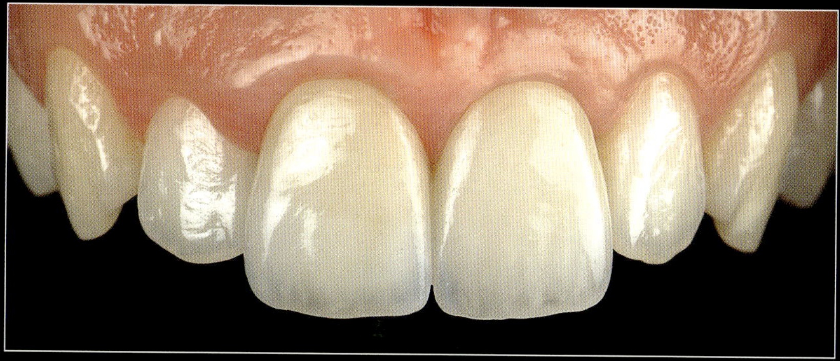

A feldspathic veneer on the maxillary right central incisor and an alumina crown with the corresponding zirconia abutment on the maxillary left central incisor implant were fabricated to complete the case. The staged provisional approach allowed for control of the soft tissue and a stable result.

Patient situation 3: Too much pressure

When the amount of pressure from the implant restoration exceeds the resistance of the soft tissue grafted on the buccal aspect of the implant site, a recession is created that can be difficult to correct. The communication among surgeon, restorative dentist, and laboratory technician is crucial to avoid such mistakes. The restorative dentist must know the donor site whenever a CTG was placed and communicate the exact pressure intended for exertion on the soft tissue to the laboratory technician. Pressure on the soft tissue from the abutment-crown complex is directly related to the quality (density) and the volume of the tissue at the respective site. Conversely, CTG donor site selection is crucial for restorative and surgical success.

Placing an implant with CTG augmentation affects all phases of esthetic rehabilitation. Patients with a thick soft tissue biotype who do not require augmentation are very rare. Creating uncontrolled recessions through restoration overcontouring poses a high-risk situation since regaining the lost soft tissue at a later time is often a very difficult task. The patient should be seen every 10 days for the clinician to assess and immediately control the situation if needed.

Surgeon: Dr José Antonio Arruti

A CTG from the palate was placed around the maxillary right central incisor implant. A provisional restoration was inserted and re-evaluated after 10 days, at which time it was noted that the pressure exerted on the soft tissue was too high. The abutment-crown complex was unscrewed and the buccal emergence profile flattened to allow the soft tissue to regenerate more coronally. Such regeneration takes significantly longer than creating a tissue recession. The situation after 1 month is shown.

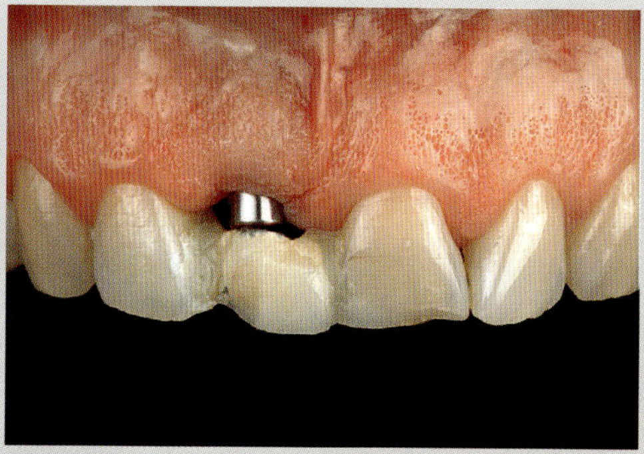
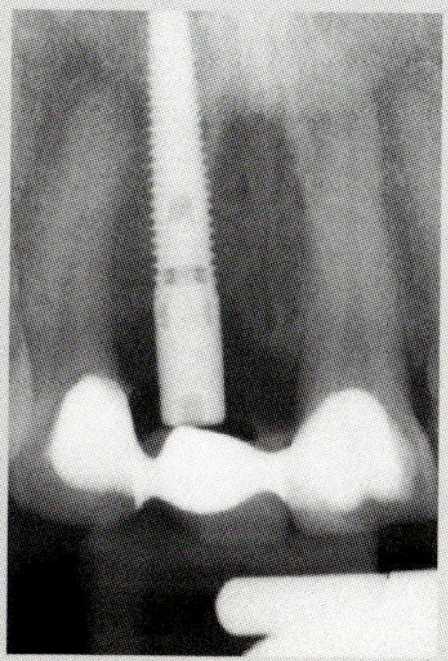
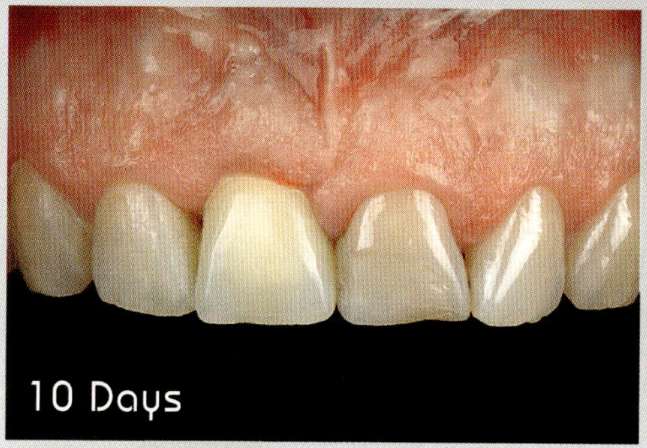

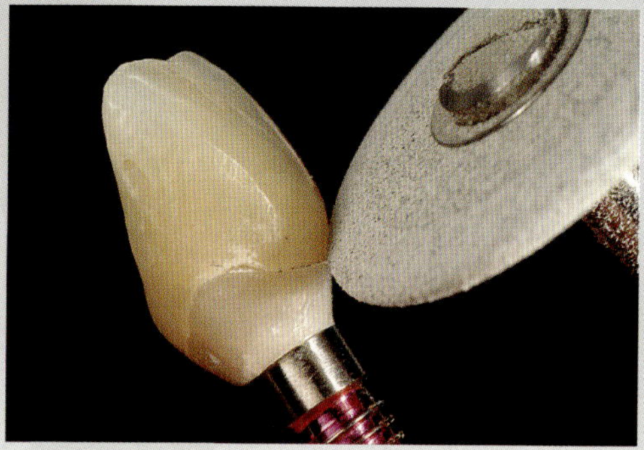
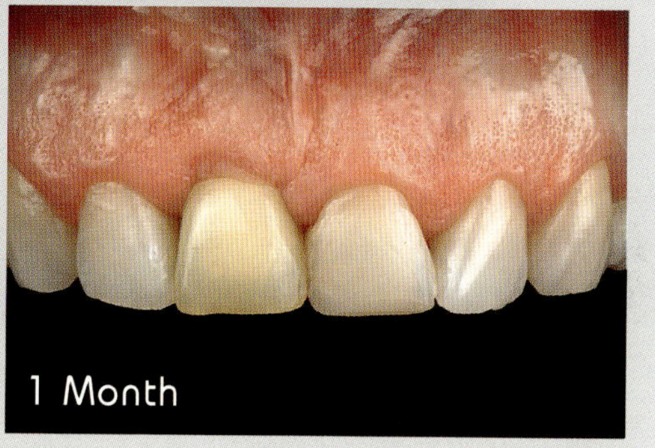

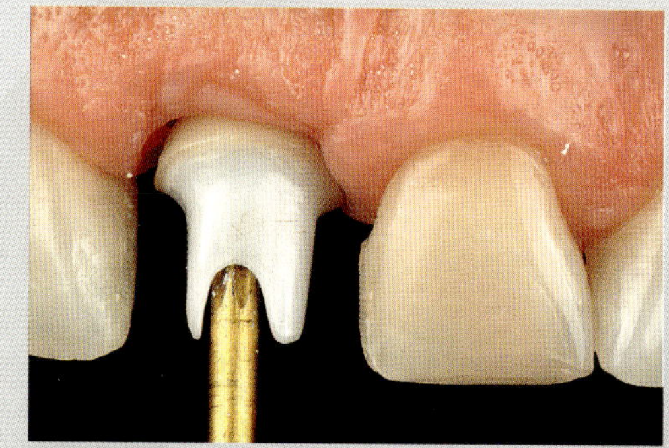
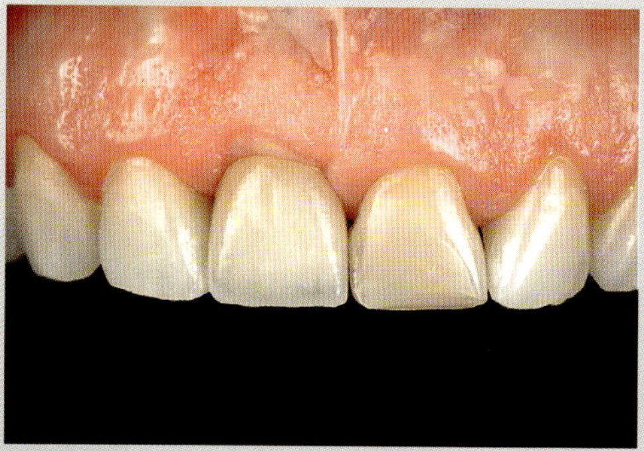
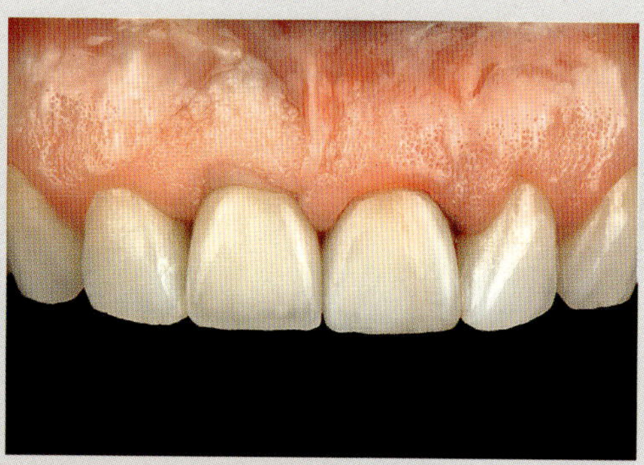

After 3 months of tissue stability, the prosthetic phase can continue. Some soft tissue recontouring on the maxillary left central incisor was necessary to level the soft tissue architecture and blend the composite veneer restoration with the adjacent zirconia implant crown and abutment restoration.

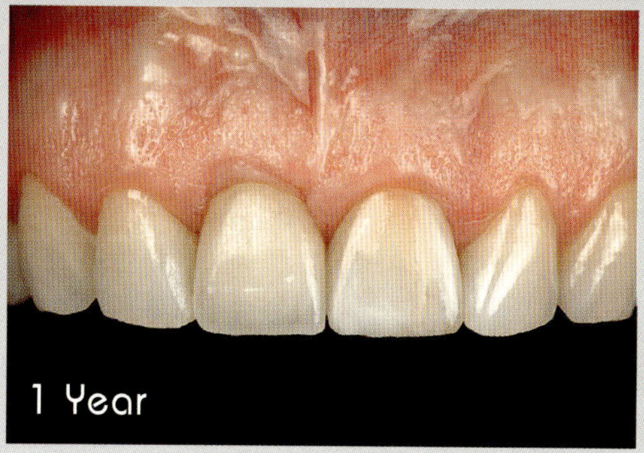

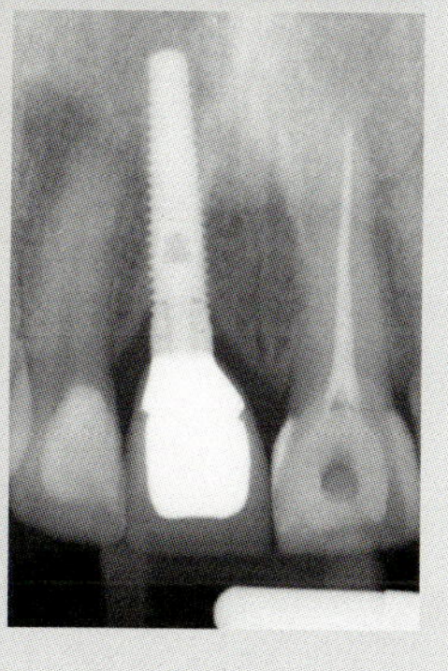

Patient situation 4: New trends for soft tissue manipulation

Current implant restoration concepts recommend placement of the definitive zirconia abutment with a provisional crown restoration on the first day of the restorative phase. The definitive restoration is only placed after an ideal soft tissue morphology has been established. Disconnection of the abutment or provisional restoration is not recommended during this stage because it could disrupt the fragile peri-implant soft tissue complex. This adds another degree of difficulty for the restorative dentist because disconnection often simplifies manipulation of the crown-margin-abutment interface. From a biologic standpoint, however, this approach is minimally invasive.

The success of this concept depends on certain prerequisites. First of all, the criteria for soft tissue evaluation must be met: interproximal heights, free gingival margin, and buccal volume. The graft tissue donor site must provide a dense, nonmobile, thick tissue as it shields the peri-implant tissue from trauma and ensures long-term tissue stability.

Implant placement occurred during orthodontic treatment. A NobelReplace Groovy NP (3.5 × 13 mm) implant with a narrow, 5-mm abutment was placed with a CTG from the tuberosity to compensate for the volume typically lost during stage-one surgery. An implant impression was made to fabricate the definitive zirconia abutment and the provisional crown restoration. After 10 days, some tissue growth was observed, requiring increased pressure on the buccal aspect of the abutment-crown complex. The problem was that the finish line was located coronally to the area of applied pressure. Therefore, pressure needed to be applied more cervically.

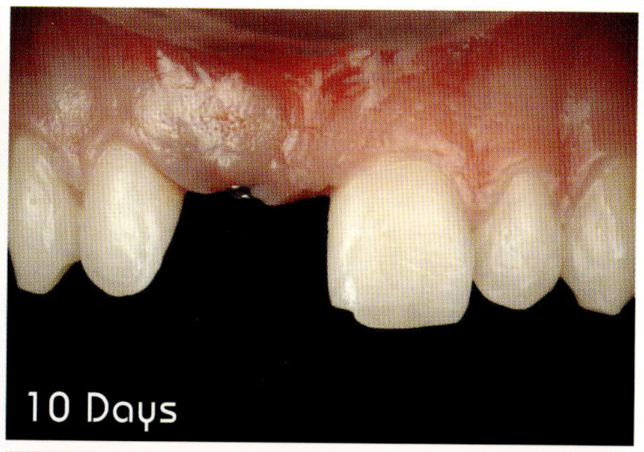

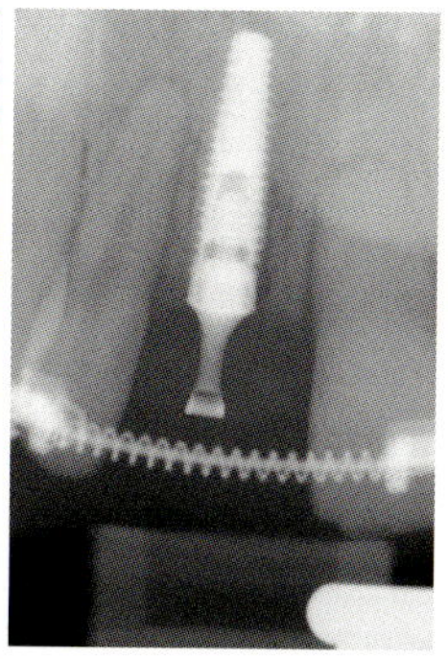

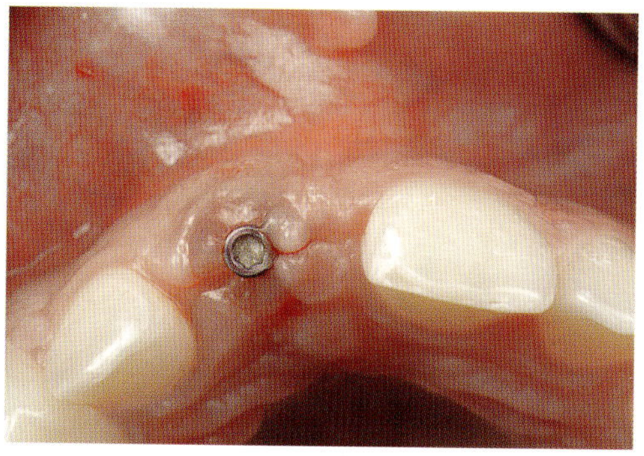

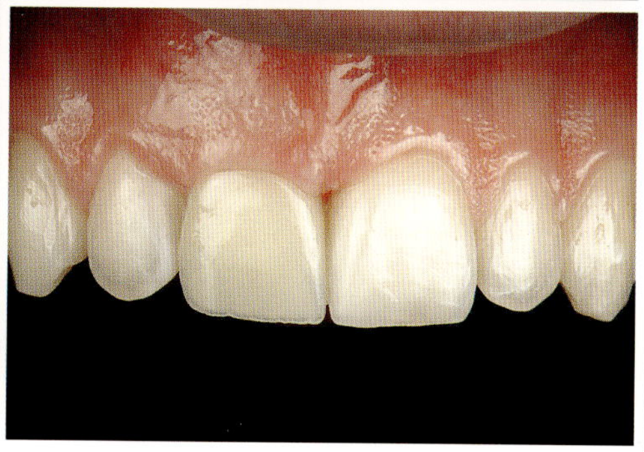

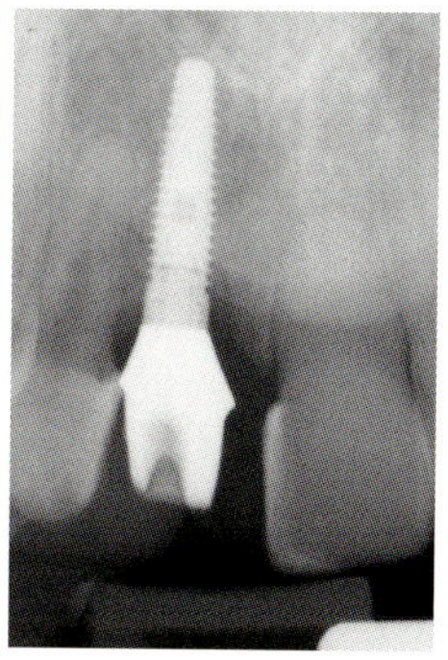

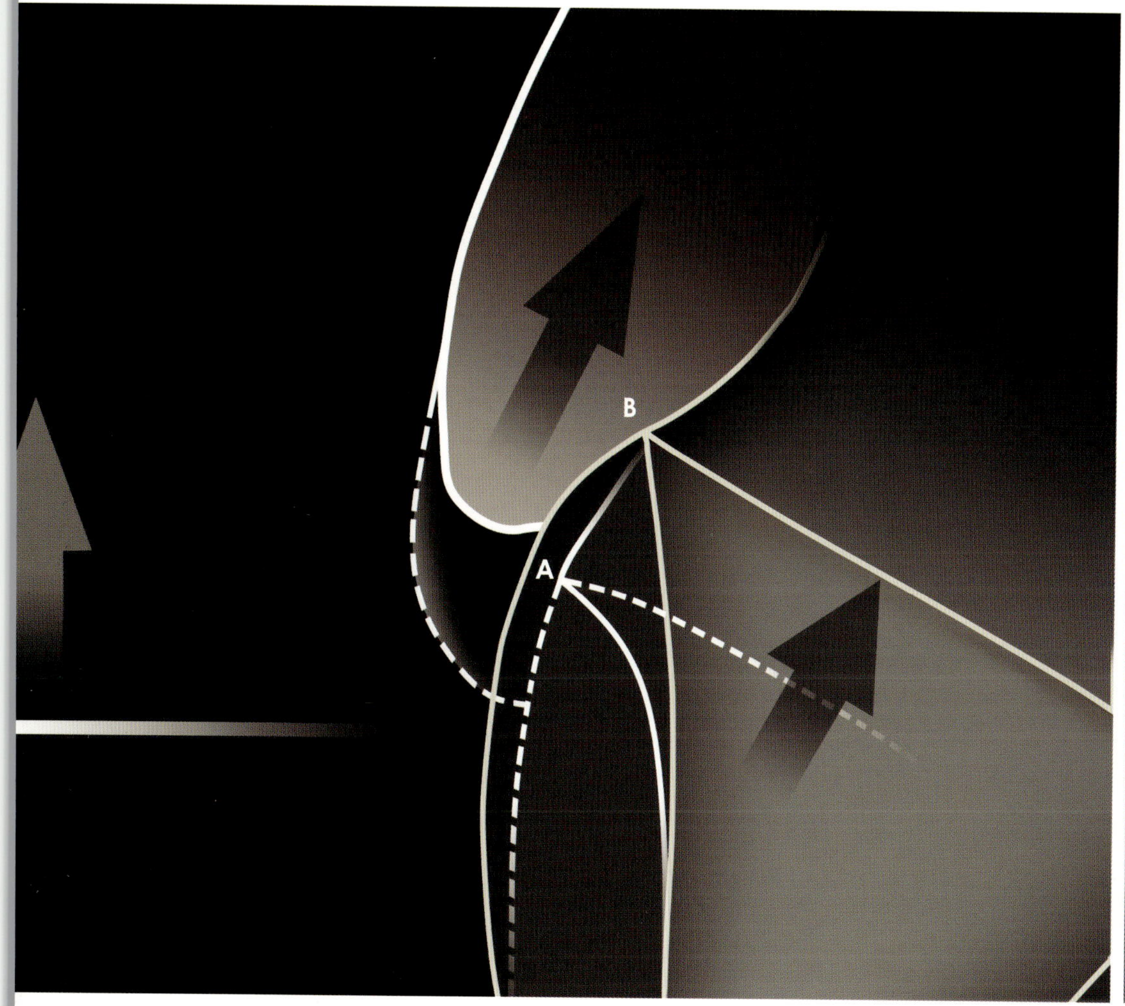

The illustration depicts the problem in respect to the location of the finish line. Position A is too coronal to allow for overcontouring of the crown and to create the recession with an ideal emergence profile. Apical repositioning of the margin to create a nice blend of the emergence profile with crown position B and the desired tissue recession will necessitate the disconnection of the abutment-crown complex. Unfortunately, the apically relocated margin of the zirconia abutment will shift the area of greatest tissue support from the abutment to the crown, which may cause difficulties with cement removal, especially with the concave design of the abutment.

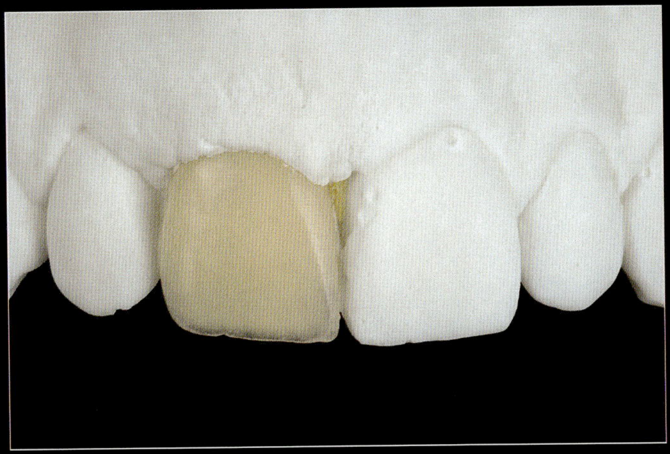

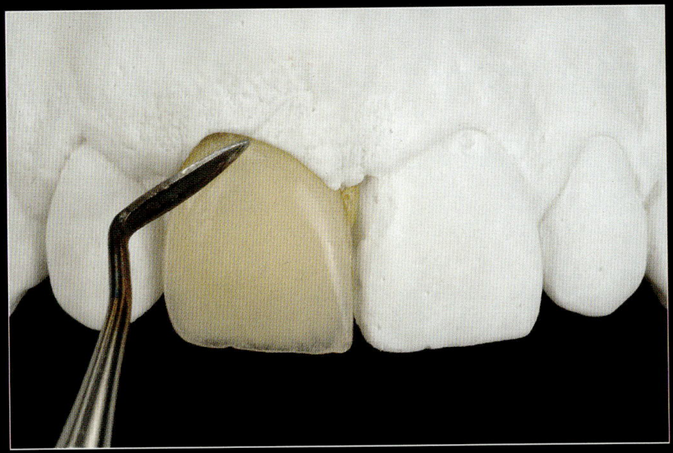

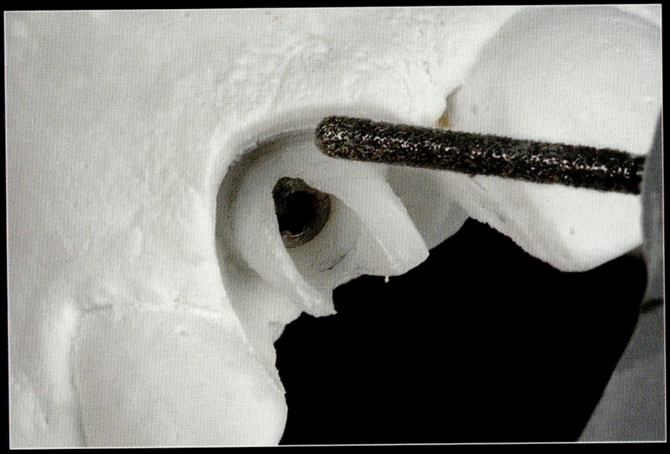

Therefore, a pickup impression was made from the provisional restoration to precisely reposition the location of the margin and create the desired tissue support and pressure. The abutment-crown complex was removed, and the abutment was disconnected. It was placed back into the polyvinyl siloxane (PVS) impression with its corresponding laboratory analog connected and poured in stone. The ideal soft tissue morphology was then carved into the master cast, creating a favorable angle that apically blended with the abutment. The preparation finish line was repositioned further apically to support the carved emergence profile. Afterward, acrylic resin was placed with a spatula into the carved emergence profile and the provisional crown restoration to re-create the emergence profile of the crown.

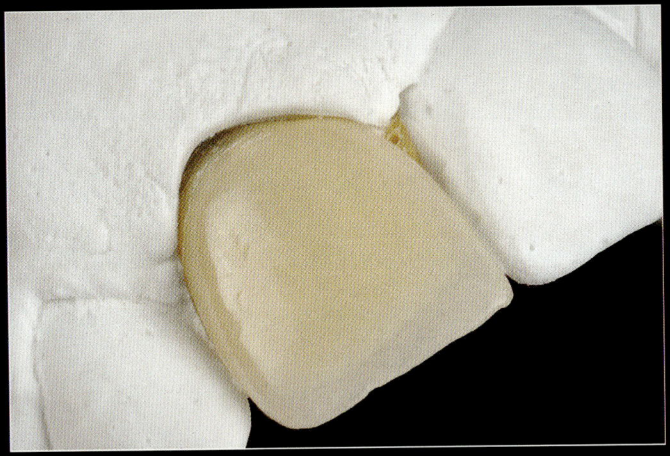

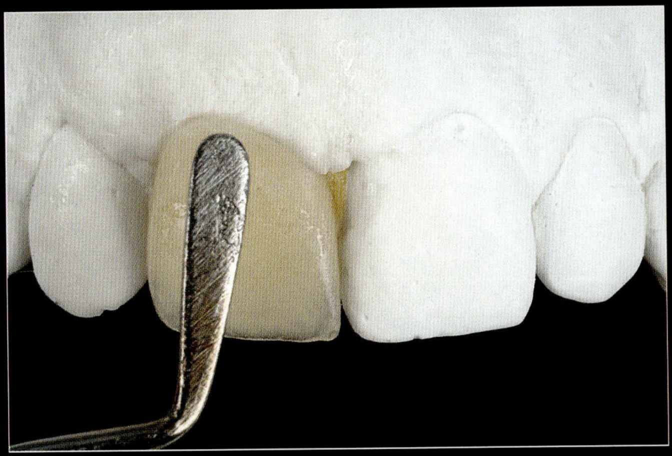

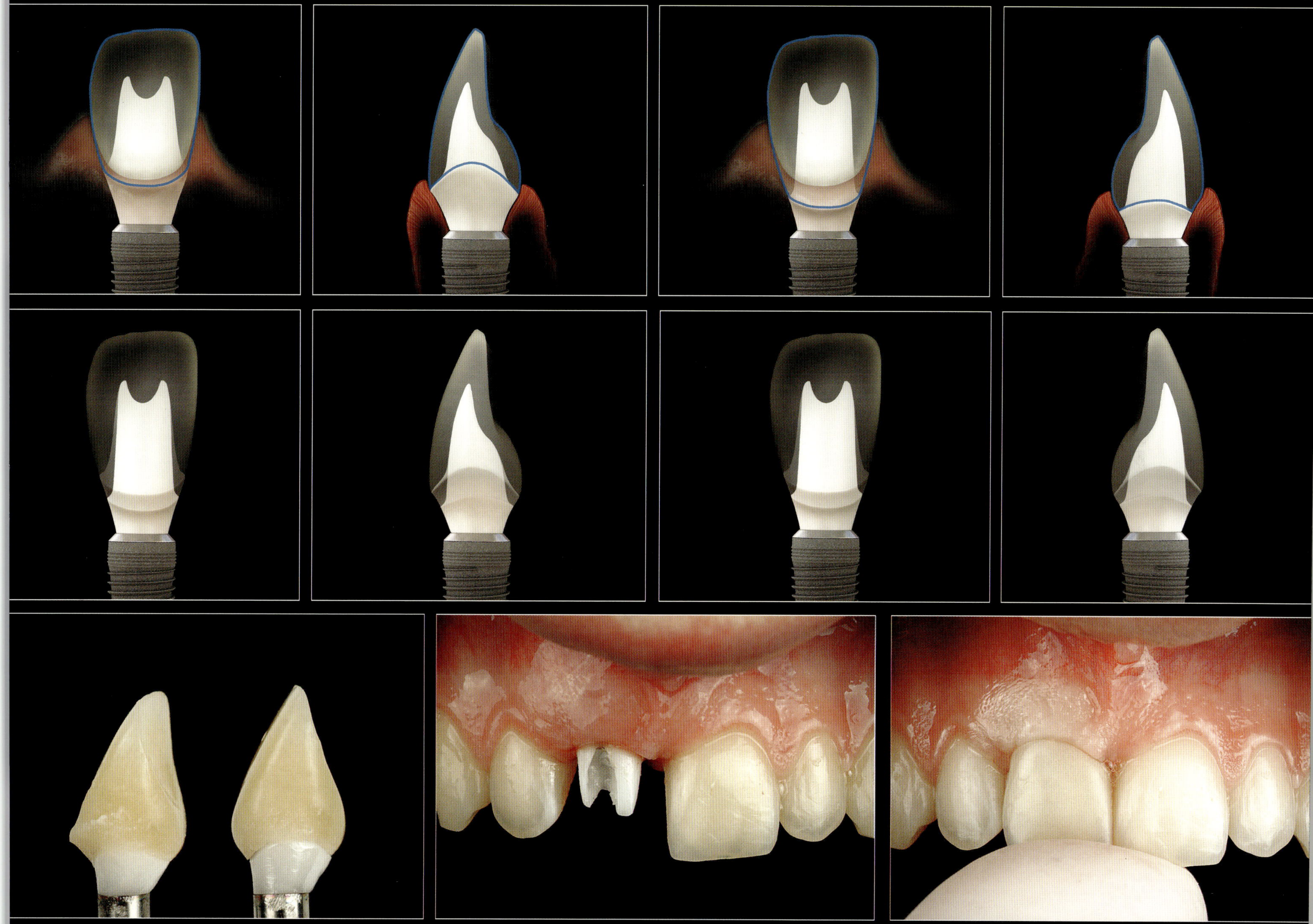

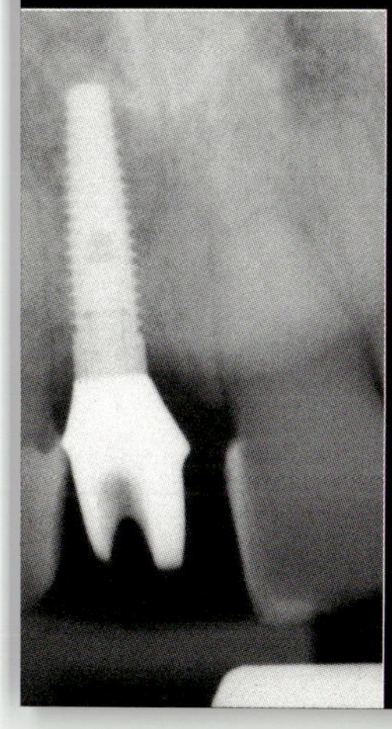

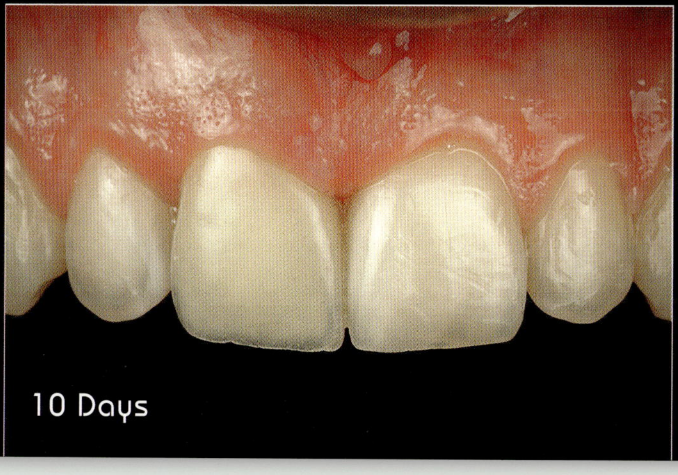

Graphic representations of the emergence profile management and finishing line with the definitive abutment in place from day 1 of the prosthetic phase. The abutment needs to be displaced apically in order to create the desired recession margin with the crown. With this technique, the soft tissue is supported more by the crown than by the abutment, which makes removal of excess cement difficult. This technique provides a predictable way to create the desired scalloping and support of the peri-implant soft tissue.

The provisional crown restoration was refined and polished. The components were reattached, and the crown was cemented. After 10 days, reevaluation of the tissue revealed a favorable tissue contour that matched the adjacent natural tooth. This pickup technique allows precise control of the emergence profile and margin location.

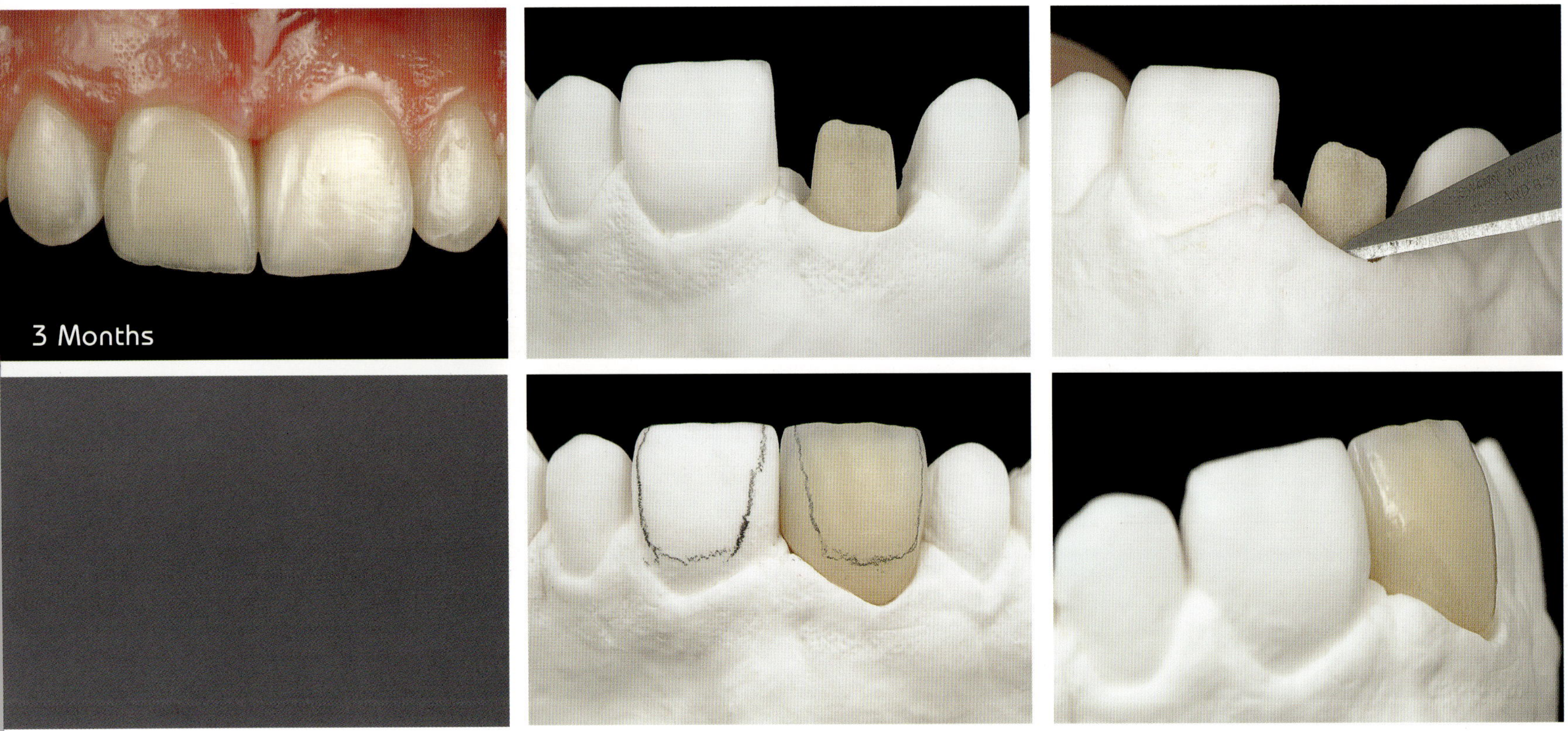

The amount of soft tissue regenerated around the recession defect during the 3-month observation period is obvious. This regeneration is due to the large amount of tissue grafted into the defect implant site. Obviously, there is a limit to the amount of overcontour a restoration should have to keep the tissue apically, and this is done with the definitive restoration. The dental technician re-creates the soft tissue contour, shifting the entire tooth outline toward the facial aspect. If the tissue continues to grow, a gingivectomy or a gingivoplasty is advised.

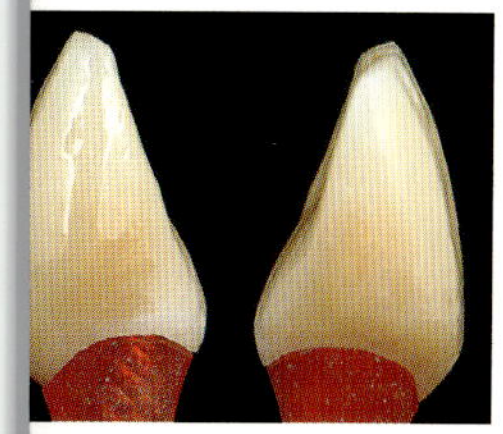

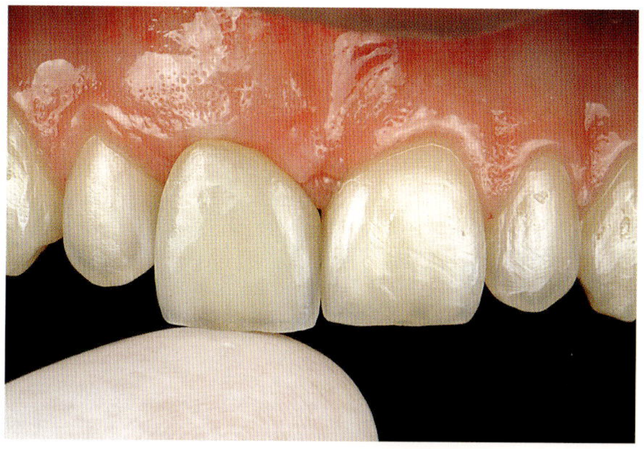

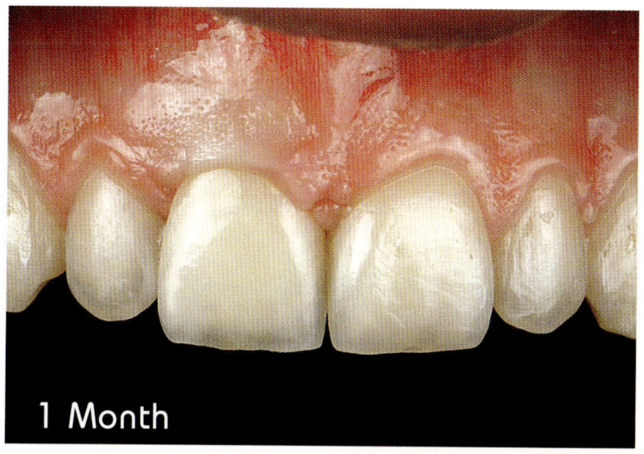

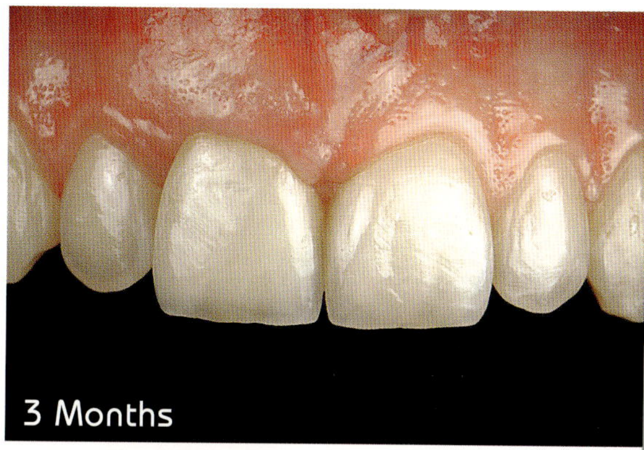

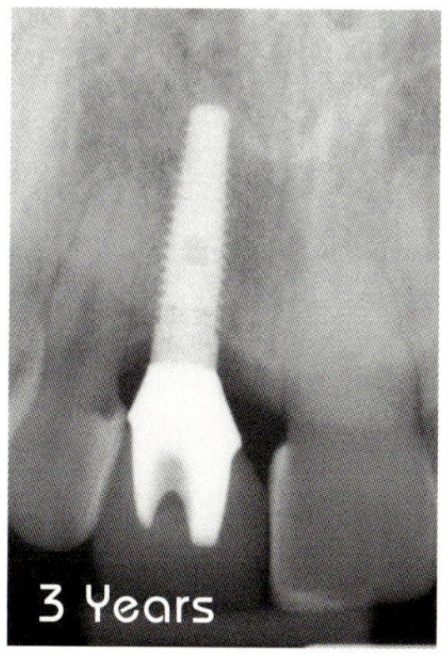

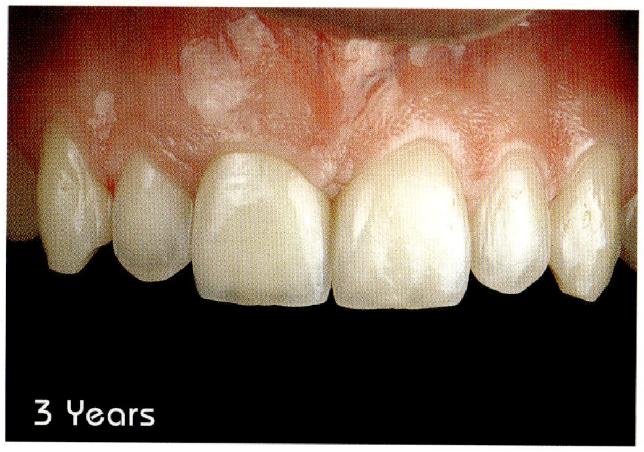

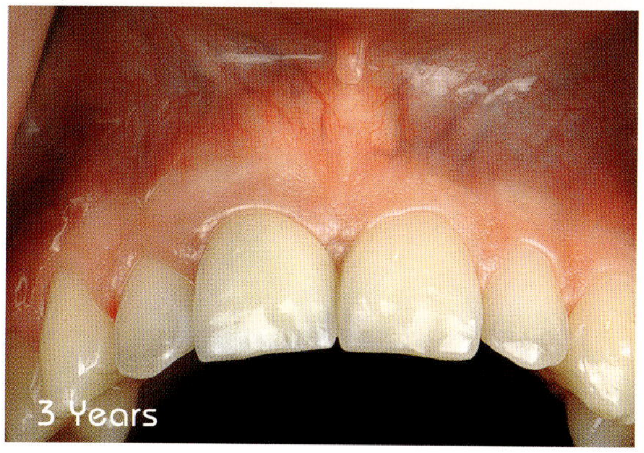

The definitive alumina crown featured the detailed emergence profile designed during the provisional stage. Try-in and cementation of the definitive crown required special attention due to the depth of the new finish line and the overcontoured restoration, which make cement removal more difficult. The situation after 3 years indicated stable soft tissue conditions.

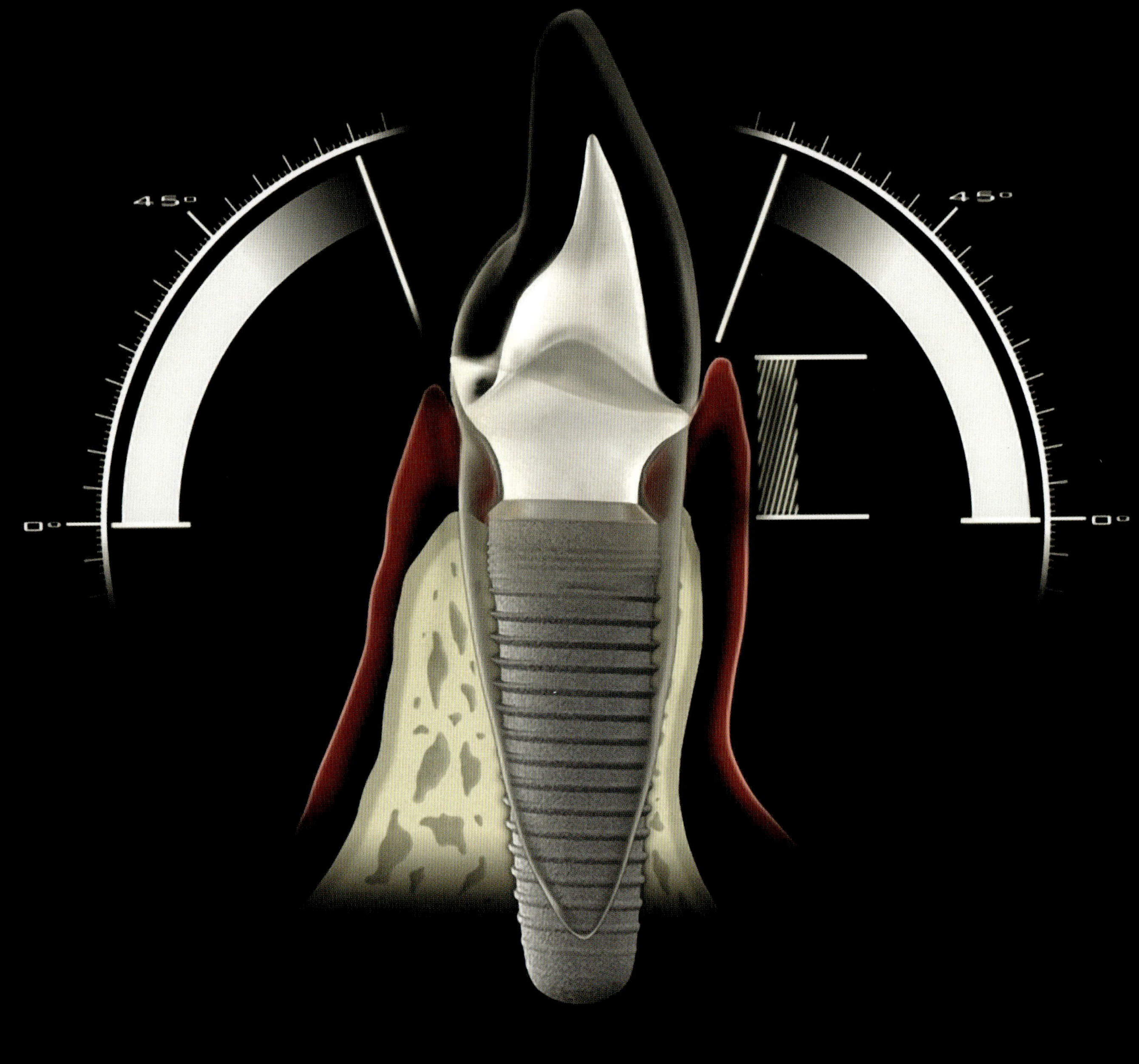
45°
0°
45°
0°

Abutment design and provisional fabrication

Previous abutment concept

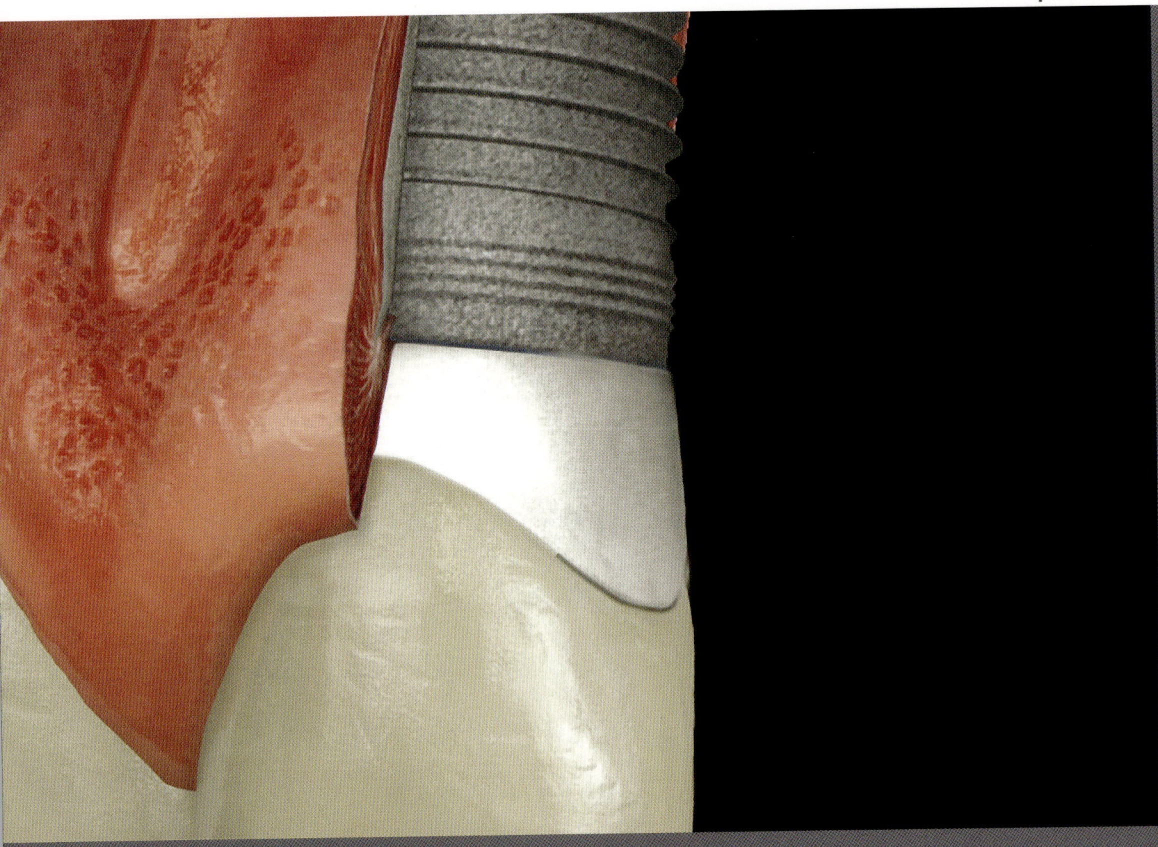

Arguably the most crucial aspect in implant prosthodontics is the fabrication of the abutment and the provisional crown to provide ideal "white esthetics." Equally important, however, they must support and sculpt the "pink esthetics," the natural frame of the definitive restoration.

Abutment design has evolved dramatically in terms of shape and form. Previous abutment designs were oversized, creating too much pressure at the implant-abutment interface; parallel or cylindric transmucosally to replicate the present root diameter from the implant neck up; and wide coronally to support the crown. The width of these designs at the abutment-implant interface created excessive pressure on the surrounding tissues and led to interproximal marginal bone loss. This phenomenon worsened under function as the tissue thinned over time and led to poor long-term esthetics.

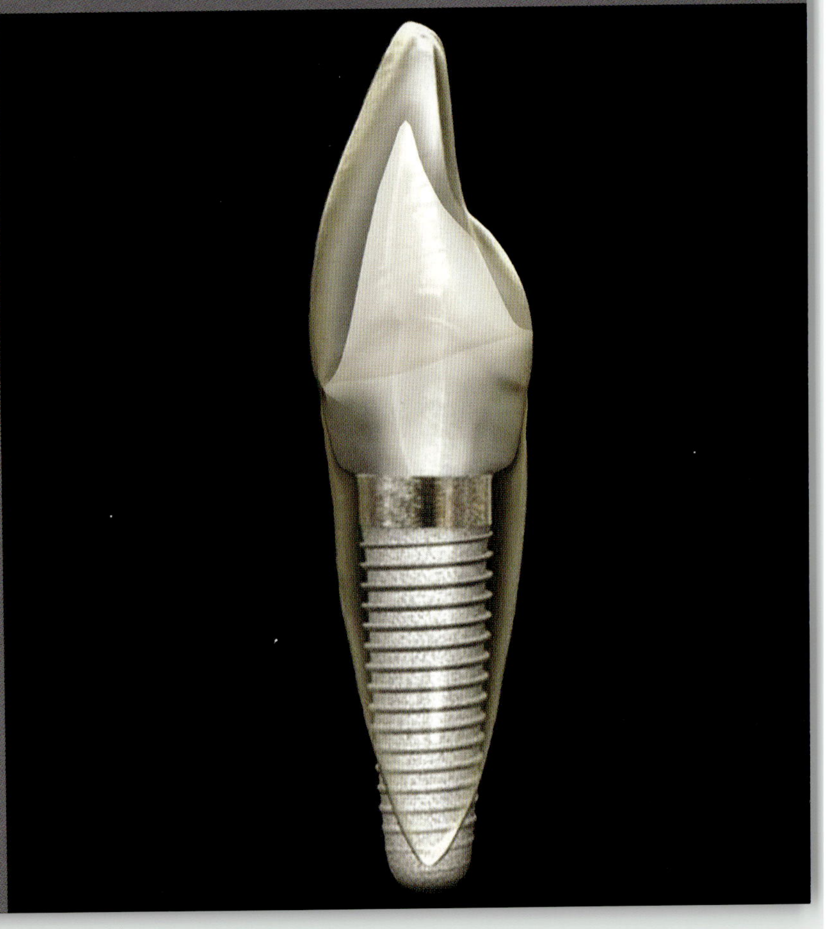

Contemporary concept

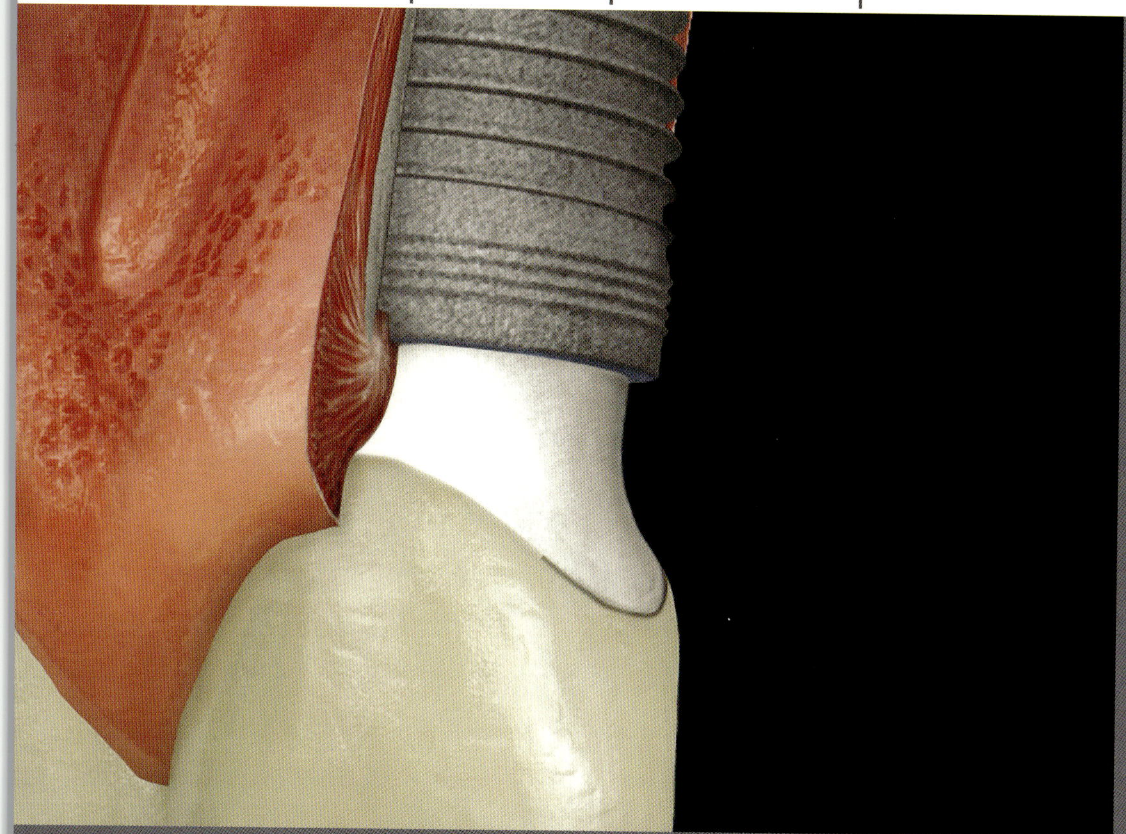

Contemporary concepts of abutment design are dramatically different. The current recommendation is to create an abutment as narrow as possible at the implant-abutment interface, concave and divergent transmucosally, and wide coronally at the finish line (replicating the diameter of the natural tooth) to support the crown contour.

The concave shape at the implant-abutment interface ensures greater thickness of the surrounding peri-implant tissues and greater stability in the long term. Another advantage is a simplified soft tissue grafting procedure around the implants due to the extra space provided by the narrow prosthetic components. This ability to thicken the biotype around dental implants has provided long-lasting and predictable results that were previously impossible.

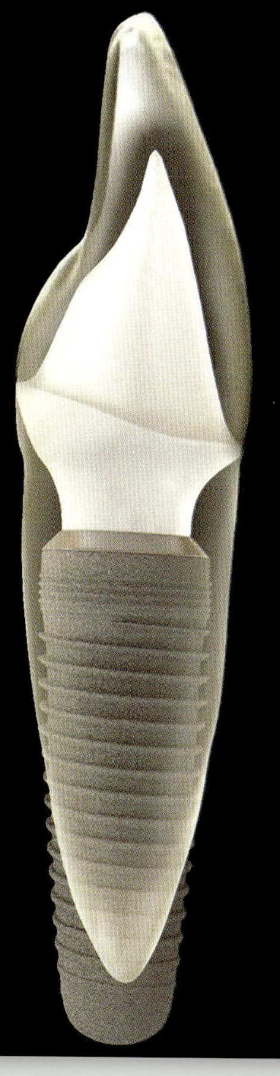

Structural design of the abutment

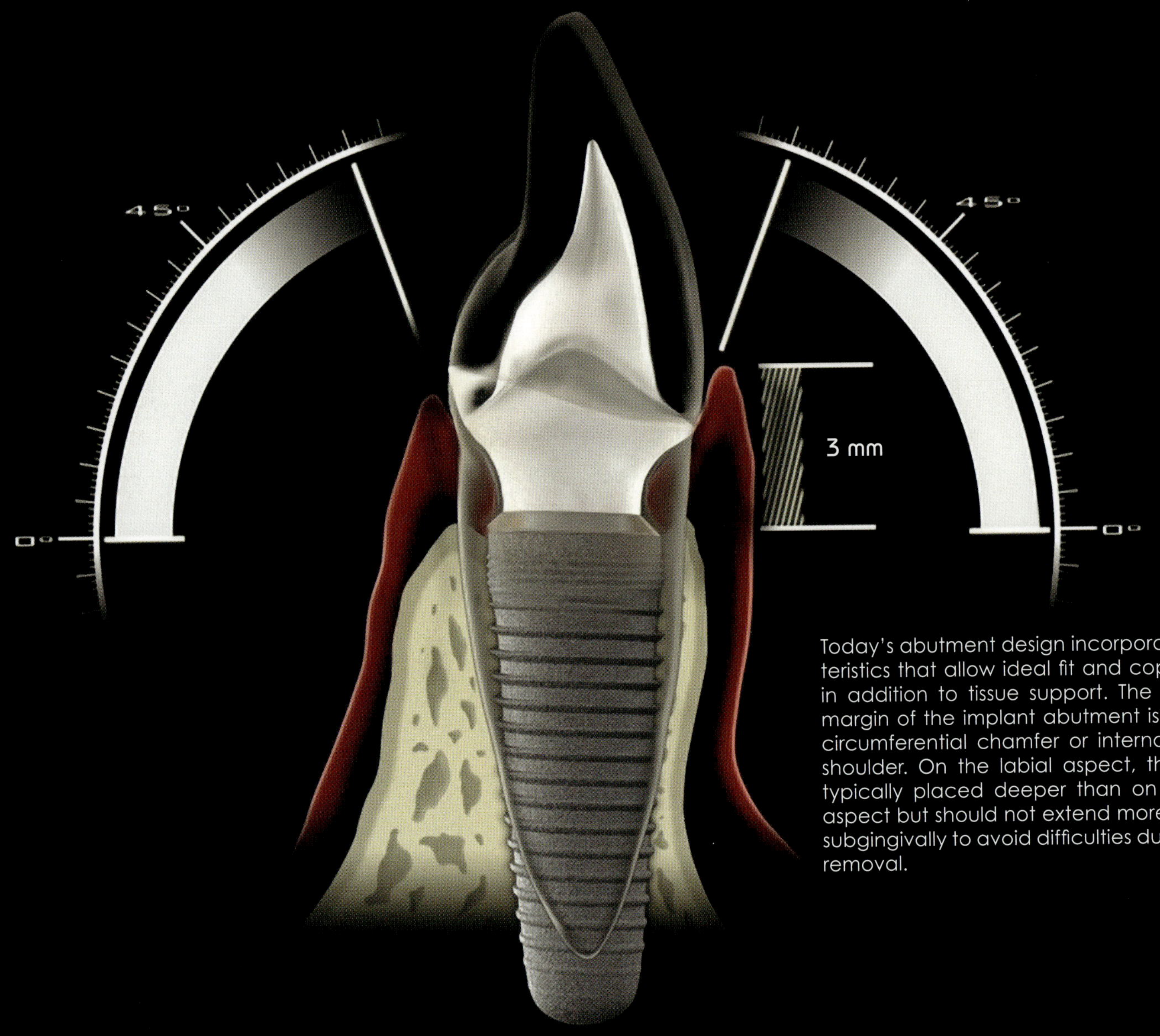

Today's abutment design incorporates characteristics that allow ideal fit and coping stability in addition to tissue support. The preparation margin of the implant abutment is generally a circumferential chamfer or internally rounded shoulder. On the labial aspect, the margin is typically placed deeper than on the palatal aspect but should not extend more than 1 mm subgingivally to avoid difficulties during cement removal.

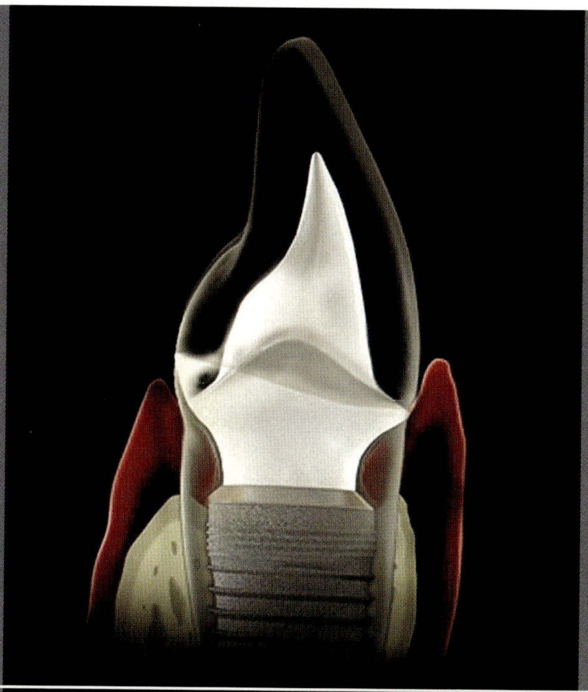

When planning abutment margins either between implants or between an implant and a tooth, they should be leveled in a symmetric manner interproximally or buccolingually to support the interproximal tissue from both sides of the emergence profile of the crowns.

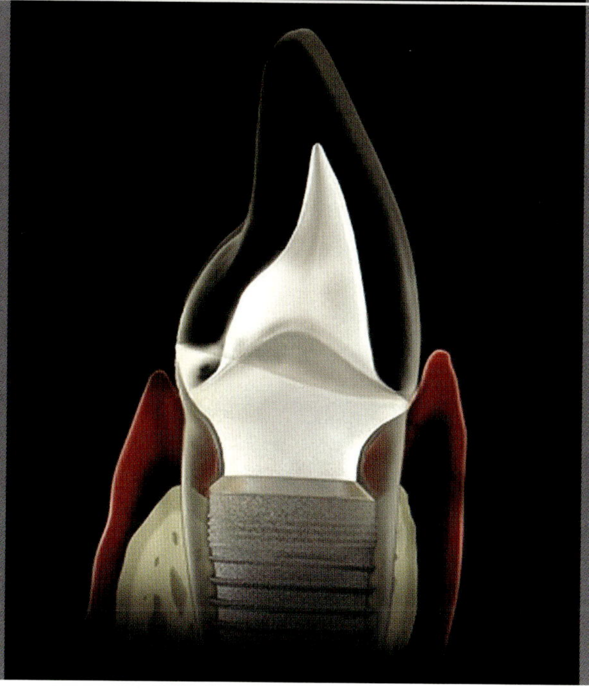

The interproximal design of the preparation (eg, flat or scalloped) is directly related to the interproximal bone contour of the adjacent tooth (more scalloped) or implant (flatter), the amount of tissue to support in terms of interproximal width or height, the actual gingival embrasure volume, and the proximity of the adjacent root or implant abutment. The abutment should support approximately 90% of the total surrounding soft tissue contour, with the crown supporting no more than 10%. Interabutment distance is a crucial aspect to take into consideration because it may limit the restorative dentist's expectations of papillary height. A minimum interabutment space of 1.5 to 2.0 mm is necessary between a tooth and an implant and 2.0 to 2.5 mm between implants.

The patient presented with a removable partial denture and a missing maxillary left lateral incisor with vertical and horizontal tissue defects. A NobelReplace Groovy RP implant (4.3 × 13 mm) was placed with a platform switching (PS) adapter and a 3.5 × 5–mm healing abutment. A CTG from the tuberosity was placed at stage-one surgery to restore the volume lost vertically and horizontally. This was achieved after 3 months.

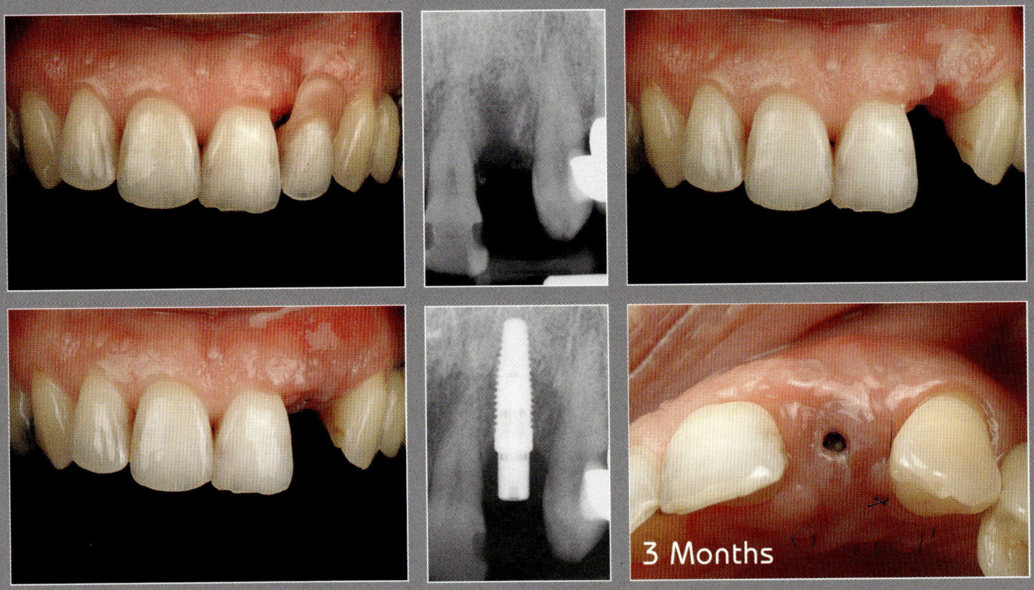

A PVS implant impression was made with the corresponding impression coping, and a master cast was fabricated. A diagnostic wax-up was made to replicate the natural tooth and duplicate its diameter especially in the gingival third. A line was drawn on the master cast following the scallop of the wax-up and desired emergence profile to carve a cone from that line to the abutment head.

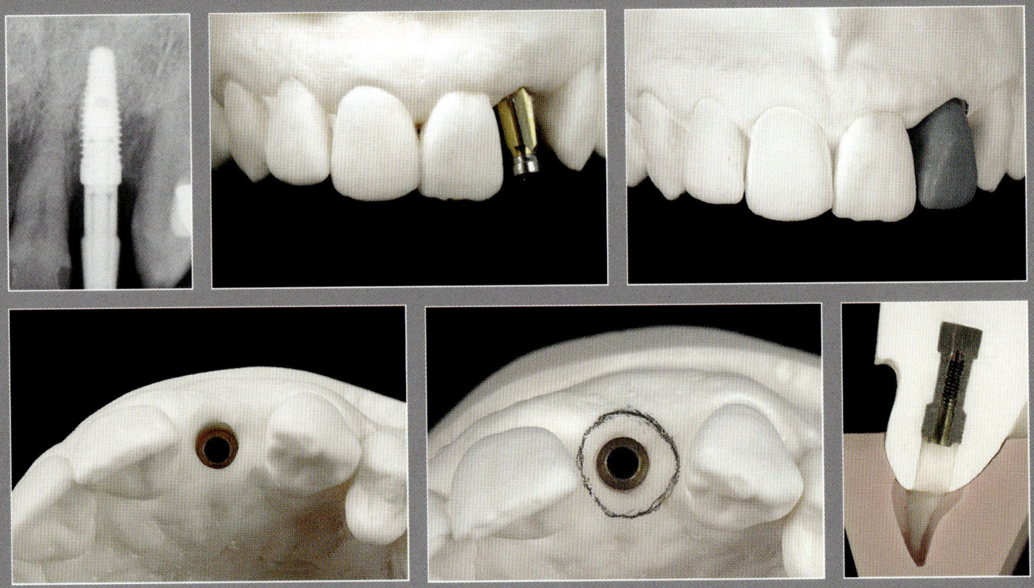

PVS matrices were made to visualize the full-contour wax-up and fabricate the composite abutment. The stone was carved with hand instruments until a divergent cone was created from the implant head to the PVS silicone matrix in such manner that the abutment would match the contour of the provisional crown restoration. Then the plastic abutment was connected to the laboratory analog, and composite resin was placed between the conically carved stone and the plastic sleeve until the ideal full-preparation contour was achieved. The composite abutment was light cured and prepared to create a 1-mm subgingival margin on the buccal aspect or supragingival margin on the palatal aspect.

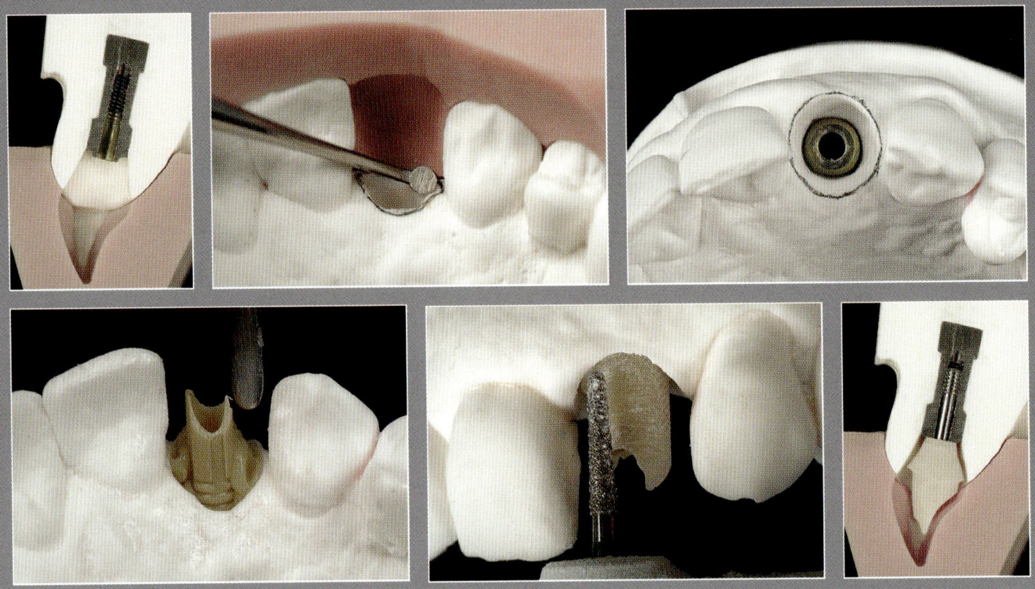

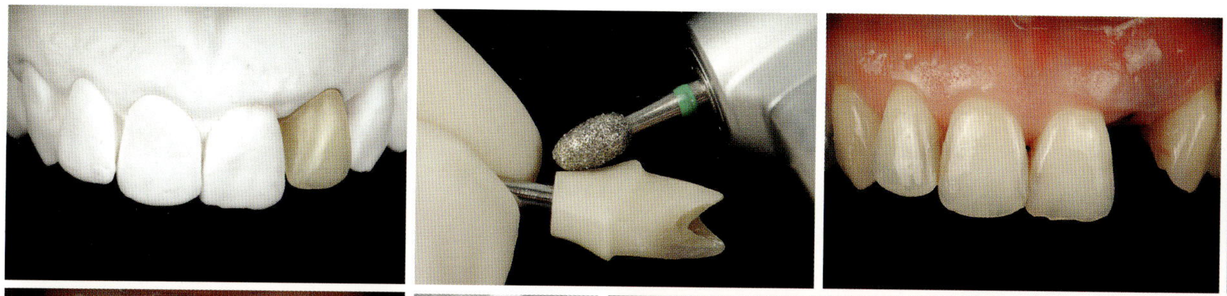

The provisional crown was fabricated with a sandwich technique on top of the composite abutment and with the PVS matrices. The subgingival aspect of the abutment was modified from a divergent to a concave design to allow a thicker band of peri-implant connective tissue. The provisional abutment was then connected and the provisional crown relined chairside to establish ideal fit and proper interproximal contact points. It is common to disconnect the abutment to adapt the margins and polish the provisional crown restoration extraorally.

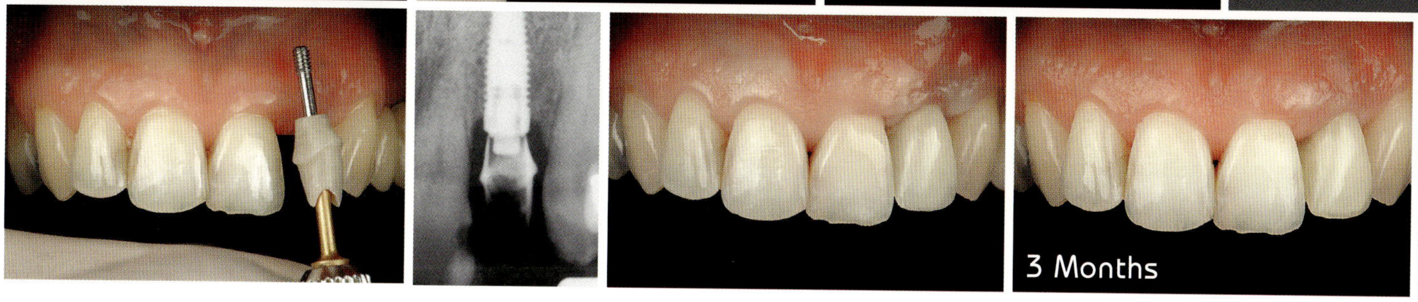

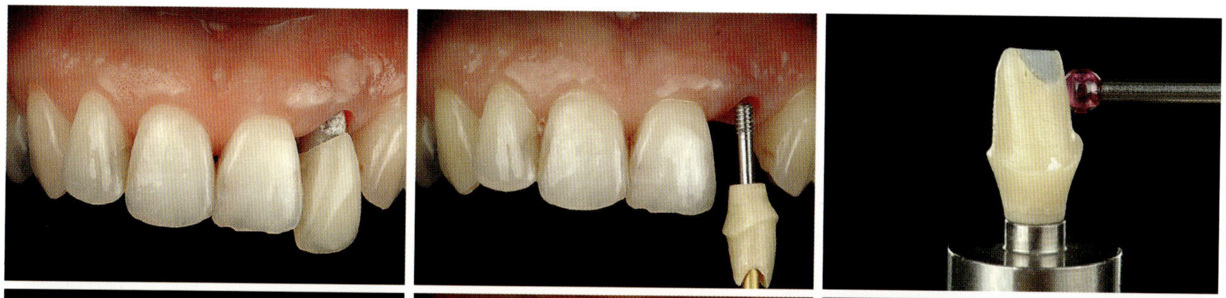

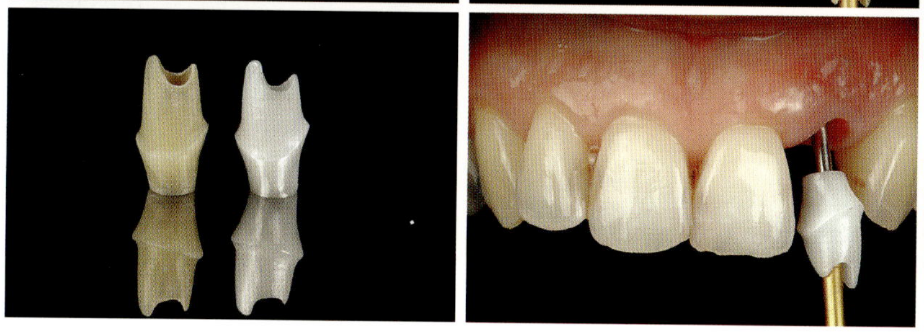

After 3 months of tissue stability, the patient was sent to the laboratory technician with an uncemented provisional crown. The technician could easily remove the crown, unscrew the abutment, and make a virtual impression with an intraoral scanner for CAD/CAM abutment fabrication. This way, the technician can order a duplicate zirconia abutment of the provisional abutment from the milling center.

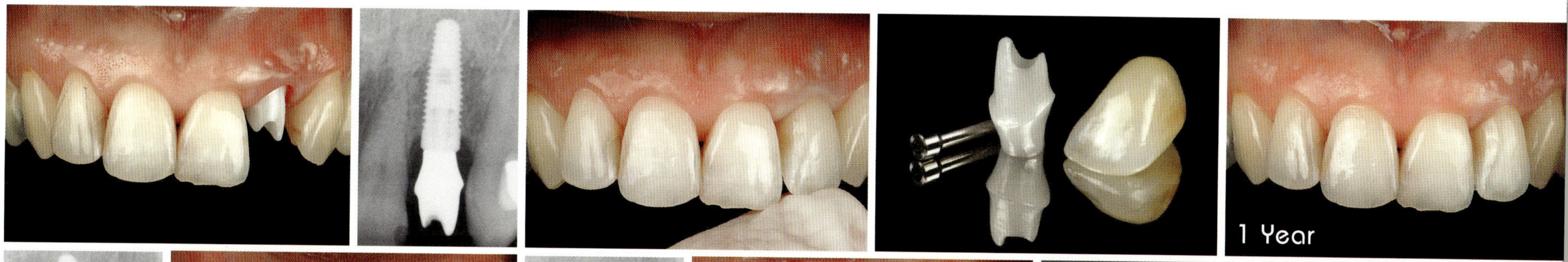

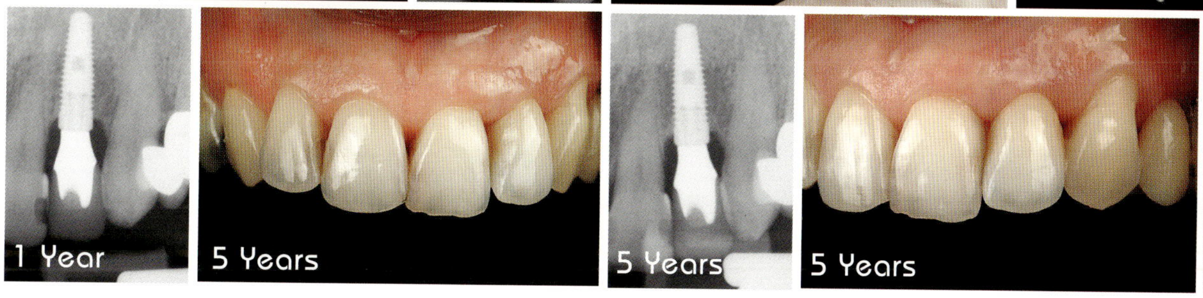

The final PVS impression was made, and the definitive crown restoration was fabricated on top of the definitive abutment. Note the bone remodeling around the implant head and how the marginal bone has receded because of the manipulation trauma during the different steps of the prosthetic phase. The soft tissue was stable for 5 years with no additional marginal bone loss.

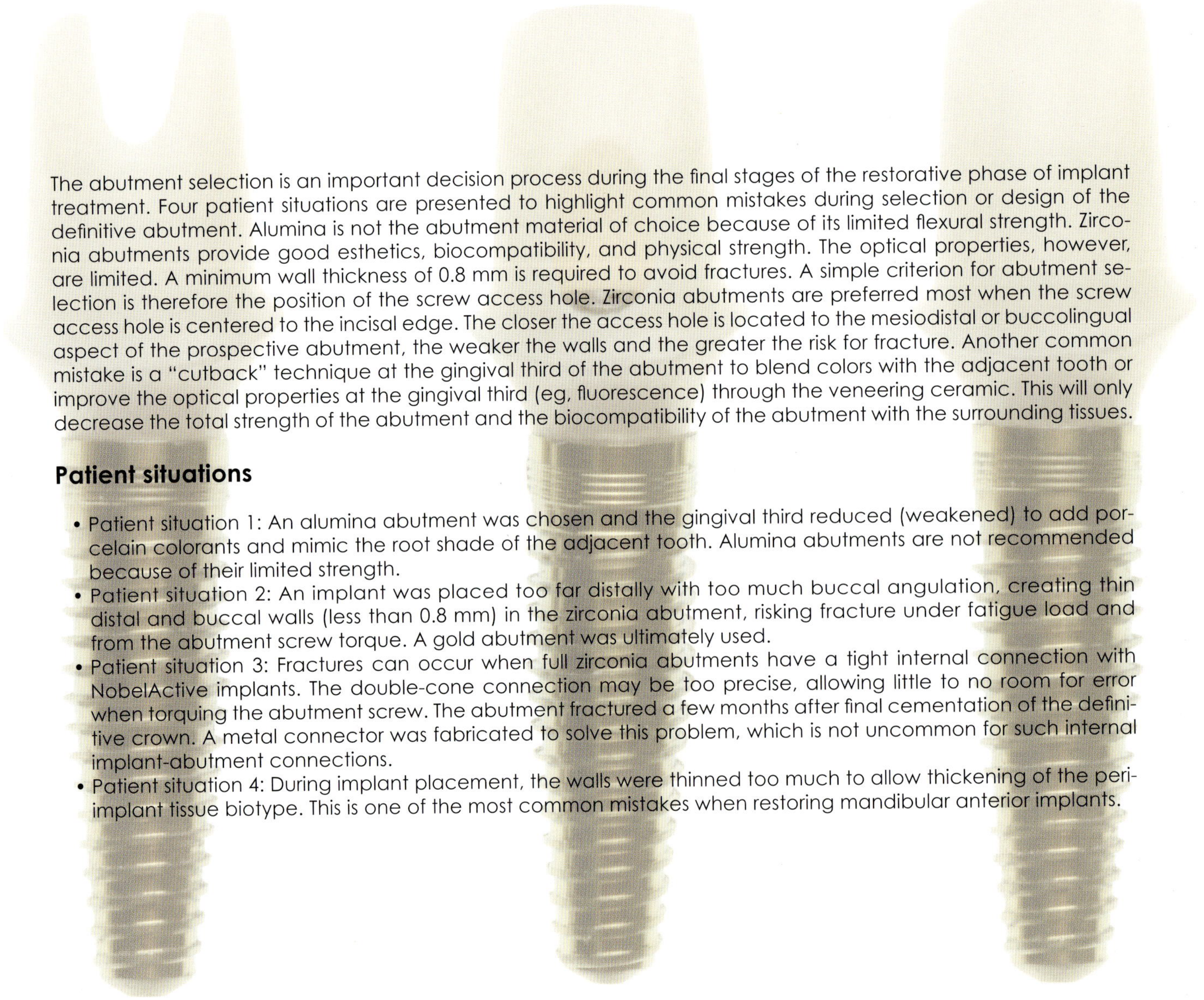

The abutment selection is an important decision process during the final stages of the restorative phase of implant treatment. Four patient situations are presented to highlight common mistakes during selection or design of the definitive abutment. Alumina is not the abutment material of choice because of its limited flexural strength. Zirconia abutments provide good esthetics, biocompatibility, and physical strength. The optical properties, however, are limited. A minimum wall thickness of 0.8 mm is required to avoid fractures. A simple criterion for abutment selection is therefore the position of the screw access hole. Zirconia abutments are preferred most when the screw access hole is centered to the incisal edge. The closer the access hole is located to the mesiodistal or buccolingual aspect of the prospective abutment, the weaker the walls and the greater the risk for fracture. Another common mistake is a "cutback" technique at the gingival third of the abutment to blend colors with the adjacent tooth or improve the optical properties at the gingival third (eg, fluorescence) through the veneering ceramic. This will only decrease the total strength of the abutment and the biocompatibility of the abutment with the surrounding tissues.

Patient situations

- Patient situation 1: An alumina abutment was chosen and the gingival third reduced (weakened) to add porcelain colorants and mimic the root shade of the adjacent tooth. Alumina abutments are not recommended because of their limited strength.
- Patient situation 2: An implant was placed too far distally with too much buccal angulation, creating thin distal and buccal walls (less than 0.8 mm) in the zirconia abutment, risking fracture under fatigue load and from the abutment screw torque. A gold abutment was ultimately used.
- Patient situation 3: Fractures can occur when full zirconia abutments have a tight internal connection with NobelActive implants. The double-cone connection may be too precise, allowing little to no room for error when torquing the abutment screw. The abutment fractured a few months after final cementation of the definitive crown. A metal connector was fabricated to solve this problem, which is not uncommon for such internal implant-abutment connections.
- Patient situation 4: During implant placement, the walls were thinned too much to allow thickening of the peri-implant tissue biotype. This is one of the most common mistakes when restoring mandibular anterior implants.

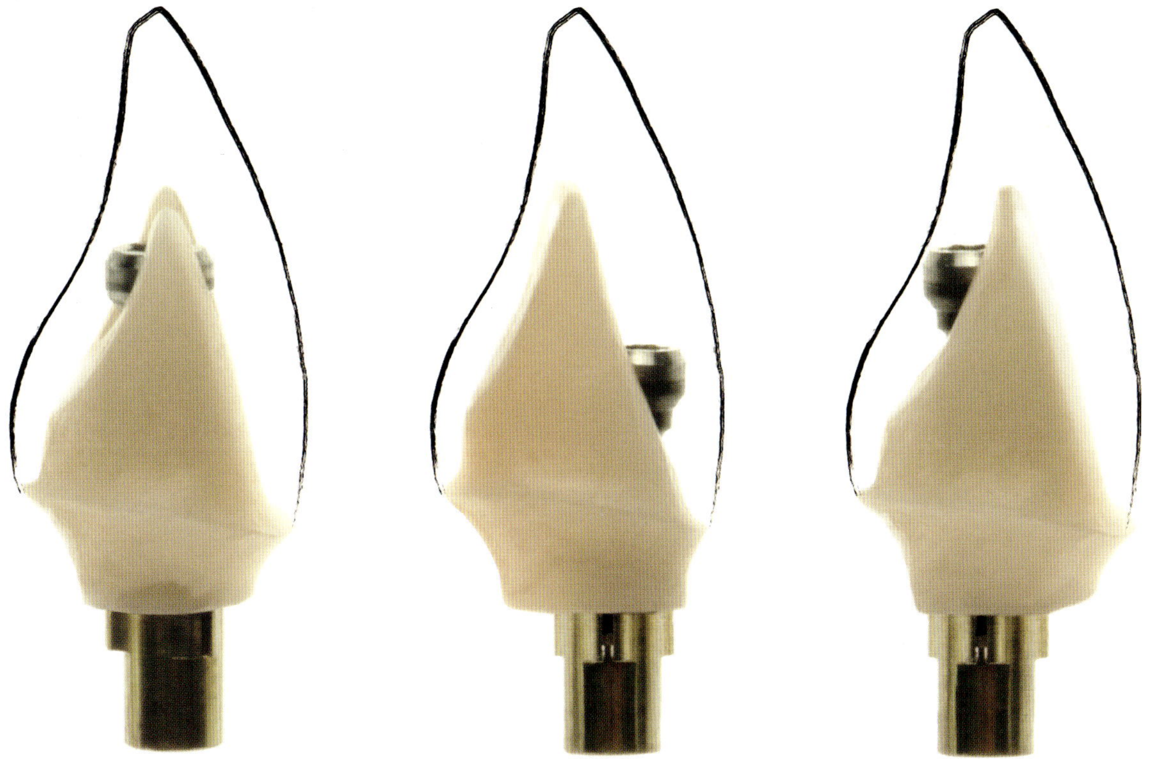

Implant abutment selection

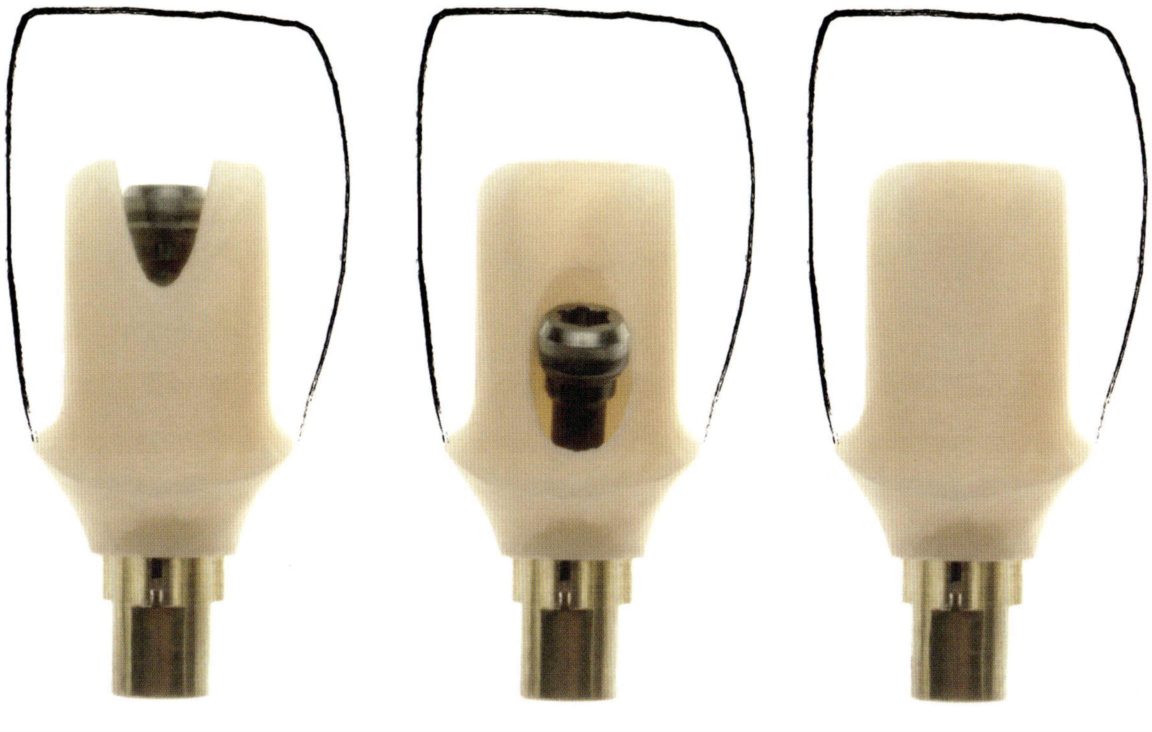

Research

Implant abutments

Systematic literature reviews indicate no significant differences in survival and success rates between screw- and cement-retained implant-supported restorations.[1,2] The cement-retained option, however, allows for placement of a definitive abutment at the earliest possible stage. Soft tissue and tooth esthetics may then be optimized with a provisional restoration but without unnecessary removal of the abutment.[3] The implant abutment, as the submucosal part of the prosthetic complex, shapes the soft tissue contour and emergence profile. It supports the restoration and may compensate for less-than-ideal implant positions and angulations.

Based on the current evidence, abutment material (eg, gold, titanium, or ceramic) does not significantly influence clinical implant success[1] but greatly affects esthetics.[4] Animal studies demonstrate greater soft tissue recessions around gold-alloy than around titanium or ceramic abutments,[5,6] with no significant differences between the latter two in respect to collagen fiber orientation and mucosal attachment.[7,8] Histologically, however, soft tissues around titanium healing caps tend to undergo a higher rate of possibly destructive remodeling and regenerative processes than around zirconia.[9,10] In addition, zirconia ceramic abutments are less prone to bacterial adhesion.[11] Surface roughness is crucial and should be about 0.2 µm,[4,12] which is approximately the roughness found on machined surfaces. Ultrapolished zirconia abutments showed greater probing depths,[4,12] indicating that submucosal zirconia aspects should not be polished excessively.

Systematic reviews of clinical studies did not find significant differences in technical or biologic outcomes between metal and ceramic abutments.[13] A recent randomized clinical trial compared zirconia and titanium abutments in canine and posterior areas and found survival rates for both materials at 100% after 5 years in function.[14] Of the high-strength ceramic materials used for implant abutments, zirconia has the most favorable physical properties.[15,16] To prevent fractures, however, zirconia abutment wall thickness is critical and recommended to be at least 0.5 mm.[14]

The greatest advantages of ceramic abutments are their optical and esthetic properties. Metal abutments and porcelain-fused-to-metal restorations cause significantly greater soft tissue discoloration than all-ceramic abutments and crowns, especially in thin soft tissue up to 2 mm in thickness.[17,18] With soft tissue thickness of 3 mm or greater, however, there are no detectable differences.[18] A light orange and pink abutment shade has the least influence on soft tissue color.[19,20] A very light or white abutment shade, however, may actually improve the oftentimes grayish appearance of the soft tissue and increase the overall value of the restoration and tissue.[3] Adding a higher degree of fluorescence with specific veneering ceramics or infiltrated modifiers adds to that effect.[4] With ceramic abutments, the inevitable soft tissue recession after prosthetic connection will not expose any metal margins.[3] However, the position of the abutment finish line has to be carefully planned. It depends on the intended soft tissue height but also on tissue biotype, as thin tissues are more prone to recession.[3]

According to systematic reviews, there is no significant difference between internal and external implant connections in respect to implant survival or technical or biologic complications.[1,13] Abutments made entirely from zirconia may cause wear of titanium implants at the connection interface.[21] Exceptions are internal conical connections with high precision of fit. For other internal and especially external connections, titanium inserts or bases at the connection interface are recommended.

References

1. Wittneben JG, Millen C, Brägger U. Clinical performance of screw- versus cement-retained fixed implant-supported reconstructions—A systematic review. Int J Oral Maxillofac Implants 2014;29(suppl):84–98.

2. Weber HP, Sukotjo C. Does the type of implant prosthesis affect outcomes in the partially edentulous patient? Int J Oral Maxillofac Implants 2007;22(suppl):140–172.

3. Blatz MB, Bergler M, Holst S, Block MS. Zirconia abutments for single-tooth implants—Rationale and clinical guidelines. J Oral Maxillofac Surg 2009;67(11 suppl):74–81.

4. Happe A, Körner G. Biologic Interfaces in esthetic dentistry. Part II: The peri-implant/restorative interface. Eur J Esthet Dent 2011;6:226–251.

5. Abrahamson I, Berglundh T, Glantz PO, Lindhe J. The mucosal attachment at different abutments. An experimental study in dogs. J Clin Periodontol 1998;25:721–727.

6. Welander M, Abrahamson I, Berglundh T. The mucosal barrier at implant abutments of different materials. Clin Oral Implants Res 2008;19:635–641.

7. Tetè S, Mastrangelo F, Bianchi A, Zizzari V, Scarano A. Collagen fiber orientation around machined titanium and zirconia dental implant necks: An animal study. Int J Oral Maxillofac Implants 2009;24:52–58.

8. Kohal RJ, Weng D, Bächle M, Strub JR. Loaded custom-made zirconia and titanium implants show similar osseointegration: An animal experiment. J Periodontol 2004;75:1262–1268.

9. Degidi M, Artese L, Scarano A, Perrotti V, Gehrke P, Piattelli A. Inflammatory infiltrate, microvessel density, nitric oxide synthase expression, vascular endothelial growth factor expression, and proliferative activity in peri-implant soft tissues around titanium and zirconium oxide healing caps. J Periodontol 2006;77:73–80.

10. Degidi M, Artese L, Franceschini N, et al. Matrix metalloproteinases 2, 3, 8, 9, and 13 in the peri-implant soft tissues around titanium and zirconium oxide healing caps. Int J Oral Maxillofac Implants 2013;28:1546–1551.

11. Rimondini L, Cerroni L, Carrassi A, Torricelli P. Bacterial colonization of zirconia ceramic surfaces: An in vitro and in vivo study. Int J Oral Maxillofac Implants 2002;17:793–798.

12. Bollen CM, Papaioanno W, Van Eldere J, Schepers E, Quirynen M, van Steenberghe D. The influence of abutment surface roughness on plaque accumulation and peri-implant mucositis. Clin Oral Implants Res 1996;7:201–211.

13. Zembic A, Kim S, Zwahlen M, Kelly R. Systematic review of survival rate and incidence of biologic, technical, and esthetic complications of single implant abutments supporting fixed prostheses. Int J Oral Maxillofac Implants 2014;29(suppl):99–116.

14. Zembic A, Bosch A, Jung RE, Hämmerle CH, Sailer I. Five-year results of a randomized controlled clinical trial comparing zirconia and titanium abutments supporting single-implant crowns in canine and posterior regions. Clin Oral Implants Res 2013;24:384–390.

15. Att W, Kurun S, Gerds T, Strub JR. Fracture resistance of single-tooth implant-supported all-ceramic restorations after exposure to the artificial mouth. J Oral Rehabil 2006;33:380–386.

16. Att W, Kurun S, Gerds T, Strub JR. Fracture resistance of single-tooth implant-supported all-ceramic restorations: An in vitro study. J Prosthet Dent 2006;95:111–116.

17. Jung RE, Sailer I, Hämmerle CH, Attin T, Schmidlin P. In vitro color changes of soft tissues caused by restorative materials. Int J Periodontics Restorative Dent 2007;27:251–257.

18. Jung RE, Holderegger C, Sailer I, Khraisat A, Suter A, Hämmerle CH. The effect of all-ceramic and porcelain-fused-to-metal restorations on marginal peri-implant soft tissue color: A randomized controlled clinical trial. Int J Periodontics Restorative Dent 2008;28:357–365.

19. Park SE, Da Silva JD, Weber HP, Ishikawa-Nagai S. Optical phenomenon of peri-implant soft tissue. Part I. Spectrophotometric assessment of natural tooth gingiva and peri-implant mucosa. Clin Oral Implants Res 2007;18:569–574.

20. Ishikawa-Nagai S, Da Silva JD, Weber HP, Park SE. Optical phenomenon of peri-implant soft tissue. Part II. Preferred implant neck color to improve soft tissue esthetics. Clin Oral Implants Res 2007;18:575–580.

21. Stimmelmayr M, Edelhoff D, Güth JF, Erdelt K, Happe A, Beuer F. Wear at the titanium-titanium and the titanium-zirconia implant-abutment interface: A comparative in vitro study. Dent Mater 2012;28:1215–1220.

Patient situation 1: Incorrect abutment and design choice

The maxillary right central incisor was restored with an implant, but an alumina abutment was chosen. The gingival third of the abutment was also cut back to add shoulder porcelain and thereby increase the fluorescence and match the color of the abutment with the root shade of the adjacent tooth. The alumina crown was cemented, and the patient returned on the following day with the fractured abutment. A zirconia abutment, which was just introduced to the market at that time, was selected and fabricated without cutback to avoid weakening the zirconia abutment structure. Eight-year follow-up revealed the clinical and radiographic outcome.

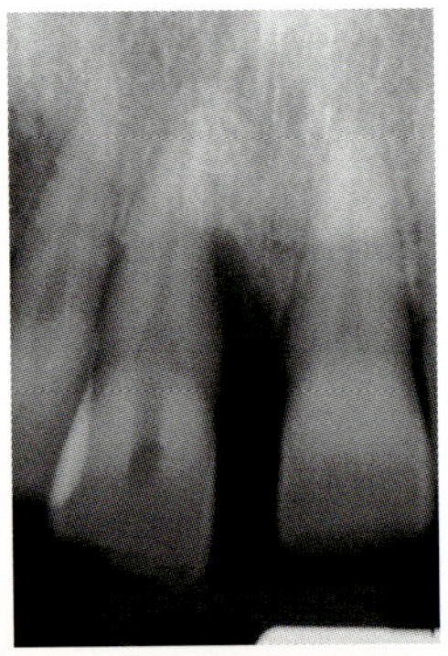
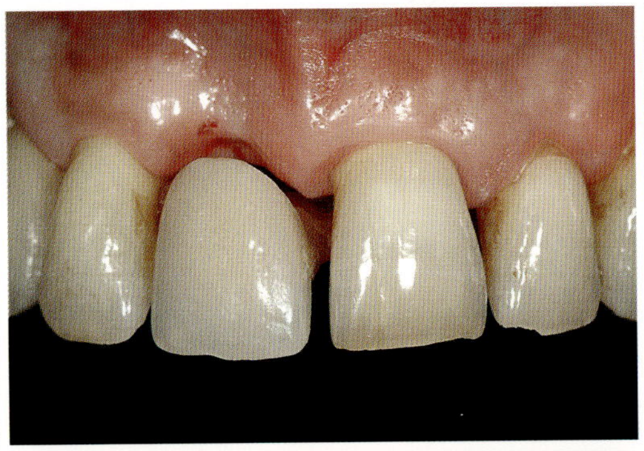
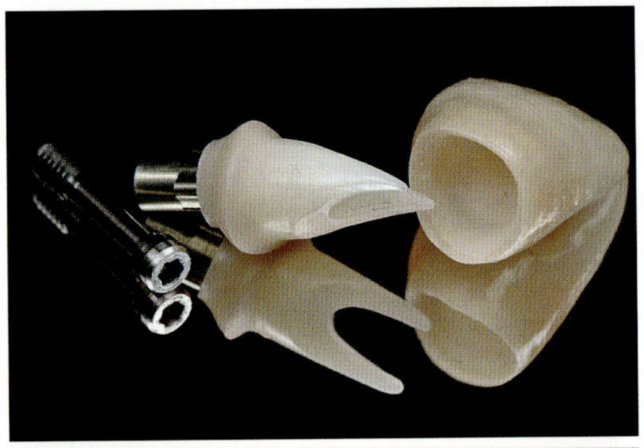
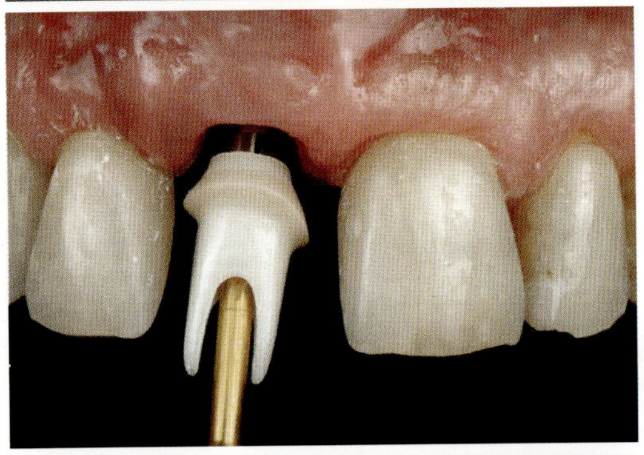
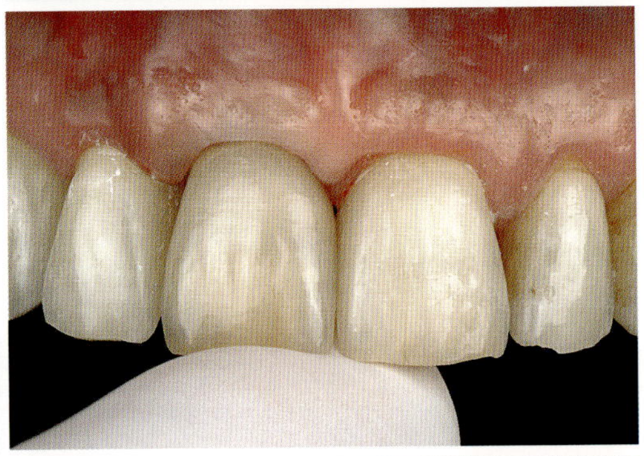
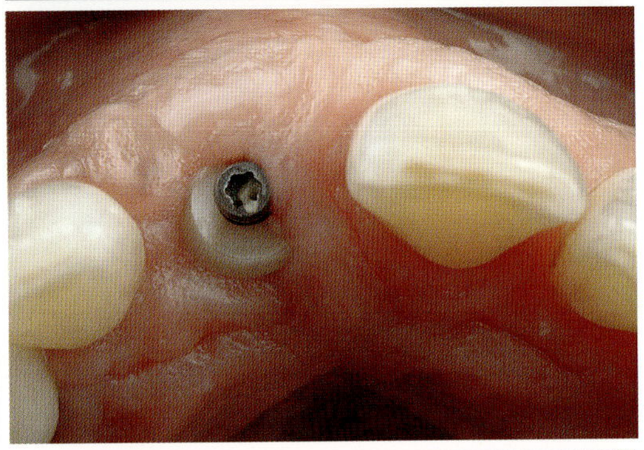
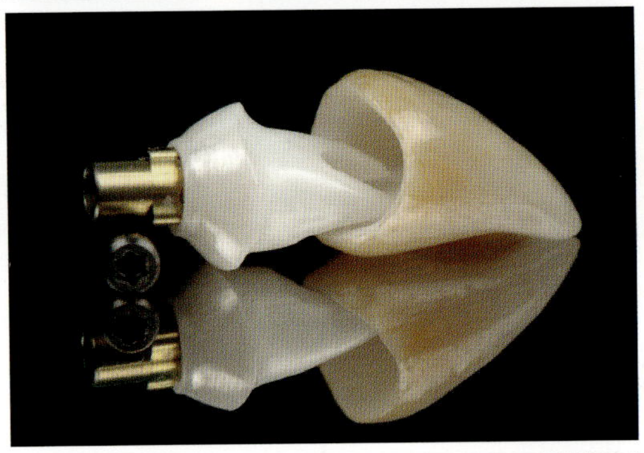
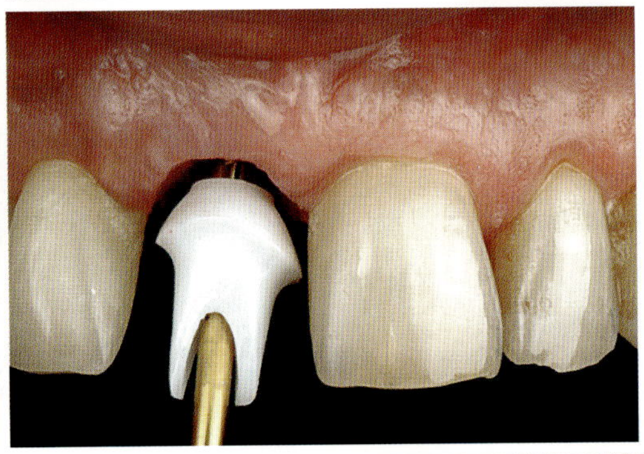
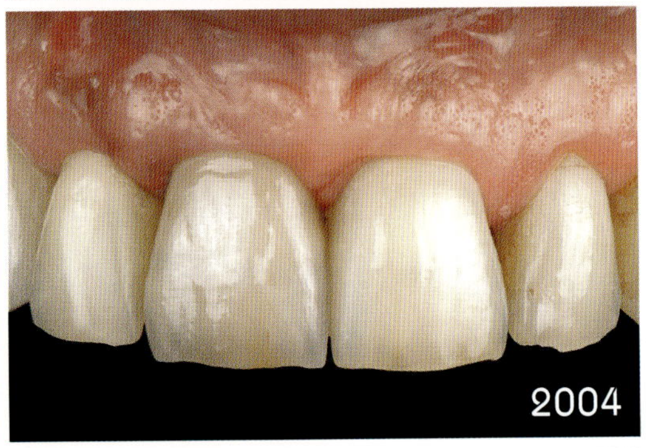

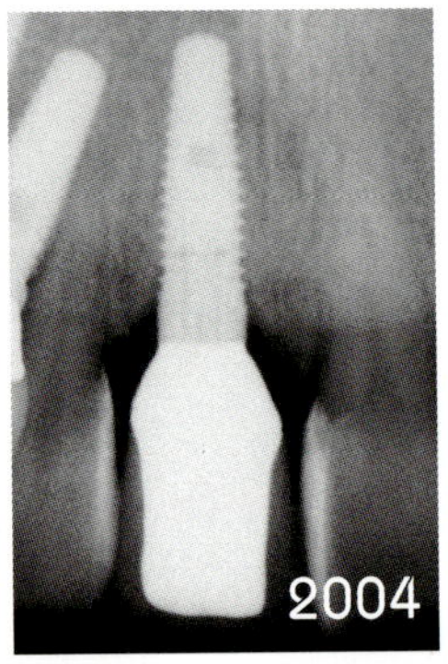

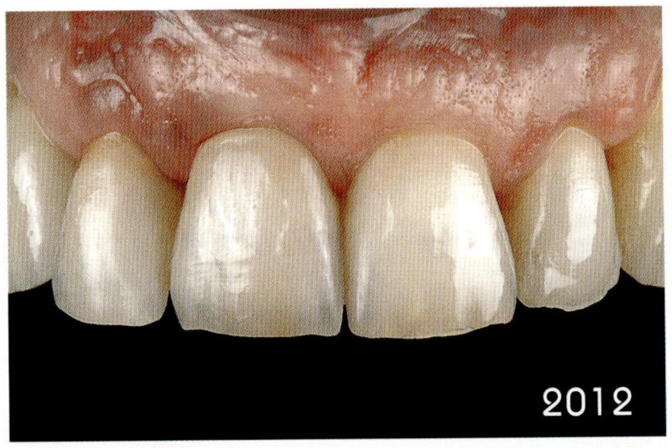

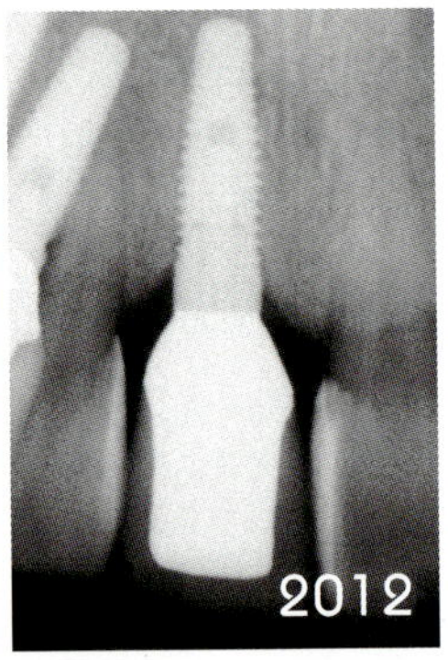

Patient situation 2: Compromised implant placement and incorrect abutment selection

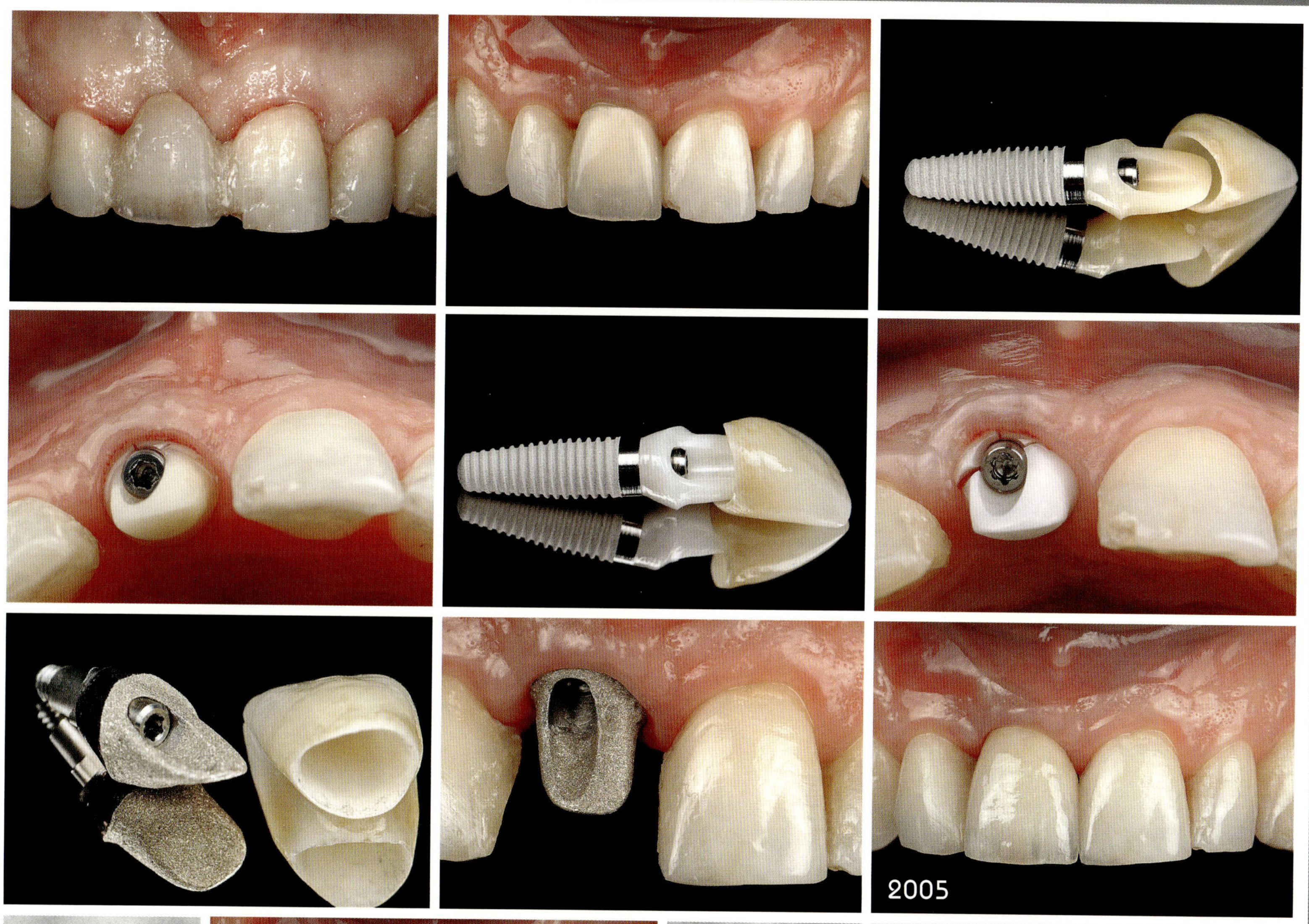

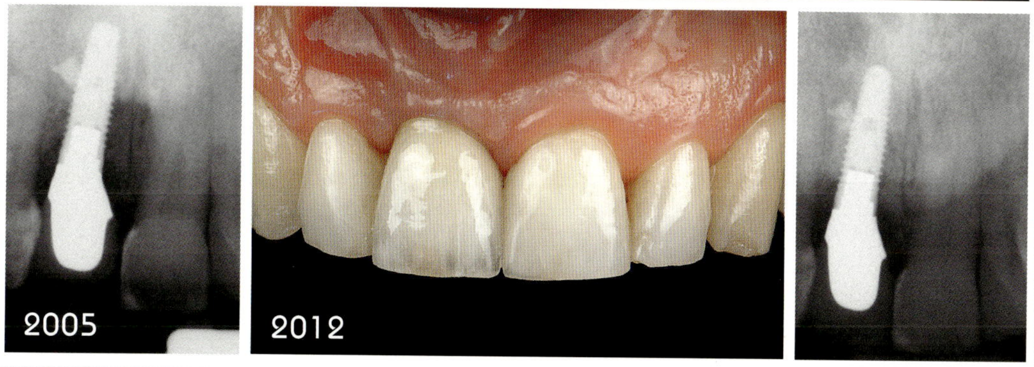

The maxillary right central incisor was restored with an implant placed too far to the distal and buccal aspects, compromising the fracture resistance of the abutment because of the thin walls surrounding the screw access hole. Alumina and zirconia abutments fractured under torque, so a gold-alloy abutment was chosen. Bone remodeling was observed at 7-year follow-up.

Patient situation 3: Internal connection implants with zirconia abutments

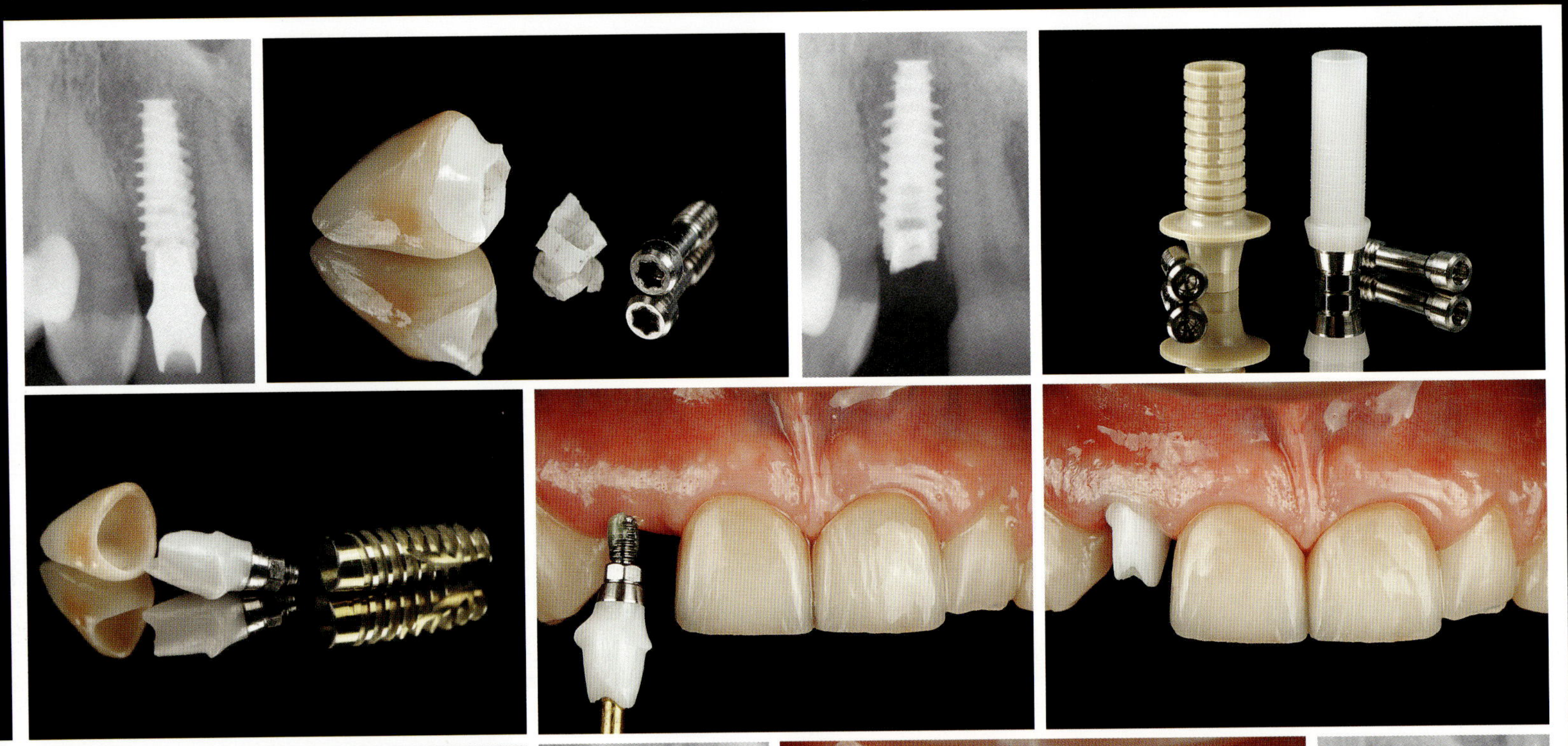

The patient received a NobelActive implant on the maxillary right lateral incisor with a full zirconia abutment and alumina crown restoration. Two months after final cementation, the abutment fractured at the base of the internal connection. A metal insert was fabricated to counteract the tight implant-zirconia connection and allow use of a zirconia abutment. The composite abutment bonded to the plastic sleeve was scanned and then cemented into the metal insert, which has an external hex for this purpose. An internal thread designed into the metal insert facilitates the removal of the abutment from the tight connection.

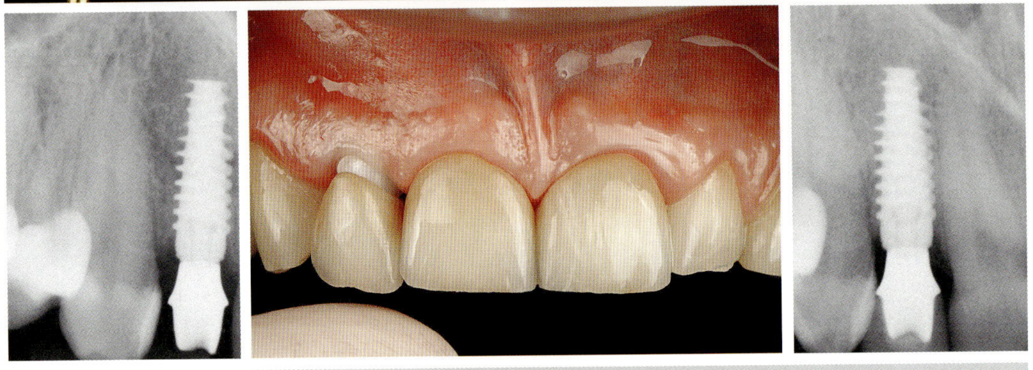

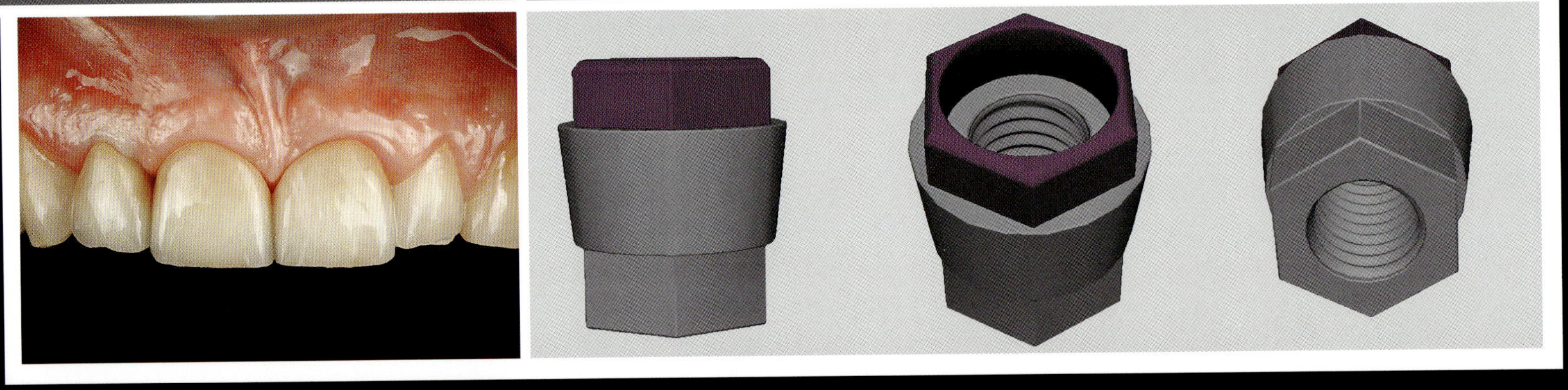

Patient situation 4: Small teeth and zirconia abutments

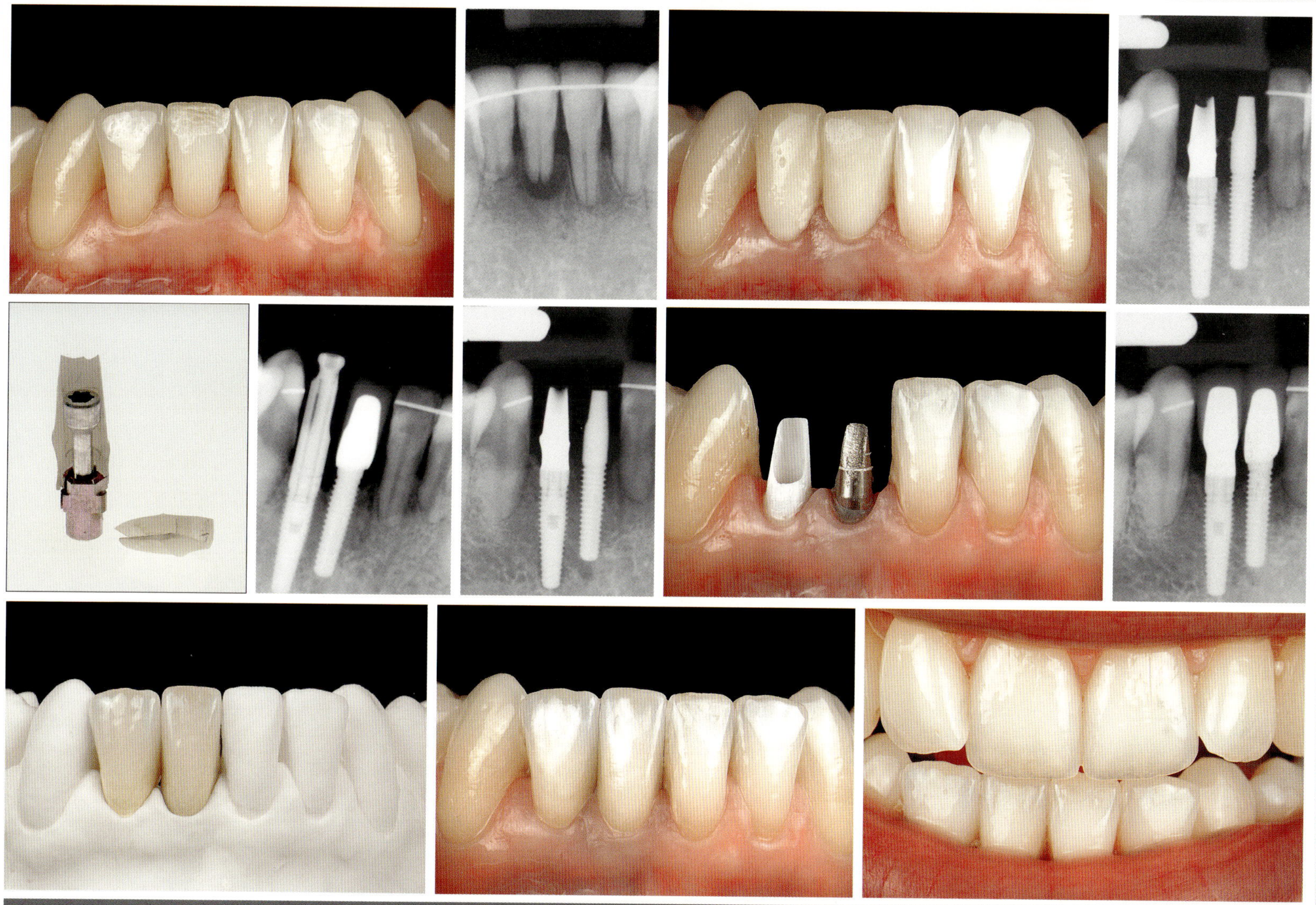

Replacing mandibular anterior teeth with implants is one of the most difficult challenges in dentistry. Here, two adjacent anterior mandibular implants were placed. During restoration, the zirconia abutment fractured because the walls were thinned excessively to create more space for the grafting procedures and to improve tissue thickness around the dental implants. In this type of clinical situation, where small-diameter teeth need to be restored, space is crucial. Therefore, the abutment was adjusted with respect to the necessary thickness of the walls. A titanium abutment is recommended in the initial stages to create the desired tissue thickness. Once the emergence profile has been acceptably modified and sufficient tissue volume has been achieved, a definitive zirconia abutment can be placed to control the tissue topography and support the intended esthetics.

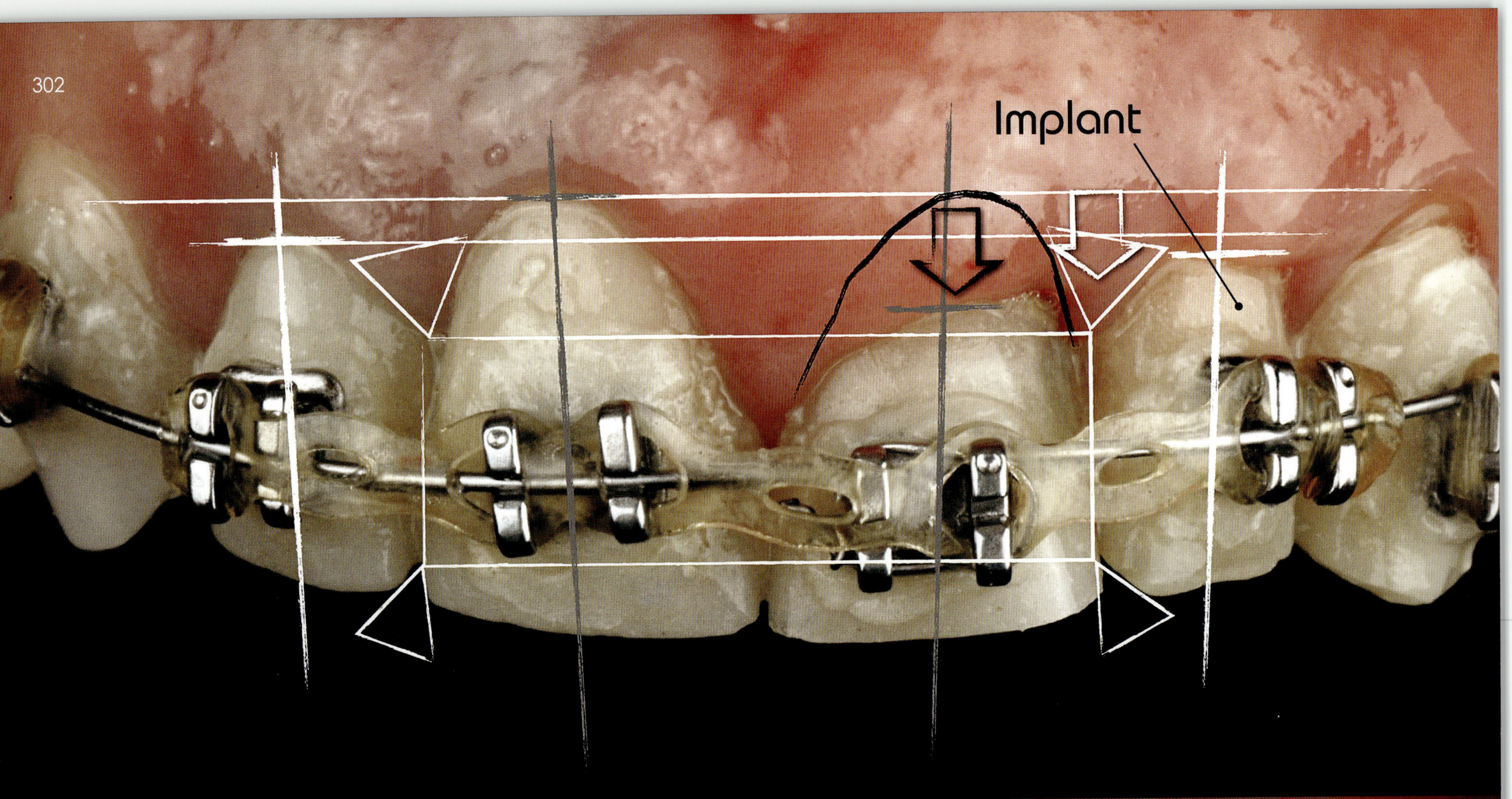
Implant

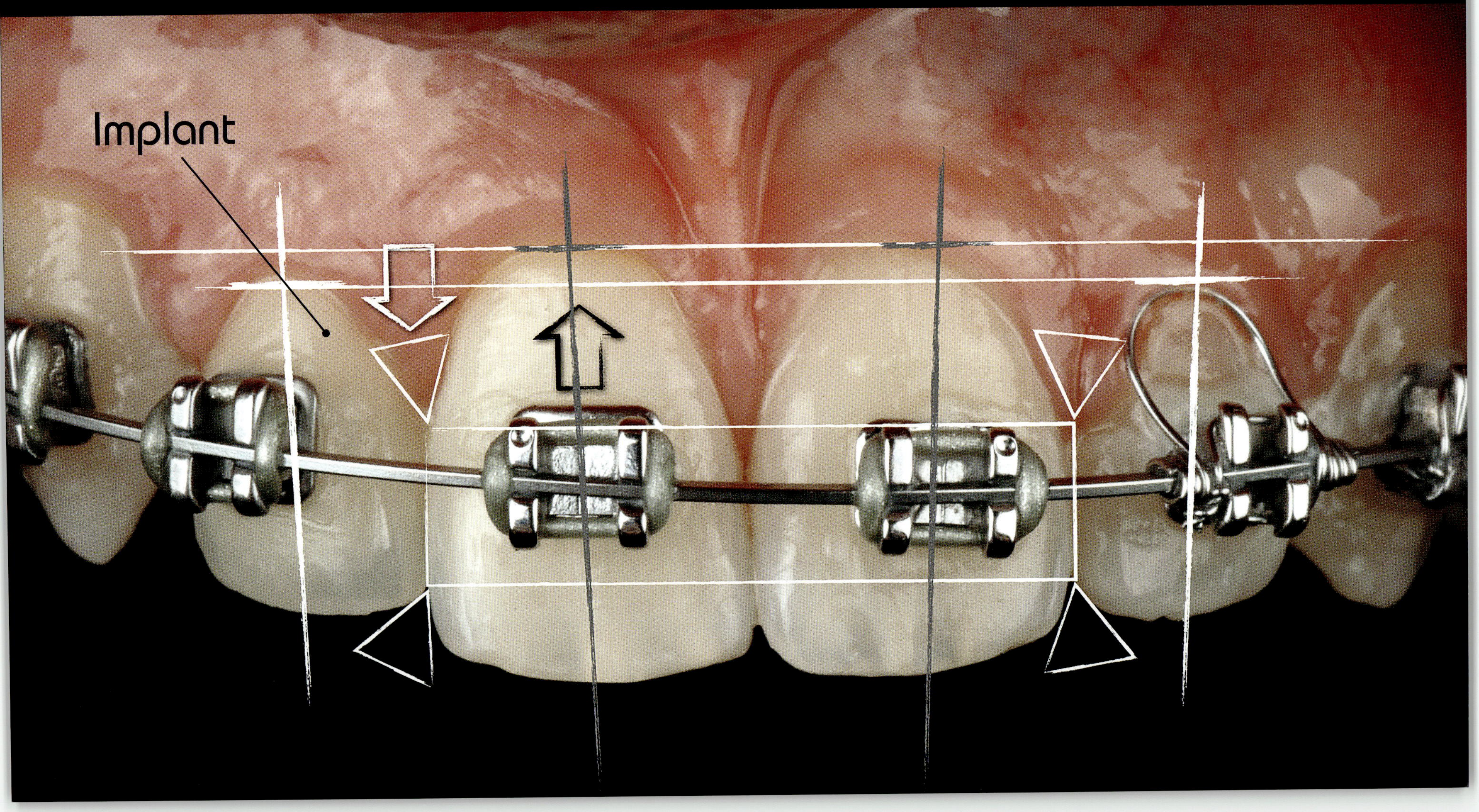
Implant

Orthodontics to Maximize Soft Tissue Esthetics

Research

Orthodontics

Orthodontics are an important treatment tool and should be preferred over more invasive treatment options whenever possible.[1] Publications on orthodontic pretreatment of single-tooth implant sites are mostly descriptive in nature, and there is little scientific evidence to suggest one procedure over another in terms of providing better long-term success. The decision-making process is therefore mostly guided by clinical parameters and the individual patient situation, and the "treatment of choice should be the least invasive option that satisfies the expected esthetic and functional objectives."[2]

Orthodontic tooth movements facilitate positioning and alignment of teeth in a most functional and esthetic manner[3] and are critical for creating and maintaining space for implant placement.[1] One clinical study on post-orthodontic root approximation after space was opened for maxillary lateral incisor implants recommends a minimum intercoronal space of 6.3 mm and interradicular space of 5.7 mm between the adjacent central incisor and canine.[4] It also suggested maintaining the space with a bonded wire or resin-bonded bridge until implant placement and restoration to reduce root approximation, which occurred in 11% of the cases. Space opening may reduce width and height of the alveolar ridge in newly created lateral incisor sites in the adolescent patient.[5,6] However, these changes are minimal 2 years after space opening.[7]

Orthodontic tooth movements allow for targeted manipulation and enhancement of the supporting bone and soft tissues.[8] If a tooth cannot be maintained, they may be used for implant site development, especially in immediate implant cases.[9,10]

The concept of orthodontic extrusion, or *forced eruption*, was first described by Ingber[11–13] to treat infraosseous bone defects[14] and restore severely compromised teeth.[15]

Controlled vertical extrusion results in bone formation at the apex and within the alveolar crest as the attachment apparatus follows the tooth during this movement.[16,17] As the mucogingival junction remains stable, the width of keratinized gingiva is increased. Therefore, extrusion and other tooth movements may be applied to regain lost or deficient tissues, even interproximal papillae.[18] They may limit the need for surgical augmentation procedures,[9] which are more complicated, very invasive, and less predictable. While comparative clinical data is missing, the viability and excellent success of orthodontic extrusion was demonstrated in systematic and narrative reviews.[19–21] A recent clinical study provided additional evidence for the efficacy of orthodontic implant site development for bone regeneration, soft tissue augmentation, and increased keratinized gingiva.[22] Slow tooth movement (1 mm per month) with forces as low as 15 g for anterior teeth, depending on the amount of surrounding bone, and a stabilization phase of up to 8 to 10 months have been recommended.[19–21]

Other orthodontic tooth movements, root tipping,[23] torque, intrusion, and combinations thereof are equally instrumental for nonsurgical augmentation or alteration of bone and soft tissue levels.

References

1. Kinzer GA, Kokich VO Jr. Managing congenitally missing lateral incisors. Part III: Single-tooth implants. J Esthet Restor Dent 2005;17:202–210.

2. Kokich VO Jr, Kinzer GA. Managing congenitally missing lateral incisors, Part I: Canine substitution. J Esthet Restor Dent 2005;17:1–6.

3. Nold SL, Horvath SD, Stampf S, Blatz MB. Analysis of select facial and dental esthetic parameters. Int J Periodontics Restorative Dent 2014;34:623–629.

4. Olsen TM, Kokich VG Sr. Postorthodontic root approximation after opening space for maxillary lateral incisor implants. Am J Orthod Dentofacial Orthop 2010;137:158–159.

5. Uribe F, Chau V, Padala S, Neace WP, Cutrera A, Nanda R. Alveolar ridge width and height changes after orthodontic space opening in patients congenitally missing maxillary lateral incisors. Eur J Orthod 2013;35:87–92.

6. Uribe F, Padala S, Allareddy V, Nanda R. Cone-beam computed tomography evaluation of alveolar ridge width and height changes after orthodontic space opening in patients with congenitally missing maxillary lateral incisors. Am J Orthod Dentofacial Orthop 2013;144:848–859.

7. Nováčková S, Marek I, Kamínek M. Orthodontic tooth movement: Bone formation and its stability over time. Am J Orthod Dentofacial Orthop 2011;139:37–43.

8. Atherton JD. The gingival response to orthodontic tooth movement. Am J Orthod Dentofacial Orthop 1970;58:179–186.

9. Salama H, Salama M. The role of orthodontic extrusive remodeling in the enhancement of soft and hard tissue profiles prior to implant placement: A systematic approach to the management of extraction site defects. Int J Periodontics Restorative Dent 1993;13:312–333.

10. Holst S, Hegenbarth EA, Schlegel KA, Holst AI. Restoration of a nonrestorable central incisor using forced orthodontic eruption, immediate implant placement, and an all-ceramic restoration: A clinical report. J Prosthet Dent 2007;98:251–255.

11. Ingber JS. Forced eruption: Part I. A method of treating isolated one and two wall infrabony osseous defects—Rationale and case report. J Periodontol 1974;45:199–206.

12. Ingber JS. Forced eruption: Part II. A method of treating nonrestorable teeth—Periodontal and restorative considerations. J Periodontol 1976;47:203–216.

13. Ingber JS. Forced eruption: Alteration of soft tissue cosmetic deformities. Int J Periodontics Restorative Dent 1989;9:416–425.

14. Brown IS. The effect of orthodontic therapy on certain types of periodontal defects. J Periodontol 1973;44:742–756.

15. Blatz MB. Comprehensive treatment of traumatic fracture and luxation injuries in the anterior permanent dentition. Pract Proced Aesthet Dent 2001;13:273–279.

16. Mantzikos T, Shamus I. Forced eruption and implant site development: Soft tissue response. Am J Orthod Dentofacial Orthop 1997;112:596–606.

17. Mantzikos T, Shamus I. Forced eruption and implant site development: An osteophysiologic response. Am J Orthod Dentofacial Orthop 1999;115:583–591.

18. Lin CD, Chang SS, Liou CS, Dong DR, Fu E. Management of interdental papillae loss with forced eruption, immediate implantation, and root-form pontic. J Periodontol 2006;77:135–141.

19. Korayem M, Flores-Mir C, Nassar U, Olfert K. Implant site development by orthodontic extrusion: A systematic review. Angle Orthod 2008;78:752–760.

20. Brindis MA, Block MS. Orthodontic tooth extrusion to enhance soft tissue implant esthetics. J Oral Maxillofac Surg 2009;67:49–59.

21. Borzabadi-Farahani A, Zadeh HH. Adjunctive orthodontic applications in dental implantology [epub ahead of print 31 October 2013]. J Oral Implantol doi:10.1563/AAID-JOI-D-13-00235.

22. Amato F, Mirabella AD, Macca U, Tarnow DP. Implant site development by orthodontic forced extraction: A preliminary study. Int J Oral Maxillofac Implants 2012;27:411–420.

23. Uribe F, Taylor T, Shafer D, Nanda R. A novel approach for implant site development through root tipping. Am J Orthod Dentofacial Orthop 2010;138:649–655.

Orthodontic extrusion

Orthodontic tooth movement can increase papillary height and re-create lost interproximal papillae. This is typically achieved through orthodontic extrusion of the teeth adjacent to the implant site or through intrusion and torque, depending on the type of implant placement and the distribution and position of the adjacent teeth. In general, the teeth are positioned more buccally and coronally in reference to the implant.

Four patient cases are presented to illustrate the potential and versatility of orthodontic therapies in optimizing soft tissue topography around dental implants and adjacent teeth.

The height of the interproximal papillae around implants is determined by the bone height around the adjacent teeth. It is critical to understand that trauma to the bone of the adjacent teeth during surgery will negatively affect papillary height and may lead to interproximal defects and poor peri-implant soft tissue esthetics. Preservation of the adjacent bone during delayed implant placement is therefore crucial to treatment success.

Vertical extrusion

Vertical extrusion is one of the orthodontic treatment options to re-establish bone lost during surgical intervention or from previous trauma. Several aspects of the orthodontic movement must be considered: the force applied to the tooth, the timing or pace of the movement, and any occlusal trauma during the orthodontic extrusion.

The applied orthodontic force should be as small as possible to ensure adequate bone formation. Lightweight wires and 1 mm or less of movement per month are recommended. Another general rule is the bigger the defect, the lighter the force and the slower the movement should be. The clinician should see the patient about every 15 days during extrusion to verify the occlusion and ensure that there are no contacts during static and dynamic occlusion. The tooth should be stabilized after completion of the extrusion to allow for adequate bone remineralization, which occurs within 8 to 10 months. A splinting device is recommended to provide the necessary stability.

The implant can be placed or restored once the tooth is stable. When an implant is placed adjacent to an extruded tooth, care must be taken with the design of the incision for implant placement. Generally, a flapless implant placement technique is recommended on the extruded bone site due to compromised tissue thickness and stability. No or only partial-thickness flaps are recommended to limit bone resorption. Noninvasive surgical techniques enhance the long-term success of orthodontic treatment.

Vertical bone height through tooth extrusion

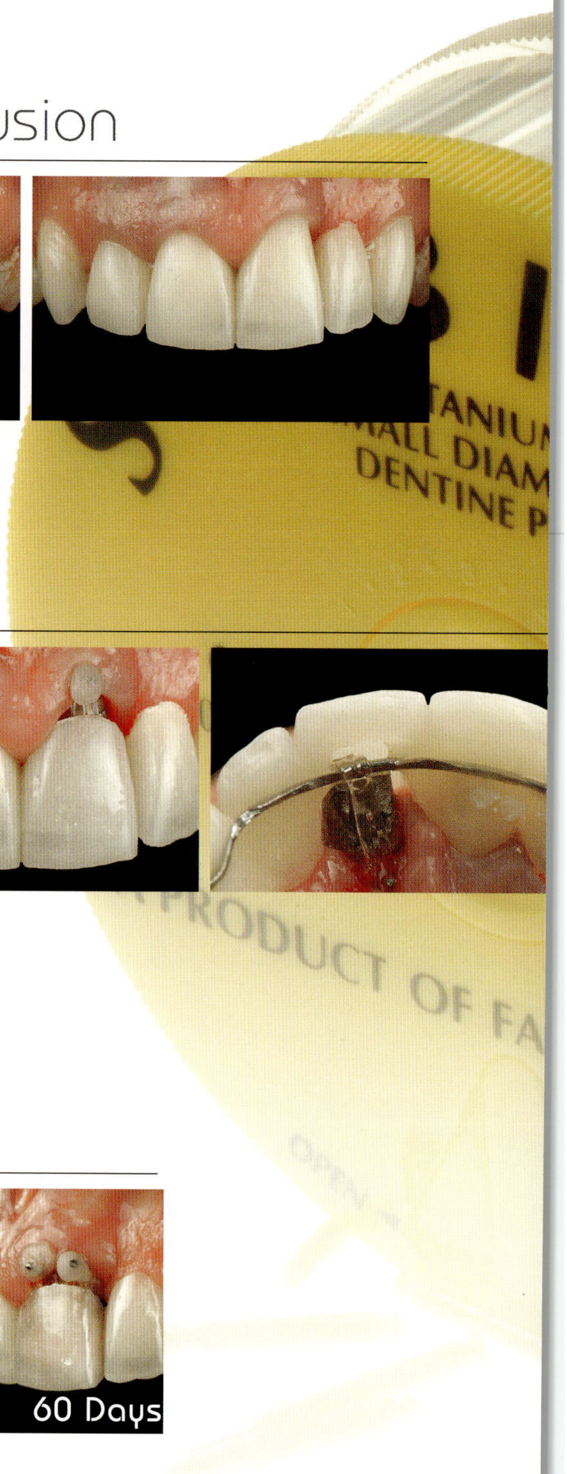

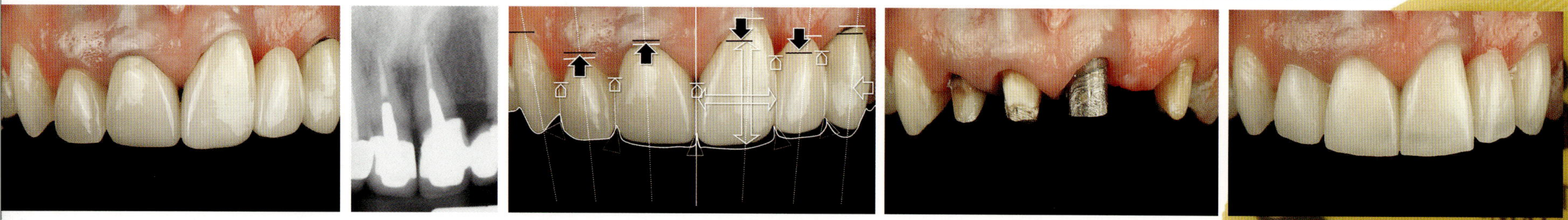

Patient 1 The patient presented with two failing crowns and a three-unit FPD that were neither functional nor esthetically pleasing. A large bony defect was present on the buccodistal aspect of the maxillary left central incisor, which made it difficult to create symmetry between the gingival embrasures and papillary heights. Provisional restoration restored tooth proportions, provided tissue support, and allowed for re-evaluation of the magnitude of the bone defect.

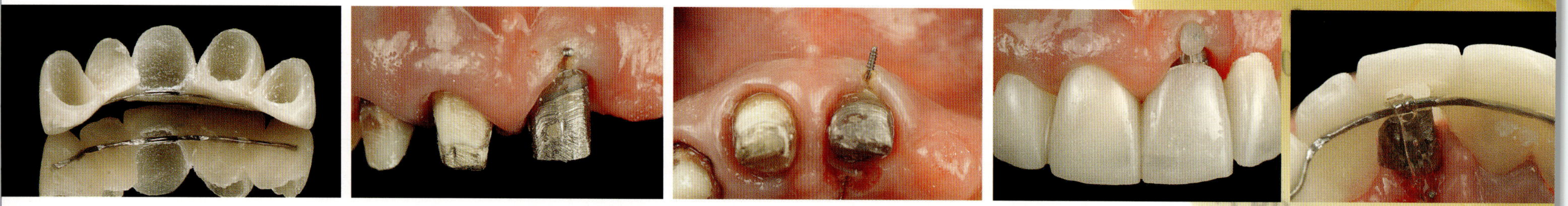

With support of the provisional restoration, orthodontic treatment was performed to extrude the tooth and improve the bone defect as well as papillary height and soft tissue topography. The provisional restoration for the maxillary left central incisor was hollowed, leaving just a buccal veneer for esthetic purposes. Intracoronal amalgam pins were then screwed into the buccal and palatal aspects of the root as anchorage for elastics, using the reinforcing wire of the provisional restoration as a lever arm. The elastics were changed every 15 days until the desired level of extrusion was accomplished. Only small extrusion forces were created to allow the adjacent bone to follow the extruded root.

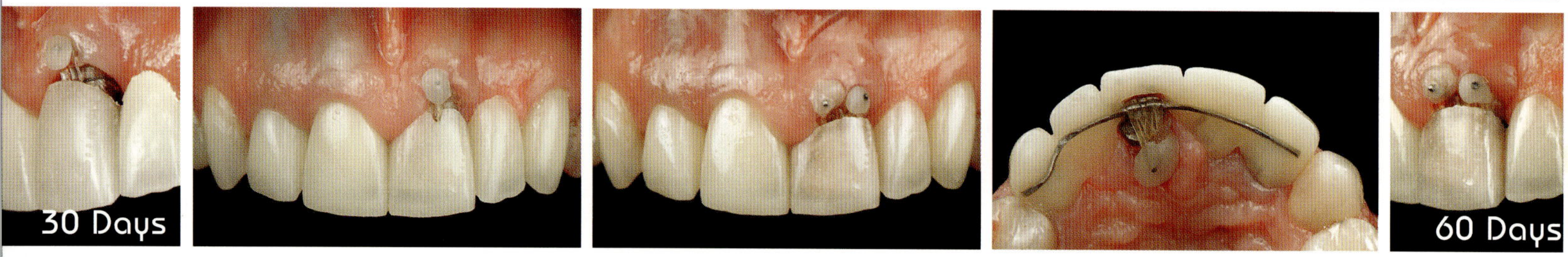

Comparison of the situation during orthodontic extrusion at 30 and 60 days reveals that an extra pin was placed on the buccal aspect of the root to ensure better 3D control over the tooth movement. Composite was placed on the tips of the intracoronal pins to protect the mucosa and tongue from laceration.

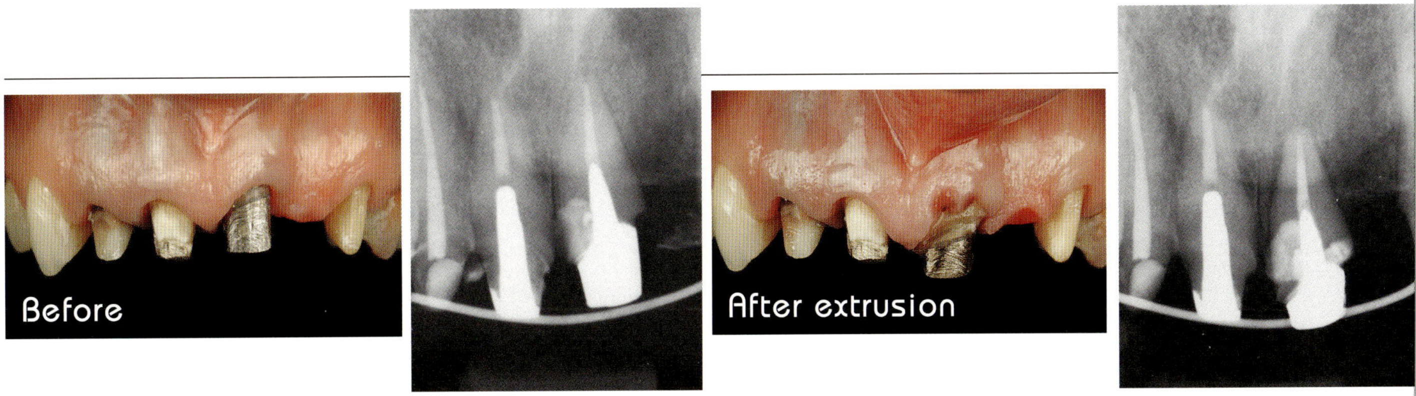

Clinical situations before and after orthodontic extrusion. A total of 3 mm of tooth extrusion was achieved, which is apparent when comparing the differences in heights between the incisal edges of the two central incisor abutments. Radiographs confirm the amount of extrusion. The increase of distal papillary height on the maxillary left central incisor creates an ideal scenario for implant placement.

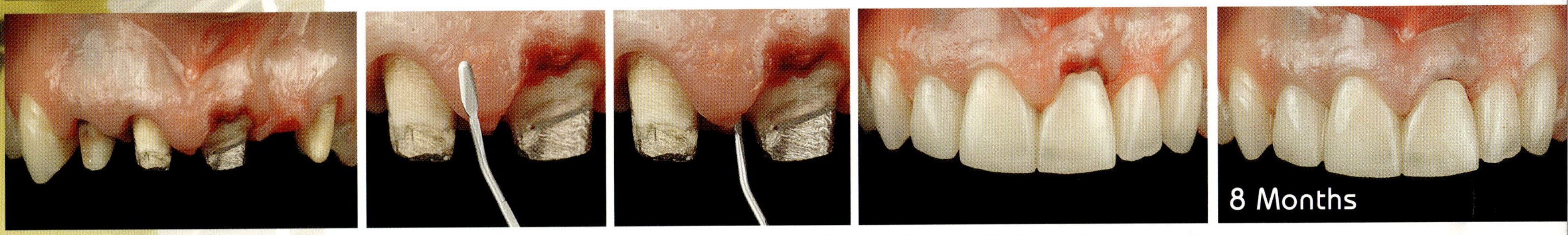

The tooth was re-prepared to level the extruded abutment with the adjacent tooth, following the same gingival scallop. Vertical fibrotomy was performed on the mesial aspect of the interproximal area of the maxillary left central incisor to maintain the same bone level and to prevent the central papilla from becoming too dominant after completion of the treatment. The provisional restoration was then relined to fit the re-prepared abutment and functioned as a retainer for tooth stability for 8 months.

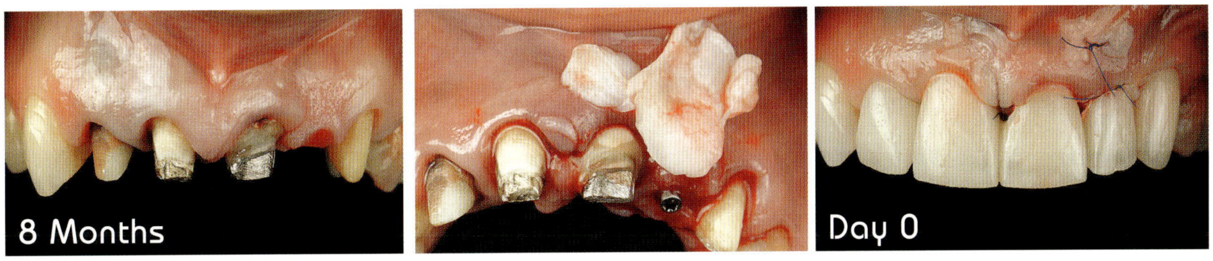

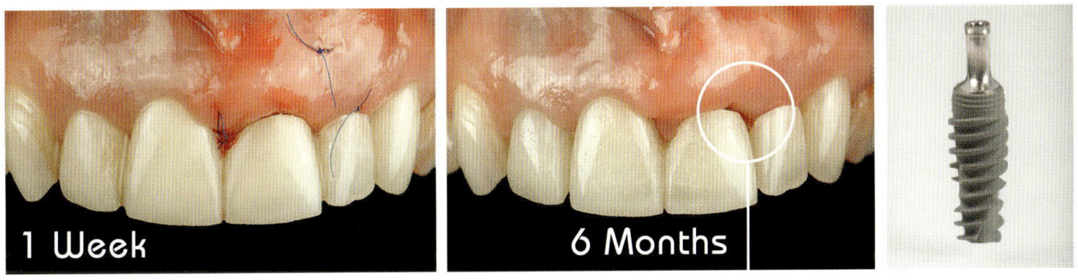

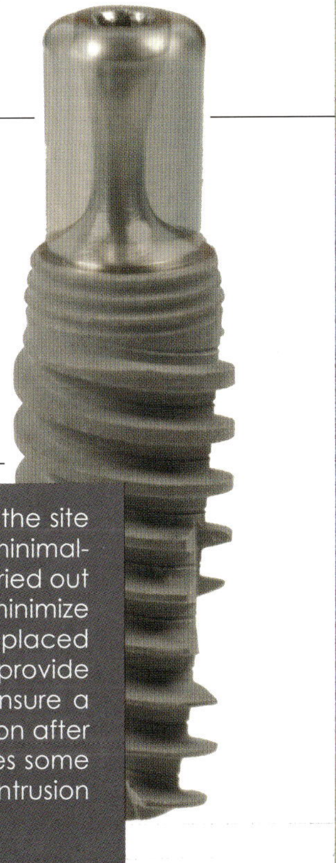

After 8 months of abutment stability, the site was ready for implant placement. A minimally invasive incision technique was carried out on the site of the extruded tooth to minimize postsurgical resorption. A CTG was placed concurrently with the implant to provide additional volume at the site and ensure a long-lasting esthetic result. The situation after a healing phase of 6 months indicates some resorption *(circle)*. This is due to the intrusion of the maxillary left central incisor.

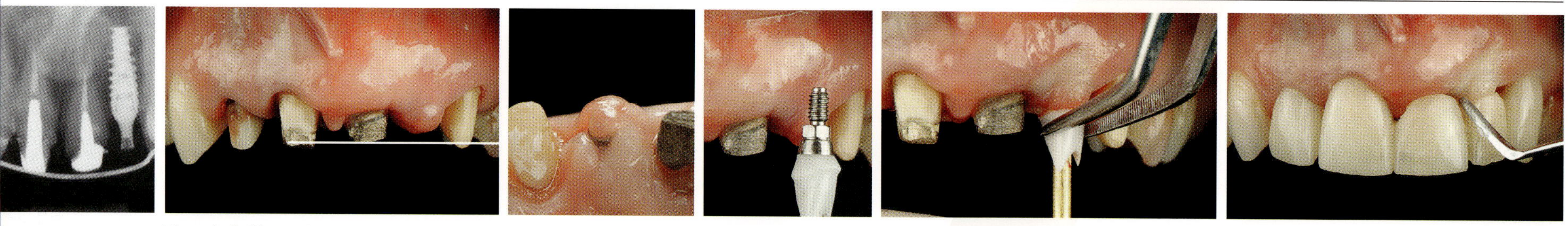

The definitive abutment was placed; note the amount of volume obtained at the tooth and implant sites. The provisional restoration was relined chairside to create an ideal emergence profile.

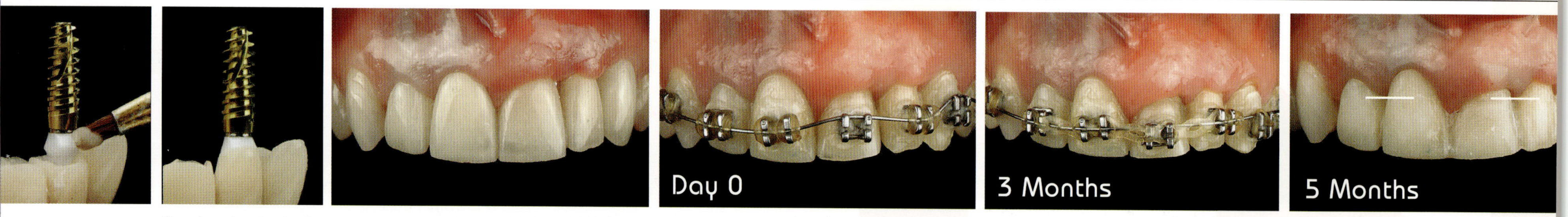

The implant abutment and provisional restoration were disconnected and adjusted in the laboratory to create the desired accuracy of fit. The provisional restoration was then repositioned in the mouth to place the orthodontic appliances and re-create the orthodontic extrusion of the maxillary left central incisor to level the interproximal papilla between the left central and lateral incisors. After completion of the orthodontic treatment, a 3-month stabilization period was observed before removal of the orthodontic appliances. Subsequently, the provisional crown restorations were splinted together with acrylic resin and kept stable for another 5 months to allow for a remineralization and bone maturation period of a total of 8 months.

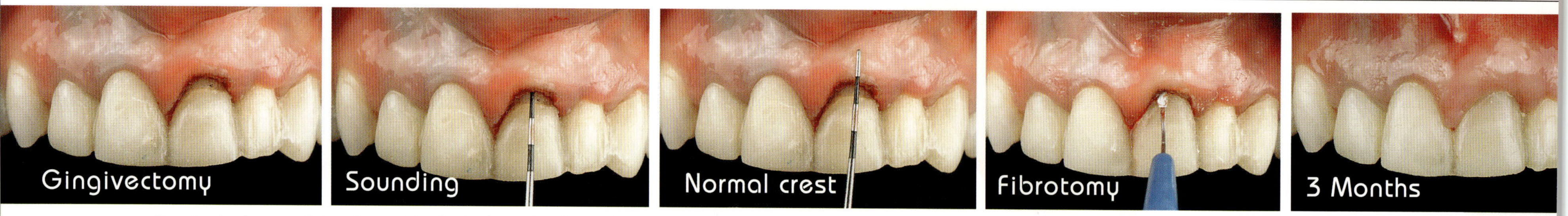

The last phase of treatment included evaluation of the bone levels through careful sounding. A gingivectomy was performed through electrosurgery to provide a symmetric gingival scallop of the maxillary right central incisor and was followed by a fibrotomy to re-establish a new dentogingival complex. A 3-month follow-up period was observed for healing and tissue maturation before fabrication of another provisional restoration to re-create the support and proportions of the teeth.

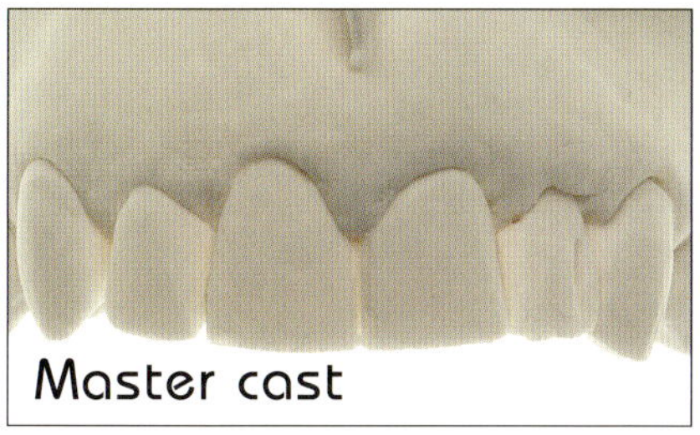

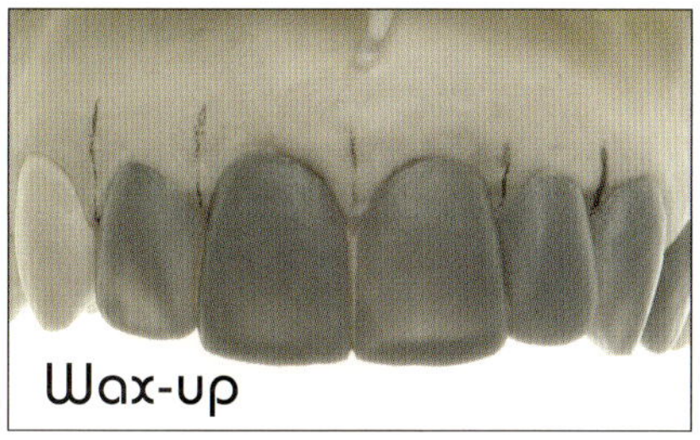

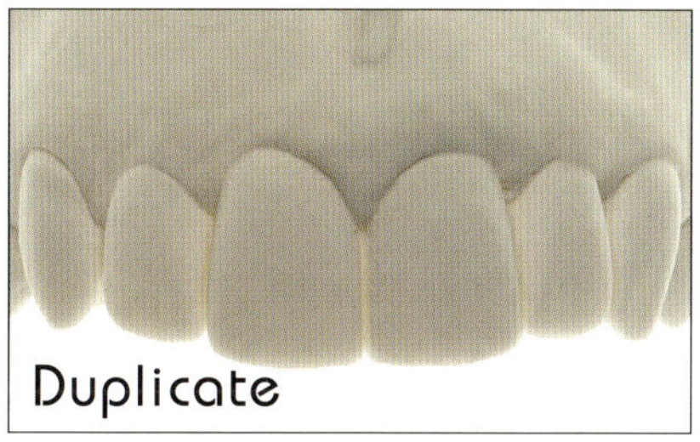

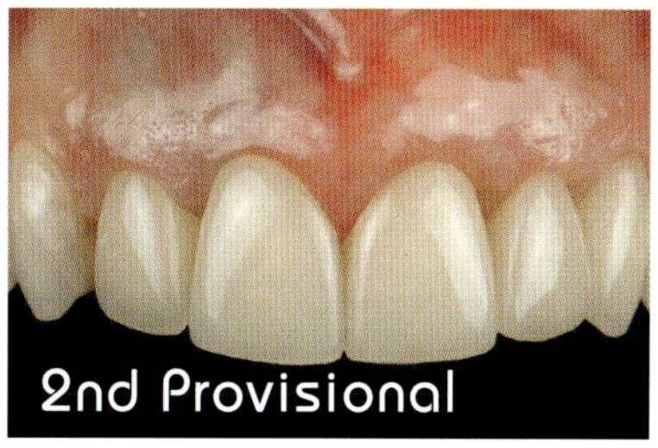

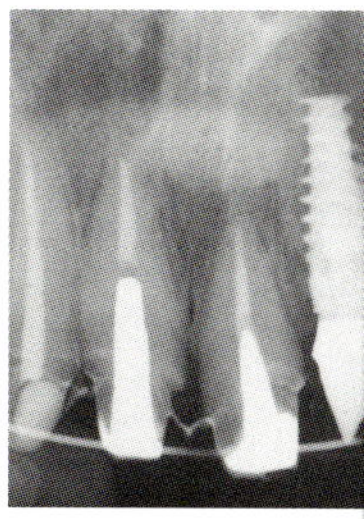

An alginate impression was made to assist with the final wax-up and redistribution of tooth proportions, axes, and emergence profiles. Typically, a line is drawn on the cast to indicate papillary heights and maintain a reference during the wax-up. Other features such as surface texture and morphology also become more obvious on a duplicate stone cast. The final wax-up served as a matrix for another set of provisional restorations.

Some modifications had to be implemented to provide the same appearance of both gingival embrasures from the distal of the left central incisor to the mesial of the left lateral incisor as well as from the distal of the right central incisor to the mesial of the right lateral incisor. It was decided to reduce the diameter of the left central incisor interproximally and blend it to the buccal and palatal aspect to create additional space for the gingival embrasure and allow the papilla to grow and fill the space, creating an ideal symmetric appearance.

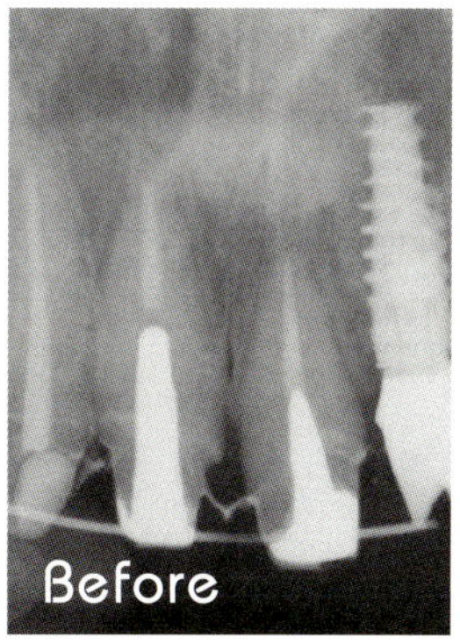

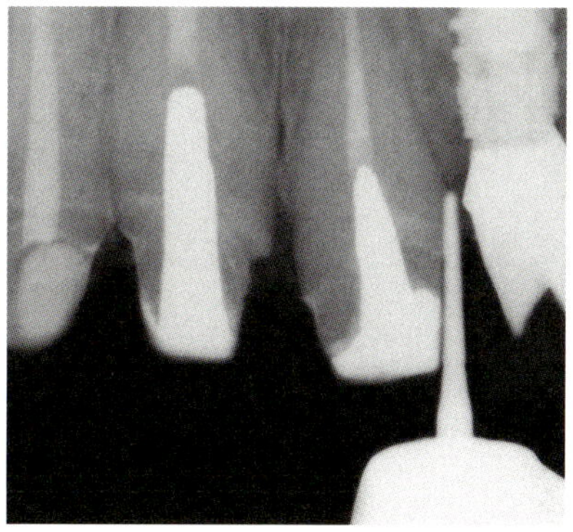

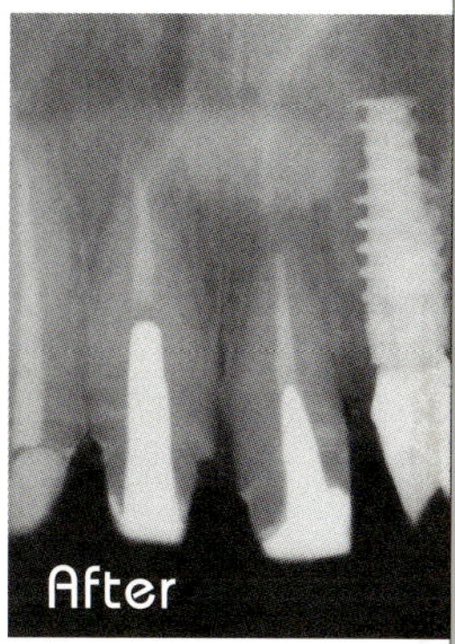

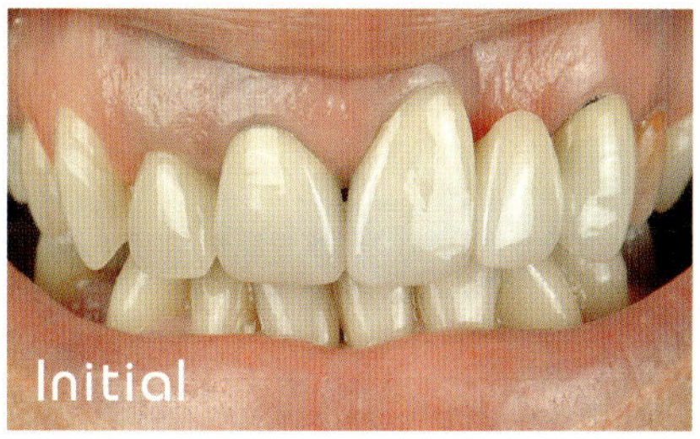

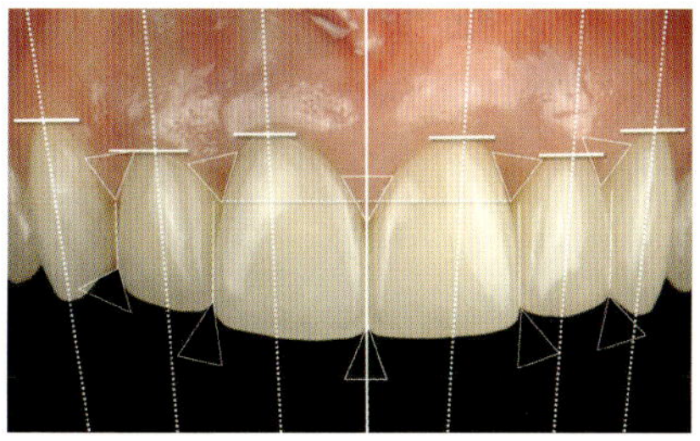

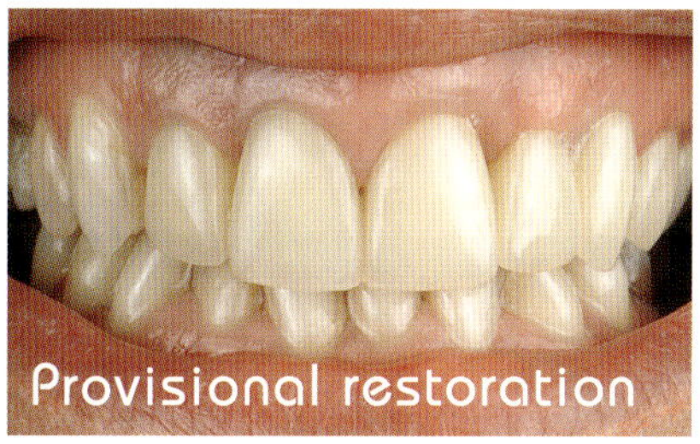

This provisional stage is intended to reestablish function, tooth alignment, and proportion while protecting and supporting the carefully created soft tissue architecture and morphology.

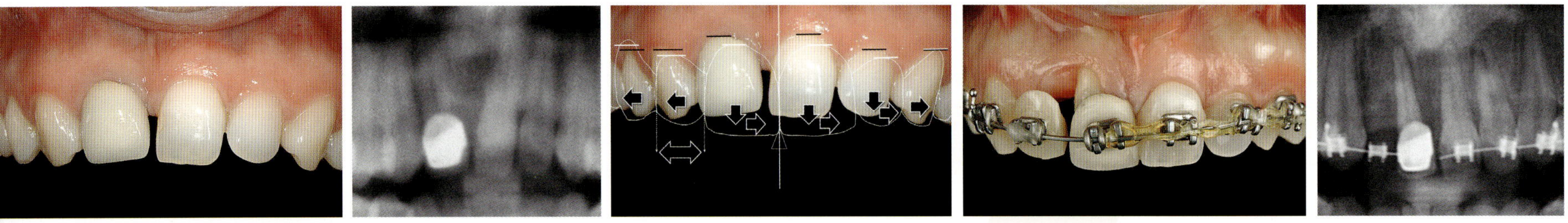

Orthodontist:
Dr Domingo Martín

Patient 2 A 38-year-old woman presented with agenesis of the maxillary right central incisor, which was camouflaged with an overcontoured crown on the right lateral incisor. Orthodontic therapy consisted of centering the midline, moving the right lateral incisor into the position of the right central incisor, extruding both teeth in the central incisor positions, leveling the interproximal and gingival heights, and creating space for an implant in the area of the right lateral incisor. The ultimate restorative treatment plan was to place an implant-supported restoration in the right lateral incisor site and a conventional crown in the right central incisor site.

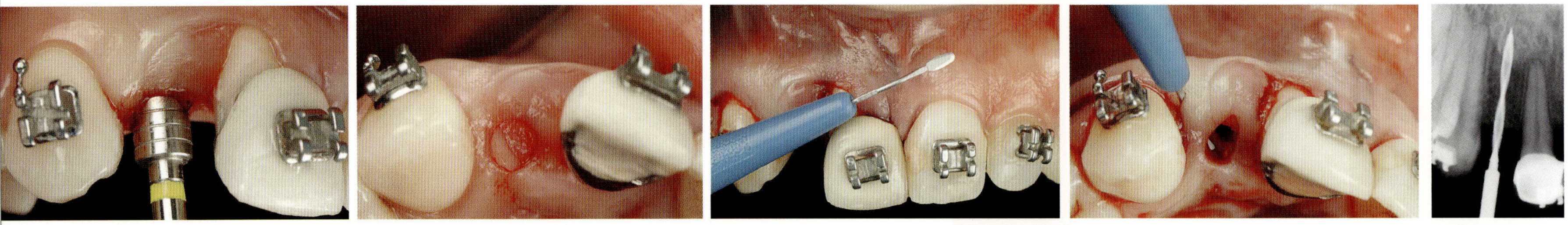

A recession was created during movement of the right lateral incisor into the position of the central incisor. Periodontal treatment therefore included augmentation of not only the implant site but also the mesially relocated tooth. A crestal circular incision was performed more distally to allow more space on the mesial aspect for tissue grafting. A partial-thickness flap was elevated with ophthalmic microsurgical blades, creating a tunnel that involved the adjacent teeth and continued apically above the mucogingival line.

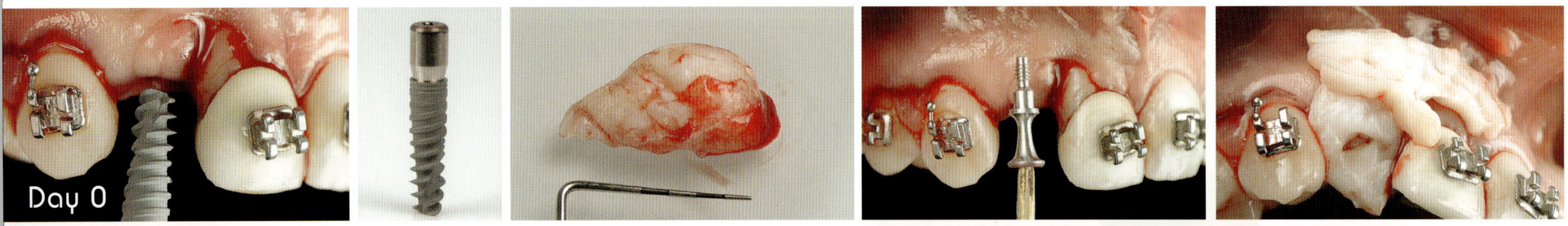

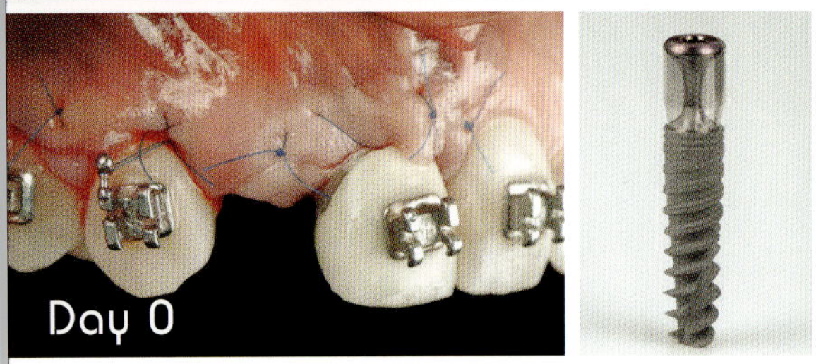

An implant (NobelActive 3.5 × 13 mm) was placed with a narrow, concave healing abutment to allow for maximal augmentation with a CTG on the implant site. The tuberosity served as the donor site for the CTG, which was adapted to the defect. An extra incision was performed at the base of the papilla between the maxillary right canine and the first premolar to allow placement of the graft into the prepared tunnel. A double CTG layer was designed on the mesial papilla of the implant to create an even greater tissue volume.

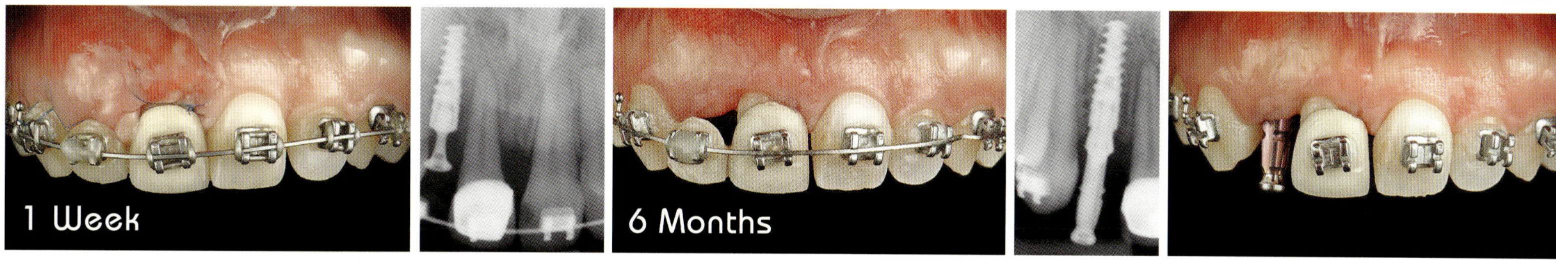

Volumetric shrinkage of the augmented site is obvious during the different stages of the healing process from 1 week to 6 months. An impression of the implant was made to fabricate the definitive abutment.

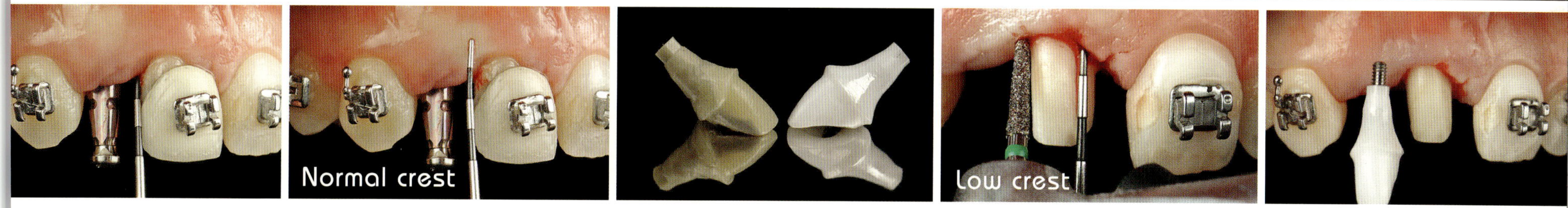

Bone sounding was performed to assess the distance between the bone and the free gingival margin. The measured distance of 4.5 mm provides a favorable prospect of complete interproximal papilla regeneration between the implant and the tooth. After fabrication of the definitive abutment and provisional restoration, the tooth was re-prepared. The preparation margin was placed more apically on the mesial aspect to allow for overcontouring of the restoration and to create the same emergence profile as that of the adjacent central incisor.

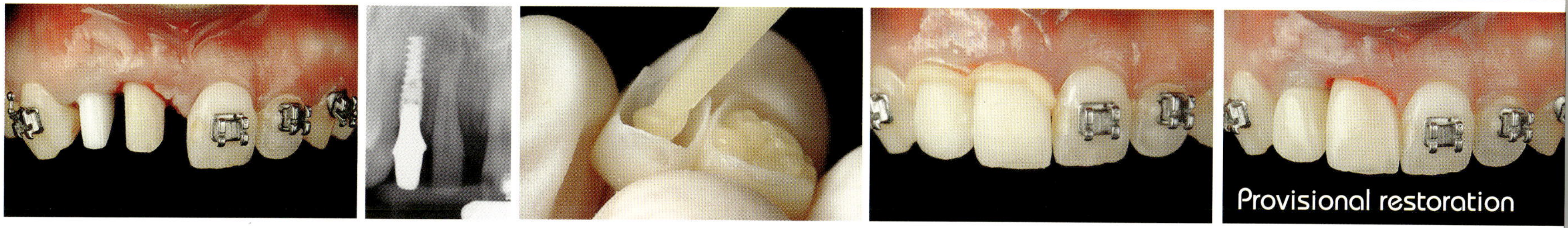

The definitive abutment was placed, and the seating was verified with a periapical radiograph. The provisional restorations were relined to fit the implant abutment and the tooth and designed to create an ideal emergence profile for both restorations. Individual restorations were fabricated to allow for orthodontic movement of the tooth to improve interproximal tissue heights, especially on the distal aspect of the right central incisor and mesial aspect of the implant.

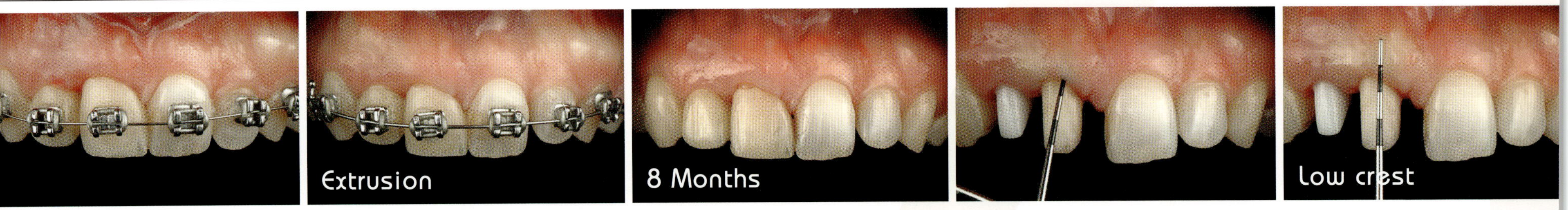

Orthodontic appliances were placed on the provisional restorations to extrude the right central incisor and improve the height of the distal papilla. After splinting the restorations for 8 months, a bone sounding was performed for diagnostic purposes and to optimize position of the preparation finishing line for the ideal emergence profile support. The intent was to create a recession on the buccal and mesial aspect of the right central incisor to duplicate the gingival scallop on the maxillary left central incisor with the definitive restoration.

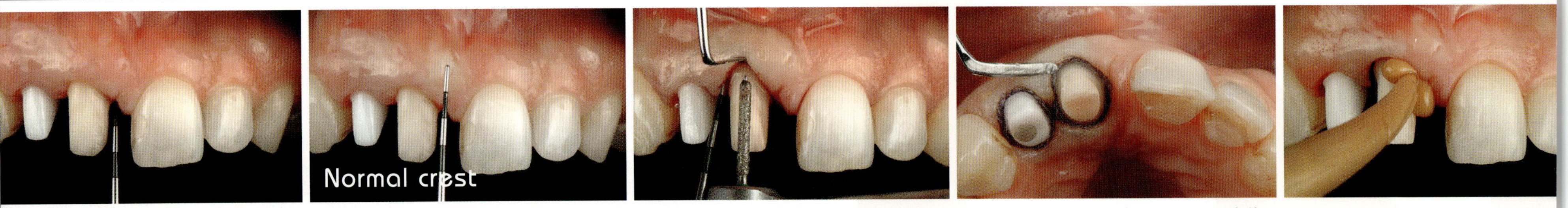

Consequently, the preparation finish line was placed more apically. A triple-cord technique around the prepared tooth as well as spatulas were used to deflect and protect the surrounding soft tissue and expose the margin. A single cord was placed on the implant abutment site to obtain an accurate PVS impression.

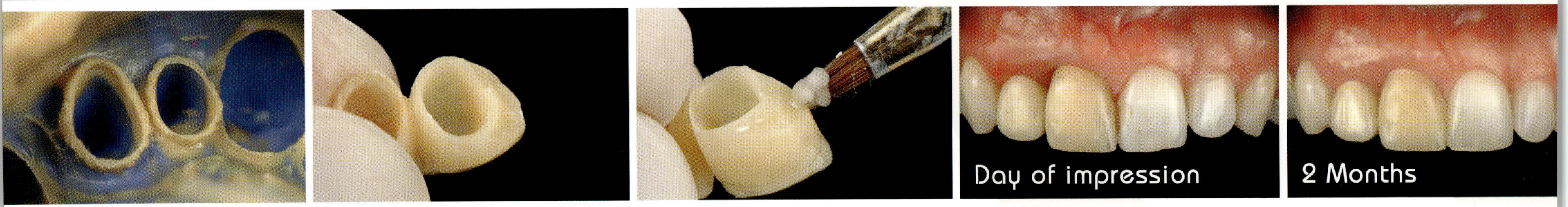

The provisional restorations were relined and modified to add a horizontal component on the mesial aspect of the central incisor. The differences in gingival architecture between the original clinical situation and the provisional stage are noticeable during the 2-month follow up.

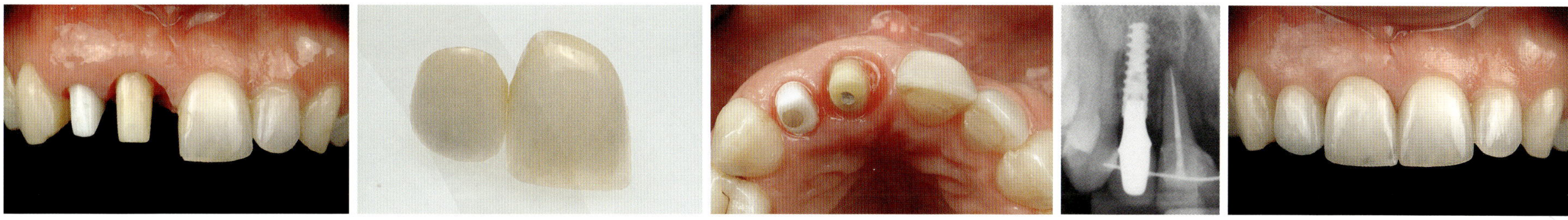

The blend of soft tissue architecture on the mesial aspect of the right central incisor and the support achieved through provisional management and relocation of the finishing line are apparent. Two alumina crowns were fabricated to blend with the surrounding teeth.

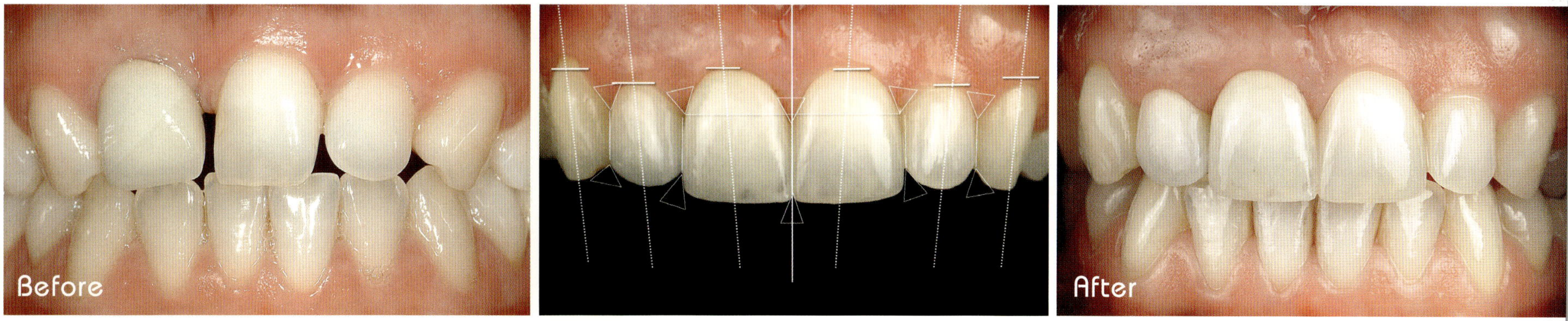

The final result supports the prosthetic goals: alignment of the soft tissues and teeth.

Intrusion and torque

This orthodontic combination tooth movement may be applied in situations where the anterior teeth or incisal plane are extruded compared with the posterior occlusal plane and buccally displaced or protruded, sometimes even out of the alveolar support structure. Intrusion and torque movements provide the ability to reposition the interproximal bone from being too palatal to a more centered position buccopalatally or horizontally, re-creating the appearance of the papillae due to the tooth position in respect to the implant position. The implant may sometimes be used as anchorage for more controlled orthodontic tooth movements. Implants may also be placed during the orthodontic treatment to reduce the overall treatment time. Obviously, the surgeon must closely evaluate the adjacent tooth position to place the implant in an ideal position and visualize the definitive crown restoration in respect to the other anterior teeth and the orthodontic treatment goal. This type of combined treatment necessitates very specific protocols to provide predictable outcomes. One of the key references for ideal implant placement is the final location of the dental midline or mediolateral position. Failure to refer to this location as a reference will affect the overall treatment outcome and compromise the esthetic result. Other crucial aspects are depth of the implant to create a similar emergence profile of the tooth of reference, mesiodistal position to avoid root perforation and obtain adequate papillary heights, and angulation so that it matches the final angulation of the adjacent teeth.

Vertical bone height through intrusion and torquing

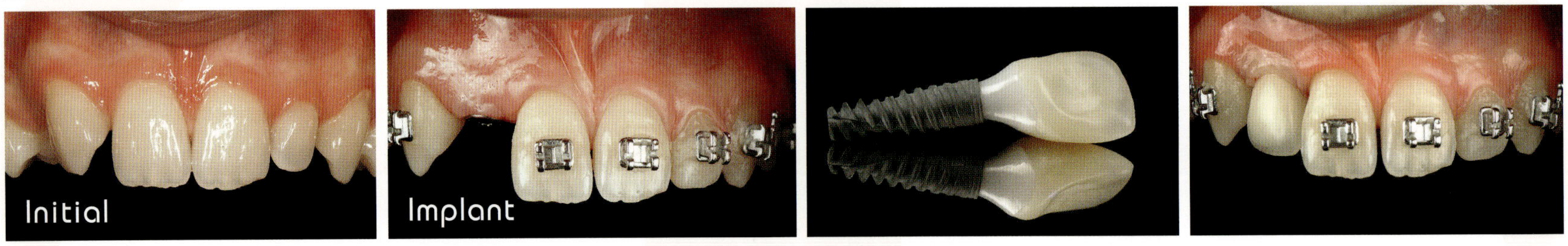

A 29-year-old man presented with agenesis of the maxillary right lateral incisor. Orthodontic treatment was performed to open the space. An implant (NobelActive 3.5 × 13 mm) was placed with a CTG and concave healing abutment. The implant was placed during orthodontic treatment, and the definitive zirconia abutment and provisional restoration were subsequently inserted to determine the final tooth position.

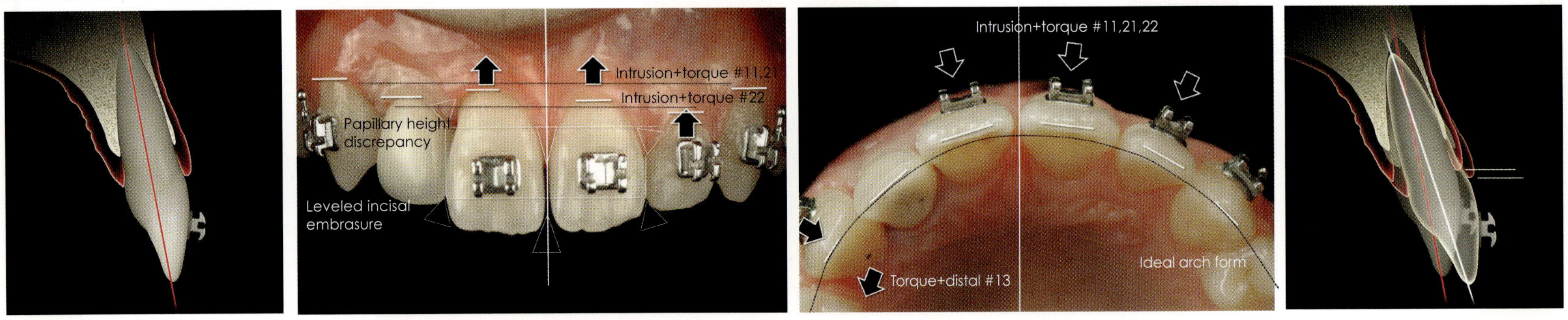

The difference in papillary height between the mesial aspects of the lateral incisors as well as the buccal soft tissue recession around the implant compared with the contralateral lateral incisor are apparent. This is a typical "counteracting movement" in which a space is created for implant placement; teeth are sometimes extruded and buccally displaced while opening the space. The depth and angulation of the implant are critical and must be determined in context with the other anterior teeth. In this situation, the implant in the area of the right lateral incisor was restored more palatally to provide the orthodontist with sufficient anchorage for intrusion and torque to the root as well as the prerequisites to create an ideal arch form.

Orthodontist:
Dr Domingo Martín

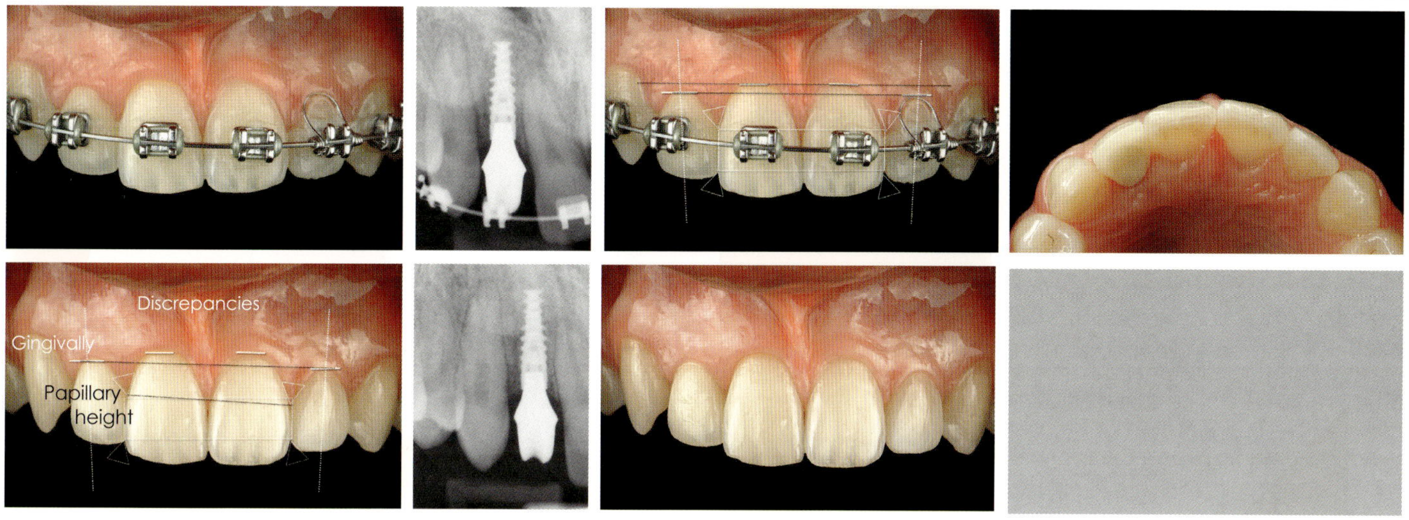

Bone and tissue leveling was accomplished with an interdisciplinary team approach (surgeon, orthodontist, restorative dentist). Arch form and tooth axes were idealized with papillary heights, and the soft tissue morphology was symmetric and even throughout the anterior teeth.

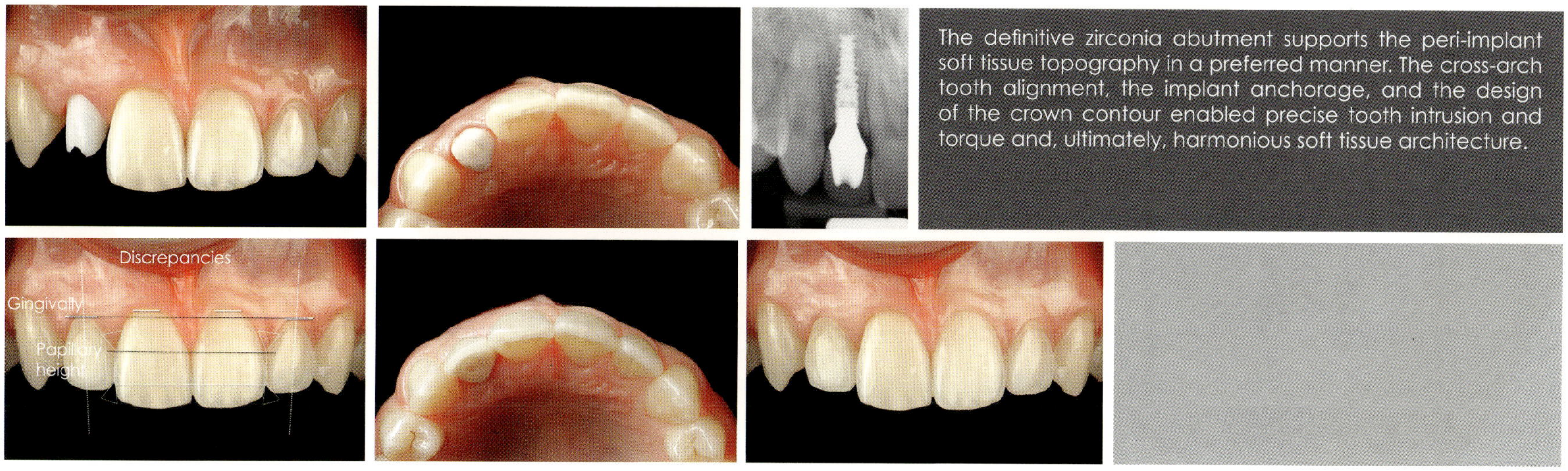

The definitive zirconia abutment supports the peri-implant soft tissue topography in a preferred manner. The cross-arch tooth alignment, the implant anchorage, and the design of the crown contour enabled precise tooth intrusion and torque and, ultimately, harmonious soft tissue architecture.

Combination movements

Orthodontist:
Dr Domingo Martín

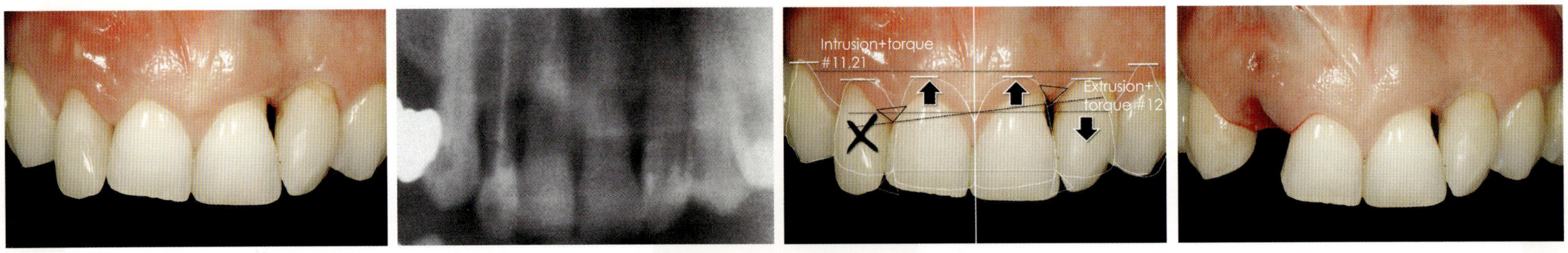

A 49-year-old woman presented with a fractured maxillary right lateral incisor and a three-wall periodontal defect on the distal of the maxillary left central incisor and mesial of the maxillary left lateral incisor but without increased tooth mobility. Combination orthodontic tooth movements were planned to be carried out during the healing period after extraction of the fractured tooth. First, extrusion of the left lateral incisor was planned to level the interproximal defect between the left central and lateral incisors. Slight extrusion of the left central incisor was also part of the treatment plan. The implant would then be placed, followed by final intrusion of the central and lateral incisors and re-creation of the interproximal bone between the implant and the tooth.

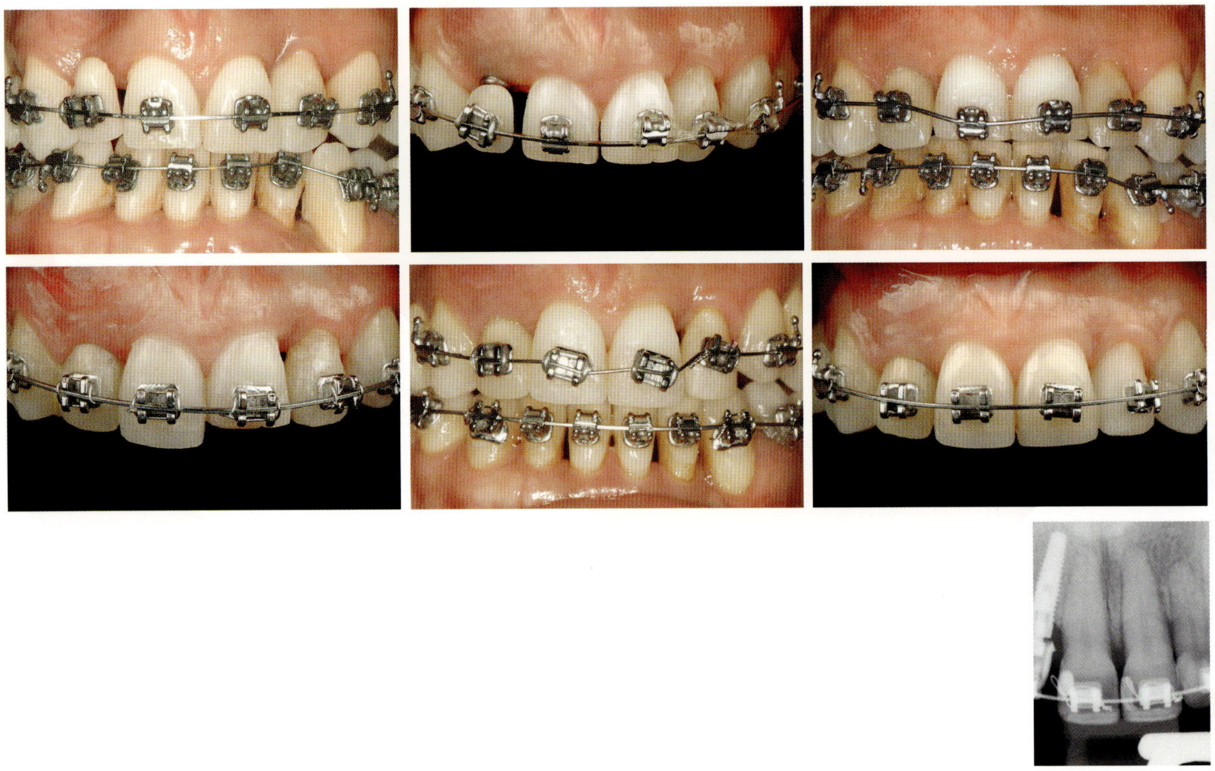

The orthodontic treatment during the healing phase of the extracted right lateral incisor was staged differently. Extrusion of the left lateral incisor reduced the black space considerably, and an implant was placed based on the papillary height achieved between the left central and lateral incisors. Four months later, this implant was restored with a provisional restoration to be used as anchorage for slow intrusion of both central incisors. Subsequently, composite restorations were placed to communicate the final tooth proportions to the orthodontist and finalize tooth positions. A few combination movements of intrusion-extrusion-torque were necessary to level interproximal tissue height in reference to the adjacent papilla.

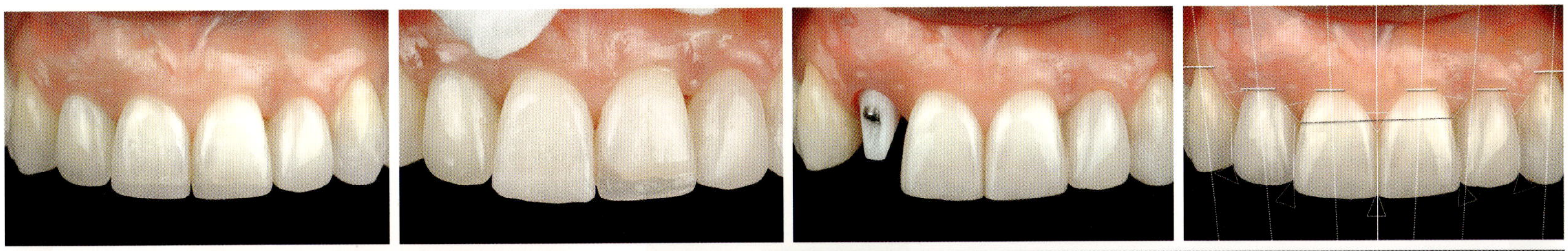

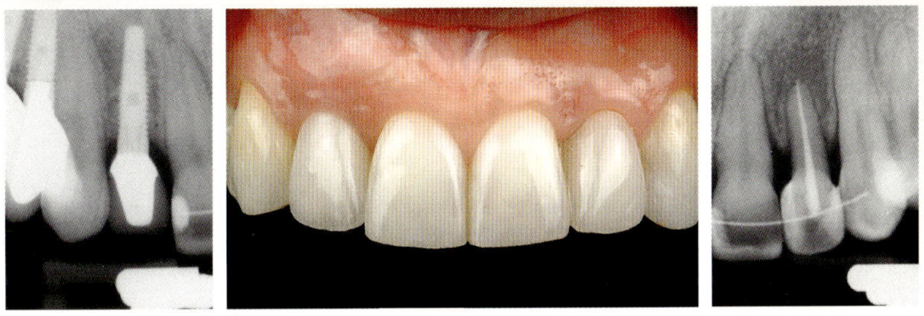

After final orthodontic treatment, the teeth were splinted for 8 months before the definitive restorations were placed. Meanwhile, new provisional composite restorations were placed on the incisal edges of the central incisors to better blend with the rest of the dentition. A composite veneer was fabricated to verify the idealized tooth proportion and morphology of the left lateral incisor. A definitive zirconia abutment and alumina crown restoration were then cemented. Symmetric and level soft tissue contours were achieved with this individually staged combination treatment approach.

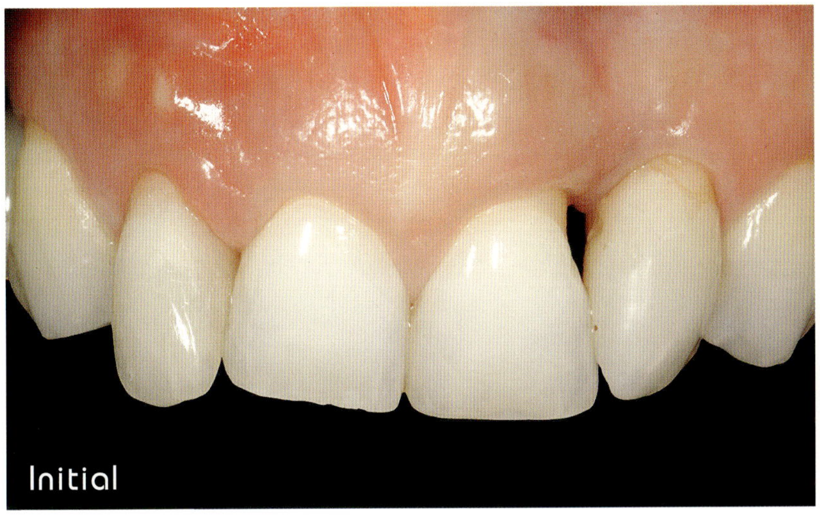

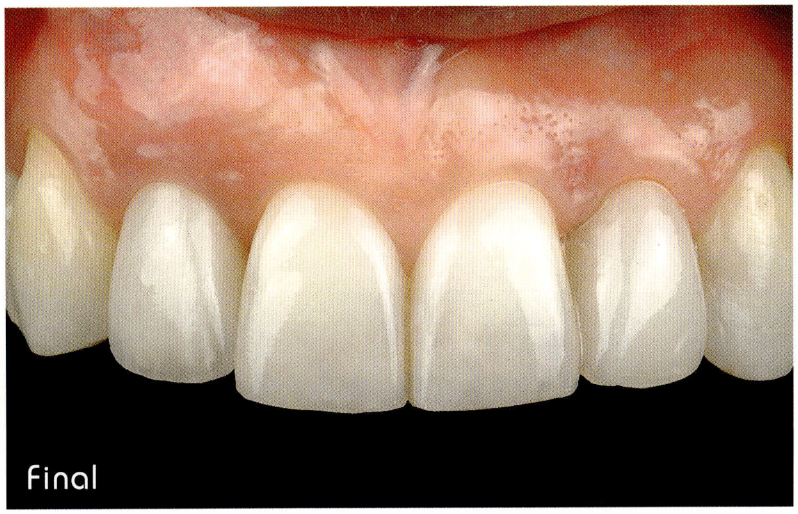

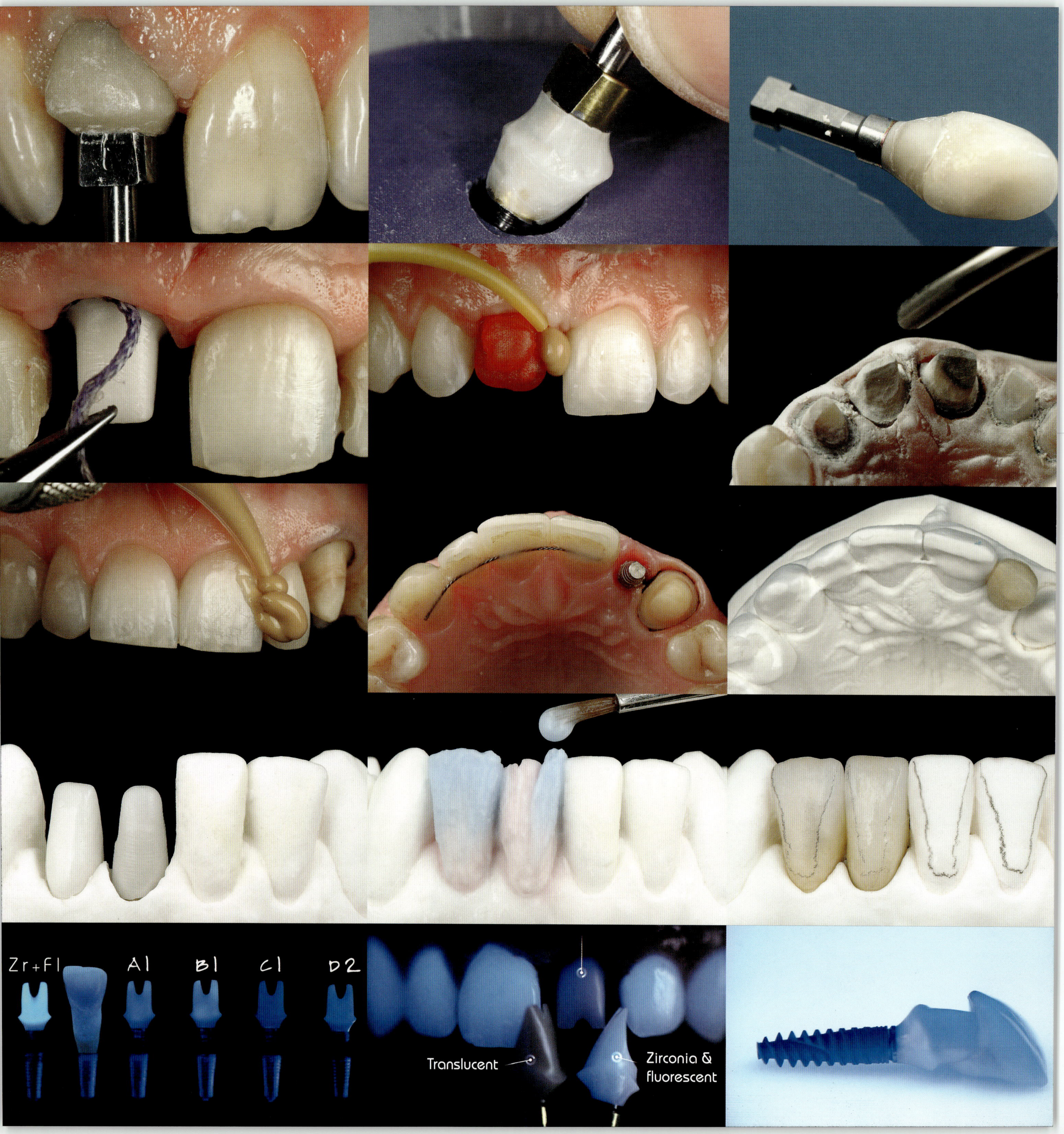
Zr+F1
A1
B1
C1
D2
Translucent
Zirconia &
fluorescent

Laboratory Communication for Definitive Restoration

- Impressions
  - Customized impression coping
  - Impression coping fabrication
  - Provisional pickup impression
- Without Removing the Abutment
  - Retraction cord
  - Impression coping
  - Digital scanner/intraoral scanning
- 3D Emergence Profile and Tooth Contour
- Color and Coping Selection
  - → Research: Definitive crown material
  - Zirconia coping
  - Alumina coping
- Abutment Material Selection
  - → Research: Fluorescence

Chapter 5

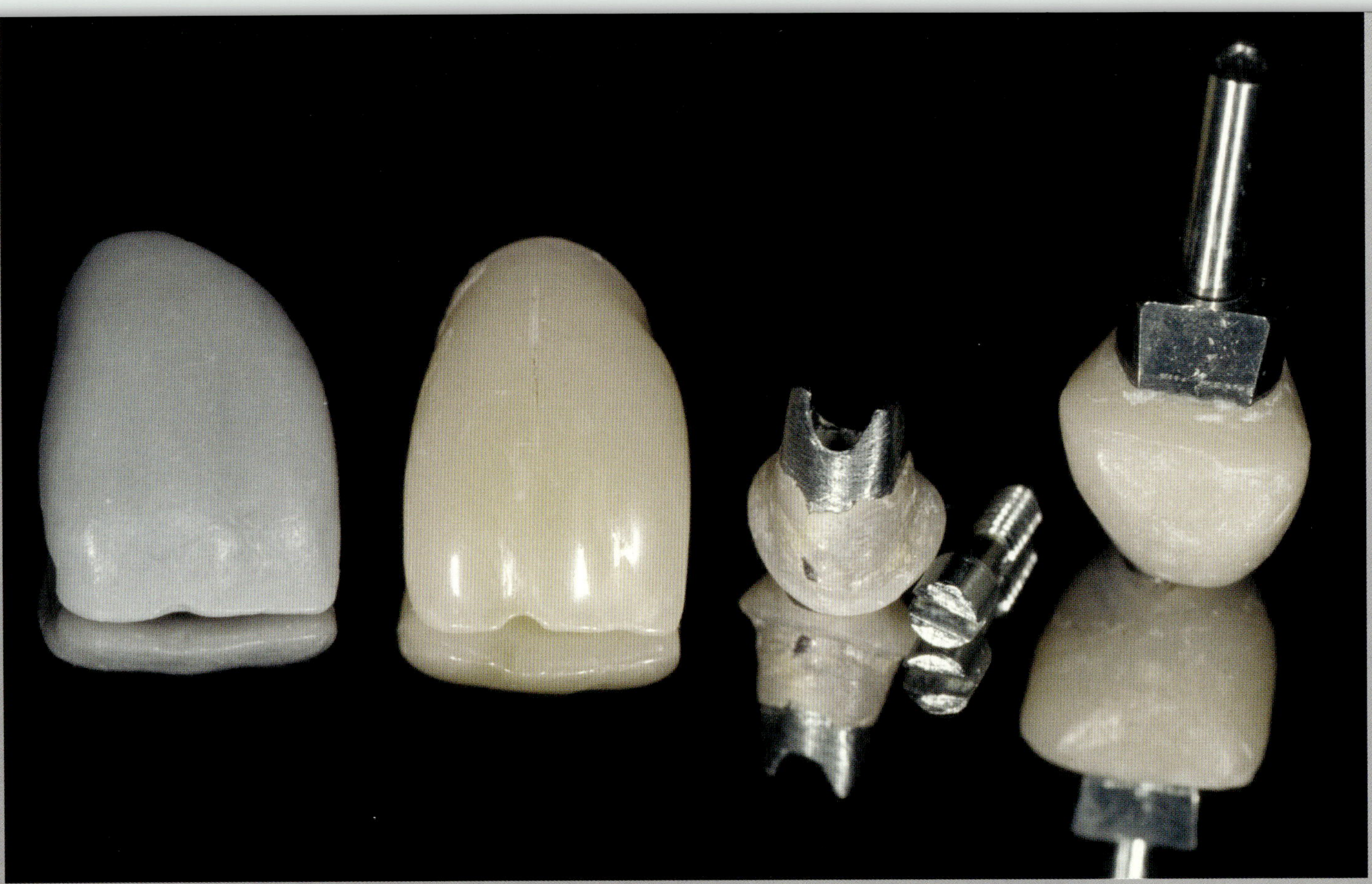

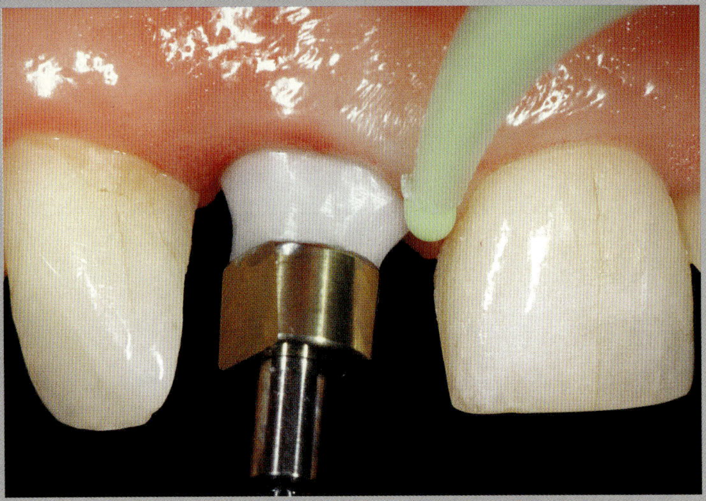

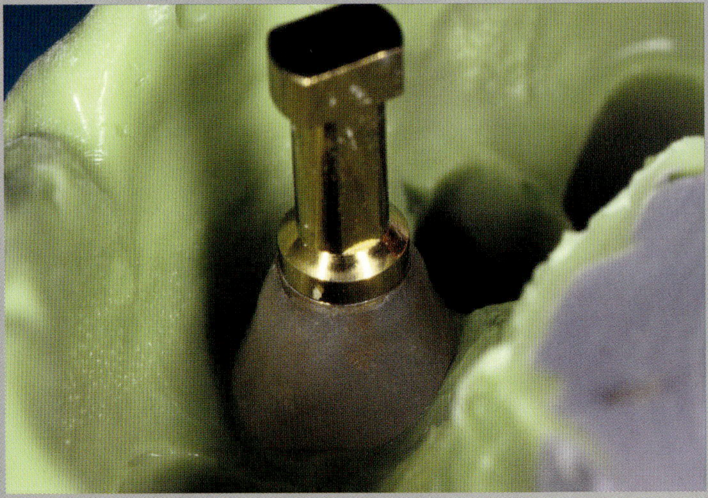

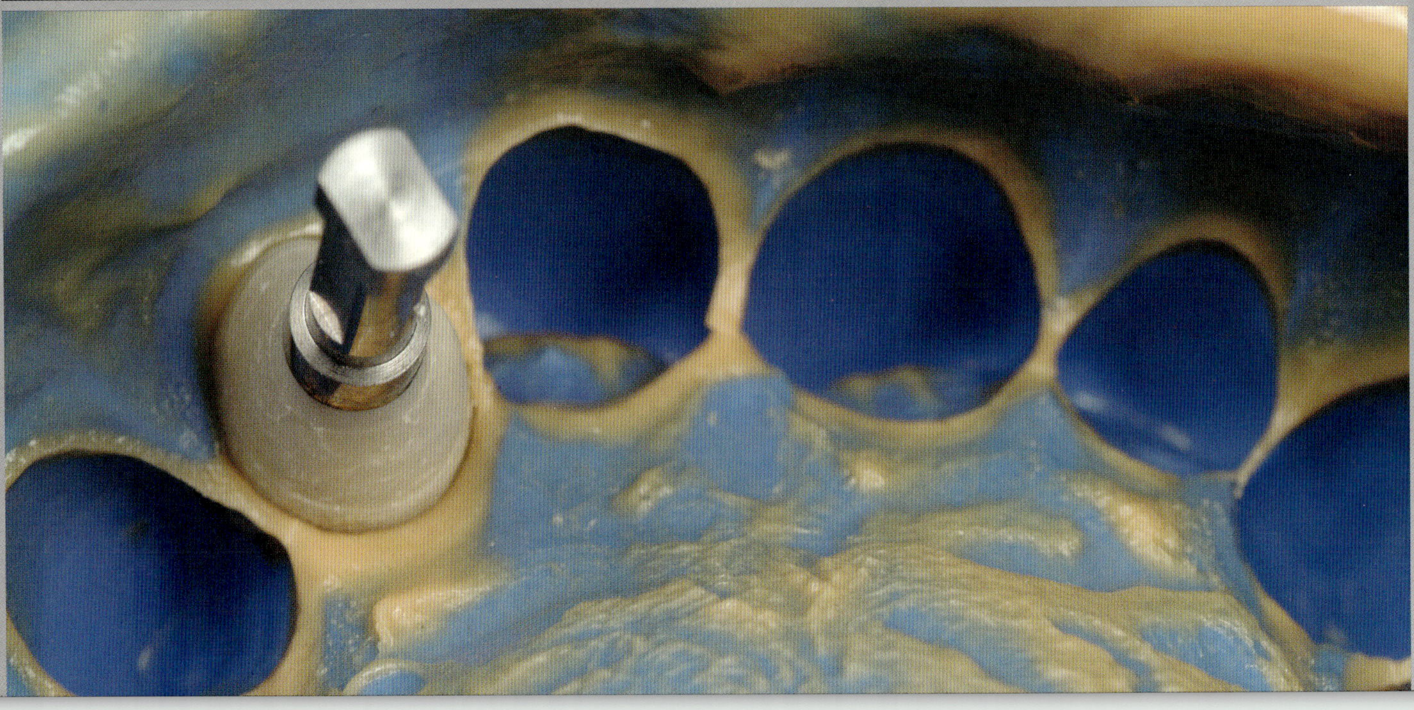

Impressions

Implant-supported provisional restorations play a key role in achieving the esthetic and functional goals of the definitive restorations. There are many techniques available to maximize not only the prosthetic result but also the appearance of the soft tissues around dental implants through alteration of the provisional restoration. The ideal emergence profile and the morphology of the peri-implant soft tissues should be determined during the pre-prosthetic laboratory phase and then modified chairside. A proper impression technique is key for an accurate transfer of the peri-implant soft tissue contour from the intraoral situation to the definitive cast. This section describes three techniques for transferring the peri-implant soft tissues in different clinical scenarios that are common in daily practice:

1. Transfer of the original emergence profile established with a provisional restoration to the definitive restoration through a customized impression coping
2. Transfer of a modified emergence profile established through subsequent modification of a provisional restoration to the definitive restoration through a customized impression coping
3. Transfer of the final emergence profile to the definitive restoration through a provisional polyvinyl siloxane (PVS) pickup impression

Customized impression coping

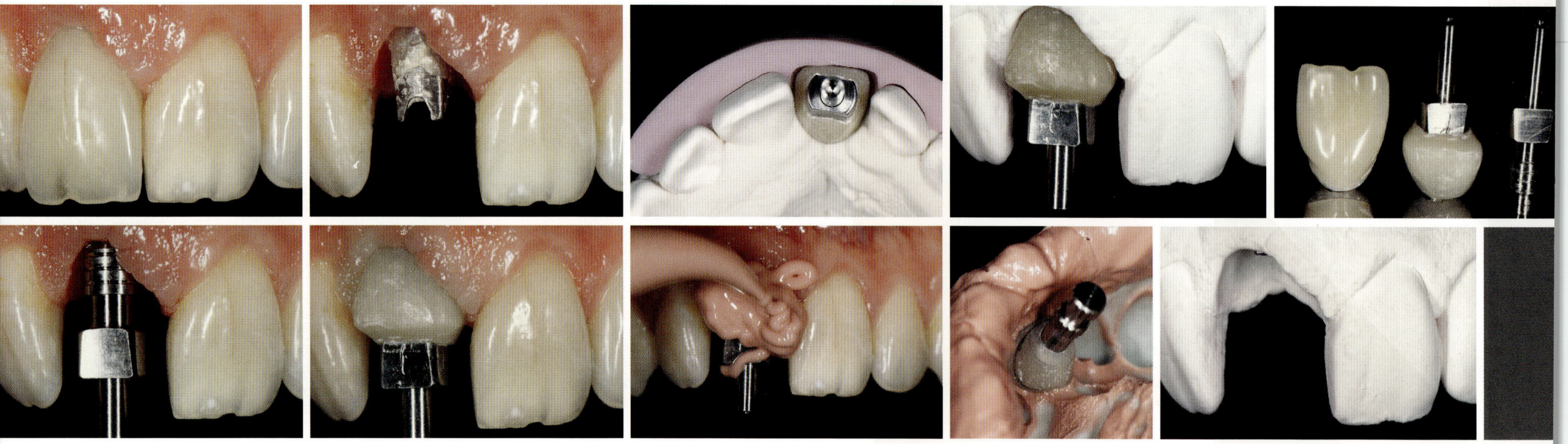

Provisional restoration 3 months after insertion with a provisional abutment made from a 3.25-mm implant carrier and modified with composite resin at the gingival third. The customized impression coping was fabricated on the initial master cast with composite resin, filling the space between the machined impression coping and the carved emergence profile.

A PVS impression was made while the custom impression coping supported the surrounding tissues. Comparison of the initial cast on which the provisional restoration and the impression coping were fabricated and the definitive cast reveals favorable soft tissue changes, particularly on the distal aspect.

A UCLA-type abutment was veneered with feldspathic ceramic.

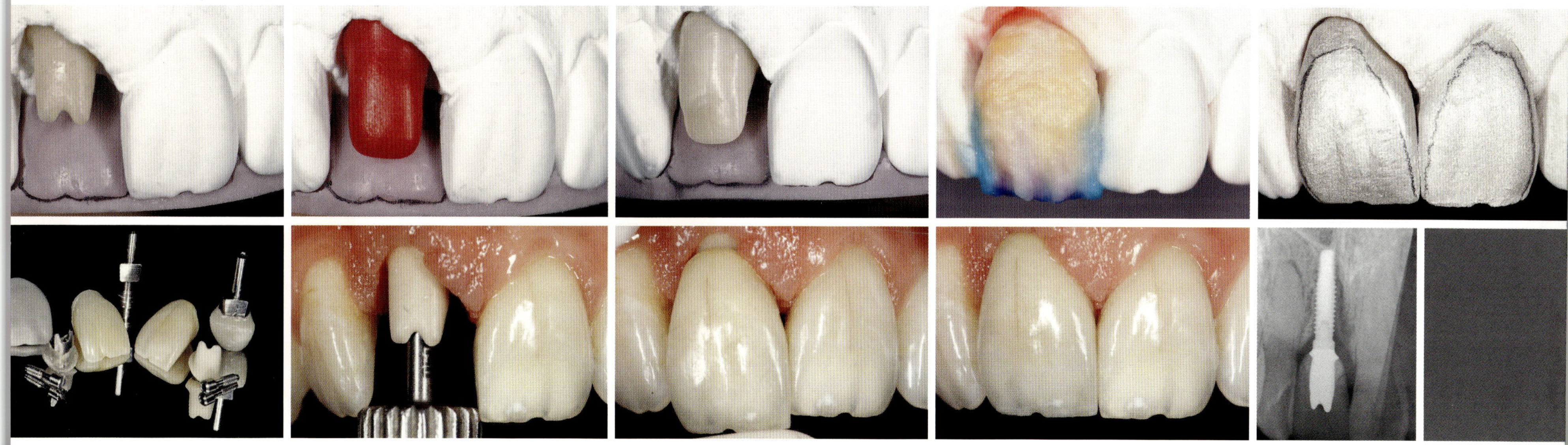

A silicone matrix of the full-contour wax-up served as a reference during waxing of the coping to ensure the desired dimensions and adequate porcelain support. An alumina coping was fabricated with a double-scan of the abutment and the waxed-up coping. The feldspathic veneering ceramic was applied subsequently.

The definitive all-ceramic crown and abutment duplicate the emergence profile established with the provisional restoration. The postoperative situation after 1 year is shown with its corresponding periapical radiograph.

Impression coping fabrication

The maxillary left central incisor had been replaced with a removable partial denture. A 3-mm healing abutment and a CTG were inserted simultaneously at the time of implant placement to increase the soft tissue height and labial bulk. At stage-two surgery, a 5-mm healing abutment was placed.

A diagnostic wax-up and silicone matrices served as references for fabrication of the provisional abutment and crown. The cervical third was designed to create an emergence angle from the implant head to the gingival margin and carved in the solid stone cast. A provisional abutment was fabricated with an implant carrier and composite resin. The abutment was prepared with the silicone matrix as a reference. The preparation finish line was located 1 mm supragingivally on the palatal aspect. The provisional crown was cemented to the provisional abutment with temporary cement.

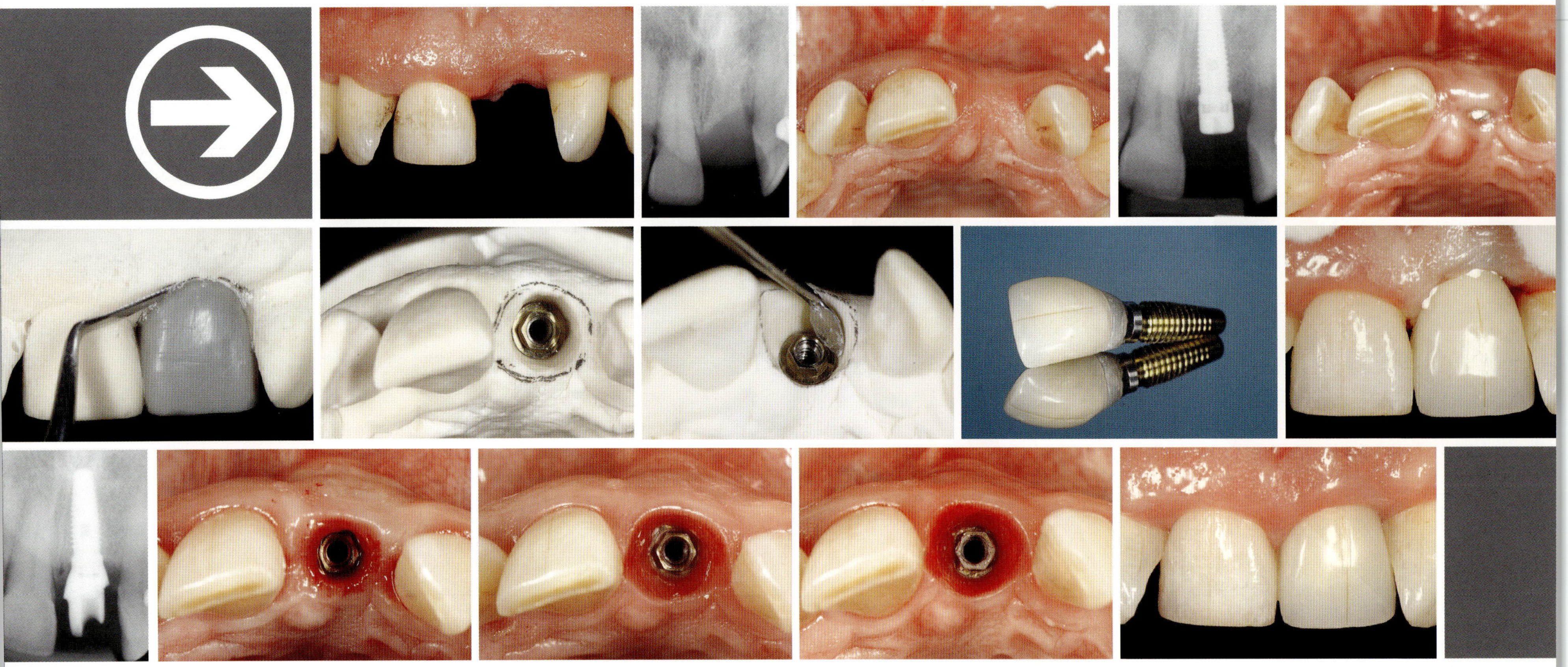

Over a period of 1 month, acrylic resin was added to the cervical aspect of the provisional restoration every 10 days to modify the emergence profile, to close open spaces (black triangles), and to stimulate interproximal tissue growth. The intraoral situation 3 months after placement of the provisional crown reveals improved conditions.

The provisional abutment-crown complex was connected to an implant analog and embedded in impression material (polyether in a plastic cup) to duplicate the cervical aspect of the restoration. Close-up view of the trimmed polyether mold depicts the cervical contour of the provisional restoration emergence profile.

A standard impression coping was screwed to the implant analog fixed in the impression material. Flowable composite resin was injected into the space between the coping and the impression material. After light curing, the customized impression coping was used to accurately transfer the emergence profile topography of

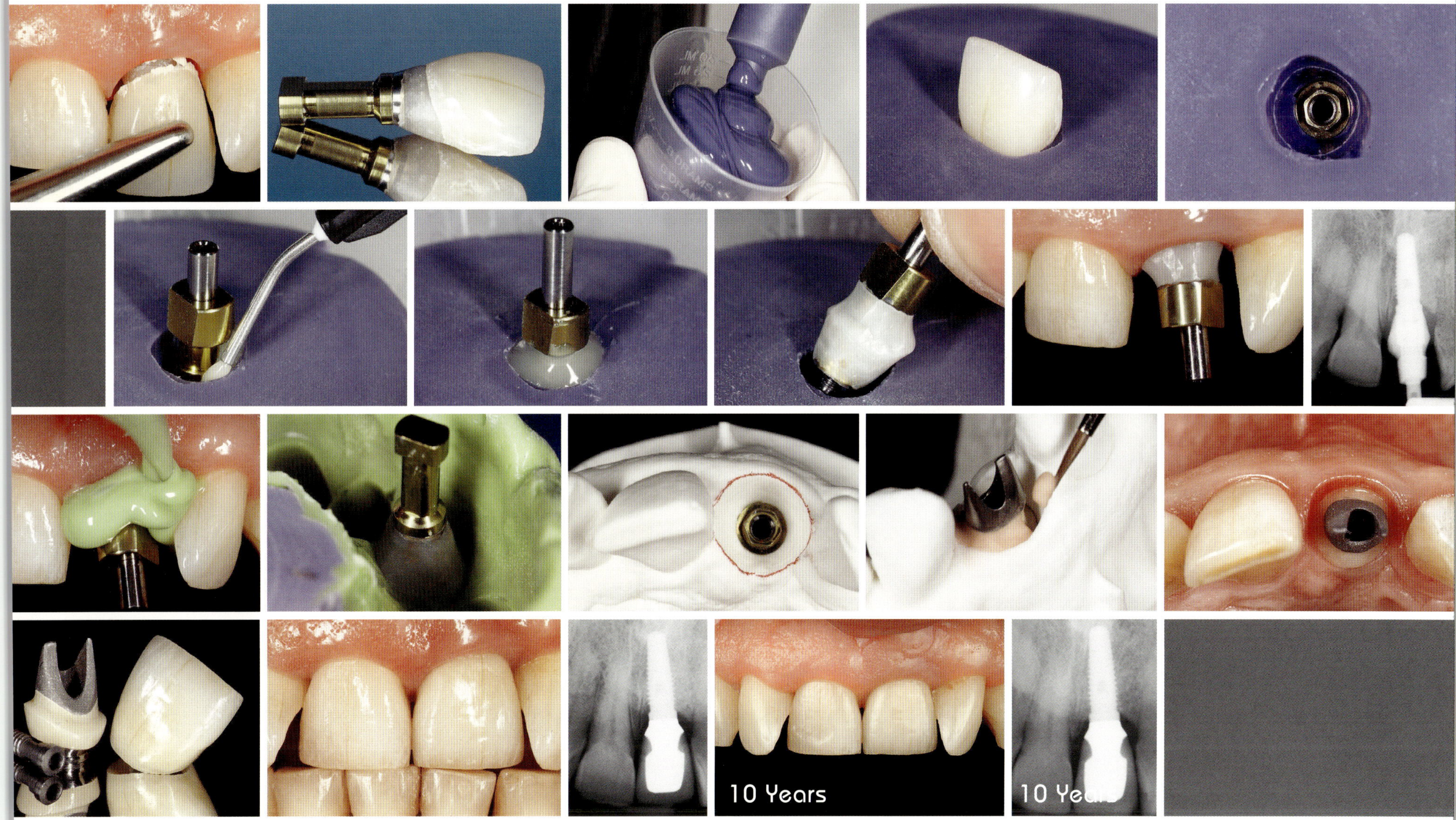

the provisional crown. It is important to provide sufficient interproximal height to support the interproximal tissue. Seating of the customized impression coping was verified with a radiograph.

The final impression was made with a customized impression coping and low-viscosity impression material around the coping for maximum detail and to transfer the peri-implant tissue morphology to the definitive cast. A UCLA-type abutment was fabricated with the lost-wax technique and cast with high-noble alloy. After finishing and polishing of the metal, porcelain shoulders were applied between the abutment and the transferred cervical contour to prevent discolorations by the underlying metal.

An alumina crown was fabricated with the exact emergence profile established during the provisional phase. Situation of the implant restoration with its corresponding radiograph after 10 years is shown.

Provisional pickup impression

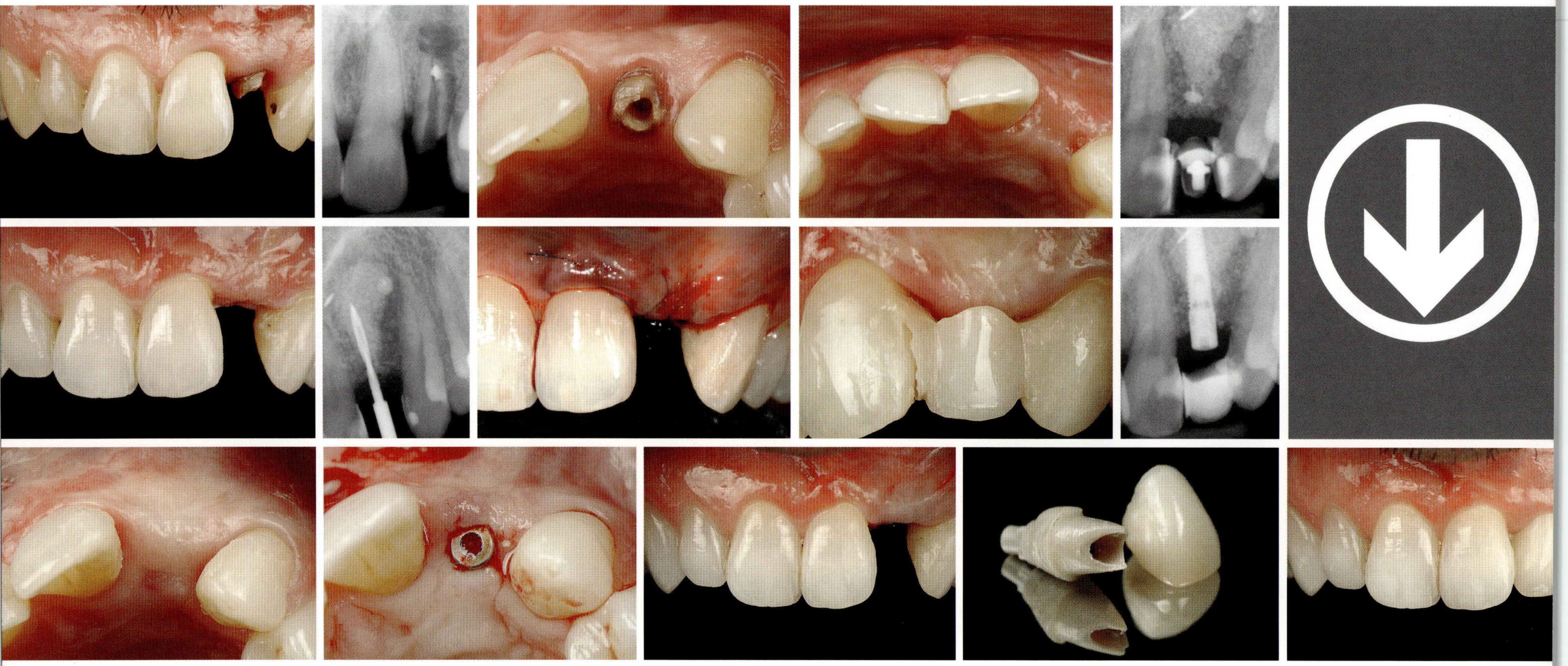

A maxillary left lateral incisor had been restored with a severely compromised porcelain-fused-to-metal (PFM) crown in a 46-year-old man. The clinical and radiologic examination suggested extraction of the tooth due to the root fracture, recurrent caries, and extensive hard tissue loss beyond the buccal crestal bone. Because of the severe loss of buccal bone, a socket grafting technique was performed with Bio-Oss (Geistlich) and membranes prior to implant placement.

Eight months later, a NobelReplace 3.5 × 13–mm implant was inserted with a CTG and 5-mm healing abutment. Six months after the surgery, a PVS impression was made to fabricate the provisional crown and abutment restorations. The provisional crown was relined on the provisional abutment for optimal fit and cemented with temporary cement.

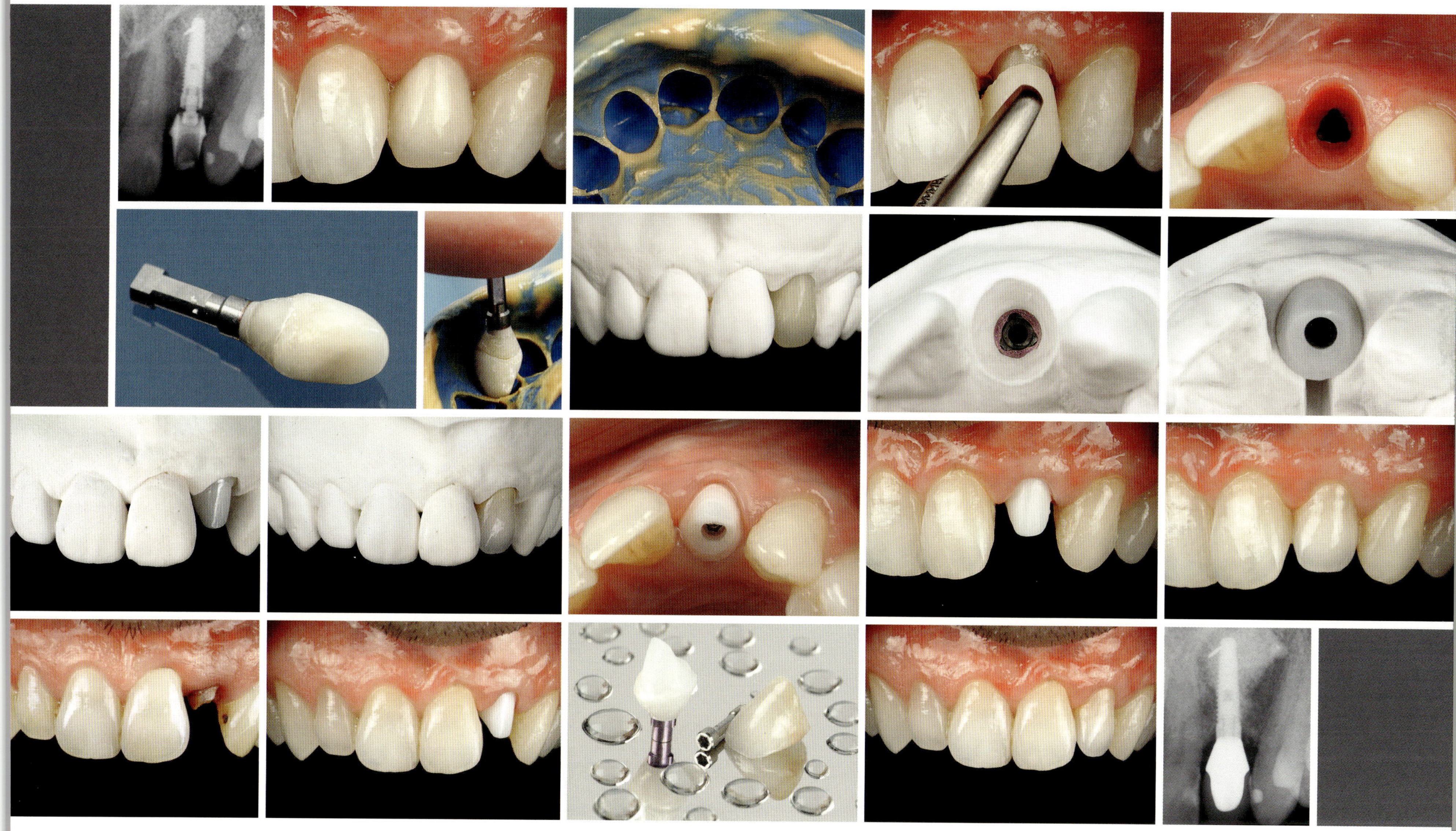

The clinical situation and soft tissue topography were examined every 10 days. Periapical radiographs were taken to verify implant integration. Once the ideal soft tissue topography was achieved, a final impression was made with the provisional restoration as a custom impression coping. A single-impression double-mix technique was applied with low-viscosity PVS material injected around the provisional restoration and adjacent teeth and with heavy-body material in the impression tray. After setting, the provisional restoration was removed, and the provisional abutment was unscrewed. The crown was placed on the abutment and connected to an implant analog and then inserted into the final impression. A thin layer of wax was placed around the cervical aspect of the crown to avoid damage of the restoration with the die stone. The final cast was poured, and the provisional restoration was placed in the patient's mouth immediately after setting of the stone. A definitive abutment and an alumina crown were fabricated and inserted.

The postoperative view and periapical radiograph are shown.

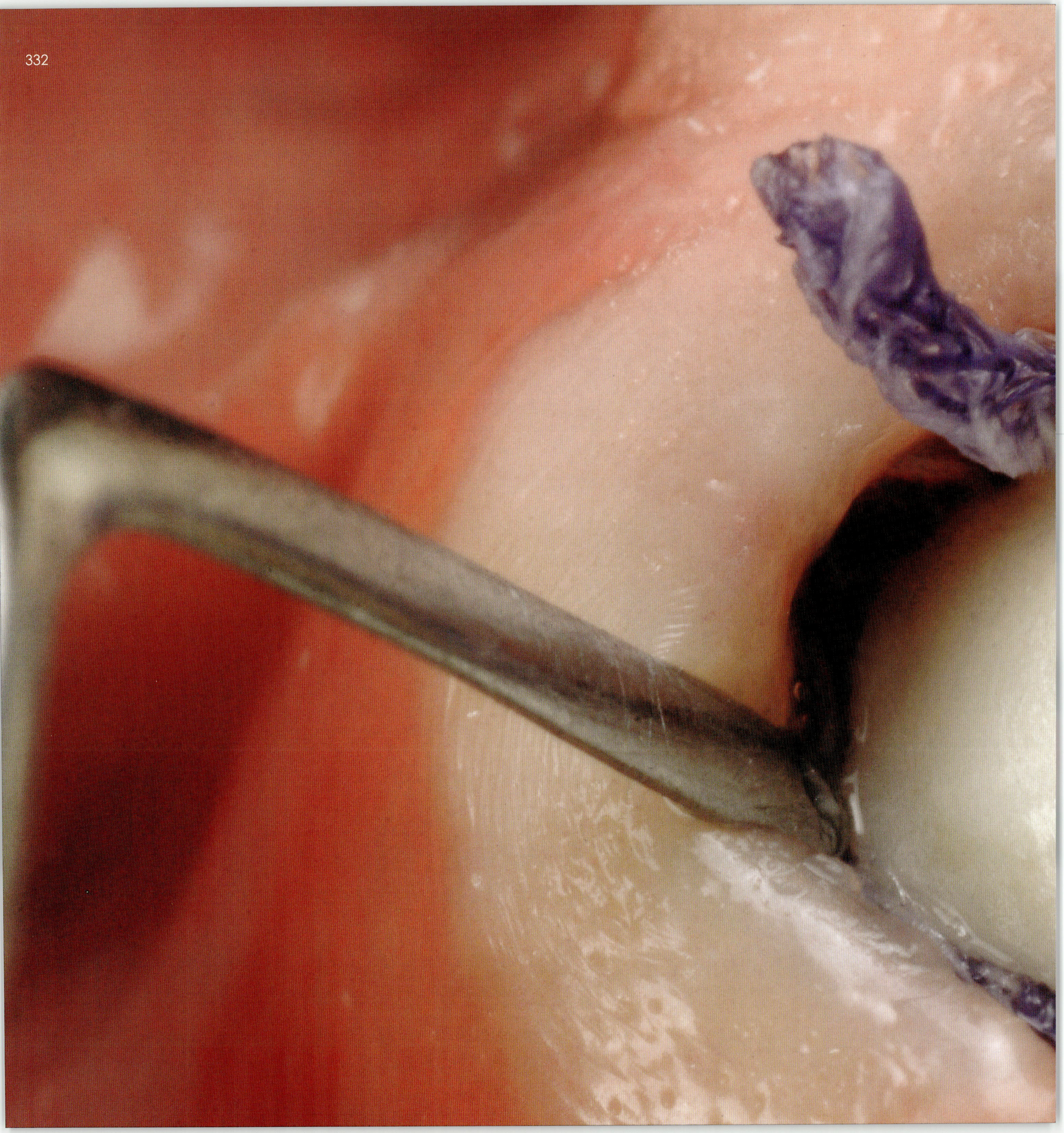

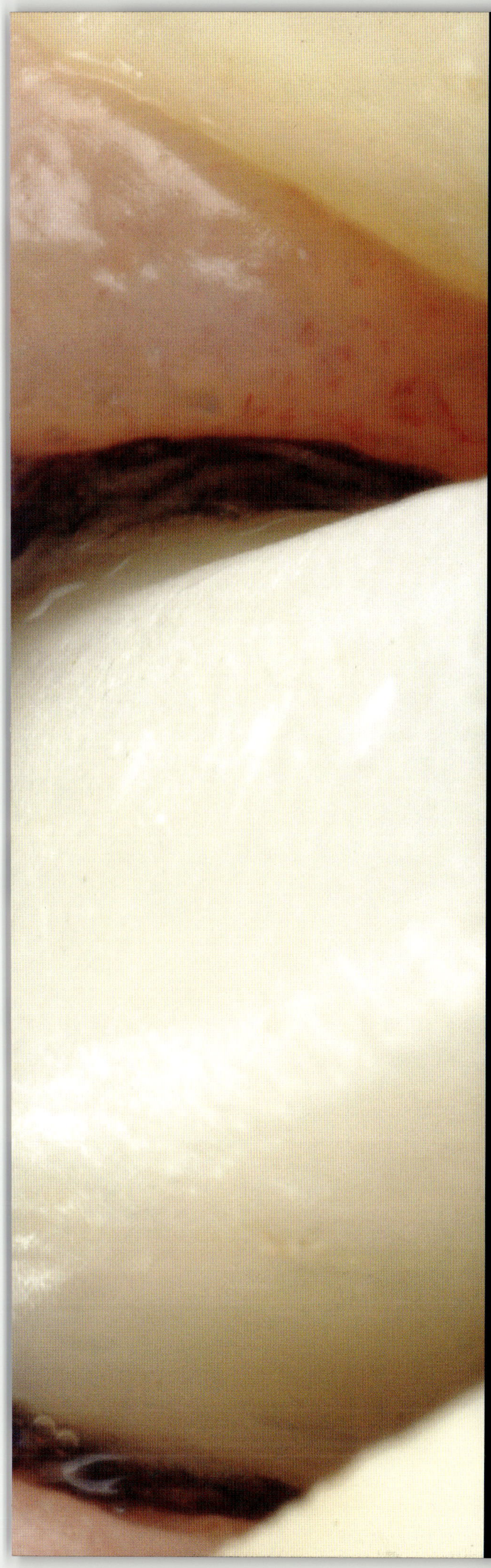

Without Removing the Abutment

The new trend of restoring implants is to:

- Provide soft tissue thickness for long-term stability and success
- Place a definitive zirconia abutment from day 1 of the prosthetic phase
- Avoid dis- and reconnection of the prosthetic components
- Understand the importance of the shape and contours of the abutment and crown

These new trends in restoring implants require some adjustments by the restorative dentist who has traditionally been educated to use a multistep approach for implant restoration. The idea is to avoid multiple steps as much as possible in order to reduce the trauma to the fragile biologic bone-implant–soft tissue complex. These concepts suggest placement of the definitive zirconia abutment on the first day of the prosthetic phase to provide ideal biologic integration of the abutment material (ie, zirconia). This step represents a challenge for the restorative dentist and laboratory technician because the fabricated abutment may not support the desired emergence profile as anticipated. In this section, three patient scenarios demonstrate the different techniques and criteria to communicate the emergence profile created with the provisional restoration to the laboratory without removing the abutment:

1. **Retraction cord (treated like a tooth)**: One retraction cord is placed to expose the prepared finishing line of the zirconia abutment and to communicate the soft tissue topography created with the provisional crown and abutment. The disadvantage of this technique is that retracted tissue impressions cannot perfectly reflect the outline of the soft tissue scalloping created with the provisional restoration.
2. **Coping impression:** A coping impression is made before placement of the definitive abutment with a PVS impression. Then, through duplication of the abutment, a coping impression with retentive elements is fabricated for use in the final PVS pickup impression. This coping impression technique accurately records the soft tissue topography while placing the duplicate abutment and pouring the stone. A great advantage of this technique is that the tissues remain undisturbed. Acrylic can be added to the impression coping to support the soft tissue in the same way as the provisional crown, thereby communicating the exact soft tissue scalloping created with the provisional restoration.
3. **Intraoral scanning:** Cords are still necessary: double-cord technique for natural teeth and single-cord technique for implant restorations. Depending on the intraoral scanning system, antireflection powder must be sprayed on top of the prepared abutment for the scanner to capture the three-dimensional (3D) preparation morphology. Some disadvantages of intraoral scanning include digital intraoral handling and a steep learning curve for the clinician. Smaller sensors, faster digital impressions, and picture-type recording instead of video will speed up the process. The cord packing also causes a distorted soft tissue topography, which necessitates a PVS pickup impression of the bisque bake try-in to communicate the emergence profile and gingival embrasure design.

Retraction cord

An implant was placed in the area of the maxillary left central incisor in combination with a CTG. The definitive abutment was placed on day 1 of the restorative phase with its corresponding provisional restoration. Conventional gingival retraction (single-cord technique) was used to communicate with the laboratory via PVS impression. In the laboratory, the emergence profile and ideal gingival contour were redesigned for definitive crown fabrication, which was controlled by spectrophotometry before sending it for bisque bake try-in.

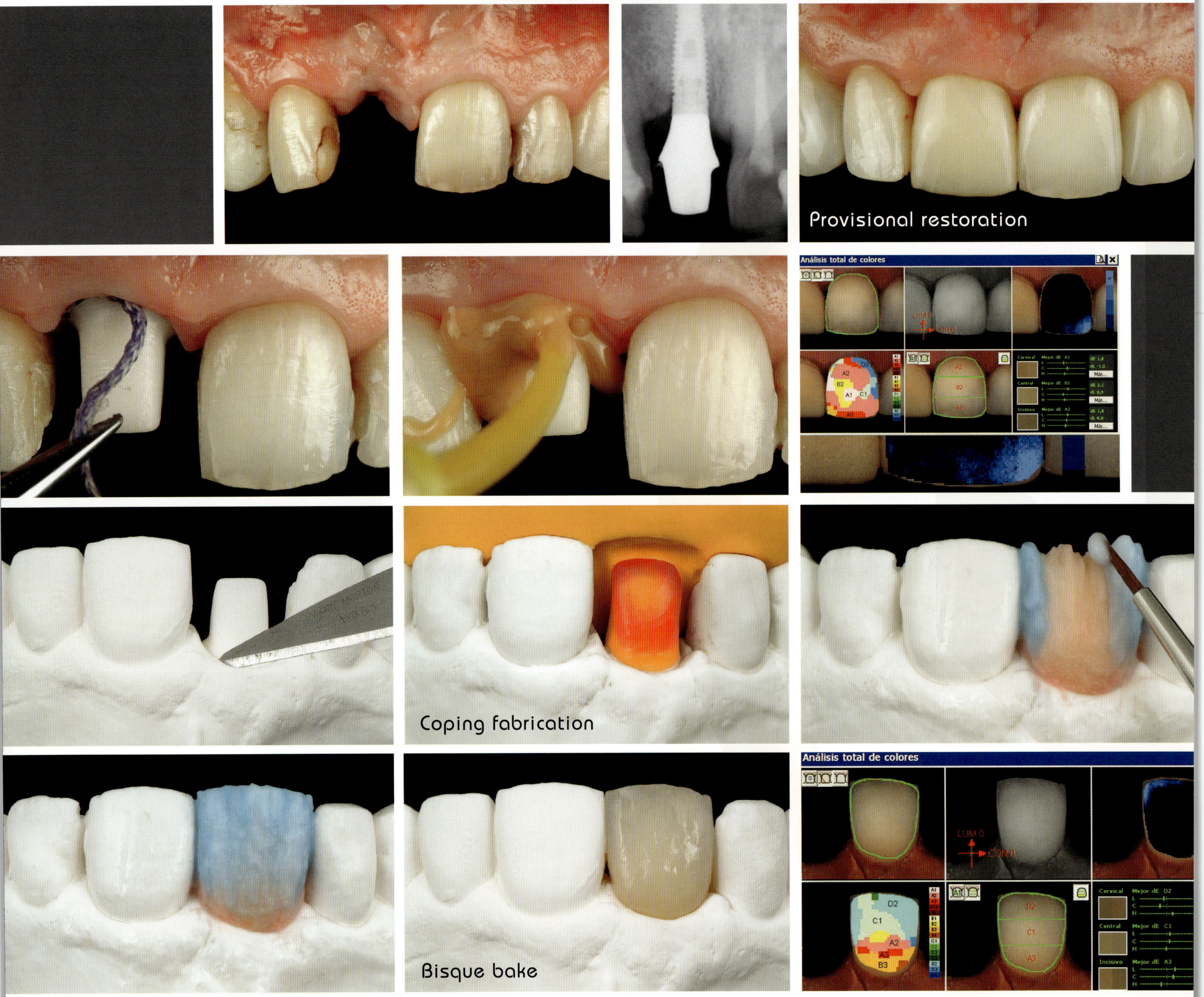

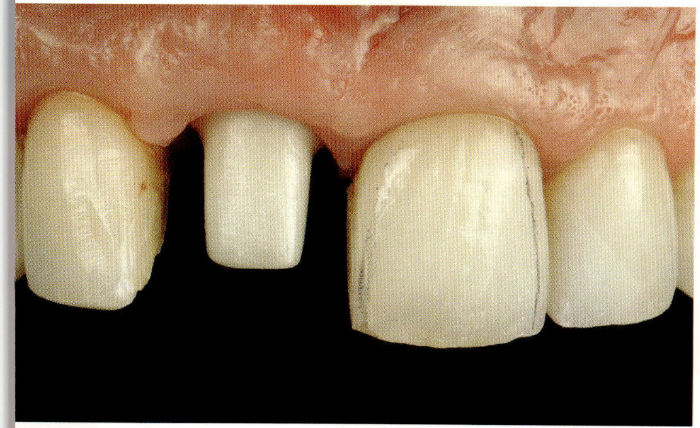

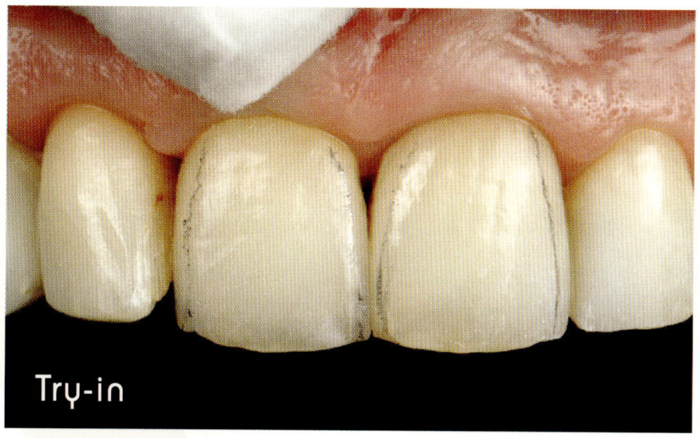

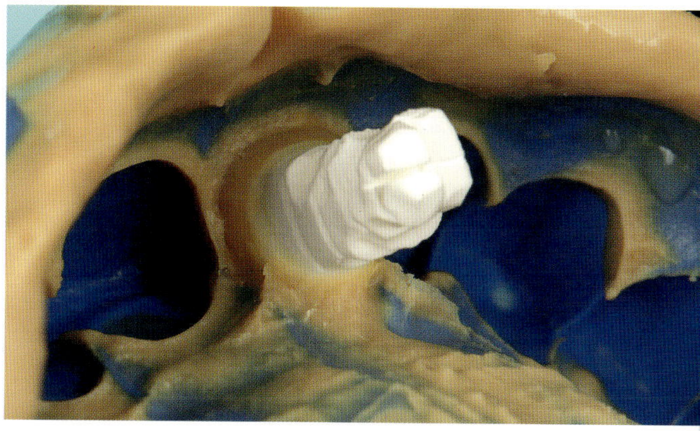

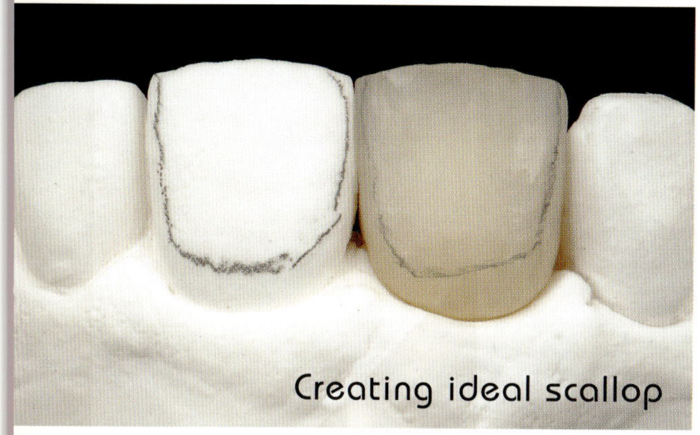

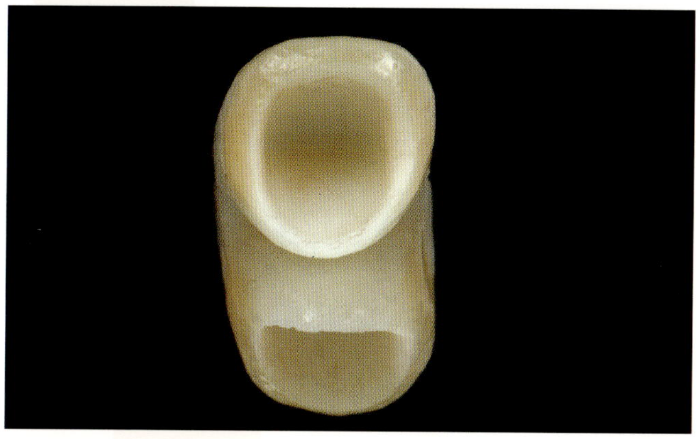

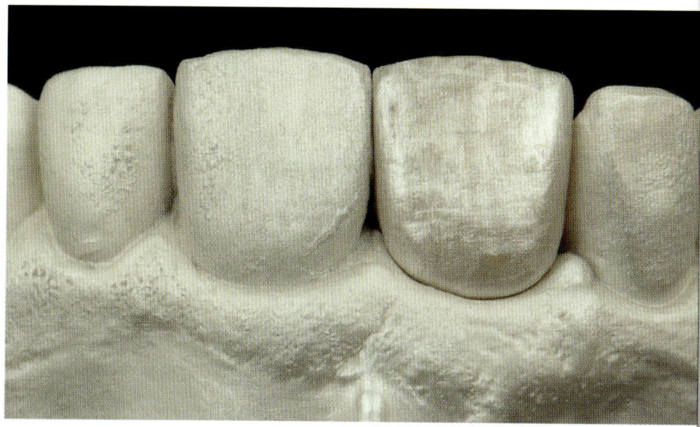

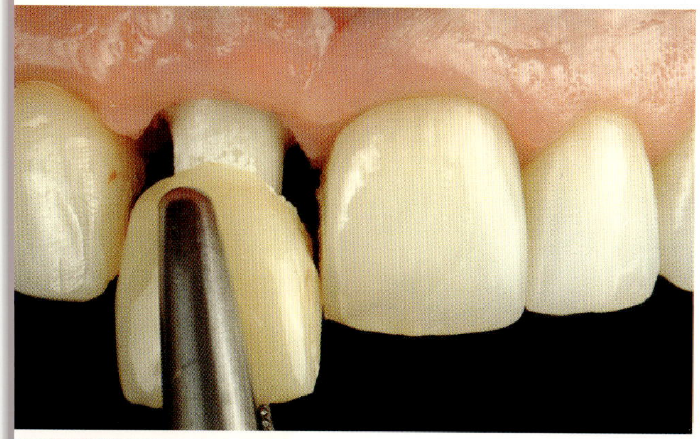

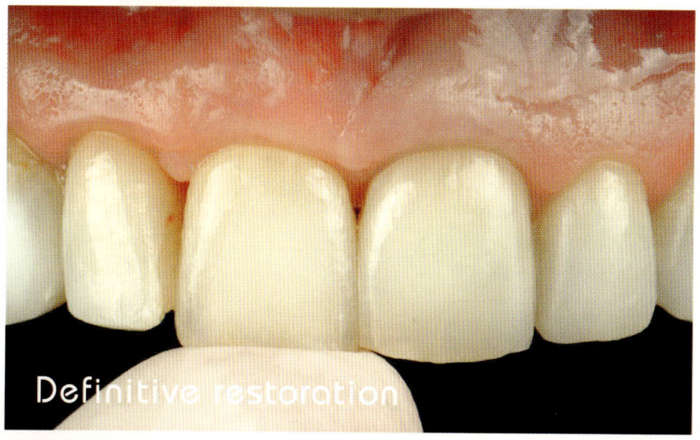

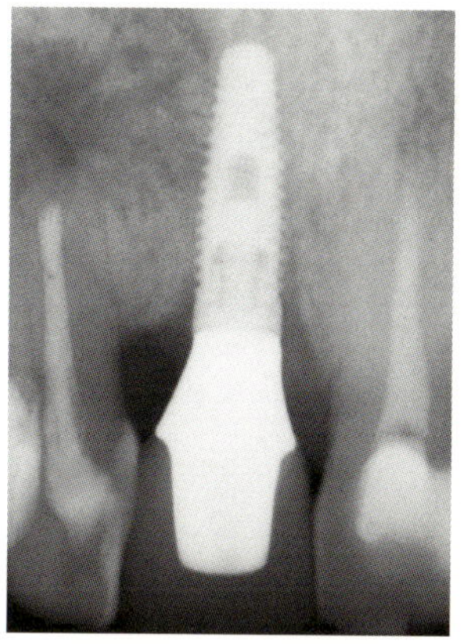

During bisque bake try-in, the need for a redesign of the emergence profile to match the soft tissue contour of the adjacent tooth was verified. A PVS pickup impression was made to transfer the emergence profile. Try-in of the definitive alumina crown and result 4 years after cementation are shown.

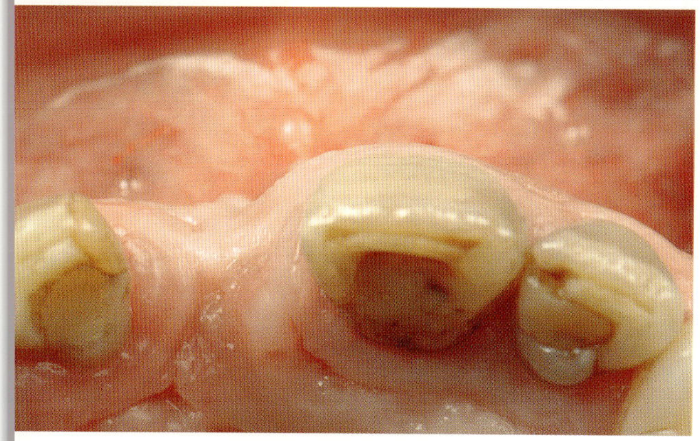

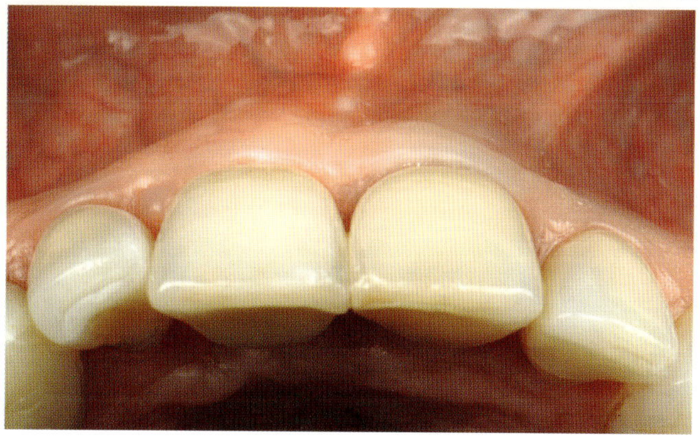

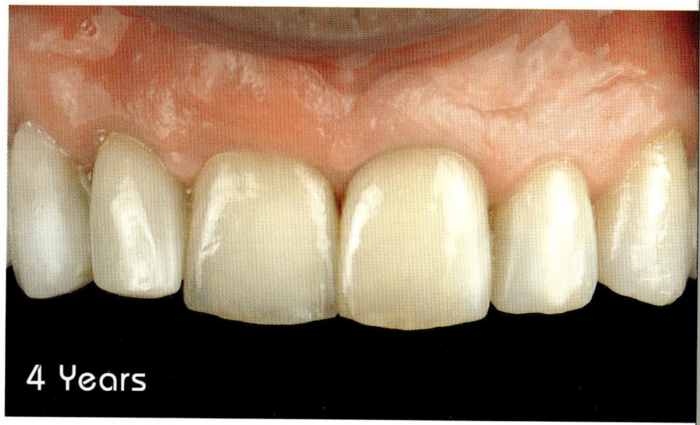

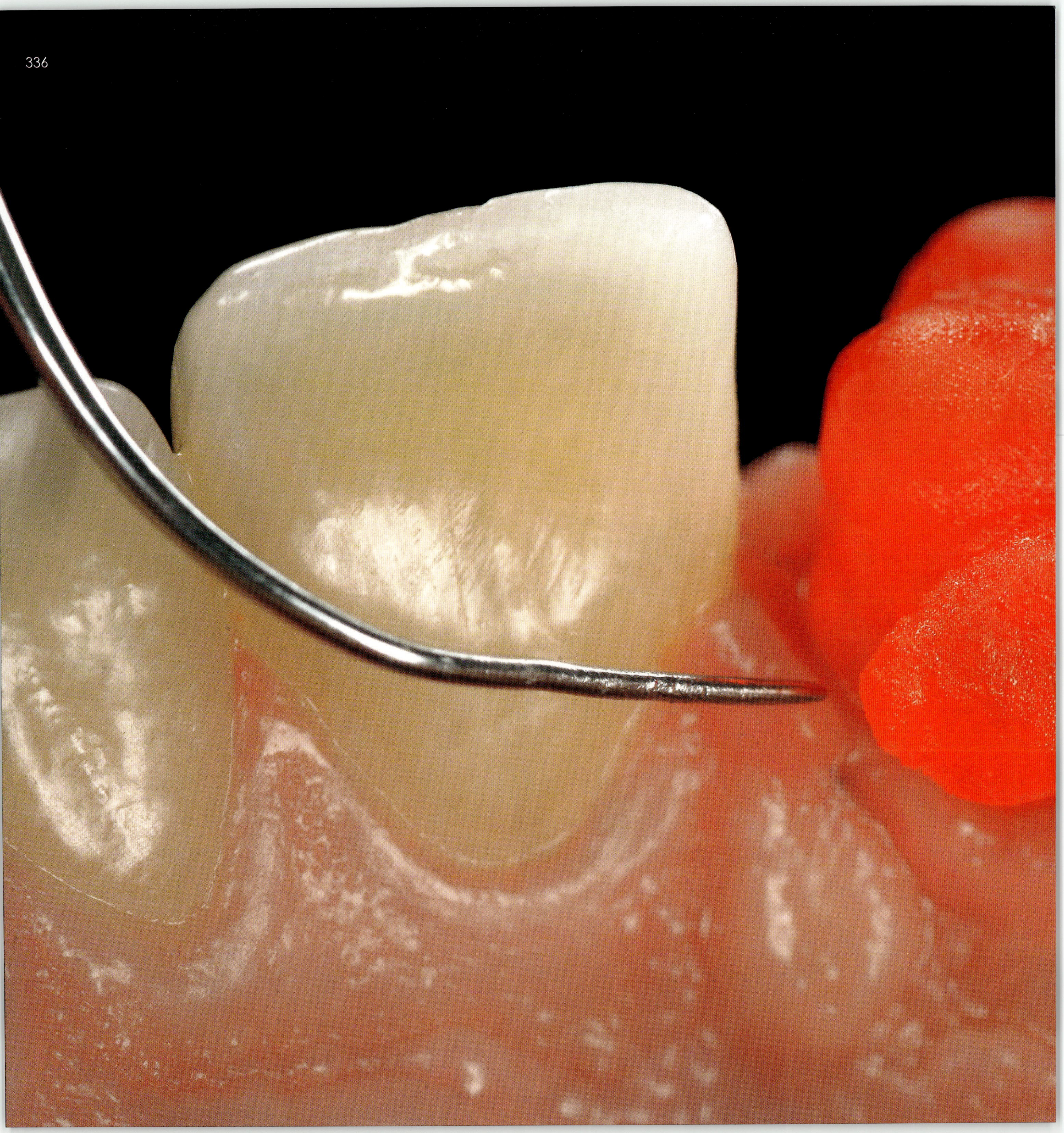

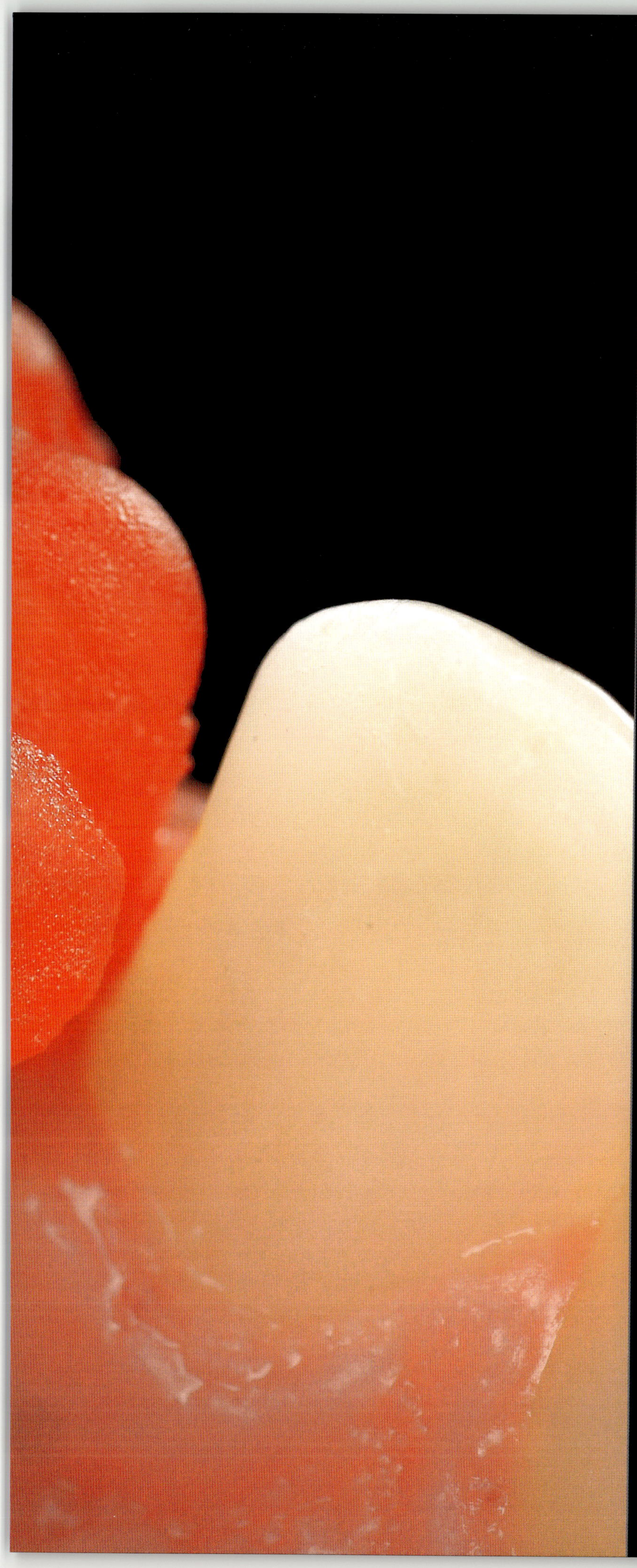

Impression coping

Soft tissue was managed around the implant in the area of the maxillary right lateral incisor. Through the process of modification of the provisional crown and zirconia abutment margin, a PVS impression was made to avoid subsequent disconnection of the abutment. An abutment replica and coping impression were fabricated. Buccal and palatal retentive elements in the coping enable precise capturing of the undisturbed soft tissue topography with a pickup impression.

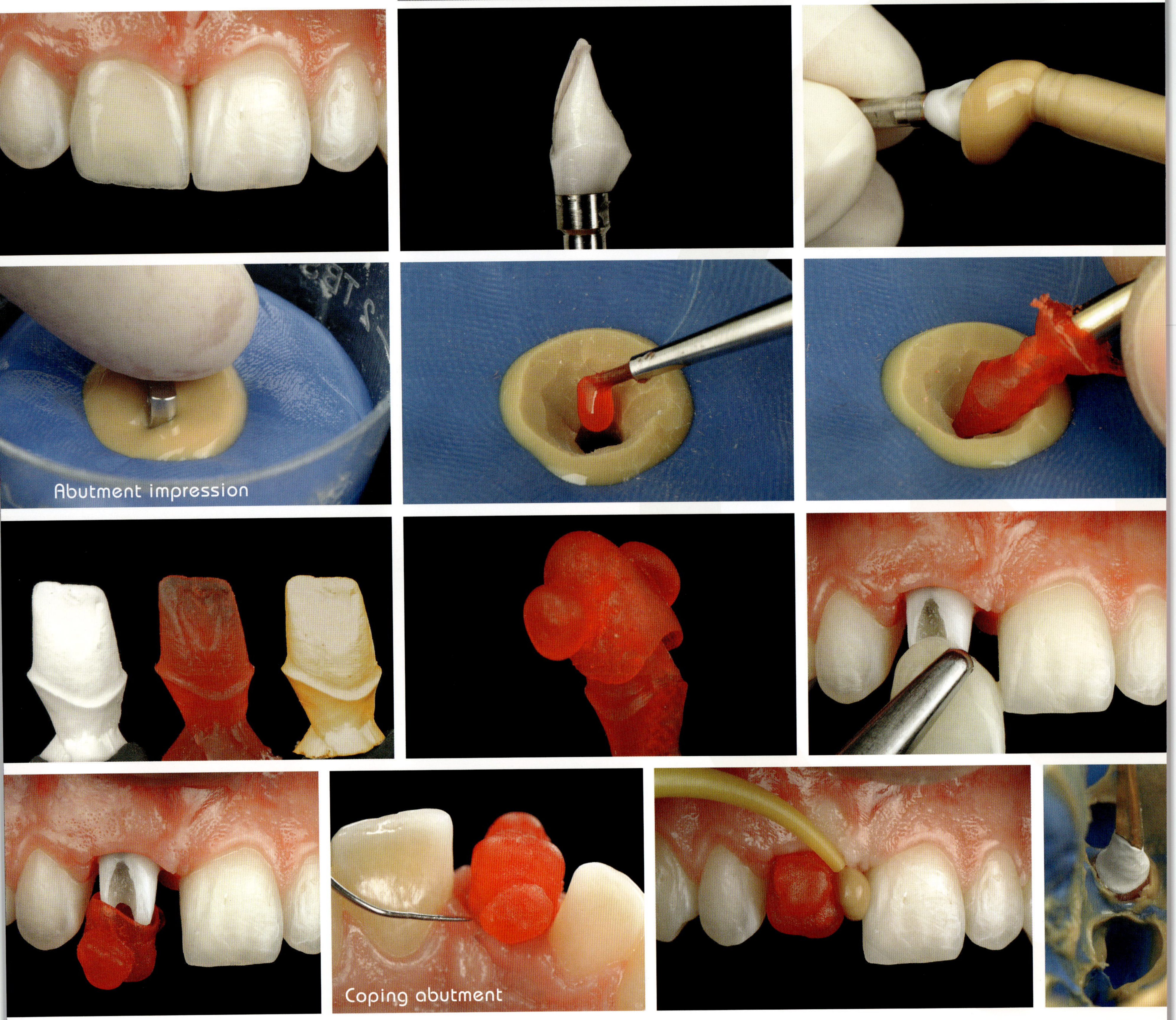

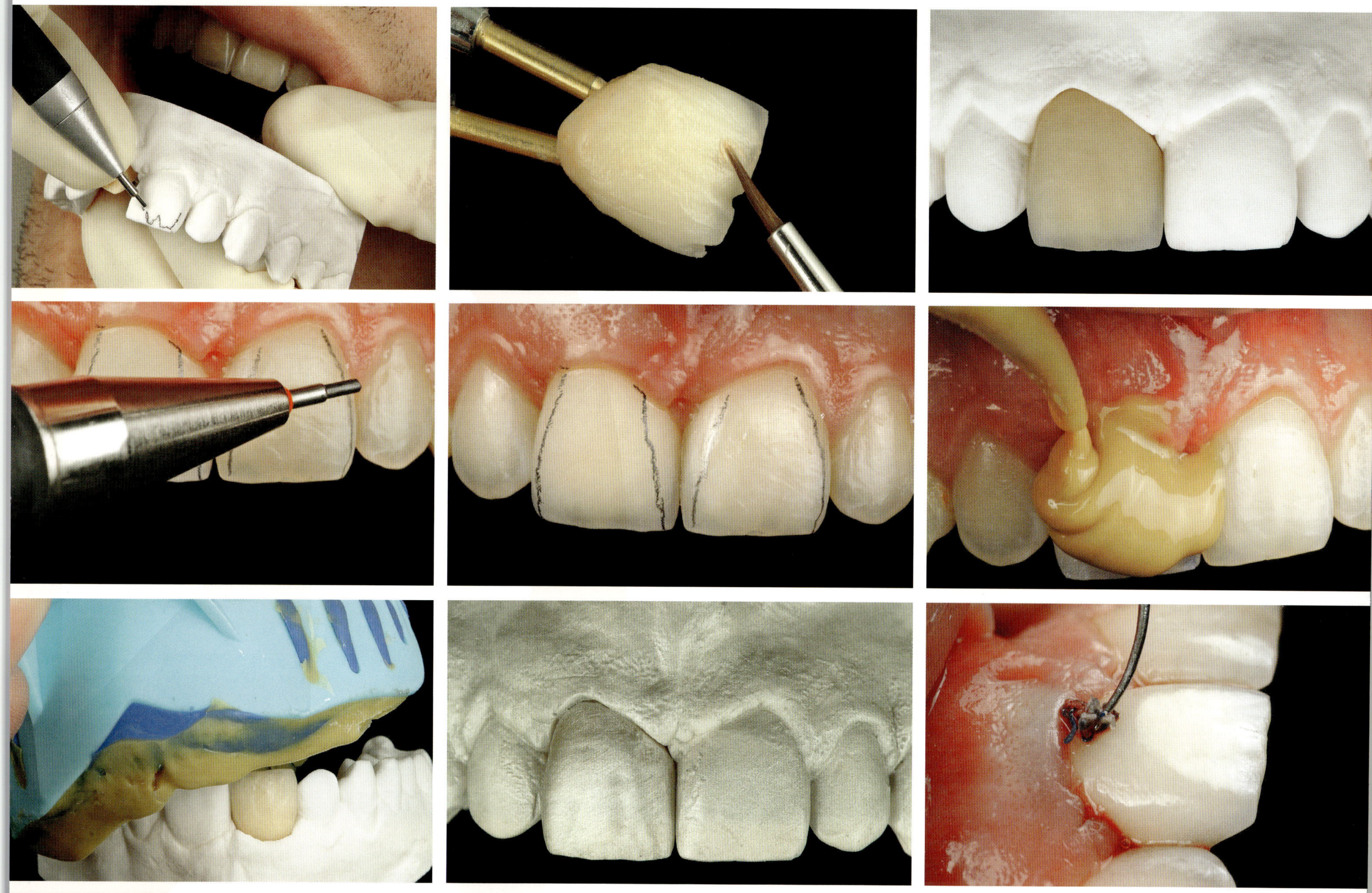

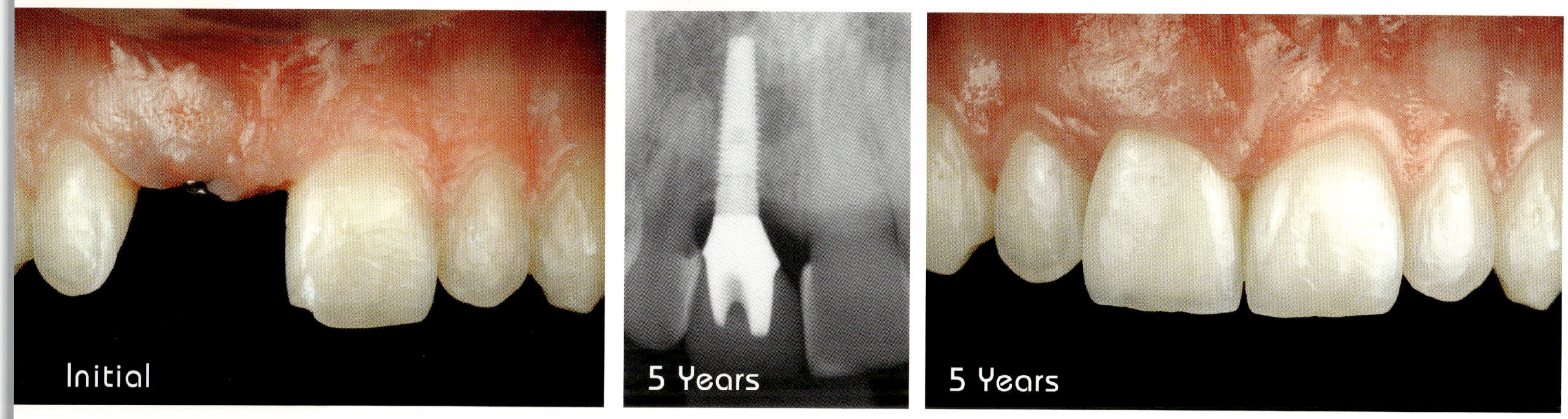

Mamelons were transferred and indicated so they could be visualized during fabrication of the definitive restoration. Then the bisque bake was tried in, and a pick-up impression was made to finalize the restoration. Note the balance between the restoration contour and the grafted site after 5 years.

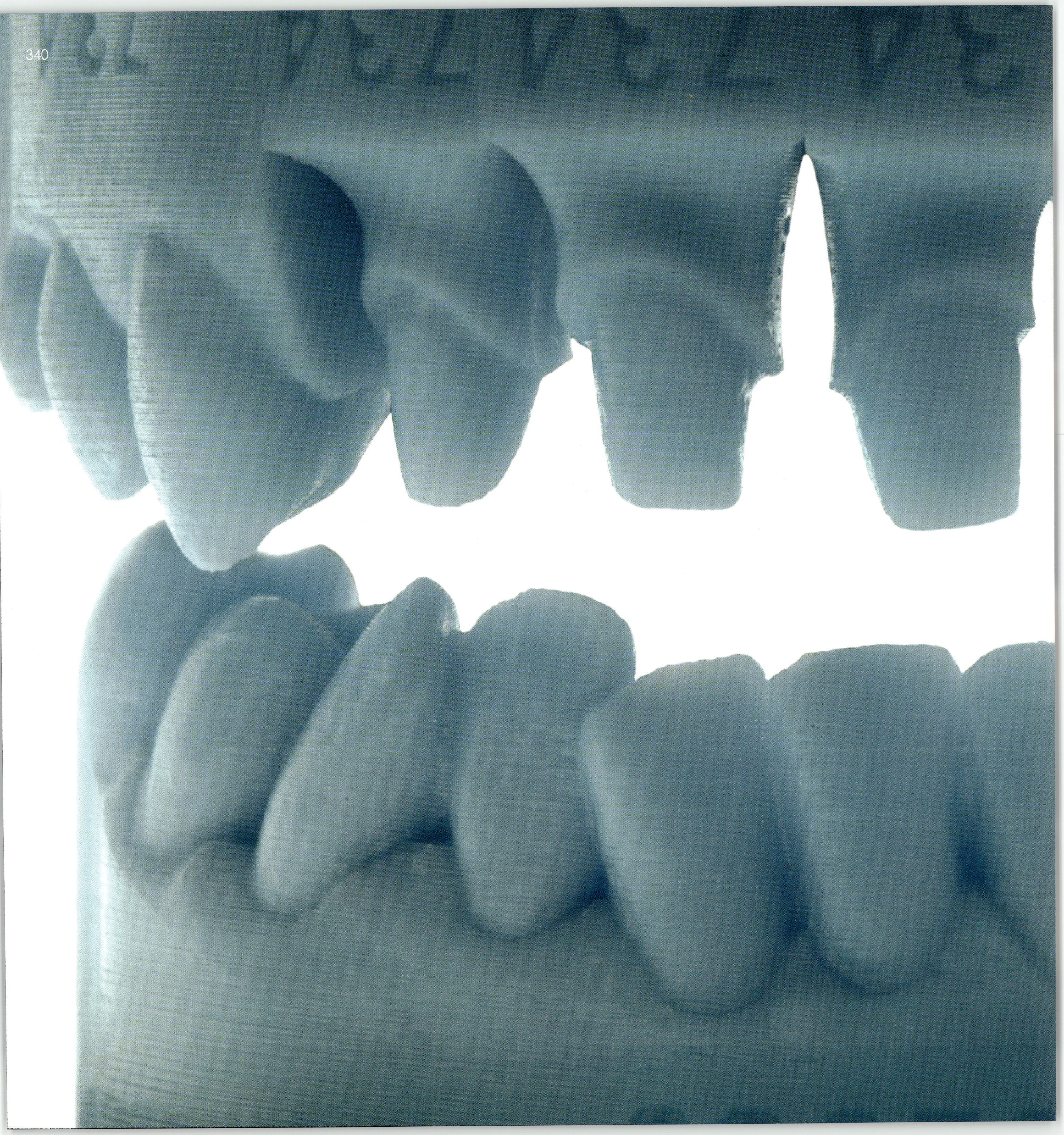

Digital scanner/ intraoral scanning

The final impression should be made without removing the abutment, following the biologic concept of implant restoration. Conventional cords were used on teeth and implants, and an intraoral scanner transferred the preparations to the laboratory with a digital impression.

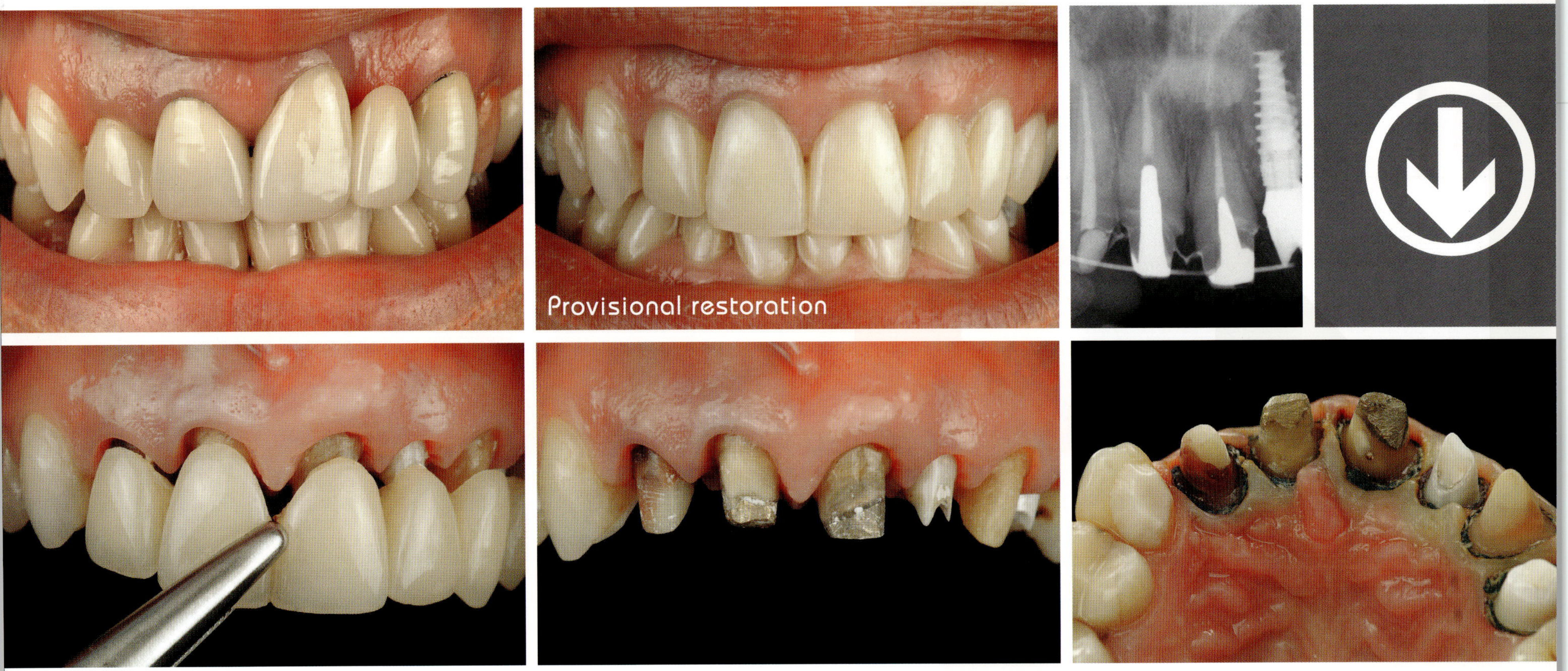

The retraction cord was removed, and titanium oxide powder was sprayed over the preparations for the 3D intraoral digital scan.

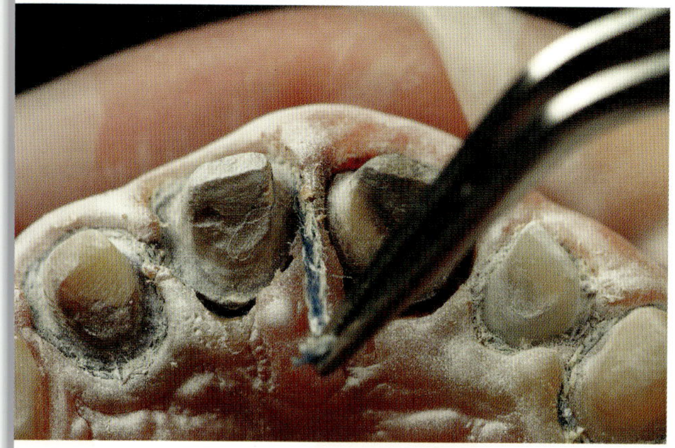

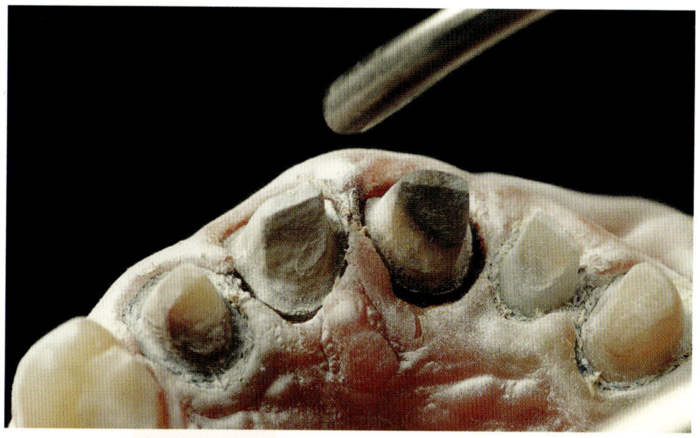

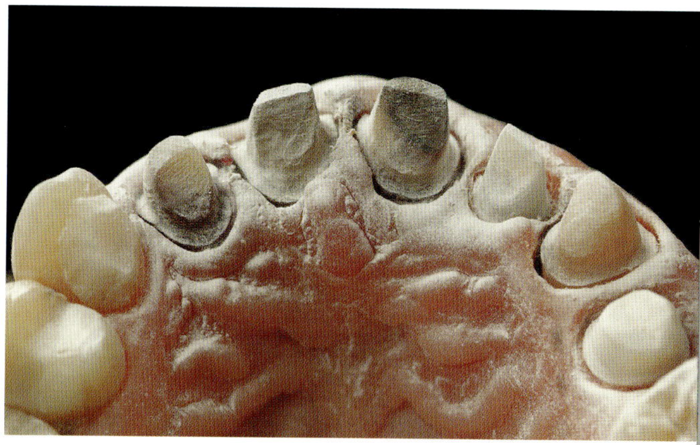

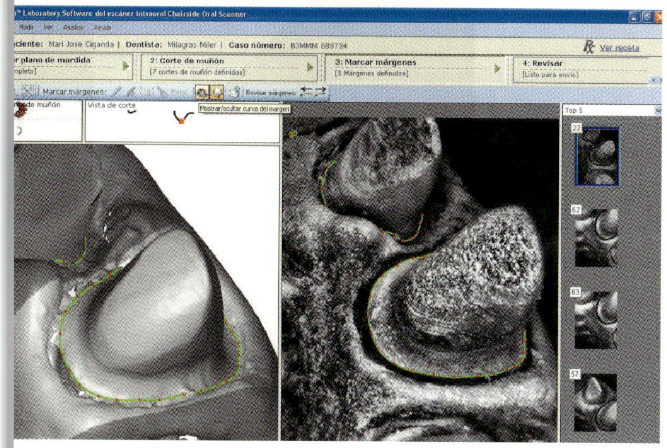

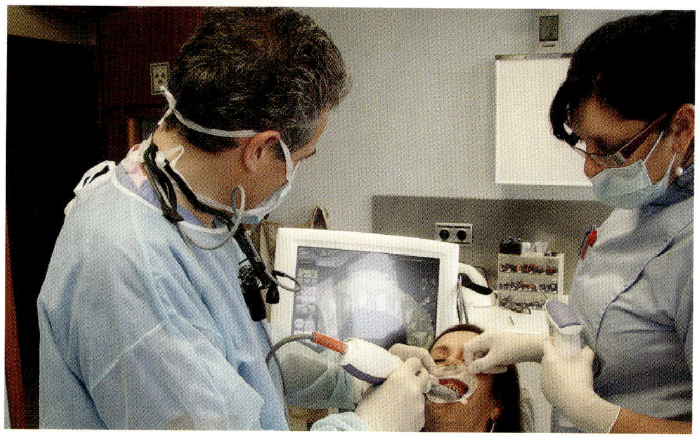

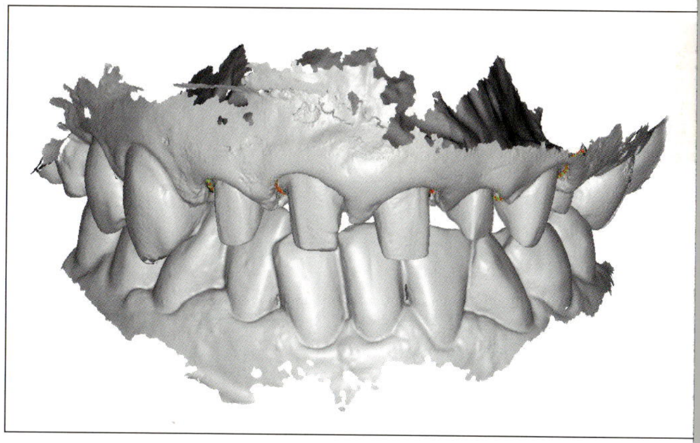

With the digital file, the laboratory technician was able to design the copings to optimally support the veneering porcelain. The manufacturer fabricated the stereolithographic master cast and crown coping. The technician then layered the veneering porcelain on the coping. The crown was tried in at bisque bake stage and adjusted before completion. Another pickup impression was made to communicate the emergence profile and create the prosthetic soft tissue support. The cast was sectioned, and the dies were inserted into the pickup impression for the final master cast. Note the volume acquired around the maxillary left central and lateral incisors.

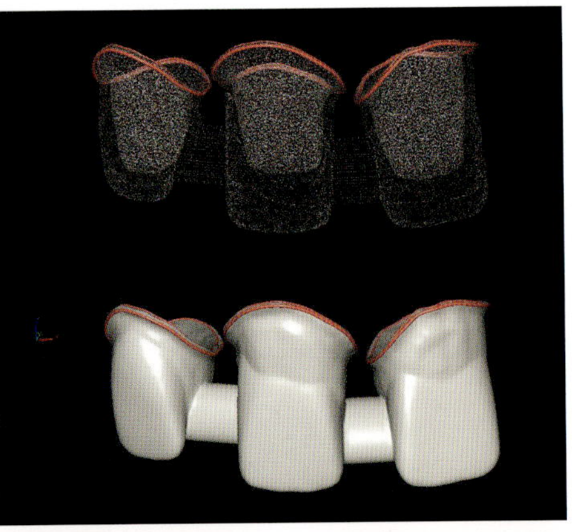
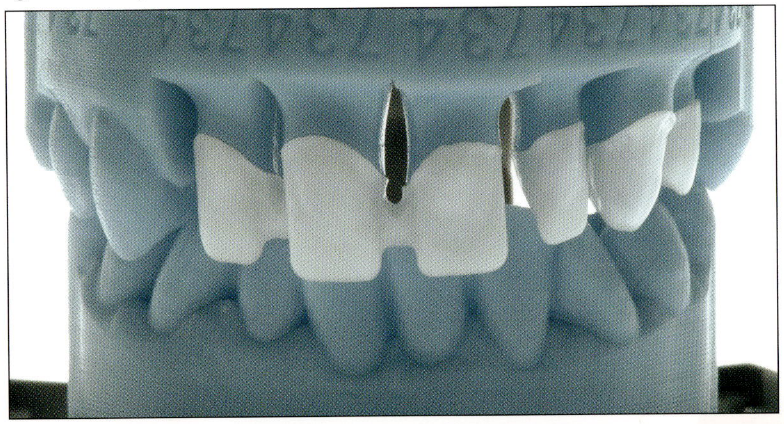
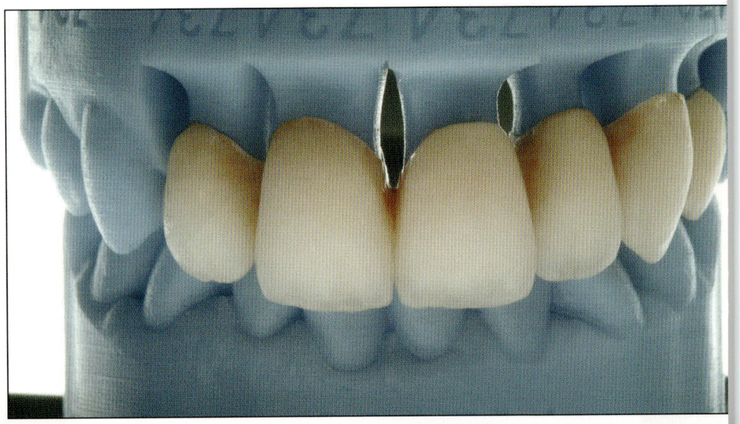
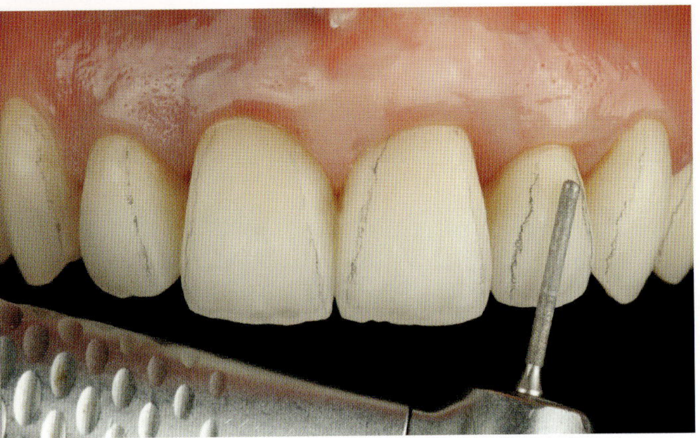
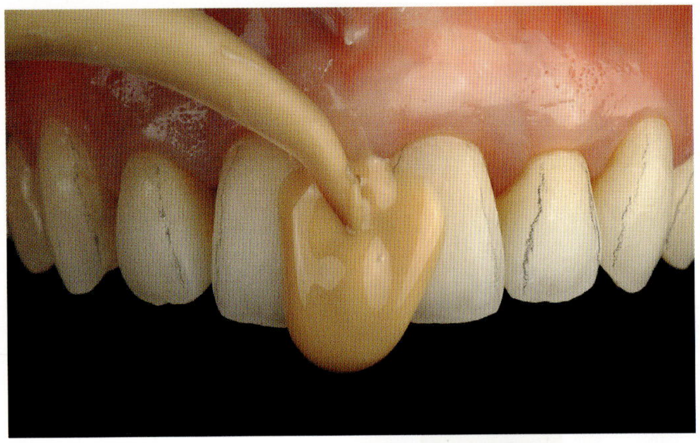
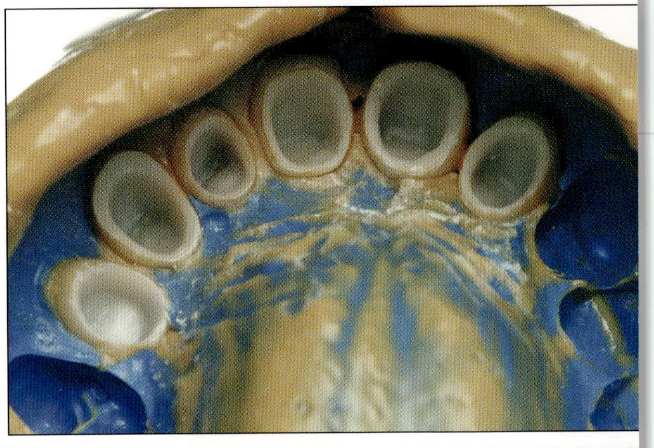
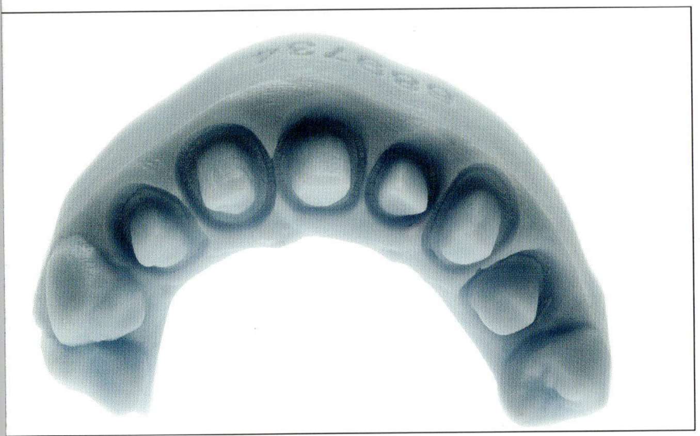
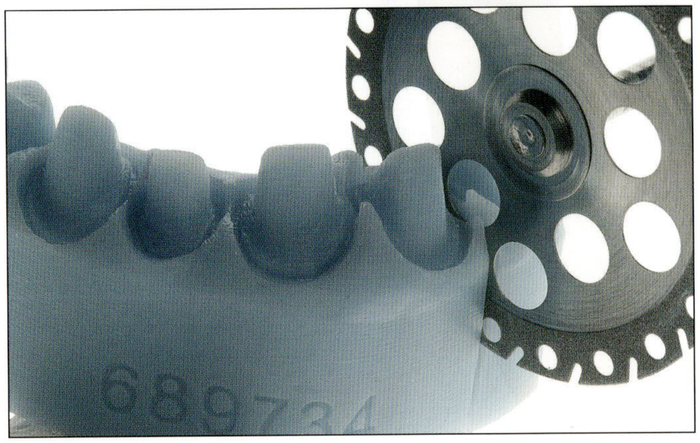

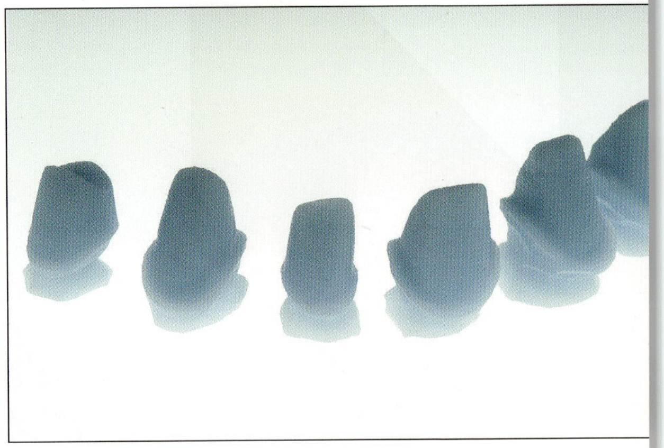
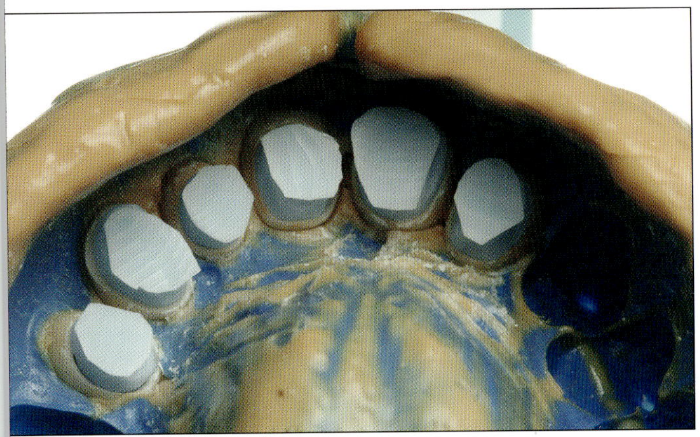
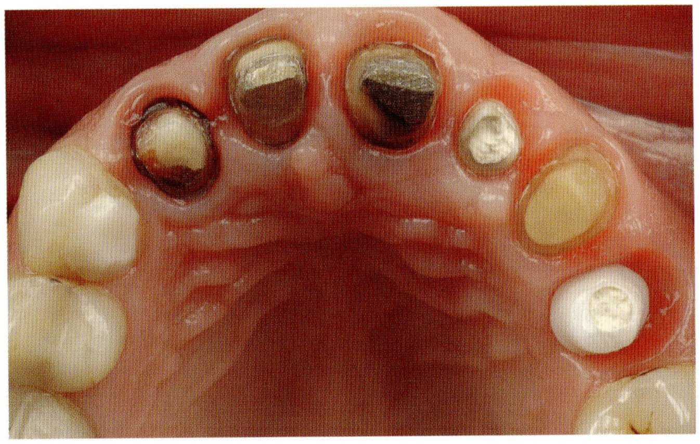
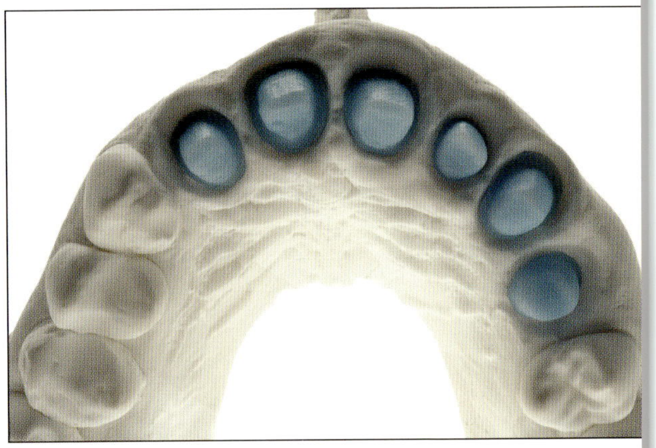

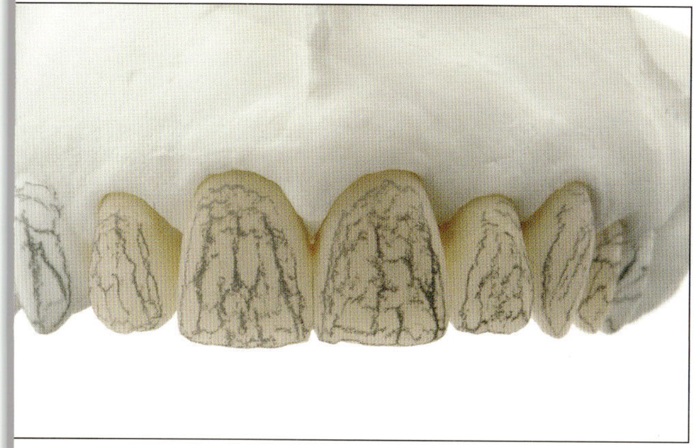

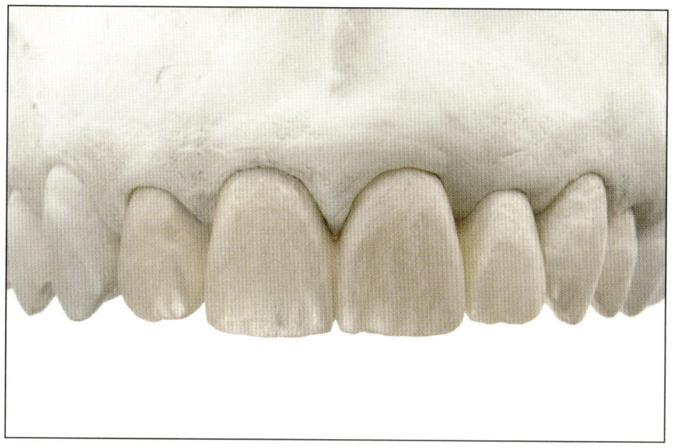

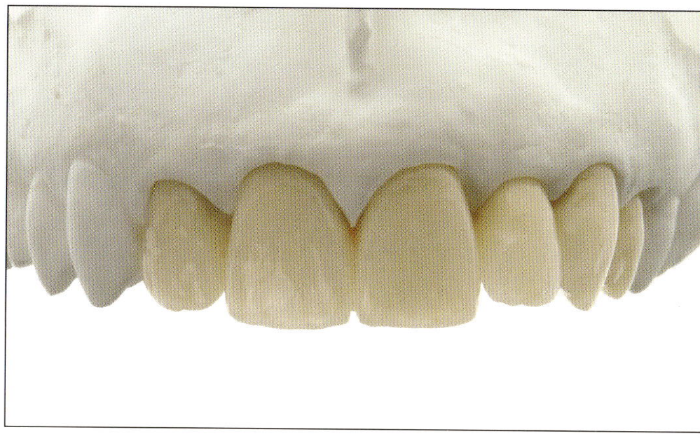

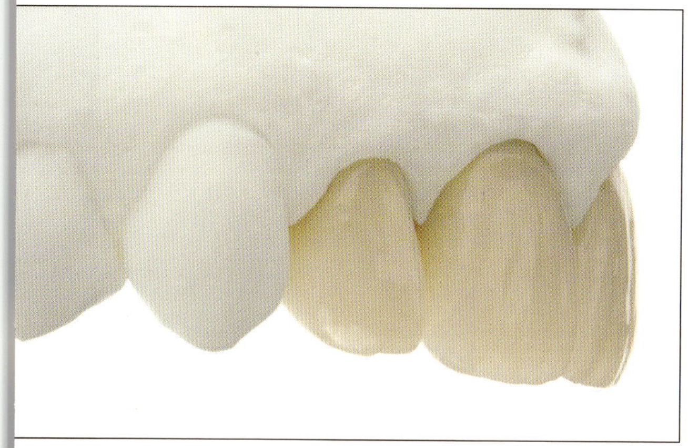

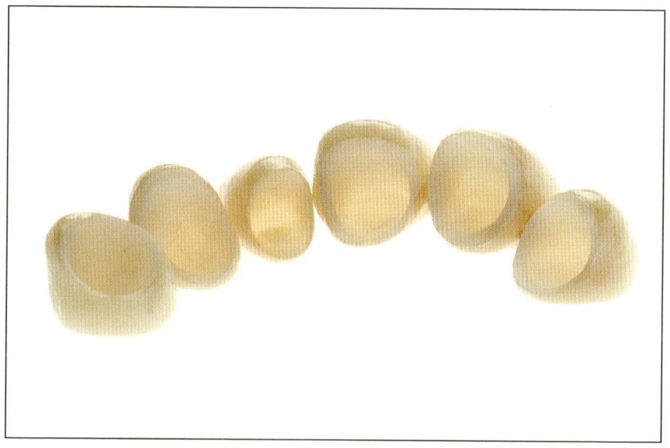

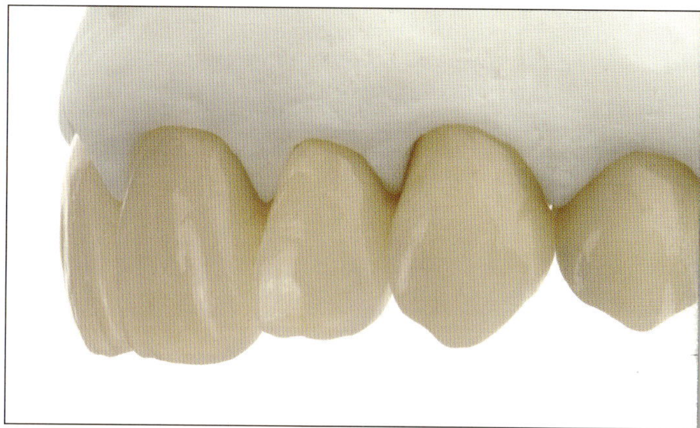

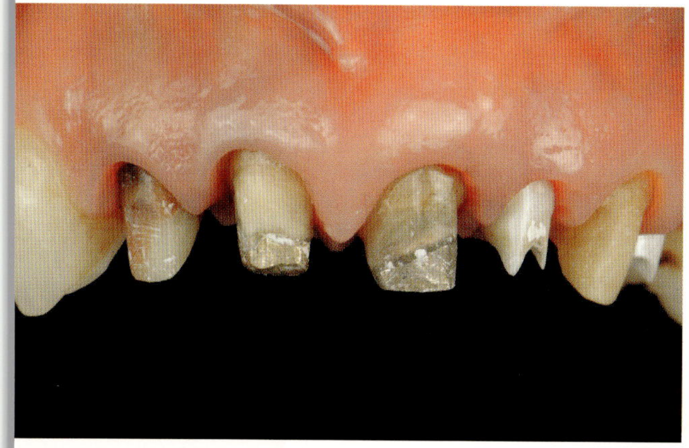

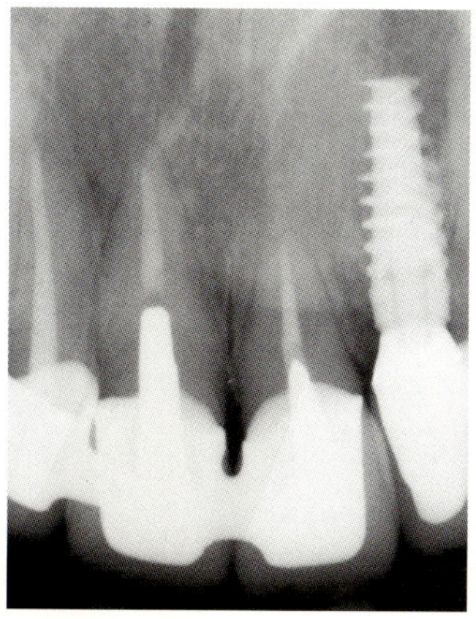

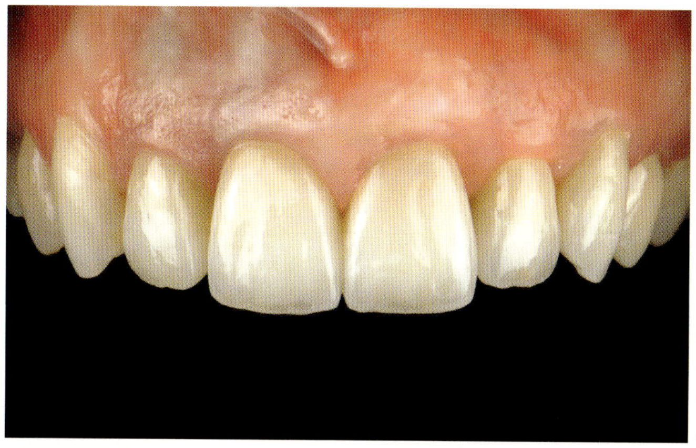

The technician completed the recontouring, surface texture, and luster. Final outcome after 2 years.

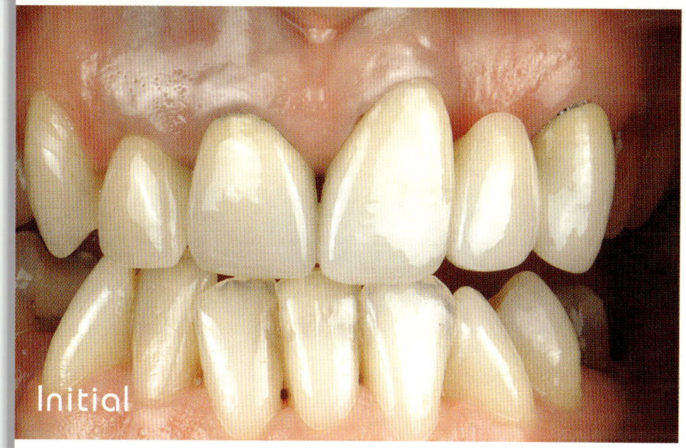

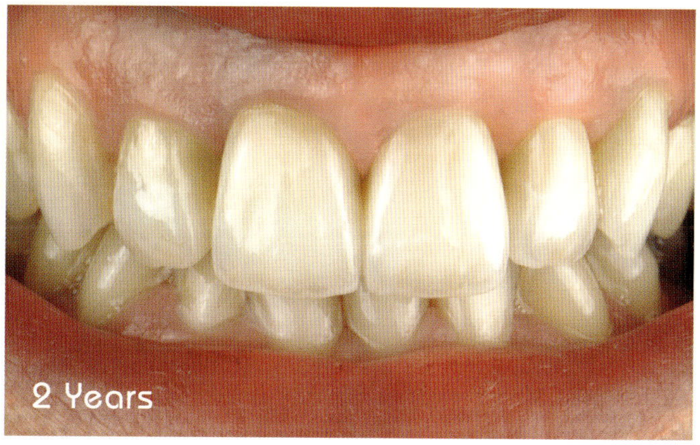

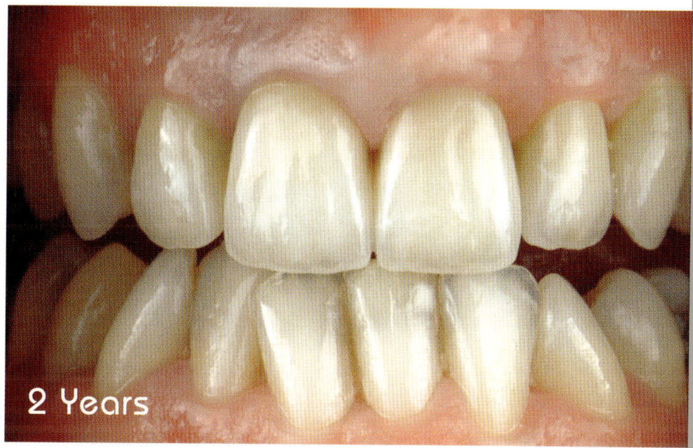

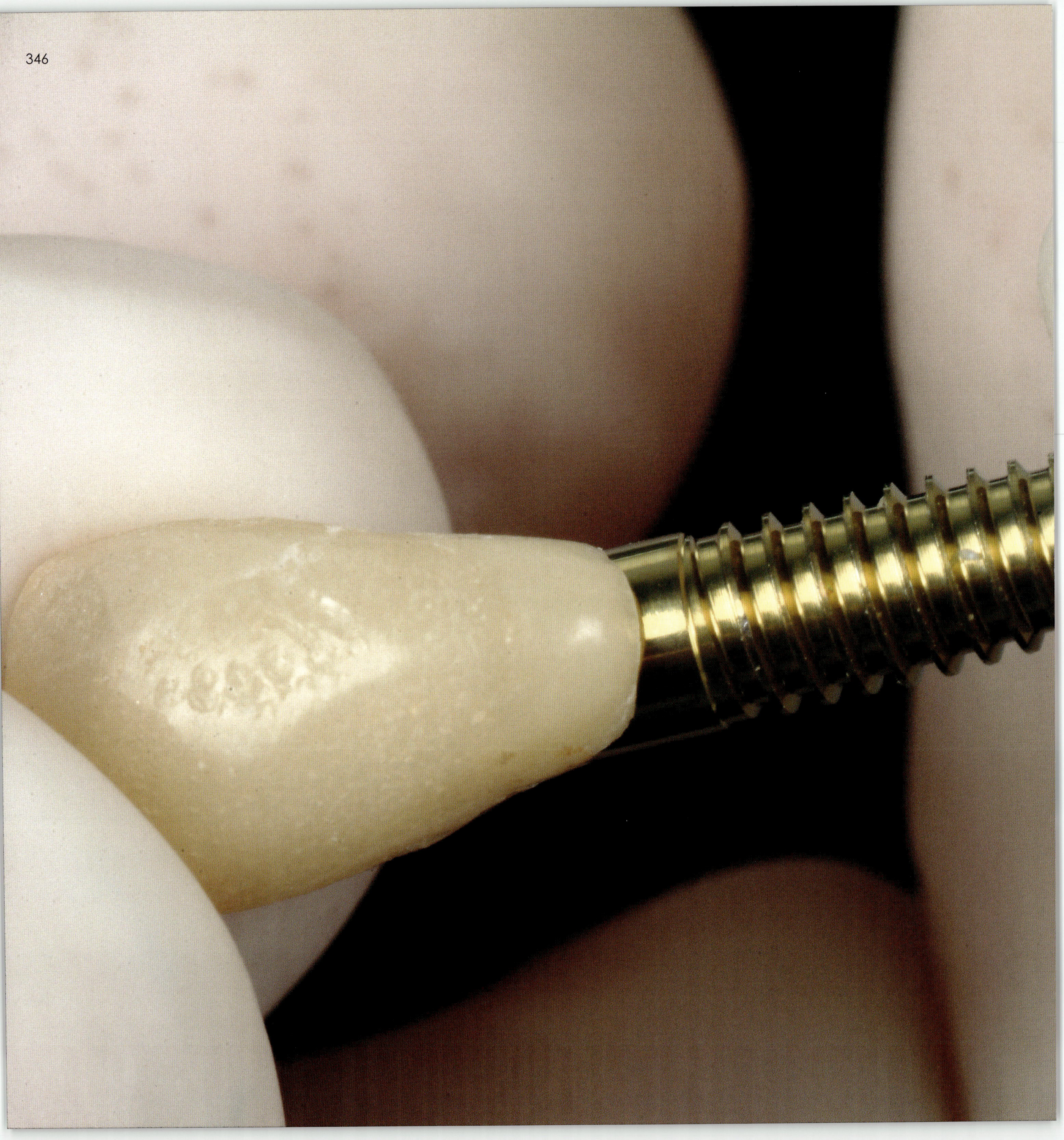

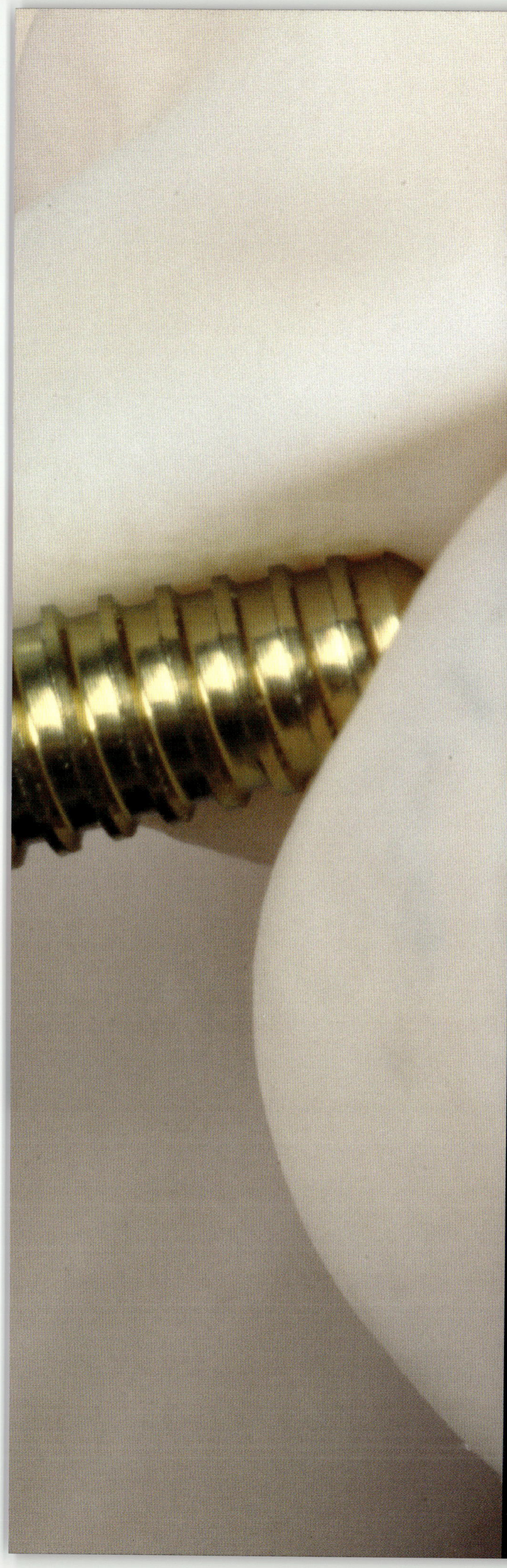

3D Emergence Profile and Tooth Contour

When tight spaces are encountered during restoration of teeth and implants, the best way to communicate mesiodistal space to the laboratory technician is the pickup impression of the provisional restorations. Pickup impression technique for the provisional restoration is chosen to communicate the exact mesiodistal space available for the reconstruction of the definitive zirconia restorations and ensure close replication of the contralateral esthetics. This pickup impression was chosen to communicate the undisturbed peri-implant soft tissues. With a one-piece implant, it is difficult to create and allocate the subgingival finish line and emergence profile, which should be performed on the day of implant placement. This allows the clinician to visualize the final outcome of the prosthetic design and gingival support. It is important that, once the one-piece implant is placed, the coronal part of the implant is never prepared. This way, a replica of the implant can be used chairside to create the emergence profile and determine the location of the preparation finish line based on the desired emergence profile. Usually, the final preparation of the abutment is performed and designed by the laboratory technician to create more space for the definitive coping and crown.

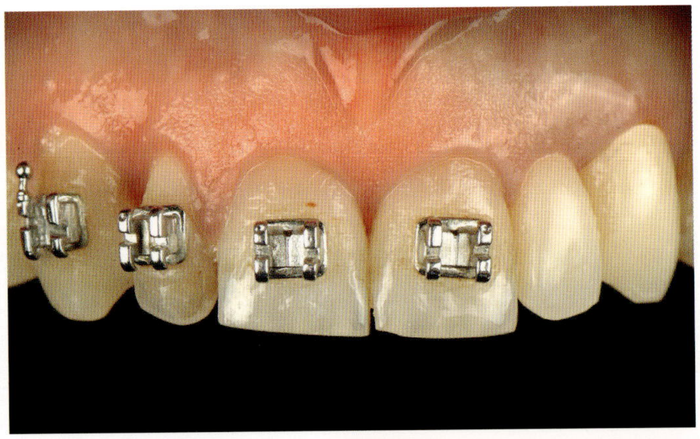
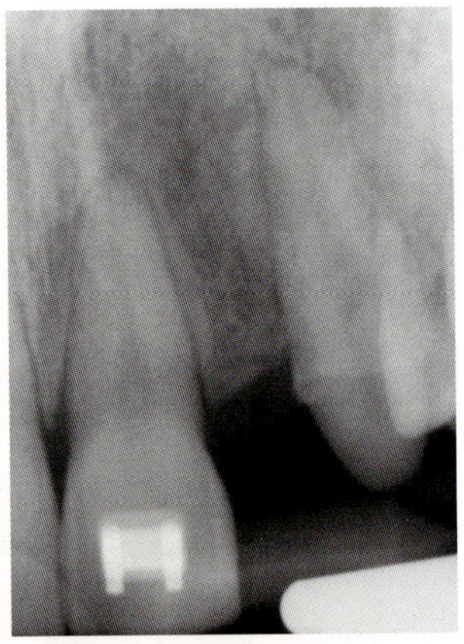
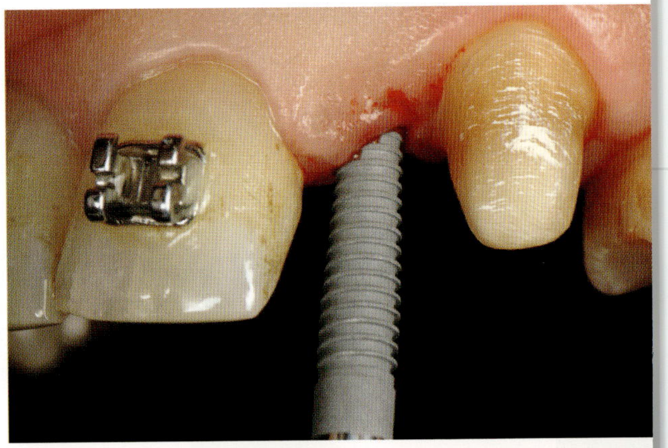

The patient was referred by an orthodontist. No additional space could be provided. A 3.0 × 13–mm NobelDirect implant was placed, and a provisional restoration was relined to fit the top of the implant.

Orthodontist:
Dr Domingo Martín

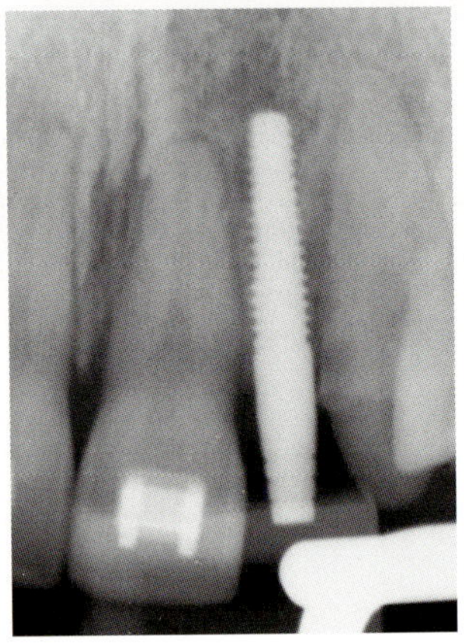
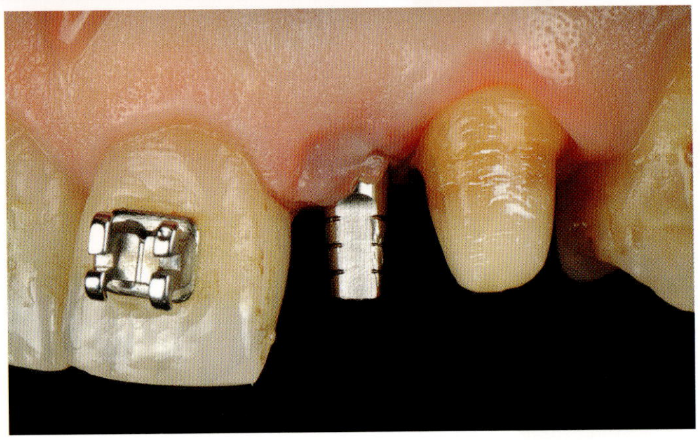
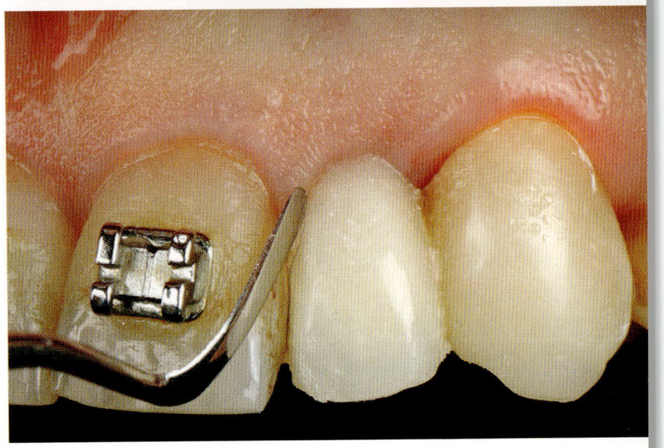

A NobelDirect 3.0 replica was used for the provisional restoration to create the ideal emergence profile from the implant abutment to the desired crown. The provisional crowns were separated to allow minor orthodontic adjustments of the canine.

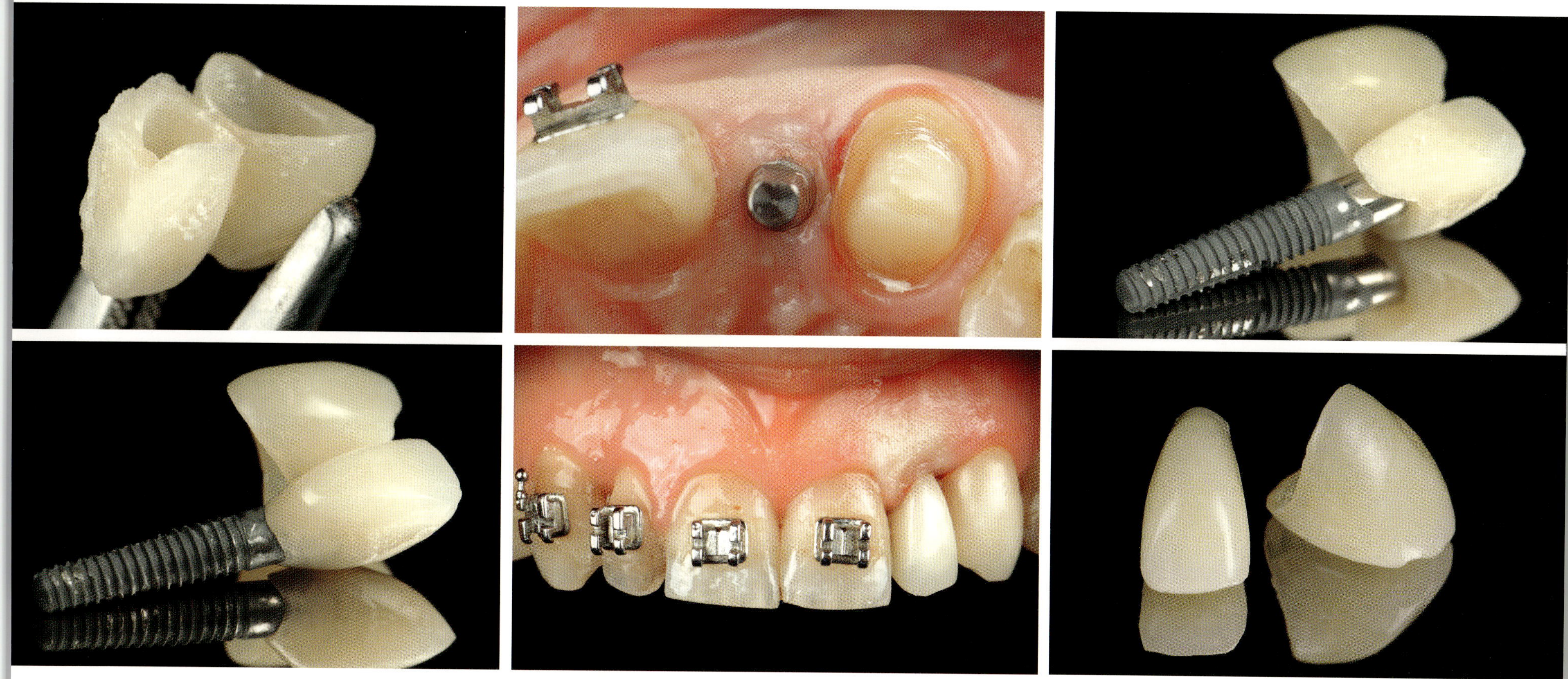

After orthodontic treatment, the six anterior teeth were splinted for 6 months to obtain stability. The final impression was made with an alternative technique. The double-cord technique was used on the natural maxillary left canine while leaving the provisional crown on the maxillary left lateral incisor, allowing for a pickup impression of the provisional crown. Stone was poured in the master impression following placement of the implant replica on the provisional crown. This allowed for adequate soft tissue contour of the definitive crown as well as the mesiodistal space. A reduction coping was fabricated with acrylic resin to create more space for the lateral incisor crown restoration, and the coronal aspect of the implant was reduced with a bur.

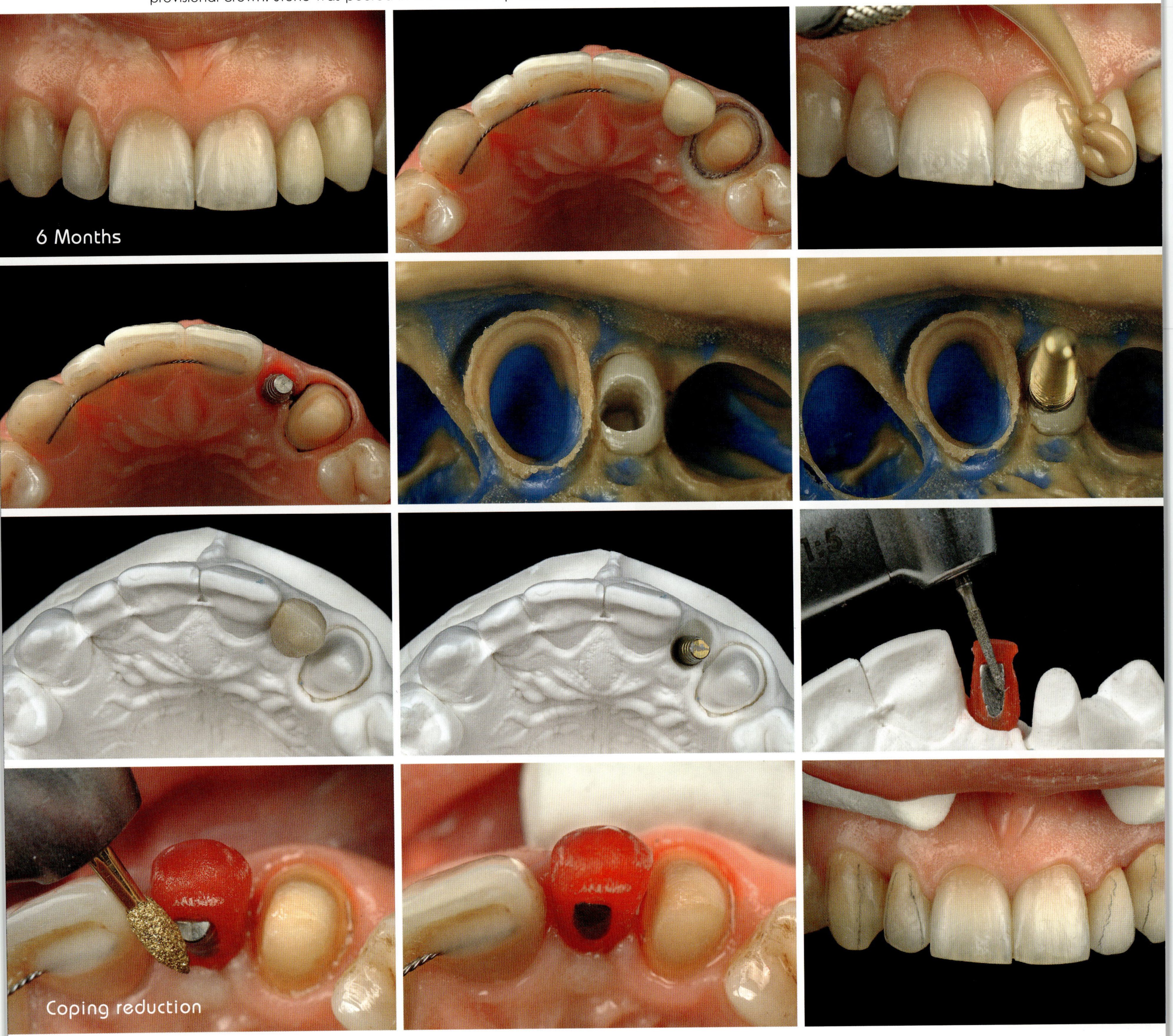

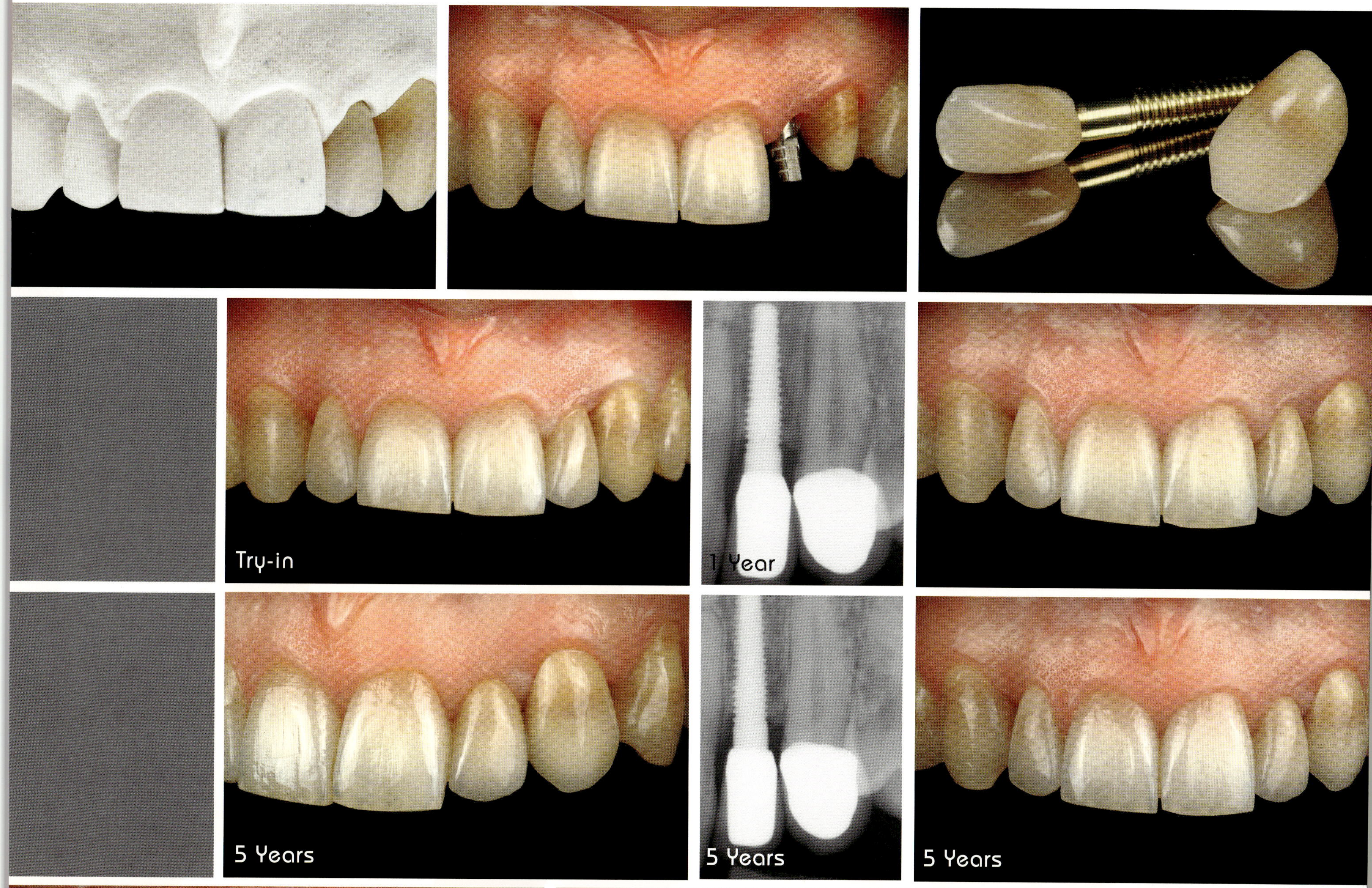

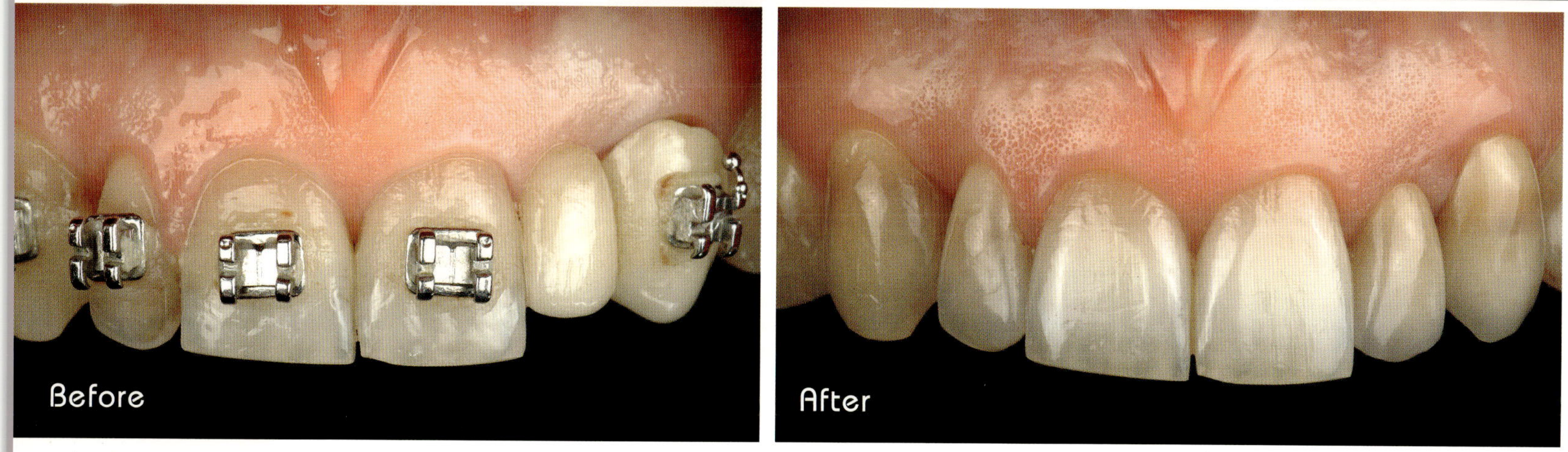

Zirconia crowns were fabricated and cemented on the implant with a universal self-adhesive resin cement and on the natural tooth with a glass-ionomer cement. The double-cord technique was used for cement removal. Postoperative situation 1 and 5 years later.

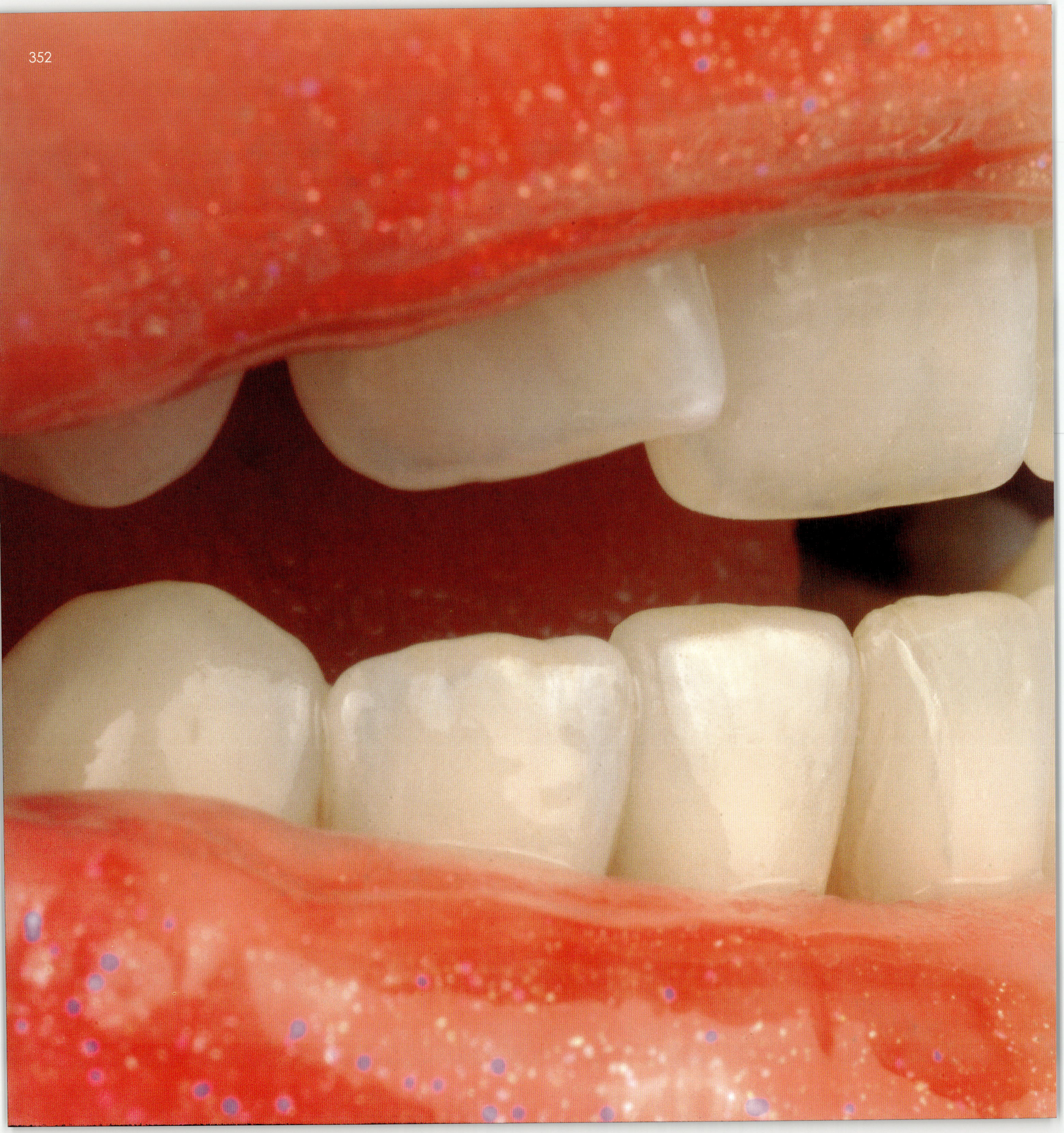

Color and Coping Selection

Research

Definitive crown material

The selection of materials for definitive implant-supported restorations is based on physical and optical properties and therefore may differ substantially depending on location of the restoration in the oral cavity as well as esthetic and functional requirements.[1–3] Single anterior implant restorations present a specific challenge because they must perfectly blend with the existing dentition and soft tissue conditions.[4] While there is little guidance through systematic literature reviews due to inconsistent outcome measures and evaluation tools,[5] there are numerous clinical and laboratory studies that are instrumental in the material selection process.

An all-ceramic approach is beneficial for natural esthetic outcomes.[6,7] Monolithic all-ceramic crowns, especially ones made from lithium disilicate, have become very popular.[8] However, a customized layered crown veneered with feldspathic ceramics is needed to perfectly mimic the individual esthetic and optical intricacies (ie, mamelons, translucency patterns, shaded layers, fluorescence) of individual natural teeth in the anterior region and blend them with the adjacent dentition. High-strength ceramics, especially alumina and zirconia, are preferred coping materials for layered crowns.

Densely sintered high-purity aluminum-oxide (> 99.9%) ceramics[1–3] with a flexural strength of 610 MPa[9] are mainly used for single-crown copings (eg, NobelProcera alumina crown). Long-term clinical studies have demonstrated excellent success rates of veneered alumina crowns on natural teeth.[10–13] Galindo et al[13] estimated the 10-year survival rate of alumina crowns at 95%. Alumina is more translucent than zirconia[14] and is therefore preferred in some esthetically demanding situations.[1,2]

Zirconium dioxide (zirconia) offers several advantages as a core material due to its esthetic characteristics, mechanical properties (flexural strength over 1,000 MPa), and biocompatibility.[15] In dentistry, it is most commonly used in forms of Yttria-stabilized tetragonal polycrystals, which provide high flexural strength and a distinctive crack-resisting property called *transformation toughening*. Early studies on bilayer zirconia-based fixed partial dentures indicated a high incidence of chipping in the veneering ceramic.[15] However, recent clinical studies, extrapolated in several systematic reviews, indicate no difference in clinical success rates between tooth-supported PFM and porcelain-fused-to-zirconia (PFZ) crowns but suggest studies with longer observation times.[16–18] A practice-based long-term study did not find any difference in clinical survival of over 2,000 PFZ and PFM crowns on posterior teeth after a mean 7.4 years of follow up.[19]

Selection of adequate veneering ceramics in respect to coefficient of thermal expansion, modulus of elasticity, flexural strength, and fracture toughness as well as modified firing and cooling parameters are key for clinical longevity of PFZ restorations.[19,20] CAD/CAM technology facilitates a customized and anatomical design of the coping for optimal support of the veneering ceramic and increased reliability.[21,22] Also, alternative veneering materials may become more popular in the future.[23]

The precision of fit achieved with modern laboratory-based CAD/CAM systems such as NobelProcera is excellent[24] and, especially for multiunit implant-supported restorations, significantly exceeds traditional fabrication methods.[25,26]

The long-term clinical performance of implant-supported all-ceramic crowns still needs further scientific validation but seems promising, especially in the anterior region.

References

1. Blatz MB. Long-term clinical success of all-ceramic posterior restorations. Quintessence Int 2002;33:415–426.

2. Sadan A, Blatz MB, Lang B. Clinical considerations for densely sintered alumina and zirconia restorations: Part 1. Int J Periodontics Restorative Dent 2005;25:213–219.

3. Sadan A, Blatz MB, Lang B. Clinical considerations for densely sintered alumina and zirconia restorations: Part 2. Int J Periodontics Restorative Dent 2005;25:343–349.

4. Sadan A, Blatz MB, Bellerino M, Block M. Prosthetic design considerations for anterior single-implant restorations. J Esthet Restor Dent 2004;16:165–175.

5. Martin WC, Pollini A, Morton D. The influence of restorative procedures on esthetic outcomes in implant dentistry: A systematic review. Int J Oral Maxillofac Implants 2014;29(suppl):142–154.

6. Jung RE, Sailer I, Hämmerle CH, Attin T, Schmidlin P. In vitro color changes of soft tissues caused by restorative materials. Int J Periodontics Restorative Dent 2007;27:251–257.

7. Büchi DL, Sailer I, Fehmer V, Hämmerle CH, Thoma DS. All-ceramic single-tooth implant reconstructions using modified zirconia abutments: A prospective randomized controlled clinical trial of the effect of pink veneering ceramic on the esthetic outcomes. Int J Periodontics Restorative Dent 2014;34:29–37.

8. Pieger S, Salman A, Bidra AS. Clinical outcomes of lithium disilicate single crowns and partial fixed dental prostheses: A systematic review. J Prosthet Dent 2014;112:22–30.

9. Zeng K, Oden A, Rowcliffe D. Flexure tests on dental ceramics. Int J Prosthodont 1996;9:434–439.

10. Oden A, Andersson M, Krystek-Ondracek I, Magnusson D. Five-year clinical evaluation of Procera AllCeram crowns. J Prosthet Dent 1998;80:450–456.

11. Odman P, Andersson B. Procera AllCeram crowns followed for 5 to 10.5 years: A prospective clinical study. Int J Prosthodont 2001;14:504–509.

12. Fradeani M, D'Amelio M, Redemagni M, Corrado M. Five-year follow-up with Procera all-ceramic crowns. Quintessence Int 2005;36:105–113.

13. Galindo ML, Sendi P, Marinello CP. Estimating long-term survival of densely sintered alumina crowns: A cohort study over 10 years. J Prosthet Dent 2011;106:23–28.

14. Costello RV, Thompson J, Sadan A, Burgess JO, Blatz MB. Light transmission of high-strength ceramics with four curing lights. J Dent Res 2004;83(special issue A):1813.

15. Komine F, Blatz MB, Matsumura H. Current state of zirconia-based fixed restorations. J Oral Sci 2010;52:531–539.

16. Larsson C, Wennerberg A. The clinical success of zirconia-based crowns: A systematic review. Int J Prosthodont 2014;27:33–43.

17. Wang X, Fan D, Swain M, Zhao K. A systematic review of all-ceramic crowns: Clinical fracture rates in relation to restored tooth type. Int J Prosthodont 2012;25:441–450.

18. Takeichi T, Katsoulis J, Blatz MB. Clinical outcome of single porcelain-fused-to-zirconium dioxide crowns: A systematic review. J Prosthet Dent 2013;110:455–461.

19. Ozer F, Mante FK, Chiche G, Saleh N, Takeichi T, Blatz MB. A retrospective survey on long-term survival of posterior zirconia and porcelain-fused-to-metal crowns in private practice. Quintessence Int 2014;45:31–38.

20. Blatz MB, Bergler M, Ozer F, Holst S, Phark JH, Chiche GJ. Bond strength of different veneering ceramics to zirconia and their susceptibility to thermocycling. Am J Dent 2010;23:213–216.

21. Rosentritt M, Steiger D, Behr M, Handel G, Kolbeck C. Influence of substructure design and spacer settings on the in vitro performance of molar zirconia crowns. J Dent 2009;37:978–983.

22. Larsson C, El Madhoun S, Wennerberg A, Vult von Steyern P. Fracture strength of yttria-stabilized tetragonal zirconia polycrystals crowns with different design: An in vitro study. Clin Oral Implants Res 2012;23:820–826.

23. Taguchi K, Komine F, Fushiki R, Blatz MB, Kamio S, Matsumura H. Fracture resistance of single-tooth implant-supported zirconia-based indirect composite-layered molar restorations. Clin Oral Implants Res 2014;25:983–991.

24. Limkangwalmongkol P, Chiche GJ, Kee E, Blatz MB. Comparison of marginal fit between all-porcelain margin vs alumina supported margin on Procera alumina crowns. J Prosthodont 2009;18:162–166.

25. Katsoulis J, Mericske-Stern R, Rotkina L, Zbaeren C, Enkling N, Blatz MB. Precision of fit of implant-supported screw-retained 10-unit computer-aided-designed and computer-aided-manufactured frameworks made from zirconium dioxide and titanium: An in vitro study. Clin Oral Implants Res 2014;25:165–174.

26. Katsoulis J, Mericske-Stern R, Yates D, Izutani N, Enkling N, Blatz MB. In-vitro precision of fit of computer-aided design and computer-aided manufacturing titanium and zirconium dioxide bars. Dent Mater 2013;29:945–953.

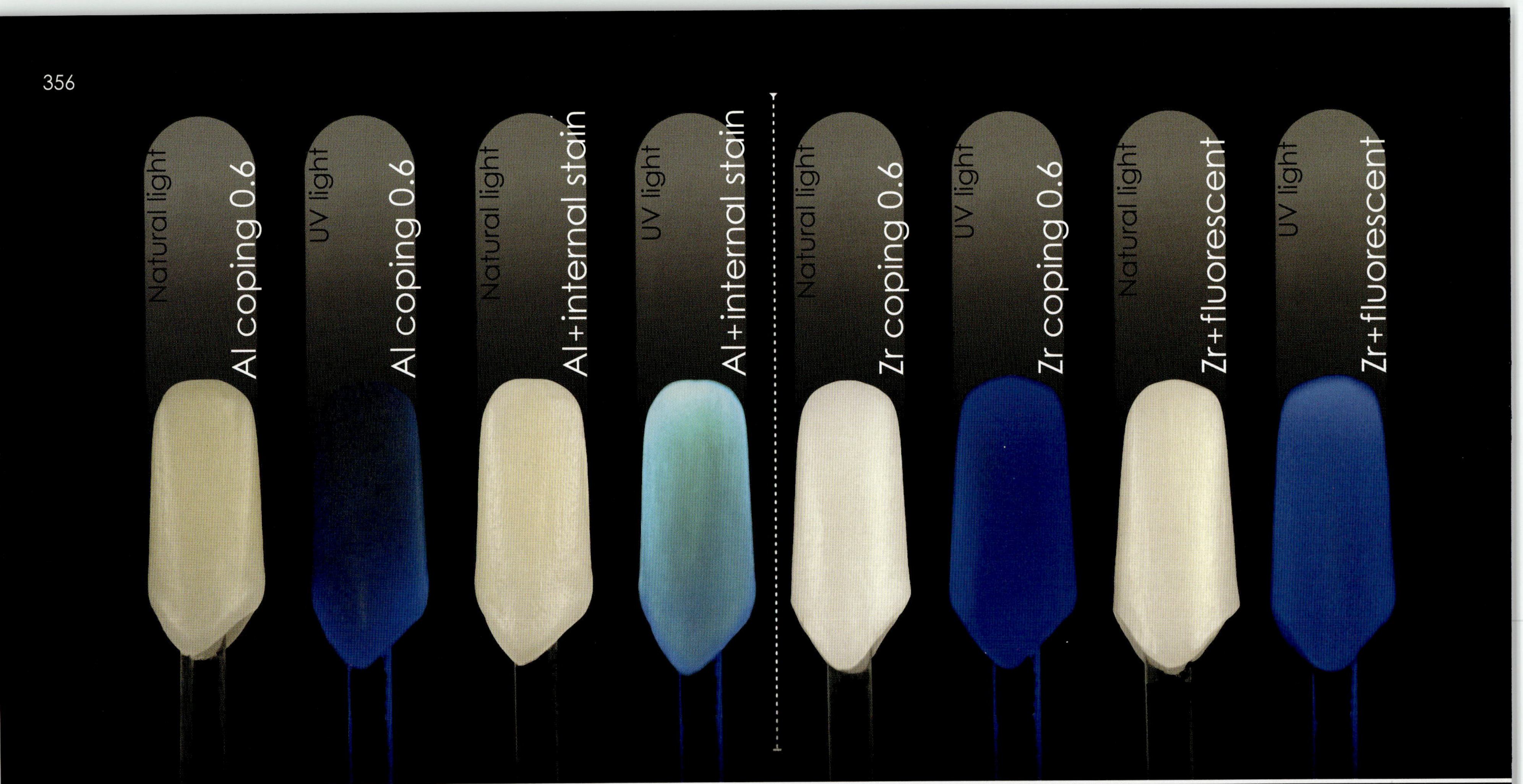
Natural light
Al coping 0.6
UV light
Al coping 0.6
Natural light
Al+internal stain
UV light
Al+internal stain
Natural light
Zr coping 0.6
UV light
Zr coping 0.6
Natural light
Zr+fluorescent
UV light
Zr+fluorescent

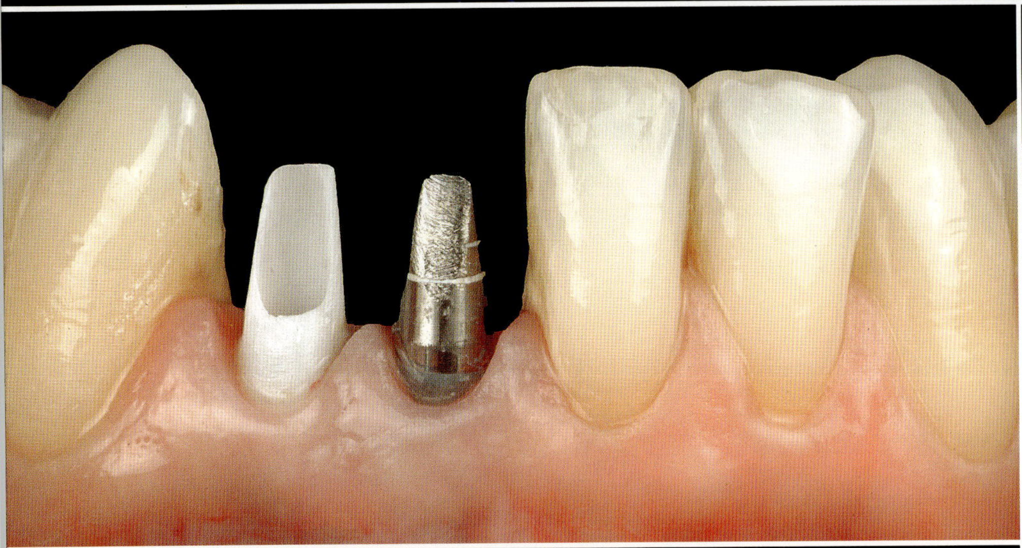

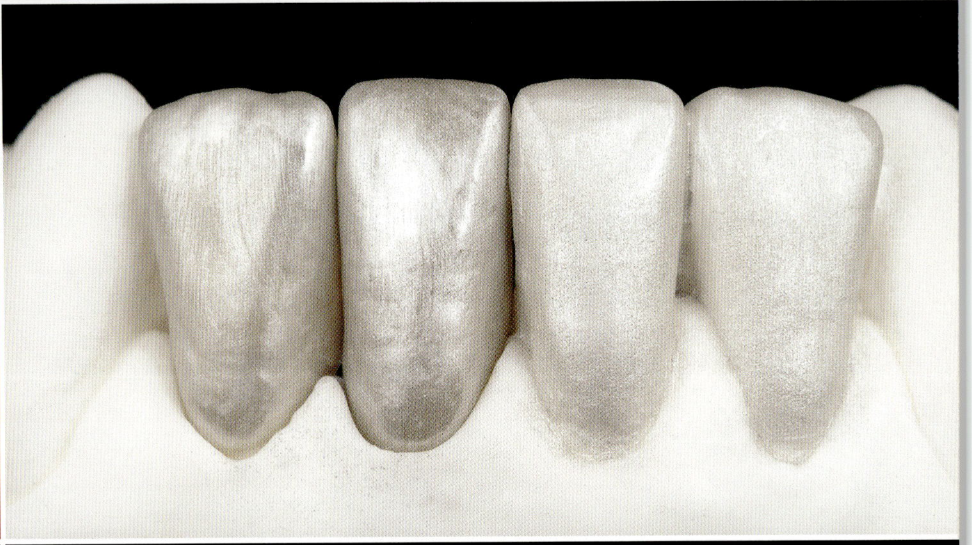

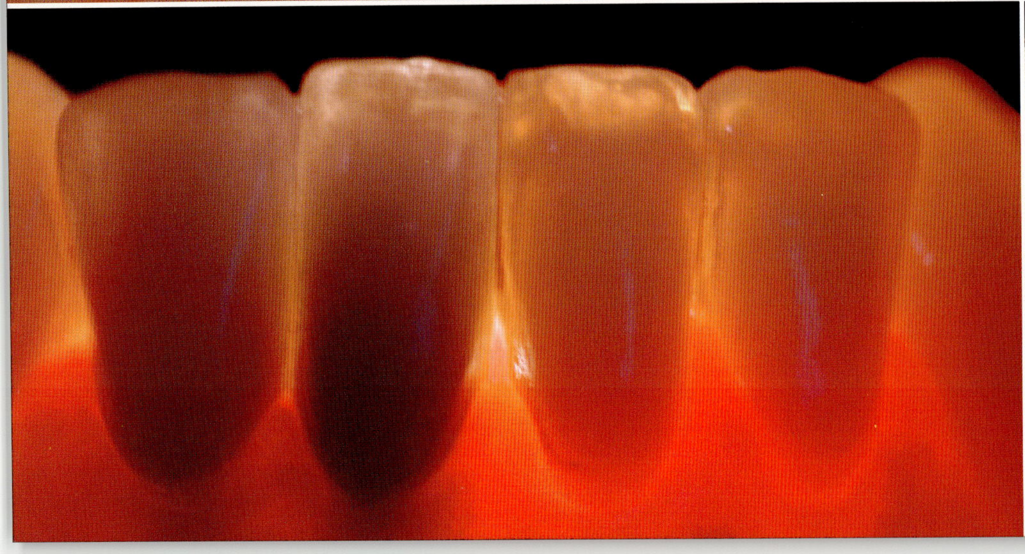

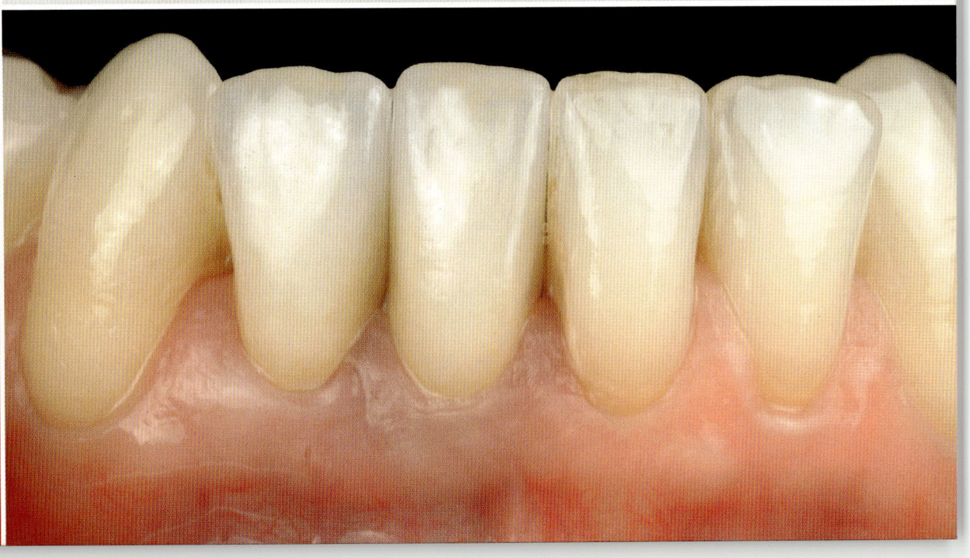

The definitive crown material is selected based on the core structure to enhance the optical characteristics of the intended restoration by closely mimicking the optical properties of natural teeth. The coping is chosen for its ability either to mask underlying structures if necessary or to complement the restoration with the underlying abutment color. Zirconia is a favorable coping material because of its versatility in respect to strength, thickness, color, and translucency but also because of its inherent brightness and fluorescence options through infiltration.

Ceramic coping materials such as alumina and zirconia are selected based on the color of the intended crown, the interocclusal space, and the color of the abutment. Zirconia is usually selected to mask dark substructures; the thickness of the coping—about 0.6 mm—is also essential for masking the substructure. Alumina is used with a thinner coping—0.4 mm—to allow a higher degree of translucency and blend with the supporting abutment.

Two patient scenarios are shown. The first requires a zirconia coping (0.6-mm thick) crown to mask the dark titanium of a 3.0 NobelDirect one-piece implant. In the second, an ideal fluorescent zirconia abutment had been fabricated, and an alumina coping was selected for increased translucency and to blend with the color of the substructure.

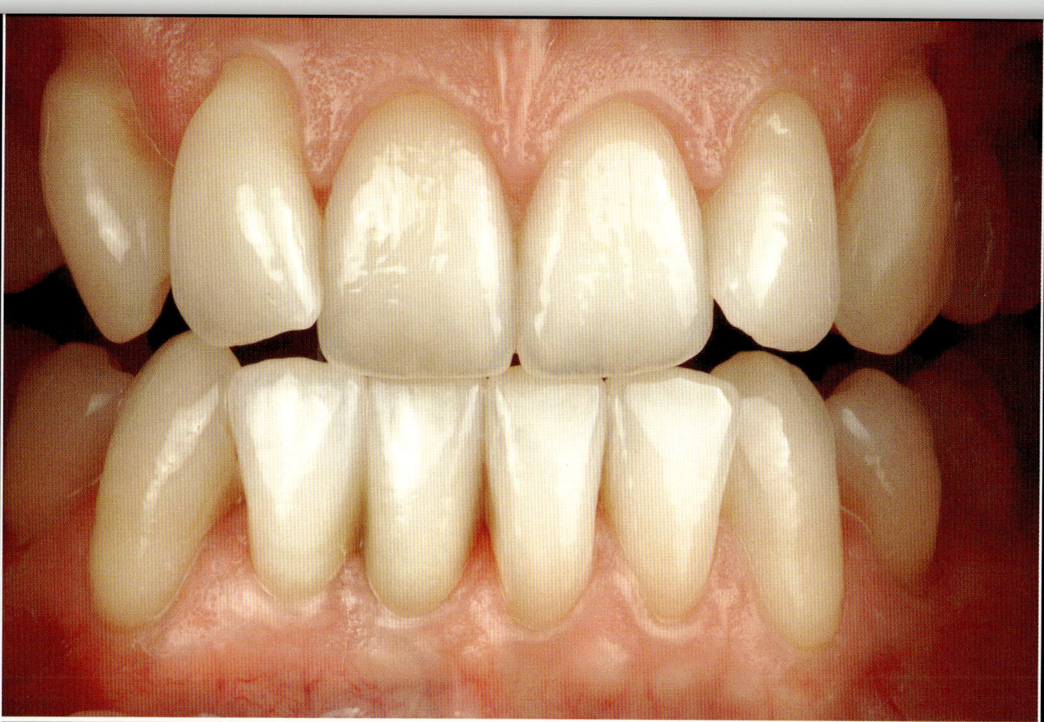

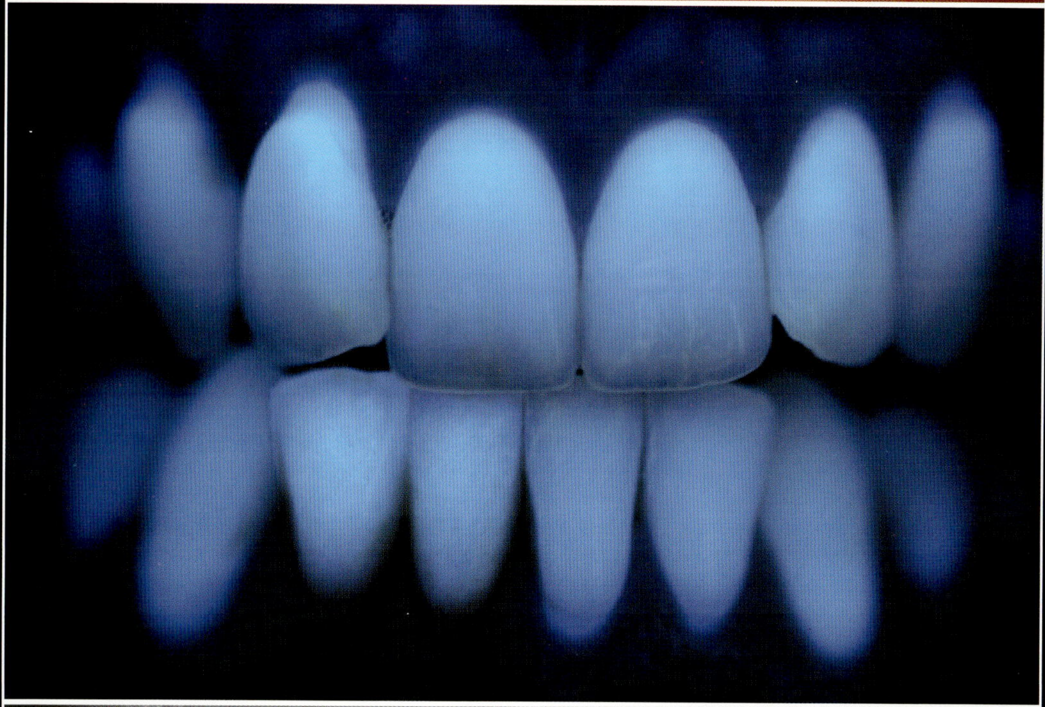

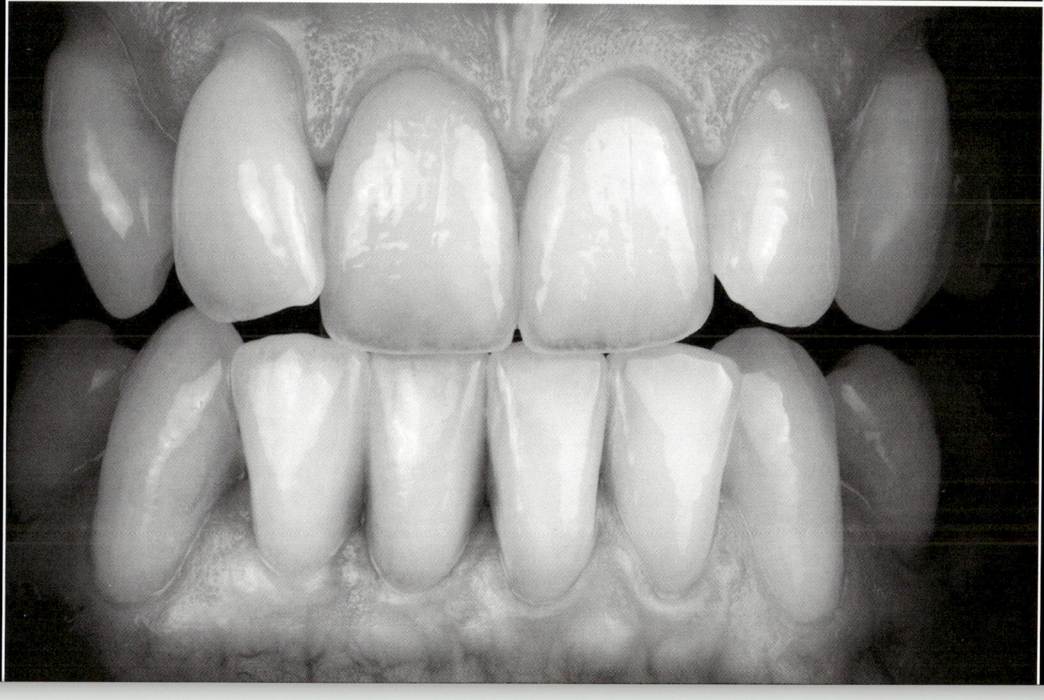

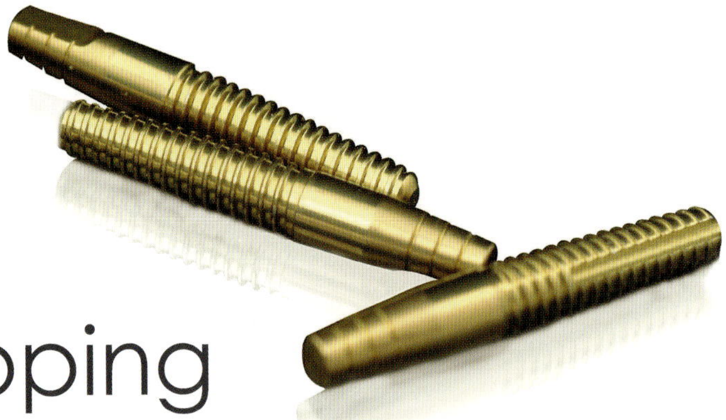

Zirconia coping

A mandibular central incisor was failing because of periodontal pathology. The tooth was extracted, and a CTG was placed to compensate for lost bone volume. After 3 months, the ridge had matured, and a NobelDirect 3.0 × 13–mm implant was placed together with a provisional crown restoration. A CTG was not necessary because of the adequate tissue volume. The coronal part of the implant was not prepared to allow for insertion of the implant analog and to define the subgingival finishing line and the correct emergence profile for the implant placement.

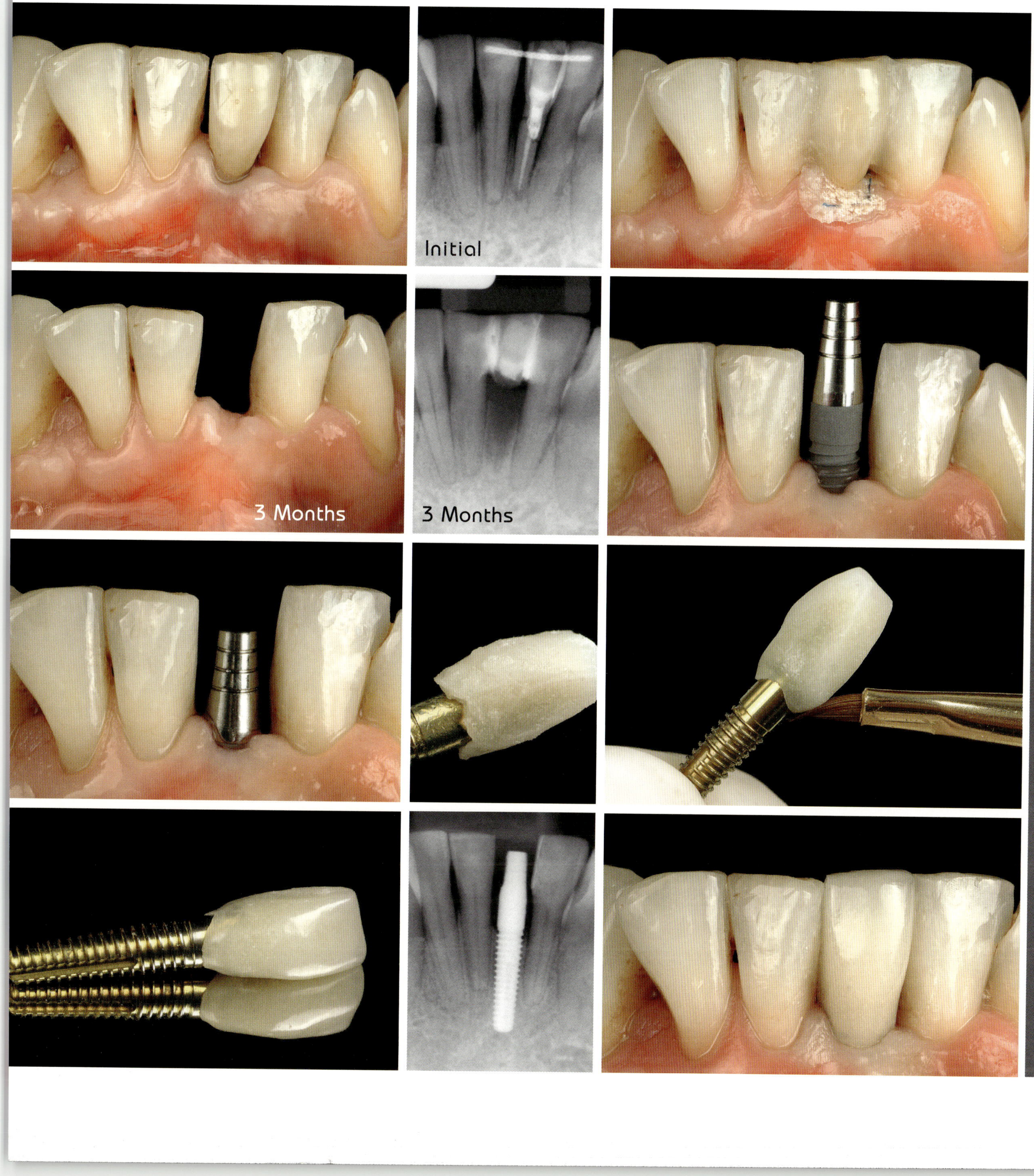

After 3 months of healing, the implant had integrated, and a pickup impression of the provisional restoration was performed with PVS impression material to communicate the established finishing line as well as the emergence profile to the laboratory.

A PVS matrix was fabricated on a duplicate model to design the definitive coping and crown. The existing space for the coping and porcelain was minimal, so the abutment needed to be reduced. A 0.6-mm zirconia coping was chosen to mask the dark metal substructure and blend with the adjacent teeth. The laboratory technician created a reduction coping with self-curing acrylic resin. The emergence profile was improved by carving the stone master cast and creating a better blend with the gingival levels at the adjacent teeth. The abutment was reduced intraorally through the coping reduction, and a PFZ crown with a 0.6-mm coping was tried in at the bisque bake stage.

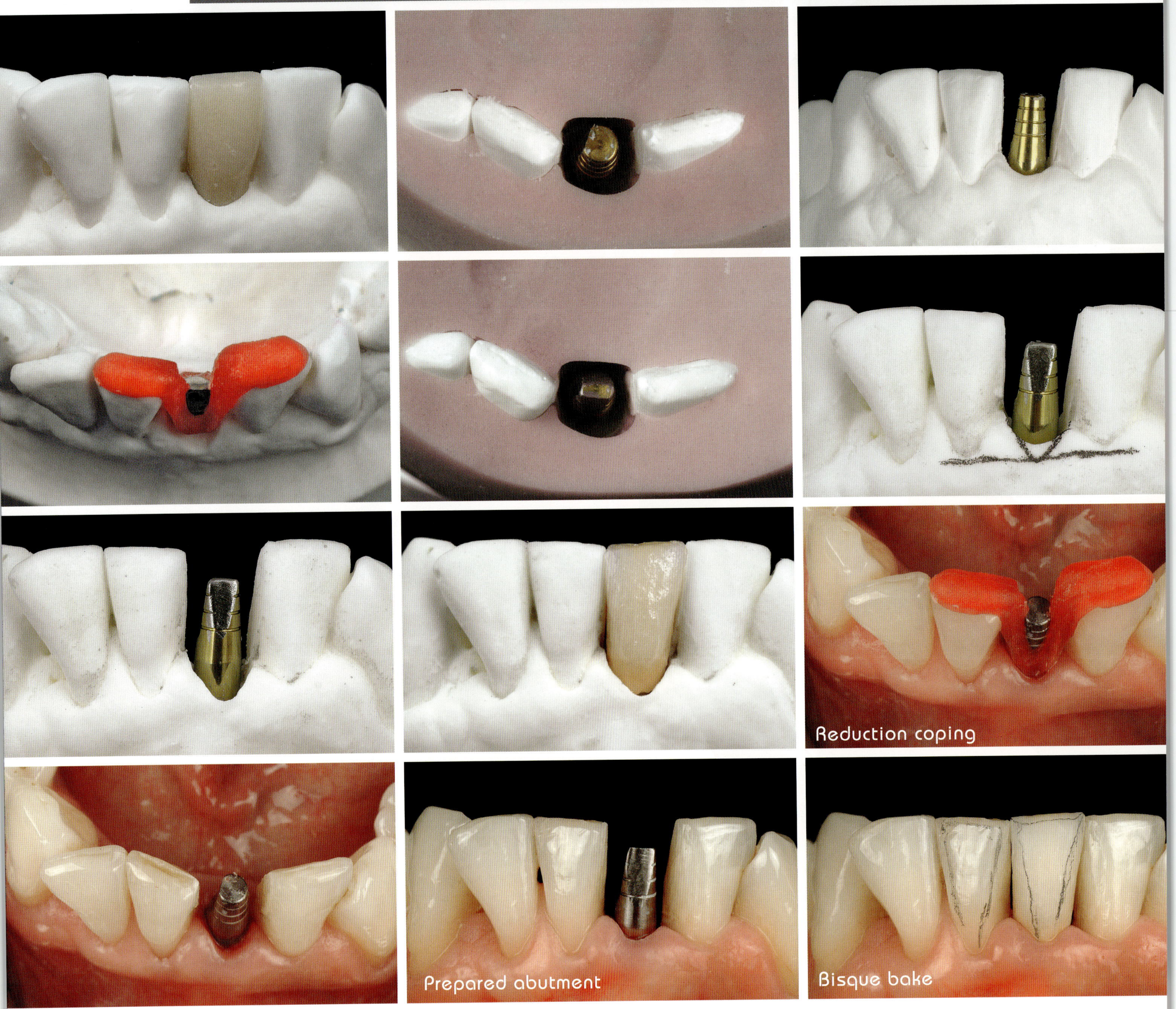

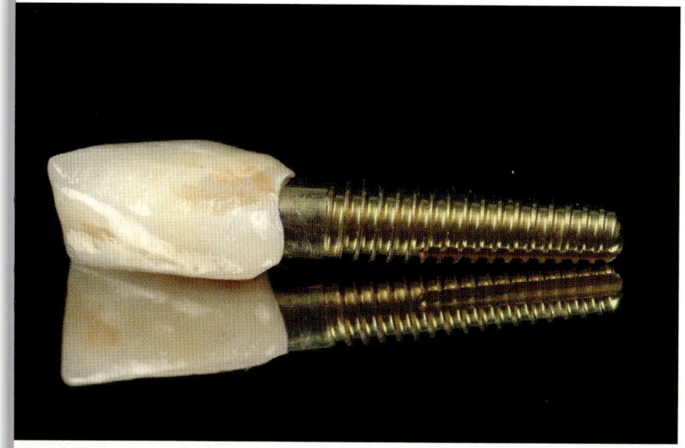

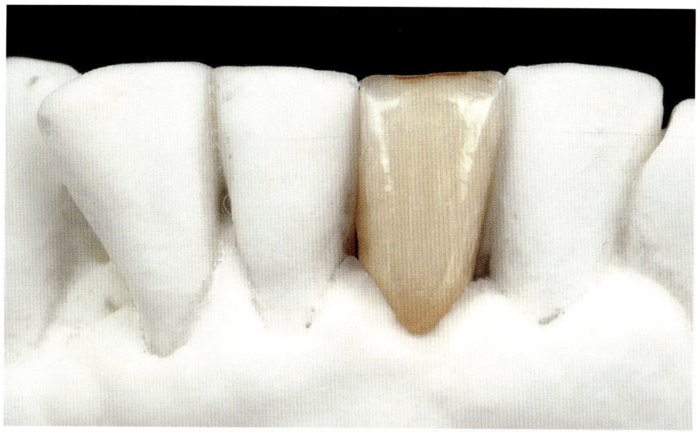

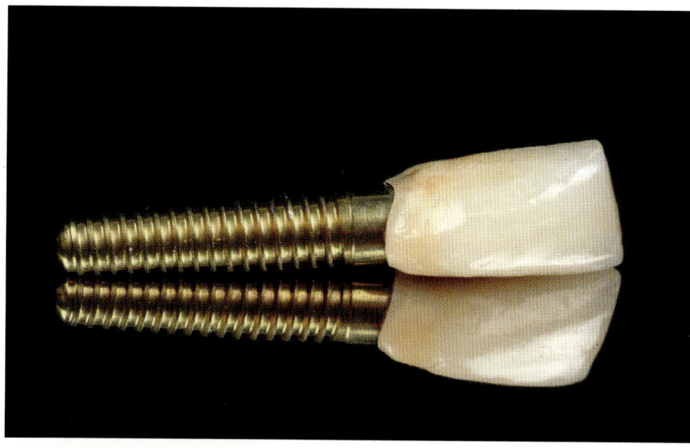

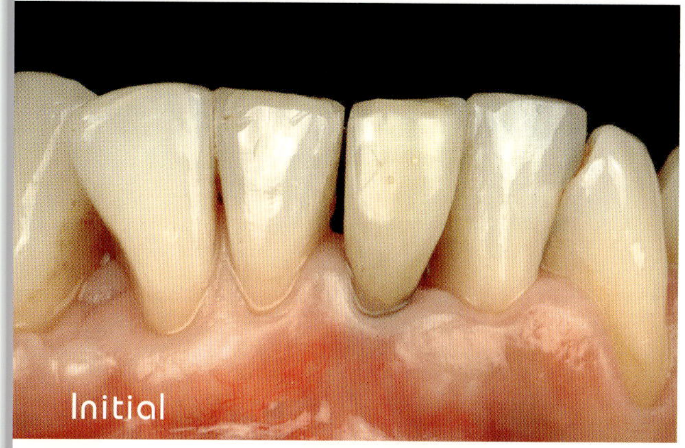

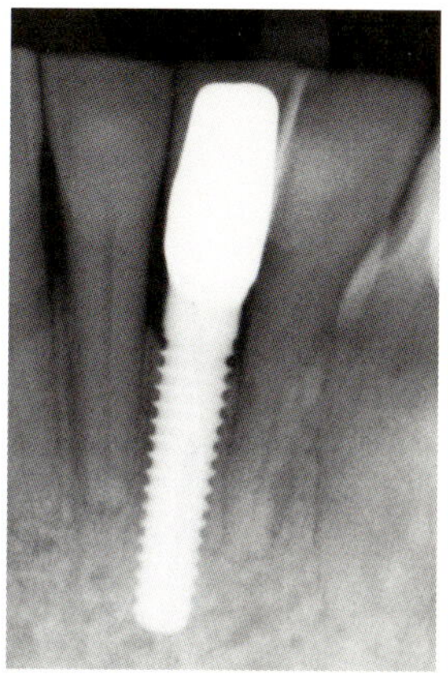

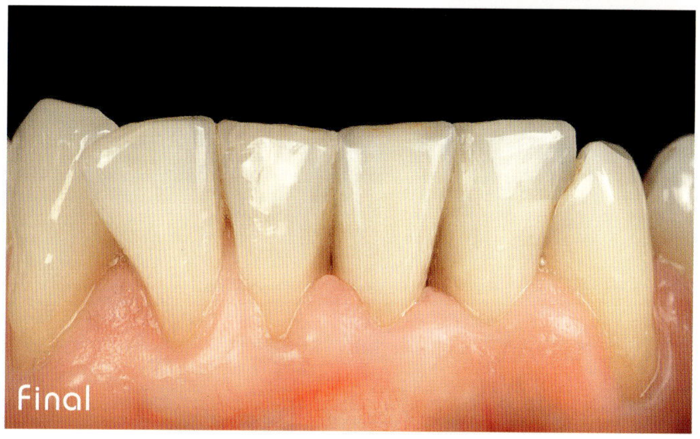

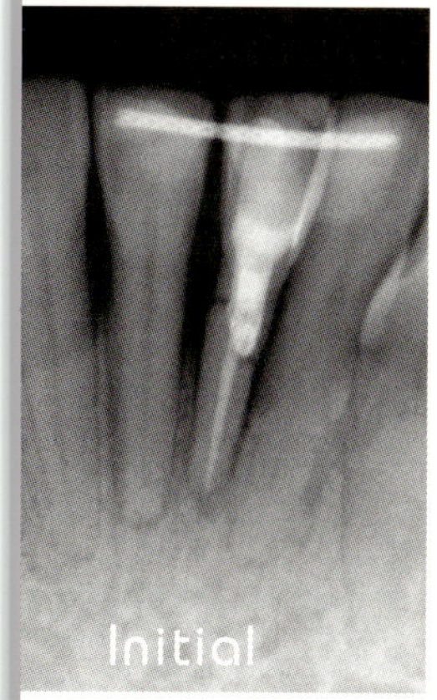

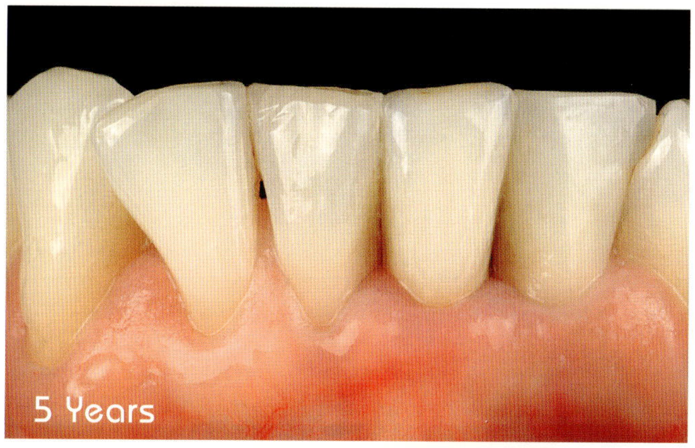

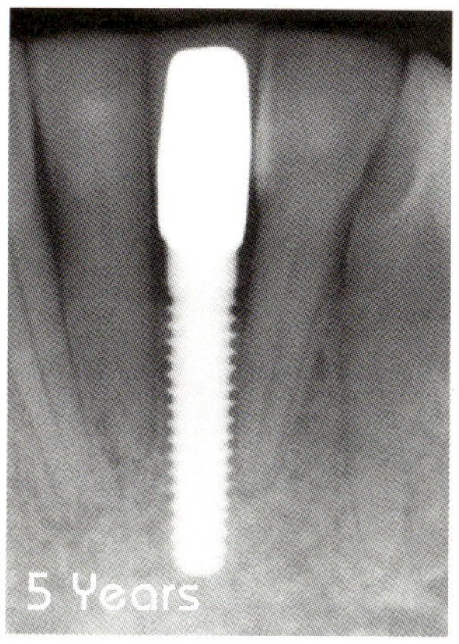

The definitive zirconia crown was refined to completion and cemented to the implant with a universal self-adhesive resin cement. Note the close proximity of the implant to the adjacent teeth, which influences the loss of papillary height over time. Also note the blend of the crown in respect to value and masking abilities.

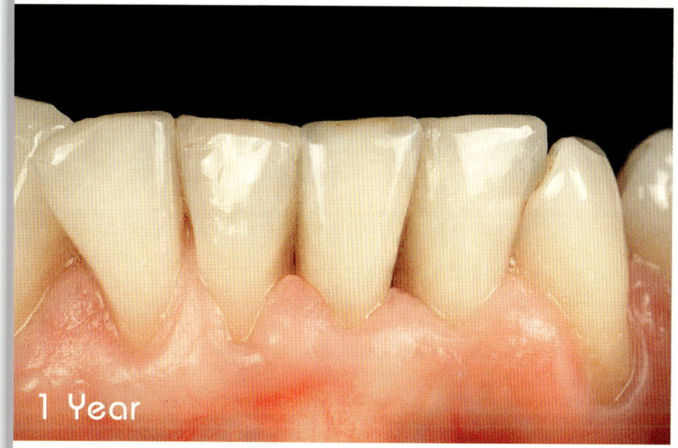

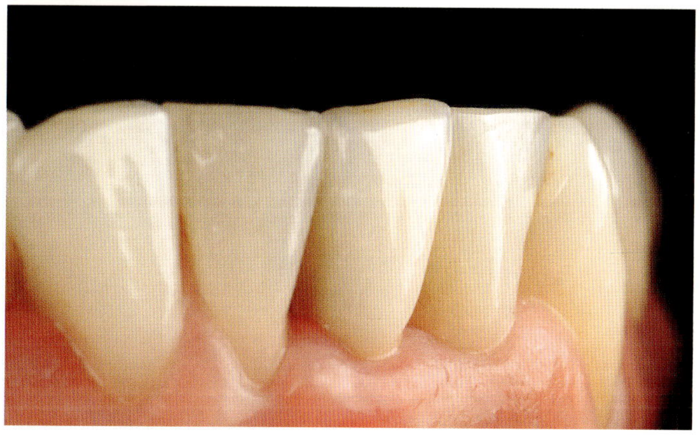

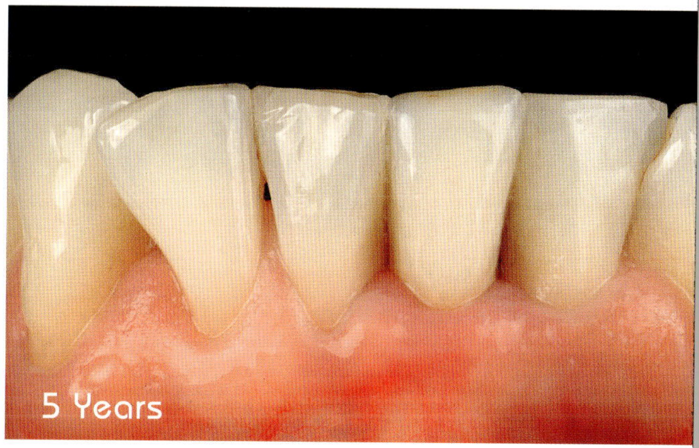

Alumina coping

The densely sintered alumina coping is one of the best materials when it comes to blending with the underlying abutment color substructure because of its index of reflection and light-transmission properties.

The thickness of alumina copings is typically 0.4 mm to maximize the blend with the abutment and create esthetic integration.

The patient presented with a fractured crown on her maxillary left central incisor implant. The implant had a ceramic-veneered, screw-retained abutment and a feldspathic ceramic crown cemented on top. Because of the grayish appearance of the peri-implant tissue and the lack of adequate soft tissue thickness, a CTG from the tuberosity was placed to hide the prosthetic implant interface. A crestal tunnel incision technique was performed, and the same abutment was used as a provisional solution with an acrylic crown to provide the patient an esthetically pleasing situation on the first day of the surgical phase. After 6 months of tissue healing, a PVS impression was made to fabricate the definitive zirconia abutment and a corresponding provisional crown.

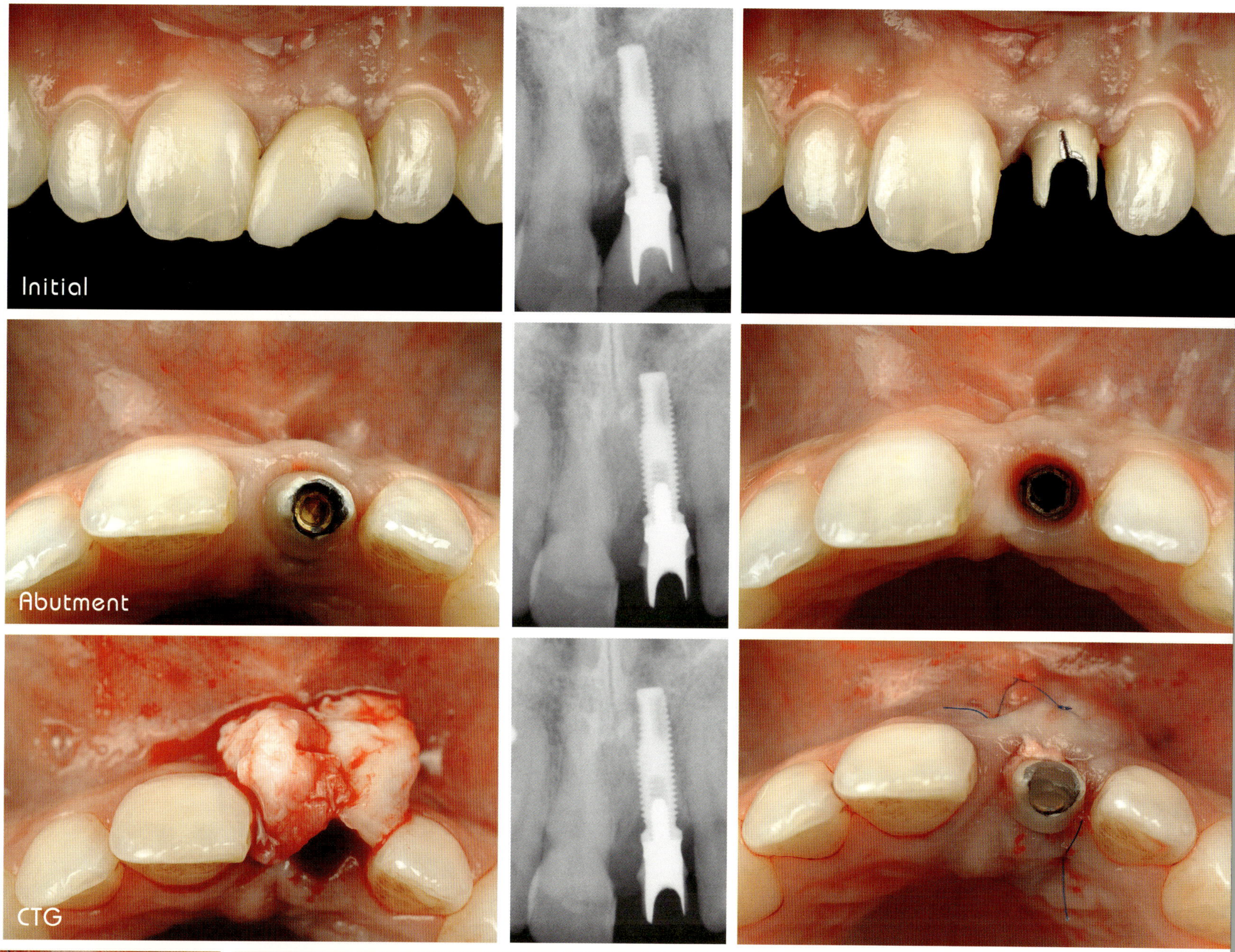

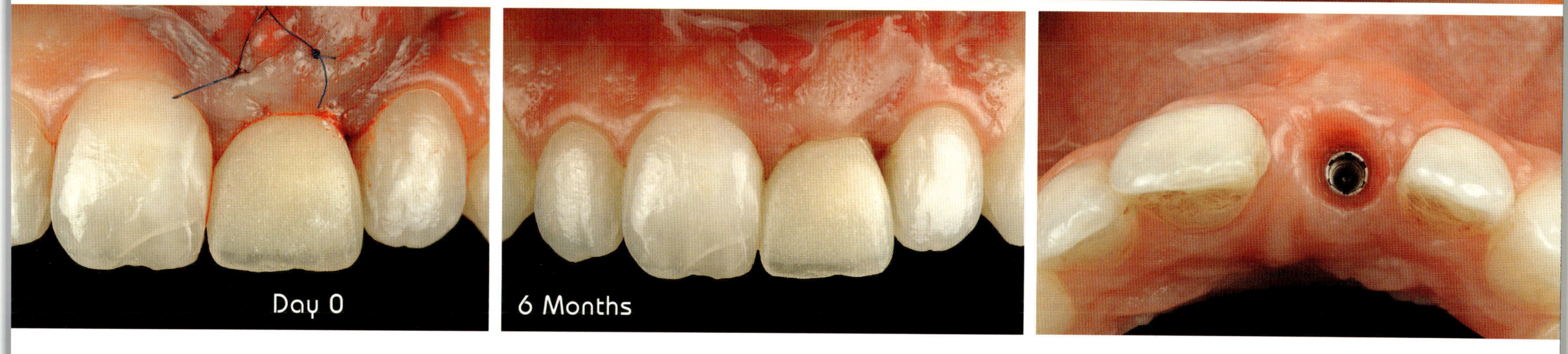

The definitive fluorescent zirconia abutment was delivered to the patient together with the corresponding provisional crown. After 1 month, the soft tissue scallop around the provisional restoration did not blend with the soft tissue contour of the adjacent teeth. A pickup impression of the provisional crown was made to transfer the soft tissue morphology of the adjacent tooth to the master cast. To achieve that, the crown was removed and the abutment unscrewed. An implant analog was attached in the laboratory to the crown-abutment-analog assembly in the pickup impression, and the stone was poured. The resulting master cast provided an exact representation of the clinical situation and critical information for carving of the cast around the implant analog for customized soft tissue conditioning. When the idealized soft tissue situation was carved into the cast, the abutment finish line was located coronally to the desired intracrevicular depth. The finish line was therefore prepared further apically to provide better support for the desired emergence profile. The provisional restoration was relined with acrylic to fill the newly carved space and extended further apically to the prepared finish line.

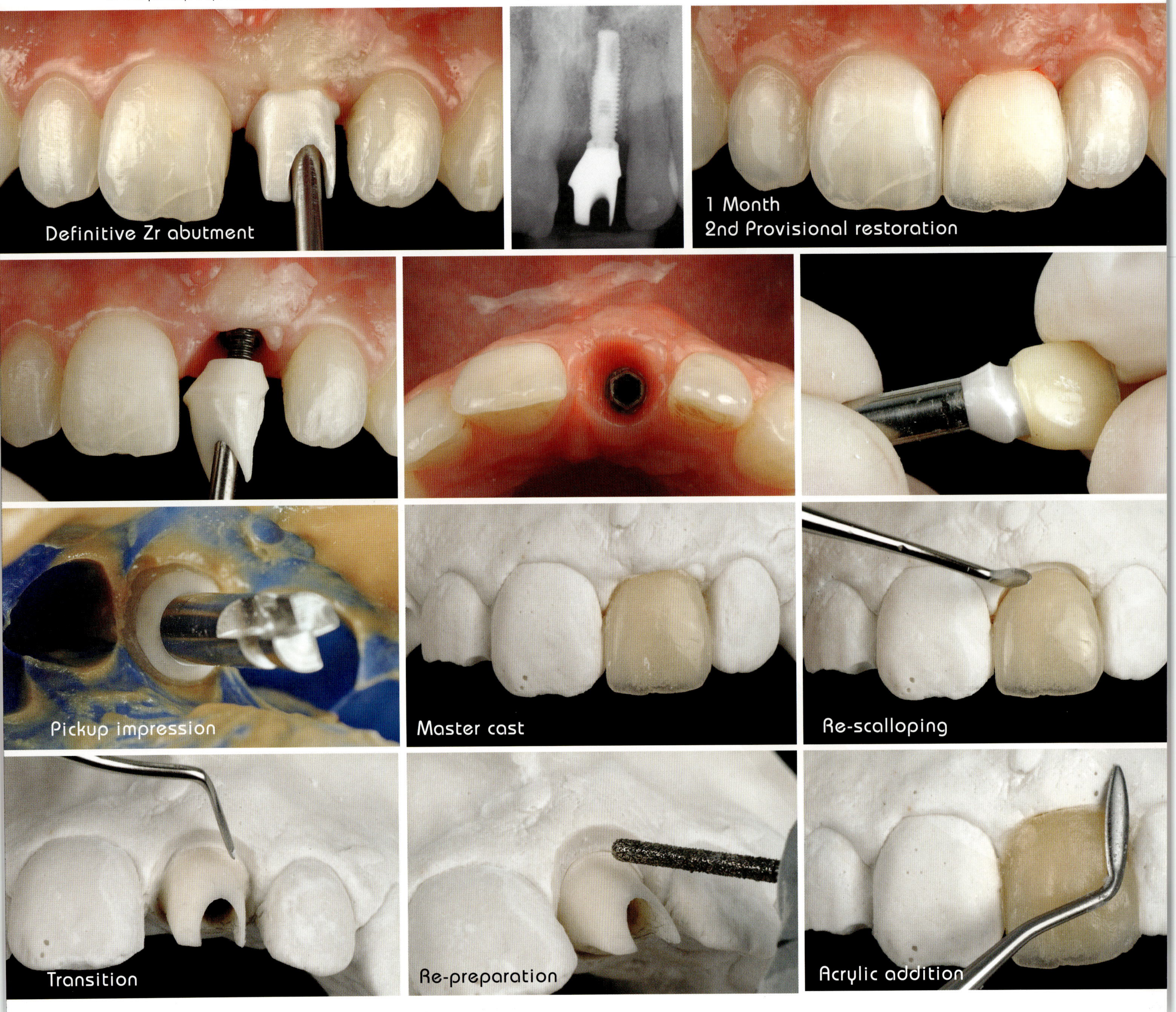

The tissue aspect of the relined provisional restoration was polished, and the transition areas were blended to provide a seamless surface. The abutment was then screwed back onto the implant, and the provisional restoration was cemented, providing improved soft tissue pressure and support. Three months later, the similarity between the soft tissue contour around the implant and the one around the adjacent natural teeth is obvious. An alumina coping was selected for the definitive crown. The higher translucency provides a better blend with the supporting fluorescent abutment. The favorable optical properties of the fluorescent definitive abutment and the crown restoration are obvious under ultraviolet (UV) light and natural light. The idealized soft tissue morphology is stable at the 5-year follow-up.

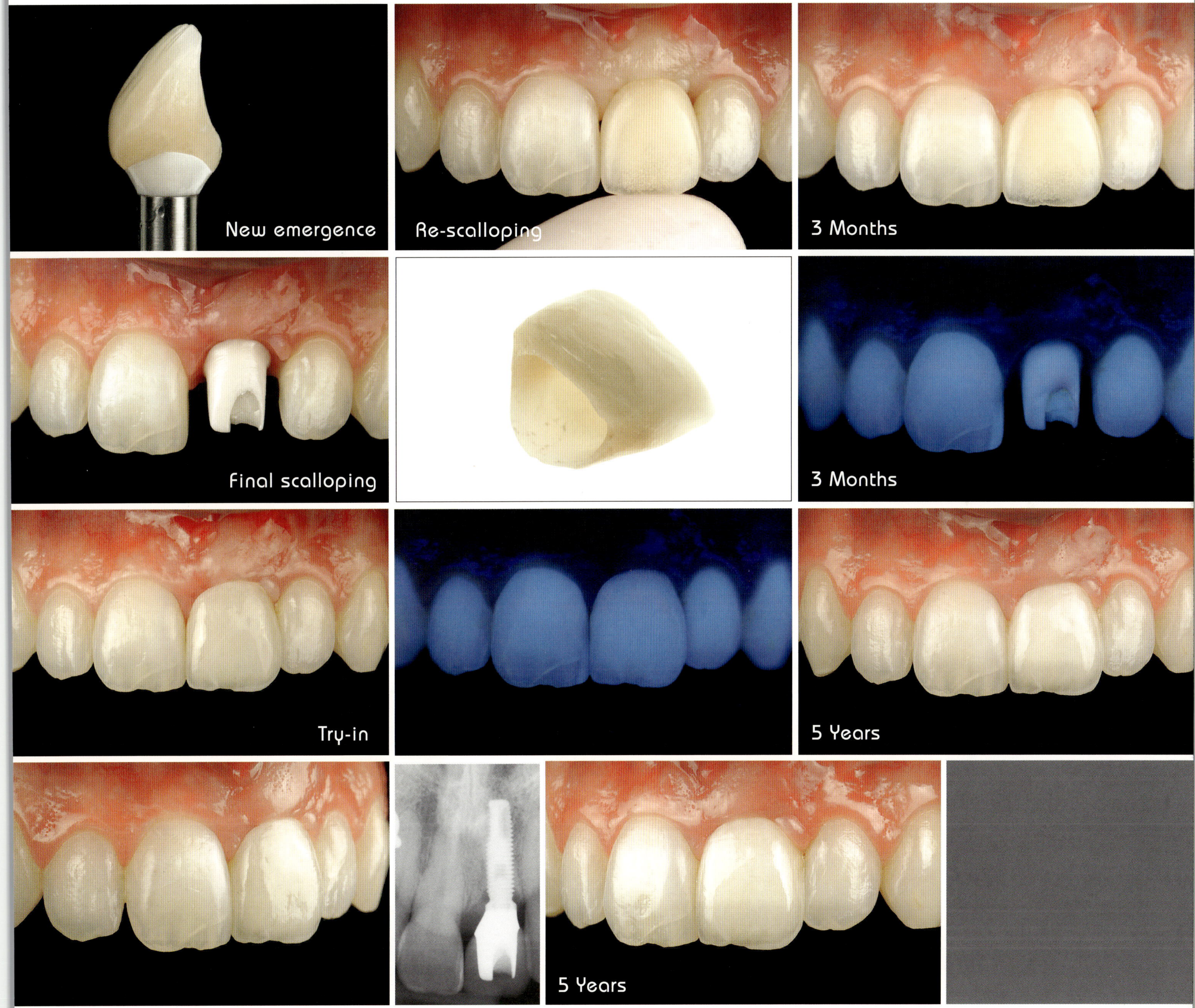

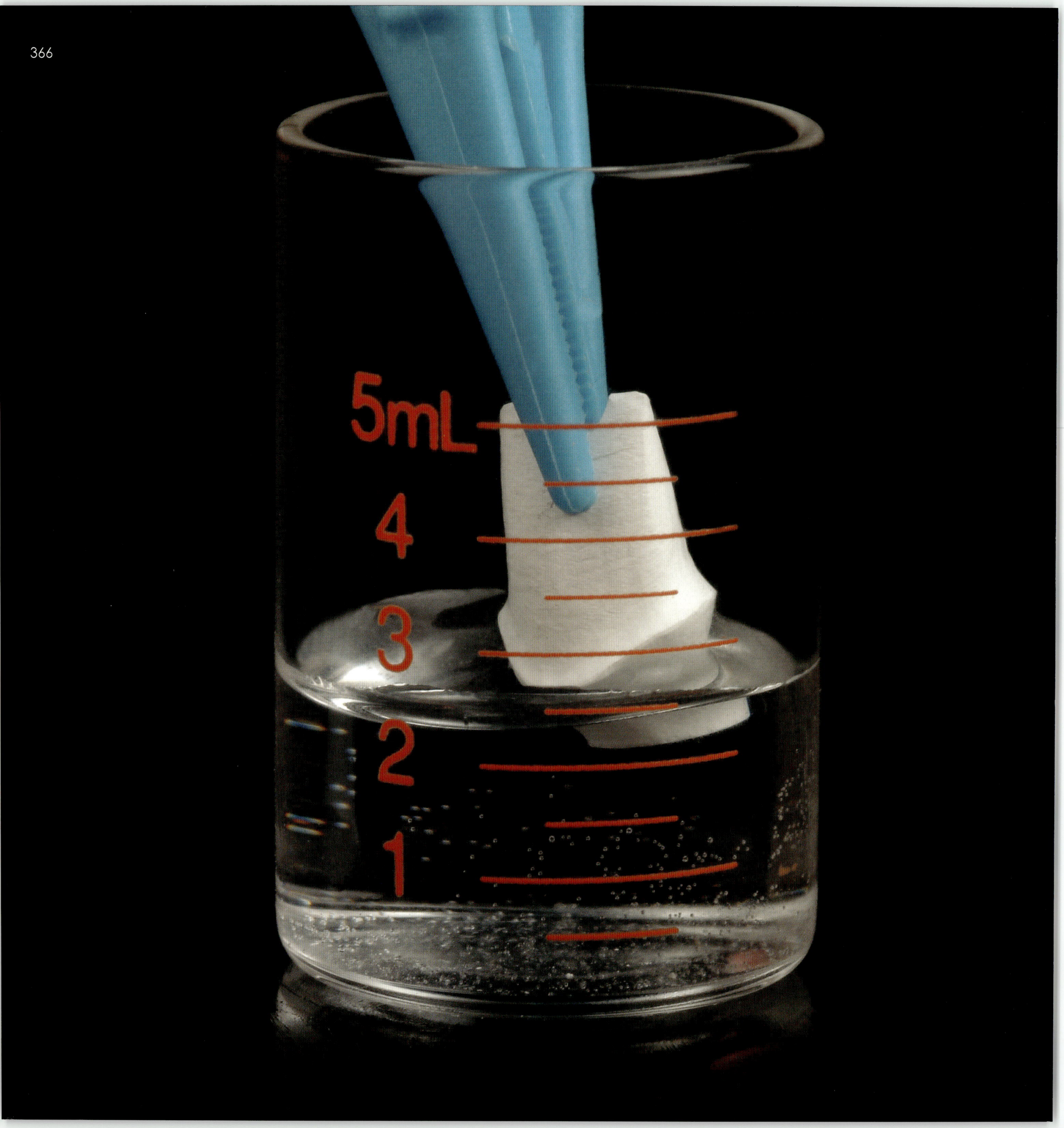
5mL
4
3
2
1

Abutment Material Selection

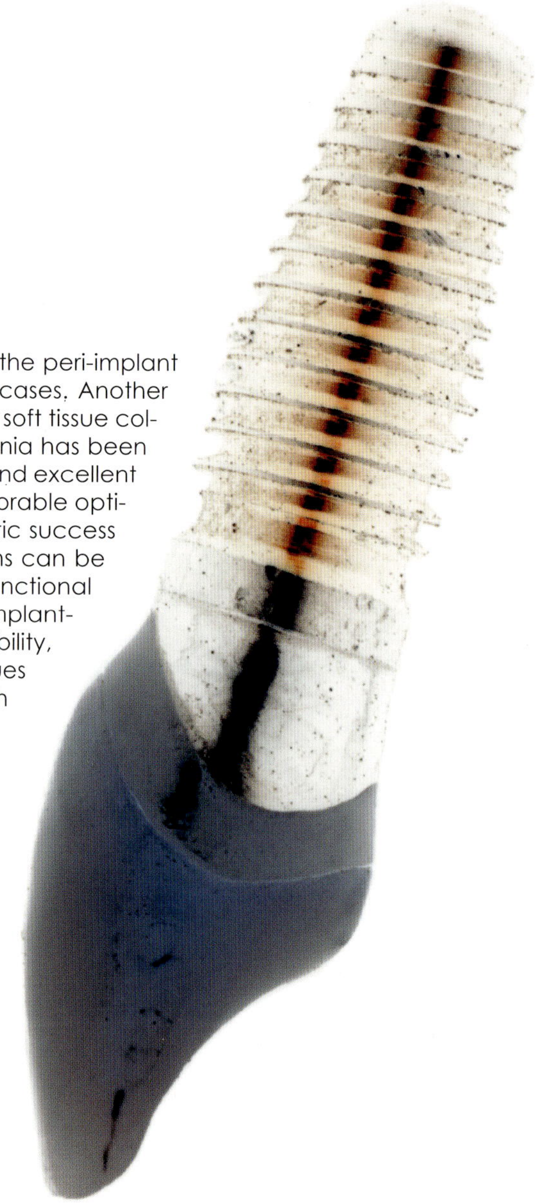

In an evaluation of the soft tissue around single-tooth implant crowns, the color of the peri-implant soft tissue matched that of the reference tooth in no more than one-third of the cases. Another study found that all-ceramic implant abutment and crown materials provide better soft tissue color match with neighboring teeth than conventional metal-alloy components. Zirconia has been shown to be the preferred implant abutment material because of its high strength and excellent biocompatibility. Traditional shortcomings of zirconia include higher cost and unfavorable optical properties regarding color and fluorescence. Influencing parameters for esthetic success and clinical guidelines to avoid the "gray zone" around dental implant restorations can be summarized and categorized into five key factors: *(1)* 3D implant placement for functional and esthetic long-term implant success; *(2)* soft tissue thickness to conceal the implant-restorative interface; *(3)* abutment selection to improve biocompatibility, tissue stability, color, translucency, and fluorescence to provide perfect blend with surrounding tissues and teeth; *(4)* crown restoration to imitate natural teeth; and *(5)* the lip line, which may greatly influence the final outcome. Mimicking the inherent optical properties, especially fluorescence, of natural teeth with idealized prosthetic implant components and crown materials is fundamental for ultimate restorative and soft tissue esthetics.

A simple but essential guideline is to position the implant as close as possible to where the natural tooth was or ideally would be. If a line were to be drawn at the center of the implant along its long axis and extended through the tooth restoration, it should run through the center of the incisal edge of the prospective tooth. The greater the 3D mismatch between the crown and the implant body positions, the poorer and less stable the final outcome will be.

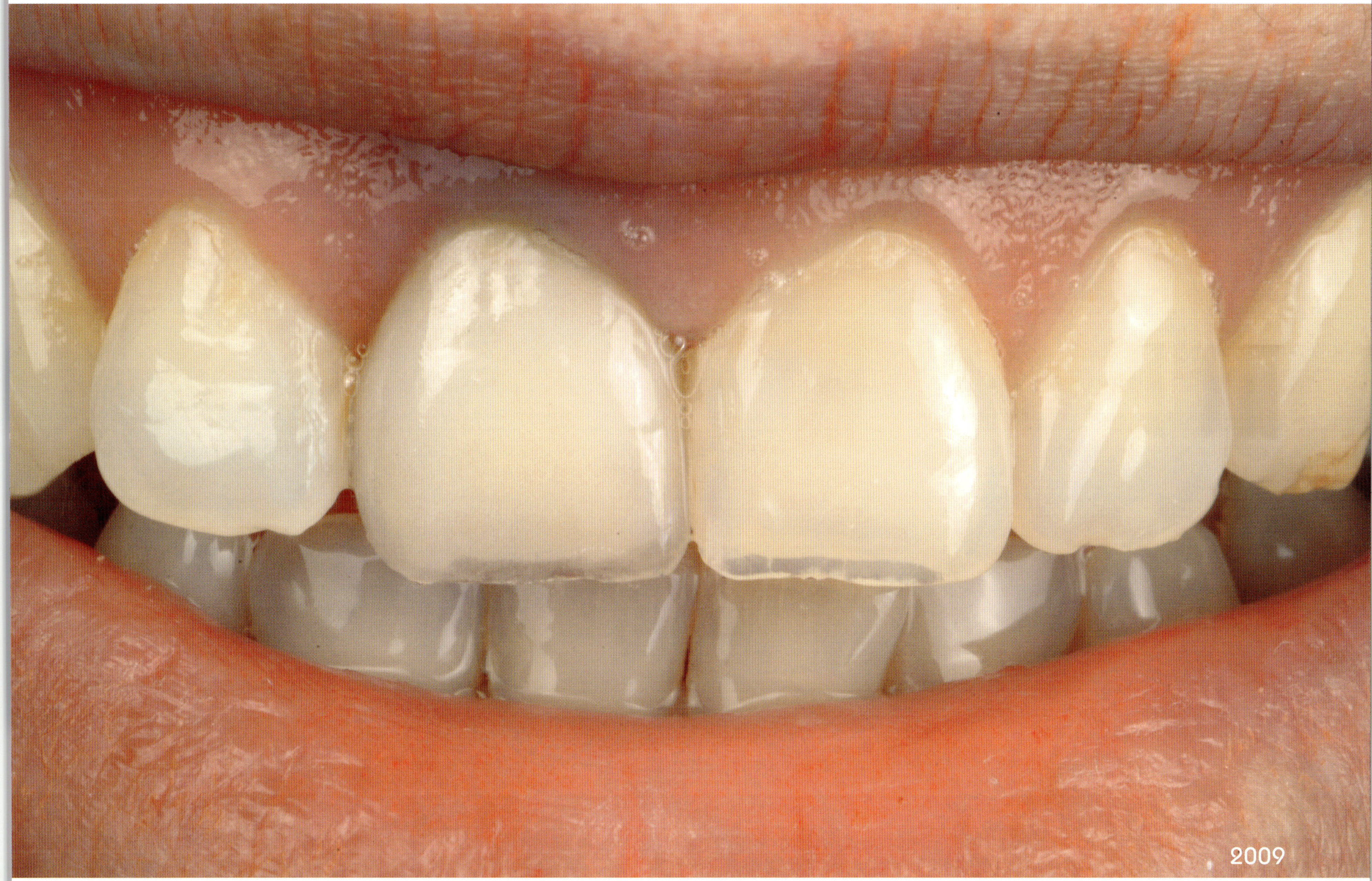

A single implant was placed immediately after extraction of the maxillary right central incisor and without any hard or soft tissue augmentation. A modified metal-alloy abutment was fabricated, and the definitive restoration was inserted in 1999. A smile photograph taken 10 years postoperatively reveals a grayish appearance of the soft tissue surrounding the implant restoration.

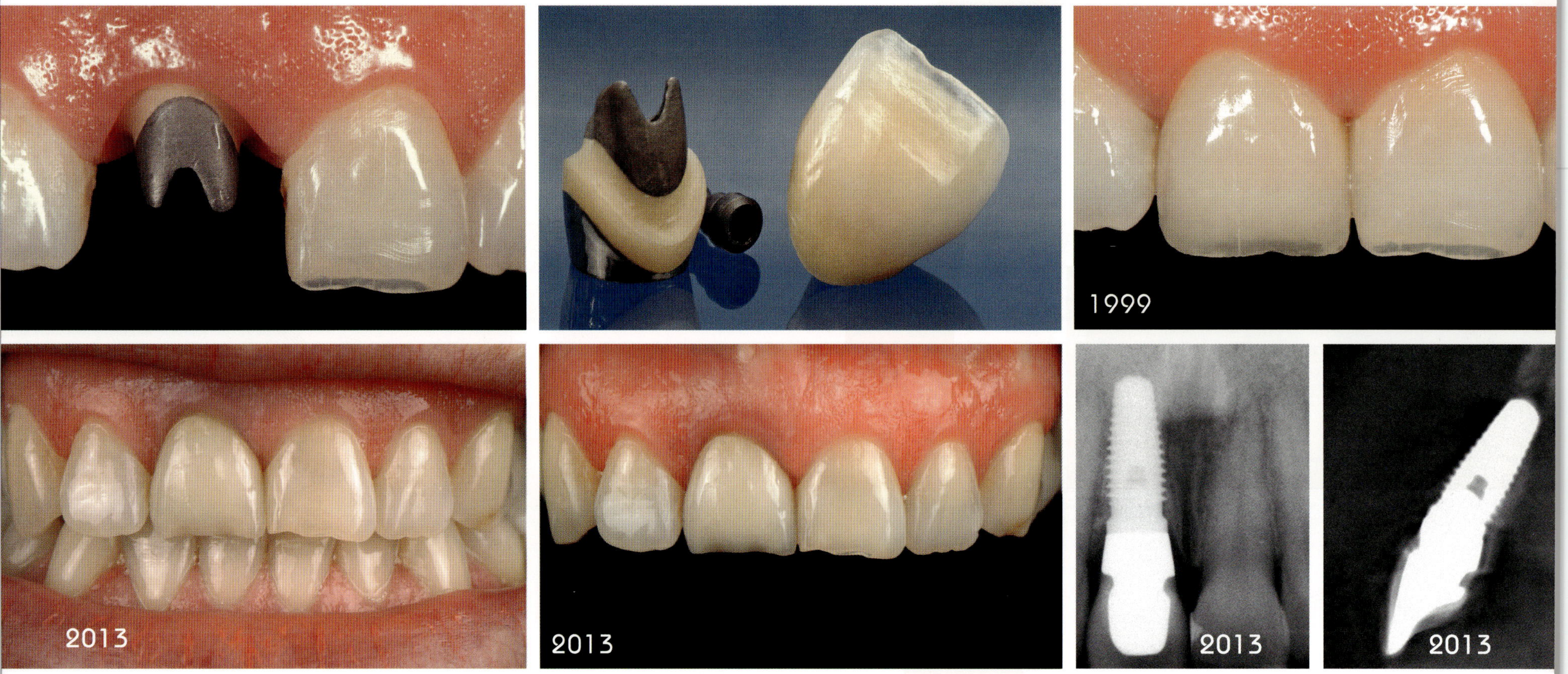

Even when the implant was placed in an ideal manner, the esthetic outcome may become increasingly compromised over time because of subsequent resorption of the marginal bone and soft tissues. This seems to have occurred here, where, 14 years after completion, the surrounding soft tissues reveal the unfavorably gray color of the metal implant abutment.

It is therefore advisable to maximize tissue thickness in every case and for both delayed and immediate implant placement. In fact, the mucosal characteristics of the peri-implant tissues necessitate connective tissue grafting.

Thicker peri-implant soft tissue masks the implant-abutment-restoration interface and provides a better color match between the soft tissues around the implant and those around the neighboring teeth.

Evolution of the case completed 14 years earlier is shown. At that time, a UCLA-type PFM abutment was used to create the best gingival integration of the restoration. Subsequently, the tissues have thinned and bone resorption has taken place, leading to the dark appearance of the tissue, which is also due to the metal collar of the abutment and the umbrella effect provided by the upper lip when smiling.

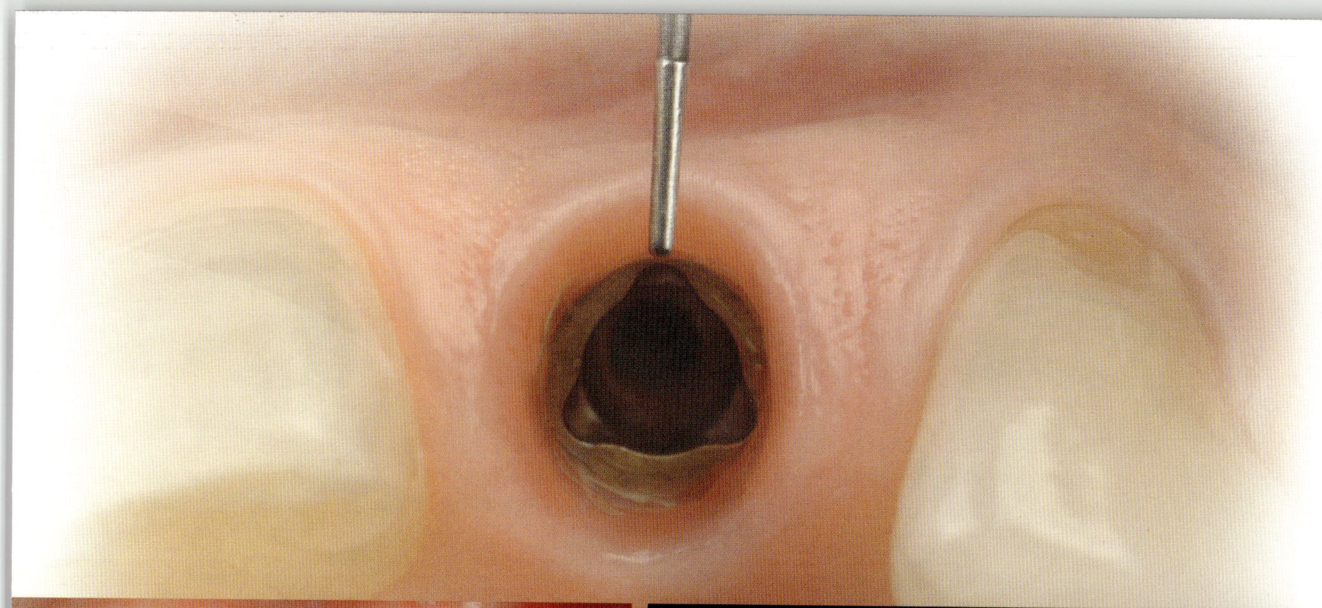

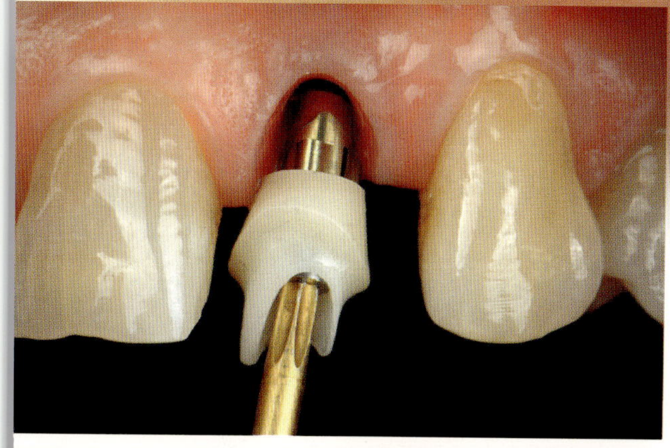

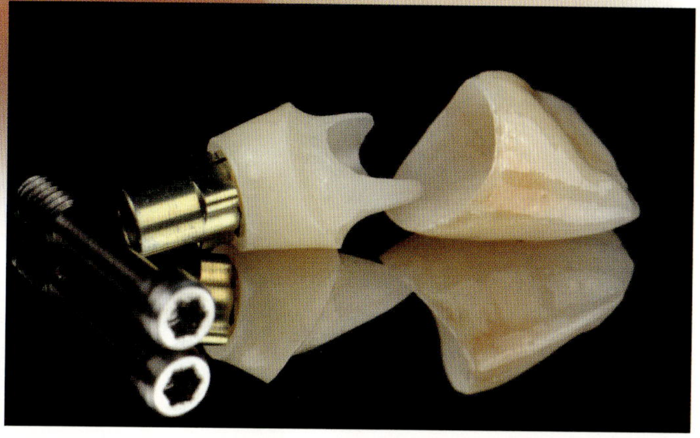

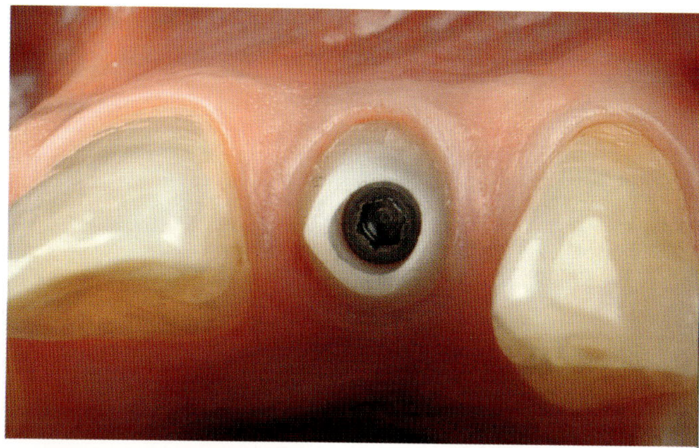

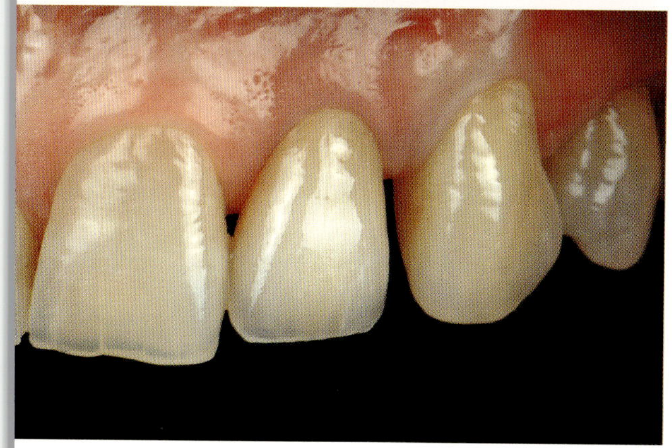

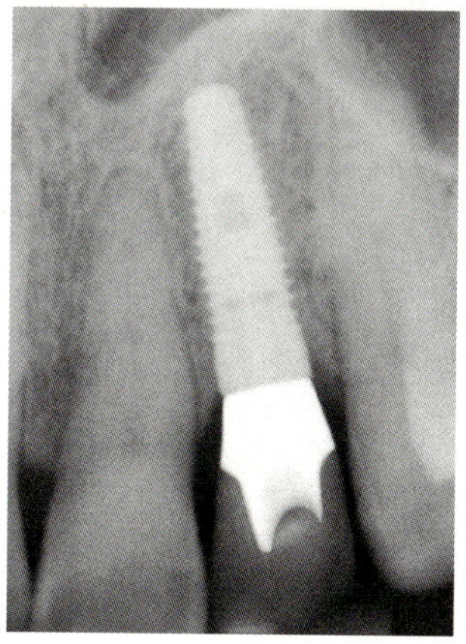

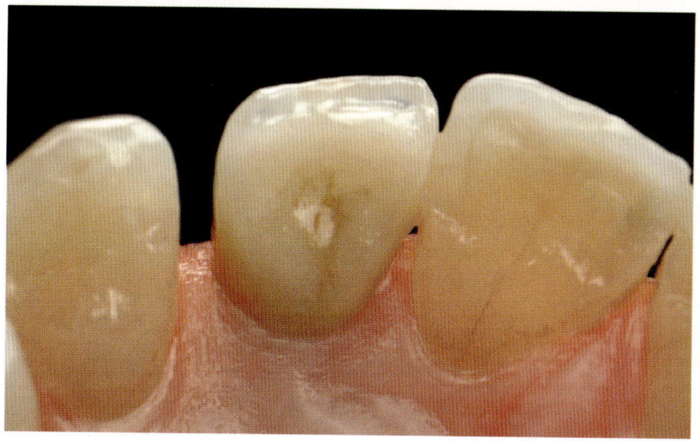

A colored instead of a white zirconia abutment was placed because of the thin labial soft tissue, which was less than 1 mm in thickness. This approach combined with adequate soft tissue support and contour provided a satisfying outcome.

Colored zirconia abutments in different shade ranges further improve esthetic outcomes over the conventional white zirconia. In situations with thin soft tissue, however, fluorescence may actually play a greater role than color.

Some basic guidelines for tissue thickness and abutment selection include the following:

- Soft tissue thickness greater than 3 to 4 mm allows for the use of titanium or zirconia abutments without esthetic implications
- Thin tissue of less than 3 mm requires either a CTG or a zirconia abutment
- Dentin-colored abutments are possible

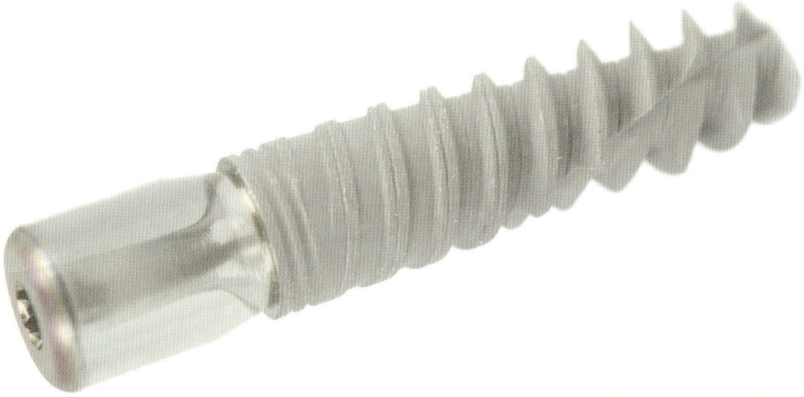

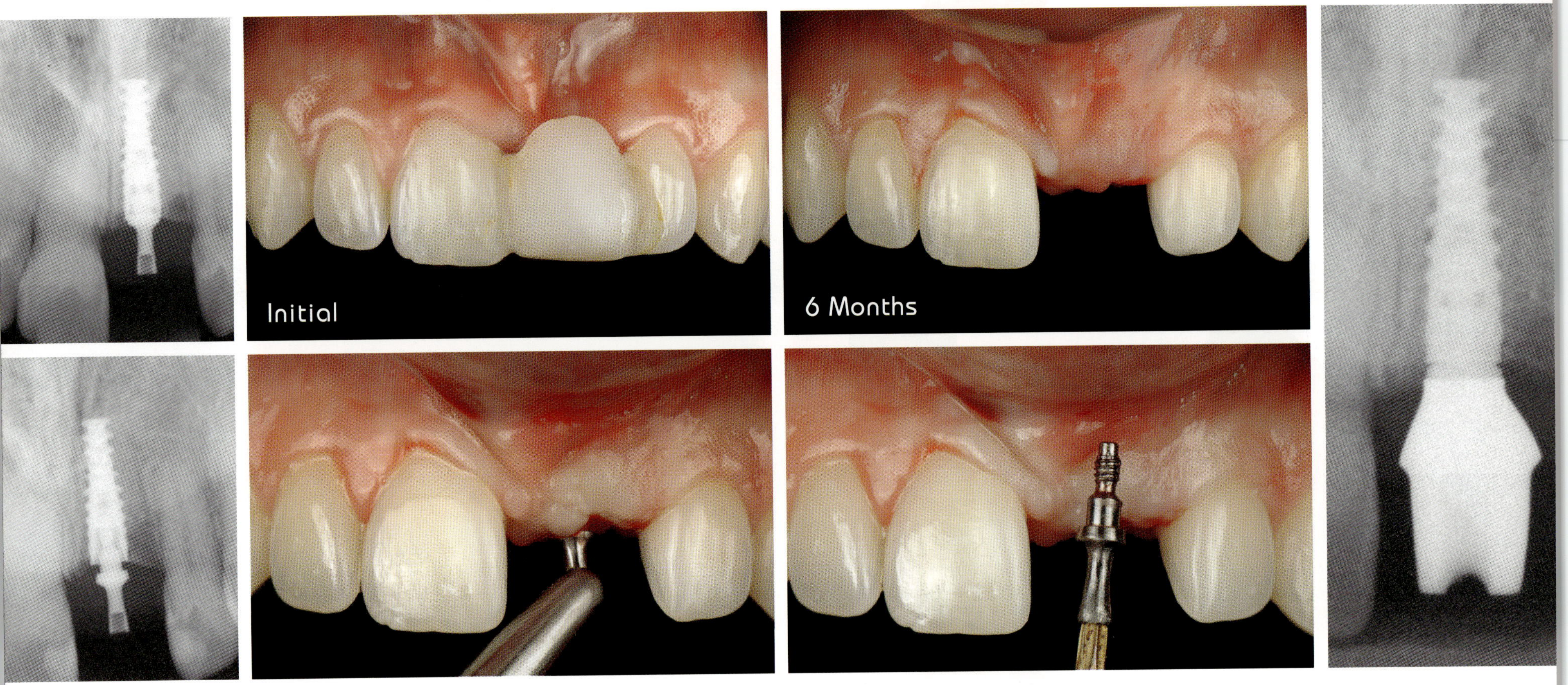

The missing maxillary left central incisor was replaced with a dental implant. An ideal 3D implant placement was planned during stage-one surgery, and the implant (3.5 × 13–mm NobelActive) was inserted with a straight 5-mm healing abutment to be able to coronally suture the CTG, which was harvested from the maxillary tuberosity and placed to increase tissue thickness. The photograph shows the augmented edentulous ridge 6 months post-operatively and the massive tissue thickness that was created.

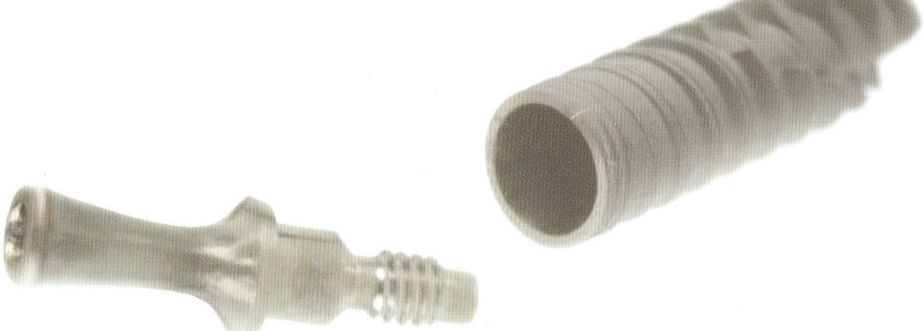

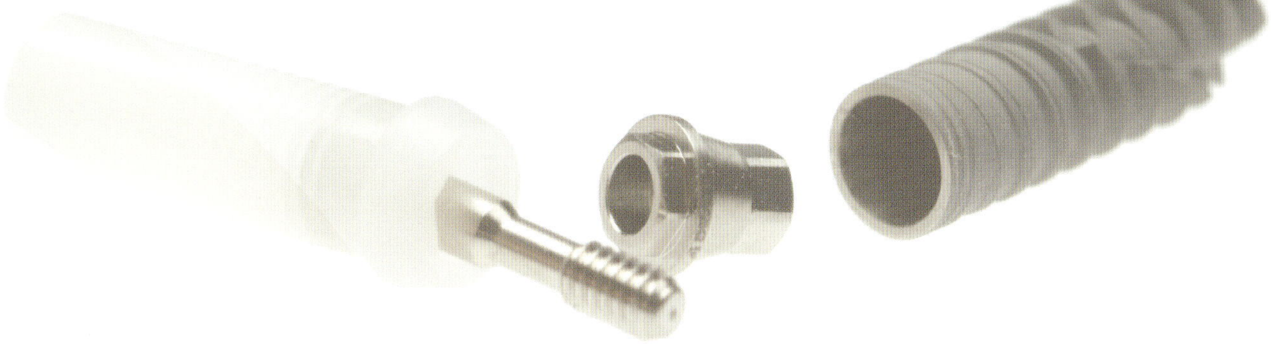

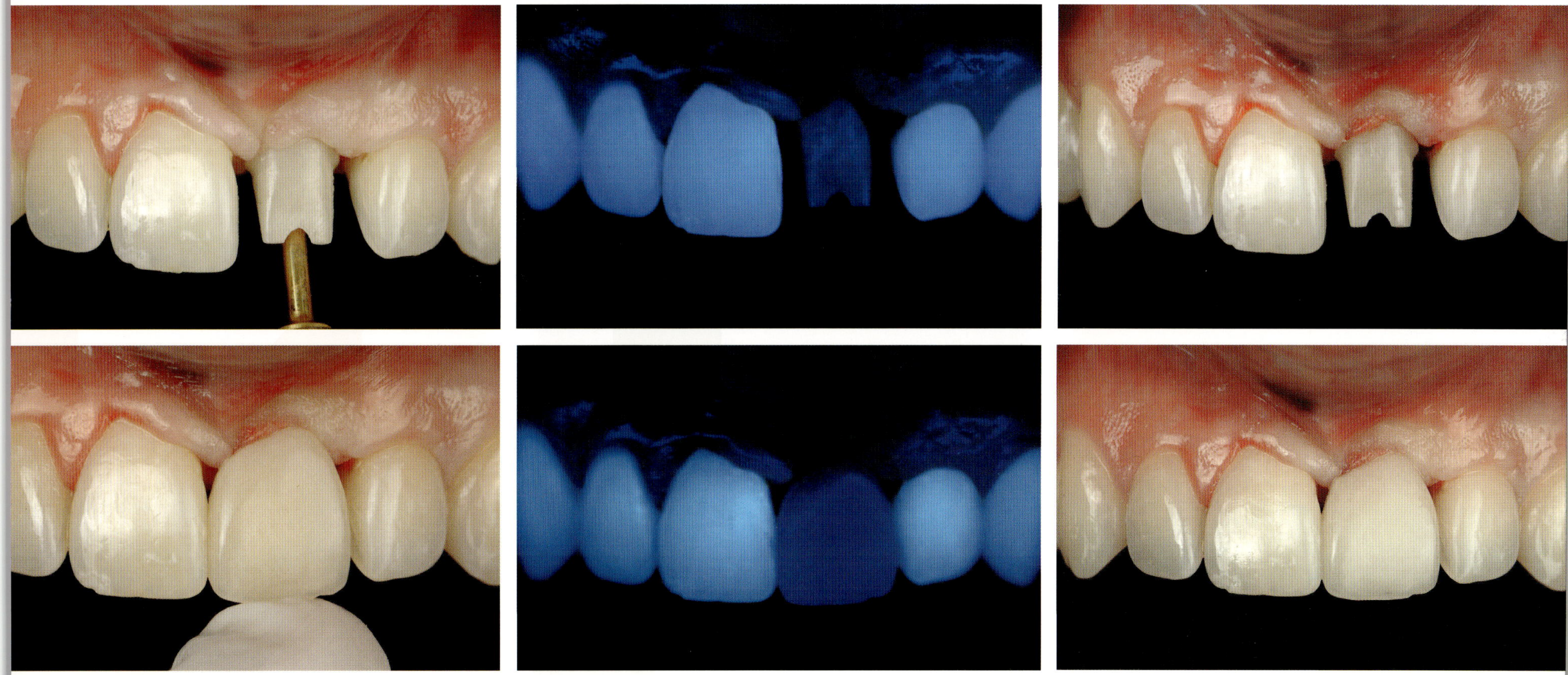

A zirconia abutment was connected to the implant, and a provisional restoration was fabricated, relined in the oral cavity, and cemented with provisional cement on day 1 of the prosthetic phase. The choice of metal connection for the zirconia abutment is preferred in situations in which maximum load is exerted on the connection while the abutment is screwed in place and large amounts of soft tissue are displaced. Different light conditions (natural and UV light) reveal the optical shortcomings of these materials, especially lack of natural fluorescence.

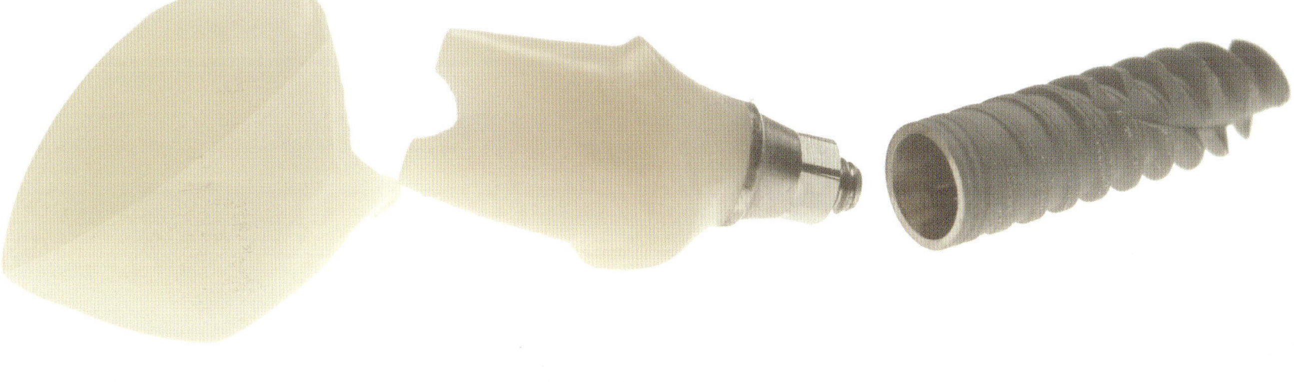

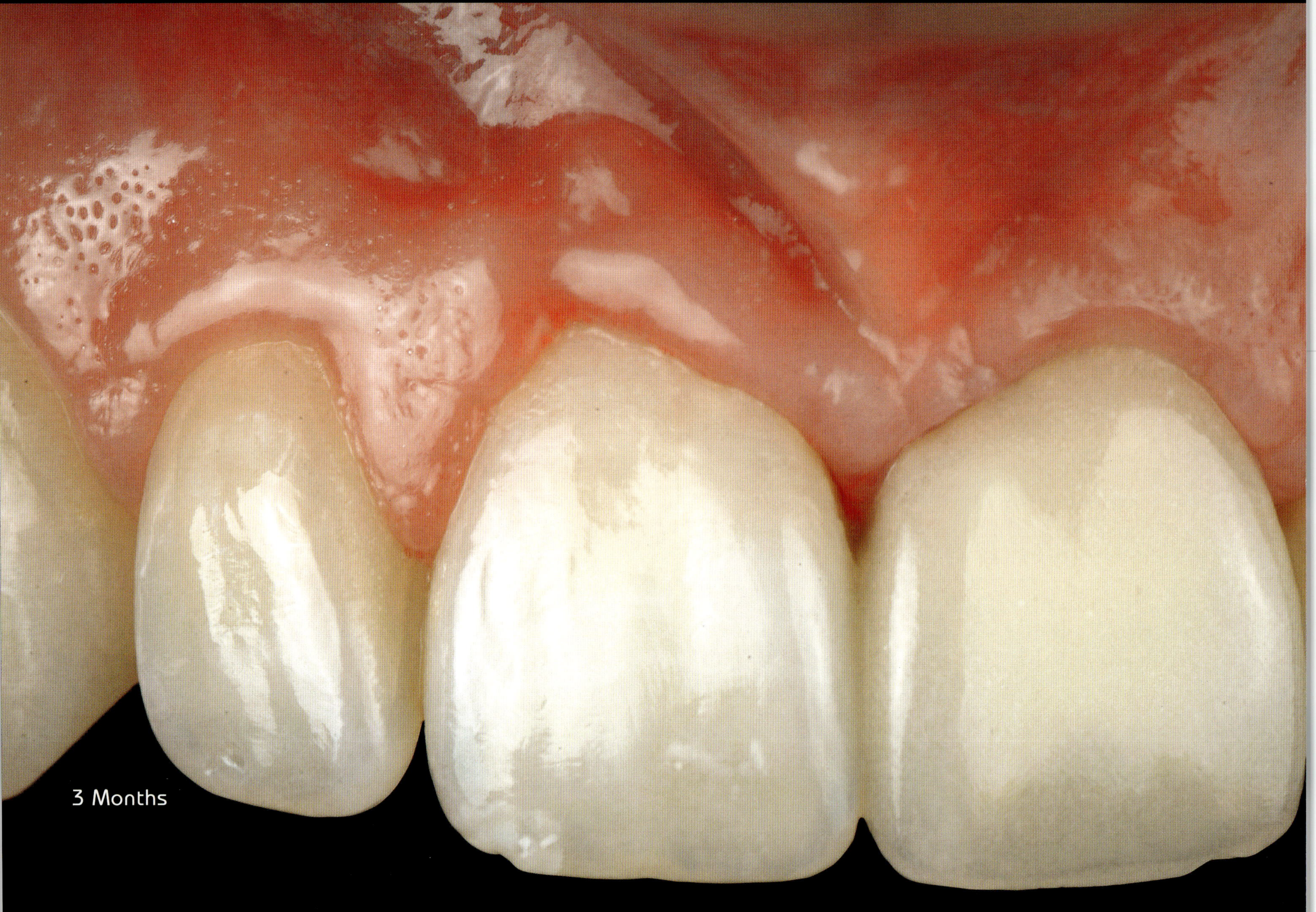

3 Months

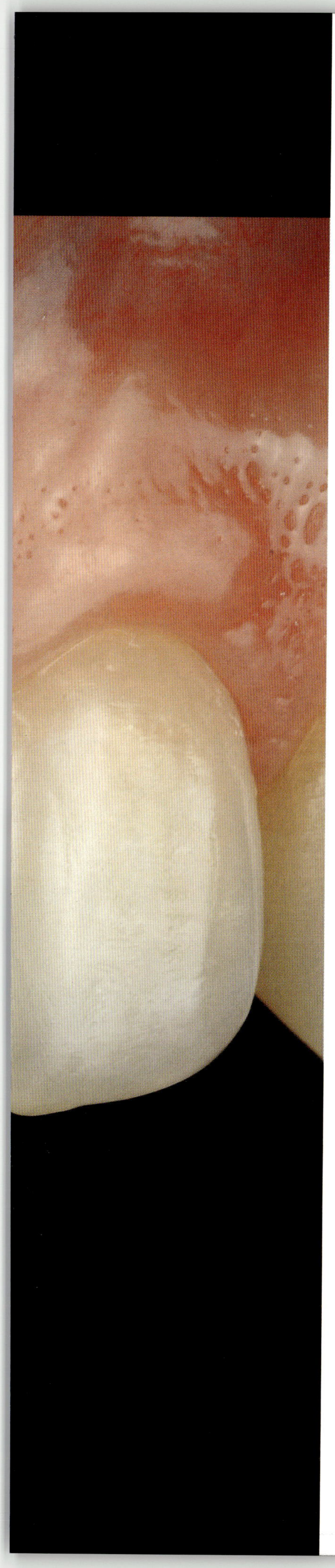

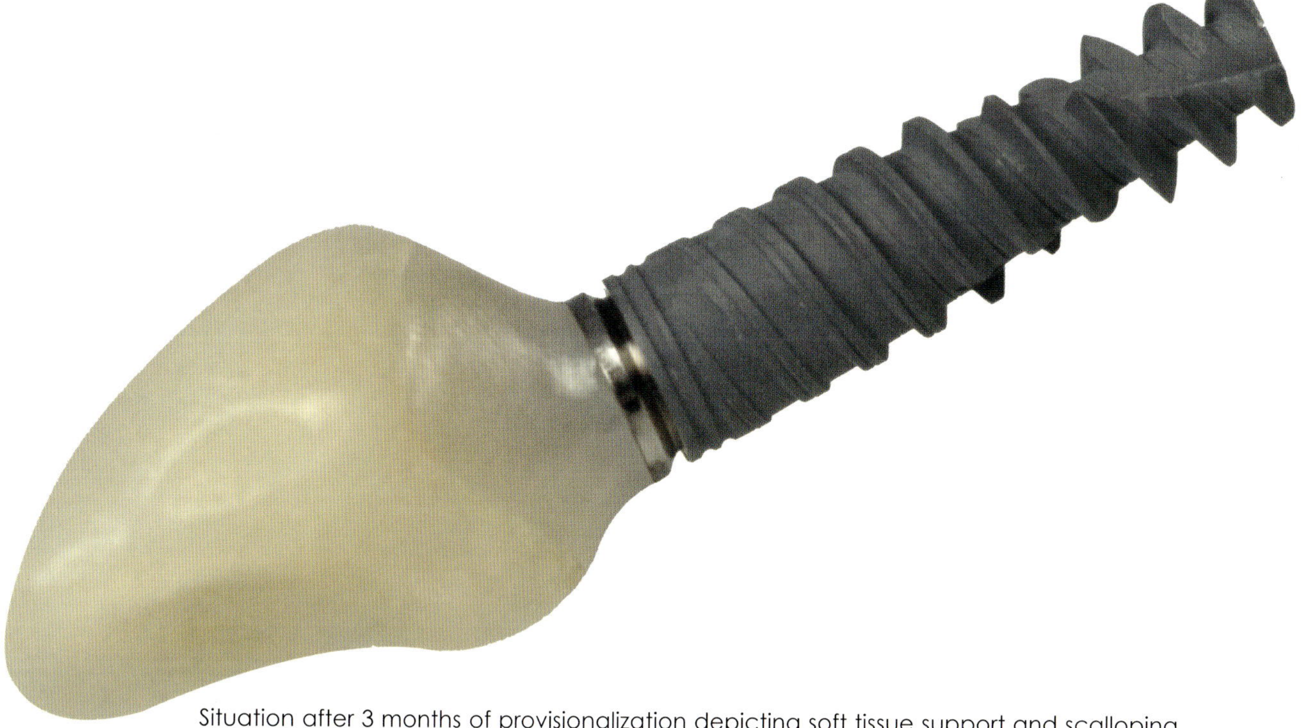

Situation after 3 months of provisionalization depicting soft tissue support and scalloping. A minimum of a 3-month waiting period should be observed.

The image on this page shows cross sections of natural teeth with a polarizing filter.

A goal in esthetic restorative dentistry is to mimic the optical properties of natural teeth. Modern veneering porcelains and ceramic coping materials are intended to mimic the optical qualities of natural teeth: translucency, color (hue, chroma, value), fluorescence, and opalescence. These characteristics are crucial not only for the restoration itself but also to reduce a "shadowing effect" at the restorative-gingival interface and to provide a healthy-looking gingival architecture. In fact, the creation of an inconspicuous dental restoration starts with well-designed prosthetic contours and natural, healthy integration within the surrounding soft tissues.

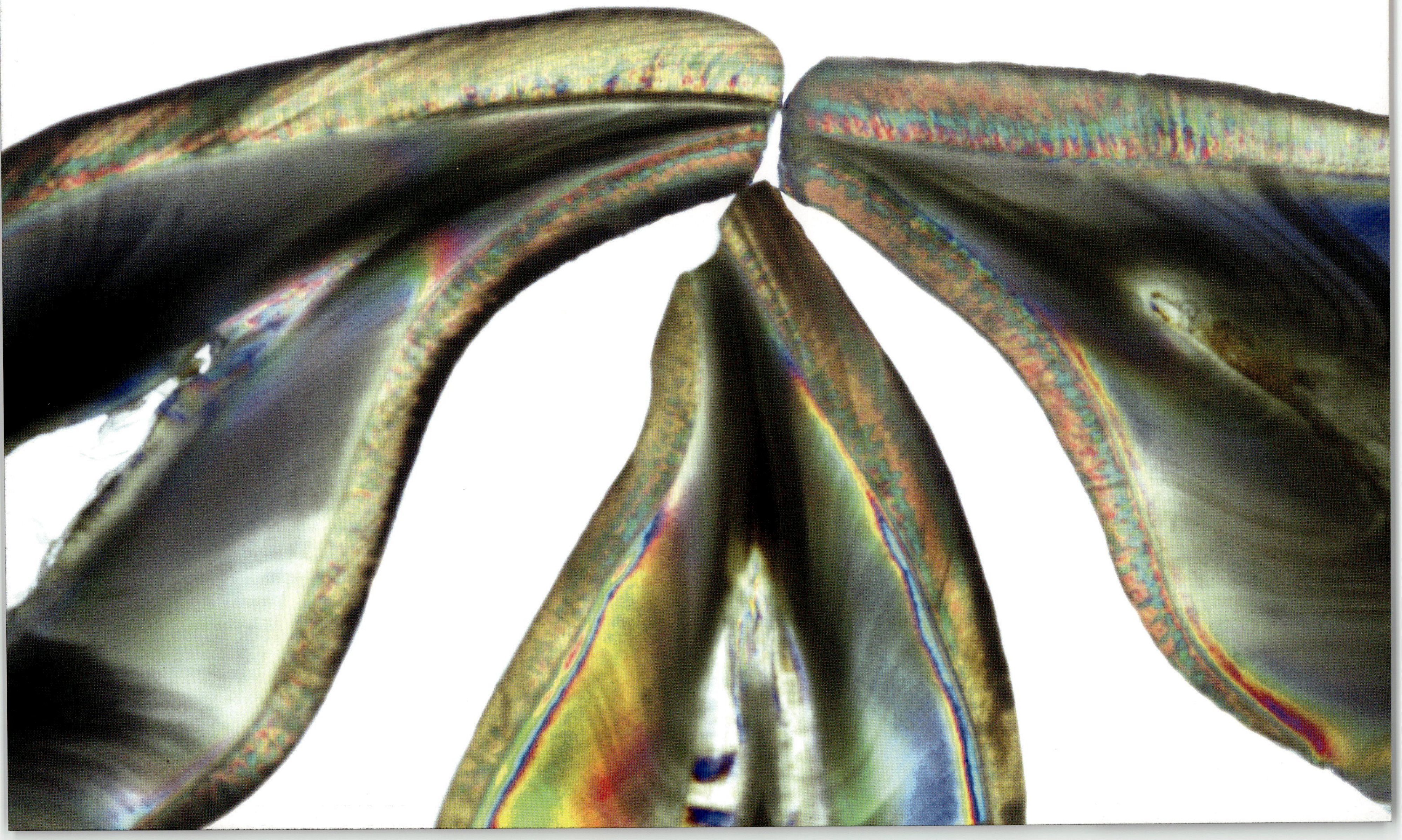

Tooth characteristics under various lighting conditions. Natural teeth provide a certain degree of fluorescence, meaning that they emit visible light when exposed to UV light. However, this important feature is greatly overlooked in restorative dental materials. Fluorescence adds to the vitality of a restoration and minimizes the metameric effect between teeth and restorative materials under various lighting conditions.

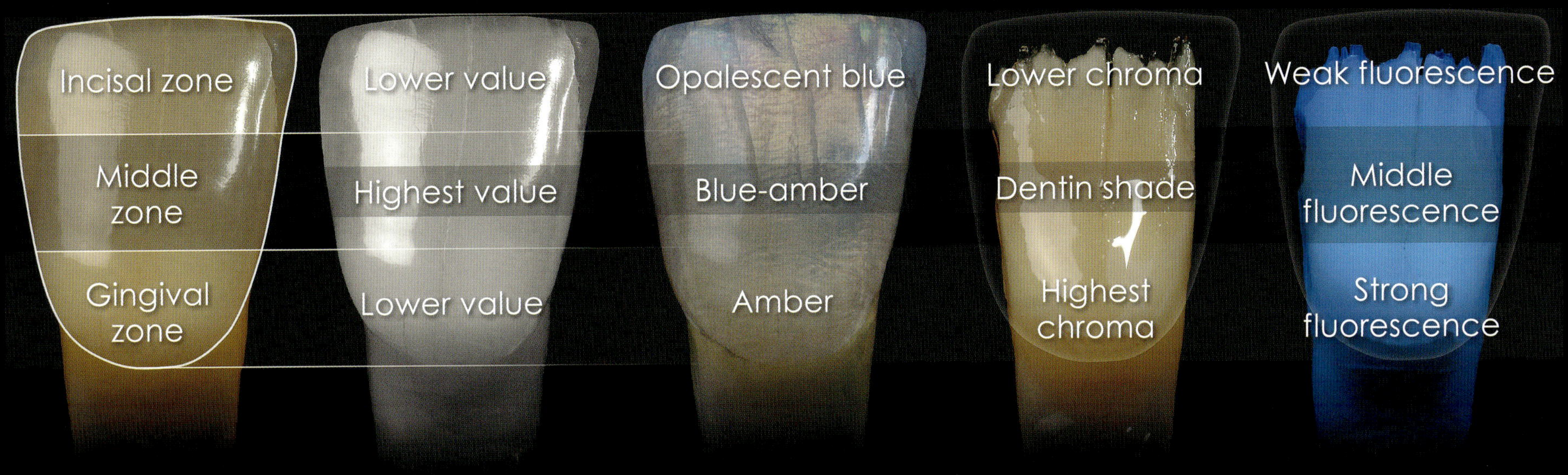

Detailed optical characteristics of natural enamel and dentin under different light sources. Three zones are present on the tooth, showing the three basic zones of color. The base shade is usually on the center of the tooth or middle third of the tooth, which in most situations is the brightest area of the tooth. The gingival zone is usually higher in chroma and lower in value than the incisal zone, which is lower in value, higher in translucency, and lower overall in chroma. Different lighting conditions and different areas of the tooth include the following:

- Natural light
- Black-and-white light
- Polarizing light (only enamel)
- Natural light (only dentin)
- Fluorescent light (only dentin)

Under a polarizing filter, the opalescence of the enamel changes to a bluish color toward the incisal and a more amber color toward the gingival aspect. Looking at the dentin zones only, three distinct zones are evident, with higher chroma in the gingival third and a basic shade on the middle third and in the incisal zone. Under fluorescent light, the dentin has the higher degree of fluorescence, especially in the gingival third due to the higher organic content of the dentin, which explains the vivid look of the teeth in that gingival zone.

Research

Fluorescence

The fact that natural teeth are fluorescent when irradiated with UV light (max = 450 nm) was first described by Stuebel in 1911.[1,2] Subsequent studies demonstrated that dentin has much greater fluorescent properties than enamel,[3,4] due to its higher organic content.[3,5,6] Cementum reveals similar but less intense fluorescence than dentin. Carious enamel and dentin lack fluorescence and appear black or dark brown under UV light,[7–9] making fluorescence a reliable and noninvasive indicator for caries detection.[9–12] It even serves as a screening method for oral cancer because abnormal oral mucosa lesions appear dark brown or black under UV light.[13]

The fluorescent intensity of dentin increases with tooth age. Fluorometric investigations revealed that a complex of cross-linked collagen with hydroxyapatite is a possible fluorescing compound within the tooth tissue.[2,6] When the organic structure of a tooth is affected by, for example, caries or pulpal necrosis, the tooth loses its vitality and appears dark brown in both natural and UV light. Therefore, less fluorescence correlates with lesser value.

Fluorescence is one of several key optical properties to create dental restorations that match the appearance of natural teeth. Modern resin composites for anterior tooth restorations contain fluorescent pigments to simulate the optical properties of natural teeth in all types of light.[14–16] Like natural dentin, many composites have fluorescence wavelength peaks at 440 to 450 nm, while others lack this important feature.[14,15]

Modern ceramic veneering and coping materials are intended to mimic all optical qualities of natural teeth: translucency, color (hue, chroma, value), fluorescence, and opalescence. Feldspathic veneering porcelains and stains typically contain particles that provide fluorescence.[17] However, fluorescence is often not homogenous within the same or among different porcelain systems.[17] Various techniques and contents have been suggested to achieve natural tooth–like fluorescence in ceramic materials.[18–20]

Proper positioning of varying degrees of fluorescence between enamel and dentin and in different areas of the tooth is crucial for natural esthetics. Fluorescence is the strongest in root cementum and gingival areas[3–6] and therefore a key factor in implant dentistry, where these areas are entirely replaced by dental materials. Zirconia has gained tremendous popularity as an implant abutment material in the esthetic zone because it prevents the grayish appearance of the surrounding soft tissues often seen with titanium or other metal-alloy abutments.[21] The availability of colored zirconia abutments in different shade ranges further adds to its esthetic potential. In thin soft tissue situations, however, fluorescence may actually play a greater role than shade. Fluorescence may provide natural illumination and light transmission of the peri-implant soft tissue at the abutment-crown interface and eliminate the shadowing effect often seen in conventional implant-supported restorations. The importance of fluorescence for ceramic restorations, especially in implant dentistry, has been largely ignored in the dental literature. Some case reports have demonstrated the positive effects of fluorescent implant abutments and crowns on natural esthetic outcomes and soft tissue color,[22,23] which were confirmed by a recent clinical study.[24]

References

1. Stuebel H. The fluorescence of animal tissues in ultraviolet light [in German]. Arch Ges Physiol 1911;142:1–14.

2. Araki T, Miyazaki E, Kawata T, Miyata K. Measurements of fluorescence heterogeneity in human teeth using polarization microfluorometry. Appl Spectrosc 1990;44:627–631.

3. Hartles RL, Leaver AG. The fluorescence of teeth under ultraviolet irradiation. Biochem J 1953;54:632–638.

4. Benedict HC. A note on the fluorescence of teeth in ultra-violet rays. Science 1928;67:442.

5. Dickson G, Forziati AF, Lawson ME Jr, Schoonover IC. Fluorescence of teeth; A means of investigating their structure. J Am Dent Assoc 1952;45:661–667.

6. Booij M, ten Bosch JJ. A fluorescent compound in bovine dental enamel matrix compared with synthetic dityrosine. Arch Oral Biol 1982;27:417–421.

7. Armstrong WG. Fluorescence characteristics of sound and carious human dentine preparations. Arch Oral Biol 1963;8:79–90.

8. Armstrong WG. The presence of ultra violet absorbing material and its relation to fluorescence "quenching" effects in carious dentine. Arch Oral Biol 1963;8:223–231.

9. Buchalla W. Comparative fluorescent spectroscopy shows differences in noncavitated enamel lesions. Caries Res 2005; 39:150–156.

10. Terrer E, Koubi S, Dionne A, et al. A new concept in restorative dentistry: Light-induced fluorescence evaluator for diagnosis and treatment: Part 1—Diagnosis and treatment of initial occlusal caries. J Contemp Dent Pract 2009;10:1–12.

11. Rodrigues JA, Hug I, Diniz MB, Lussi A. Performance of fluorescence methods, radiographic examination and ICDAS II on occlusal surfaces in vitro. Caries Res 2008;42:297–304.

12. Adeyemi AA, Jarad FD, Pender N, Higham SM. Comparison of quantitative light-induced fluorescence (QLF) and digital imaging applied for the detection and quantification of staining and stain removal on teeth. J Dent 2006;34:460–466.

13. Poh CF, Williams PM, Zhang L, Rosin MP. Heads up!—A call for dentists to screen for oral cancer. J Can Dent Assoc 2006;72:413–416.

14. Lee YK, Lu H, Powers JM. Fluorescence of layered resin composites. J Esthet Restor Dent 2005;17:93–100.

15. Tani K, Watari F, Uo M, Morita M. Discrimination between composite resin and teeth using fluorescence properties. Dent Mater J 2003;22:569–580.

16. Sant'Anna Aguiar Dos Reis R, Casemiro LA, Carlino GV, et al. Evaluation of fluorescence of dental composites using contrast ratios to adjacent tooth structure: A pilot study. J Esthet Restor Dent 2007;19:199–206.

17. Monsénégo G, Burdairon G, Clerjaud B. Fluorescence of dental porcelain. J Prosthet Dent 1993;69:106–113.

18. Komine F, Blatz MB, Yamamoto S, Matsumura H. A modified layering technique to enhance fluorescence in glass-infiltrated aluminum oxide ceramic restorations: Case report. Quintessence Int 2008;39:11–16.

19. Nik Mohd Polo Kinin NM, Wan Mohd Arif WI, Zainal Arifm A. Study on the effect of Y_2O_3 addition to the fluorescent property of dental porcelain. Med J Malaysia 2004;59(suppl B):23–24.

20. Ferreira Zandoná AG, Kleinrichert T, Analoui M, Schemehorn BR, Eckert GJ, Stookey GK. Effect of two fluorescent dyes on color of restorative materials. Am J Dent 1997;10:203–207.

21. Blatz MB, Bergler M, Holst S, Block M. Zirconia abutments for single-tooth implants—Rationale and clinical guidelines. J Oral Maxillofac Surg 2009;67:74–81.

22. Gamborena I, Blatz MB. Fluorescence—Mimicking nature for ultimate esthetics in implant dentistry. Quintessence Dent Technol 2011;34:7–23.

23. Gamborena I, Blatz MB. The grey zone around dental implants—Keys to esthetic success. Am J Esthet Dent 2011;1:26–46.

24. Happe A, Schulte-Mattler V, Fickl S, Naumann M, Zöller JE, Rothamel D. Spectrophotometric assessment of peri-implant mucosa after restoration with zirconia abutments veneered with fluorescent ceramic: A controlled, retrospective clinical study. Clin Oral Implants Res 2013;24(suppl A100):28–33.

Zirconia has gained tremendous popularity as an implant abutment material in the esthetic zone because it prevents the grayish appearance of the surrounding soft tissues often seen with titanium or other metal-alloy abutments. The lack of fluorescence of the zirconia abutment makes it a poor choice when it comes to copying the optical properties of the natural tooth, as shown in the side-by-side images of different zirconia abutments without fluorescence compared with a natural tooth.

Fluorescence is a crucial optical property for natural esthetics in dentistry. Fluorescence provides natural illumination and light transmission of the soft tissue at the implant-restorative interface and eliminates a shadowing effect often seen in implant-supported restorations even when tooth-colored abutments are being used. Colorants and fluorescent modifiers that can be applied to zirconia abutments even after milling and finishing have been developed.

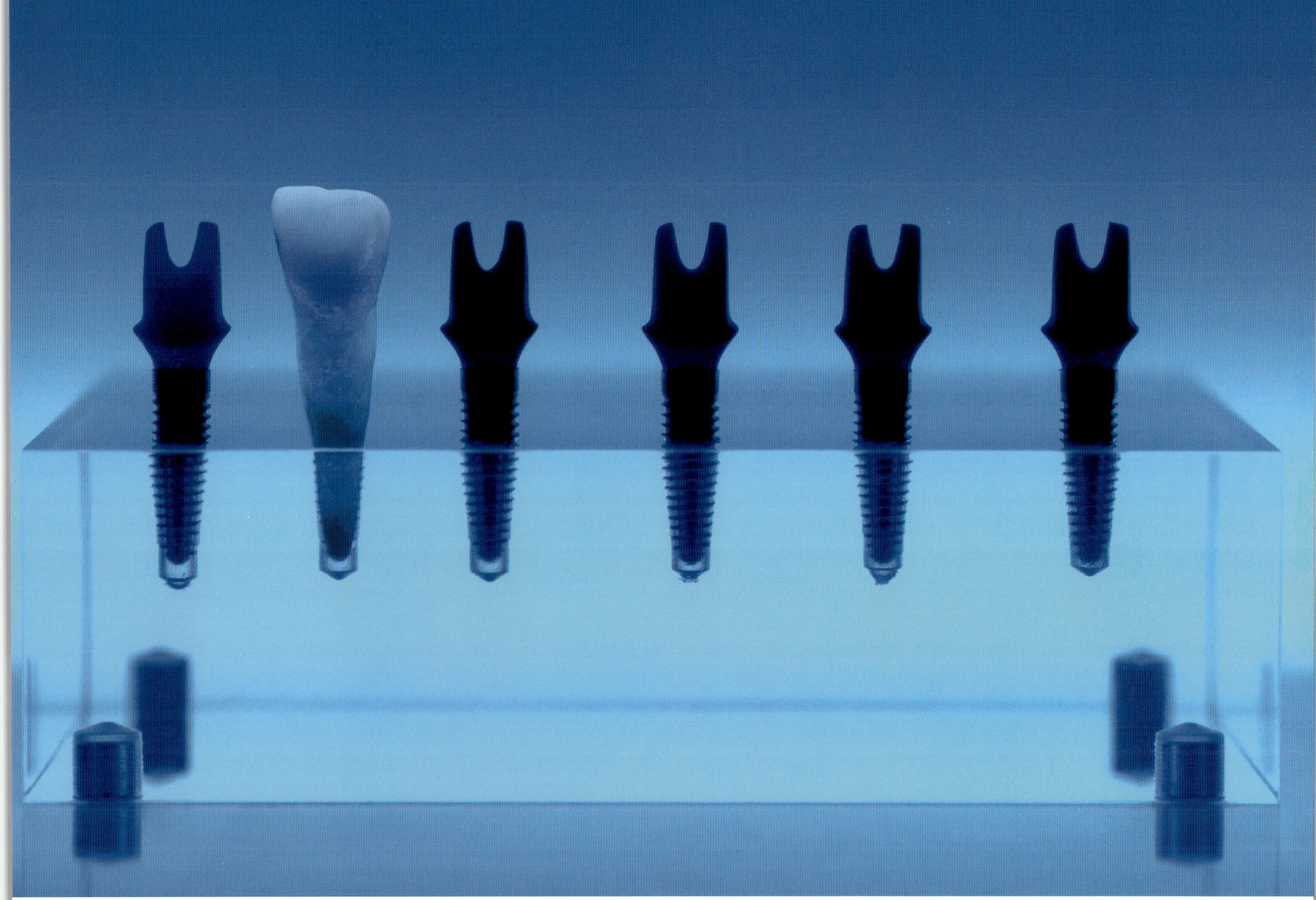

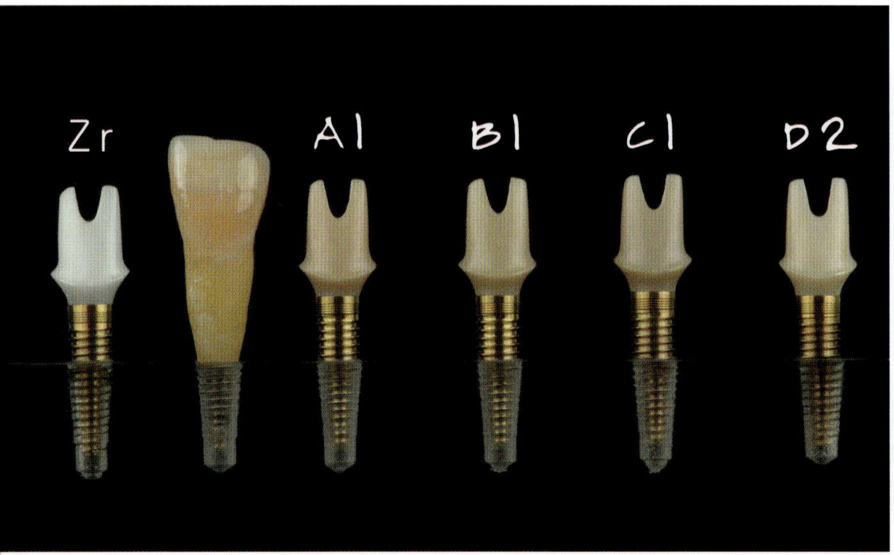

The abutment or framework is dipped into a fluorescent coloring liquid before sintering to infiltrate the zirconia with the liquid (Colour Liquid Fluoreszenz, Zirkonzahn). The abutment is blow-dried after the dipping process to remove any excess liquid and placed under a drying lamp to prevent damage to the heating elements of the sinter furnace.
The infiltration process and its effect on the optical appearance under different light sources is shown.

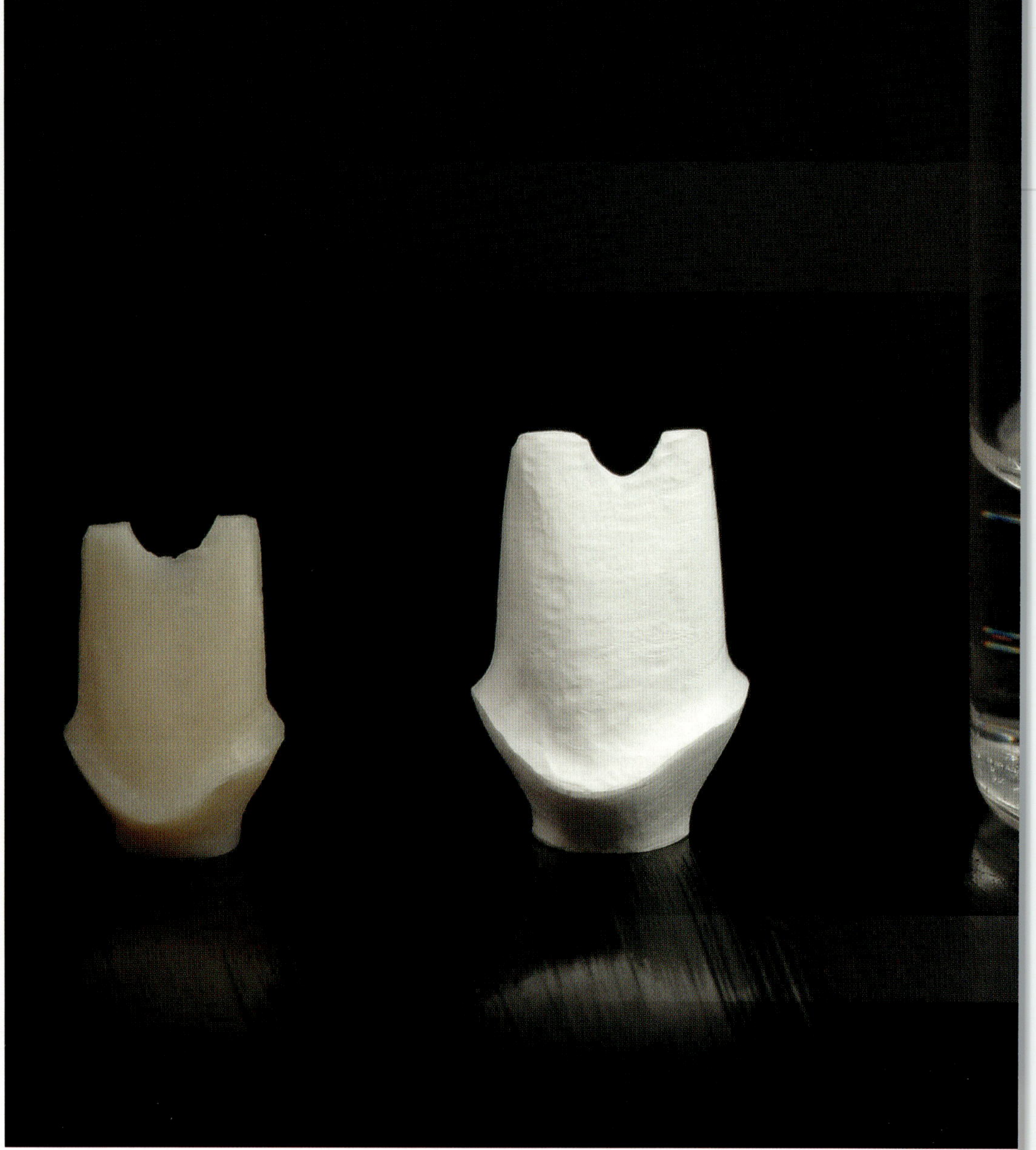

Five different abutments were fabricated: zirconia conventional color with fluorescence and zirconia with the four representative colors of the VITA shade guide (Vita Zahnfabrik) without fluorescence. Comparison under natural light and fluorescent light from conventional zirconia versus colored zirconia without UV light are shown. Note the lack of fluorescence and how the colors of the abutments do not match the colors of the VITA shade guide, demonstrating the challenges when trying to achieve a certain base color.

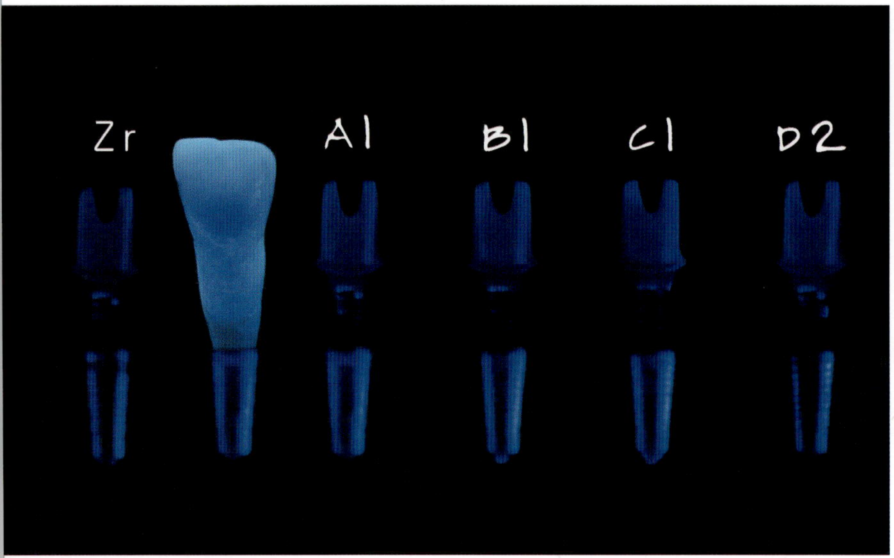

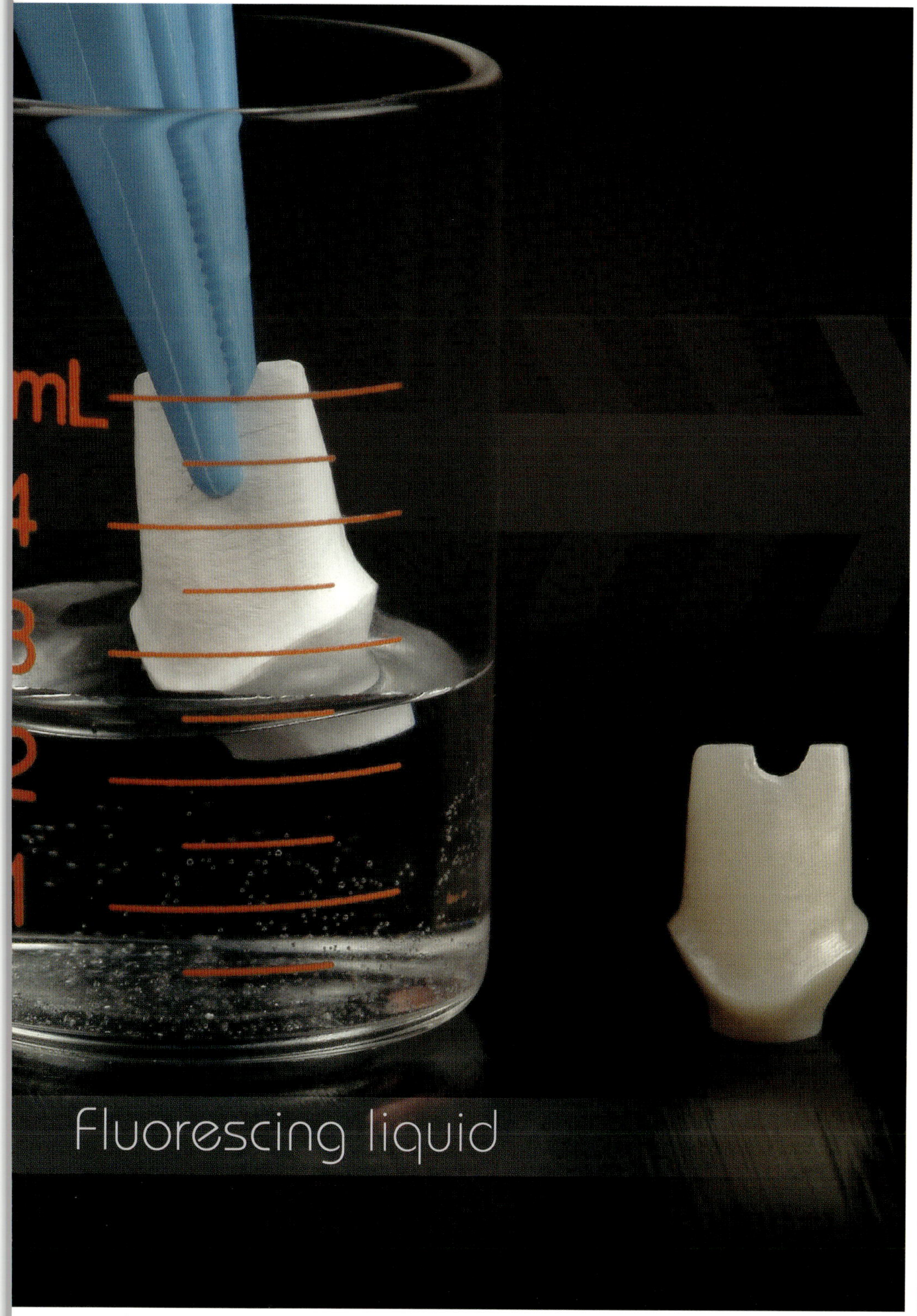

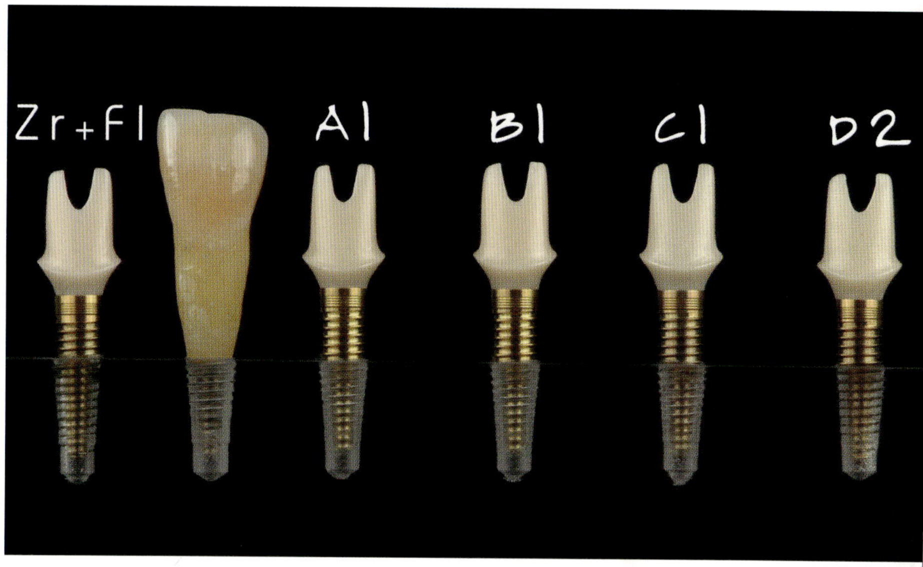

Zirconia abutments after application of fluorescence (Zr + Fl) under natural light. In addition to fluorescence, shade-modifying colorants were applied. Fluorescence and color can be added to zirconia to a certain degree. It is still difficult to create a dark shade with a high degree of fluorescence, because the dark color pigments may overshadow the fluorescent properties. Therefore, strong fluorescence of the implant abutment may actually be more important for overall and especially gingival esthetics than its actual shade.

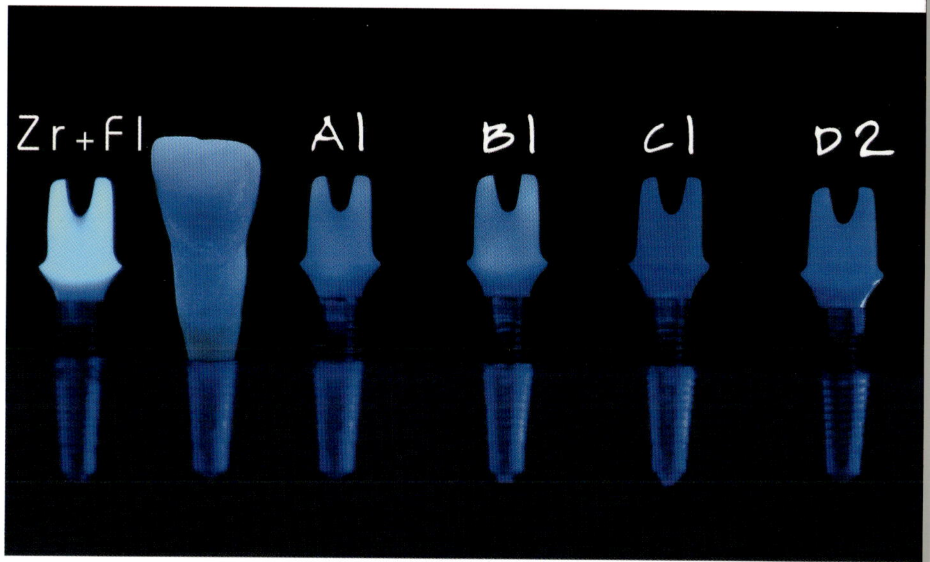

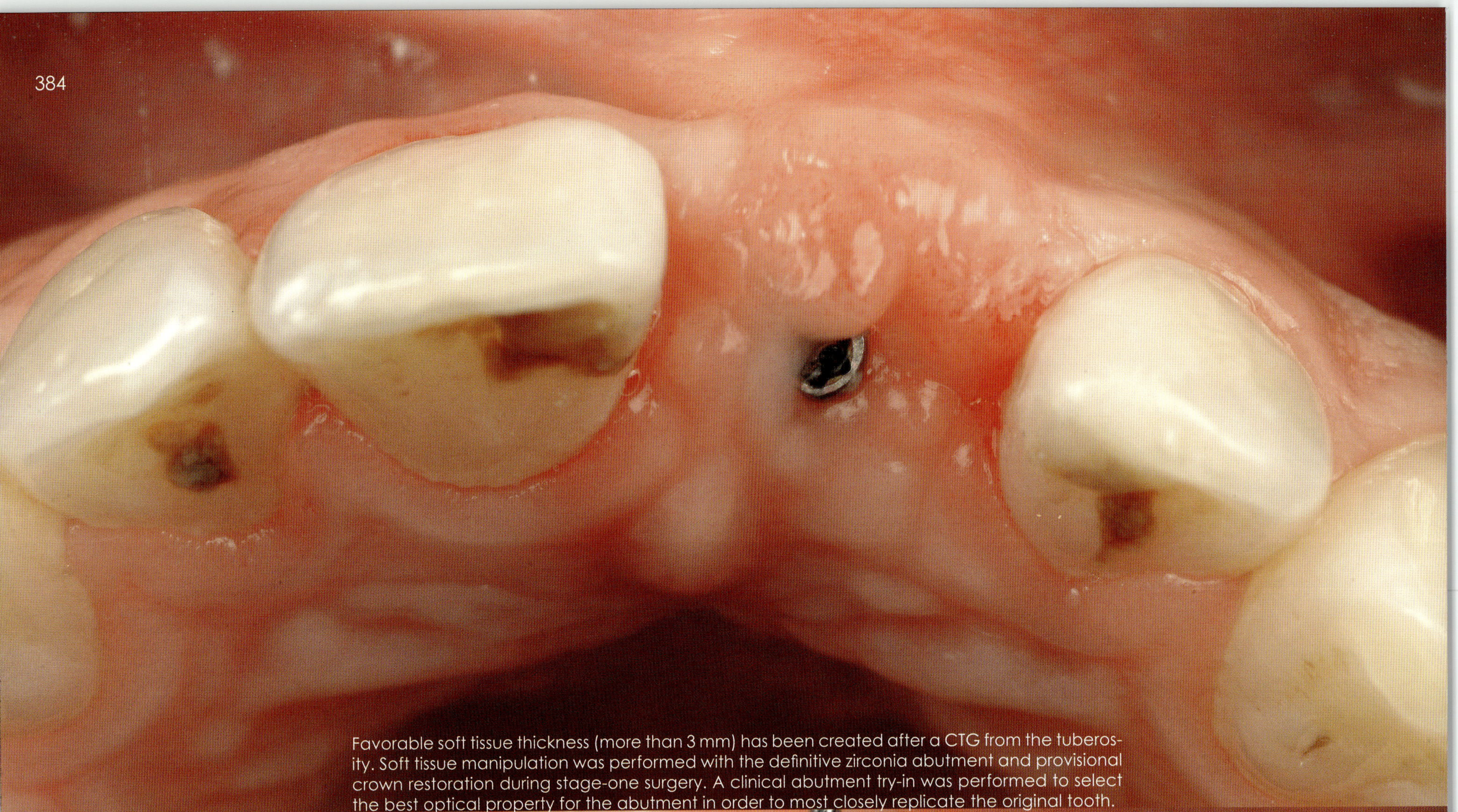

Favorable soft tissue thickness (more than 3 mm) has been created after a CTG from the tuberosity. Soft tissue manipulation was performed with the definitive zirconia abutment and provisional crown restoration during stage-one surgery. A clinical abutment try-in was performed to select the best optical property for the abutment in order to most closely replicate the original tooth.

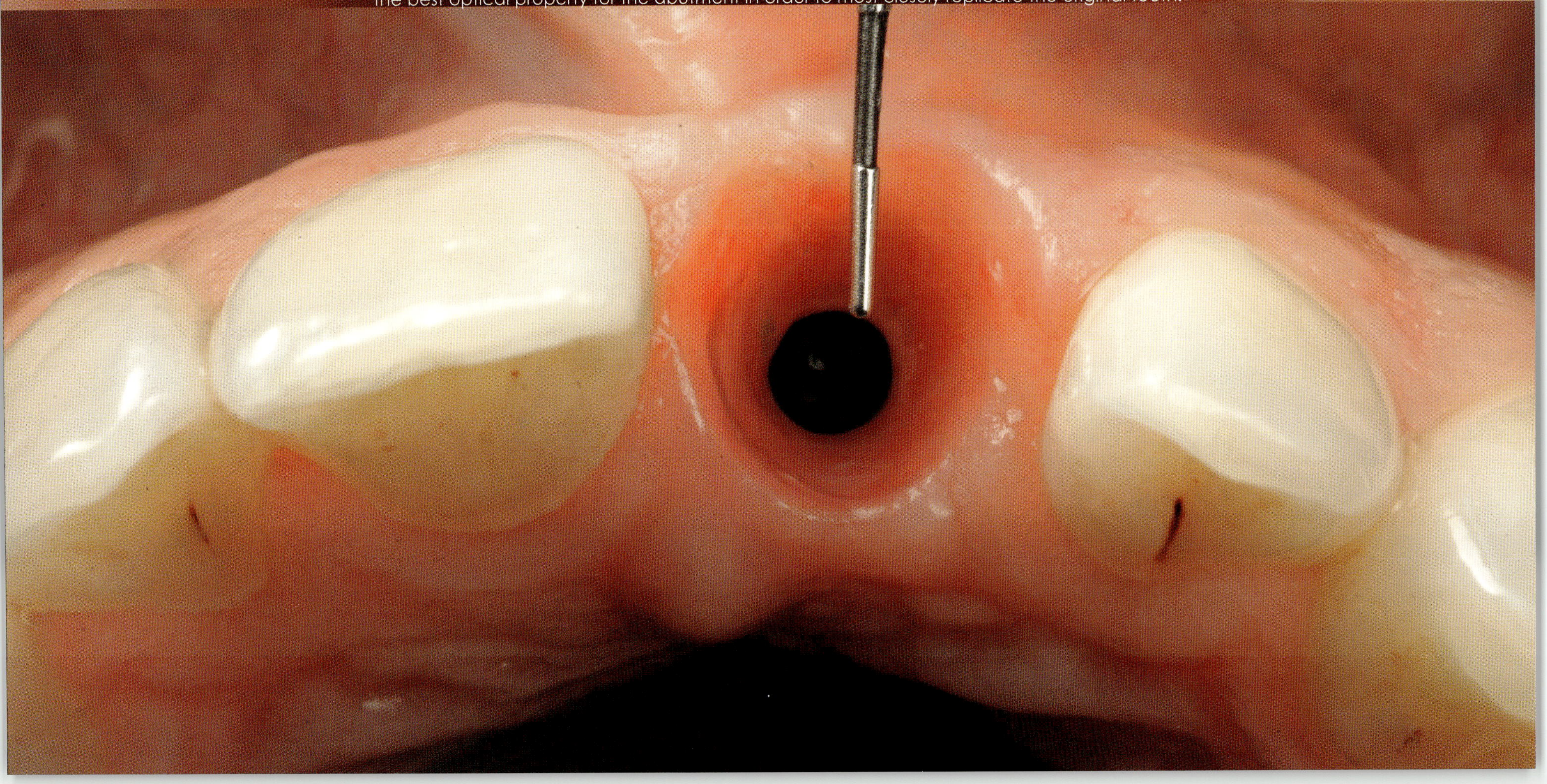

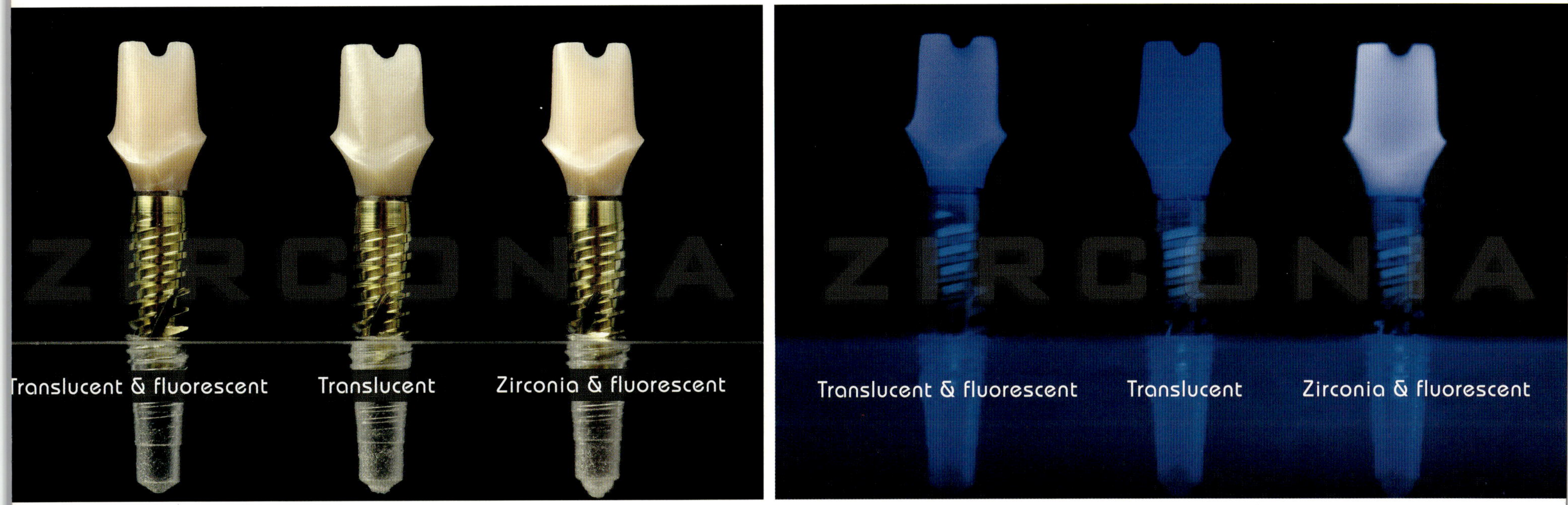

Three different zirconia abutments were fabricated and assessed under different lighting conditions (natural and UV light). In addition to the regular zirconia, a more translucent type was compared with the original zirconia and fluorescence. The optical differences between a conventional translucent and fluorescent abutment are evident under different lighting conditions. Interestingly, a higher degree of translucency translates to a lower value and influences the ultimate amount of fluorescence.

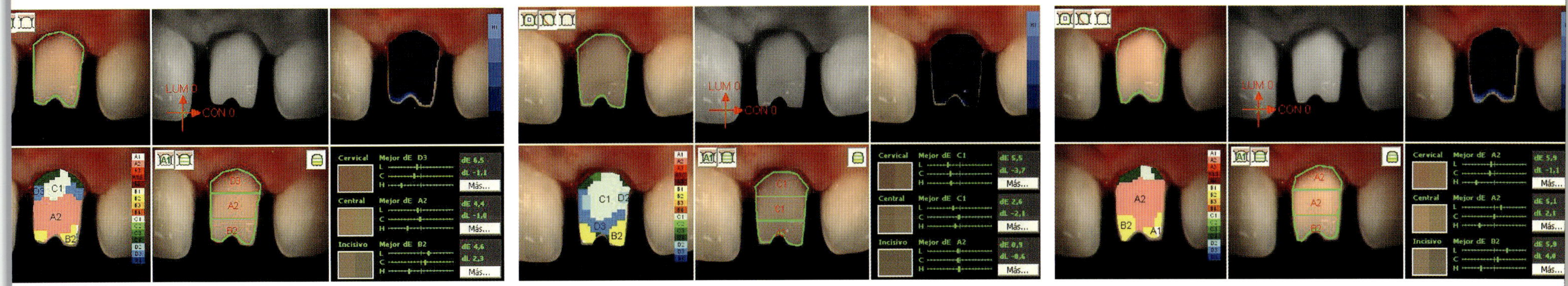

Digital shade selection of the three different abutments was performed with the Spectroshade (MHT Optic Research) to objectively record the color shade of each one. The translucent and fluorescent abutment had an overall A2-B3 color, while the translucent one had a C1 color because of its low value. The fluorescent abutment had the highest value of A2-B2.

Intraorally, the translucent abutment provided the best match in natural light but the worst under UV light. The translucent and fluorescent abutment had a better optical effect than the translucent one, with higher value and a closer match to the real tooth. The most favorable fluorescent effect was achieved with colored conventional zirconia and fluorescing liquid. Note the perfect value match under UV light and natural light.

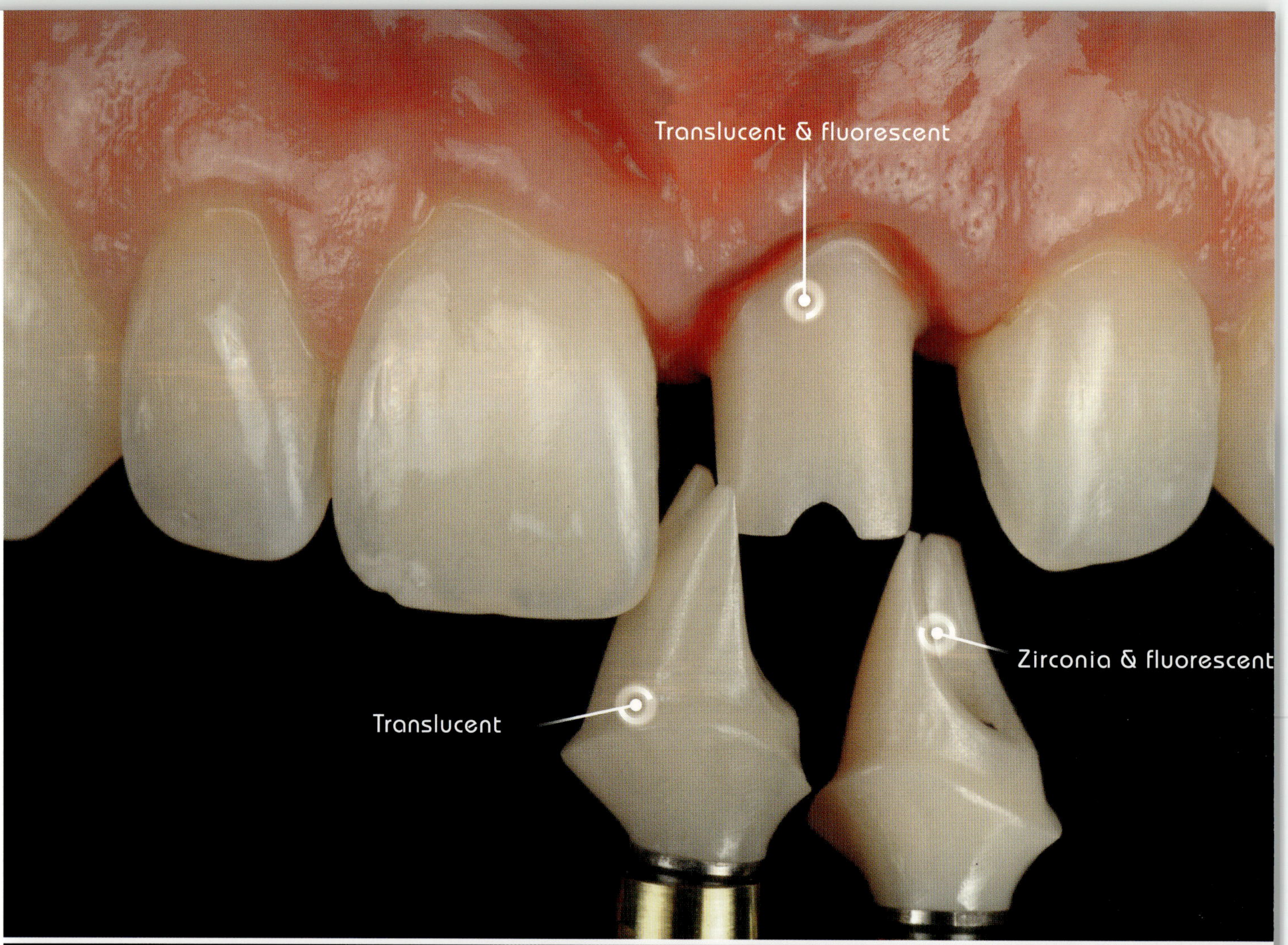

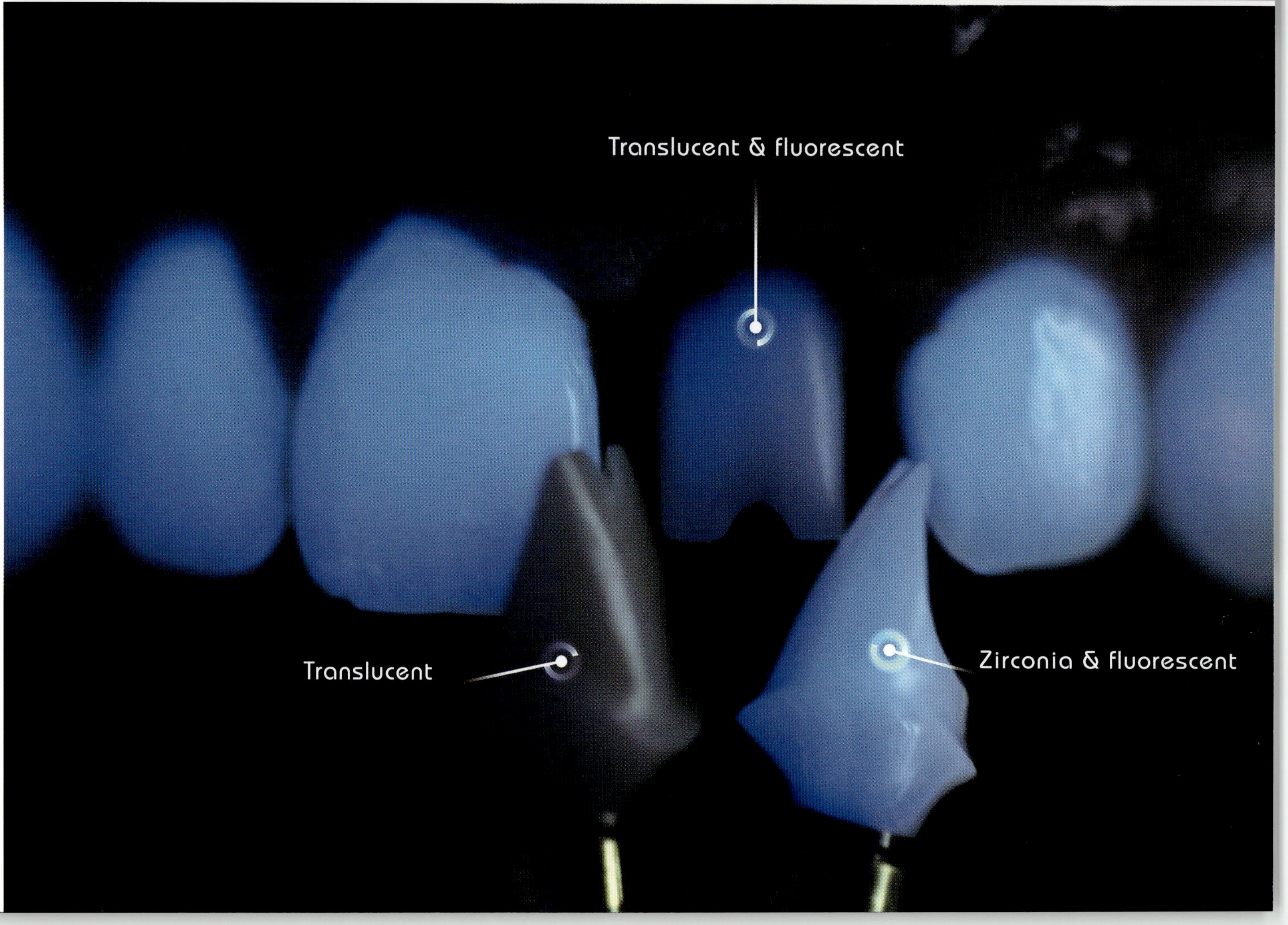

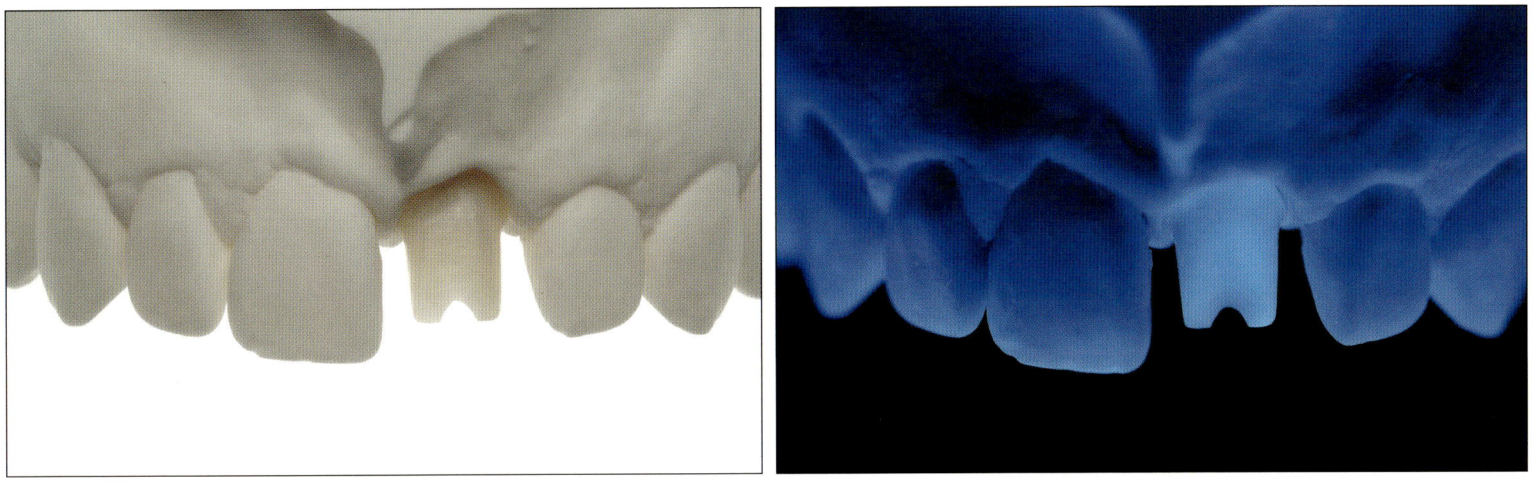

The fluorescent abutment on the master cast under natural light and UV light reveals the dramatic effects of fluorescence on the surrounding peri-implant soft tissue of the master cast, creating brightness and the vitality exhibited by natural teeth. Fluorescence is an inherent property of natural teeth but is rarely found even in "esthetic" dental materials, so adding it to the abutment seems only logical.

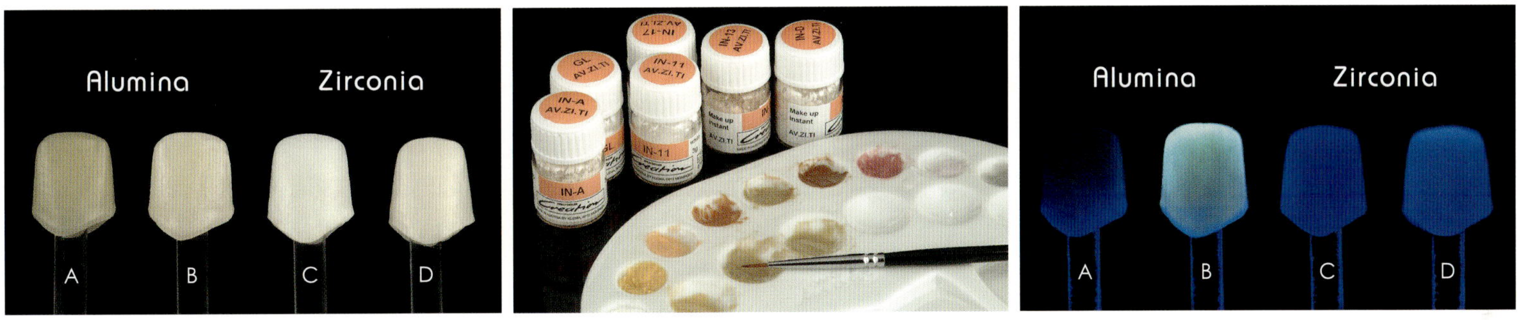

The definitive crown material is selected based on the core structure to enhance the optical characteristics of the intended restoration. The coping is chosen for its ability either to mask underlying structures if necessary or to complement the restoration by the underlying abutment color. Note the difference between alumina and zirconia copings with no liner whatsoever (A and C), with a porcelain internal stain (B) represented in the middle image by In Nova stains (Creation Willi Geller) and an infiltrated coping (D) with fluorescence that appears less fluorescent because of the thickness of the coping.

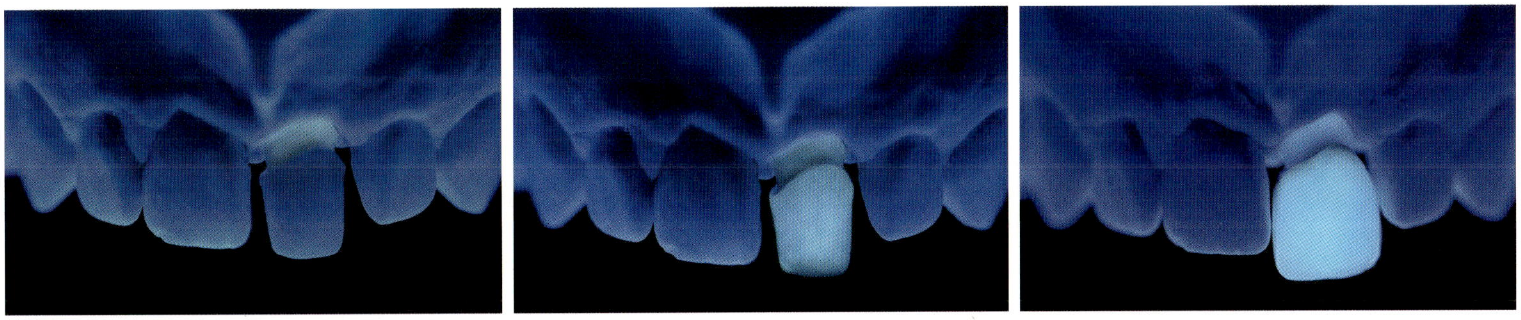

Different views of the definitive crown and coping restoration under UV light. It is important to evaluate the optical properties of the coping in relation to the remaining natural dentition under different light sources. UV light can reveal the dramatic effects of fluorescence, which provides the vitality and brightness exhibited by natural teeth.

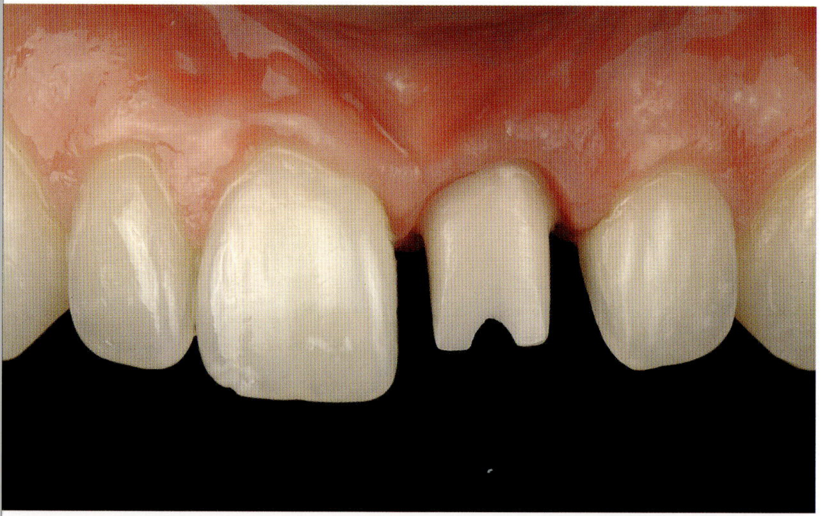

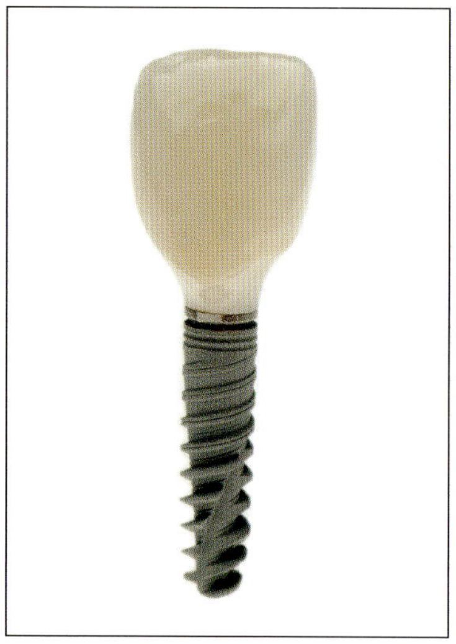

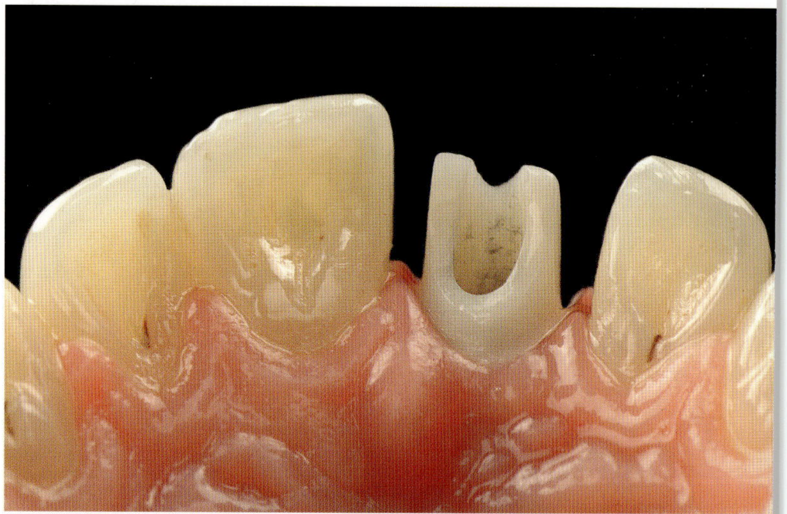

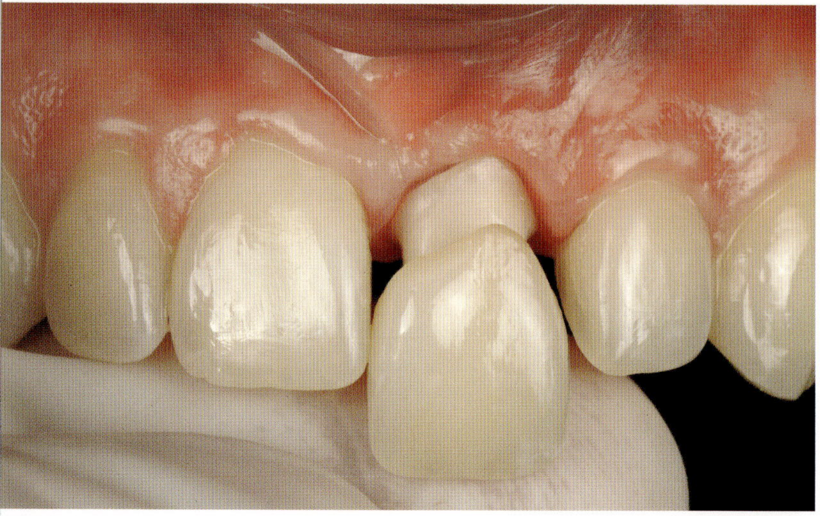

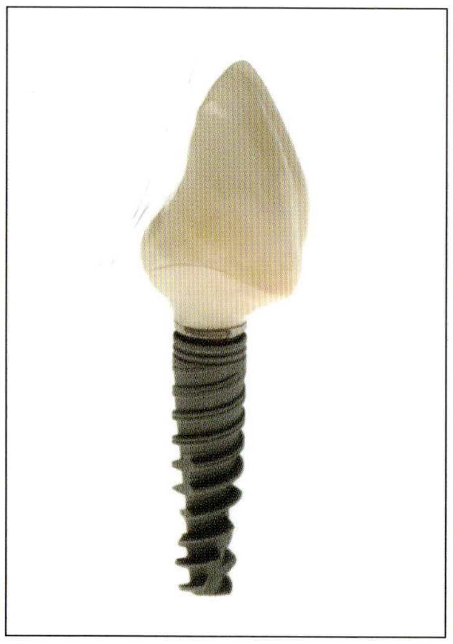

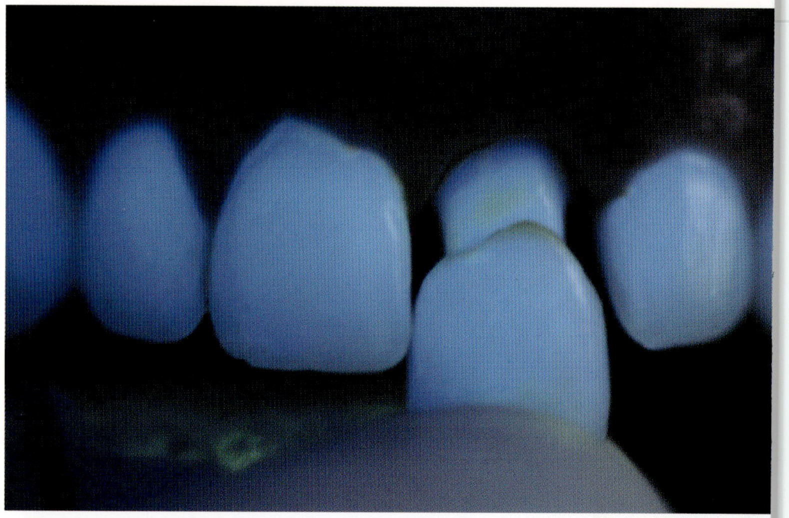

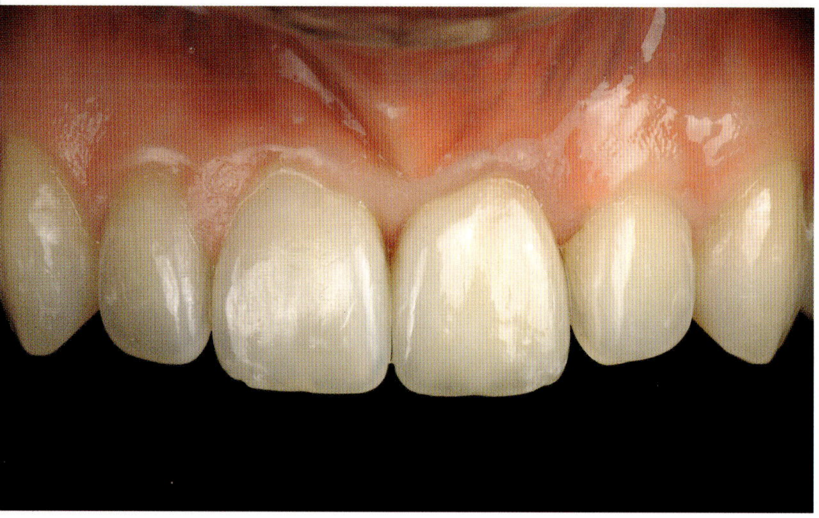

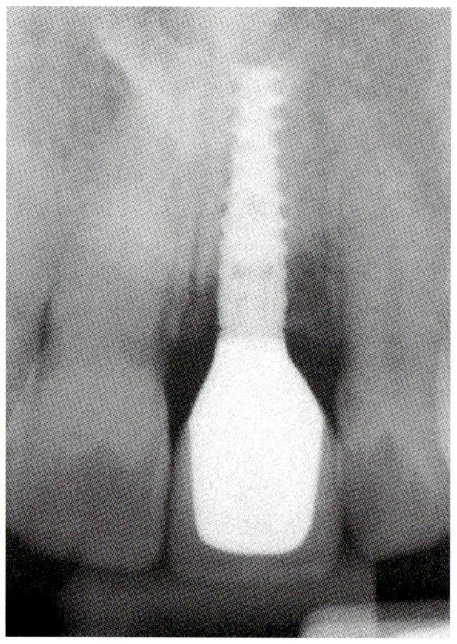

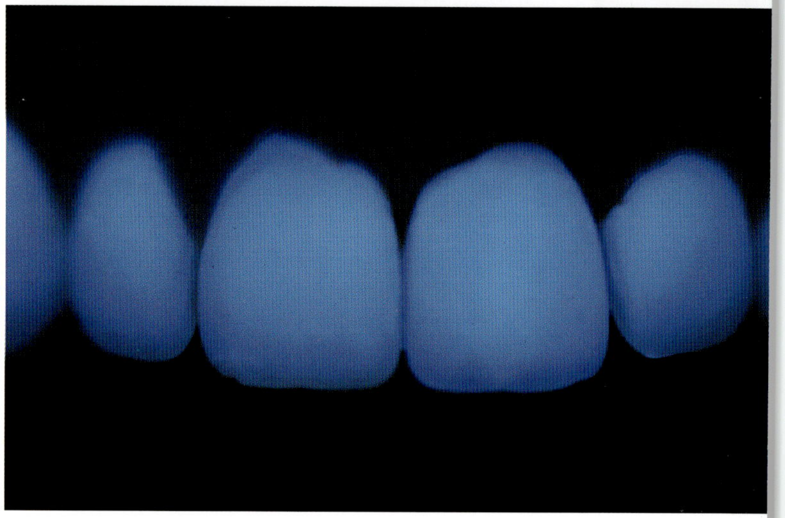

In natural teeth, the root and coronal dentin show the highest degree of fluorescence, especially in the gingival third, while enamel has only low fluorescent properties. Ceramic coping materials such as alumina and zirconia do not provide natural fluorescence and, therefore, are treated with fluorescent modifiers and/or veneered with fluorescent dentin stains, liners, and shoulder porcelains. The fluorescent effect is, congruent to the natural tooth, most prominent in the gingival third of the restoration. Therefore, natural fluorescence does not only influence the optical effects of the restoration itself but greatly influences the color and appearance of the surrounding soft tissues. The definitive implant-supported crown has optical and fluorescent properties that ideally match the existing natural dentition under various light sources.

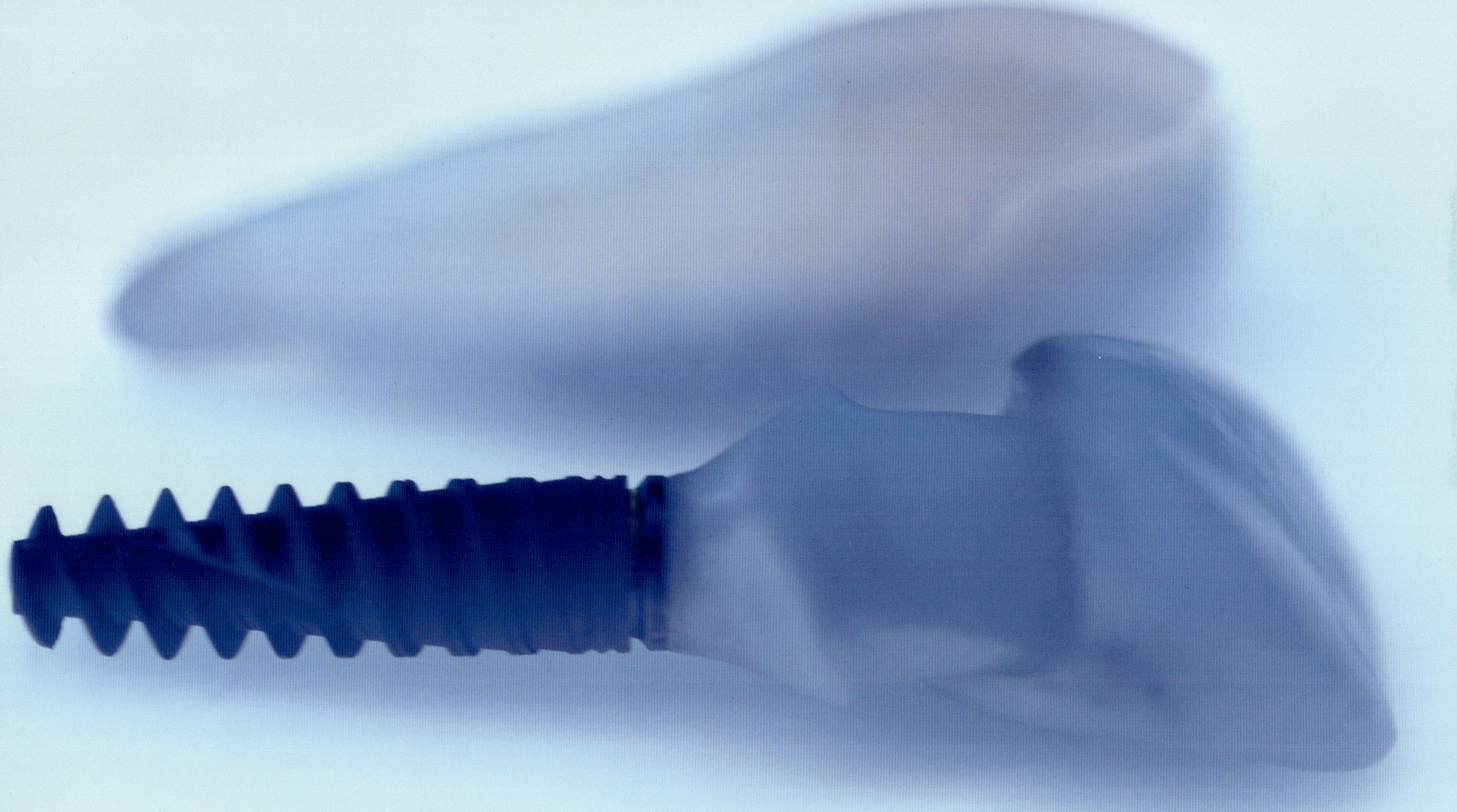

A provisional implant crown was placed in the area of the maxillary left central incisor to condition the soft tissue morphology after implant placement. The provisional restoration remained in place for 3 months until the position of the soft tissue was stabilized. Afterward, the definitive abutment was designed and fabricated. The optical differences between a conventional and a fluorescent abutment are evident under different lighting conditions. Alumina was selected as the coping material for the definitive crown on the zirconia abutment for better light transmission with the underlying fluorescent abutment. The images here demonstrate and compare the preoperative and postoperative situation after implant placement and fabrication of an implant-supported restoration with natural fluorescence.

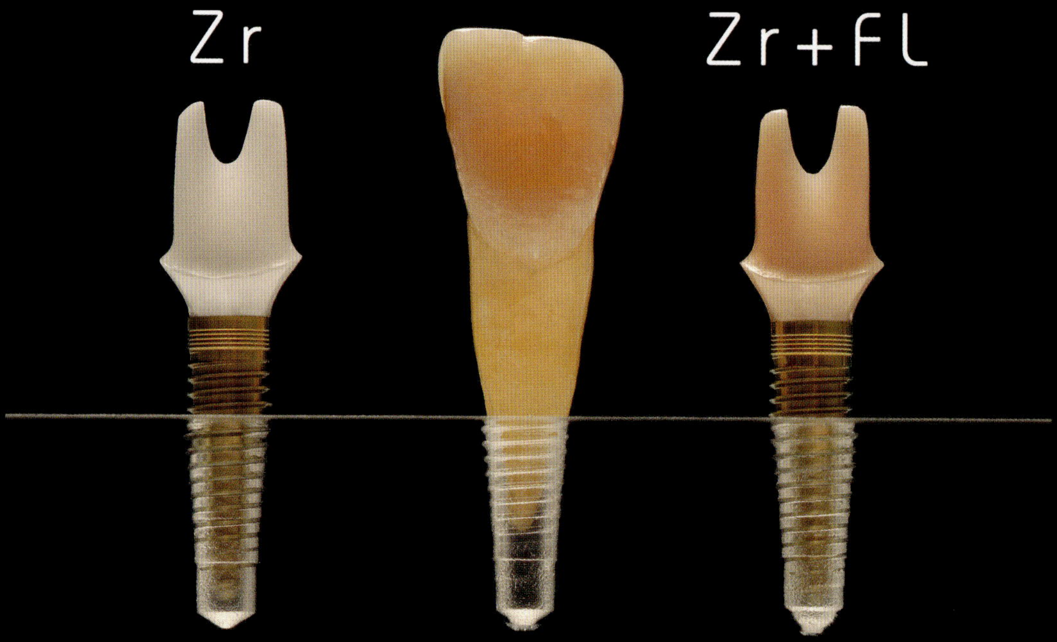

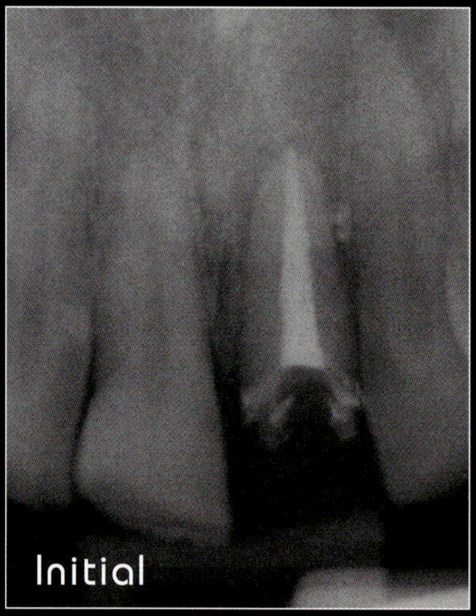

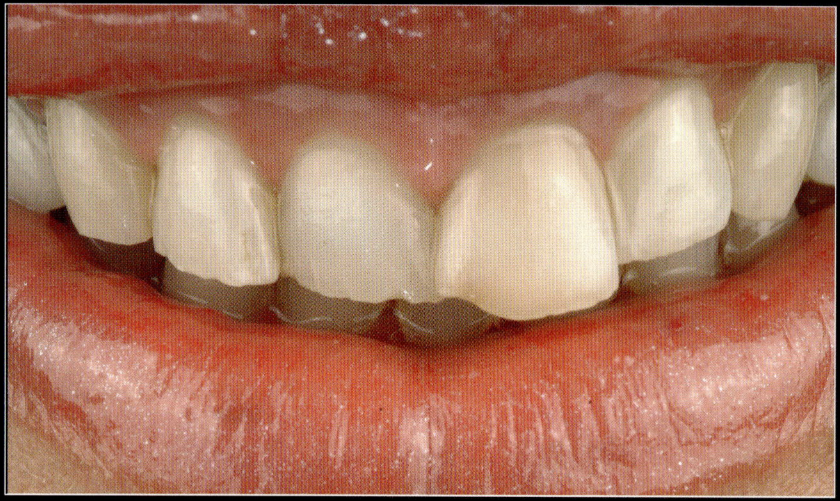

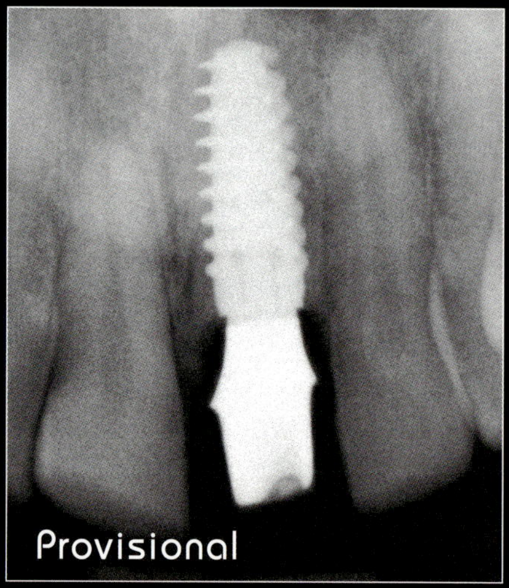

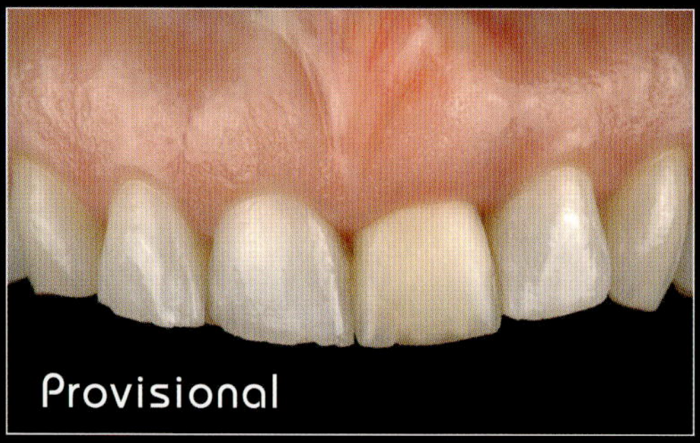

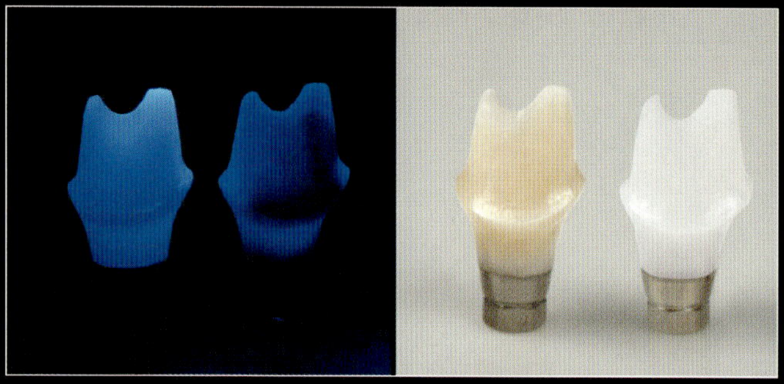

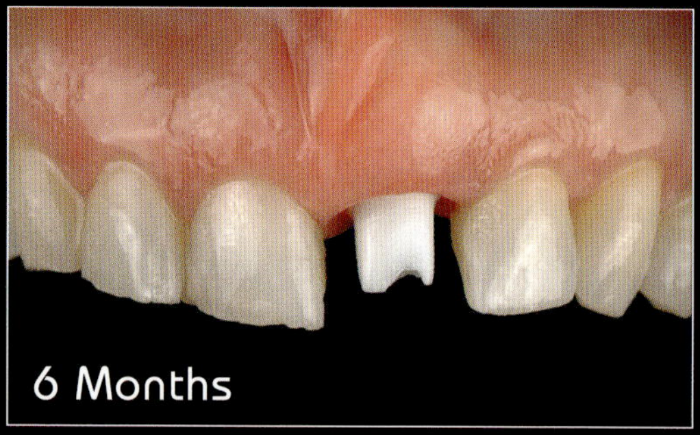

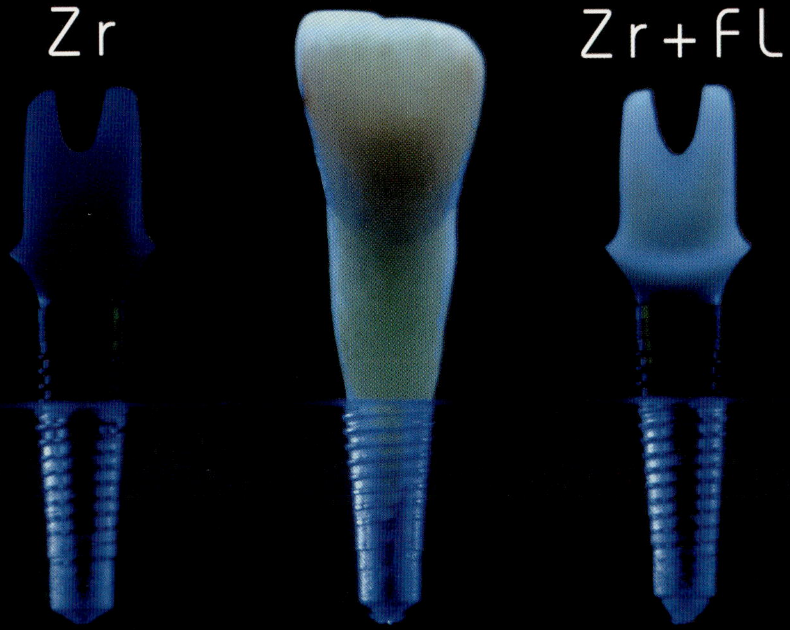

Comparison of zirconia versus zirconia with fluorescence demonstrates the proximity of the coloring with fluorescence to the root of the natural tooth with great matching characteristics.

The integration of a high degree of fluorescence is especially important in patients with a high smile line, as presented here, to reduce the so-called umbrella shadowing effect. The fluorescent abutment under UV light shows the favorable fluorescent properties in this particular case.

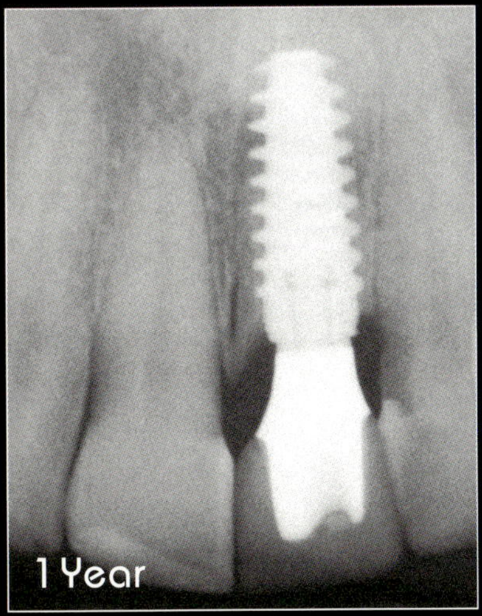

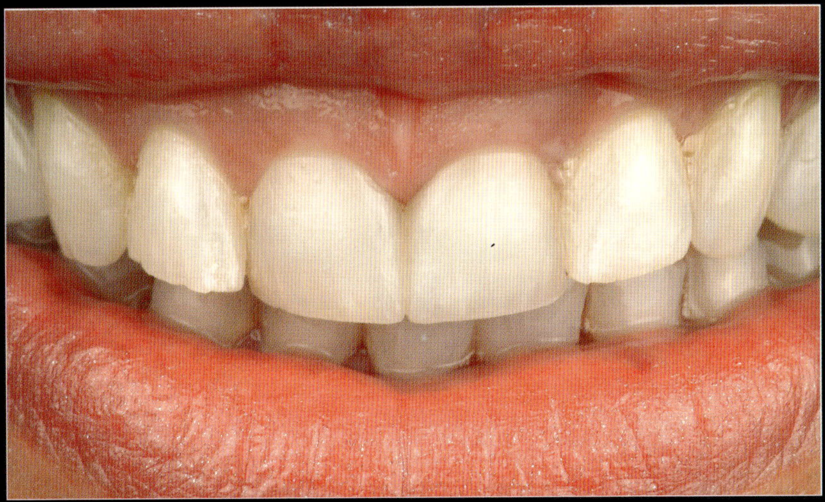

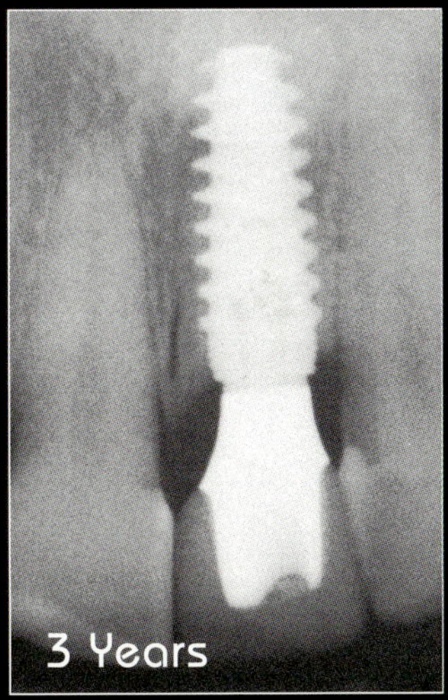

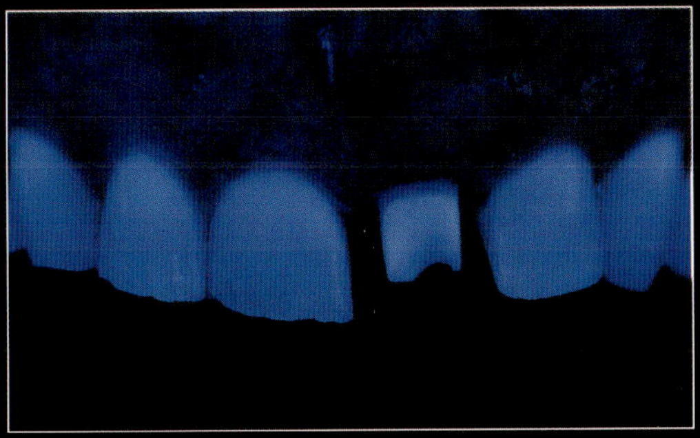

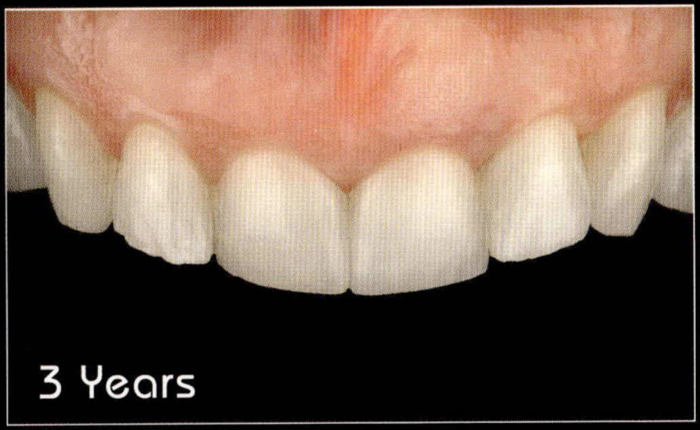

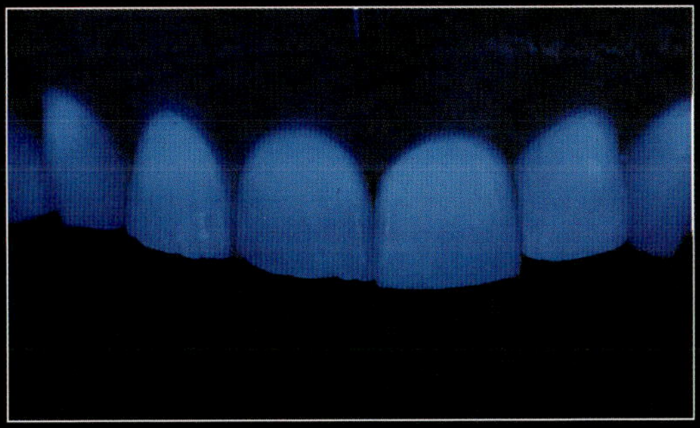

Some challenging patient situations may require shaded or translucent types of zirconia or further coloring of the implant abutment to achieve the ideal abutment esthetics. The degree of translucency, however, translates to a lower value and influences the ultimate degree of fluorescence; more important, it influences the color of the crown that is cemented on top, resulting in a lower value.

To achieve an optimal match between the two restorations, the color of the severely destructed maxillary left central incisor abutment tooth must be taken into consideration. In addition to conventional shade tabs, a digital spectrophotometer (SpectroShade) was used to select the "stump shade" of the abutment tooth (VITA shade C3).

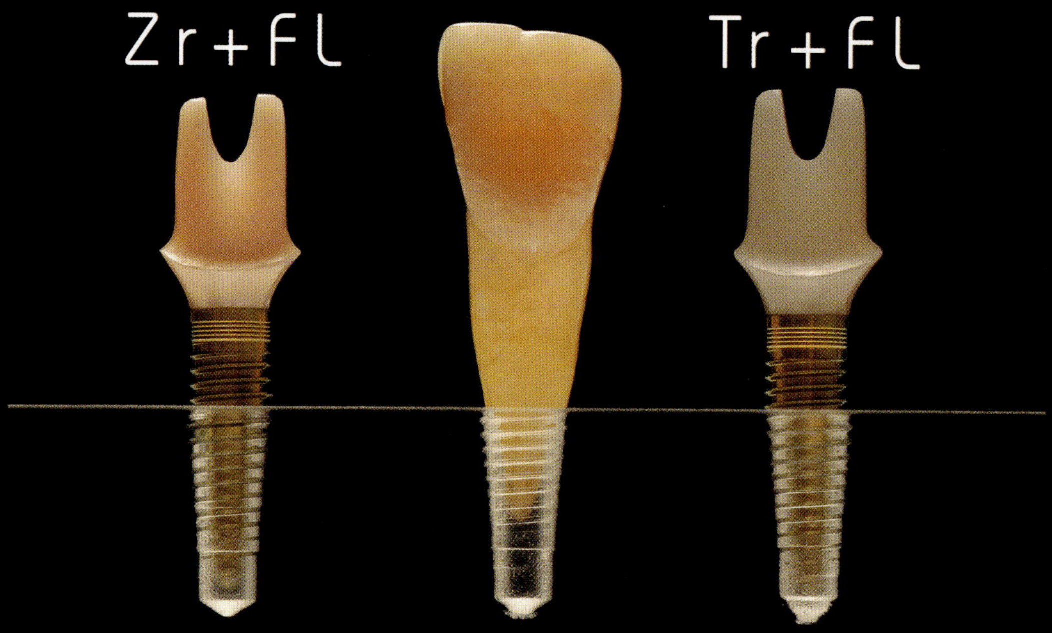

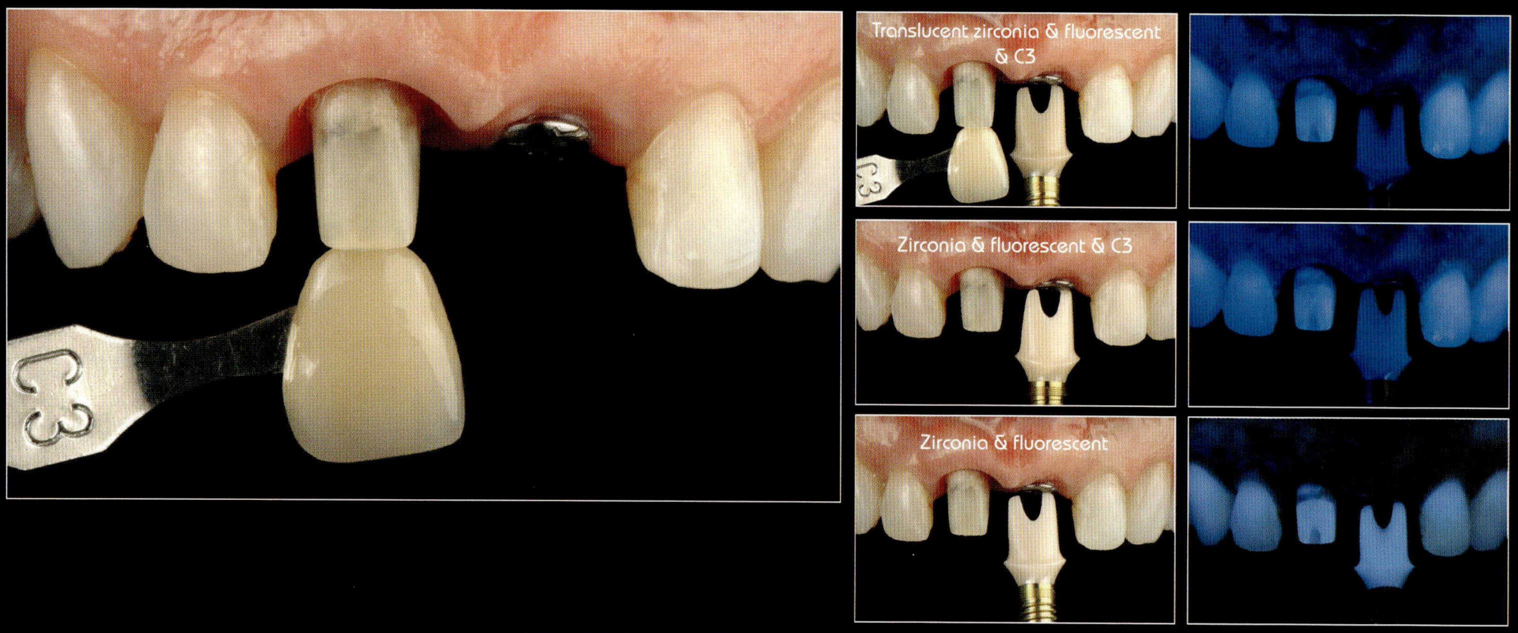

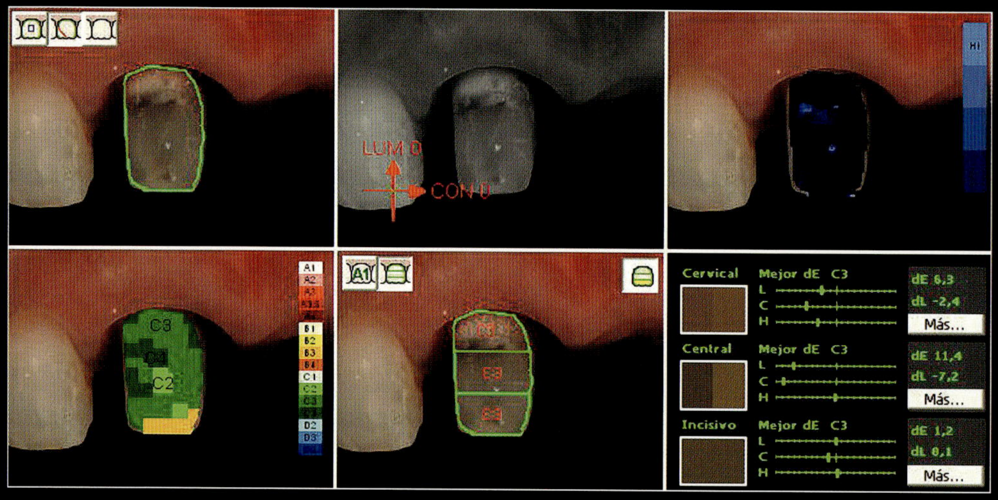

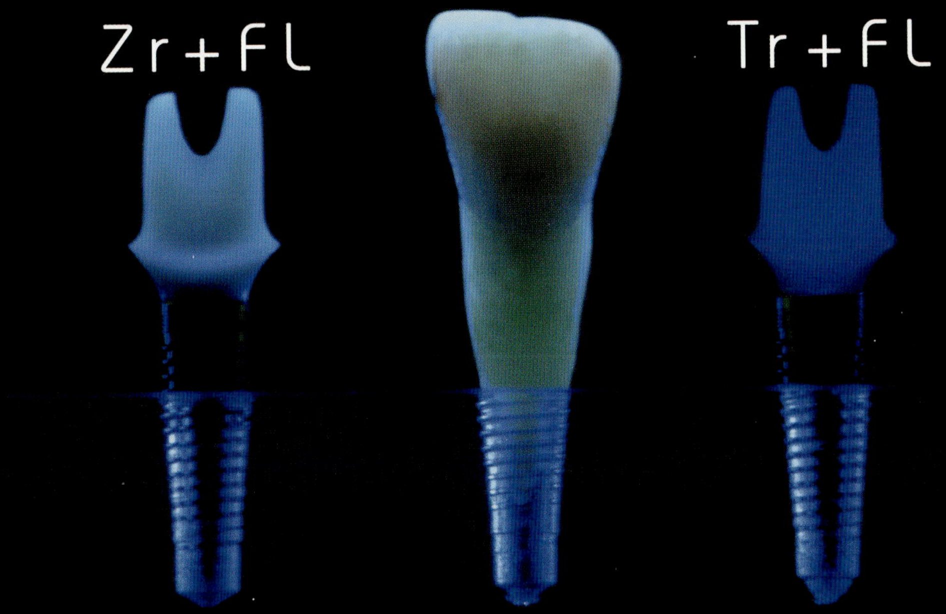

At first, it was attempted to match the shade of the implant abutment with that of the natural abutment tooth. However, this picture depicts the negative effects of different shade and translucence colorants on the ultimate degree of fluorescence. A preferred soft tissue appearance with new provisional restorations was only achieved with a noncolored but fluorescent zirconia abutment that matched the fluorescence and value but not necessarily the shade (chroma and hue) and translucency of the natural abutment tooth. Therefore, in such situations, fluorescence/value matching takes priority over translucency and shade matching.

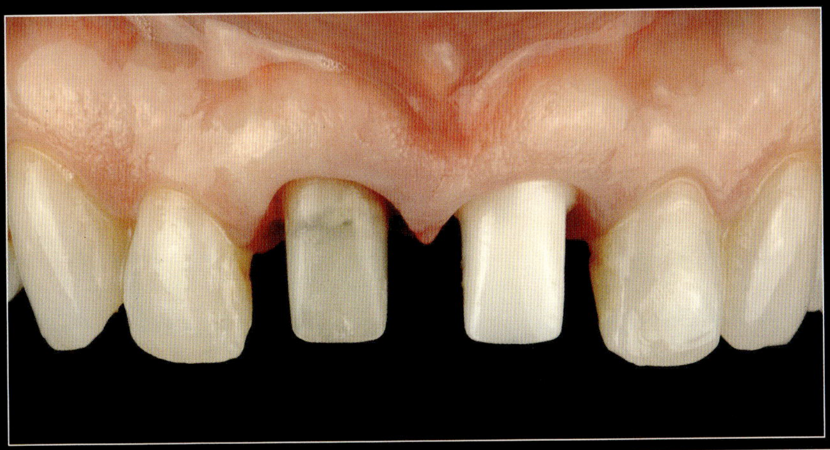

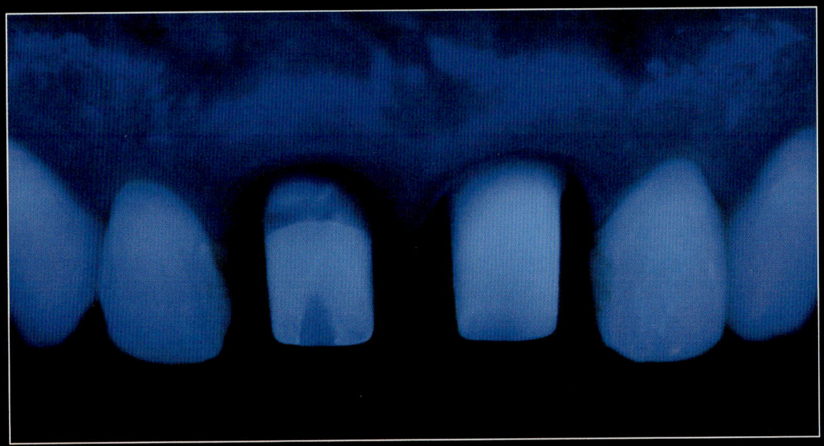

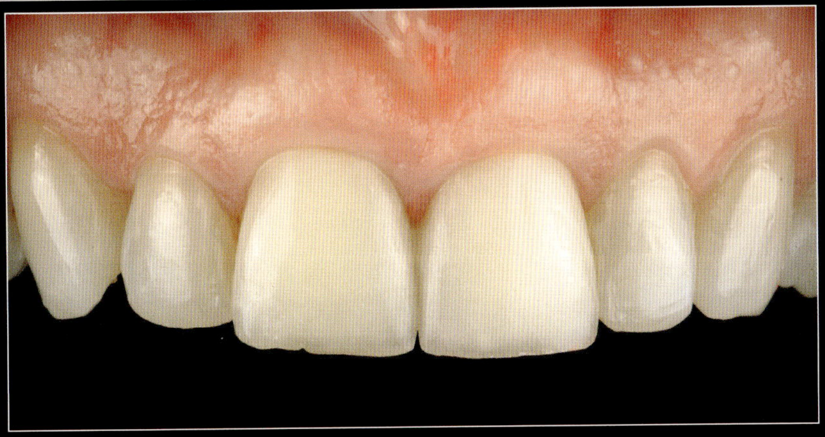

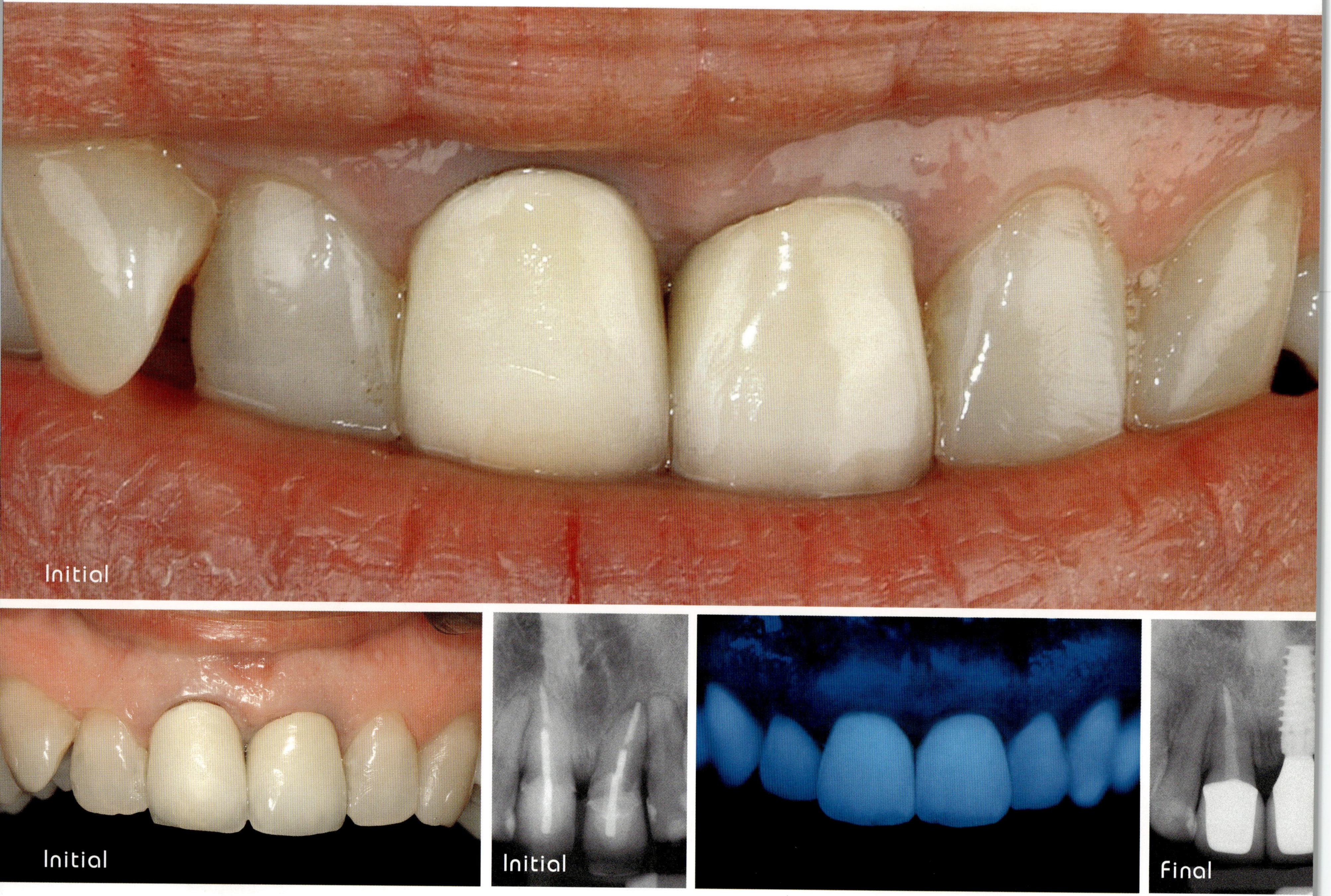

The importance of mimicking natural fluorescence to achieve optimal esthetics in implant dentistry is exemplified in the preoperative and postoperative views of the treatment and demonstrated in a patient with a high smile line.

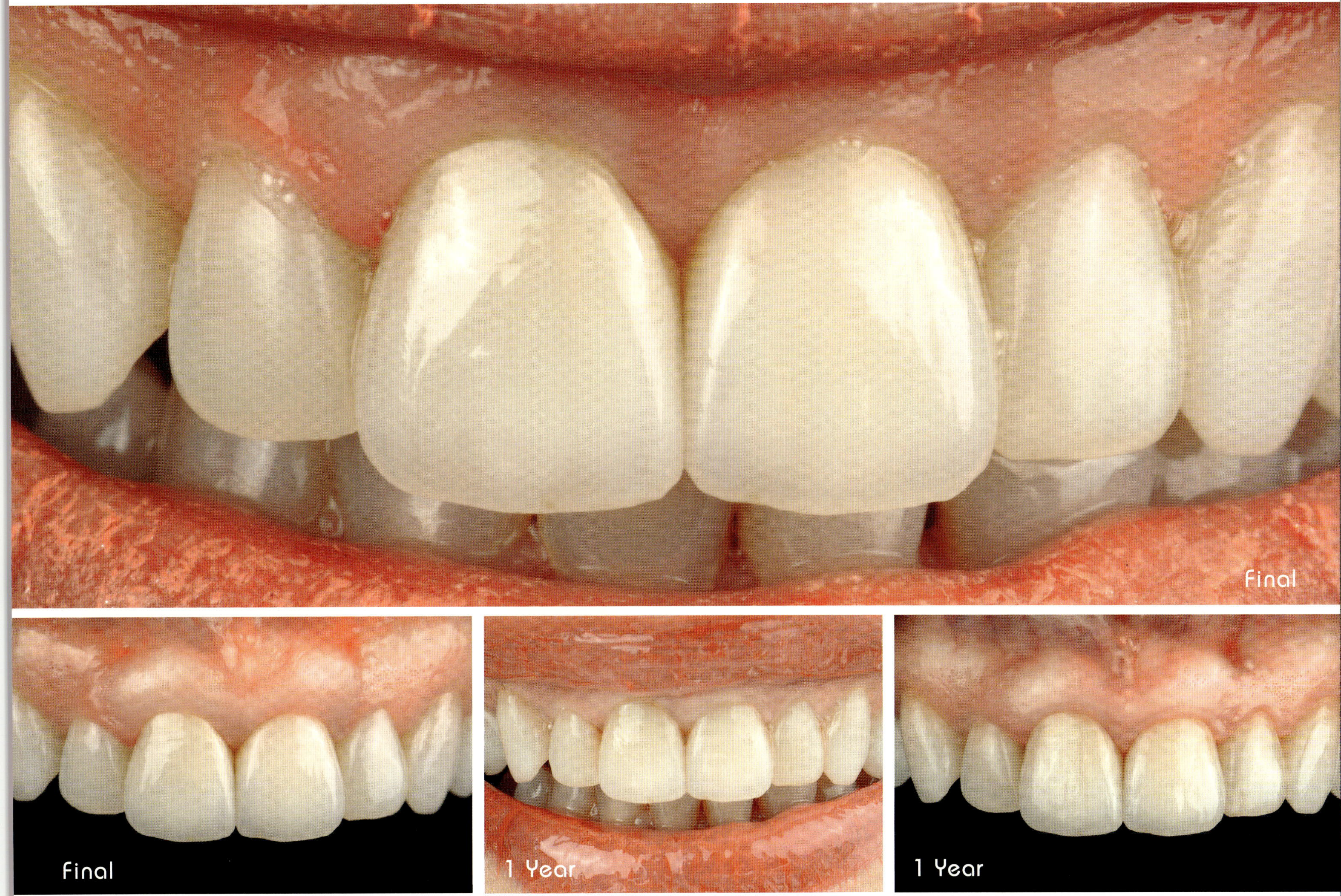

Images from the preoperative smile to the final combined treatment of orthodontic therapy and implant placement at the left central incisor, which was required because of mechanical and structural problems, to the final intraoral view of the definitive zirconia crowns under UV light, depict the favorable fluorescent properties and esthetic outcome.

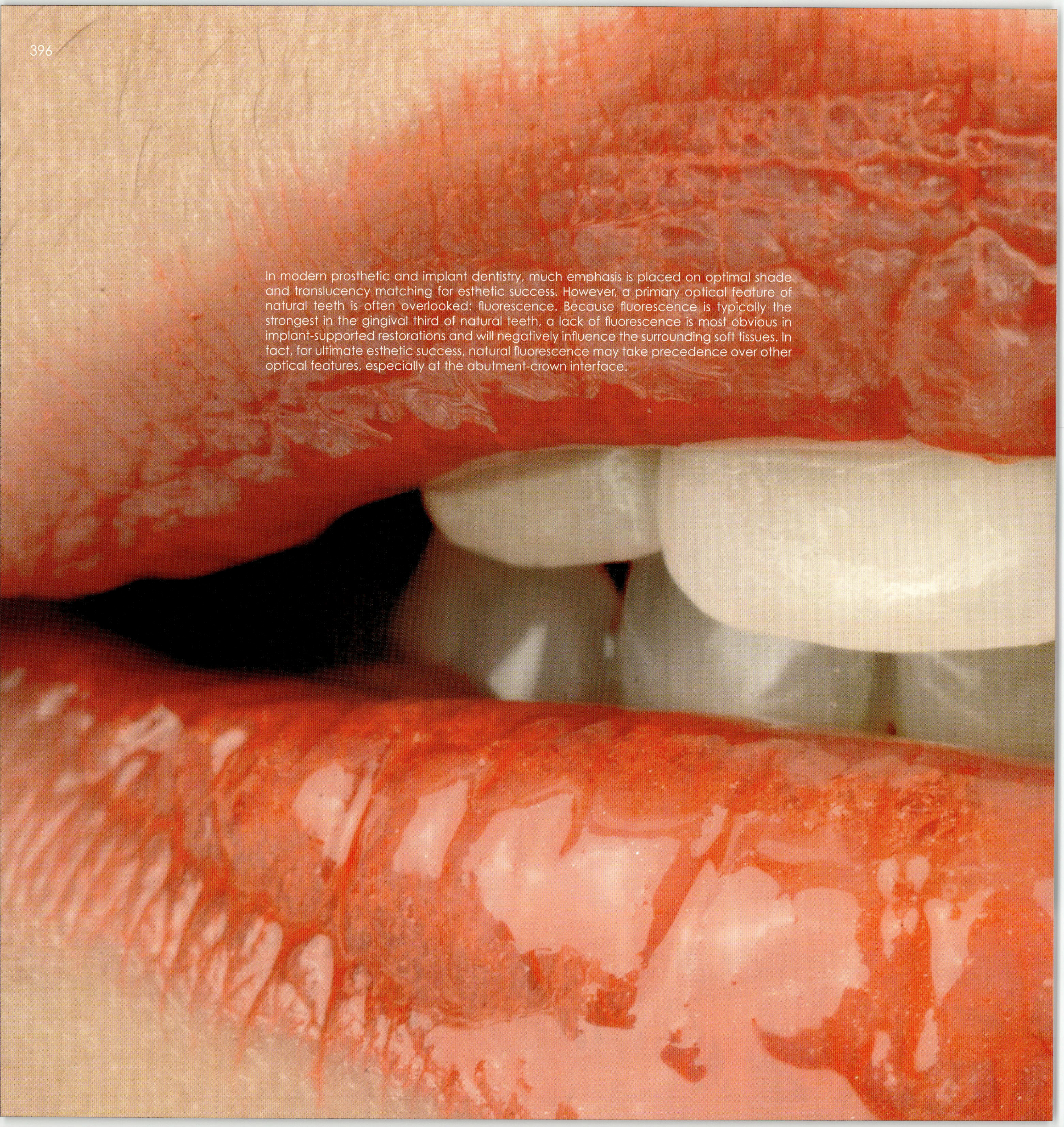

In modern prosthetic and implant dentistry, much emphasis is placed on optimal shade and translucency matching for esthetic success. However, a primary optical feature of natural teeth is often overlooked: fluorescence. Because fluorescence is typically the strongest in the gingival third of natural teeth, a lack of fluorescence is most obvious in implant-supported restorations and will negatively influence the surrounding soft tissues. In fact, for ultimate esthetic success, natural fluorescence may take precedence over other optical features, especially at the abutment-crown interface.

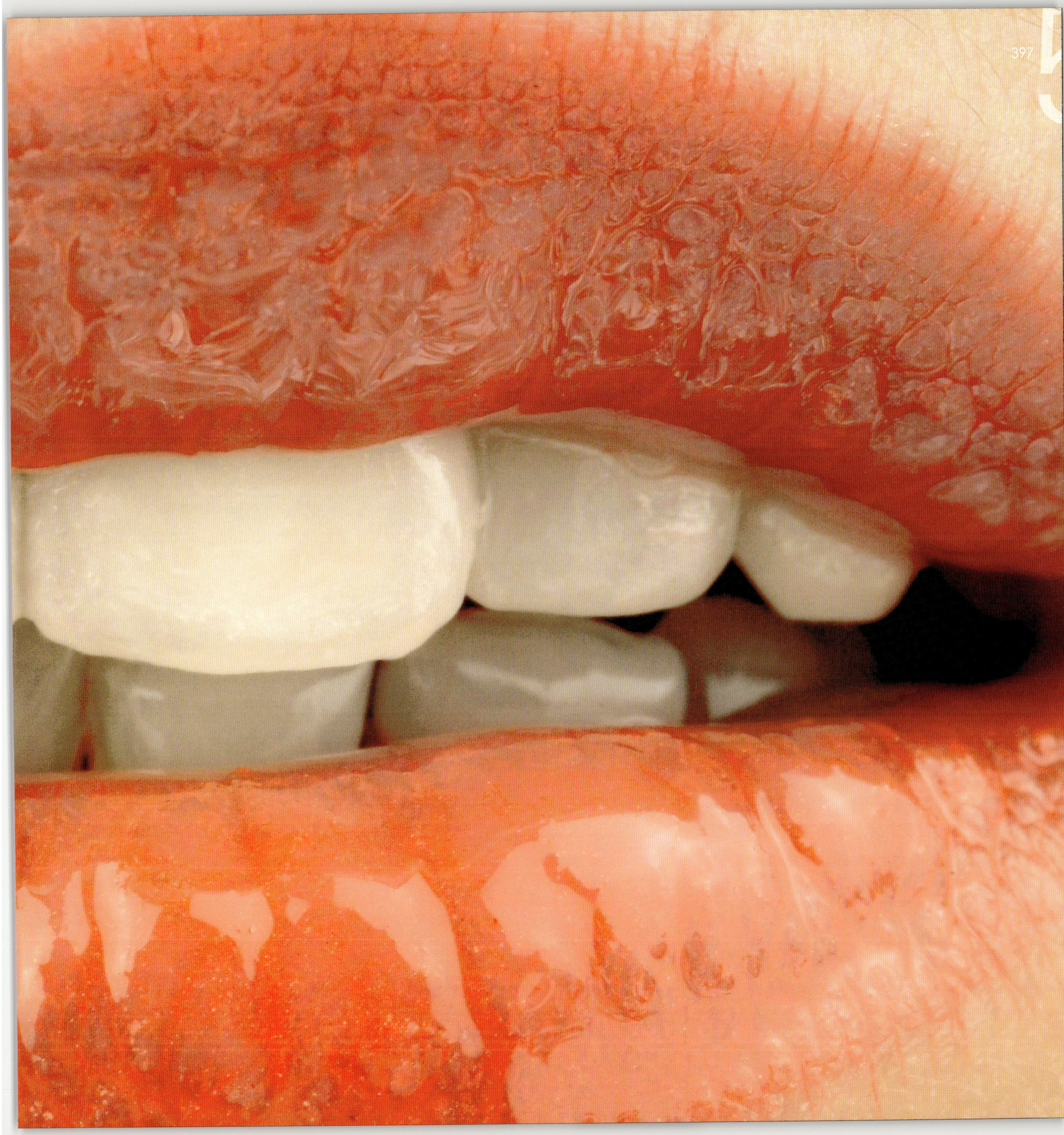

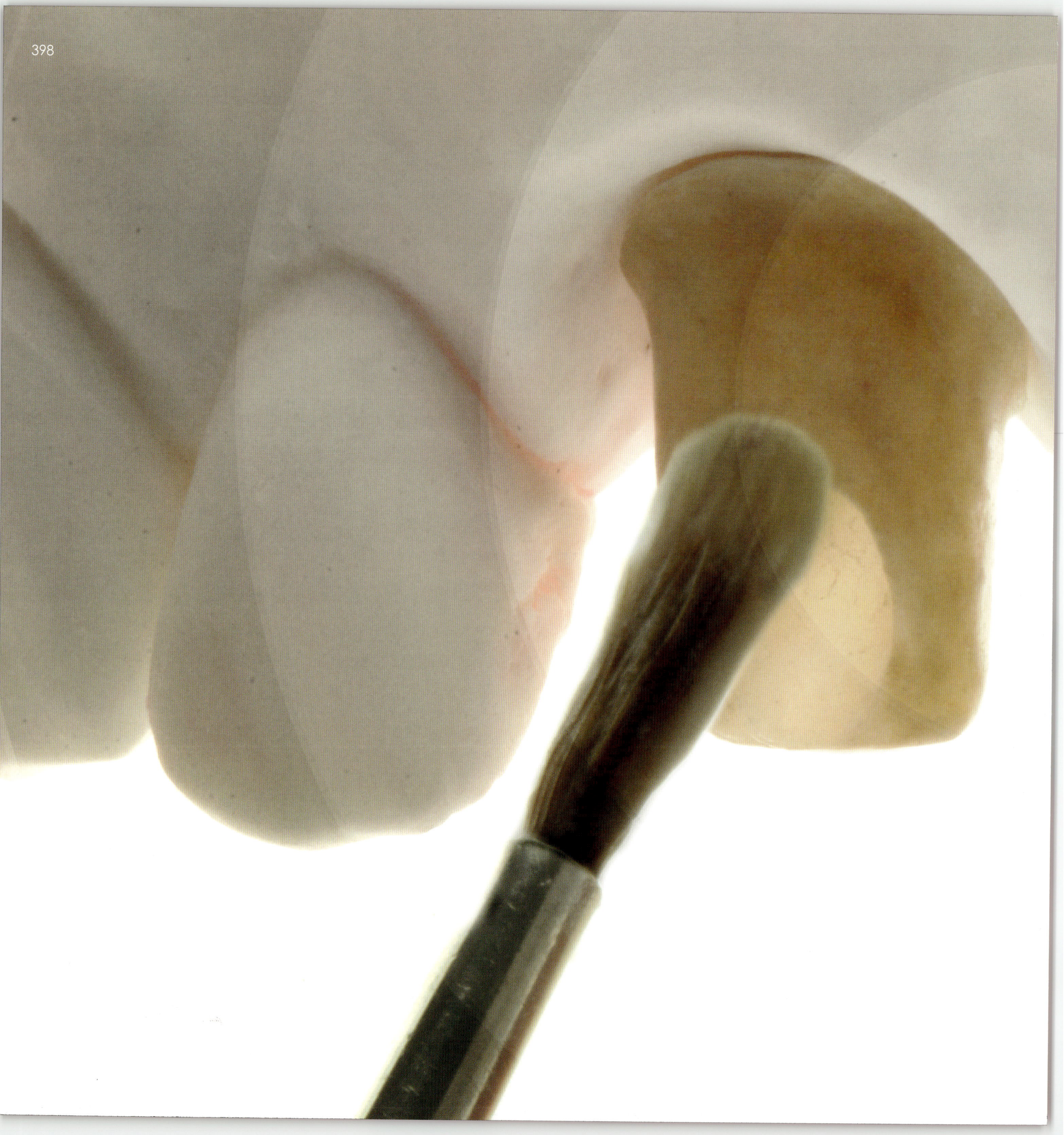

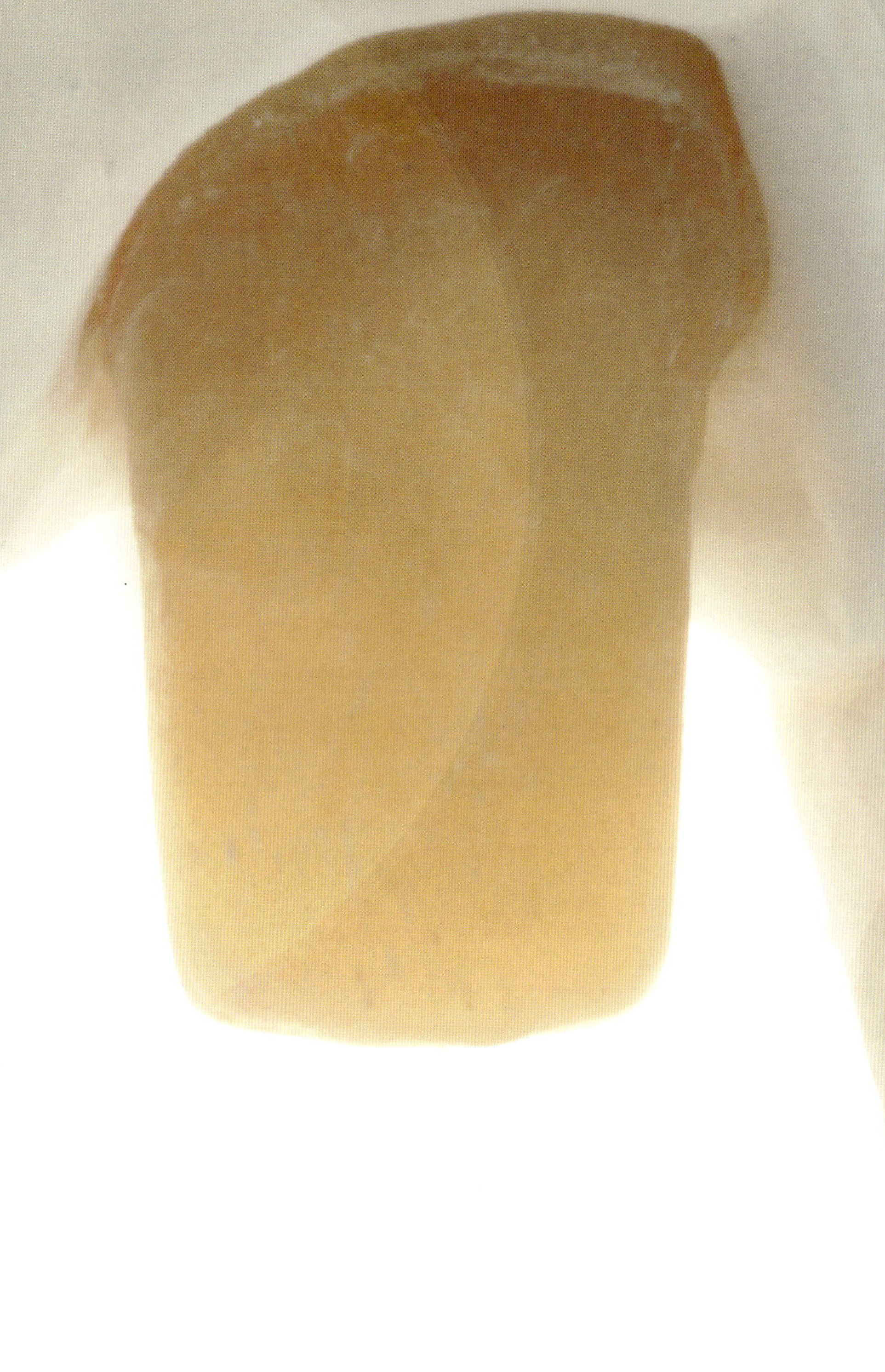

This patient situation demonstrates the difficulty of matching a natural dark-color abutment tooth adjacent to an implant-abutment restoration when restoring both central incisor crowns.

Unlike in the previous cases, the staining colors did not create the intended shade and, once color and fluorescence were mixed, the result was poor and did not match the clinical situation of the patient.

An advanced approach and technique was chosen to create a definitive implant abutment that matched the natural abutment tooth and an inconspicuous definitive crown restoration. Communication between the clinician and the laboratory technician is often a great challenge in such situations as technicians usually have to work only with images, digital shade data, and shade tabs, unless they have an opportunity to personally assess the shade and intraoral situation.

One of the preferred ways to communicate the shade of the abutment tooth (stump shade) to the laboratory technician is for the clinician to perform an extra step: the fabrication of a colored die with composite to replicate the shade of the abutment tooth. Once the final impression of both abutments is made, flowable composite resins are mixed with composite stains until the color of the mixture matches the shade of the natural abutment tooth. The mixture is then poured into the impression and light cured to create a customized, shaded die. Some retentions are carved into the composite to allow the stone to mechanically attach to it. The master cast now features a die of the prepared tooth that matches the shade of the natural abutment tooth and allows the dental technician to select the necessary materials and shade to mask the underlying tooth structure. In this situation, a customized impression coping was used to communicate the emergence profile from the previous provisional crown restoration and abutment. It is recommended to fabricate the definitive abutment at the same time as the definitive crowns to better control the ceramic powders, the shade and value of both restorations, and the fit of the coping on the custom-stained definitive abutment.

The definitive abutment was selected based on the fluorescence that could match the adjacent abutment restoration. In this situation, a zirconia abutment with fluorescent staining was selected but customized at the coronal aspect with internal porcelain staining to match the color of the adjacent natural tooth.

After shade selection, a zirconia plus fluorescence abutment was selected as the definitive abutment and inserted together with a provisional crown restoration. The natural abutment could not be bleached internally with the conventional methods (sodium perborate and hydrogen peroxide). This provided a great challenge since the stump shade of the natural abutment tooth was significantly darker than the implant abutment.

Meanwhile, the provisional crown-abutment unit was instrumental in modifying the peri-implant soft tissue topography to match the natural teeth.

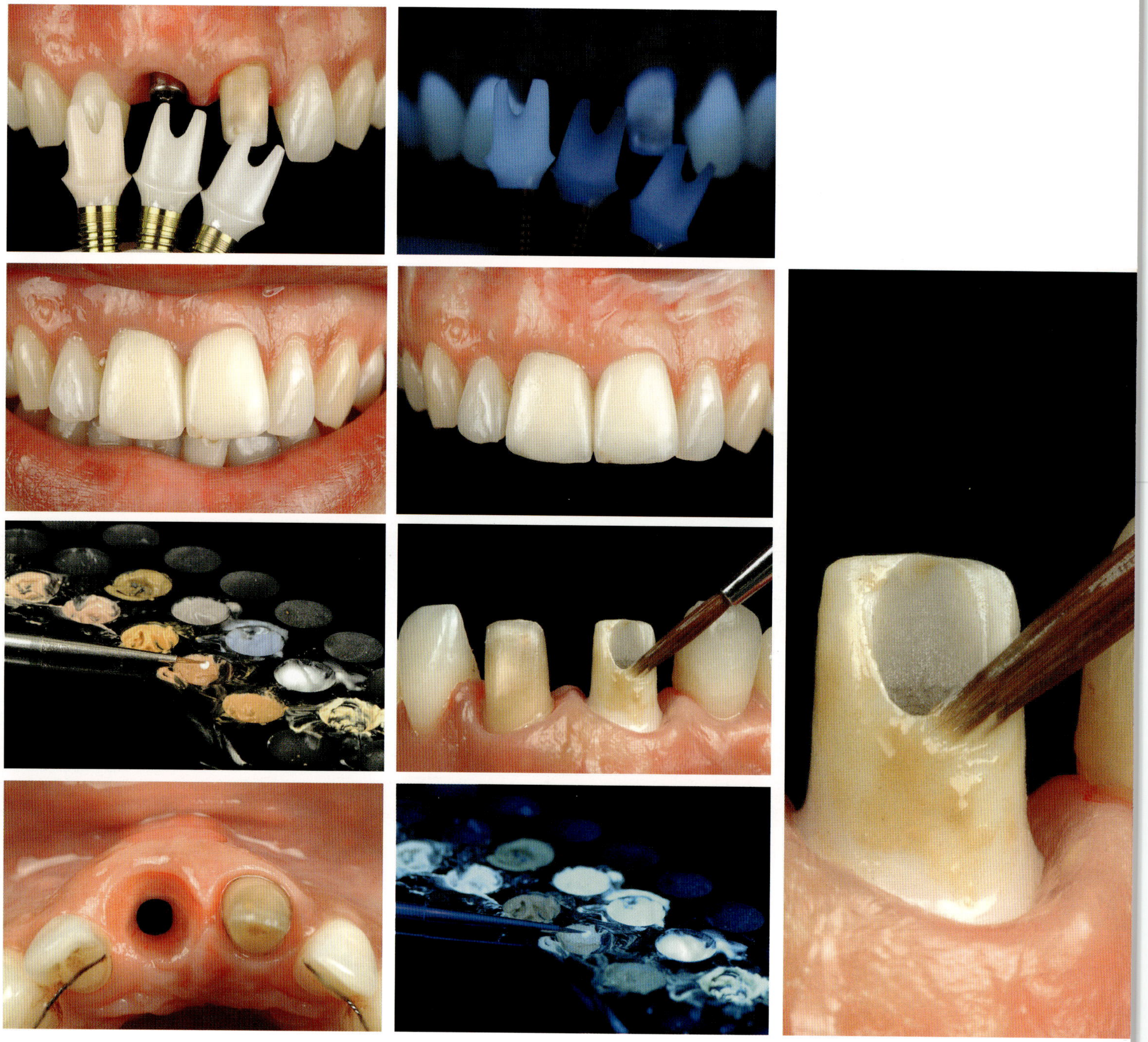

A new zirconia plus fluorescence abutment was fabricated to support the peri-implant soft tissue topography in the same way. The abutment was stained intraorally with internal porcelain stains (In Nova) to match the adjacent natural abutment color. Notice the differences in fluorescence/value once the chroma is increased.

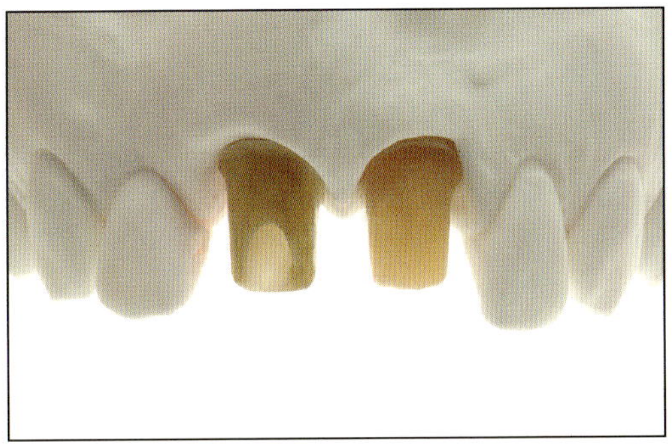

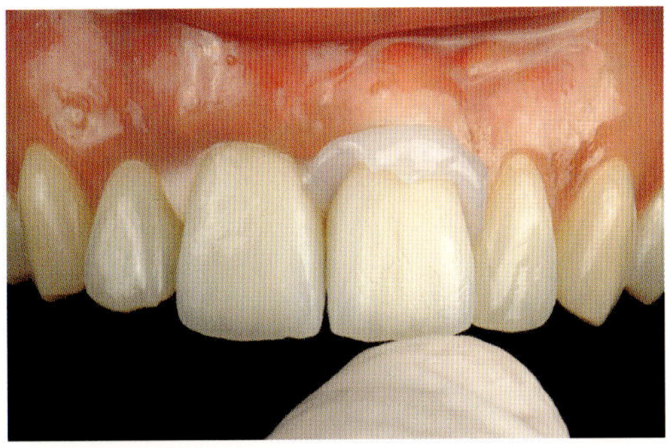

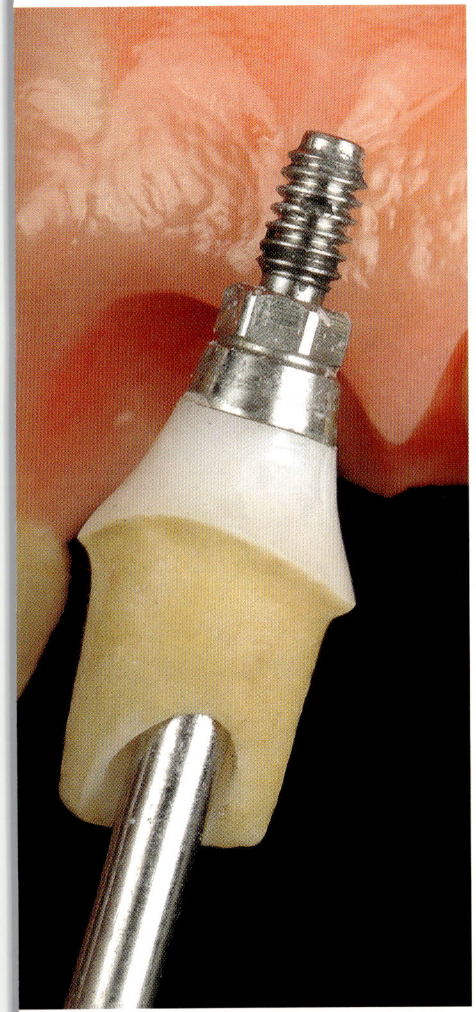

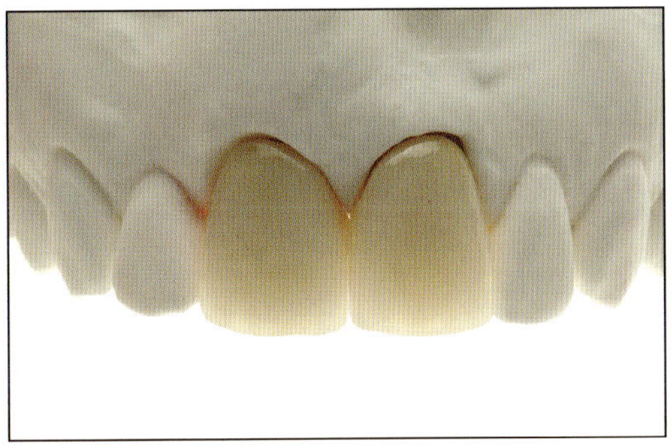

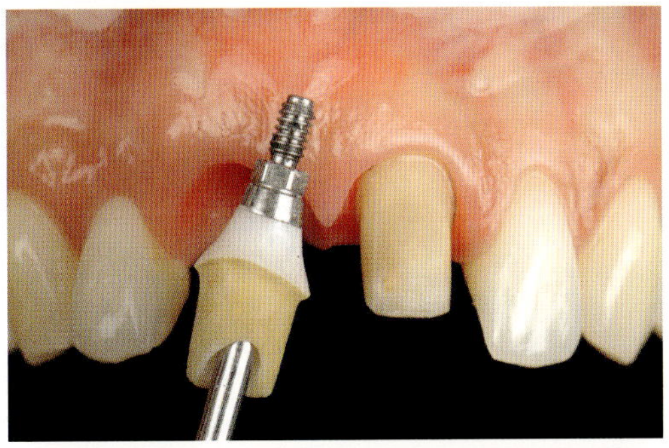

The stain was fired onto the abutment in the ceramic furnace and resulted in a customized abutment that presented optical properties and shade similar to those of the natural abutment tooth when viewed under different light sources (natural and UV light). Two zirconia crown restorations with 0.6-mm copings were then fabricated to mask the dark uniformed abutments. Different intraoral views illustrate the increased volume achieved through the surgical procedures, the tissue support achieved through the restorations, and masking of the dark substructures. Final outcome with radiographic confirmation are also shown.

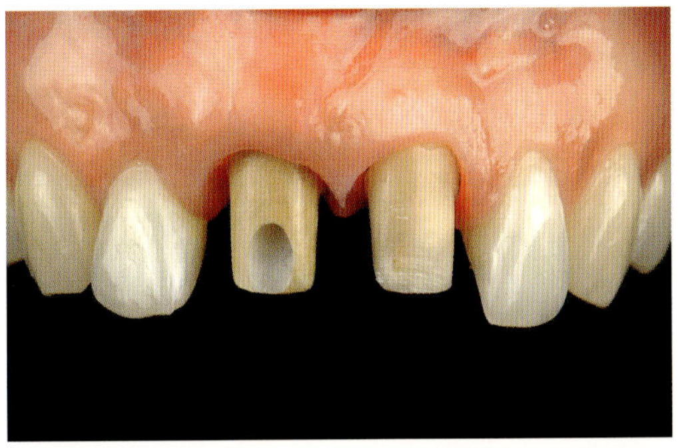

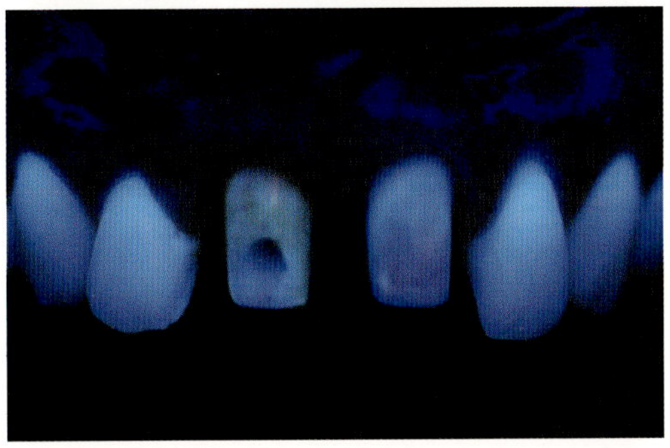

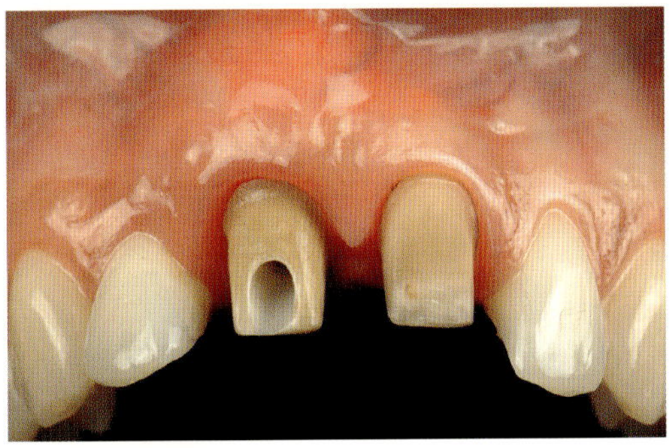

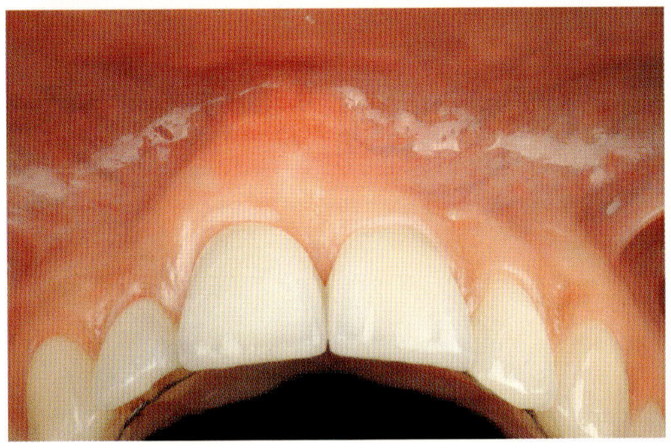

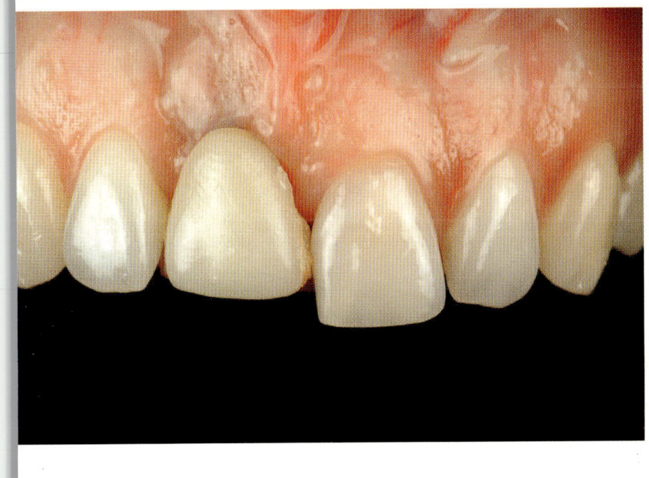

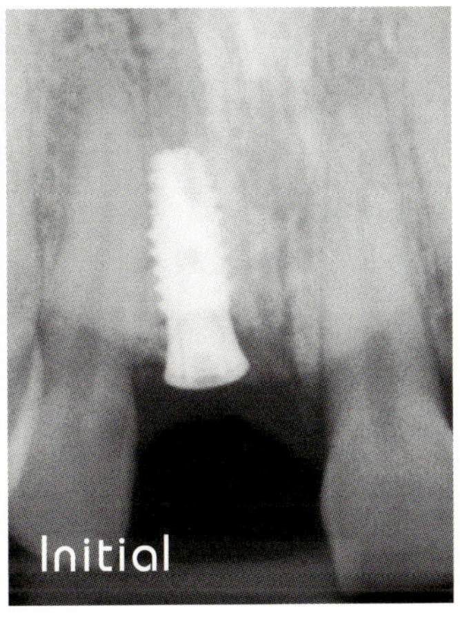

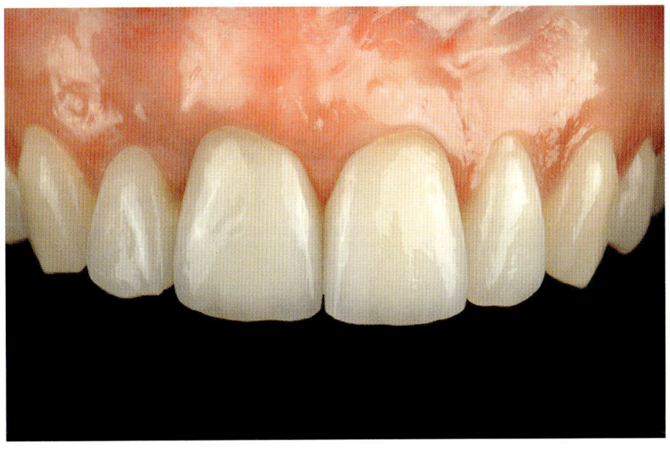

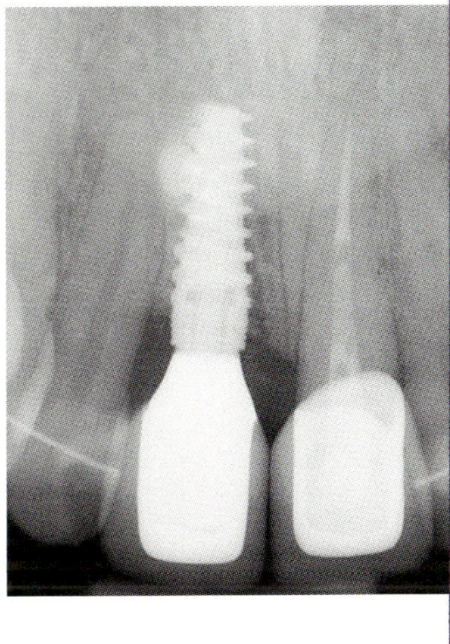

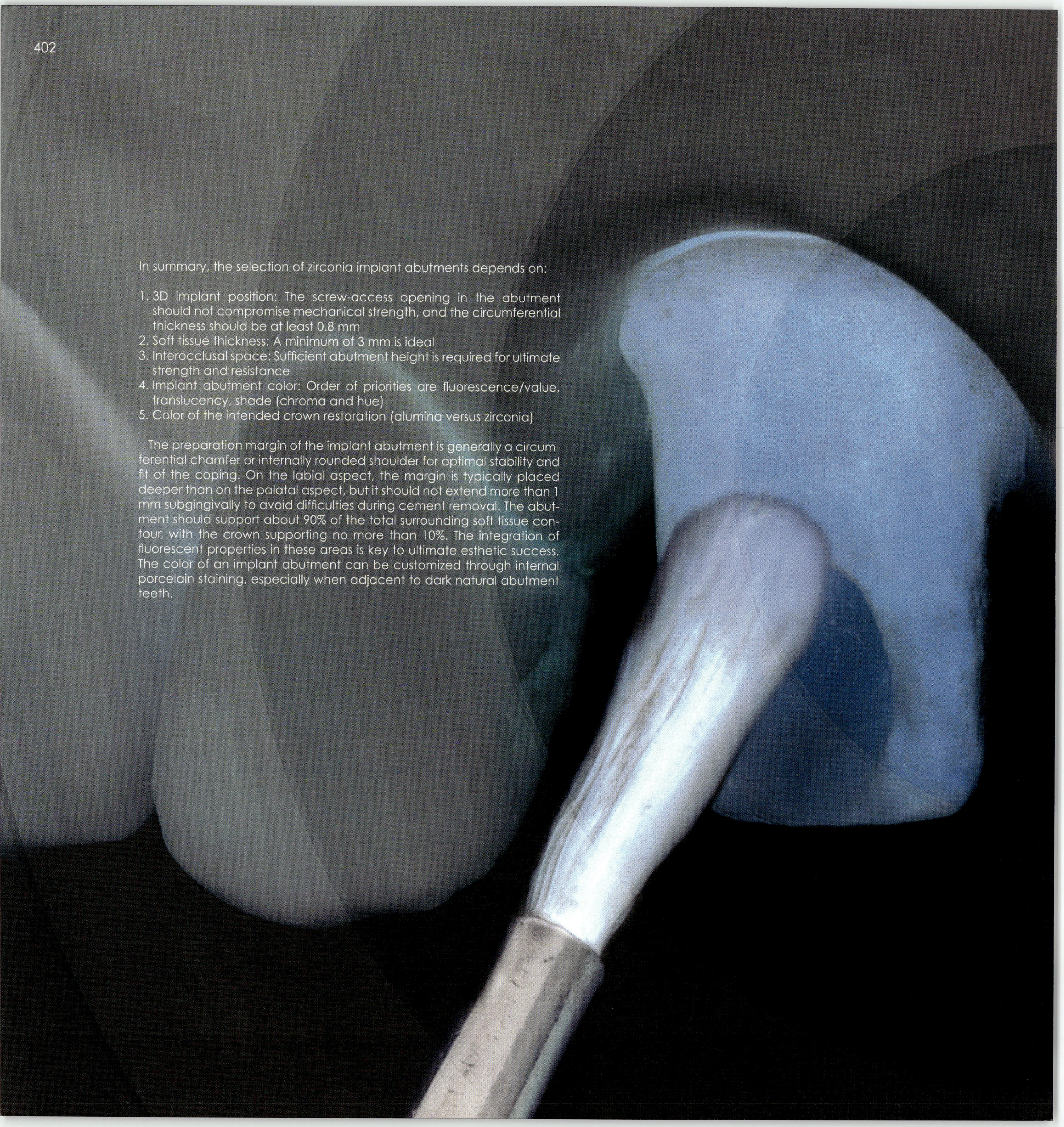

In summary, the selection of zirconia implant abutments depends on:

1. 3D implant position: The screw-access opening in the abutment should not compromise mechanical strength, and the circumferential thickness should be at least 0.8 mm
2. Soft tissue thickness: A minimum of 3 mm is ideal
3. Interocclusal space: Sufficient abutment height is required for ultimate strength and resistance
4. Implant abutment color: Order of priorities are fluorescence/value, translucency, shade (chroma and hue)
5. Color of the intended crown restoration (alumina versus zirconia)

The preparation margin of the implant abutment is generally a circumferential chamfer or internally rounded shoulder for optimal stability and fit of the coping. On the labial aspect, the margin is typically placed deeper than on the palatal aspect, but it should not extend more than 1 mm subgingivally to avoid difficulties during cement removal. The abutment should support about 90% of the total surrounding soft tissue contour, with the crown supporting no more than 10%. The integration of fluorescent properties in these areas is key to ultimate esthetic success. The color of an implant abutment can be customized through internal porcelain staining, especially when adjacent to dark natural abutment teeth.

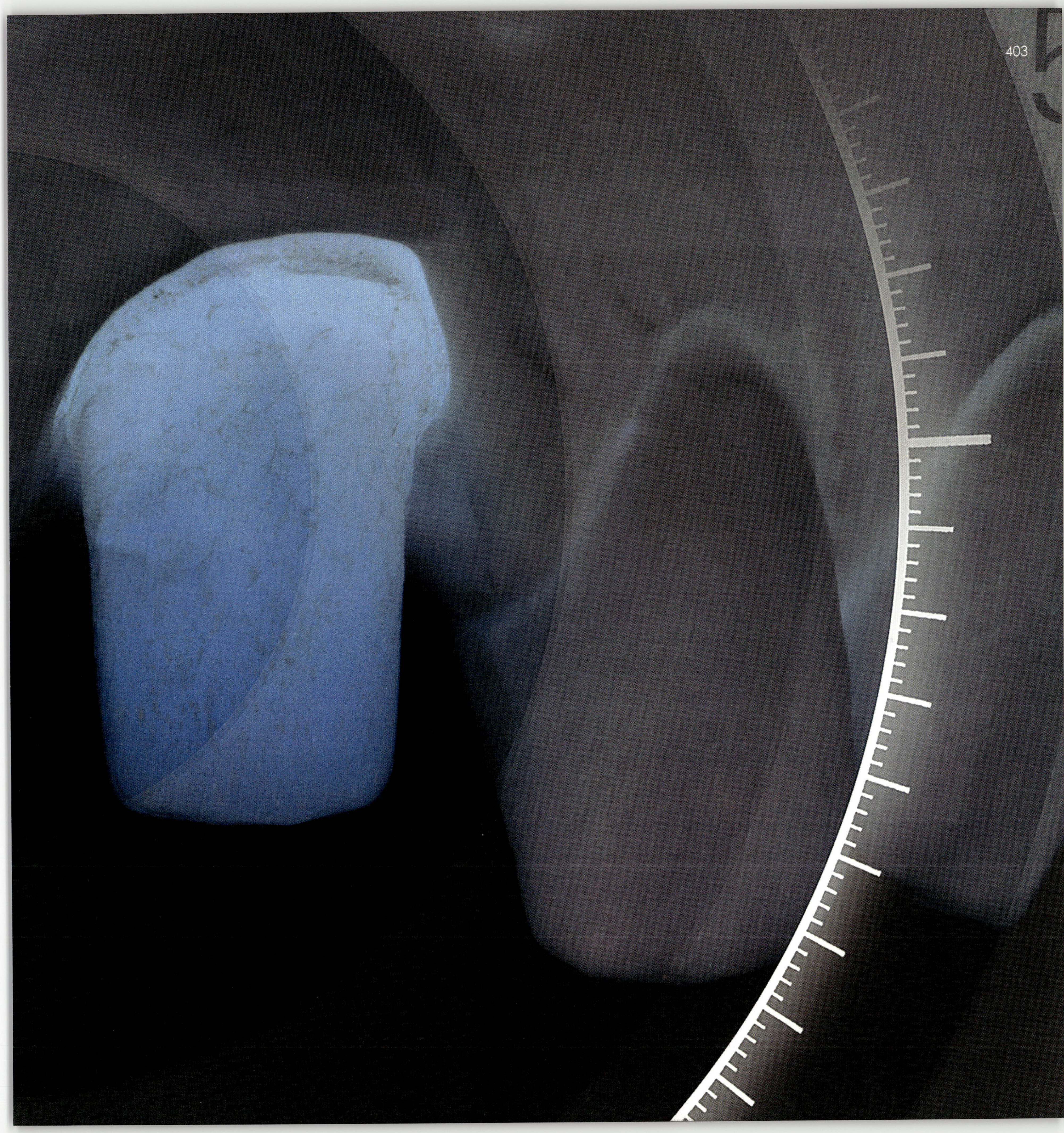

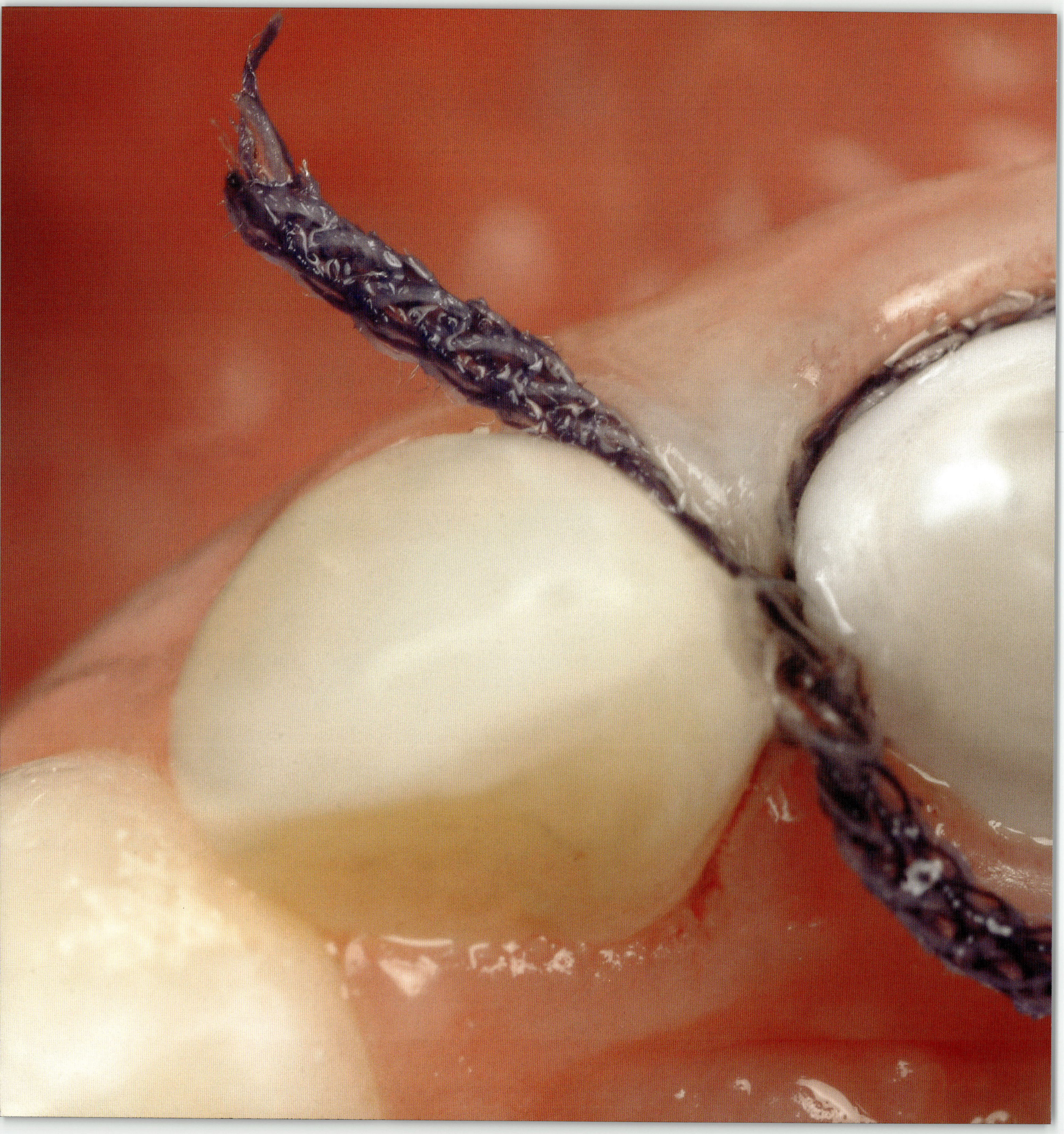

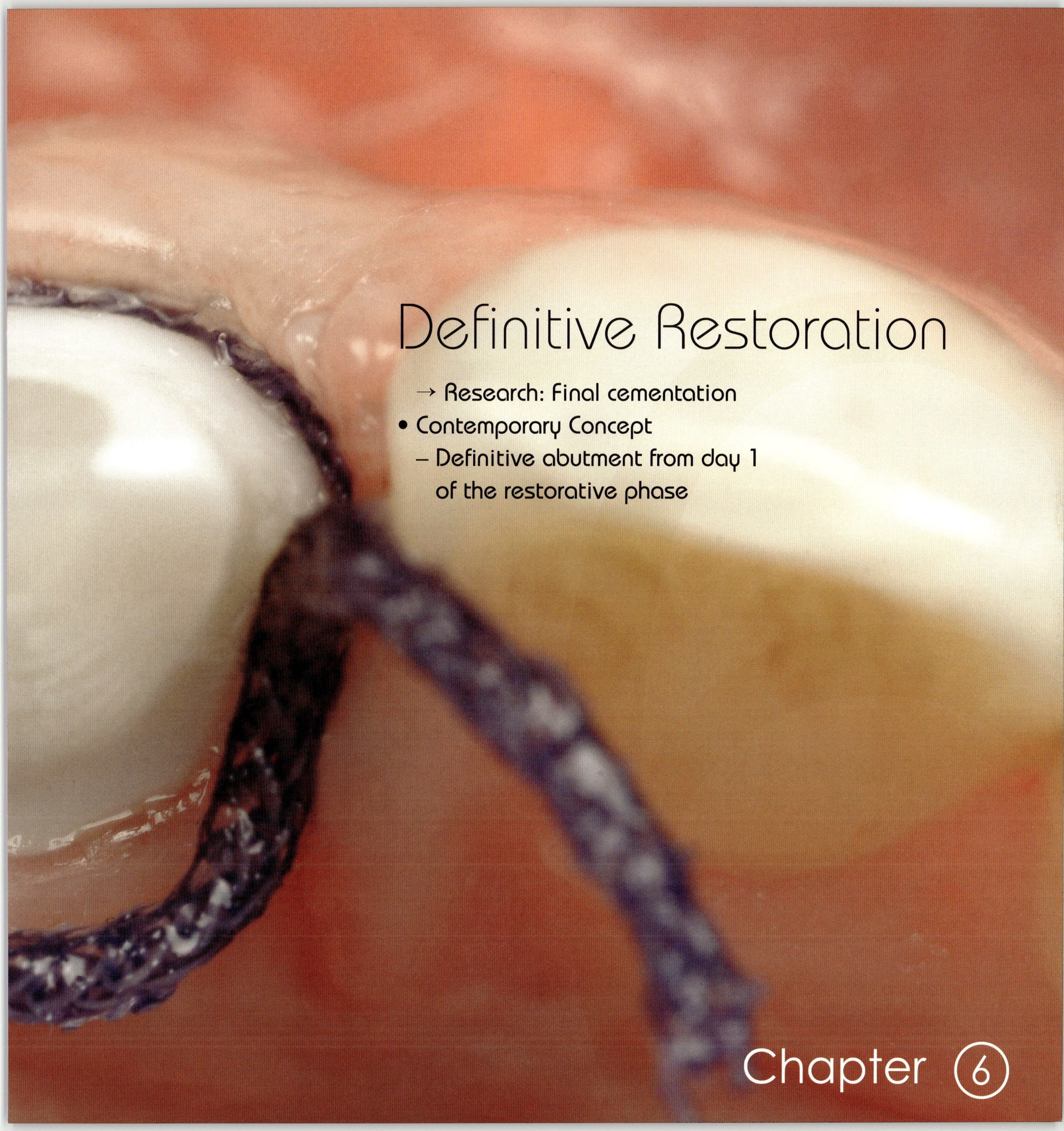

Definitive Restoration

→ Research: Final cementation

- Contemporary Concept
  - Definitive abutment from day 1 of the restorative phase

Chapter 6

Research

Final cementation

The cement-retained implant-supported crown has some technical and biomechanical advantages over the screw-retained restoration[1,2] and is necessary for many protocols described in this book. However, the importance of the definitive cementation step is often underestimated, and systematic reviews of clinical data fail to identify superior cementation protocols or materials.[1–4] Conversely, growing evidence indicates the detrimental biologic effects of careless implant crown cementation and incomplete cement removal.[3–5]

There is little guidance in the scientific literature regarding cement selection for implant crowns.[6,7] Therefore, this decision is mainly based on clinical parameters and needs. Many clinicians favor provisional cements for implant crowns to allow retrieval in the event of technical complications such as screw loosening,[1–5] which has become a rare incidence with internal implant connections.[3,4] Zinc oxide eugenol or non-eugenol cements are preferred for retrievable cementation of provisional or definitive restorations. For permanent cementation of implant crowns, zinc phosphate cements seem more popular than polycarboxylate, glass-ionomer, or composite resin cements.[1]

The concept of "provisional cementation" is questionable for all-ceramic crowns and abutments because it is quite difficult to retrieve all-ceramic restorations without damaging the ceramic structure, even when provisional cement was used. In addition, most ceramic materials, especially the ones at the lower end of the flexural strength spectrum, benefit from adhesive cementation with composite resin luting agents, which increases their fracture strength, retention, and marginal seal.[8,9] There are several in vitro studies on various implant cement properties and influencing parameters.[10–14] Provisional cements provide the lowest retentive forces between CAD/CAM all-ceramic abutments and crowns, closely followed by resin-modified glass-ionomer cement, while resin cements ensure the highest retention.[13] Abutment surface, size, height, and taper and size of the cement gap also have a direct influence on retention.[11–14] One clinical study demonstrated the advantage of a composite resin luting agent over zinc phosphate cement for all-ceramic implant-supported restorations.[15]

The high fracture strength of crowns and abutments made from oxide-based ceramics may allow for conventional cementation.[7] However, resin bonding with composite resin luting agents provides maximum retention and further increases fracture strength, especially for alumina-based crowns.[9] Both crown and abutment bonding interfaces must be treated adequately to yield maximum bond strengths. According to the current literature,[16] air-particle abrasion with aluminum-oxide particles and application of a ceramic primer containing special adhesive monomers is a highly effective and simple method to pretreat alumina and zirconia bonding surfaces.[16–23] A self- or dual-curing composite resin luting agent is recommended.[8]

Self-adhesive resin cements have become very popular because they provide decent bond strengths without time-consuming and technique-sensitive bonding steps.[24] Their application is as simple as conventional cementation, so these cements are therefore the material of choice in many clinical situations.[24] Air abrasion with aluminum-oxide particles further enhances their bond strength to oxide-based high-strength ceramics.[24]

A key part of the cementation protocol, thorough surface cleaning and decontamination of the definitive abutment before final insertion improves soft tissue integration[25,26] and increases cement bond strength.

References

1. Chaar MS, Att W, Strub JR. Prosthetic outcome of cement-retained implant-supported fixed dental restorations: A systematic review. J Oral Rehabil 2011;38:697–711.
2. Nissan J, Narobai D, Gross O, Ghelfan O, Chaushu G. Long-term outcome of cemented versus screw-retained implant-supported partial restorations. Int J Oral Maxillofac Implants 2011;26:1102–1107.
3. Wismeijer D, Brägger U, Evans C, et al. Consensus statements and recommended clinical procedures regarding restorative materials and techniques for implant dentistry. Int J Oral Maxillofac Implants 2014;29(suppl):137–140.
4. Morton D, Chen ST, Martin WC, Levine RA, Buser D. Consensus statements and recommended clinical procedures regarding optimizing esthetic outcomes in implant dentistry. Int J Oral Maxillofac Implants 2014;29(suppl):216–220.
5. Sailer I, Mühlemann S, Zwahlen M, Hämmerle CH, Schneider D. Cemented and screw-retained implant reconstructions: A systematic review of the survival and complication rates. Clin Oral Implants Res 2012;23(suppl 6):163–201.
6. Abt E, Carr AB, Worthington HV. Interventions for replacing missing teeth: Partially absent dentition. Cochrane Database Syst Rev 2012;(2):CD003814.
7. Selz CF, Strub JR, Vach K, Guess PC. Long-term performance of posterior InCeram Alumina crowns cemented with different luting agents: A prospective, randomized clinical split-mouth study over 5 years. Clin Oral Investig 2014;18:1695–1703.
8. Blatz MB, Sadan A, Kern M. Resin-ceramic bonding—A review of the literature. J Prosthet Dent 2003;89:268–274.
9. Blatz MB, Oppes S, Chiche GJ, Holst S, Sadan A. Influence of cementation technique on fracture strength and leakage of alumina all-ceramic crowns after cyclic loading. Quintessence Int 2008;39:23–32.
10. Sheets JL, Wilcox C, Wilwerding T. Cement selection for cement-retained crown technique with dental implants. J Prosthodont 2008;17:92–96.
11. Bernal G, Okamura M, Muñoz CA. The effects of abutment taper, length and cement type on resistance to dislodgement of cement-retained, implant-supported restorations. J Prosthodont 2003;12:111–115.
12. Pan YH, Ramp LC, Lin CK, Liu PR. Retention and leakage of implant-supported restorations luted with provisional cement: A pilot study. J Oral Rehabil 2007;34:206–212.
13. Carnaggio TV, Conrad R, Engelmeier RL, et al. Retention of CAD/CAM all-ceramic crowns on prefabricated implant abutments: An in vitro comparative study of luting agents and abutment surface area. J Prosthodont 2012;21:523–528.
14. Gultekin P, Gultekin BA, Aydin M, Yalcin S. Cement selection for implant-supported crowns fabricated with different luting space settings. J Prosthodont 2013;22:112–119.
15. Sorrentino R, Galasso L, Tetè S, De Simone G, Zarone F. Clinical evaluation of 209 all-ceramic single crowns cemented on natural and implant-supported abutments with different luting agents: A 6-year retrospective study. Clin Implant Dent Relat Res 2012;14:184–197.
16. Kern M. Bonding to oxide ceramics—Laboratory testing versus clinical outcome [epub ahead of print 21 July 2014]. Dent Mater doi:10.1016/j.dental.2014.06.007.
17. Blatz MB, Sadan A, Arch GH Jr, Lang BR. In vitro evaluation of long-term bonding of Procera AllCeram alumina restorations with a modified resin luting agent. J Prosthet Dent 2003;89:381–387.
18. Sadan A, Blatz MB, Soignet D. Influence of silanization on early bond strength to sandblasted densely sintered alumina. Quintessence Int 2003;34:172–176.
19. Blatz MB, Sadan A, Blatz U. The effect of silica coating on the resin bond to the intaglio surface of Procera AllCeram restorations. Quintessence Int 2003;34:542–547.
20. Blatz MB, Sadan A, Soignet D, Blatz U, Mercante D, Chiche G. Long-term resin bond to densely sintered aluminum oxide ceramic. J Esthet Restor Dent 2003;15:362–368.
21. Blatz MB, Sadan A, Martin J, Lang B. In-vitro evaluation of shear bond strengths of resin to densely-sintered high-purity zirconium-oxide ceramic after long-term storage and thermocycling. J Prosthet Dent 2004;91:365–362.
22. Blatz MB, Chiche G, Holst S, Sadan A. Influence of surface treatment and simulated aging on bond strengths of luting agents to zirconia. Quintessence Int 2007;38:745–753.
23. Koizumi H, Nakayama D, Komine F, Blatz MB, Matsumura H. Bonding of resin-based luting cements to zirconia with and without the use of ceramic priming agents. J Adhes Dent 2012;14:385–392.
24. Blatz MB, Phark JH, Ozer F, et al. In-vitro-comparative bond strength of contemporary self-adhesive resin cements to zirconium-oxide ceramic with and without air-particle abrasion. Clin Oral Investig 2010;14:187–192.
25. Rompen E, Domken O, Degidi M, Pontes AE, Piattelli A. The effect of material characteristics, of surface topography and of implant components and connections on soft tissue integration: A literature review. Clin Oral Implants Res 2006;17(suppl 2):55–67.
26. Rompen E. The impact of the type and configuration of abutments and their (repeated) removal on the attachment level and marginal bone. Eur J Oral Implantol 2012;5(suppl):S83–S90.

From bisque bake to final cementation, there are a few stages that require caution to avoid problems with fit and biocompatibility. Many articles and textbooks stress the importance of cement removal and the ability to control the situation while cementing crown restorations on top of implants. This section explains a preferred cementation protocol.

Adjusting and cementing crowns should be done in a specific sequence:

1. Adjust interproximal contacts to verify proper seating and fit of the crown.
2. Check occlusion in centric and excursive movements.
3. Check shape (line angles), proportions, tissue support, emergence profile, surface texture, and shade (value, chroma, hue).

One of the most important aspects is control of the contact areas between implants and adjacent natural teeth or crowns, because dental implants do not feature the biologic resistance to food impaction and periodontal disease found in the gingival attachment apparatus around natural teeth. One of the major esthetic peri-implant soft tissue failures is an open contact, which may result in bone loss at the interproximal bone due to food impaction and, consequently, loss of papillary height. Replacing single teeth with dental implants presents a great challenge because of the adjacent teeth shapes, positions, prosthetic path of insertion, and, especially when the interproximal bone was affected, undercuts and long contact areas. Interproximal recontouring of the adjacent teeth with direct composite restorations, for example, is required in a high percentage of cases. The goal is to restore the interproximal contact point, which should actually be a surface area rather than a point. Almost 80% of the cases in this book necessitated some sort of recontouring with composite resin to create a satisfactory contact area between the adjacent tooth and the definitive implant crown restoration and to re-create support for the interproximal papilla.

Composite resin recontouring should be performed on the day of the final cementation of the implant restoration to allow for precise soft tissue support. It will also simplify the cementation process since a path of insertion has already been established. After recontouring, a specific protocol for decontamination and cleaning of the implant abutment should be followed.

Two patient situations are presented in this section in which the abutments were fabricated following different concepts. In the first patient, a provisional abutment was made from composite to create ideal soft tissue support and emergence profile of the prosthetic restoration. In the second one, the definitive abutment was inserted on the first day of the restorative phase, representing a more contemporary approach. Both scenarios follow the same cementation protocol. The only difference is that the more contemporary approach includes removal of the definitive abutment to check for excess provisional cement on the abutment surface. After removal of the abutment, the soft tissue is cleaned with chlorhexidine, and the abutment is wiped with sterile gauze and saline to remove any debris.

The maxillary left lateral incisor was extracted because of root fracture and localized periodontitis. After 3 months of healing, a NobelReplace Select NP 3.5 × 13–mm implant was placed with a connective tissue graft (CTG) harvested from the tuberosity. After 4 more months of healing, a provisional crown restoration and composite abutment were fabricated to support the peri-implant soft tissue and copy the soft tissue topography of the contralateral tooth.

Subsequently, a definitive zirconia abutment was designed following the outline of the composite provisional abutment. Glutaraldehyde (2%) was applied for 5 minutes to disinfect the abutment, which was then rinsed with water and inserted. The abutment screw was torqued with 35 Ncm, and the screw access hole was filled with polytetrafluoroethylene and Fermit (Ivoclar).

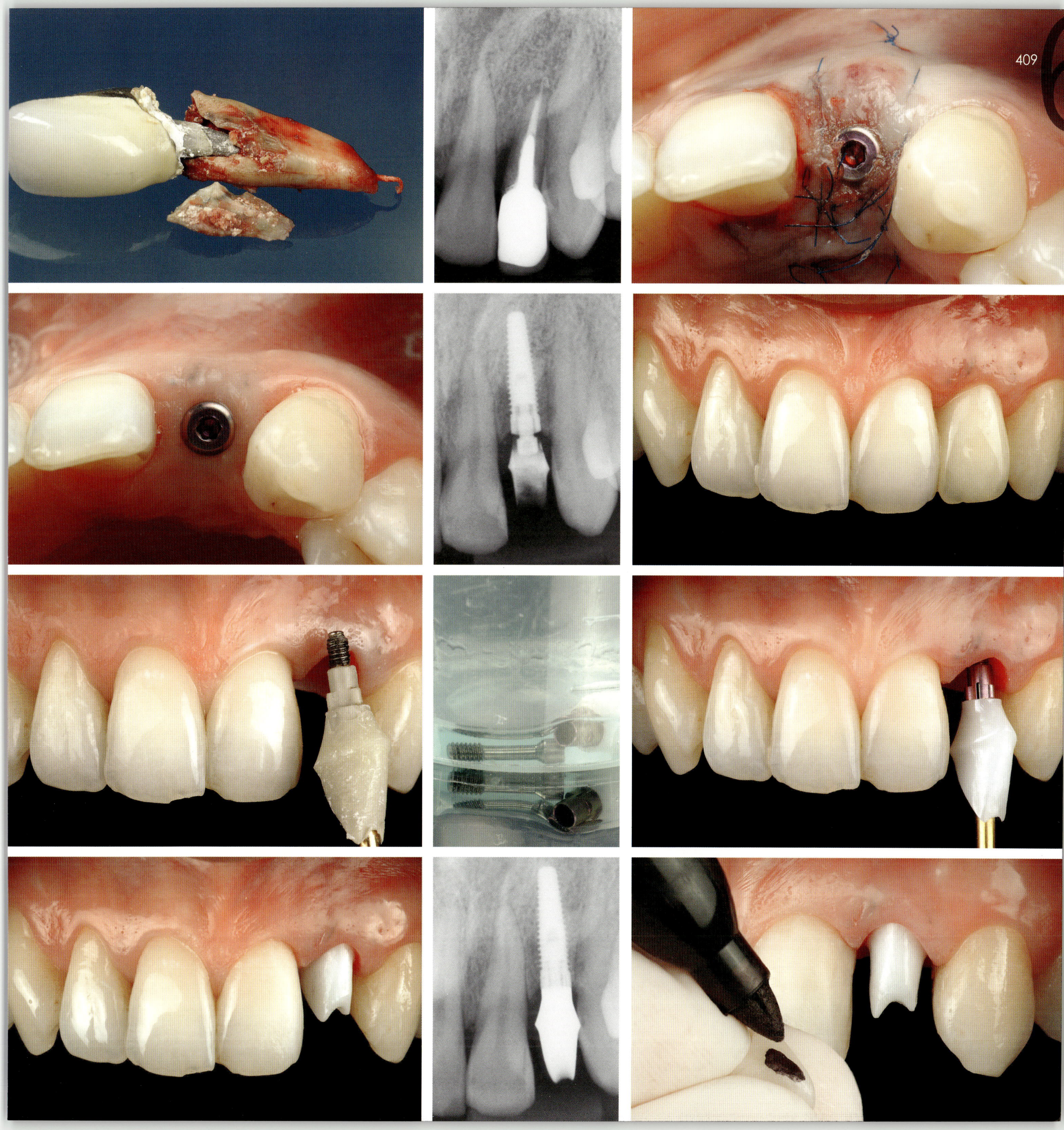

The definitive alumina crown restoration was tried in. Composite resin was applied on the distal of the maxillary left central incisor before cementation to support the mesial short papilla (due to previous bone loss) and the gingival embrasure and to provide a more defined interproximal contact area with the crown restoration. Before the final impression was made, retraction cords were placed to simplify cement removal. Two independent retraction cords, one buccal and one palatal, were placed in a 180-degree fashion. The viscosity of the cement is also crucial: Higher viscosity creates greater hydraulic pressure, pushing the cement further apically below the preparation finish line. A cement of lower viscosity is therefore recommended.

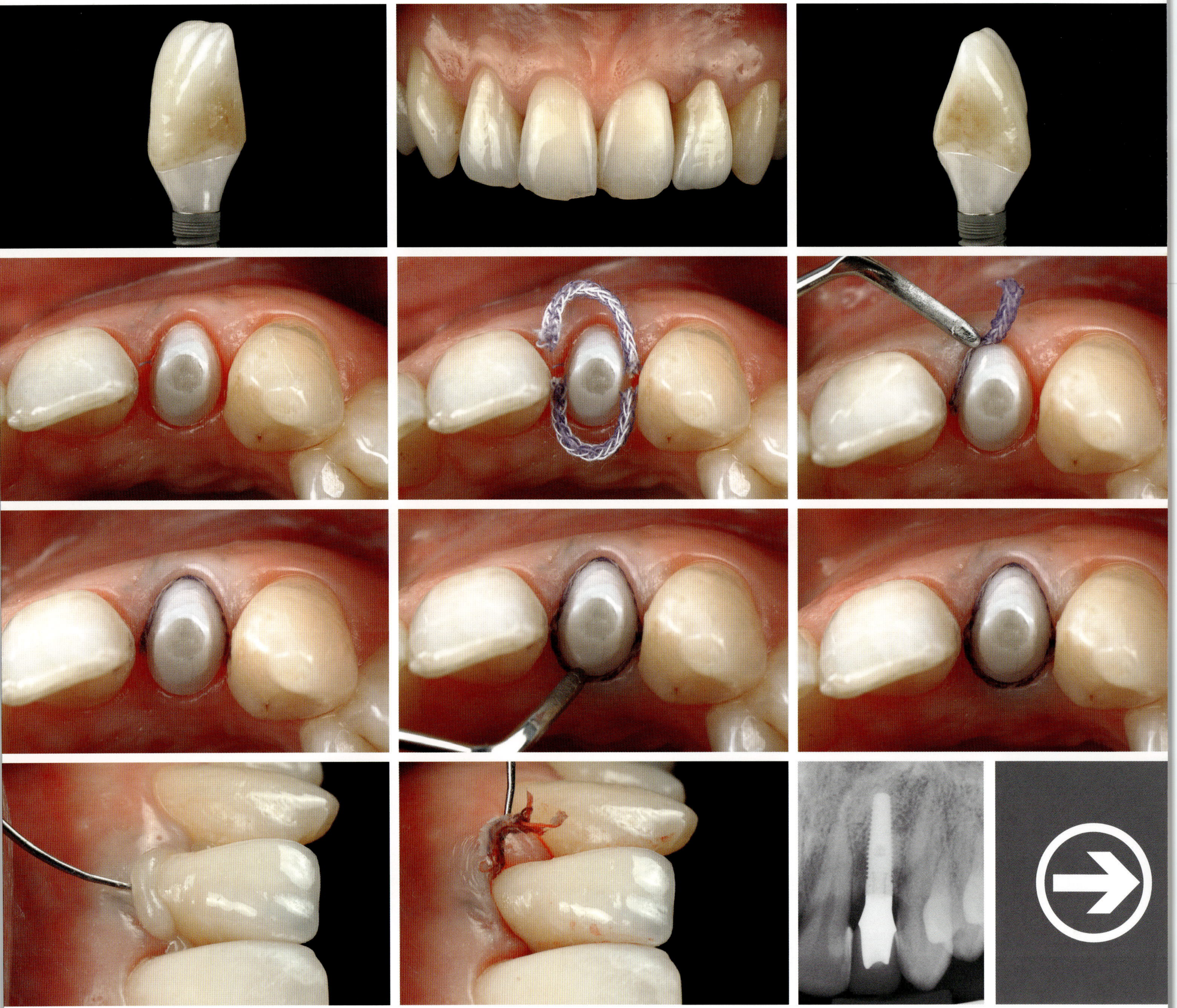

Different aspects of the restoration 1 to 5 years postoperatively with corresponding radiographs demonstrate bone remodeling and stability. The composite resin restoration on the distal aspect of the central incisor allowed for ideal maturation of the interproximal papilla and long-term stability.

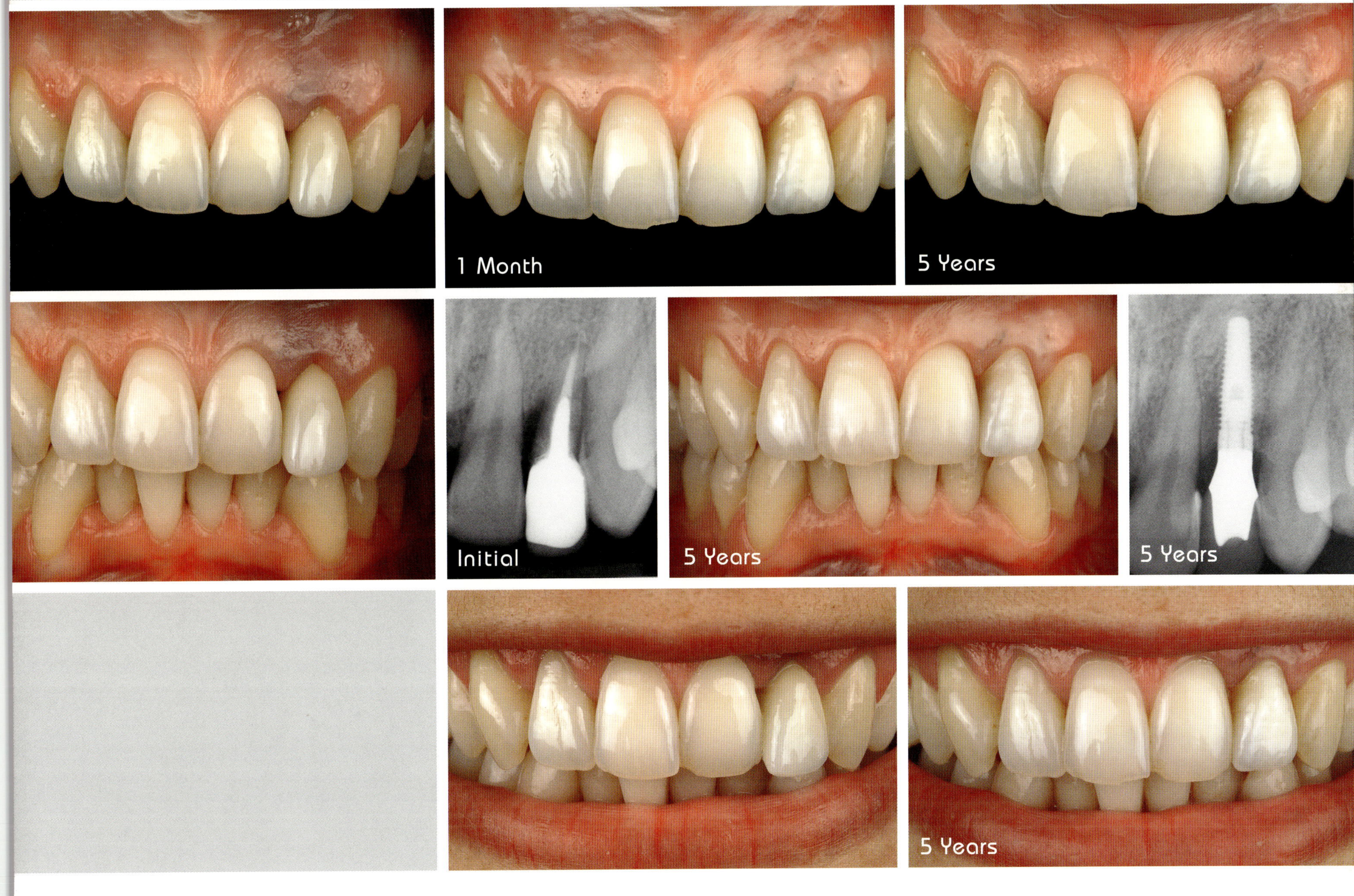

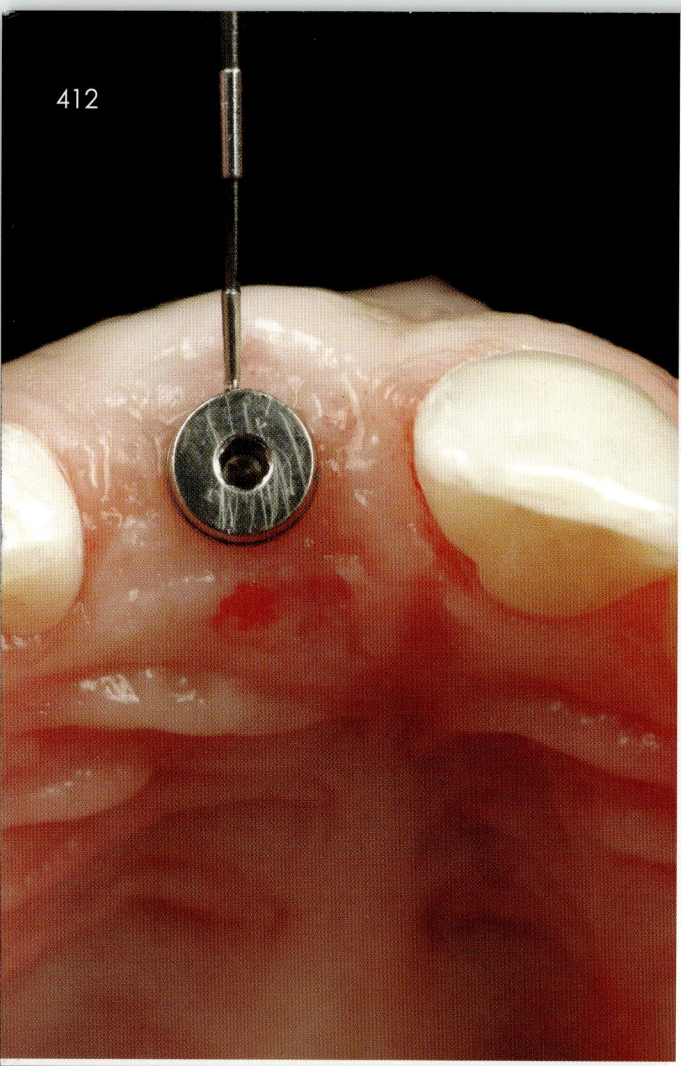

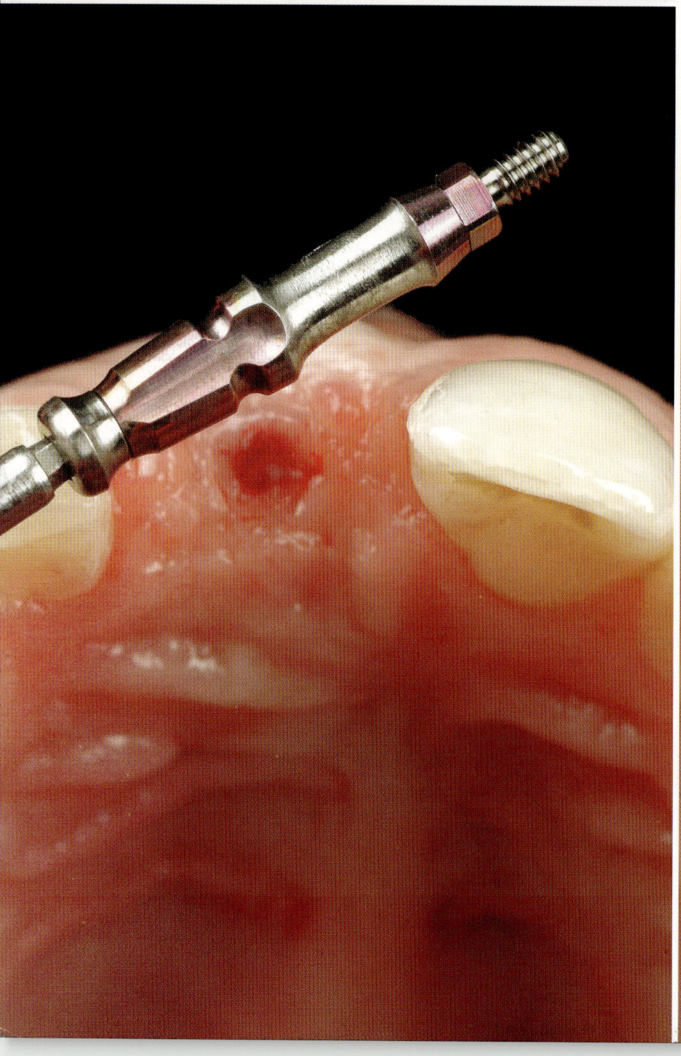

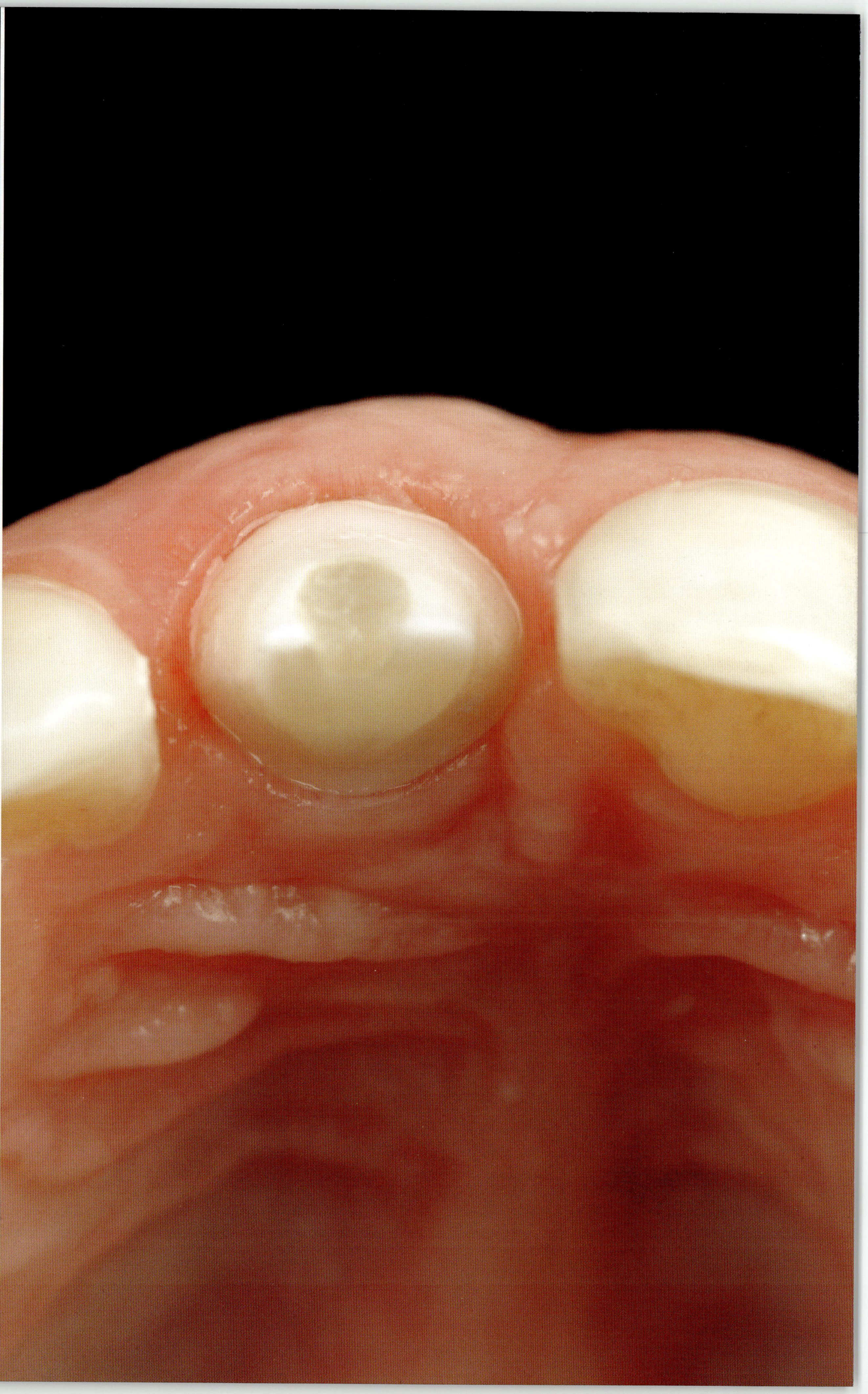

Contemporary Concept

Definitive abutment from day 1 of the restorative phase

The maxillary right central incisor had to be extracted because of periodontal inflammation and bone destruction. An epithelialized-subepithelial CTG was placed to seal the extraction socket and to prevent tissue collapse but also create a thicker tissue at the crestal aspect. A NobelActive 3.5 × 13–mm implant was inserted, and a second CTG from the tuberosity was placed to further increase soft tissue volume. A slim temporary healing abutment was connected to the implant to provide physical space and to allow suturing of the CTG in a coronal position. After 4 months of healing, the slim temporary abutment was removed, and an implant impression was made for abutment and provisional crown fabrication.

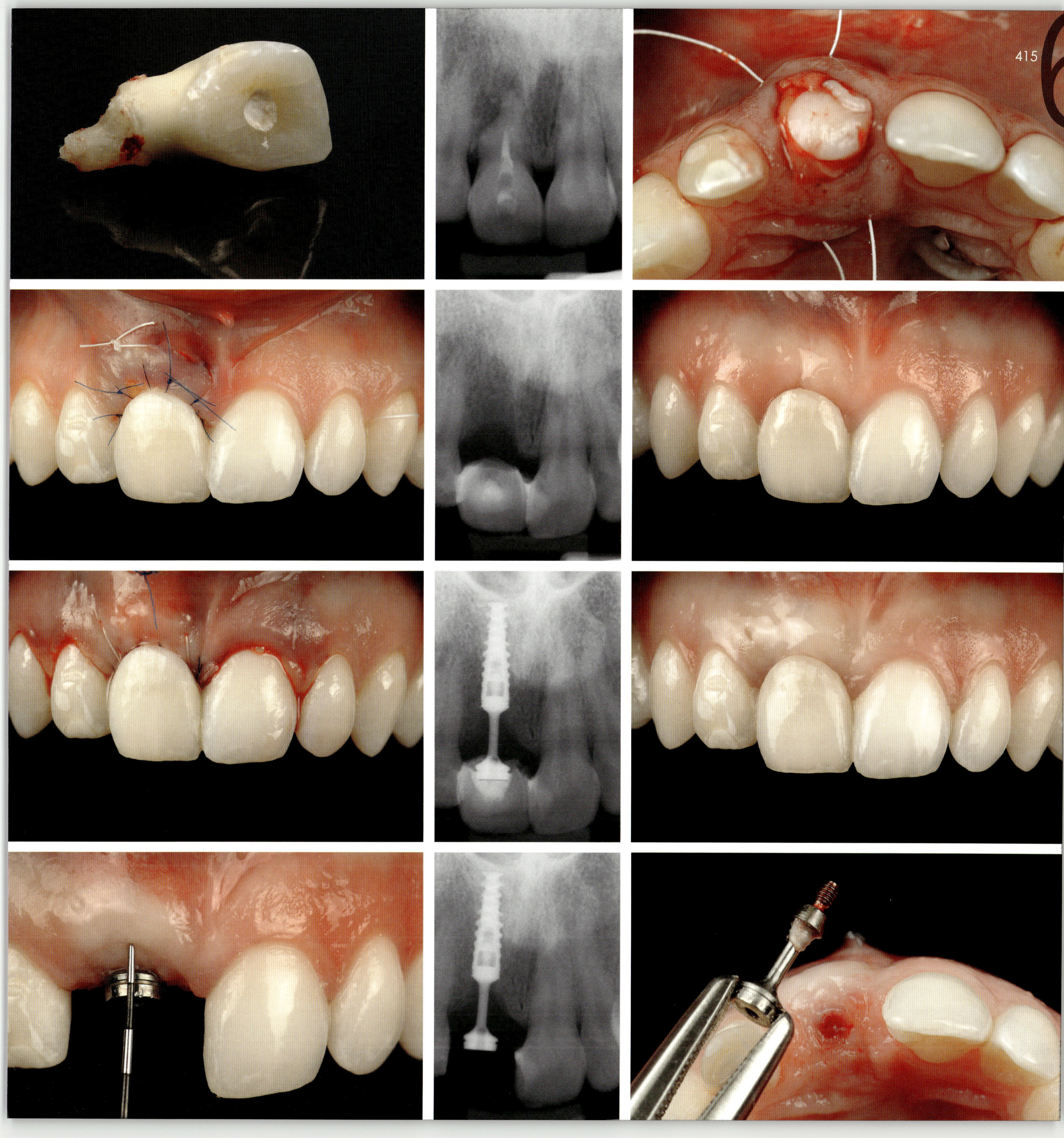

The definitive abutment was disinfected with 2% glutaraldehyde for 5 minutes before its insertion and intraoral relining of the crown. The abutment was thoroughly rinsed with water and then tightened onto the implant with 35 Ncm. The customized crown-abutment unit created a preferred soft tissue topography by the 3-month re-evaluation. A final impression was made, and the crown restoration was finalized. Fit and occlusal contacts were examined and adjusted before final cementation. Matching fluorescence between the implant restoration and the adjacent natural teeth is shown under ultraviolet light.

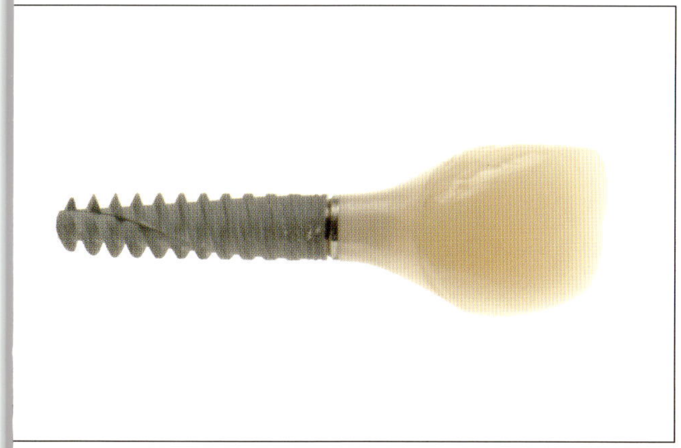

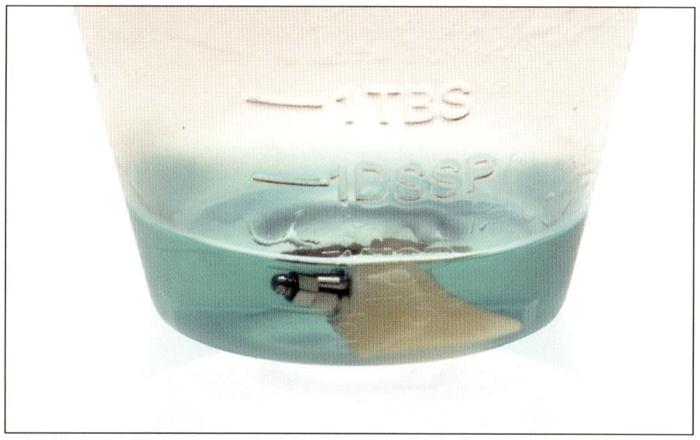

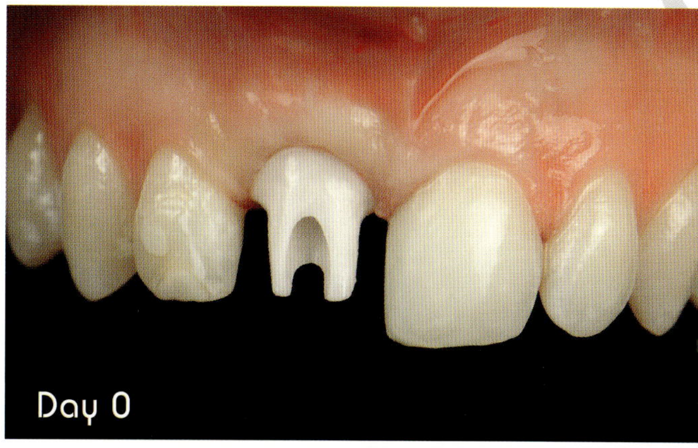
Day 0

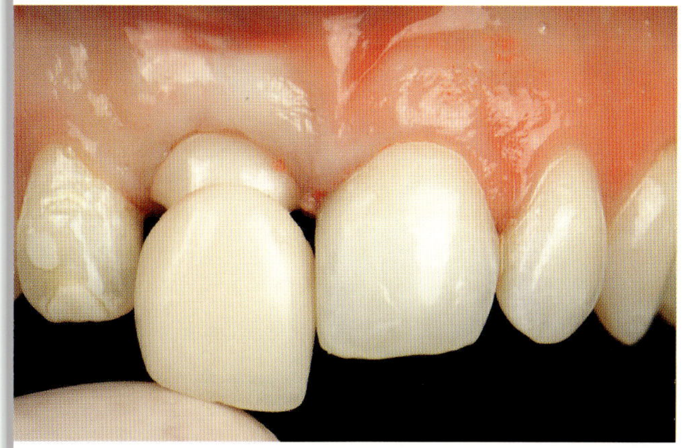

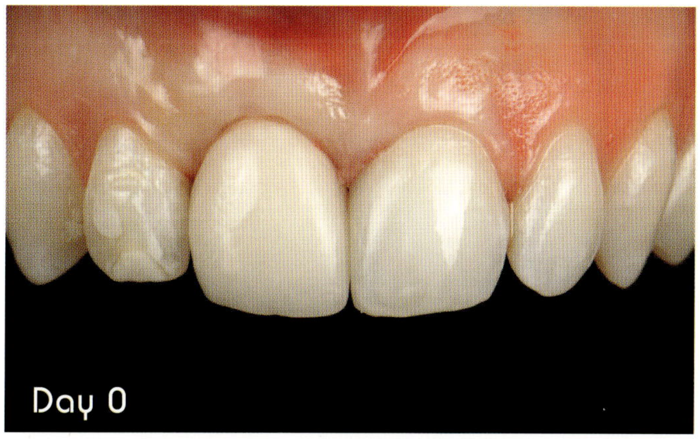
Day 0

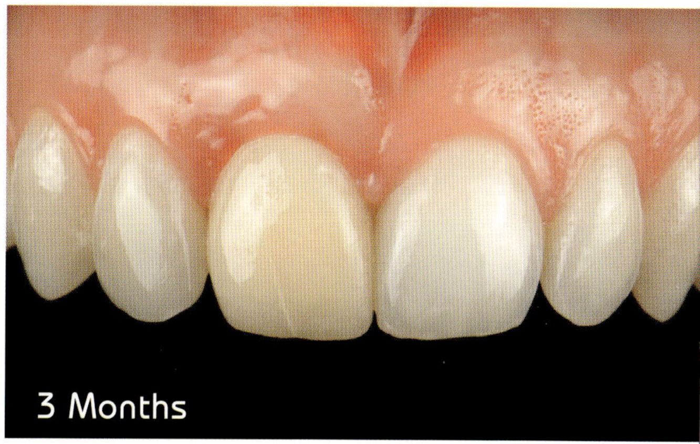
3 Months

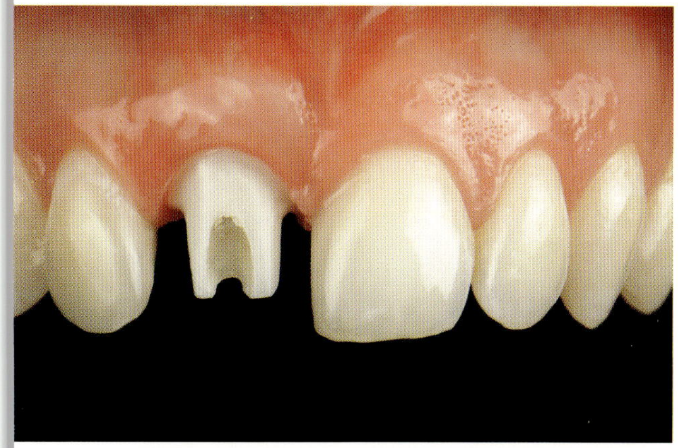

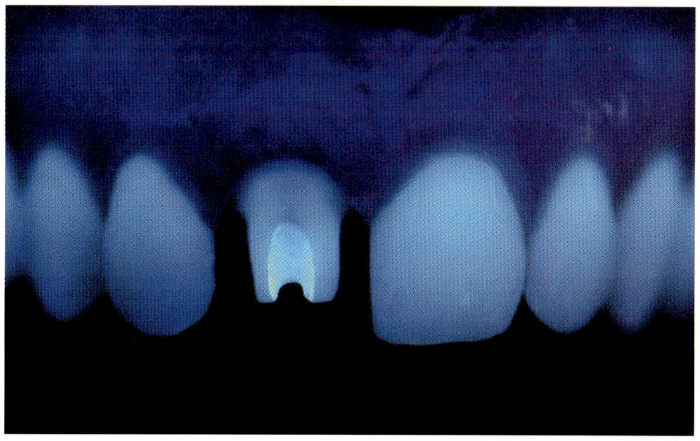

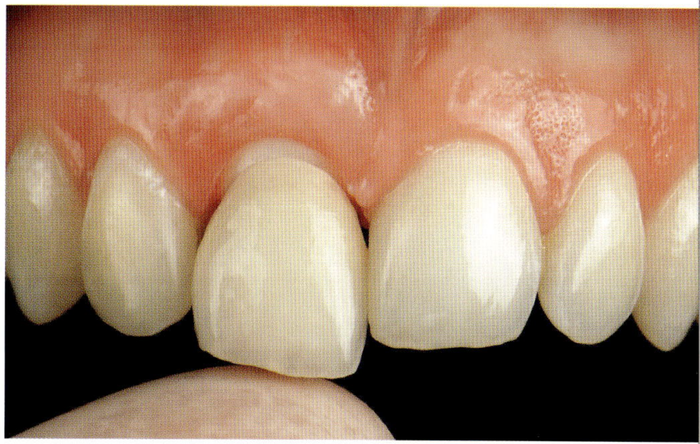

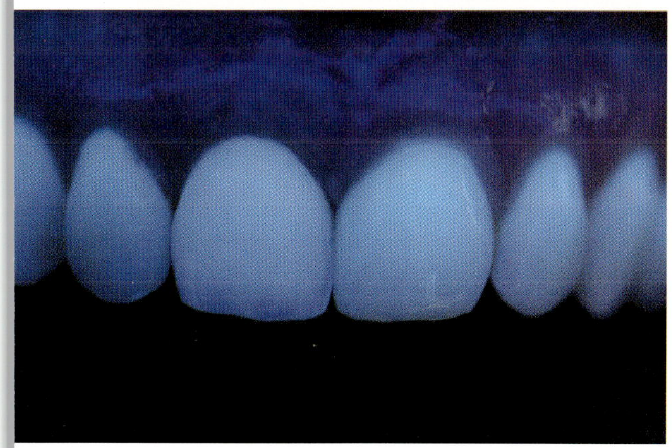

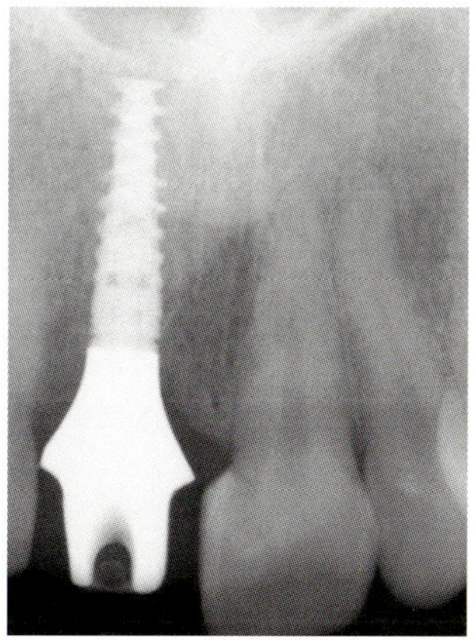

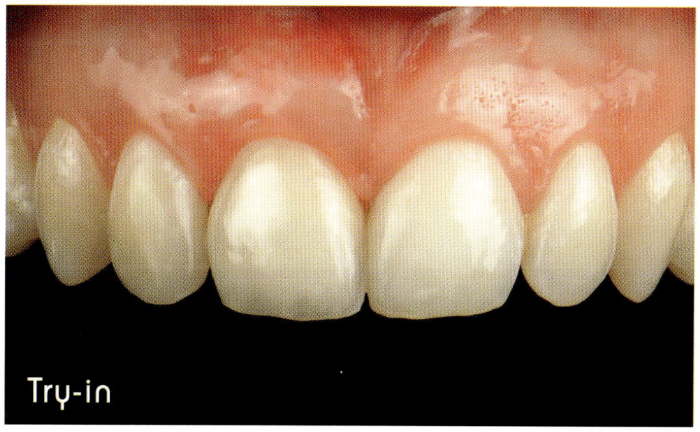
Try-in

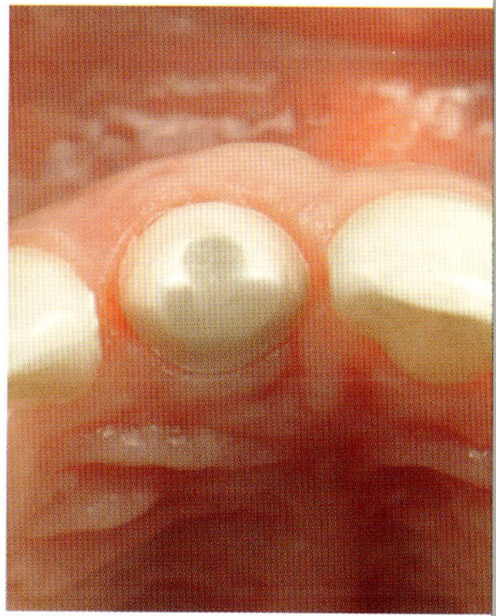

After respective try-ins and adjustments, the definitive crown was cemented. Periapical radiographs are always recommended to verify proper seating and fit of the prosthetic components and to identify possible excess cement. Whenever a definitive abutment is placed together with a provisional restoration, it should be completely removed before final cementation of the definitive restoration to check for any excess cement that may have remained on the soft tissue or abutment surface. If necessary, cement remnants should be removed by thorough rinsing of the tissue with saline and chlorhexidine. The abutment should be cleaned with sterile gauze and saline to remove all cement and debris remnants. After cleaning, two retraction cords were placed independently, one on the buccal and the other on the palatal aspect of the abutment. The cords were extended into the sulci of the adjacent teeth, which allows for easy retrieval of the cords and control of cement removal from both sides, buccally and palatally, in an independent manner. A periapical radiograph was taken after cleaning of the cementation site with dental floss.

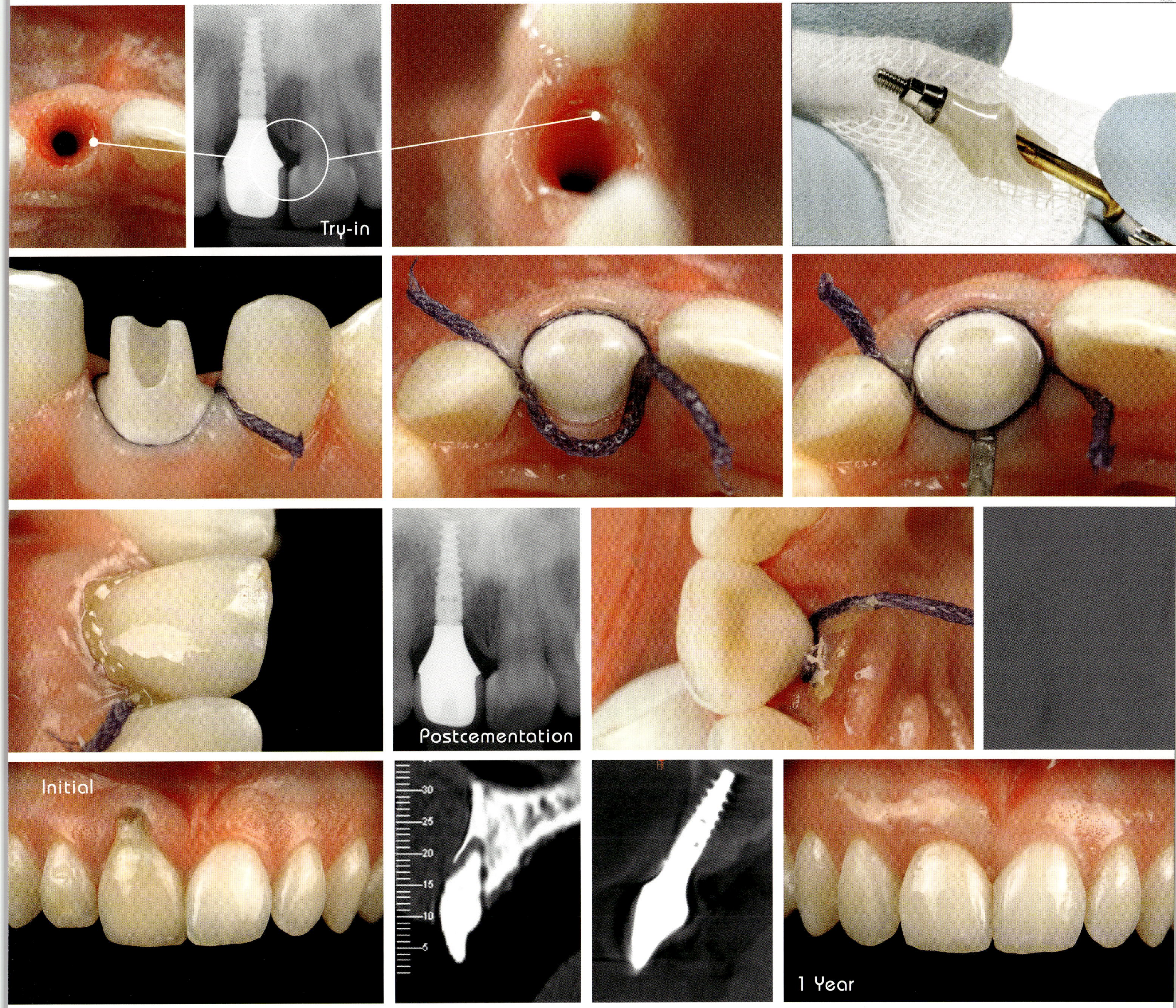
Try-in
Postcementation
Initial
30
25
20
15
10
5
1 Year

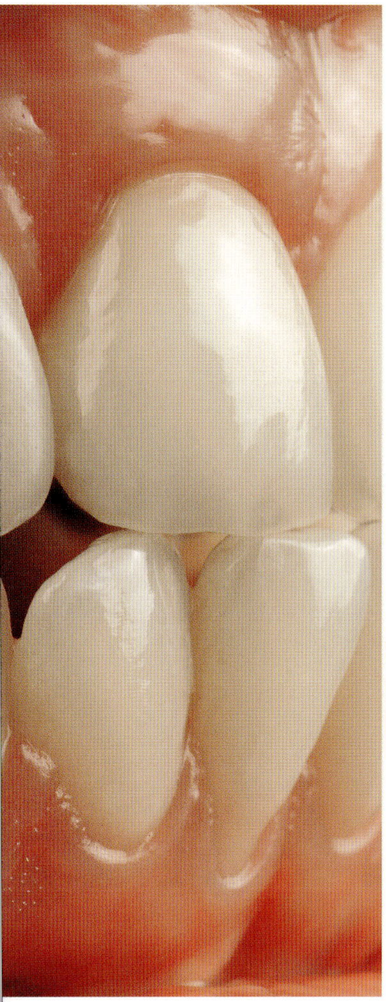

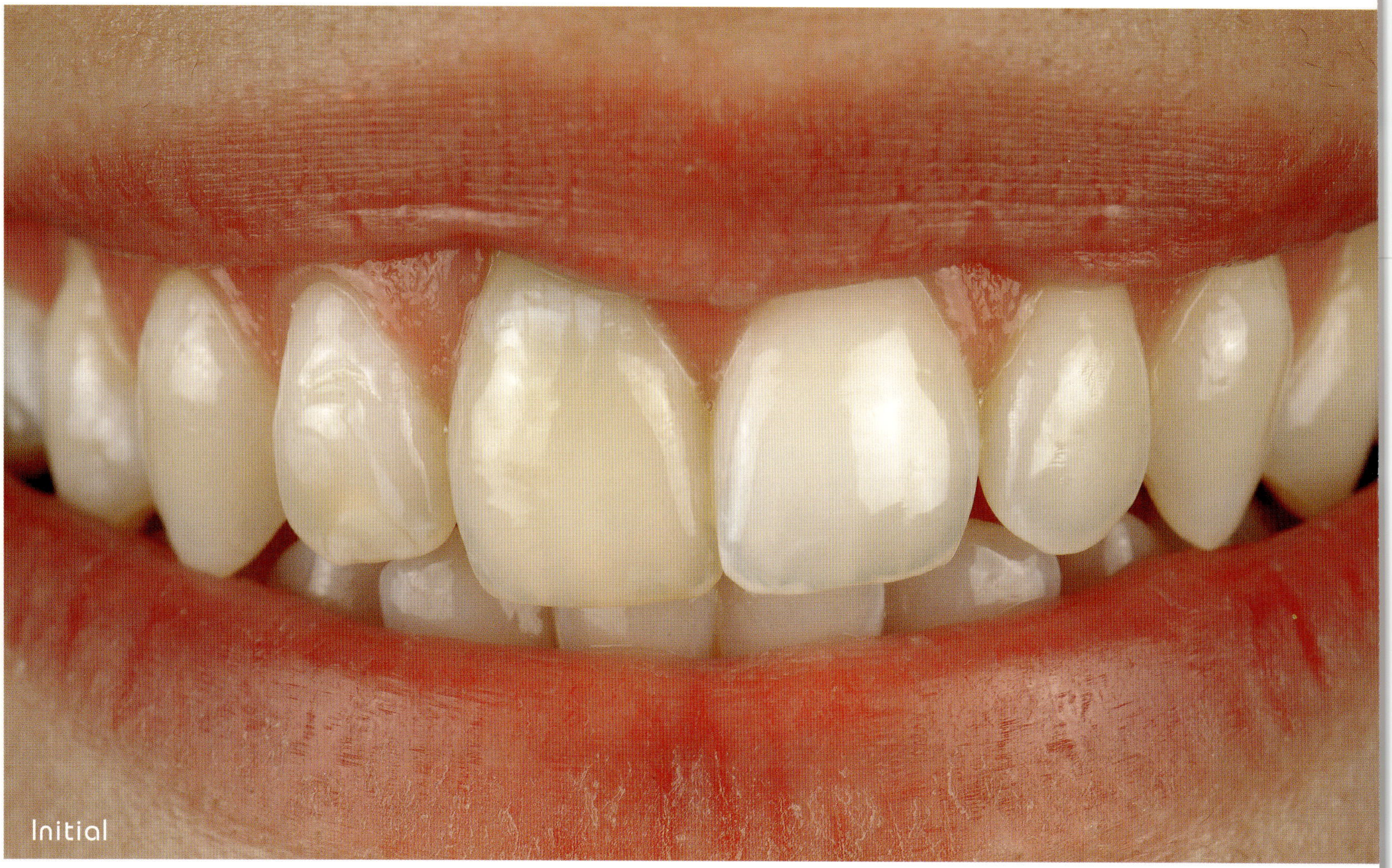
Initial

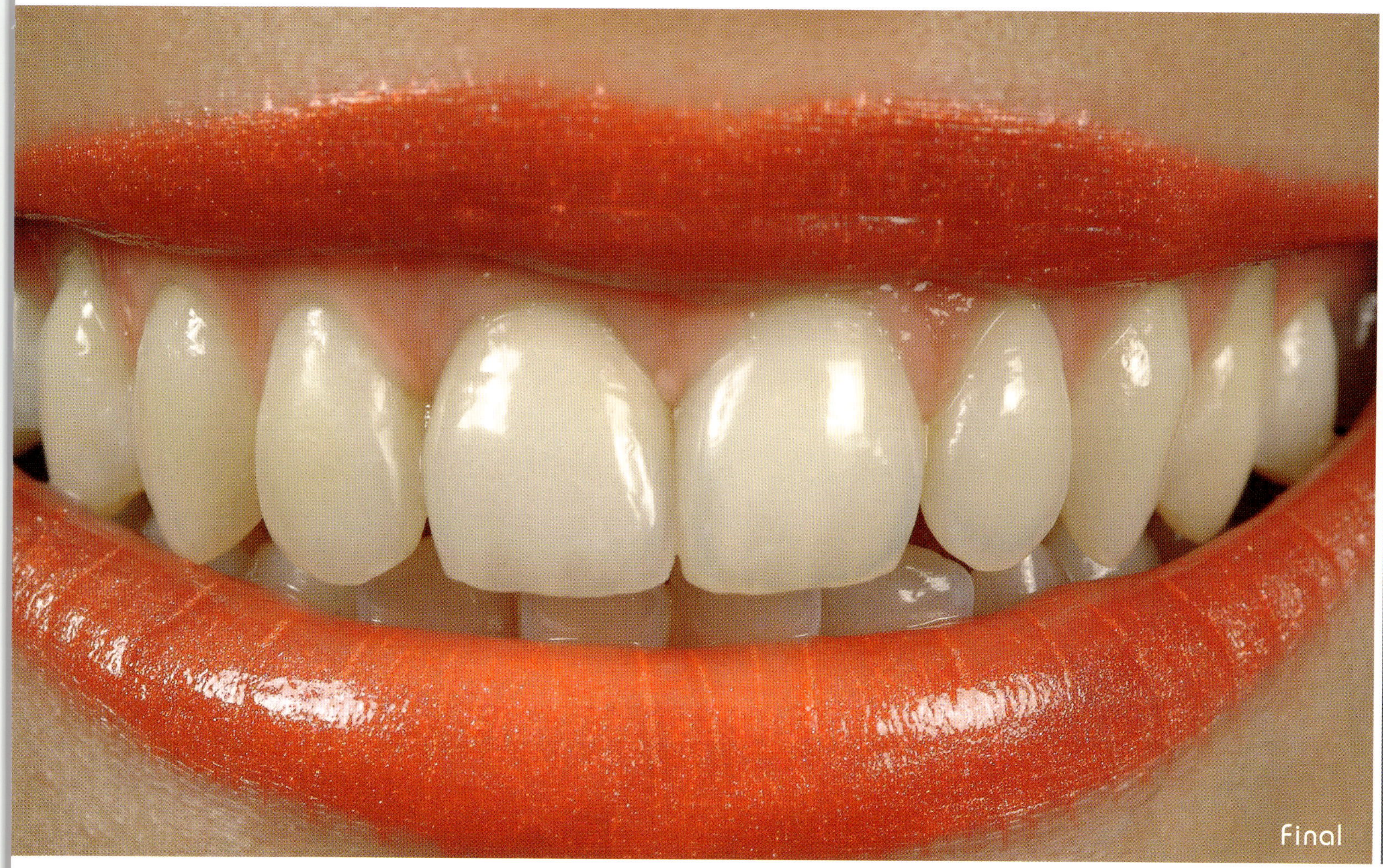

Comparison of the preoperative and postoperative intraoral situations. The final outcome 1 year after implant crown cementation. The CTG ensured a long-term esthetic result.

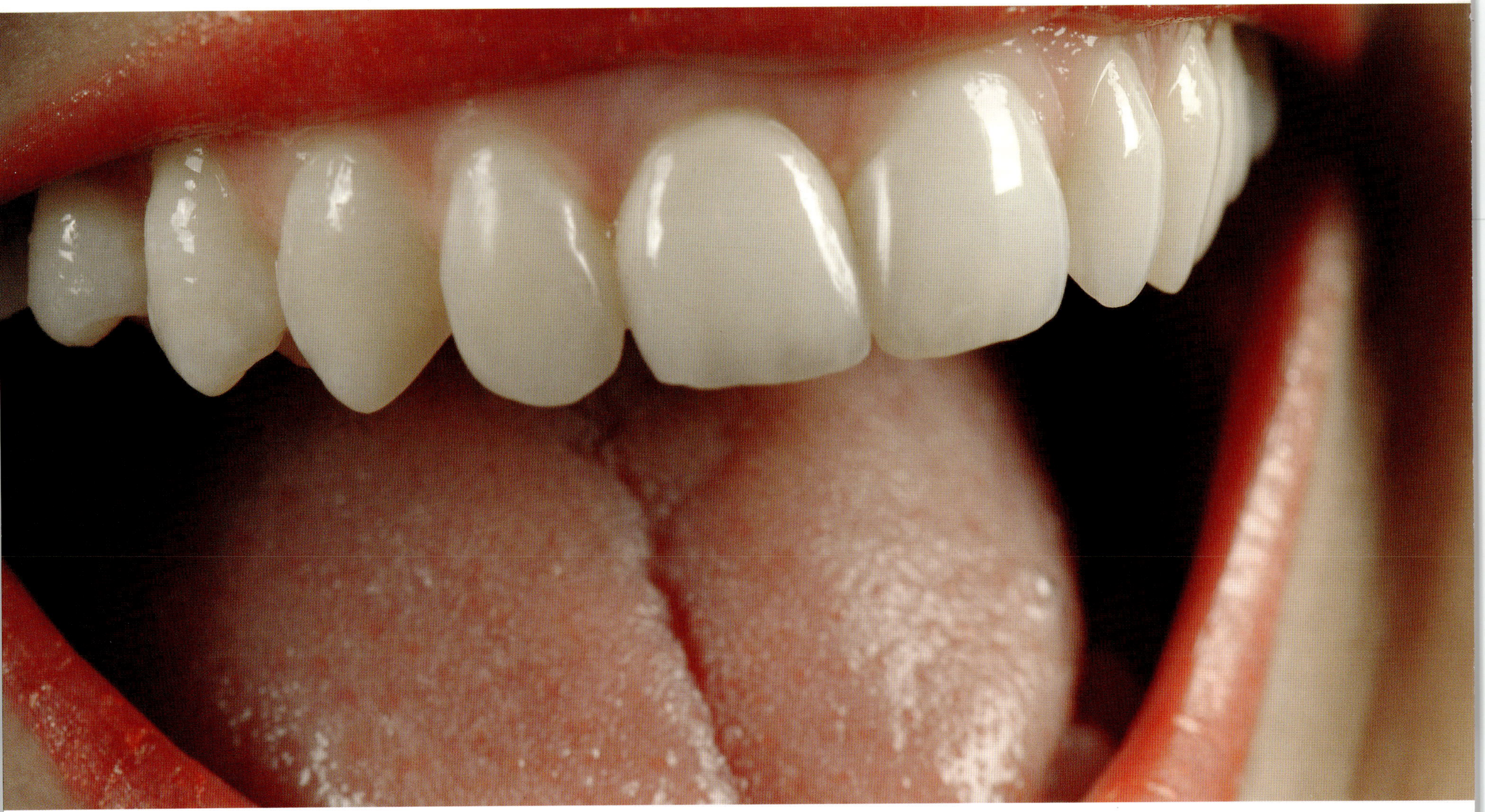

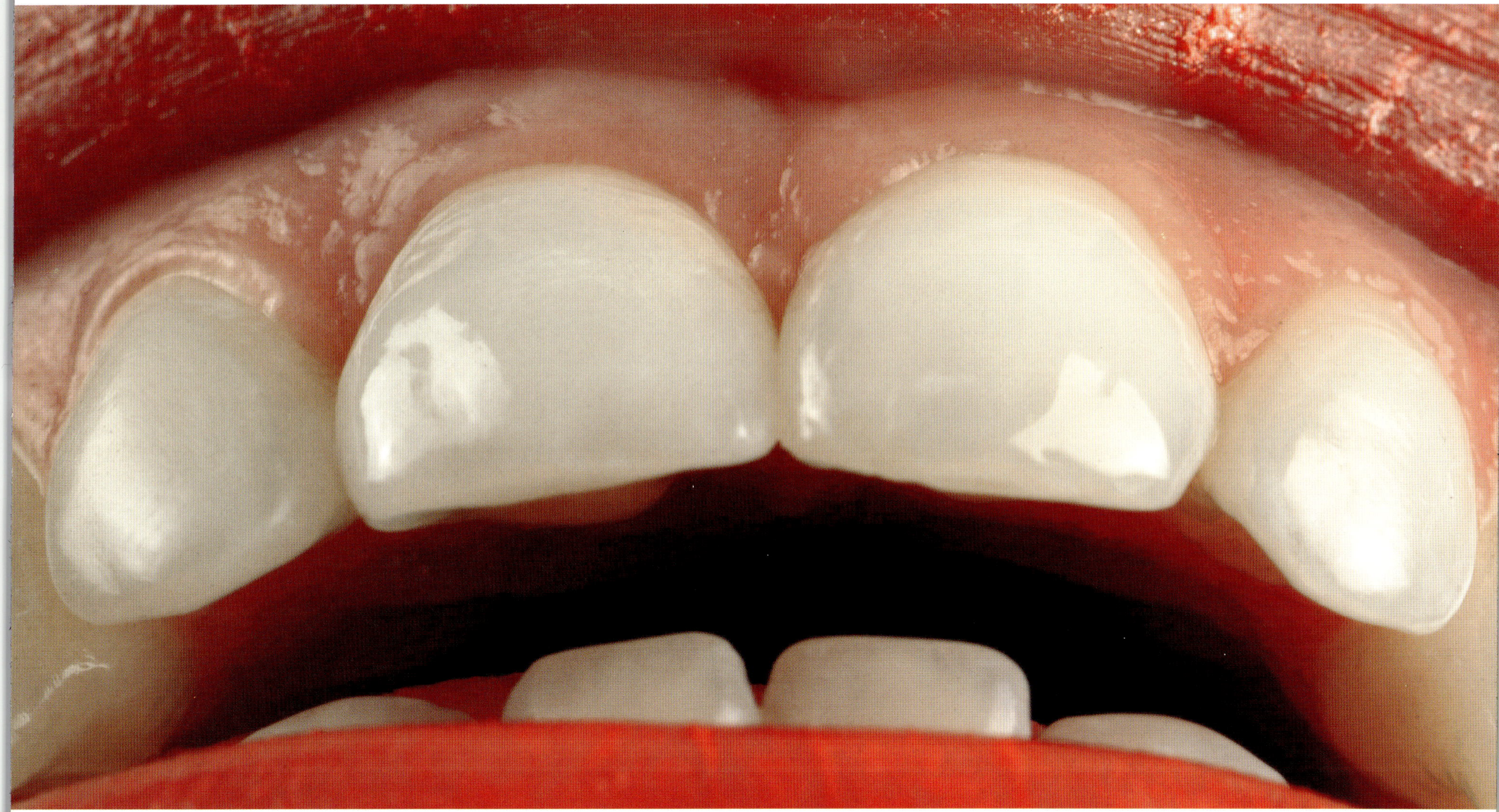

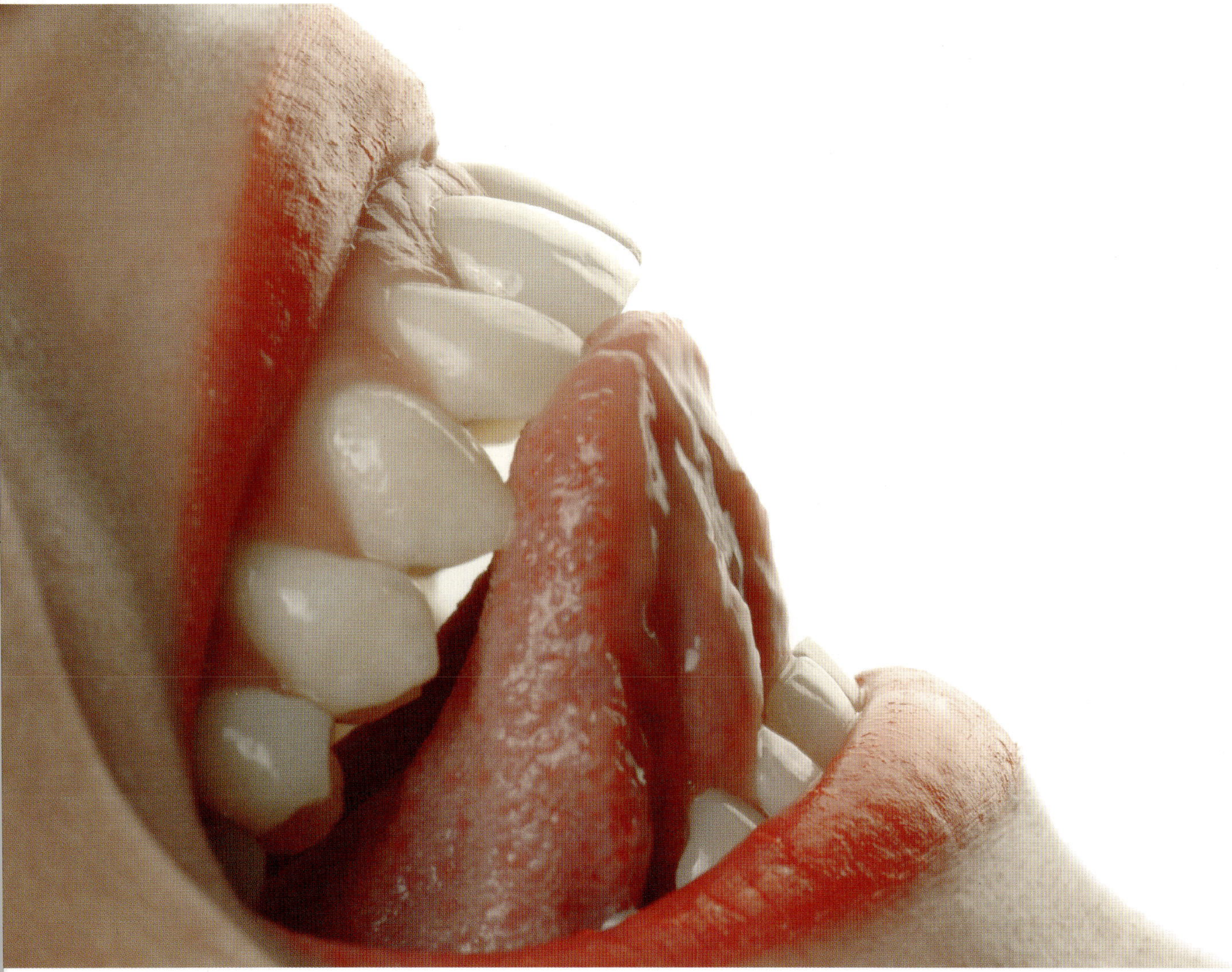